MANUAL THERAPY

of

the

SPINE

an integrated approach

■

MANUAL THERAPY

of

the

SPINE

an integrated approach

MARK DUTTON, PT

Human Motion Rehabilitation
Allegheny General Hospital
Pittsburgh, PA

McGraw-Hill
Medical Publishing Division

New York / Chicago / San Francisco / Lisbon / London
Madrid / Mexico City / Milan / New Delhi / San Juan
Seoul / Singapore / Sydney / Toronto

McGraw-Hill

A Division of The McGraw·Hill Companies

Manual Therapy of the Spine: An Integrated Approach

Copyright © 2002 by The **McGraw-Hill Companies**, Inc. All rights reserved. Printed in the United States of America. Except as permitted under the United States Copyright Act of 1976, no part of this publication may be reproduced or distributed in any form or by any means, or stored in a data base or retrieval system, without the prior written permission of the publisher.

1 2 3 4 5 6 7 8 9 0   KGP/KGP   0 9 8 7 6 5 4 3 2 1

ISBN 0-07-137582-1

This book was set in New Baskerville by TechBooks.
The editors were Stephen Zollo and Barbara Holton.
The production supervisor was Rick Ruzycka.
The cover designer was Aimée Nordin.
The index was prepared by Deborah Tourtlotte.

Quebecor World Kingsport was printer and binder.

This book is printed on acid-free paper.

Library of Congress Cataloging-in-Publication Data

Dutton, Mark.
    Manual therapy of the spine: an integrated approach / author, Mark Dutton.
       p. ; cm.
    Includes bibliographical references and index.
    ISBN 0-07-137582-1
    1. Spine—Diseases—Physical therapy. 2. Spinal adjustment. 3. Manipulation (Therapeutics) I. Title.
    [DNLM: 1. Spine—physiopathology. 2. Manipulation, Orthopedic. 3. Physical Examination. 4. Spinal Diseases—rehabilitation. WE 725 D981m 2001]
RD768 .D88 2001
617.5'6062—dc21
                                        2001030679

*This book is dedicated to the memory of
David W. Lamb, a major contributor to the
field of manual medicine worldwide, and
an inspiration to all who aspire
to teach, and treat patients.*

Contents

Preface

There is a vast amount of information available on the spine. As an undergraduate, and later, as a practicing clinician, I was frustrated that the material I required was scattered throughout a multitude of texts. This usually resulted in long hours of searching, and so I began compiling this information, including the pertinent information I had obtained from a wide variety of continuing education courses, and the peer-reviewed articles I had collected.

What began as a fairly modest task, resulted in this book, which I feel has achieved my original goal of having a text containing the information required to provide a high level of care to a varied outpatient population.

With the recent advances in technology, the tendency has been for an increased reliance on the findings from imaging studies such as computed axial tomography (CAT) and magnetic resonance imaging (MRI), and a decreased reliance on the clinical findings and diagnosis. This often results in the physician having to rely on the imaging study results and not on the clinician's opinion.

A systematic approach is imperative for the provision of an accurate clinical, and biomechanical, diagnosis. This book, aimed at all clinicians who use manual therapy techniques, including physical therapists, osteopaths and chiropractors, covers the functional anatomy, clinical examination, pathology and intervention of the spine, pelvis, and temporomandibular joint. Although each area is dealt with separately, they should be considered as being interrelated. The temporomandibular joint is included because of its functional relationship to the upper quadrant. The Whiplash Associated Disorder (WAD) is afforded its own chapter, as this syndrome produces impairments in multiple body systems, and the treatment approach thus incorporates attention to each of these systems simultaneously.

The sequential flow of the subjective and objective examinations is outlined, with explanations given as to the rationale, allowing a clinician of any proficiency level to use this book as a resource for an accurate biomechanical examination. Working from this foundation, detailed explanations for each of the various areas are given, enabling the clinician to differentially diagnose, and to integrate the results gleaned from the examination, in order to formulate a working hypothesis. The working hypothesis is based on the findings from the comprehensive examination, and helps to plan the intervention, focusing on the cause of the problem in addition to alleviating the symptoms. Recognizing the varying abilities between clinicians, most of the evaluation and treatment techniques are described with the patient in different positions.

Therapeutic exercise is a major component of the intervention plan for spinal impairments, and the exercises for each of the areas are covered in detail, with special emphasis on stabilization exercises.

The approaches drawn upon for this book stem from the teachings of the North American Institute of Orthopaedic Manual Therapy (NAIOMT).[1,2,3,4,5,6] About ten years ago I began a series of NAIOMT courses, and the standards and philosophy of the faculty impressed me. Perhaps the most refreshing characteristic of their philosophy was an eclectic approach, a sort of 'best of the best'. This eclectic approach was founded upon a vast amount of experience in attempting the various examination and intervention techniques that existed in the field of manual therapy. From these trials, an amalgam of doctrines and techniques, that had proved successful in the clinic, and were supported by a credible scientific foundation, emerged. The techniques incorporate the biomechanical concepts of the Norwegians,[7,8,9] the selective tissue tension principles of James Cyriax MD,[10] the muscle energy concepts of the American osteopaths,[11,12] the manipulative techniques of Alan Stoddard, DO,[13] the stability therapy exercises of the Australians,[14] the exercise protocols of McKenzie,[15] the muscle balancing concepts of Janda Jull, and

Sahrmann[16,17,18] and the movement re-education principles of the neurodevelopment and sensory integrationist physical therapists.

The numerous case studies in this book serve a variety of functions. At times they are used to illustrate the clinical presentation, examination and intervention of common musculoskeletal impairments. At other times they give an in-depth description of the underlying pathologic processes of commonly encountered conditions. In addition, the case studies reinforce the contents of this book, guiding the clinician through the necessary thought processes and evaluation sequences. The chapter entitled Differential Diagnosis for the Manual Therapist—Systems Review emphasizes and expands upon Grieve's work on the masqueraders of musculoskeletal pain.[19] In the chapter entitled the Subjective Examination, illustrative case studies are used to highlight the clinical presentation of the more serious pathologies that can mimic a musculoskeletal dysfunction to help the inexperienced clinician recognize these pernicious signs and symptoms.

While it would be nice to be able to give myself credit for the contents of this book, that would be a gross misrepresentation. A huge debt is owed to all those practitioners who continue to publish their findings for the benefit of the rest of us. I am merely serving as a conduit for that information and to select those techniques and principles that have worked for me as practicing clinician.

REFERENCES

1. Fowler C. Muscle energy techniques for pelvic dysfunction. In: Grieve GP. (ed). *Modern Manual Therapy of the Vertebral Column.* Churchill Livingstone, Edinburgh, 1986;57:781.
2. Lee DG, Walsh MC. A Workbook of Manual Therapy Techniques for the Vertebral Column and pelvic girdle, 2nd ed. Nascent, Vancouver, 1996.
3. Lee D. *The Pelvic Girdle: An Approach to the Examination and Treatment of the Lumbo-Pelvic-Hip Region.* 2nd ed. Churchill Livingstone, 1999.
4. Lee DG. Clinical manifestations of pelvic girdle dysfunction. In: Boyling JD, Palastanga N. (eds). Grieve's Modern Manual Therapy: The Vertebral Column, 2nd ed. Edinburgh, Churchill Livingstone, 1994.
5. Meadows JTS. *Orthopedic Differential Diagnosis in Physical Therapy,* McGraw-Hill, 1999.
6. Pettman E. In: Boyling JD, Palastanga N. (eds). Grieve's Modern Manual Therapy: The Vertebral Column, 2nd ed. Edinburgh, Churchill Livingstone, 1994.
7. Kaltenborn F. *The Spine: Basic Evaluation and Mobilization Techniques.* New Zealand University Press, Wellington, 1993.
8. Kaltenborn F. *Manual Therapy for Extremity Joints.* Bokhandel, Oslo, 1974.
9. Evjenth O, Hamberg J. *Muscle Stretching in Manual Therapy; A Clinical manual, Vol 1; The Extremities; Vol 2, The Spinal Column and the TMJ.* Alfta, Sweden, Alfta rehab Forlag, 1980.
10. Cyriax J. *Textbook of Orthopedic Medicine,* vol 1, 8th ed. London, Balliere Tindall and Cassell, 1982.
11. Mennell JM. *Back Pain.* Little Brown, Boston, 1960.
12. Mitchell F, Moran PS, Pruzzo NA. *An Evaluation and Treatment Manual of Osteopathic Muscle Energy Procedures,* 1979.
13. Stoddard A. Manual of Osteopathic Technique. London, Hutchinson, 1983
14. Maitland GD. *Vertebral Manipulation.* 5th ed. Butterworths, London, 1986.
15. McKenzie RA. The Lumbar Spine: Mechanical Diagnosis and Therapy. Waikanae, New Zealand: Spinal Publications Limited, 1989.
16. Jull GA, Janda V. Muscle and Motor control in low back pain, In: Twomey LT, Taylor JR. (eds). Physical Therapy of the Low Back: Clinics in Physical Therapy, New York, Churchill Livingstone, 1987;259–276.
17. Janda V. *Muscle Function Testing,* London, Butterworths, 1983;163–167.
18. Sahrmann SA. Diagnosis and Treatment of Movement Impairment Syndromes. Mosby, St. Louis, 2001.
19. Grieve GP. The Masqueraders. In: Boyling JD. Palastanga N. (eds). Grieve's Modern Manual Therapy, 2nd ed. Edinburgh, Churchill Livingstone, 1994.

Acknowledgments

It is my firm belief that our accomplishments in life are due to a number of personal characteristics such as perseverance and motivation, and to a supporting cast of people, who help shape, direct and inspire. Most of the time, these people are unaware of the effect that they have, and the opportunity to thank them never arises, until such a time as this. I would like to thank the following:

- The faculty of the North American Institute of Manual and Manipulative Therapy (NAIOMT)—especially the late Dave Lamb, Jim Meadows, Erl Pettman, Cliff Fowler and Diane Lee, who provided me with the inspiration to pursue a specialization in manual therapy. My enthusiasm for manual therapy was ignited following the first NAIOMT course that I attended, and I highly recommend these courses. It was Jim Meadows who gave me the confidence, and provided me with the impetus, to write this book.
- My family—my wife Beth, and my two daughters, Leah and Lauren. Whenever a task of this size is undertaken, certain sacrifices are necessary. I am convinced that time spent with the family is irreplaceable, and so I attempted to minimize those sacrifices as much as possible.
- The production team of McGraw-Hill—Steve Zollo for his confidence in this project, Julie Scardiglia and Barbara Holton for their patience, guidance, and support.
- My parents, Ron and Brenda, for teaching me the importance of hard work and perseverance, and for giving me my independence. My Dad, a talented abstract artist, prepared the initial illustrations for this book.
- Bob Davis for the photography
- Phil and Shari Vislosky for agreeing to be the photographic models
- The staff of Human Motion Rehabilitation, Allegheny General Hospital
- Marianne Tomnay and Nancy Drakulic for generously giving up their personal time to help in the preparation of this manuscript
- Ted Laska, PT and Richard Lambie, PT for introducing me to the NAIOMT courses
- To the countless manual therapists throughout the world who continually strive to improve their knowledge and clinical skills

MANUAL THERAPY

of

the

SPINE

an integrated approach

CHAPTER ONE

PRINCIPLES

HISTORICAL PERSPECTIVE[1,2]

The history of the spine, its pathology, and its biomechanics, is a long and fascinating one. The earliest clinical accounts of a spinal injury date back to when the great pyramids were being built. These accounts were contained in the Edwin Smith surgical papyrus, originally written during the Egyptian Old Kingdom (2600–2200 BC).[3–8] It is clear that the ancient Egyptians recognized that misalignment of the bony vertebral column could have disastrous consequences, and that a fracture–dislocation was associated with a poorer prognosis than a simple fracture of the spine. There is also good evidence that the Egyptians realized that the appropriate intervention for extremity fractures was reduction and immobilization, although there is no evidence to suggest that this was practiced with spinal fractures. Uncarthed splints, dating from the Fifth Dynasty, suggest that bone setting was an established art in ancient Egypt.[9]

The first account of an intervention for spinal dysfunction is recorded in the *Srimad Bhagwat Mahapuranam*, an ancient Indian epic written between 3500 and 1800 BC.[10,11]

Hippocrates (460–361 BC) is probably the most celebrated physician in history, although judged against modern standards, his knowledge of anatomy was poor. Hippocrates did, however, realize that the bony column was held together by the discs, ligaments, and muscles. He also noted that the spinous process could be broken without ill effect, but that injury to the vertebral body was often fatal.

Spinal manipulation, as an intervention for spinal dysfunction, was an accepted practice at the time of Hippocrates. Hippocrates recommended subjecting the body to traction, and applying pressure locally to the area of the kyphosis to treat kyphotic deformities.[12] Later physicians, such as Henri de Mondeville (1260–1320) and Guy de Chauliac (1300–1368), commonly used Hippocrates' methods through the Middle Ages.

"Succussion," a procedure that involved flinging a patient to the ground in an upside-down position while attached with ropes to an elevated ladder, was practiced through the 15th century AD. It was hoped that the jerk produced by the sudden deceleration would realign any spinal deformity.[12]

The Middle Ages, aside from Galen, were almost devoid of any advancement in biomechanics. Galen (AD 131–201) was a firm believer in the Hippocratic teachings and used spinal manipulation to treat spinal problems. He was the first to use the terms "kyphosis," "lordosis," and "scoliosis."[13] Unlike Hippocrates, Galen had a keen interest in anatomy, and he correctly identified many anatomic features of the spinal column, including the number of vertebrae in each segment of the spinal column (7 cervical, 12 thoracic, and 5 lumbar),[14] and the correlation of neurologic findings with specific spinal levels.[15] Galen was also the first to describe the ligamentum flavum as a ligamentous structure distinct from the underlying dura and pia mater.[15]

Many ancient Greek and Roman texts on medicine, philosophy, and the natural sciences were rediscovered in Italy during the 15th and 16th centuries. The study of mechanics was revived, and several scientists began to contemplate the relationship between anatomy, mathematics, and mechanics.[16]

Leonardo da Vinci (1452–1519) was a master artist, engineer, and anatomist. His uncompleted work on human anatomy, *De Figura Humana*, reveals that he embraced a mechanistic approach to the study of the human body.[17] Da Vinci was the first to accurately describe the spine with the correct curvatures and articulations. He was also the first to suggest that stability to the spine was provided, in part, by the cervical musculature.[18] In his later works, da Vinci began to wonder how the body moved, and how geometry and mechanics could further unlock the secrets of human physiology.

Vesalius (1514–1564) deserves a place in the history of spinal biomechanics because of his accurate descriptions of spinal anatomy.

Giovanni Alfonso Borelli (1608–1679) was one of the founders of "iatromechanics," or the application of mechanics to physiology—the forerunner of what we now call biomechanics. Borelli, who was not a physician, worked with Marcello Malphigi, professor of theoretical medicine at the University of Pisa, to ensure that his mechanical calculations made biologic sense. Although Borelli's knowledge of mechanics was restricted to the principle of levers and the triangle of forces, he was able to generate an accurate and comprehensive account of muscle action.[19]

His work, *De Motu Animalium*,[20] published posthumously in 1680, is the first comprehensive text devoted to biomechanics. Borelli noted that the muscles act with short lever arms, so that the intervening joint transmits a force of a greater magnitude than the weight of the load. This concept overturned the older posits of muscle action, which stated that long lever arms allowed weak muscles to move heavy objects.[21] In addition, Borelli realized that the intervertebral discs acted like a viscoelastic substance, by both cushioning the bones and acting like springs, and that the discs must perform some load sharing because of an inability of the spinal musculature alone to support heavy weights.

In 1646, Fabricus Hildanus, a German surgeon, proposed a method of spinal reduction that was very advanced for his time. He also described a method for reducing cervical fracture–dislocations, similar in principle to modern cervical traction.[22]

Leonhard Euler (1707–1783), one of the founders of pure mathematics, noted that the mathematical stability of a column was a function of column height and stiffness,[23,24] and although Euler did not address spinal biomechanics per se, his studies had a direct bearing on biomechanical models of the spine.

Eduard Weber is reported as being the first to study cadaveric spines with the specific intention of determining mechanical properties. Using observational methods, he assessed the range of movement in various regions, correlating the results with his observations of spinal movement in vivo. He stated that the lumbar spine could flex only in the sagittal and coronal planes, it being devoid of any axial rotation.[25,26] More recently this latter statement has been challenged by Fisk,[27] and actual recordings of transverse plane movements in the lumbar spine have been recorded by Murray[28] and Thurston.[29–31]

In 1872, Hughes related the rotations of one vertebra to those of the adjacent vertebrae.[31,32] In 1873, von Meyer[33,34] determined the axis of movement in lateral flexion and rotation, and Guérin described centers of lateral inclination and their relationship to articular and muscular systems.[35] Morris, in studying facet joint movements, claimed that the superior and inferior facets in the lumbar spine did not contact, and that the intervening space provided for rotation.[26,36]

Julius Wolff (1836–1902), a German orthopedic surgeon, was engrossed with the relationship between the form and function of bone.[37] Based on his own experiments and the work of others, he detailed Wolff's law: "Every change in the function of a bone is followed by certain definite changes in internal architecture and external conformation in accordance with mathematical laws." Wolff's law has important implications for the clinician, and it explains why an intervertebral bone graft will fuse when subjected to loading.

Strasser, Krammer, and Novogrodsky were the first to study the effects of external forces on two adjacent vertebrae.[33,38] They attempted to systematize and classify spinal movements by defining frames of reference, so that each movement could be expressed in terms of three angular values.[33,39]

Until recently, attempts to measure spinal movement in vivo have been, at best, approximate. Löhr's method involved the measurement of spine movement from shadows thrown onto a screen. He measured sagittal plane movement of the thoracic and lumbar spines in 47 subjects.[26,40] McKendrick, in 1916, measured the interspinous distances in flexion and extension.[41] This marked the beginning of the appearance of many ingenious devices to record the range of movement of the spine in vivo. Cyriax produced a spinal torsionometer,[42] Dunham produced a spondylometer,[43] and Asmussen used an inclinometer to assess spinal movement in the sagittal plane.[44] Israel and Goff both introduced special instruments for measuring spinal mobility.[45,46] One recent introduction is the vector stereograph, capable of measuring spinal mobility in three dimensions.[47,48]

Francis Denis[49] proposed a three-column model in 1983, and he described a middle column consisting of the posterior vertebral body, the posterior anulus fibrosis, and the posterior longitudinal ligament. Disruption of two columns was required for instability. Denis's model has undergone modification by many authors, but the concept of three columns in the spine has withstood more than a decade of scrutiny.[50]

As the understanding of spinal anatomy and its biomechanics became more refined, treatment of spinal injuries became more sophisticated, with devices being introduced that could achieve the intended therapeutic goals.[51]

MANUAL THERAPY

Together with these advances in the knowledge of spinal anatomy and biomechanics, came the methods for treating the soft tissue injuries around the spine. The field of manual therapy was born. Over the past few decades, manual therapy for the spine has become popular and has been deemed a useful intervention to spinal dysfunctions.

Many clinicians have played their part in making manual therapy a specialization within the field of physical therapy, and Cyriax,[52] Grieve,[53] Kaltenborn,[54,55] Evjenth,[56] Janda,[57] Maitland,[58] McKenzie,[59] Mennel,[60] Paris,[61] and others, have all contributed to this process. This specialization should be viewed as a positive step as it allows the manual therapist to provide a comprehensive, and conservative, approach to the management of spinal and peripheral joint pain of musculoskeletal origin. From the selfish viewpoint, this increase in competence provides the profession with added kudos, and, altruistically, the patients benefit from this increase in knowledge and expertise.

Traditionally, the manual therapist has had to be a highly motivated clinician, as very little of this specialized area is covered in the average physical therapy curriculum. This has placed the responsibility on individuals to pursue their development through a series of continuing education courses or through a training institution. To acquire the necessary skill to be good manual therapists, clinicians must practice constantly, and continually build upon their knowledge base.

The manual therapy approach described in this book is based on a systematic examination and the utilization of sound biomechanical principles. The causes of spinal dysfunction are multifactorial and cannot just be ascribed to a simple alteration in the position of the various mechanical structures that compose the functional unit of the spine.[62,63]

Unfortunately, too many physical therapists with no training in manual therapy are treating patients in the outpatient setting. These generalists place too much emphasis on the alleviation of a patient's pain and not enough emphasis on eliciting the correct diagnosis of a patient. This lack of a specific diagnosis, or clinical knowledge, forces a clinician to rely on the "shotgun" approach to an intervention, resulting in the use of a host of nonspecific techniques and modalities, only to find that the patient's condition does not improve. This approach has done little to promote the profession. Although the intention to alleviate the patient's sufferings is honorable, the patient is being shortchanged. Clinicians have no business treating patients for whom there is no specific, or clinically tested diagnosis, or treating a patient by blindly following a prescription.

It is imperative that the clinician determine the cause of the patient's symptoms so that the optimum level of care can be delivered, and any recurrence of symptoms prevented. This is especially true for symptoms with an insidious onset where the cause may be more serious, or systemic in nature. The tools for a very specific and accurate examination are available, but, as with any skill, time and work are needed to master their use.

In simplistic terms, most articular pathologies of the musculoskeletal system that are treated in physical therapy clinics result from the joint, or joints, moving too much (being hypermobile), or too little (being hypomobile). Either macrotrauma or microtrauma induces this change in motion status. Macrotrauma occurs when the musculoskeletal system receives a direct physical insult. This insult may be controlled, as occurs with surgery, or uncontrolled, as occurs during a high-speed collision. Microtrauma, often the result of faulty biomechanics or overuse, is induced by a repeated absorption of daily stresses. These stresses eventually cause a gradual breakdown of the joint, slowly reducing its adaptive potential and increasing its vulnerability.

The breakdown of the joint results in anomalies of motion, modifying the normal arthrokinematics and increasing the shear forces across the joint, resulting in arthrotic destruction. What begins as a painful, but mild, degree of hypermobility in the early stages of arthrosis becomes a gradual fibrosis and thickening of the joint, reducing its motion and decreasing the pain. Contiguous regions are coupled functionally, and changes in one component of the complex result in compensation of the other components; thus, a secondary joint dysfunction occurs. These changes result in a level of pain sufficiently high for the patient to seek help.

One of the objectives of the musculoskeletal examination is to determine whether the clinician is confronted with a hypomobility, or hypermobility, problem and then to locate the specific structure at fault. If a patient's symptoms are reproduced with a motion that is found to be limited, the clinician needs to determine which structure is producing the limitation: Is a restriction within the joint limiting the motion, or is surrounding soft tissue causing the limitation? If, on the other hand, the patient's symptoms are reproduced with a motion that appears to be excessive, the clinician needs to determine if a hypermobility, or instability, exists and whether that hypermobility, or instability, is ligamentous or articular in origin.

A specific intervention requires a specific biomechanical diagnosis. Damage to the spinal unit can produce inflammation, pain, abnormal tissue texture, and muscle splinting. The pain, with its own characteristics, is either felt locally or referred in a predictable pattern.[64,65] As one can appreciate, merely reproducing a patient's pain with a movement does not implicate the structure involved, unless the clinician has a sound knowledge of anatomy and function, and an appreciation of all the structures that can produce pain in, or refer pain to, that area. Armed with this knowledge, and through use of specific techniques to correctly isolate a structure, either for palpation purposes or for applying stresses through it, the clinician can deduce that the symptoms are being reproduced by the structure under scrutiny.

On the surface this would seem to utilize nothing more than a simple and common sense approach to the intervention of orthopedic problems. However, upon reflection, it is clear that although the approach is simple, it demands a level of knowledge in anatomy, biomechanics, and differential diagnosis that is well beyond that of the average clinician.

Cyriax[52] devised a sequential scheme of systematic analysis to provide the clinician with a portrait of the joint dysfunction in relation to signs and symptoms. He coined the expression "selective tissue tension tests" and reasoned that if one isolated, and then applied stress to a structure, one could make a conclusion as to the integrity of that structure. Put more simply, reproducing the pain while stressing a particular structure implicates that structure. Thus, the intervention should involve techniques geared toward alleviating the stresses from that structure. His scanning examination is the foundation on which additional information can be built. Several other methods of analysis are employed by the manual therapist; these include testing of intervertebral joint motion, compression and distraction techniques, application of specific pressures on bony landmarks, analysis of joint position, and passive stretching of the neural system.[63]

Each examination is a new experience. There will be times when different patients relate the same symptoms, but each one will have subtle differences. Every patient perceives pain differently, heals at a different rate, and uses his or her joints differently. Although manual therapists expect to treat only musculoskeletal dysfunctions, knowledge of referred or systemic pain is essential, because many nonmusculoskeletal impairments mimic musculoskeletal ones.

One of the roles of the manual therapist is to confirm a physician's diagnosis. This is not an attempt by our profession to belittle the knowledge of the prescribing physician. On the contrary, we are merely acting as a second pair of eyes and ears and are working *with* the physician in the patient's best interest. Most primary care physicians would admit that their knowledge of the musculoskeletal system is scant at best, and that they occasionally rely on the manual therapist to arrive at a more definitive diagnosis. When used correctly, manual therapy can save the patient from having to go through a battery of unnecessary diagnostic imaging tests or a course of unnecessary drug therapy.

The examination of the musculoskeletal system falls into three parts:

1. The *subjective examination,* which utilizes the information gained from the replies to questions to screen for clues to the patient's condition. (Refer to Chapter 9)
2. The *scanning examination,* which screens for diagnoses that need medical intervention or that can be treated without further examination. (Refer to Chapter 10)
3. The *biomechanical examination,* which looks for specific motion problems, or imbalances. (Refer to Chapter 11) The biomechanical examination is performed if the scanning examination does not indicate either the presence of any serious signs or symptoms, or a diagnosis.

THE DISABLEMENT PROCESS

The main aim of the clinician is the prevention of disability whenever possible, and to help the patient regain a meaningful level of function. The outcomes of the treatments must not only measure objective improvements, but also subjective ones. The vast majority of the tests used in our clinics, such as range of motion and strength, are not measures of function and do not truly reflect a patient's quality of life. Even the assessment of pain, which is subjective, affords little information as to functional improvement, unless the pain is removed entirely. That is not to say that these measurements should be discontinued, as there is a clear link between deficits in motion and strength and the level of function.

Disability can be defined as a difficulty performing activities in any domain of life (from hygiene to hobbies, errands to sleep) due to a health or physical problem. Disability can be assessed as perceived difficulty in different activities, or as a level of dependence on personal help. As Jette[66] pointed out, the rating of perceived difficulty in performing various activities can be considered the primary assessment of disability, whereas the rating of actual dependence on assistance is an assessment of the consequence of disability. Both types of assessment are useful in increasing our understanding of the disablement process.

The disablement process proposed by Jette and Verbrugge[66] describes how a chronic and acute condition can affect the functioning of specific body systems, generic physical and mental actions, and activities of daily life. It also describes the personal and environmental factors that speed or slow disablement, namely, risk factors, interventions, and exacerbators.

Other models or schemes have been proposed to describe the disablement process,[67–70] each with slight variations. Like the Jette and Verbrugge model, these models postulate a main disease–disability pathway, which consists of a series of consecutive, linked events as follows:

> Pathology → Impairment → Functional limitations → Disability.

In this sequence, the term *pathology* is self-explanatory and encompasses any diagnosed disease, injury, or abnormal condition.[66]

Impairment represents a pathologic dysfunction or structural abnormality in a specific body system that leads to a loss of function, and includes pain, loss of motion, loss of strength, or any other impairment diagnosis.[71,72] Factors not directly related to impairment have been shown to contribute to patient disability in patients with rheumatoid arthritis, and it is clear that these factors would have a similar impact on any significant impairment. The factors include quality of life issues such as the patients' physical status, economic status, psychological status,[73,74] educational background,[75] social support,[76] and coexistent morbidity.[77–80] The interactions among the various factors that can cause disability in the individual patient often make it difficult to determine which ones are the most suitable targets for intervention.

Functional limitations are restrictions in performing basic physical and mental actions at the level of the whole organism. Examples of functional limitations include gait abnormalities and an inability to put on shoes.

Disability is defined as difficulty in the performance of socially defined roles and tasks within a sociocultural and physical environment.[66,81] There are a number of measures of physical disability. The physical-function scale of the Short Form 36 (SF-36) questionnaire,[82] which measures perceived limitations in a variety of physical activities, and

the disability index of the modified Health Assessment Questionnaire (M-HAQ),[83] which measures the amount of difficulty in performing eight activities of daily living, are two examples. The Functional Independence Measure (FIM) is another tool designed to measure functional disability.[84] The FIM assesses self-care, sphincter management, mobility, locomotion, communication, and social cognition on a seven-level scale.

The main disease–disability pathway outlined earlier is itself modified by contextual variables, which are innate characteristics or secondary conditions of a person that are not considered amenable to modification. The external modifiers are factors that can influence the level of disability but are not directly related to the disease process itself (Fig. 1–1).

Reducing the possibility of disability is critical when treating patients with a spinal impairment. Disability as a result of spinal impairment is multifactorial. Articular pain and tenderness, muscle weakness, impairment duration, and the presence of deformities (e.g., scoliosis), all contribute to the disablement process. The aim of the intervention plan is to change the direction of travel along the pathway whenever possible. Thus interventions can work anywhere along the continuum from pathology to disability.

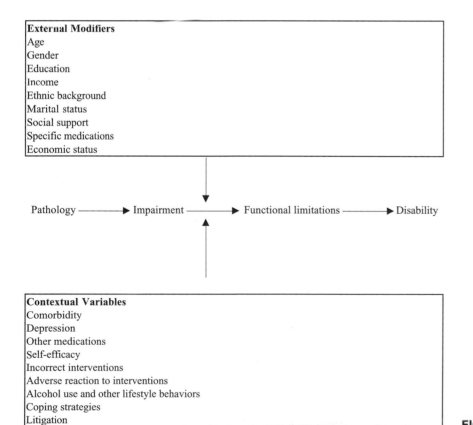

External Modifiers
Age
Gender
Education
Income
Ethnic background
Marital status
Social support
Specific medications
Economic status

Pathology ——▶ Impairment ——▶ Functional limitations ——▶ Disability

Contextual Variables
Comorbidity
Depression
Other medications
Self-efficacy
Incorrect interventions
Adverse reaction to interventions
Alcohol use and other lifestyle behaviors
Coping strategies
Litigation

FIGURE 1–1 The disablement process.

Low back pain (LBP) provides a good example of the disablement pathway as it takes its toll on the individual in multiple ways.

Pathology

The etiology of LBP remains elusive, although a number of structures have been implicated, including the intervertebral disc, the zygapophysial joints, and the surrounding soft tissues. As in any disease with which the body is confronted, the forces to counteract the injury are mobilized and the body attempts to return to its normal, prepathological state.[85]

Impairments

The primary physical impairments that can be associated with LBP are pain, loss of range, and loss of strength. Psychological and social impairments also develop. The degree of impairment from LBP depends on a number of factors related to the pathology itself such as:

- The extent of the disease process
- The chronicity of the pathology
- The number of intervertebral segments involved
- Which structures are involved and to what extent
- The presence of radiculopathy

Factors not directly involved with the pathology also have a part to play and include:

- The patient's perception
- The compensatory and coping strategies of the patient
- The patient's pain tolerance and motivation
- Comorbidity
- The patient's personal and health habits
- The level of social support
- Marital status
- Obesity
- Litigation

Functional Limitations

The functional limitations associated with LBP depend largely on the degree of impairment and the extent and severity of the pathology. The disease pathway in LBP is highly individual in clinical presentation and progression. The progression along the pathway can be slowed or halted by proper medical care, lifestyle changes, and rehabilitation interventions.[85] Ideally, the clinical presentation should be classified according to the musculoskeletal impairments producing certain functional limitations; the intervention plan is then designed to address those limitations rather than just the musculoskeletal impairments.

Relationships need to be founded that establish the required amount of motion and strength at each joint to perform functional tasks. For example, Badley and associates[86] found that at least 70 degrees of knee flexion was needed by the majority of their subjects to perform such activities as walking to a toilet, getting in and out of a bathtub, and walking up and down steps.[85] This linking of range of motion with functional ability is to be commended and must become the central focus for physical therapy practice and research. Unfortunately, all of the tests that have been traditionally used in the outpatient clinics to obtain objective measures have little, if any, correlation with function. Perhaps physical therapists should change their examination process to focus on (1) assessing the patients' ability to perform such functional tasks as transfers, dressing, activities of daily living, or other tasks that they feel are important, and (2) grading them on how difficult these tasks are to complete. Each of these functional tasks could then be broken down to the physical requirements necessary to perform each task. Regaining these requirements would constitute the short-term goals, while the completion of the task would be the long-term goal. The functional outcome measures would then be a reflection of how successful the clinician was at returning the patient to the desired level of function, for it is the ability of the patient to function in his or her environment that is the true test of treatment effectiveness. It is no longer acceptable to use objective measures such as improvement in range of motion or strength, or both, as a means of assessing effectiveness of treatment. All of the outcomes need to evaluate functional improvement as perceived by the patient.

In the case studies throughout this book, the reader should be able to determine the pathology, impairment, and functional limitations of each patient and the interventions that are undertaken to counteract them. The challenge for the clinician appears to be the identification of those factors that may assist in predicting which patients have a propensity toward disability, so that the provision of an appropriate intervention strategy can be made.

WORKING HYPOTHESIS

The clinician's plan of care should be based on the clinical evidence formulated from both the signs observed and the symptoms reported. From this clinical evidence, a working hypothesis should be sought. This working hypothesis is not rigid, and needs to remain responsive to any emerging information. The working hypothesis is based on the following information:

- The physician's diagnosis. The diagnosis given by the physician may be vague, as in the case of LBP, or specific, as in L4-5 disc herniation. The clinician must determine the accuracy of the diagnosis
- Severity, irritability, and stage of the condition
- Location, nature, and extent of the condition
- Cause of the pain. Is it due to a loss or to an excess of motion?
- Relationship of end feel and resistance to passive motion
- Reliability of the patient's subjective information

At the end of the examination, an evaluation is performed to determine a specific diagnosis. The evaluation is an interpretation of the data collected in the examination process.[87] The diagnosis is based on:

- A summation of all the relevant findings
- The recognition of a clinical syndrome or preferred practice pattern[87]

Based on the diagnosis, a prognosis is made and a plan of care is established. The prognosis includes the predicted optimal level of improvement in function and amount of time needed to reach that level.[87] In designing the plan of care, the clinician integrates all of the previous data, incorporates the prognostic predictions, and determines the degree to which the interventions are likely to achieve the anticipated goals and desired outcomes.[87] The goals should relate to the remediation of the impairments, and the outcomes should relate to the minimization of functional limitations.[87]

INTERVENTION

Once the specific diagnosis, prognosis, and plan of care have been determined, the intervention is initiated. As part of the plan of care, the clinician needs to ascertain his or her expectations for the patient's progress, including the estimated changes expected, the natural progression of the condition, and the rate of change.

The intervention may involve the use of a certain protocol for the recognized clinical syndrome, or it may be based on the stage of healing (the principles of protection, rest, ice, compression, and elevation [PRICE] for the patient with an acute condition).

In these days of managed care and overall cost containment, the clinician needs to be both efficient and cost effective. Efficiency, a function of time taken and

effectiveness, can be divided up according to the degree of specificity of the technique used, and the time taken to achieve the desired result—the contact time with the patient. The ultimate goal should be to use the most appropriate and specific intervention that achieves the desired result in the least amount of time. Clearly, the selection criteria need to be based on the best interests of the patient and not just on cost-effectiveness, and are necessarily based on the findings from the examination. Ideally, the two should coincide—an efficient clinician can be both expeditious and cost-effective if his or her expertise permits the correct diagnosis to be made at the initial visit. Once the clinician has determined if the injured structure is a contractile or inert tissue, and whether the aberration of motion is angular or linear, subsequent treatments can be targeted at the specific dysfunction, and the home exercise program tailored to reinforce those activities performed in the clinic.

As the knowledge of the evaluation and treatment of the musculoskeletal system advances, the clinician faces a number of choices as to which intervention should be used. Clinicians now have a continuum of tools at their disposal, from general to specific techniques (Table 1–1).

The least efficient technique is a general technique that is time and labor intensive, whereas the most efficient

TABLE 1–1 THE SPECIFICITY OF VARIOUS INTERVENTIONS

SPECIFICITY	TECHNIQUE EXAMPLES
General	Deep myofascial releases
	Exercise that involves muscle groups with more than one action (cervical rotation)
	Modality applied to a general area
Semi-specific	Strain–counterstrain & trigger-point therapy—are you treating the symptoms rather than the cause?
	Muscle energy techniques that use minimal stabilization
	Symmetric mobilization techniques
	3D exercises involving muscle groups with the same actions (e.g., cervical side flexion and rotation)
Specific	Myofascial techniques to specific muscles, or stretching of specific muscles when angular motion is found to be restricted
	Asymmetric mobilizations (grades I–V)
	Manipulations
	Exercises involving one muscle, or one joint (VMO, atlanto-axial rotation, supraspinatus, etc.)
	Specific traction to a particular level (grades I–II)
	Modalities—ES, ice, massage, US applied to a specific structure

ES, Electrical stimulation; US, Ultrasound; VMO, Vastus medialis obliquus.

technique is a specific technique that requires little contact time, yet is effective. The more experienced and skilled clinicians rely heavily on the specific techniques, and less on the general and semispecific techniques, although there are times when the latter are useful. The term *specific* should not be interpreted as complicated. Many specific techniques are simple in their execution and, wherever possible, the clinician should ensure that their intervention remains as simple as possible for the patient's sake. Fortunately, most musculoskeletal lesions respond well to a combination of heat, ice, and specific strengthening and stretching exercises. The skill involves an accurate selection. This selection is based on the following factors:

- Identification of the structure, or structures, at fault
- Stage of healing
- Reasons for the aberration in movement
- Prognosis
- The ability to aid the healing process, while simultaneously working toward the prevention of recurrences
- Selection and intent of technique
- Comorbidity
- Age
- Severity of symptoms

PATIENT-RELATED INSTRUCTION

Two people will typically affect the outcome of a plan of care, the clinician and the patient. Patients need to be encouraged to become active participants in their own recovery so they do not rely solely on the intervention sessions to improve their outcome. Every therapy session needs to include an educational component as well as a therapeutic one, and the prescribed home exercise program must be carefully explained to ensure that the patient:

- Performs the exercises precisely
- Is aware of the rationale for the exercises
- Is knowledgeable about the types of pain that might be encountered during and after the exercises
- Can use the simple modalities of heat and cold to assist in the healing process
- Modifies certain postures or activities

The exercises prescribed as home exercises should first be demonstrated by the clinician. As the patient performs each exercise, questions should be asked about changes in symptoms. By increasing each patient's knowledge about his or her own condition and the rationale behind the intervention, the clinician is empowering them for the future.

REEVALUATIONS

The treatment plan is dynamic. At each subsequent visit, the clinician needs to determine what has changed. This determination is made by assessing:

- *The quantity and quality of motion.* Often the quantity increases before the quality. Has the end feel changed?
- *The pain.* An increase in the patient's localized pain following an intervention should not be viewed as a negative, and is better than no change as it indicates that the clinician was working on the correct structure, albeit too aggressively. An increase in peripheral symptoms is not a good sign.
- *The effect of the last intervention.* How much relief occurred immediately after, and how did the patient feel the day after?
- *Functional changes.* Are there any activities of daily living that the patient can now perform?

Based on an assessment of the last intervention session, the clinician determines what modifications, if any, are necessary. If there is no change in the patient's status after one or two visits, some modification is imperative. If a particular exercise or manual technique appears to be irritating the condition, it should be modified or discontinued. If the patient appears to be making progress, additions to the plan may be required.

DISCHARGE

A discharge is the process of discontinuing interventions and is based on the clinician's analysis of the dynamic interplay between the achievement of anticipated goals and the achievement of desired outcomes.[87] Before discharging the improving patient, a number of questions must be addressed:

- Is the patient completely or partly recovered?
- Is a recurrence of the impairment likely and, if so, how is the patient going to prevent these recurrences?
- Which exercises must the patient continue to perform at home, and for how long?
- What modifications must the patient make in his or her lifestyle?
- Is an external support necessary?

EXAMINATION FLOW

The flow diagram in Figure 1–2 outlines the examination sequence used throughout this book. The various components of the flow diagram will be described in the various chapters, and its logical sequence is employed for each joint, with the pertinent details for those joints explained. The flow sequence is dependent on the clinical findings and provides a framework for the clinician to work from.

In the absence of criterion validity, most of the theories behind the examination and treatment approaches are based on construct validity. However, in the absence of convincing evidence to refute the construct, this validity is preferable to no validity, and is stronger than the unvalidated attacks on the theory.

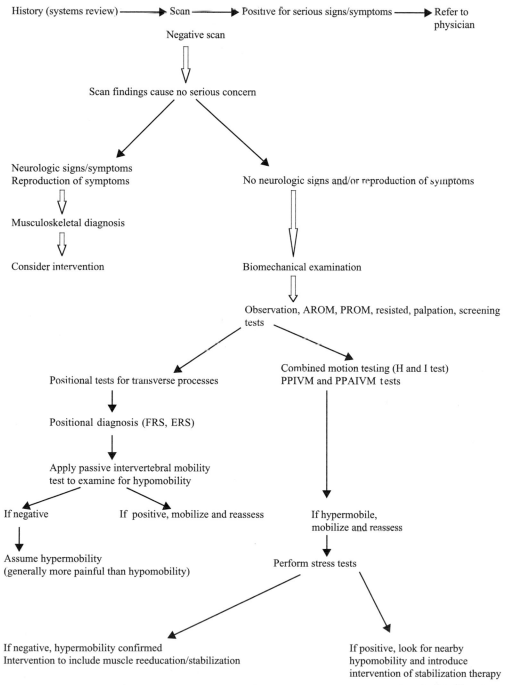

FIGURE 1–2 General examination sequence for the spine. (*Abbreviations:* AROM, Active range of motions; H and I, 'H' and 'I' Tests; PPAIVM, Passive physiological articular intervertebral motion; PPIVM, Passive physiological intervertebral motion; PROM, Passive range of motion)

REFERENCES

1. Sanan A, Rengachary SS. The history of spinal biomechanics. Neurosurgery 1996;39(4): 657–668; discussion 668–669.
2. Thurston, J. Giovanni Borelli and the study of human movement: An historical review. Aus N Zeal J Surg 1999;69:276–288.
3. Breasted JH. The Edwin Smith papyrus: An Egyptian medical treatise of the seventeenth century before Christ. N Y Hist Soc Q Bull 1922;6:5–31.
4. Breasted JH. The Edwin Smith Surgical Papyrus [facsimile and hieroglyphic transliteration with translation and commentary, in two volumes]. Chicago, Ill: The University of Chicago Press; 1930.
5. Dawson WR. The earliest surgical treatise. Br J Surg 1932;20:34–43.
6. Elsberg CA. The Edwin Smith Surgical Papyrus and the diagnosis and treatment of injuries to the skull and spine 5000 years ago. Ann Med Hist 1931;3: 271–279.
7. Elsberg CA. The anatomy and surgery of the Edwin Smith Surgical Papyrus. Mt Sinai Hosp J 1945;12: 141–151.
8. Majno G. *The Healing Hand: Man and Wound in the Ancient World.* Cambridge, Mass: Harvard University Press; 1975.
9. Smith GE. The most ancient splints. Br Med J 1908;1: 732–734.
10. Kumar K: Historical perspective: Spinal deformity and axial traction. Spine 1996;21:653–655.
11. Subramaniam K. *Srimad Bhagavatam.* Bombay, India: Bharatiya Vidya Bhavan; 1979.
12. Hippocrates. *The Genuine Works of Hippocrates* [Adams F, trans]. Baltimore, Md: Williams & Wilkins; 1939: 231–241.
13. Galen. *On the Affected Parts* [Siegel RE, trans]. Basel, Switzerland: S Karger; 1976:114.
14. Shapiro R. Talmudic and other ancient concepts of the number of vertebrae in the human spine. Spine 1990;15:246–247.
15. Galen. *On the Anatomical Procedures: The Later Books* [Duckworth WLH, trans]. Cambridge, England: University Press; 1962:24.
16. Novell JR. From Da Vinci to Harvey: The development of mechanical analogy in medicine from 1500 to 1650. J R Soc Med 1990;83:396–398.
17. Soutas-Little RWM. Louisa Burns memorial lecture: Biomechanics and osteopathic manipulative treatment. J Am Osteopath Assoc 1983;83:126–128.
18. Kumar K. Did the modern concept of axial traction to correct scoliosis exist in prehistoric times? J Neurol Orthop Med Surg 1987;8:310.
19. Alexander RM. The progress of animal mechanics. Fortschr Zool 1977;24:3–11.
20. Borelli GA. *De Motu Animalium.* Rome: Angeli Bernabo; 1680.
21. Borelli GA. *On the Movement of Animals* [Maquet P, trans]. Berlin, Germany: Springer-Verlag; 1989.
22. Hildanus WF. *Opera quae Extant Omnia.* Francofurti ad Moenum: J Beyeri; 1646.
23. Crisco JJ, Panjabi MM. The intersegmental and multisegmental muscles of the lumbar spine: A biomechanical model comparing lateral stabilizing potential. Spine 1991;16:793–799.
24. Euler L. *Leonhardi Euleri Opera Omnia.* Lipsiae: BG Teubneri; 1911.
25. Weber EH. Anatomisch-physiologische Untersuchung über einige Einrichtungen im Mechanismus der Menschlichen Wirbelsäule. Archiv Anat Physiol 1827; 240–271.
26. Elward JF. Motion in the vertebral column. Am J Roentgenol 1939;42:91–99.
27. Fisk GR. The influence of hip rotation upon the gait. Aust N Z J Surg 1979;49:7–12.
28. Murray MP. Gait as a total pattern of movement. Am J Phys Med Rehabil 1967;46:290–333.
29. Thurston AJ. Pelvic and lumbar spinal movement during walking in a group of normal males. Annu Rep Oxf Orthop Eng Centre 1980;7:33–37.
30. Thurston AJ, Whittle MW, Stokes IAF. Spinal and pelvic movement during walking—a new method of study. Eng Med 1981;10:219–222.
31. Thurston AJ. *Kinematics of the Lumbar Spine and Pelvis.* Oxford, England: University of Oxford; 1981. MSc Thesis.
32. Hughes AW. Die Drehbewegungen der menschlichen Wirbelsäule und die segenaunten Musculi rotatores. Arch Anat Entwicklungsgeschichte 1892;265–280.
33. Andersen N, Ekström T. Uber die Beweglichkeit der Wirbelsäule. Gegenbaurs Morph Jabuch 1940;85:135–185.
34. von Meyer GH. *Die Stat und Mechanische d. Menschlichen.* Leipzig, Germany: Knochenger; 1873.
35. Guérin J. Mémoire sur les mouvments de flexion et l'inclinaison e la colonne vertebrale. Bull Acad Med 1876;5:936.
36. Morris H. *The Anatomy of the Joints of Man.* London, England: 1879.
37. Wolff J. Concerning the interrelationship between form and function of the individual parts of the organism [Scheck M, trans]. Clin Orthop 1988;228:2–11.
38. Novogrodsky M. *Die Bewegungsmöglichkeit in d. menschlichen Wirbelsäule.* Bern, Switzerland: 1911.
39. Strasser H. *Lehrb. d. Muskel-u, Gelenmech.* Berlin, Germany: 1913.

40. Löhr C. Untersuchungen über de Bewegungen der Wirbelsäule nach vorn und hinten. Munch Med Wochenschr 1890;37:73–97.
41. Troup JDG, Hood CA, Chapman AE. Measurements of sagittal mobility of lumbar spine and hips. Ann Phys Med 1968;9:308.
42. Cyriax JH. An apparatus for estimating degree of rotation in the spinal column. BMJ 1924;2:958.
43. Dunham WF. Ankylosing spondylitis: Measurement of hip and spine movements. Br J Phys Med 1949; 12:126.
44. Asmussen E. Heeboll-Neilsen. Posture, mobility and strength of the back in boys 7–16 years old. Acta Orthop Scand 1959;28:174–189.
45. Israel M. A quantitative method of estimating flexion and extension of the spine; a preliminary report. Mil Med 1959;124:181–186.
46. Goff CF. Postural evolution related to back pain. Clin Orthop 1955;5:8–15.
47. Thurston AJ, Stokes IAF. Measurement of spinal movement in 3-dimensions using the vector stereograph. Annu Rep Oxf Orthop Eng Centre 1980;7:27–28.
48. Grew ND, Harris JD. A method of measuring human body shape and movement. The Vector Stereograph. Eng Med 1979;8:115–118.
49. Denis F. The three column injury and its significance in the classification of acute thoracolumbar spinal injuries. Spine 1983;8:817–831.
50. Panjabi MM, Oxland TR, Kifune M, Arand M, Wen L, Chen A. Validity of the three-column theory of thoracolumbar fractures: A biomechanic investigation. Spine 1995;20:1122–1127.
51. Taylor AS. Fracture dislocation of the cervical spine. Ann Surg 1929;90:321–340.
52. Cyriax J. *Textbook of Orthopedic Medicine.* vol 1, 8th ed. London, England: Balliere Tindall and Cassell; 1982.
53. Grieve GP. *Common Vertebral Joint Problems.* 2nd ed. New York, NY: Churchill Livingstone; 1988:159–209.
54. Kaltenborn F. *Mobilization of the Spinal Column.* Wellington, New Zealand: New Zealand University Press; 1970.
55. Kaltenborn F. *Manual Therapy for Extremity Joints.* Oslo; Sweden: Bokhandel; 1974.
56. Evjenth O, Hamberg J. *Muscle Stretching in Manual Therapy; A Clinical manual. Vol 1, The Extremities. Vol 2, The Spinal Column and the TMJ.* Alfta, Sweden: Alfta rehab Forlag; 1980.
57. Janda V. *Muscle Function Testing.* London, England: Butterworths; 1983:163–167.
58. Maitland GD. *Vertebral Manipulation.* 5th ed. London, England: Butterworths; 1986.
59. McKenzie RA. *The Lumbar Spine: Mechanical Diagnosis and Therapy.* Waikanae, New Zealand: Spinal Publications Limited; 1989.
60. Mennel JM. *Back Pain.* Boston, Mass: Little Brown; 1960.
61. Paris SV. *The Spinal Lesion.* Christchurch, England: Pegasus; 1965.
62. Schmorl G, Junghanns H. *The Human Spine in Health and Disease.* 2nd American ed. New York, NY: Grune & Stratton; 1971.
63. Lamb D. A review of manual therapy for spinal pain. In: Boyling, JD, Palastanga N eds. *Grieve's Modern Manual Therapy: The Vertebral Column.* 2nd ed. Edinburgh, Scotland: Churchill Livingstone; 1994.
64. Bogduk N, Jull G. The theoretical pathology of acute locked back: A basis for manipulative therapy. Man Med 1985;1:78.
65. April C, Dwyer A, Bogduk N. Cervical zygapophyseal joint pain patterns II: A clinical evaluation. Spine 1990;15:458–461.
66. Verbrugge LM, Jette AM. The disablement process. Soc Sci Med 1994;38:1–14.
67. Nagi S. Some conceptual issues in disability and rehabilitation. In: Sussman M, ed. *Sociology and Rehabilitation.* Washington, DC: American Sociological Association; 1965:100–113.
68. Nagi S. Disability concepts revisited: Implications for prevention. In: Pope A, Tartov A, eds. *Disability in America: Toward a National Agenda for Prevention.* Washington, DC: National Academy Press; 1991:309–327.
69. *International Classification of Impairments, Disabilities, and Handicaps.* Geneva, Switzerland: World Health Organization; 1980.
70. Pope A, Tartov A, eds. *Disability in America: Toward a National Agenda for Prevention.* Washington, DC: National Academy Press; 1991.
71. Sahrmann SA: Diagnosis by the physical therapist. Phys Ther 1988;68:1703–1706.
72. Jette AM. Diagnosis and classification by physical therapists. Phys Ther 1989;69:967–969.
73. Cavalieri F, Salaffi F, Ferraccioli GF. Relationship between physical impairment, psychological variables and pain in rheumatoid disability: An analysis of their relative impact. Clin Exp Rheumatol 1991;9:47–50.
74. Parker J, Smarr K, Anderson S, et al. Relationship of changes in helplessness and depression to disease activity in rheumatoid arthritis. J Rheumatol 1992;19:1901–1905.
75. Callahan LF, Pincus T. Formal education level as a significant marker of clinical status in rheumatoid arthritis. Arthritis Rheum 1988;31:1346–1357.
76. Fitzpatrick R, Newman S, Archer R, Shipley M. Social support, disability and depression: A longitudinal study of rheumatoid arthritis. Soc Sci Med 1991;33:605–611.
77. Berkanovic E, Hurwicz ML. Rheumatoid arthritis and comorbidity. J Rheumatol 1990;17:888–892.

78. Mitchell JM, Burkhauser RV, Pincus T. The importance of age, education, and comorbidity in the substantial earnings losses of individuals with symmetric polyarthritis. Arthritis Rheum 1988;31:348–357.

79. Callahan LF, Bloch DA, Pincus T. Identification of work disability in rheumatoid arthritis: Physical, radiographic and laboratory variables do not add explanatory power to demographic and functional variables. J Clin Epidemiol 1992;45:127–138.

80. Pincus T, Callahan LF. Formal education as a marker for increased mortality and morbidity in rheumatoid arthritis. J Chronic Dis 1985;38:973–984.

81. Verbrugge LM. Disability. Rheum Dis Clin North Am 1990;16:741–761.

82. Ware JR Jr. *SF-36 Health Survey: Manual and Interpretation Guide.* Boston, Mass: The Health Institute, Nimrod Press; 1993.

83. Pincus T, Summey JA, Soraci SA Jr, Wallston KA, Hummon NP. Assessment of patient satisfaction in activities of daily living using a modified Stanford Health Assessment Questionnaire. Arthritis Rheum 1983;26:1346–1353.

84. Heinemann AW, Linacre JM, Wright BD, et al. Relationships between impairment and physical disability as measured by the Functional Independence Measure. Arch Phys Med Rehabil 1993;74:566–573.

85. Guccione AA. Arthritis and the process of disablement. Phys Ther 1994;74:408–414.

86. Badley EM, Wagstaff S, Wood PHN. Measures of functional ability (disability) in arthritis in relation to impairment of range of joint movement. Ann Rheum Dis 1984;43:563–569.

87. Guide to physical therapist practice, Phys Ther. (Suppl) 1997;77:1163–1650.

CHAPTER TWO

MUSCULOSKELETAL TISSUE

Chapter Objectives

At the completion of this chapter, the reader will be able to:

1. Describe the composition properties and function of bone.
2. List the differences between osteoporosis and osteomalacia.
3. Describe the composition properties and function of articular cartilage.
4. Describe the composition properties and function of the synovial membrane, and list the different theories of joint lubrication.
5. Describe the disease process of osteoarthritis and its affect on function.
6. Describe the function and location of joint receptors.
7. Describe the composition properties and function of skeletal muscle.
8. Describe the three phases of soft tissue healing and their implications for treatment.

THE STRUCTURE AND GROWTH OF BONE[1]

The function of bone is to provide support, enhance leverage, protect vital structures, and store calcium. From the manual clinician's perspective, it would appear that the most important function of the bones is that they serve as useful landmarks during the palpation phase of the examination, and that they serve as the attachment for both tendons and ligaments. However, although it is true that most of the manual clinician's caseload involves the examination and treatment of the soft tissues, including the tendons, muscles, ligaments, and joints, the ability to detect the presence of an injury to the bone is vital, especially in the spine.

The injury sustained to a bone depends largely on three factors:

1. *The magnitude of the force.* The force may be large, such as that occurring with blunt trauma or a traction injury (macrotrauma), or it may be small but cumulative (microtrauma). Cumulative forces may strengthen the bone or cause it to fracture.
2. *The location of the injury.* Thicker bones can resist larger forces.
3. *The presence of an underlying disease process.* Two such disease processes are osteoporosis and osteomalacia.

OSTEOPOROSIS

Based on World Health Organization criteria, it is estimated that 15% of postmenopausal Caucasian women in the United States and 35% of women older than 65 years of age have osteoporosis.[2] As many as 50% of women have some degree of low bone density in the hip. One of every two Caucasian women will experience an osteoporotic fracture at some point in her lifetime. There is a significant risk, although lower, for men and non-Caucasian women to also sustain osteoporotic fractures. Patients with fragility fractures create a significant economic burden with more than 400,000 hospital admissions and 2.5 million physician visits per year.[2]

Riggs and Melton[3,4] in 1983 proposed that involutional osteoporosis could be divided into two distinct types, although it has always been acknowledged that this model is an oversimplification and that overlap exists. The first type, type I postmenopausal osteoporosis, characterized by the accelerated phase of bone loss in the early postmenopausal period, affects primarily cancellous bone and therefore particularly affects the spine.[5] This rapid phase of bone loss (usually 1% to 2% per year) generally lasts 4 to 8 years and is related to estrogen deficiency.[5] Estrogen seems to control the local production of bone-resorbing cytokines and other factors.[6] Reduced estrogen seems to result in osteoclastic activation and bone resorption.[5] The reduction of estrogen also seems to allow for an increase in bone sensitivity to the bone-resorbing effect of parathyroid hormone (PTH).[5] The mobilization of calcium from bone tends to suppress serum PTH levels.[5] Increased loss of urinary calcium and reduced gastrointestinal calcium absorption maintains normal serum calcium levels.[4]

The second phase of bone loss, type II osteoporosis (age-related or senile osteoporosis), occurs 10 to 20 years after menopause (late menopause), is associated with a more gradual loss of bone (about 0.5% to 1% per year), and affects cancellous and cortical bone loss in both women and men.[4,5] During this phase of bone loss, a variety of age-related alterations in calcium metabolism result in secondary hyperparathyroidism.[7] PTH levels tend to rise (although generally stay within the normal range), leading to increased bone turnover.[5] Age-related declines in the renal function, intestinal malabsorption of calcium, and altered vitamin D metabolism have all been attributed to the rise in PTH.[5] In addition, senescent changes in osteoblast function cause reduced bone formation.[8]

Osteoporosis is characterized by a decrease in bone mass, microarchitectural deterioration of the matrix, and fragility fractures,[9] whereas osteomalacia is characterized by a failure to mineralize the matrix. Osteomalacia is often associated with a vitamin D deficiency, although there are other causes, including hereditary causes such as vitamin D–resistant rickets.

When the mineralized matrix disintegrates, calcium is inevitably lost. The negative calcium balance observed with matrix loss has given rise to erroneous beliefs that the calcium requirements of postmenopausal women are higher than those of premenopausal women, and that osteoporosis could be prevented by calcium supplementation.[10] Although calcium is certainly critical during the development of bone, it cannot replace the disintegrating matrix or prevent its loss.[11] Calcium is a nutrient, not a drug, and the only disorder it can be expected to alleviate is a calcium deficiency.[12] In addition, excess calcium supplementation suppresses the secretion of PTH, retarding the natural turnover of bone, and increasing its risk for microfractures. Thus, the focus on preventing osteoporosis should be on preserving bone matrix, rather than on calcium therapy.

Bone turnover is maintained by osteoclasts, which dig pits in mineralized matrix, and osteoblasts, which refill the pits. Osteoclastic activity is constrained by the action of sex steroids, and coordination with the osteoblasts is normally maintained such that there is no net change in bone mass during early adult life. After menopause, estrogen concentrations fall rapidly and osteoclastic activity accelerates. The net result is bone loss that over a period of years, may amount to 20% or more of the skeleton.

Hui and colleagues[13] related fracture risk to bone density in different age groups, finding that, for the same bone density, the risk of fracture rose eightfold to 10-fold from age younger than 45 years to 80 years or older. In a sample of 5800 Dutch men and women more than 55 years of age, the risk of hip fracture rose 13-fold with age, to which the decrease in bone density contributed only 1.9 in women and 1.6 in men.[14] These observations indicate that something very important in the aging process influences fracture risk, independently of bone density. Because of this rise in the frequency of impact fractures with age, intervention should be focused on infirm older people, irrespective of their bone density.

It is highly likely that bone depends more on architecture than on mass for its strength. Whereas bone in a younger person is structurally normal, its architecture in older people is compromised in two ways:

1. The progressive erosion of trabeculae, the internal scaffolding of bone, leaves them weakened.[15,16]
2. The rate of bone turnover in women who are deficient in estrogen inevitably is higher, mass for mass, than in women who are estrogen replete.

Osteoporosis is also common in alcoholics, drug addicts, and individuals who undertook severe dieting during their teenage years.

Vertebral fracture resulting from minimal trauma is a classical manifestation of osteoporosis. The epidemiology and risk factors of vertebral fractures are difficult to study because significant proportions of the fractures are asymptomatic. The acute pain of a compression fracture superimposed on chronic discomfort, often in the absence of a history of trauma, may be the only presenting symptom. The patient may recall a "snap" associated with mild back pain that occurred when bending over to pick up a small object. More intense pain may not develop for hours or until the next day.[17]

The differential diagnosis between osteomalacia and osteoporosis can be made certain only by using bone biopsy.[18] Figure 2–1 lists the conditions thought to provoke osteoporosis or osteomalacia.[19]

The significance of osteoporosis to the clinician is twofold:

● *The link to patient falls.* Falls and osteoporotic fractures are highly prevalent, interrelated conditions in older adults.[20] Each year, approximately 30% of community-dwelling older people in developed countries fall at least once and 10% to 20% fall twice or more.[21–24] Although less than 5% of falls among older adults lead to a bone fracture, multiple falling is clearly a marker of physical frailty.[21–24] Accumulating evidence indicates that activities that help to maintain mobility, physical functioning, bone mineral density, muscle

Cushing's syndrome—this syndrome occurs as a result of large doses of cortisol in some patients. Patients with Cushing's syndrome of long duration almost always demonstrate demineralization of bone. In severe cases, this may lead to pathologic fractures, but more commonly it results in wedging of the vertebrae, kyphosis, bone pain, and back pain (secondary to bone loss).

- Hypogonadism
- Hypercalciuria
- Hyperparathyroidism
- Hyperthyroidism
- Vitamin D deficiency
- Osteogenesis imperfecta
- Renal tubular acidosis

FIGURE 2–1 Conditions that promote osteoporosis.

strength, and balance, may prevent falls and osteoporotic fractures.[25–27]

- *The potential for spinal fractures.* The location can vary, but these fractures are particularly significant if they occur in the upper cervical spine, where their proximity to vital structures can have disastrous consequences following an overzealous manual technique.

ARTICULAR CARTILAGE[28]

The development of bone is usually preceded by the formation of cartilage, a type of connective tissue. Body cartilage exists in three forms: elastic, hyaline, and fibrocartilage.

- Elastic cartilage is a very specialized connective tissue, primarily found in the symphysis pubis and the larynx.
- Hyaline cartilage covers the ends of long bones and, along with the synovial fluid that bathes it, provides a smoothly articulating, slippery, friction-free surface when two bones move against each other.
- Fibrocartilage basically acts as a shock absorber in both weight-bearing and non–weight-bearing joints. Its large fiber content makes it ideal for bearing large stresses in all directions.

Articular cartilage plays a vital role in the function of the musculoskeletal system by allowing almost frictionless motion to occur and distributing the loads of articulation over a larger contact area, thereby minimizing the contact stresses, and dissipating the energy associated with the load.[29,30] These properties allow the potential for articular cartilage to remain healthy and fully functional throughout decades of life, despite the very slow turnover rate of its collagen matrix.

Normal articular cartilage is comprised of chondrocytes and an extracellular matrix that consists primarily of collagen and proteoglycans. The chondrocytes, which make up approximately 10% of the wet weight of articular cartilage, are specialized cells that are responsible for the development of articular cartilage, and the maintenance of the extracellular matrix.[31] The extracellular matrix also contains additional, but quantitatively minor, glycoproteins and lipids.[32] Water and dissolved electrolytes comprise 60% to 85% of the wet weight of normal cartilage.

Collagen is found in numerous tissues, including articular cartilage, bone, muscles, tendons, ligaments, menisci, and blood vessels. Collagen makes up 10% to 30% of the wet weight of normal articular cartilage. While collagen fibers do not offer much in the way of resistance to compression, they do, however, possess great tensile strength.[33,34]

Three distinct zones, with differing collagen orientations, are found in articular cartilage: the superficial zone (zone I), the transitional or middle zone (zone II), and the deep zone (zone III).[35,36] In the superficial zone, the collagen fibrils are arranged parallel to the surface. In the middle zone, the collagen fibril orientation is less organized, and in the deep zone, the fibrils are perpendicular to the surface of the joint. The tidemark delineates the boundary between zone III and the zone of calcified cartilage.

Proteoglycans comprise 3% to 10% of the wet weight of articular cartilage.[29] To the proteoglycans are attached many extended polysaccharide units called glycosaminoglycans,[37] of which there are two types: chondroitin sulfate and keratin sulfate. Chondrocytes produce aggrecan, link protein, and hyaluronan, which are extruded into the extracellular matrix where they aggregate spontaneously.[37] The aggrecans form a strong, porous-permeable, fiber-reinforced composite material with collagen.

Viscoelasticity is defined as the time-dependent response of a material that has been subjected to a constant load or deformation. Viscoelastic structures are capable of responding in one of two ways, creep and stress relaxation. Creep occurs when a viscoelastic material undergoes constant loading, and responds by initially deforming rapidly and then deforming more slowly over time until the load is balanced and deformation ceases. Stress relaxation occurs when a viscoelastic material undergoes constant deformation, and responds with a high initial stress that progressively decreases over time, until equilibrium is reached. Articular cartilage has been shown to exhibit both creep and stress relaxation behaviors.[38]

Understanding the compressive properties of articular cartilage is vital to understanding its overall function. As it is compressed, articular cartilage undergoes a change in volume that causes a pressure change in the tissue, and results in the flow of interstitial fluid.[38]

The primary functions of cartilage are threefold:

1. Wear resistance, with the collagen providing strength, and the matrix providing smoothness and firmness.
2. Low coefficient of friction owing to the smoothness, elasticity, and viscoelasticity. Cartilage is 10 times smoother than the surface of a ball bearing.
3. Compression force attenuation is afforded by the elastic and viscoelastic properties of the cartilage. Cartilage is 10 times more effective than bone at reducing compression, but there is much less of it.

Synovial Membrane

The synovial membrane is derived from the embryonic mesenchyme and is found as the nonarticular component of joints, in bursae, and in tendon sheaths. It is formed in two layers:

1. *Lamina intima* consists of one to four layers of synovial cells embedded in a granular fiber free matrix. It produces synovial fluid and absorbs substances from the joint cavity.
2. *Lamina subintima* is formed by a vascular fibrous layer where the collagen and elastin run parallel to the surface and contains fibroblasts, macrophages, and fat cells. Its elasticity prevents excessive folding of the synovial membrane during movement, thereby preventing pinching. The fat imparts firmness, deformability, and elastic recoil.

Joint Lubrication

The function of synovial fluid is to provide nutrition, lubrication, and heat dissipation.

The friction between the articular surfaces is greatest during sliding, and lubrication is necessary to minimize frictional resistance between the weight-bearing surfaces. Fluid lubrication happens when a film is established and maintained between the two surfaces as long as movement occurs. There are a number of theories with regard to joint lubrication:

1. *Boundary lubrication.*[39] The hyaluronate molecules adhering to the joint surfaces provide this and keep a very thin film of fluid between the two moving surfaces.
2. *Hydrostatic (weeping) lubrication.*[40] Under compression, the cartilage weeps water and small ions between the surfaces. This maintains a lubricating layer under weight-bearing conditions.
3. *Hydrodynamic lubrication.* The motion of the lubricant in the tapered gaps of the primary and secondary contours generates the pressure required to support the load.
4. *Elastohydrodynamic lubrication.* The pressure generated by the moving fluid deforms the elasticity of the weight-bearing surfaces (i.e., it flattens the ridges) and so smoothes the surfaces.
5. *Boosted lubrication.* Under very heavy loads, small molecules pass into the cartilage, leaving large hyaluronate molecules in the hollows. This increases the viscosity of the synovial fluid and so improves its lubricating abilities.

Disease, Damage, and Repair[41]

Diseases such as osteoarthritis (OA) that affect articular cartilage and other joint structures represent some of the most common and debilitating diseases encountered in orthopedic practice. Yelin[42] estimated the cost of OA in the United States at $15.5 billion (in 1994 dollars), roughly three times the cost of rheumatoid arthritis. More than half of the OA costs are a result of work loss. Admissions to hospitals for conditions directly related to OA were the third most common form of admission between 1985 and 1988.[43] It is estimated that approximately 123,000 hip arthroplasties and 95,000 total knee replacements were performed annually during this time; the majority of these arthroplasties were performed to treat OA.[43] Moreover, diseases of cartilage cause activity limitations in an even greater numbers of patients, limiting their performance of sports, and even adversely affecting normal activities of daily living.

OA is the most common articular disease of older adults. Reported incidence and prevalence rates of OA in specific joints vary widely, however, because of differences in the contributing risk factors and the case definition of OA.[44–47] OA may be defined by radiographic abnormalities (radiographic OA) alone, by typical symptoms (symptomatic OA), or by both.[48] The distal and proximal interphalangeal joints of the hand are the most prevalent location of radiographic abnormalities but are least likely to be symptomatic.[45,46,49–51] The knee,[50,52] and hip,[46,52] are the second and third most common locations of radiographic abnormalities, respectively, and, in contrast to the hand, are frequently symptomatic.[49,50,53,54]

OA is diagnosed by typical symptoms, physical findings, and radiographic changes.[55] Patients early in the disease process experience localized joint pain that worsens with activity and lessens with rest, whereas those with severe disease may have pain at rest.[56] Weight-bearing joints may "lock" or "give way" as a result of internal derangement that is a consequence of advanced disease. Morning stiffness and stiffness following inactivity, also known as *gel phenomena*, rarely exceed 30 minutes.[56] Physical findings in osteoarthritic joints include bony prominence, crepitus, and deficits in range of motion. Tenderness on palpation at the joint line and pain on passive motion are also common, although not unique to OA.[56] Progressive cartilage destruction, malalignment, joint effusions, and subchondral bone collapse contribute to irreversible deformity.[55] Radiographic findings in OA include osteophyte formation, joint space narrowing, subchondral sclerosis, and cysts.[57–60]

Both systemic and local factors affect the likelihood that a joint will develop OA.[61] Systemic factors probably make cartilage more vulnerable to daily injuries and less capable of repair. Many mechanisms could explain this process, including the effects of growth factors and cytokines on chondrocytes and their synthesis of cartilage matrix. Other systemic factors including bone factors, might accelerate enzymatic destruction of the matrix, and reduce its repair capabilities. Once the systemic vulnerability factors are in place, local biomechanical factors begin to play a role.

It is well established that damaged articular cartilage has a very limited potential for healing, and articular defects larger than 2 to 4 mm in diameter rarely heal, even with such advances as the use of continuous passive motion.[62–64] Damage to articular cartilage is a common problem. In one study, it was associated with 16% (21) of 132 injuries of the knee that were sufficient to cause intraarticular bleeding.[65] Furthermore, damage to a joint surface can lead to premature arthritis.[66] Elderly patients (those who are 65 years of age or older), who have an arthritic condition can obtain dramatic relief from pain and restoration of function after total joint replacement.[56] However, such procedures have higher rates of failure in young and early-middle-aged patients (those who are younger than 40 years old and those who are 40 to 60 years old, respectively), than in elderly patients.[67]

Articular cartilage in adults possesses neither a blood supply nor lymphatic drainage. In fact, after they are surrounded by their extracellular matrix, articular chondrocytes are sheltered even from immunologic recognition.

Risk Factors for Osteoarthritis

Age Although specific risk factors for OA differ by anatomic joint region, age is the most consistently identified demographic risk factor for all articular sites.[46,47] The incidence of OA has been reported to be 0.2 per 100 males and 0.4 per 100 females under 20 years of age, and 17.0 per 100 males and 29.6 per 100 females over 60 years of age.[43] Before the age of 50 years, men have a higher prevalence and incidence of this disease than women, but after age 50, women have a higher prevalence and incidence.[68] Both incidence and prevalence appear to level off or decline in both sexes at around age 80.[49] However, survivor bias may falsely lower estimates of prevalence and incidence of hip OA in the oldest age group.[49,69]

The increase in the incidence and prevalence of OA with age is likely a consequence of several biologic changes that occur with aging, including a decreased responsiveness of chondrocytes to growth factors that stimulate repair; an increase in the laxity of ligaments around the joints, making older joints relatively unstable and, therefore, more susceptible to injury; and a gradual decrease in strength and a slowing of peripheral neurologic responses,[71] both of which protect the joint. The question arises as to whether OA is a disease or a natural consequence of aging, as increasing age does not appear to be an absolute risk factor, for not every elderly person develops osteoarthritis.[72,73] OA and normal aging cartilage are distinguished by relative differences in water content and the ratio of chondroitin sulfate to keratan sulfate constituents.[74,75] Another distinction is that degradative enzyme activity is increased in OA but not in normal aging cartilage.[72] Even over many decades, the accumulated damage in normal articular cartilage is usually minimal, indicating that an effective mechanism for protecting the cartilage from supporting loads must exist.

Degenerative changes in diarthrodial joints, occurring gradually over time, probably result from an initial reduction in the ability of the solid matrix to support loads, which causes a breakdown of the matrix, further reducing its load-bearing capacity.[76–78] Eventually, loss of the articular surface may occur. If the rate of this kind of damage exceeds the rate at which the cartilage cells can repair the tissue, the accumulated damage may eventually lead to bulk tissue failure.[30,77]

Racial Characteristics Cross-national and cross-racial studies can often produce insights about disease etiology. With respect to OA, there is conflicting evidence as to whether blacks have different rates of OA than whites.[81,82]

The higher relative weight of black women may predispose them to high rates of knee OA.

Genetic Susceptibility Generalized OA, an entity common in elderly women, consists of concurrent OA in the hand joints, including the distal interphalangeal (DIP), proximal interphalangeal, and first carpometacarpal (CMC) joints; the cervical and lumbosacral spine; the knees; and, possibly, the hips. There are two types of generalized OA, nodal OA (Heberden's nodes) and non-nodal OA.[83]

Several studies have confirmed that OA in the general population is inherited. Thus, for risk-profiling purposes, persons whose parents had OA, especially if the disease was polyarticular, or if the onset was in middle age or earlier, are at high risk of OA themselves.

Osteoporosis Radin[86] has suggested that subchondral bone deformation during impact loading of the joint protects articular cartilage from damage. Those with more deformable bone may be less susceptible to OA. Dequeker and associates[87] recently found that osteoporosis and OA were inversely associated in 53 of the 67 (mostly cross-sectional) studies reviewed. Individuals with osteoporosis exhibit a lower-than-expected rate of OA.[88] Furthermore, bone density in patients with OA is greater than in age-matched controls, even at sites distant from the joint affected by OA.[89,90]

Estrogen In addition to the high incidence of OA in women after age 50, which is the approximate age of menopause, some women develop "menopausal arthritis," that is, rapidly progressive hand OA at the time of menopause. These sex- and age-related prevalence patterns are consistent with the role of postmenopausal hormone deficiency in increasing the risk of OA.

Nutritional Factors Damage from reactive oxygen species has been implicated as pathogenic in a variety of human diseases, including OA,[93] and there is evidence that antioxidants from diet or other sources may prevent or delay the occurrence of some of these diseases.

Obesity Obesity clearly plays a role in the development of OA. Epidemiologic studies, for example, the Framingham study,[54] demonstrated a temporal link between obesity and the development of OA. Cohort studies have demonstrated a clear association of obesity with the development of radiographic OA of the knee in older women and a weaker association with OA of the hip.[54] There are several theories about the link between obesity and the development of OA. One theory holds that obesity causes an abnormally increased load across the joint

that predisposes it to OA. Another theory postulates that there is a biologic mediator of obesity that in some way also causes cartilage degeneration, although such a mediator has yet to be found.[95]

Immobility Joint immobility is also suspected as a factor that can lead to eventual cartilage OA, and studies in animals have, in fact, shown that the immobilization of a joint can lead to cartilage degeneration. For example, a decrease in cartilage thickness, and a change in the mechanical properties of articular cartilage, have been noted in dogs that were immobilized using a cast or external fixator.[97–99] Compositional changes in articular cartilage resulting from immobilization have also been demonstrated. Proteoglycan content has been shown to decrease, while an increase in water content has been observed.[100] Such compositional changes may result in decreased cartilage stiffness and an associated reduced capacity for it to bear normal loads.[101] Although remobilization generally can restore the cartilage to normal composition and function, prolonged immobilization may result in permanent changes.[102]

Repetitive Activities While studies have shown that normal loading of the joint is required to sustain healthy articular cartilage, repetitive activities over a long period of time have been associated with cartilage degeneration, and occupations that involve repetitive actions have been shown to be correlated with increased rates of osteoarthritis. Farmers, for example, have high rates of OA of the hip,[103] and epidemiologic studies have shown that firefighters, farmers, construction workers, and miners have a higher prevalence of OA of the knee than the general population.[95] In fact, workers whose jobs require knee bending, as well as lifting or regularly carrying loads of 25 lbs or more, have increased radiologic evidence of OA in the knee compared with those workers who do not.[81] This trend has also been shown to hold true for the upper extremity, as jackhammer operators exhibit an increased prevalence of OA of the upper extremity when compared with the general population.[95] Complete avoidance of repetitive motions at work may prove extremely difficult, especially if they are requirements for the job. However, the identification of those activities which are the most harmful to articular cartilage is important.

Impact In addition to the long-term accumulation of fatigue damage to the matrix that may eventually lead to bulk tissue failure, it has been observed that transarticular impact may result in the development of OA in the traumatized joint. A single episode of joint impact, if sufficiently large, may cause cracks at or near the junction of cartilage and the zone of calcified cartilage–subchondral bone,[79,107–109] often without immediate disruption to the joint surface. As indicated, the solid matrix of cartilage is normally shielded from the high stresses of joint loading through the presence of interstitial fluid pressurization. In cartilage with a perforation in the zone of calcified cartilage-subchondral bone, however, the solid matrix stresses and strains are significantly increased owing to the diminished fluid pressurization in the region of the defect.[110]

Repetitive Injury and Physical Trauma   Although the prevalence of OA in the knee is greater in adults who have engaged in repetitive bending and strenuous activities, an association with intense exercise or physical activity has not been as easy to establish.[113] This difficulty may partly arise from the high prevalence of OA in the knees of older adults. The Framingham study provides the first longitudinal association between level of physical activity and incident knee OA of the OA.[114] In contrast, studies have not associated low-impact recreational activities[115] with OA of the knee.

Sports   As a risk factor for osteoarthritis, sports is an area of debate,[116] particularly because so many people engage in athletic activities. Studies performed on runners have presented conflicting evidence of an increased incidence of OA of the hip,[85,117] and have not shown an increased incidence of OA of the knee.[95,115,118,119] To the contrary, studies suggest that older adults who engage in running and vigorous activities have slower development of disability than more sedimentary individuals.[120] However, epidemiologic studies have shown that athletes in certain sports may be predisposed to OA of particular joints. For example, soccer and football players have been shown to have an increased prevalence of OA of the knee,[121–123] whereas baseball pitchers may be predisposed to degenerative changes of the shoulder and elbow.[124] However, these degenerative changes may be related to traumatic injuries that participants undergo as a result of their activities,[125] rather than from performing the activity itself. Studies have demonstrated that sudden and extreme loading of the joint may be responsible for superficial damage to the cartilage (fissures, flaps and fragmentation),[116] and that if the loading is sufficiently severe, cracks can occur at or near the junction of cartilage and the zone of calcified cartilage–subchondral bone.[79,107,108,126] It is possible that these cracks predispose the traumatized joint to OA.

Weight Bearing   To examine whether long-term weight-bearing exercise predisposes the joints to osteoarthritis, Newton and colleagues[127] studied the effects of lifelong running in dogs and concluded that regular lifelong exercise does not necessarily predispose the joint to OA. Exercise in the setting of an abnormal joint, however, may predispose the joint to degenerative changes. Epidemiologic studies show that runners who have an anatomic abnormality, such as genu varum, or who have had a prior injury are predisposed to degenerative changes of the knee.[128,129]

Temperature[130]   The enzymatic processes in cartilage breakdown involves the production of degradative enzymes and protease inhibitors. Matrix pH and physical factors, such as temperature, influence enzymatic activity. For example, collagenase is more active at high joint temperatures ($36°C$ versus $33°C$). If cells are even mildly heated, they synthesize a substance called a heat shock protein, which is found in the synovia of arthritic joints. Heat shock proteins are molecules produced in response to various stimuli with an ability to bind to, and influence, the intracellular function and distribution of other proteins. They appear to provoke a cellular stress response. It is believed that the temperature of an inflamed joint has the adverse effect of inducing synthesis of these proteins.[131,132] In rheumatoid arthritis, serum antibodies to these proteins are present. Such data support the use of cold over heat in acutely inflamed joints.

Inflammation[130]   The typical inflammatory response to injury or pathology is more visible in the most vascular joint tissue, the synovial lining tissue. Synovitis may result from a variety of stimuli and creates an environment that is hostile to articular cartilage.

The enzymatically degraded cartilage releases proteoglycans. This initiates a vicious cycle resulting in synovial intimal cells releasing more collagenase and proteinases, cytokines, and interleukin-1, which further weakens the cartilage and enhances mechanical damage.[134–136] Type B synovial cells may be primarily involved in this reaction, while Type A synovial cells are believed to release cytokines (chemical messengers), such as interleukin-1 and prostaglandin E_2, which may play a major role in the perpetuation of synovitis.[138] Interleukin-1 is an inflammatory mediator that can cause chondrocytes to decrease matrix synthesis and resorb their surrounding matrix.

Not until the subchondral bone is penetrated does the usual inflammatory wound-healing response occur in a damaged joint surface. This involves cells from the bone marrow, which attempt to fill the defect with new tissue. The extent to which the new tissue resembles articular cartilage depends on the age and species of the host, as well as the size and location of the defect. However, complete restoration of the hyaline articular cartilage and the subchondral bone to a normal status is rarely seen.

The options for operative intervention after a joint surface has been damaged, or a portion has been lost, can be grouped according to four concepts or principles. The articular cartilage can be restored, replaced, relieved, or resected (the four R's). Restoration refers to healing or regeneration of the joint surface, including the hyaline articular cartilage and the subchondral bone. Replacement can be accomplished with use of an allograft or a prosthesis. The pressures through a damaged joint surface can be relieved by an osteotomy that unloads and decreases the stresses on it. The final option is resection with or without an interposition arthroplasty.

JOINT RECEPTORS

Periarticular receptors, highly specialized cells within the nervous system, detect the presence of, and changes in, different forms of energy, and convert these forms of energy into proprioceptive information.[139,140] The periarticular receptors are mechanoreceptors that are sensitive to mechanical deformation of the tissue and cell membranes.[141] This deformation can arise in a number of ways including indentation, compression, relaxation, and stretch, and each nerve ending serves as a filter for a specific kind of stimulus. The information received by each of these mechanoreceptors must be conveyed rapidly and accurately to the central nervous system in order to regulate joint position and angulation, thereby protecting the joint from damage.

Most of the mechanoreceptors are only active near the end of range of motion.[142] Four of these mechanoreceptors are discussed next.[143–146]

Type I receptors consist of small, thinly encapsulated globular corpuscles located in the peripheral layers of the fibrous joint capsule. These are low-threshold, slowly adapting mechanoreceptors whose frequency of discharge is a continuous function of the prevailing tension in the region of the joint capsule where they are located. They have an inhibitory effect on the nociceptive activity from the type IV articular receptor system, and their activity exerts powerful influences on the motor neuronal pool of the muscles. Type I mechanoreceptors also contribute to the reflex regulation of postural tone, to coordination of muscle activity, and to the perceptional awareness of joint position.

Type II receptors operate as low-threshold, rapidly adapting mechanoreceptors that fire off brief bursts of impulses only at the onset of changes in tension in the joint capsule. They are thickly encapsulated and myelinated. Their behavior suggests their role as a control mechanism to regulate motor-unit activity of the prime movers of the joint, giving information with regard to acceleration and deceleration of quick joint movements.

Type III mechanoreceptors, located in the intrinsic and extrinsic joint ligaments, except the longitudinal ligaments of spine, may be regarded as high threshold. They are thinly encapsulated and similar to Golgi tendon organs in function, evoking discharges only during strong capsular tension.

The type IV receptor system, located in the joint capsule, fibrocartilage, fat pads, ligaments, blood walls (vessels), periosteum, and synovium, consists of high threshold, nonadapting, nociceptor and non-nociceptor receptors. The system is activated when its nerve fibers are depolarized by the generation of high mechanical or chemical stresses in the joint capsule. These receptors are usually controlled by gate inhibition.

A knowledge of receptors is important in the application of treatment.

- Rest prevents mechanical irritation, thereby decreasing type IV input.
- Joint mobilizations (grades I to IV), help to control pain through the stimulation of type I and II receptors, thereby increasing large A fiber input.
- Active range of motion stimulates the mechanoreceptors, acts as a muscle pump, and stimulates an inhibition of the antagonists.
- Joint distraction techniques, which are maximum and sustained, produce muscle inhibition through the type III mechanoreceptors.

SKELETAL MUSCLE[147]

Skeletal muscle, unlike cardiac and smooth muscle, can operate only under neural control.

Muscle Fibers

The nod of the head, the handshake, and the gesture are all brought about by muscular actions. The mechanism behind these muscle actions was first discovered from early studies of living skeletal muscle, when it was noted that stripes were localized in long fibrous cylinders called myofibrils that ran the length of the muscle cell. It is the myofibrils that contain the machinery of the muscles. Each myofibril is punctuated with alternating light and dark bands called A and I bands, which are arranged so that an A band on one myofibril is closest to an A band on its neighbor. When a muscle contracts, the I band shortens, but the A band does not change size.

Each myofibril contains many fibers called filaments, which run parallel to the myofibril axis. Some filaments, the thick ones, are confined to the A band; the other, thinner ones seem to arise in the middle of the I band, at the Z line (a structure that runs perpendicular to the myofibril through the I band, connecting neighboring my-ofibrils). The thin filaments run the course of the I band and partway into the A band, where they overlap with the thick filaments.

When the protein actin is extracted from muscle tissue, the thin filaments disappear, and when the protein myosin is extracted, the thick filaments disappear. Moreover, when the cell membrane is destroyed and substances other than these two proteins are removed, the muscle can still contract. These results imply that the thick and thin filaments are the contractile machinery, and that the thick filaments are made of myosin, and the thin ones are actin.

The thick A band consists of a lighter middle region (the H zone), with denser regions on each side. The denser edges are where the thick myosin and thin actin filaments overlap. The middle (H zone) contains only myosin. The I bands contain only actin. Whenever a muscle or myofibril changes length, either by contracting or stretching, neither myosin nor actin filaments change length. Thus, they must slide past each other, increasing their area of overlap during contraction, and decreasing it during stretching. During contraction, the I band and the H zone decrease. The A band cannot change because it represents the length of the myosin filaments, which do not change.

Structures, called cross-bridges, serve to connect the actin and myosin filaments. When a muscle is relaxed, the cross-bridges are detached from the actin filaments. During contraction, they attach and provide the contractile force. The thick filaments contain two flexible hinge-like regions that allow the cross-bridges to attach and detach from the actin filament. This attaching and detaching is asynchronous, so that some are attaching while others are detaching. Thus, at each moment, some of the cross-bridges are pulling, while others are releasing. The movement is not jerky, and there is no tendency for the filaments to slip backward.

A muscle contraction involves mechanical, chemical, or electrical processes, or a combination, producing force as a result of the interaction of the cross-bridges of the myosin with the actin. The force produced requires energy. The immediate source of this energy is adenosine triphosphate (ATP). It is ATP that energizes the myosin, but in doing so, it loses a phosphate, and becomes adenosine diphosphate (ADP). The energized cross-bridge is now ready for action. If the muscle is stimulated, the cross-bridge will move the actin along (the power stroke). Following the power stroke, the myosin and actin remain attached until the beginning of the next cycle, when ATP once again binds, releases the attachment, and de-energizes the myosin cross-bridge. The ATP splitting is not directly involved in the power stroke. Its energy is used to

"prime" the myosin head so that it can attach to the myosin and repeat the cycle.

An additional substance, calcium (Ca^{2+}), which is required for the attachment phase of the cycle, serves to prevent the muscle continuing to contract until all the ATP is used up. If there is sufficient Ca^{2+}, attachment can occur, but at lower levels, it cannot. Refer to Figure 2–2.

Motor Unit

Within a given muscle, the smallest motor units have the lowest thresholds for recruitment. That is, they are the easiest to call into play and the hardest to prevent from responding, so they are generally considered to be active whenever the muscle is producing any force at all.[148] By contrast, the largest units within the muscle have the highest thresholds, and so are recruited only for the maximum force. This is the size principle of motor unit recruitment.[149] This principle applies in all types of contractions.

For the purpose of this text, three types of contraction are discussed:

1. *Concentric.* A concentric contraction occurs when the tension generated within the muscle exceeds the load to be moved, and is one in which the prime mover produces a shortening of the muscle.
2. *Isometric.* An isometric contraction occurs when the tension generated within the muscle is equal to the load, and no movement of the limb or trunk occurs. Consequently, there is no overall change in the muscle length.
3. *Eccentric.* An eccentric contraction occurs when the load exceeds the tension generated by the muscle and the muscle is forced to lengthen. There is some evidence to suggest that the large motor units are preferentially selected for eccentric actions.[150]

When stimulated, all the fibers of the motor units recruited attempt to shorten. Although this contraction is all-or-none, it is obvious that body movements are not. Sometimes they are forceful, at other times, slight. This is because body movements are brought about by whole muscles and not by single cells acting alone.

Increasing the force of movement may simply be a matter of recruiting more and more cells into cooperative action. However, the maximum tension that is created within a fully activated muscle is not a constant and depends on a number of factors:

● *Speed and type of muscle action.* During a concentric or isometric muscle contraction, the maximum tension generated decreases with increasing speeds of shortening. During slow eccentric muscle actions, a small increase

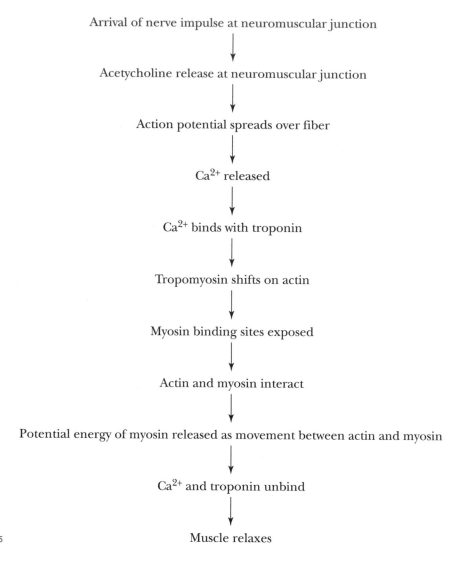

Arrival of nerve impulse at neuromuscular junction

Acetycholine release at neuromuscular junction

Action potential spreads over fiber

Ca^{2+} released

Ca^{2+} binds with troponin

Tropomyosin shifts on actin

Myosin binding sites exposed

Actin and myosin interact

Potential energy of myosin released as movement between actin and myosin

Ca^{2+} and troponin unbind

Muscle relaxes

FIGURE 2–2 Muscle contraction.[145]

in the speed of lengthening results in a disproportionately large increase in maximum muscle tension.[151] In this action, because the load exceeds the bond between the actin and myosin filaments, it probably results in some of the myosin being torn from the binding sites on the actin filament while the remainder are completing the cycle.[152] The resulting force is substantially larger for a torn cross-bridge than for one being created during a normal cycle. Consequently, the combined increase in force per cross-bridge and the number of active cross-bridges results in a maximum eccentric muscle tension that is greater than that which could be created during a concentric muscle action.[152] A comparison of the three types of muscle actions shows that:

Eccentric maximum tension > Isometric maximum tension > Concentric maximum tension

- *Force–length relationship of muscle.* The number of cross-bridges that can be formed is dependent on the extent of the overlap between the actin and myosin filaments.[153] At the natural resting length of the muscle, there is near optimal overlap of the filaments, allowing for the generation of maximum tension at this length. If the muscle shortens, the overlap reduces the number of sites available for cross-bridge formation. If the muscle is lengthened beyond the resting length, the actin filaments are pulled away from the myosin heads such that they cannot create cross-bridges.[152]

- *Angle of pennation.* When the fibers of a muscle lie parallel to the long axis of the muscle, and act directly along the line of pull of the muscle, there is no angle of pennation. However, when the fibers are arranged such that they are angled away from the line of pull of the muscle, the angle created between the fiber direction and the line of pull of the muscle is the angle of pennation. The number of fibers within a fixed volume of muscle increases with the angle of pennation.[152] Although maximum tension can be improved with pennation, the range of shortening of the muscle is reduced. Muscles that need to have large changes in length without the need for very high tension, such as the sartorius, do not have pennate muscle fibers.[152] In contrast, pennate muscle fibers are found in those muscles in which the emphasis is on a high capacity for tension generation rather than range of motion.

● *Angle of insertion.* Not only are muscles required to move bones, but a component of the force produced is needed to maintain the integrity of the joints. The actual tension generated by a muscle is a function of its length and the speed of length change, and the angle of insertion, all of which are changing during dynamic movements.[152] Just as there are optimal speeds of length change and optimal muscle lengths, there are optimal insertion angles for each of the muscles.

With the exception of the angle of pennation, the clinician can control the factors involved with force generation. For example, the use of a verbal command can change an exercise from a concentric one ("push your arm in to my hand") to an eccentric one ("don't let me move your arm"). This has important implications in both the examination of muscle strength, and in exercise prescription.

From the clinician's perspective, movement of a joint can be both provided by, and restricted by, muscles. Joint dysfunction involves a "loss of joint play movement that cannot be produced by voluntary muscles."[154] A dysfunctional joint can be painful, and this pain can have an effect on the tone of the surrounding muscles, either inhibiting or facilitating them. Thus, a harmonic balance has to be maintained between the strength of a muscle and its flexibility in order for it to function optimally. This concept is discussed in Chapter 11.

SOFT TISSUE INJURY AND HEALING

A *wound* is the medical term for cellular damage. Wound healing includes three overlapping phases: inflammation, neovascularization, and tissue remodeling. These phases involve a complex, dynamic series of events, including clotting, inflammation, granulation tissue formation, epithelialization, neovascularization, collagen synthesis, and wound contraction.[155] Wounds may be classified as acute, which heal with an orderly and timely restoration of anatomic and functional integrity;[156] or chronic, which do not heal in a timely fashion.[157] Chronic wounds appear to be "stuck" in the inflammatory or proliferative phase, with accumulation of excessive extracellular matrix components and matrix metalloproteinases, such as collagenase and elastase, which result in premature degradation of collagen and growth factors.[158]

In a crush, sprain, or strain injury, the blood vessels are damaged and oxygenated blood is unable to reach the tissues, resulting in the death of those tissues through hypoxia. Tissue hypoxia is considered a major signal that initiates and regulates processes such as wound healing and tumor growth.[159–161] Hypoxia has been shown (in vitro) to induce several major cytokines from a wide variety of cells involved in tissue repair, including fibroblasts, endothelial cells, and macrophages. During wound healing, tissue oxygen levels are considered to be low at the center of the wound, but they increase as the wound heals.[162,163]

The other major event during early wound healing is the generation of thrombin, and the formation of a provisional fibrin matrix. The provisional fibrin matrix provides the essential scaffold for the endothelial and inflammatory cells to move into the wounded tissue. The degradation of fibrin can induce a wide array of biological effects on the invading cells, and can induce the production of cytokines to initiate repair and angiogenesis during early wound healing.

Stages of Healing

"Healing is the result of cell movement, cell division and cellular synthesis of various proteins. The end product is primarily a fibrous protein which behaves predictably and which can be manipulated according to basic principles of protein chemistry. Control of the synthesis and degradation of collagen, and manipulation of the physical properties which it imparts to scar, is the goal of therapy."[164]

Healing is related to the signs and symptoms presented rather than the actual diagnosis. It is these signs and symptoms that inform the clinician as to the stage of repair that the tissue is undergoing. Three stages of healing are recognized: acute or inflammatory, subacute or tissue formation (neovascularization), and chronic or remodeling (see Table 12.1). With only a few exceptions, bone being the chief among them, mammalian tissue repairs by replacement, rather than regeneration; that is, the original tissue is replaced by another type of tissue rather than the original type.[155]

In tissues that do not have the ability to regenerate, the repair process follows identical steps independent of the tissue undergoing healing. Healing cannot be accelerated, but if the basic mechanisms by which it occurs are known, delayed healing or a very poor repair can be prevented.

Inflammation

This is the body's reaction to infection. The extent and severity of the inflammatory response depend on the size and the type of the wound. This stage typically lasts from 0 to 5 days, providing that the tissue is not being continually damaged, and includes the release of heparin and histamine.[155] Tissue injury causes the disruption of blood vessels and extravasation of blood constituents.[155] Extravasated blood contains plasma cells and platelets, both of which are dead, owing to the lack of oxygen. The dead cells break down into cellular debris and hemoglobin. The platelets not only facilitate the formation of a hemostatic plug, but also secrete several mediators of wound healing, such as platelet-derived growth factor, that attract and activate macrophages and fibroblasts.[165] However, in the absence of hemorrhage, platelets are not essential to wound healing. The purpose of the hemostatic plug is threefold:

1. It acts as glue to hold the wound edges together.
2. It gives an immediate, albeit a very poor, mechanical protection against foreign material coming into the wound.
3. It prevents the spread of infection.

Numerous vasoactive mediators and chemotactic factors are generated by the coagulation, and by the injured cells. These substances recruit inflammatory leukocytes to the site of injury.[166] The leukocytes in the inflammatory exudate engulf the bacteria through phagocytosis and remove the dead and disruptive cells from the area, when the bacteria and debris is caught in the web or fibrin. Infiltrating neutrophils cleanse the wounded area of foreign particles.

Fibrinogen changes to fibrin, which eventually becomes organized into scar tissue. The wound is vulnerable at this point as the edges are held together only by the fibrin, which has a low tensile strength and which can be easily damaged by motion. The region of the injury produces the following clinical signs and symptoms:

- Redness
- Pain
- Swelling
- Heat

The heat and redness are caused when the lysosyme breaks, and releases its chemical, which acts on the local blood vessels, causing a dilation and an increase in the vascular bed, resulting in the area becoming pink and warm a few minutes after injury.

Pain is the result of the chemical action on the bare nerve ending of the nerve fibers. It is also the result of an increase of local tissue pressure.

Swelling is caused by the chemical acting on the local blood vessels, which increases the permeability of the vessels. This allows the proteins and lymphocytes to pass through and create the inflammatory exudate. The osmolarity is altered in the area, resulting in more fluid being drawn out, and the swelling is increased. Protein and inflammatory exudate include gamma globulins. The gamma globulins are antibodies, and are the body's defense against infection.

Subjectively, the patient complains of pain at rest that is felt over a diffused area and is aggravated by activity. Objectively, in addition to the palpable warmth over the area, passive range of motion of the involved joints is often restricted owing to pain or muscle guarding, or both.

The traditional dichotomy of acute pain, with its recent onset and short duration, and chronic pain, which persists after an injury has healed, is undergoing revision. An international task force has acknowledged that acute pain, associated with new tissue injury, may last for less than 1 month, but at times for longer than 6 months,[167] and preclinical studies show that the basis for neuronal sensitization and remodeling occurs within 20 minutes of injury. Recent clinical literature also suggests that acute pain may rapidly evolve into chronic pain. Neonatal heel lancing provokes weeks of local sensitivity to touch,[168] and infant circumcision is associated with exaggerated behavioral responses to immunization months later.[169] In adults, meticulous perioperative analgesia for radical prostatectomy lowers the analgesic requirement, and improves functional status for months afterward.[170] These observations seem to indicate that the biologic and psychological foundation for long-term persistent pain is in place within hours of injury.[171] Acute pain should therefore be viewed as the initiation phase of an extensive, persistent nociceptive and behavioral cascade triggered by tissue injury.[172]

Intervention goals during this phase are to decrease early bleeding, facilitate the removal of the inflammatory exudate and "pain-causing" chemical, while preventing further damage and inflammation to the area. Methods are along the principles of PRICE (protection, rest, ice, compression, and elevation). Modalities can include cold applications, transcutaneous electrical nerve stimulation (TENS), electroacupuncture, pulsed ultrasound, and high-voltage electrical stimulation. No manual techniques should be employed; however, gentle isometric exercises, to maintain muscle function, and passive range of motion exercises, to avoid pain and muscle guarding, may be considered.

Neurovascular Stage

The neurovascular stage begins when the nearby cells, which have been dormant, begin to divide. The basal cells of the epithelium migrate by a leap-frogging action and invade or pass through the clot. In 48 hours, a peeling and excised wound can be completely epithelized. This covering is very thin and can be easily eroded by friction. Because of the poor blood supply, pressure necrosis is easily produced.

New stroma, often called granulation tissue, begins to invade the wound space approximately 4 days after injury. The granulation tissue is red and bleeds easily when touched. Macrophages, fibroblasts, and blood vessels move into the wound space at the same time.[173] The macrophages provide a continuing source of growth factors necessary to stimulate fibroplasia and angiogenesis. The fibroblasts produce the new extracellular matrix necessary to support cell ingrowth, and blood vessels carry oxygen and nutrients necessary to sustain cell metabolism. The structural molecules of newly formed extracellular matrix, termed the *provisional matrix,*[174] contribute to the formation of granulation tissue by providing a scaffold or conduit for cell migration. These molecules include fibrin, fibronectin, and hyaluronic acid.[175,176]

The new capillaries grow toward the clot and invade it. This can start 1 to 2 hours after the injury and generally continues for 3 days. Capillary buds are formed with the growth of the capillaries, and then blood begins to flow through them.

At about the same time, the fibrocytes increase in size and migrate into wounds. Fibroblasts commence the synthesis of extracellular matrix, and begin to multiply.[177,178] The provisional extracellular matrix is gradually replaced with a collagenous matrix[177,178] by about the fifth day. This is the fibrous tissue of the repair stage, in which the wound changes from a predominately cellular area, or cellular structure, to an extracellular structure. This period lasts from 5 to 15 days, and often up to 10 weeks. Collagen, mucopolysaccharides, and glycoproteins are synthesized and deposited within the granulation tissue. The collagen fibers are small, weak, and vulnerable to tearing. Once an abundant collagen matrix has been deposited in the wound, the fibroblasts stop producing collagen, and the fibroblast-rich granulation tissue is replaced by a relatively acellular scar. Cells in the wound undergo apoptosis (programmed cell death)[179] triggered by unknown signals. Dysregulation of these processes occurs in fibrotic disorders such as keloid formation, and scleroderma. During this stage, contracture of the forming scar occurs. This contracture is the cause of scar hypomobility and results in cross-linking of the collagen fibers and bundles, and adhesions between the immature collagen and surrounding tissues.

Collagen remodeling during this transition phase is dependent on continued synthesis and catabolism of collagen. By 3 weeks, the scar is 20% less than its original size. In areas where the skin is loose and mobile, this creates minimal effect, but in the hand where there is no extra skin, wound contracture can create a disastrous result. New scar tissue must always be stretched, because it will tend to shorten. If the healing tissues are kept immobile, the fibrous repair is weak, and there are no forces influencing the collagen. This results in an abundance of poorly engineered and weak collagen which is vulnerable to breakdown.

Wounds gain only about 20% of their final strength in the first 3 weeks, during which time fibrillar collagen has accumulated relatively rapidly and has been remodeled by contraction of the wound. Thereafter the rate at which wounds gain tensile strength is slow, reflecting a much slower rate of accumulation of collagen and, more important, collagen remodeling with the formation of larger collagen bundles and an increase in the number of intermolecular cross-links.[182] Nevertheless, wounds never attain the same breaking strength (the tension at which skin breaks) as uninjured skin. At maximal strength, a scar is only 70% as strong as normal skin.[183] It seems that the fibroblasts need to be guided as to how to lay the collagen, and gentle movements provide natural tensions for the healing tissues, which results in a stronger repair.

Subjectively, the patient reports no pain at rest. With specific activities, the pain is felt over a fairly localized area, and the motion of related joints is often restricted by soft tissue tightness.

Intervention goals during this phase are to protect the forming collagen, direct its orientation to be parallel with the lines of force it must withstand, and to prevent cross linking and scar contracture. If these two aims are achieved, the scar will be strong and extensible. These may be accomplished by gentle active and passive exercises (well within the tolerance of the new collagen), and gentle transverse frictions. Modalities can include high-voltage electrical stimulation and ultrasound, which in vitro experiments have demonstrated results in the stimulation of collagen production. The manual techniques employed are based on the test of the end feel:

- If pain occurs before the motion barrier, specific traction to a single joint should be the manual intervention of choice.
- If pain occurs at the motion barrier, oscillations starting at the joint neutral should be employed, beginning with grade I and II mobilizations, before progressing to grades III and IV.

Remodeling

Although collagen production and deposition is completed after 2 months, the process of remodeling can last many years. Scar remodeling continues to take place during this period, as the scar changes in appearance, strength, size, firmness, and fold. A wound at 2 months bears no resemblance to the wound 1 year later. The orientation of the collagen bundles can still be influenced and tends to be laid down parallel to the lines of force, as it was in the substrate phase.

Intervention goals, depending on the time frame, are to encourage optimum collagen aggregation, orientation, and arrangement of collagen fibers. Modalities can include electric stimulation (ES) and continuous ultrasound. Exercises are continued, progressing as tolerated to more vigorous exercises and, if necessary, deep transverse friction massage. If during the end feel test:

- Pain occurs after the motion barrier, grade IV oscillations at the barrier and gentle muscle energy techniques should be the manual intervention of choice.
- There is a painless restriction, a prolonged stretch or grade V mobilization should be employed.

REVIEW QUESTIONS

1. Which type of joint receptor inhibits muscle function around a joint?
2. How are the type III receptors stimulated?
3. Which type of joint receptor is stimulated for pain relief?
4. Which type of joint receptor contains nociceptors?
5. Which filaments make up a myofibril?
6. Which is the thicker, actin or myosin?
7. The light bands that contain only actin are called what?
8. What are the dark bands called?
9. During a muscle contraction, what does the calcium bind with?
10. During a muscle contraction, tropomyosin shifts on what?
11. What is the function of osteoblasts?
12. What is the function of osteocytes?
13. What are the four distinct zones of cartilage (articular)?
14. Which of the four zones of cartilage is vascularized?
15. Which of the four zones of cartilage is the very active zone?
16. The "tidemark" occurs between which two zones of cartilage?
17. What are the three stages of tissue healing?
18. Which chemicals are released in the acute phase (0 to 5 days)?
19. Why is the wound vulnerable during the acute phase?
20. What type of intervention is appropriate for the acute phase?
21. How long does the subacute phase last?
22. What tissue is laid down during the subacute phase?
23. What also occurs during the subacute phase?
24. What are the intervention aims of the subacute phase?
25. How long does the chronic phase last?

ANSWERS

1. Type III.
2. The application of a maximum and sustained stretch/distraction.
3. Type I and II.
4. Type IV.
5. Actin and myosin.
6. Myosin.
7. I bands (isotropic).
8. A bands (contain actin and myosin).
9. Troponin.
10. Actin.
11. Synthesis of collagen.
12. Nutritional transport and to maintenance of architecture.
13. Tangential, transitional, radial, and calcified.
14. Calcified.
15. Transitional.
16. Radial and calcified.
17. Acute, or inflammatory; subacute, or neovascularization; chronic, or remodelling.
18. Heparin and histamine.
19. It is only held together by fibrin.
20. PRICE.
21. Five days to 6 months.
22. Granulation.
23. Scar formation (cross-linking of fibers).
24. Protection of the forming collagen with gentle exercises, and direct the orientation of the scar with gentle transverse frictional massage and ultrasound.
25. About 1 year.

REFERENCES

1. Kapit R, Macey RI, Meisami E. *The Physiology Coloring Book.* New York, NY: Harper & Row, 1987.
2. World Health Organization. Assessment of fracture risk and its application to screening for postmenopausal osteoporosis: Report of a World Health Organization Study Group. World Health Organ Tech Rep Ser 1994;843:1–129.
3. Riggs L, Melton J. Evidence for two distinct syndromes in involutional osteoporosis. Am J Med 1983; 75:899–901.
4. Riggs L, Melton J. Involutional osteoporosis. N Engl J Med 1986;314:1676–1686.

5. Rubin CD. Treatment considerations in the management of age-related osteoporosis. Am J Med Sci 1999;318(3):158–170.

6. Pacifici R. Estrogen, cytokines, and pathogenesis of postmenopausal osteoporosis. J Bone Miner Res 1996;11:1043–1051.

7. Prince RL, Dick I, Devine A, et al. The effects of menopause and age on calcitropic hormones: A cross-sectional study of 655 healthy women aged 35 to 90. J Bone Miner Res 1995;10:835–842.

8. Jilka RL, Weinstein RS, Takahashi K, et al. Linkage of decreased bone mass with impaired osteoblastogenesis in a murine model of accelerated senescence. J Clin Invest 1996;97:1732–1740.

9. Melton LJ III. Epidemiology of spinal osteoporosis. Spine 1997;22(suppl 24):2S–11S.

10. Nordin BE, Horsman A, Marshall DH, Simpson H, Waterhouse GH. Calcium requirement and calcium therapy. Clin Orthop 1979;140:216–239.

11. Kreiger N, Gross A, Hunter G. Dietary factors and fracture in post-menopausal women: A case-controlled study. Int J Epidemiol 1992;21:953–958.

12. Heaney RP. Calcium in the prevention and treatment of osteoporosis. J Intern Med 1992;231:169–180.

13. Hui SL, Slemenda CW, Johston CC Jr. Age and bone mass as predictors of fracture in a prospective study. J Clin Invest 1988;81:1804–1809.

14. DeLaet CEDH, Van Hoat BA, Banger H, Hotman A, Pols HA. Bone density and risk of hip fracture in men and women: Cross sectional analysis. BMJ 1997;315:221–225.

15. Peel N, Eastell R. Osteoporosis. BMJ 1995;310:989–992.

16. Kanis J. Treatment of osteoporotic fracture. Lancet 1984;i:27–33.

17. Wedge, JH. Differential diagnosis of low back pain. In: Kirkaldy-Willis WH ed. *Managing Low Back Pain.* New York, NY: Churchill Livingstone, 1983:129–143.

18. Kroger H, Reeve J. Diagnosis of osteoporosis in clinical practice. Ann Med 1998;30(3):278–287.

19. Kohlmeier LA, Federman M, Leboff MS. Osteomalacia and osteoporosis in a woman with ankylosing spondylitis. J Bone Miner Res 1996;11(5):697–703.

20. Gregg EW, Pereira MA, Caspersen CJ. Physical activity, falls, and fractures among older adults: A review of the epidemiologic evidence. J Am Ger Soc 2000; 48(8):883–893.

21. Tinetti ME, Speechley Ginter SF. Risk factors for falls among elderly persons living in the community. N Engl J Med 1988;319:1701–1707.

22. Nevitt MC, Cummings SR, Kidd S, Black D. Risk factors for recurrent nonsyncopal falls. A prospective study. JAMA 1989;261:2663–2668.

23. Nevitt MC, Cummings SR, Hudes ES. Risk factors for injurious falls: A prospective study. J Gerontol A Biol Sci Med Sci 1991;46:M164–170.

24. Sattin RW. Falls among older persons: A public health perspective. Annu Rev Public Health 1992;13:489–508.

25. US Department of Health and Human Services. *Physical Activity and Health: A Report of the Surgeon General.* Atlanta, Ga: US Department of Health and Human Services, Centers for Disease Control and Prevention, National Center for Chronic Disease Prevention and Health Promotion, 1996.

26. Buchner DM, Beresford SAA, Larson EB, et al. Effects of physical activity on health status in older adults. II: Intervention studies. Annu Rev Public Health 1992;13:469–488.

27. American College of Sports Medicine. ACSM position stand on exercise and physical activity for older adults. Med Sci Sports Exerc 1998;30:992–1008.

28. Cohen NP, Foster RJ, Mow VC. Composition and dynamics of articular cartilage: Structure, function, and maintaining healthy state. J Orthop Sports Phys Ther 1998;28(4):203–215.

29. Buckwalter JA, Mankin HJ. Articular cartilage. Part I: Tissue design and chondrocyte-matrix interactions. J Bone Joint Surg 1997;79A:600–611.

30. Mow VC, Ratcliffe A, Poole AR. Cartilage and diarthrodial joints as paradigms for hierarchical materials and structures. Biomaterials 1992;13:67–97.

31. Mankin HJ, Mow VC, Buckwalter JA, Iannotti JP, Ratcliffe A. Form and function of articular cartilage. In: Simon SR ed. *Orthopaedic Basic Science.* Rosemont, Il: American Academy of Orthopaedic Surgeons, 1994; 1–44.

32. Mow VC, Tohyama H, Grelsamer RP. Structure-function of knee articular cartilage. Sports Med Arthroscopy Rev 1994;2:189–202.

33. Akizuki S, Mow VC, Muller F, Pita JC, Howell DS, Manicourt DH. Tensile properties of knee joint cartilage: I. Influence of ionic condition, weight bearing, and fibrillation on the tensile modulus. J Orthop Res 1986;4:379–392.

34. Roth V, Mow VC. The intrinsic tensile behavior of the matrix of bovine articular cartilage and its variation with age. J Bone Joint Surg 1980;62A:1102–1117.

35. Bullough PG, Goodfellow J. The significance of the fine structure of articular cartilage. J Bone Joint Surg 1968;50B:852–857.

36. Clark JM. The organization of collagen in cryofractured rabbit articular cartilage: A scanning electron microscopic study. J Orthop Res 1985;3:17–29.

37. Muir H. Proteoglycans as organizers of the extracellular matrix. Biochem Soc Trans 1983;11:613–622.

38. Mow VC, Kuei SC, Lai WM, Armstrong CG. Biphasic creep and stress relaxation of articular cartilage in compression. Theory and experiments. J Biomech Eng 1980;102:73–84.

39. Swanson SA. Lubrication of synovial joints. J Physiol 1972;223:22.

40. Wright V, ed. *Lubrication and Wear in Joints.* Philadelphia, Pa: JB Lippincott, 1969.

41. O'Driscoll SW. The healing and regeneration of articular cartilage. J Bone Joint Surg 1998;80A:1795–1812.

42. Yelin E. The economics of osteoarthritis. In: Brandt K, Doherty M, Lohmander LS, eds. *Osteoarthritis.* New York, NY: Oxford University Press, 1998:23–30.

43. Praemer A, Furner S, Rice SP. *Musculoskeletal Conditions in the United States.* Rosemont, Ill: American Academy of Orthopaedic Surgeons, 1992.

44. Schouten JSAG, Valkenburg HA. Classification criteria: Methodological considerations and results from a 12-year following study in the general population. J Rheumatol 1994;22:44–45.

45. Bagge E, Bjelle A, Eden S, Svanborg A. Osteoarthritis in the elderly: Clinical and radiological findings in 79 and 85 year olds. Ann Rheum Dis 1991;50:535–539.

46. Lawrence RC, Hochberg MC, Kelsey JL, et al. Estimates of the prevalence of selected arthritic and musculoskeletal diseases in the United States. J Rheumatol 1989;16:427–441.

47. Engel A. Osteoarthritis in adults by selected demographic characteristics, United States—1960–1962. Vital Health Stat, 1966, series 11.

48. Ling SM, Bathon JM. Osteoarthritis in older adults. J Am Geriatr Soc 1998;46:216–225.

49. Oliveria SA, Felson DT, Reed JI, et al. Incidence of symptomatic hand, hip, and knee osteoathritis among patients in a health maintenance organization. Arthritis Rheum 1995;38:1134–1141.

50. Bagge E, Bjelle A, Eden S, Svanborg A. A longitudinal study of the occurrence of joint complaints in elderly people. Age Ageing 1992;21:160–167.

51. Egger P, Cooper C, Hart DJ, et al. Patterns of joint involvement in osteoarthritis of the hand: The Chingford Study. J Rheumatol 1995;22:1509–1513.

52. Mauer K. Basic data on arthritis knee, hip and sacroiliac joints in adults ages 25–74 years, United States 1971–1975. Vital Health Stat, 1979, series 11.

53. Lethbridge-Cejku M, Scott WW, Reichle R, et al. Association of radiographic features of osteoarthritis of the knee with knee pain: Data from the Baltimore Longitudinal Study of Aging. Arthritis Care Res 1995;8:182–188.

54. Felson DT, Anderson JJ, Naimark A, et al. Obesity and knee osteoarthritis, the Framingham study. Ann Intern Med 1988;109:18–24.

55. Cooke TDV, Dwosh IL. Clinical features of osteoarthritis in the elderly. Clin Rheum Dis 1986;12:155–174.

56. Ling SM, Bathon JM. Osteoarthritis in older adults. J Am Geriatr Soc 1998;46:216–225.

57. Sartoris DJ, Resnick D. Radiological changes with ageing in relation to bone disease and arthritis. Clin Rheum Dis 1986;12:181–227.

58. Altman RD. The classification of osteoarthritis. J Rheumatol 1995;22(suppl):42–43.

59. Brower AC. *Arthritis in Black and White.* Philadelphia, Pa: WB Saunders, 1988.

60. Murphy WA, Altman RD. Updated osteoarthritis reference standard. J Rheumatol 1995;43:56–59.

61. Dieppe P. The classification and diagnosis of osteoarthritis. In: Kuettner KE, Goldberg WM, eds. *Osteoarthritic Disorders.* Rosemont, Il. American Academy of Orthopaedic Surgeons, 1995;5–12.

62. Calandruccio RA, Gilmer WS Jr. Proliferation, regeneration, and repair of articular cartilage of immature animals. J Bone Joint Surg 1962;44A:431–435.

63. Convery FR, Akeson WH, Keown GH. The repair of large osteochondral defects. An experimental study in horses. Clin Orthop 1972;82:253–262.

64. Furukawa T, Eyre DR, Koide S, Glimcher MJ. Biochemical studies on repair cartilage resurfacing experimental defects in the rabbit knee. J Bone Joint Surg 1980;62A:79–89.

65. Hardaker WT Jr, Garrett WE Jr, Bassett FH III. Evaluation of acute traumatic hemarthrosis of the knee joint. Southern Med J 1990;83:640–644.

66. Mankin HJ. Current concepts review. The response of articular cartilage to mechanical injury. J Bone Joint Surg 1982;64A:460–466.

67. Rand JA, Ilstrup DM. Survivorship analysis of total knee arthroplasty. Cumulative rates of survival of 9200 total knee arthroplasties. J Bone Joint Surg 1991;73A:397–409.

68. Van Saase J, Van romunde LKJ, Cats A, et al. Epidemiology of osteoarthritis: Zoetermeer survey. Comparison of radiological osteoarthritis in a Dutch population with that in 10 other populations. Ann Rheum Dis 1989;48:271–280.

69. Felson DT, Yang Y, Hannan MT, et al. The incidence and natural history of knee osteoarthritis in the elderly. Arthritis Rheum 1995;38:1500–1505.

70. Oliveria SA, Felson DT, Reed JI, et al. Incidence of symptomatic hand, hip, and knee osteoathritis among patients in a health maintenance organization. Arthritis Rheum 1995;38:1134–1141.

71. Sharma L, Pai Y-C, Holtkamp K, Rymer WZ. Is knee joint proprioception worse in the arthritic knee versus the unaffected knee in unilateral knee osteoarthritis? Arthritis Rheum 1997;40:1518–1525.

72. Brandt KD, Fife RS. Ageing in relation to the pathogenesis of osteoarthritis. Clin Rheum Dis 1986;12:117–130.

73. Hollander AP, Heathfield TF, Webber C, et al. Increased damage to type II collagen in osteoarthritic articular cartilage detected by a new immunoassay. J Clin Invest 1994;93:1722–1732.

74. Hollander AP, Pidoux I, Reiner A, et al. Damage to type II collagen in aging and osteoarthritis starts at the articular surface, originates around chondrocytes, and extends into the cartilage with progressive degeneration. J Clin Invest 1995;96:2859–2869.

75. Moskowitz RW, Howell DS, Goldberg VM, Mankin HJ. *Osteoarthritis: Diagnosis and Medical/Surgical Management.* 2nd ed. Philadelphia, Pa: WB Saunders, 1992:761.

76. Guilak F, Ratcliffe A, Lane N, Rosenwasser MP, Mow VC. Mechanical and biochemical changes in the superficial zone of articular cartilage in a canine model of osteoarthritis. J Orthop Res 1994;12:474–484.

77. Howell DS, Treadwell BV, Trippel SB. Etiopathogenesis of osteoarthritis. In: Moskowitz RW, Howell DS, Goldberg VM, Mankin HJ, eds. *Osteoarthritis, Diagnosis and Medical/Surgical Management.* 2nd ed. Philadelphia, Pa: WB Saunders, 1992:233–252.

78. Setton LA, Mow VC, Howell DS. The mechanical behavior of articular cartilage in shear is altered by transection of the anterior cruciate ligament. J Orthop Res 1995;13:473–482.

79. Armstrong CG, Mow VC, Wirth CR. Biomechanics of impact-induced microdamage to articular surface—A possible genesis for chondromalacia patella. In: Finerman G, ed. AAOS *Symposium Sports Medicine: The Knee.* St. Louis, Mo. CV, Mosby, 1985:54–69.

80. Donohue JM, Buss D, Oegema TR Jr Thompson RC Jr. The effects of indirect blunt trauma on adult canine articular cartilage. J Bone Joint Surg 1983;65A:948–957.

81. Anderson J, Felson DT. Factors associated with osteoarthritis of the knee in the First National Health and Nutrition Examination Survey (HANES I). Evidence for an association with overweight, race, and physical demands of work. Am J Epidemiol 1988;128:179–189.

82. Jordan JM, Linder GF, Renner JB, Fryer JG. The impact of arthritis in rural populations. Arthritis Care Res 1995;8:242–250.

83. Kellgren JH, Moore G. Generalized osteoarthritis and Heberden's nodes. BMJ 1952;1:181–187.

84. Hirsch R, Lethbridge-Cejku M, Scott WW Jr, Reichle R, Plato CC, Tobin J, et al. Association of hand and knee osteoarthritis: Evidence for a polyarticular disease subset. Ann Rheum Dis 1996;55:25–29.

85. Puranen J, Ala-Ketola L, Peltokallio P, Saarela J. Running and primary osteoarthritis of the hip. BMJ 1975;2:424–425.

86. Radin EL. Mechanical aspects of osteoarthritis. Bull Rheum Dis 1976;26:862–865.

87. Dequeker J, Boonen S, Aerssens J, Westhovens R. Inverse relationship osteoarthritis-osteoporosis: What is the evidence? What are the consequences? Br J Rheumatol 1996;35:813–820.

88. Hart DJ, Mootoosamy I, Doyle DV, Spector TD. The relationship between osteoarthritis and osteoporosis in the general population: The Chingford Study. Ann Rheum Dis 1994;53:158–162.

89. Gevers G, Dequeker J, Martens M, van Audekercker, Nyssen-Behets C, Dheum A. Biochemical characteristics of iliac crest bone in elderly women according to osteoarthritis grade at the hand joints. J Rheumatol 1989;16:660–663.

90. Dequeker J, Goris P, Utterhoeven R. Osteoporosis and osteoarthritis (osteoarthrosis): Anthropometric distinctions. JAMA 1983;249:1448–1451.

91. Hannan MT, Anderson JJ, Zhang Y, Levy D, Felson DT. Bone mineral density and knee osteoarthritis in elderly men and women: The Framingham Study. Arthritis Rheum 1993;36:1671–1680.

92. Nevitt MC, Lane NE, Scott JC, Hochberg MC, Pressman AR, Genant HK, et al. Radiographic osteoarthritis of the hip and bone mineral density. Arthritis Rheum 1995;38:907–16.

93. Tiku ML, Liesch JB, Robertson FM. Production of hydrogen peroxide by rabbit articular chondrocytes. J Immunol 1990;145:690–696.

94. Lawrence JJ, Bremner JM, Bier F. Osteo-arthrosis, prevalence in the population and relationship between symptoms and x-ray changes. Ann Rheum Dis 1966;25:1–24.

95. Felson DT. The epidemiology of osteoarthritis: Prevalence and risk factors. In: Keuttner KE, Goldberg VM eds. *Osteoarthritic Disorders.* Rosemont, Il: American Academy of Orthopaedic Surgeons, 1995:13–24.

96. Hochberg MC, Lethbridge-Cejku M, Plato CC, et al. Factors associated with osteoarthritis of the hand in males: Data from the Baltimore Longitudinal Study of Aging. Am J Epidemiol 1991;134:1121–1127.

97. Behrens F, Kraft EL, Oegema TR Jr. Biochemical changes in articular cartilage after joint immobilization by casting or external fixation. J Orthop Res 1989;7:335–343.

98. Jurvelin J, Kirivanta I, Saamanen, Tammi M, Helminen HJ. Partial restoration of immobilization-induced softening of canine articular cartilage after remobilization of the knee (stifle) joint. J Orthop Res 1989;7:352–358.

99. Jurvelin J, Kiviranta I, Tammi M, Helminen HJ. Softening of canine articular cartilage after immobilization of the knee joint. Clin Orthop 1986;207:246–252.

100. Palmoski MJ, Perrione E, Brandt KD. Development and reversal of proteoglycan aggregation defect in normal canine knee cartilage after immobilization. Arthritis Rheum 1979;22:508–517.

101. Setton LA, Zhu W, Mow VC. The biphasic poroviscoelastic behavior of articular cartilage role of the surface zone in governing the compression behavior. J Biomech 1993;26:581–592.

102. Behrens F, Kraft EL, Oegema TR Jr. Biochemical changes in articular cartilage after joint immobilization by casting or external fixation. J Orthop Res 1989;7:335–343.

103. Croft P, Coggon D, Cruddas M, Cooper C. Osteoarthritis of the hip: An occupational disease in farmers. Br Med J 1992;304:1269–1272.

104. Radin EL, Schaffler M, Gibson G, Tashman S. Osteoarthrosis as the result of repetitive trauma. In: Kuettner KE, Goldberg VM, eds. *Osteoarthritic Disorders.* Rosemont, Il: American Academy of Orthopaedic Surgeons, 1995:197–204.

105. Mori S, Harruff R, Burr DB. Microcracks in articular calcified cartilage of human femoral heads. Arch Pathol Lab Med 1993;117:196–198.

106. Sokoloff L. Microcracks in the calcified layer of articular cartilage. Arch Pathol Lab Med 1993;117:191–195.

107. Burr DB, Radin EL. Trauma as a factor in the initiation of osteoarthritis. Ind: Brandt KD, ed. *Cartilage Changes in Osteoarthritis.* Indianapolis, Ind: Ciba-Geigy Symposium, University of Indiana School of Medicine Press, 1990:73–80.

108. Donohue JM, Buss D, Oegema TR Jr, Thompson RC Jr. The effects of indirect blunt trauma on adult canine articular cartilage. J Bone Joint Surg 1983;65A:948–957.

109. Urovitz EPM, Fornasier VL, Risen MI, MacNab I. Etiological factors in the pathogenesis of femoral trabecular fatigue. Clin Orthop 1977;127:275–280.

110. Mow VC, Tohyama H, Grelsamer RP. Structure-function of knee articular cartilage. Sports Med Arthroscopy Rev 1994;2:189–202.

111. Klippel JH, Dieppe, PA. *Rheumatology.* St. Louis, Mo: Mosby, 1994:1,760.

112. Croft P Coggon D, Cruddas M, Cooper C. Osteoarthritis of the hip: An occupational disease in farmers. Br Med J 1992;304:1269–1272.

113. Felson DT, Hannan MT, Naimark A, et al. Occupational physical demands, knee bending, and knee osteoarthritis: Results from the Framingham study. J Rheumatol 1991;18:1587–1592.

114. Felson DT, Zhang Y Hannan MT, et al. Risk factors for incident radiographic knee osteoarthritis in the elderly: The Framingham Study. Arthritis Rheum 1997;40:728–733.

115. Lane NE. Physical activity at leisure and risk of osteoarthritis. Ann Rheum Dis 1996;55:682–684.

116. Buckwalter JA, Lane NE. Aging, sports, osteoarthritis. Sports Med Arthroscopic Rev 1996;4:276–287.

117. Marti B, Knobloch M, Tschopp A, Jucker A, Howard H. Is excessive running predictive of degenerative hip disease? Controlled study of former athletes. Br Med J 1989;299:91–93.

118. Panush RS, Schmidt C, Caldwell JR, et al. Is running associated with degenerative joint disease? J Am Med Assoc 1986;255:1152–1154.

119. Sohn RS, Micheli LJ. The effect of running on the pathogenesis of osteoarthritis of the hips and knees. Clin Orthop 1985;198:106–109.

120. Fries JF, Singh G, Morfield D, et al. Running and the development of disability with age. Ann Intern Med 1994;121:502–509.

121. Buckwalter JA, Lane NE, Gordon SL. Exercise as a cause of osteoarthritis. In: Keuttner KE, Goldberg VM, eds. *Osteoarthritic Disorders.* Rosemont, Il: American Academy of Orthopaedic Surgeons, 1995:405–418.

122. Lindberg H, Roos H, Gardsell P. Prevalence of coxarthrosis in former soccer players: 286 players compared with matched controls. Acta Orthop Scand 1993;64:165–167.

123. Vincelette R, Laurin CA, Levesque HP. The footballer's ankle and foot. Can Med Assoc J 1972;107:873–877.

124. Adams JE. Injury to the throwing arm: A study of traumatic changes in the elbow joints of boy baseball players. Calif Med 1965;102:127–129.

125. Rall K, McElroy G, Keats TE. A study of the long-term effects of football injury to the knee. Mo Med 1984;61:435–438.

126. Urovitz EPM, Fornasier VL, Risen MI, MacNab I. Etiological factors in the pathogenesis of femoral trabecular fatigue. Clin Orthop 1977;127:275–280.

127. Newton PM, Mow VC, Gardner TR, Buckwalter JA, Albright JP. The effect of life-long exercise on canine knee articular cartilage. Am J Sports Med 1977;25:282–287.

128. Appel H. Late results after meniscectomy in the knee joint: A clinical and roentgenologic follow-up investigation. Acta Orthop Scand 1970;133(suppl):1–111.

129. McDermott M, Freyne P. Osteoarthrosis in runners with knee pain. Br J Sports Med 1983;17:84–87.

130. Walker JM. Pathomechanics and classification of cartilage lesions, facilitation of repair. J Orthop Sports Phys Ther 1998;28(4):216–231.

131. Evans CH, Brown TD. Role of physical and mechanical agents in degrading the matrix. In: Woessner JF, Howell DS, eds. *Joint Cartilage Degradation.* New York, NY: Marcel Dekker, 1993:199.

132. Zvaifler NJ. Etiology and pathogenesis of rheumatoid arthritis. In: McCarty DJ, Koopman WJ, eds. *Arthritis and Allied Conditions.* 12th ed, vol 1. Philadelphia, Pa: Lea & Febiger, 1993:723–736.

133. Rodosky MW, Fu FH. Induction of synovial inflammation by matrix molecules, implant particles, and chemical agents. In: Leadbetter WB, Buckwalter JA, Gordon SL, eds. *Sports-Induced Inflammation.* Park Ridge, Ill: American Academy of Orthopaedic Surgeons, 1990:357–381.

134. Poole AR. Cartilage in health and disease. In: McCarty DJ, Koopman WJ, eds. *Arthritis and Allied Conditions.* 12th ed, vol 1. Philadelphia, Pa: Lea & Febiger, 1993:279–333.

135. Simkin PA. Synovial physiology. In: McCarty DJ, Koopman WJ, eds. *Arthritis and Allied Conditions.* 12th ed, vol 1. Philadelphia, Pa: Lea & Febiger, 1993:199–212.

136. Brandt KD, Mankin HJ. Osteoarthritis and polychondritis. In: Kelley WN, Harris ED, Ruddy S, Sledge CB, eds. *Textbook of Rheumatology.* 4th ed, vol 2. Philadelphia, Pa: WB Saunders, 1993:1355–1373.

137. Chatham WW, Swaim R, Frohsin H Jr, Heck LW, Miller EJ, Blackburn WD Jr. Degradation of human articular cartilage by neutrophils in synovial fluid. Arthritis Rheum 1993;36:51–58.

138. Fox RI, Kang H. Structure and function of synoviocytes. In: McCarthy DJ, Koopman WJ, eds. *Arthritis and Allied Conditions.* 12th ed, vol 1. Philadelphia, Pa: Lea & Febiger, 1993:263–278.

139. Brodal A. *Neurological Anatomy.* New York, NY: Oxford University Press, 1981.

140. Wyke BD. The neurology of the cervical spinal joints. Physiother 1979;65:73–76.

141. Seaman DR. Proprioceptor: An obsolete, inaccurate word. J Manipulative Physiol Ther 1997;20:279–284.

142. Burgess PR, et al. Signaling of kinesthetic information by peripheral sensory receptors. Annu Rev Neurosci 1982;5:171.

143. Wyke BD. Articular neurology: A review. Physiotherapy 1972;58:94.

144. Wyke BD, Polacek P. Articular neurology: The present position. J Bone Joint Surg 1975;57B:401.

145. Pettman E. *Level One Course Notes from North American Institute of Orthopedic Manual Therapy.* Portland, Ore: 1990. Lecture and course notes (no publisher)

146. Meadows JTS. *Manual Therapy: Biomechanical Assessment and Treatment, Advanced Technique, Lecture and Video Supplemental Manual.* 1995. Swodeam Consulting, Alberta, Canada.

147. Kapit R, Macey RI, Meisami E. *The Physiology Coloring Book.* New York, NY: Harper & Row, 1987.

148. Spurway NC. Muscle. In: Maughan RJ, ed. *Basic and Applied Sciences for Sports Medicine.* Woburn, Mass: Butterworth-Heinemann, 1999:2.

149. Henneman E, Somjen G, Carpenter DO. Functional significance of cell size in spinal motor neurones. J Neurophysiol 1965;28:560–580.

150. Enoka RM. Eccentric contractions require unique activation strategies by the nervous system. J Appl Physiol 1996;81:2339–2346.

151. Joyce GC, Rack PMH, Westbury DR. The mechanical properties of cat soleus muscle during controlled lengthening and shortening movements. J Physiol 1969;204:461–474.

152. Lakomy HKA. The biomechanics of human movement. In: Maughan RJ, ed. *Basic and Applied Sciences for Sports Medicine.* Woburn, Mass: Butterworth-Heinemann, 1999:124–125.

153. Edman KAP, Reggiani C. The sarcomere length-tension relation determined in short segments of intact muscle fibres of the frog. J Physiol 1987;385:709–732.

154. Mennel JM. *Back Pain.* Boston, Mass: Little Brown, 1964.

155. Singer AJ, Clark RAF. Cutaneous wound healing. N Engl J Med 1999;341:738–746.

156. Lazarus GS, Cooper DM, Knighton DR, et al. Definitions and guidelines for assessment of wounds and evaluation of healing. Arch Dermatol 1994;130:489–493.

157. Eaglstein WH, Falanga V. Chronic wounds. Surg Clin North Am 1997;77:689–700.

158. American Diabetes Association. Consensus Development Conference on diabetic foot wound care. Diabetes Care 1999;22:1354–1360.

159. Dvorak HF. Tumors: Wounds that do not heal. Similarities between tumor stroma generation and wound healing. N Engl J Med 1986;315:1650–1659.

160. Folkman J. Angiogenesis in cancer, vascular, rheumatoid and other disease. Nat Med 1995;1:27–31.

161. Haroon ZA, Peters KG, Greenberg CS, Dewhirst MW. Angiogenesis and oxygen transport in solid tumors. In: Teicher B, ed. *Antiangiogenic Agents in Cancer Therapy.* Totowa, NJ: Humana Press, 1999:3–21.

162. Ninikoski J, Heughan C, Hunt TK. Oxygen and carbon dioxide tensions in experimental wounds. Surg Gynecol Obstet 1971;133:1003–1007.

163. Chang N, Goodson WHd, Gottrup F, Hunt TK. Direct measurement of wound and tissue oxygen tension in postoperative patients. Ann Surg 1983;197:470–478.

164. Peacock EE Jr. Future trends in wound healing research. Plastic Surg Nurs 1984;4:32–35.

165. Heldin C-H, Westermark B. Role of platelet-derived growth factor in vivo. In: Clark RAF, ed. *The Molecular and Cellular Biology of Wound Repair.* 2nd ed. New York, NY: Plenum Press, 1996:249–273.

166. Clark RAF, ed. *The Molecular and Cellular Biology of Wound Repair.* 2nd ed. New York, NY: Plenum Press, 1996.

167. Merskey H, Bogduk N, eds. *Classification of Chronic Pain: Descriptions of Chronic Pain Syndromes and Definition of Pain Terms.* Report by the International Association for the Study of Pain Task Force on Taxonomy. 2nd ed. Seattle, Wash: IASP Press, 1994.

168. Fitzgerald M, Millard C, McIntosh N. Cutaneous hypersensitivity following peripheral tissue damage in newborn infants and its reversal with topical anaesthesia. Pain 1989;39:31–36.

169. Taddio A, Nulman I, Koren BS, Stevens B, Koren G. A revised measure of acute pain in infants. J Pain Symptom Management 1995;10:456–463.

170. Carr DB. Preempting the memory of pain. JAMA 1998;279:1114–1115.

171. Niv D, Devor M. Transition from acute to chronic pain. In: Aronoff GM, ed. *Evaluation and Treatment of Chronic Pain.* 3rd ed. Baltimore, Md: Williams & Wilkins, 1998.

172. Carr DB, Cousins MJ. Spinal route of analgesis: Opioids and future options. In: Cousins MJ, Bridenbaugh PO, eds. *Neural Blockade in Clinical Anaesthesia and Management of Pain.* 3rd ed. Philadelphia, Pa: Lippincott-Raven, 1998.

173. Hunt TK, ed. *Wound Healing and Wound Infection: Theory and Surgical Practice.* New York, NY: Appleton-Century-Crofts, 1980.

174. Clark RAF, Lanigan JM, DellaPelle P, Manseau E, Dvorak HF, Colvin RB. Fibronectin and fibrin provide a provisional matrix for epidermal cell migration during wound reepithelialization. J Invest Dermatol 1982;79:264–269.

175. Greiling D, Clark RAF. Fibronectin provides a conduit for fibroblast transmigration from collagenous stroma into fibrin clot provisional matrix. J Cell Sci 1997;110:861–870.

176. Toole BP. Proteoglycans and hyaluronan in morphogenesis and differentiation. In: Hay ED, ed. *Cell Biology of Extracellular Matrix.* 2nd ed. New York, NY: Plenum Press, 1991:305–341.

177. Clark RAF, Nielsen LD, Welch MP, McPherson JM. Collagen matrices attenuate the collagen-synthetic response of cultured fibroblasts to TGF-(beta). J Cell Sci 1995;108:1251–1261.

178. Welch MP, Odland GF, Clark RAF. Temporal relationships of F-actin bundle formation, collagen and fibronectin matrix assembly, and fibronectin receptor expression to wound contraction. J Cell Biol 1990;110:133–145.

179. Desmouliere A, Redard M, Darby I, Gabbiani G. Apoptosis mediates the decrease in cellularity during the transition between granulation tissue and scar. Am J Pathol 1995;146:56–66.

180. Mignatti P, Rifkin DB, Welgus HG, Parks WC. Proteinases and tissue remodeling. In: Clark RAF, ed. *The Molecular and Cellular Biology of Wound Repair.* 2nd ed. New York, NY: Plenum Press, 1996:427–474.

181. Madlener M, Parks WC, Werner S. Matrix metalloproteinases (MMPs) and their physiological inhibitors (TIMPs) are differentially expressed during excisional skin wound repair. Exp Cell Res 1998;242:201–210.

182. Bailey AJ, Bazin S, Sims TJ, Le Lous M, Nicholetis C, Delaunay A. Characterization of the collagen of human hypertrophic and normal scars. Biochim Biophys Acta 1975;405:412–421.

183. Levenson SM, Geever EF, Crowley LV, Oates JF III, Berard CW, Rosen H. The healing of rat skin wounds. Ann Surg 1965;161:293–308.

CHAPTER THREE

BIOMECHANICAL IMPLICATIONS

Chapter Objectives

At the completion of this chapter, the reader will be able to:

1. Identify the differences between angular and accessory motion and their relevance to motion assessment.
2. Describe the differences between the open-packed and close-packed positions of a joint.
3. Describe the biomechanics of spinal motion.
4. Describe the biomechanics of sacral motion.
5. Identify capsular patterns of the spinal joints.
6. List Fryette's three laws of motion and their relevance in the assessment and treatment of the spine.
7. Describe the biomechanics of combined motions in the spine.
8. Describe the differences between hypomobility, hypermobility, and instability.
9. Describe the two main types of spinal locking and their respective uses.
10. Identify normal and abnormal end feels.
11. Outline the differences between conjunct, congruent and adjunct rotations.
12. Understand the significance of a concave and convex surface when mobilizing.
13. Discuss the relevance of the capsular pattern.
14. Describe the biomechanics of mechanical stress.

OVERVIEW

It has been some years now since I sat and suffered through my first exposure to biomechanics. I was an undergraduate and, although the professor did his best to hold the attention of his audience by injecting some humor, I failed to grasp the relevance of it all. Learning about the various classes of levers and pulling actions of the muscles, and memorizing numerous definitions, seemed far removed from the clinic, and the treatment of patients. Some years later I began reading *Muscles and Movements* by MacConaill and Basmajian.[1] Unfortunately, this did little to change my opinions. The book seemed to be full of chapter upon chapter of mathematical equations and yet more definitions. It was only after I had been practicing for a few years that the true importance of this information finally sunk in. What follows is my attempt to make the subject of biomechanics both interesting and clinically relevant using, ironically, the aforementioned book as a source.

If one views the human body simplistically, it is a mechanical system controlled by an electrical system. As such, it obeys the same physical laws of the universe that every other system does. It is, therefore, important that the clinician understand some of the basic concepts that underlie the conditions that will be encountered clinically. Not only will these principles be used for diagnostic purposes, but they will also add a high degree of specificity to the manual techniques used in the clinic.

ANGULAR AND ACCESSORY MOTION

All motions in the musculoskeletal system involve a combination of angular motion and accessory motion. Angular motion can be viewed as the motion that is visible, such as an arm, leg, or trunk moving through space. Accessory motion is the "invisible" motion that occurs at the joint surfaces during the visible motions.

For a joint to function completely, both of these motions have to occur normally. In fact, they are directly proportional to each other—a small increment of accessory motion represents a larger increment of angular motion. It follows, therefore, that if a joint is not functioning correctly, one or both of these motions is at fault, and the intervention to restore the complete function must be aimed at the specific cause.

In the extremities, the angular motion is produced and controlled by the contractile tissues, whereas the accessory motion is controlled by the integrity of the joint surfaces and the noncontractile (inert) tissues. This is seen clinically following a complete rupture of the anterior cruciate ligament of the knee. Upon examination of that knee, the accessory motion (joint glide) is found to be increased, illustrated by a positive Lachman's test, but the range of motion of the knee—its angular motion—is not affected. This rule changes with a joint that has undergone degenerative changes, resulting in joint glides that are increased, owing to the lack of integrity of the joint surface, but an angular motion that is decreased, demonstrated by the capsular pattern of restriction. (See later)

Spinal motions obey slightly different rules to those of the extremities. Here, contractile tissues produce the angular motion, but both the contractile *and* inert tissues control the motion.

The clinician faced with a patient who has lost motion at a joint needs to determine whether the loss of motion is the result of a contractile or inert structure. If the clinician assesses the accessory motion of the joint by performing a joint glide, information about the integrity of the inert structures will be given. There are two scenarios:

A. *The joint glide is normal (unrestricted).* An unrestricted joint glide indicates two differing conclusions:
   1. The integrity of both the joint surface and the periarticular tissue is good. If the joint surface and periarticular structures are intact, the patient's loss of motion must be due to a contractile tissue. The intervention for this patient would involve techniques designed to change the length of a contractile tissue—stretching or muscle energy techniques, or both.
   2. The joint glide is not only unrestricted, it is excessive, in which case the joint has undergone significant degenerative changes, and if there is a loss of angular motion, it is in a capsular pattern. Other clinical findings, such as x-rays and a subjective history, would be needed as confirmation in those joints that have a two-dimensional capsular pattern, involving only the relationship between flexion and extension, as in the elbow. Three-dimensional capsular patterns, like those occurring at the shoulder or hip, can help the clinician determine if the rest of the capsular pattern is present. The intervention for this patient would concentrate on stabilizing techniques.

B. *The joint glide is restricted.* If the joint glide is restricted, the joint surface and periarticular tissues are implicated as the cause for the patient's loss of motion, although the contractile tissues cannot, at this stage, be ruled out. The intervention for this patient would involve specific joint mobilizations. Distraction and compression can be used to help differentiate the cause of the restriction.
   1. Distraction: Traction is a force imparted passively by the clinician that results in a distraction of the joint surfaces.
      a. If the distraction is limited, a contracture of connective tissue should be suspected.
      b. If the distraction increases the pain, it may indicate a tear of connective tissue, and may be associated with increased range.
      c. If the distraction eases the pain, it may indicate an involvement of the joint surface.
   2. Compression: The opposite movement occurs when compared to distraction. Compression involves the pushing of joint surfaces together by the clinician.
      a. If the compression increases the pain, a loose body or internal derangement of the joint may be present.
      b. If the compression decreases the pain, it may implicate the joint capsule.

Once the joint glide is restored, the angular motion can be assessed again. If it is still reduced, the contractile tissues are at fault.

CLOSE- AND OPEN-PACKED JOINT POSITIONS

The close-packed position of a joint is that position of the joint that results in maximal tautness of the major ligaments, maximal surface congruity, least transarticular pressure, minimal joint volume, and maximal stability, allowing least distraction of the joints surfaces, and reducing the degrees of freedom to zero. It is for this reason that most fractures and dislocations occur when a joint is in its close-packed position. The close-packed position of a joint always occurs at the end of range with habitual movements (e.g., hip extension). Once the close-packed position is achieved, no further motion in that direction is possible. Therefore, movement toward the close-packed position involves some degree of compression, whereas motion out of this position involves distraction.

From a clinical perspective, this position is avoided when the clinician is attempting to assess joint play. However, if the aim is to restore motion to a joint, the close-packed position is sought first as it is this position that provides maximum stability and nutrition to the joint, and it is the position the joint uses when special effort is undertaken.

The open-packed position of a joint is that position of the joint that results in the slackening of the major ligaments of the joint, minimal surface congruity, minimal joint surface contact, maximal joint volume, and minimal stability, allowing maximal distraction of the joint surfaces.

It is for this reason that most capsular or ligamentous sprains occur when a joint is in its open-packed position. In essence, any position of the joint other than the close-packed position could be considered to be the open-packed position. It is this position that a joint tends to move into when inflamed. From a clinical perspective, this position is used for joint mobilizations when the joint is in the acute stage of healing.

SPINAL MOTION

Although the spine is divided into its anatomic regions for the purpose of this book, there are similarities between these areas. The function of the spine is to:[2]

● House and protect vital structures, especially the spinal cord.
● Provide support.
● Provide mobility.
● Provide control.

The spine is a flexible curved column, presenting a lordotic curve in the lumbar and cervical regions, and a kyphotic curve in the thoracic and sacral regions. The curvature of the lumbar and cervical regions is largely due to the wedge-shaped intervertebral discs.[3] The function of these curves is to provide the spinal column with increased flexibility and shock-absorbing capabilities, while simultaneously maintaining adequate stiffness and support at the intervertebral joints.[4] In contrast to the thoracic and sacral regions, the lumbar and cervical regions are quite mobile and yet are still capable of supporting heavy loads.

Movements of the spine, as elsewhere, are produced by the coordinated action of nerves and muscles. Agonistic muscles initiate and perform the movements, whereas the antagonistic muscles control and modify the movements. The amount of motion available at each region of the spine is a factor of:

● The disc-to-vertebral height ratio
● The compliance of the fibrocartilage
● The dimensions and shape of the adjacent vertebral end plates

The type of motion available is governed by:

● The shape and orientation of the vertebral arch articular facets
● The ligaments and muscles of the arch and its processes

Although it is convenient to describe the various motions of the spine in a certain direction, the movements that occur at the vertebral segments are complex, involving a multijoint complex, and have been studied by several authors.[5-7] Including translations and rotations around three different axes, the spine is considered by some to possess six degrees of freedom.[8] The range of motion at individual segments varies; however, the relative amount of motion that occurs at each region is well documented.[9] Because the orientation of the articular facets does not correspond exactly to pure planes of motion, pure motion occurs very infrequently.[8] Thus, motions in the spine typically occur three-dimensionally, and the phenomenon of coupling occurs, in which two or more individual motions occur simultaneously throughout the lumbar,[10] thoracic,[11] and cervical regions.[12]

Coupling involves one motion being accompanied by another. In the spine, the coupled motions are side-flexion and rotation. This coupling occurs as a result of the geometry and configuration of the spine, especially the zygapophysial joints. Coupling occurs throughout the whole spine,[13-15] and in the lumbar spine appears to vary with the level and is significantly affected by the posture of the spine.[16] There have been many opinions on the direction (ipsilateral or contralateral) of the coupling (Table 3–1), but until relatively recently, little objective evidence has been produced to support or refute any particular clinical impressions.

All normal spinal motion in the cervical, thoracic, and lumbar regions involves both sides of the segment moving simultaneously around the same axis. That is to say, a motion of the right side of a segment produces a motion on the left side of that same segment. If both sides of a vertebral segment are equally impaired (equally hypomobile or hypermobile), there is no change in the axis of motion, unless it should cease to exist due to excessive scarring, or ankylosis. Where a symmetric motion impairment exists, there is no noticeable deviation from the path of flexion or extension (impaired side-flexion and rotation), but rather the path is shortened with a hypomobility, or lengthened with a hypermobility.

SACROILIAC MOTIONS

Although various motion patterns have been proposed for the sacroiliac joint,[17-20] the precise model for sacroiliac motion has remained fairly elusive,[21-24] and no thorough

TABLE 3–1 COUPLING IN THE LUMBAR SPINE

AUTHOR	NEUTRAL	FLEXION	EXTENSION
Farfan[12]	—	Contralateral	Contralateral
Kaltenborn[76]	—	Ipsilateral	Ipsilateral
Grieve[80]	—	Ipsilateral	Contralateral
Fryette[57]	Contralateral	Ipsilateral	Ipsilateral
Evjenth[74]	—	Ipsilateral	Contralateral

evaluation is available to clarify whether a motion test can specifically identify sacroiliac joint displacements. Post-mortem analysis has shown that up to an advanced age, small movements are measurable under different load conditions.[25–27] However, little is known about movements in the sacroiliac joints in patients with posterior pelvic pain after birth and in patients with inflammatory disease.

Reliable studies on living persons have been performed with radiostereometric analysis (RSA) of implanted markers,[24,28–31] and with measurements based on implanted external Steinman rods.[32] In a study using fresh cadavers,[25] all muscular tissue and the symphysial part of the pelvis were removed. Each innominate was fixed into a block of acrylic cement. With both innominates fixed, the mean rotation of the sacrum around the x-axis was 3.2 degrees (flexion plus extension); with only one innominate fixed, the mean rotation was 6.2 degrees.[24] In another study by, Vleeming and associates,[27] both the symphysis and the ligaments around the sacroiliac joints were intact; the maximal rotation observed was 4 degrees. In an RSA of four patients, Egund and colleagues[28] demonstrated a maximal rotation of 2 degrees in the sacroiliac joints. With RSA of patients changing from supine to standing position, Sturesson and co-workers[30] demonstrated that the innominates rotate as a unit around the sacrum a mean of 2.5 degrees (range: 1.6 to 3.9 degrees).[24] During hyperextension of one hip, the sacroiliac joint on the provoked side rotated 0.5 degrees more than that on the nonprovoked side.[24] The mobility of both sides was also the same in 17 patients with unilateral symptoms.[24] Kissling and associates[33] used a stereophotogrammetric method in healthy volunteers. Using stainless steel rods in the ilia and the sacrum, they showed approximately 3 degrees of movement in the sacroiliac joints between maximal flexion and extension of the spine.

Recently, in two in vivo studies using a sustained reciprocal straddle position, Smidt and colleagues registered a sacroiliac motion of 9 degrees in one study[34] and 22 to 36 degrees in the other,[35] around "an oblique sagittal axis," by using skin landmarks. In a fresh cadaver study,[36] with computed tomography the same investigators reported a total sacroiliac joint motion between extreme hip extension and flexion of 7 degrees around the sagittal axis (x-axis) on the left side and 8 degrees on the right side. Testing in the reciprocal straddle position showed 5 degrees of sacroiliac joint movement on the left side and 8 degrees on the right side. A recent study by Sturesson and co-workers evaluated, with RSA, the movements in the sacroiliac joints during a sustained reciprocal straddle position in patients with posterior pelvic pain and compared the results with those of Smidt and colleagues. The findings from this study found the values reported by Smidt and colleagues[34] to be five times higher.

Under the premise that pelvic asymmetry is related to low back pain, clinical tests of static (positional) and dynamic (motion or functional) asymmetry have been developed and promoted in orthopedic, osteopathic, physical therapy, and chiropractic texts.[8,18,37–46] However, the assumption of the association between pelvic asymmetry and low back pain has not been validated. Indeed, the findings from a recent study[47] did not support a substantive positive association between low back pain and pelvic asymmetry. The same study reported a weak association with standing posterior superior iliac spine (PSIS) asymmetry with low back pain, at least in selected groups.

Unilateral limitation of hip rotation range of motion, in which a specific movement such as external rotation is unequal between the left and right sides, has been observed in patients with disorders of the sacroiliac joint,[48–50] which is often considered a component of low back pain.[51–53] LaBan and associates[50] noted asymmetry in unilateral hip rotation—that is, abduction and external rotation were limited unilaterally—in patients with inflammation of the sacroiliac joints. Dunn and co-workers[54] reported limited hip mobility in patients with infection of the sacroiliac joint; however, no mention was given to which movements were limited. Others have described cases in which patients with low back pain had unilateral, limited internal hip rotation and excessive external hip rotation and also exhibited signs of sacroiliac joint dysfunction.[49,52] A controversy, therefore, exists about whether hip rotation is limited in patients with signs of sacroiliac joint dysfunction. A recent study[55] attempted to determine whether a characteristic pattern of hip rotation range of motion existed in patients with low back pain, and whether those classified as having sacroiliac joint dysfunction have a different pattern of hip range of motion compared with those with unspecified low back pain. The study found that patients with low back pain, who had signs suggesting sacroiliac joint regional pain, had significantly more external than internal rotation range of motion on one side and concluded that identifying unilateral hip range of motion asymmetry in patients with low back pain may help in diagnosing sacroiliac joint regional pain.[55]

Despite the controversy surrounding this joint, certain conclusions can be drawn:

- The sacroiliac joint can be a source of pain.
- Motions occur at the sacroiliac joint. The motions that are thought to occur include rotation around the x-axis (sacral nutation/counternutation, and innominate rotation), and translations between the sacral and innominate surfaces. Sacral nutation is a forward flexion of the sacrum within the two innominates, whereas sacral counternutation is a backward extension of the sacrum within the two innominates. Innominate

rotation occurs in either a posterior or anterior direction in the same direction as the sacrum motion.
- Traditional tests for this joint that rely on position by palpation are unreliable.[56]

FRYETTE'S LAWS OF PHYSIOLOGIC SPINAL MOTION[57,58]

Although referred to as "laws," these statements are better viewed as concepts as they have undergone review and modification over time. The modifications are highlighted here and in later chapters, where relevant. However, the concepts serve as useful guidelines in the evaluation and treatment of spinal dysfunction, and are cited throughout many books when discussing spinal coupling. The term *neutral*, according to Fryette, is interpreted as any position in which the zygapophysial joints are not engaged in any surface contact, and the position in which the ligaments and capsules of the segment are not under tension.

Fryette's First Law

"When any part of the lumbar or thoracic spine is in neutral position, sidebending of a vertebra will be opposite to the side of the rotation of that vertebra."

When a lumbar or thoracic vertebra is side-flexed from its neutral position, the vertebral body will turn toward the convexity that is being formed, with the maximum rotation occurring near the apex of the curve formed. In other words, when no loading of the segment is occurring (it is in neutral), side flexion and rotation occur in opposite directions. The exception to this is the cranioverteral joints, although it could be argued that as they do not possess a disc, they are not true spinal joints.

Dysfunctions that occur in the neutral range are termed, by osteopaths, *type I dysfunctions*.

This law describes the coupling for the thoracic and lumbar spines. Lee[59] and Pettman, however, have proposed that at the T3 to T10 levels, the coupling depends on which of the two coupled motions initiates the movement (rotation or side-flexion). They propose that if rotation initiates the motion (rotexion) then ipsilateral side-flexion is produced, but if side-flexion initiates the motion (latexion) then the side-flexion produces a contralateral rotation.

The cervical spine is not included in this law, as the zygapophysial joints of this region are always engaged.

Fryette's Second Law

"When any part of the spine is in a position of hyperextension or hyperflexion, the sidebending of the vertebra will be to the same side as the rotation of that vertebra."

In other words, when the segment is under load (close packed, under ligamentous tension, or in positions of flexion or extension) the coupling of side-flexion and rotation occur to the same side.

Dysfunctions occurring in the flexion or extension ranges are described, by osteopaths, as *type II dysfunctions*.

This law describes the coupling that occurs in the C2 to T3 areas of the spine.

Fryette's Third Law

Fryette's third law tells us that *if motion in one plane is introduced to the spine, motion in the other two planes is thereby restricted.*

COMBINED MOTIONS

Combined motions are used by the clinician to increase or decrease symptoms, or to provoke the reproduction of a symptom that was not reproduced using the planar motions of flexion, extension, side-flexion, and rotation.[60–62] Care should be taken when utilizing combined motions, especially with acute and subacute patients, in whom a reduction of symptoms through modalities and gentle exercise might be preferable to exacerbating their condition.

It should be obvious that, irrespective of the coupling that occurs, there is a great deal of similarity between a motion involving flexion followed by left side-flexion, and a motion involving left side-flexion, followed by flexion. Both motions have the same end result, they merely use different methods to arrive there. The same could be said of the following combined motions:

- Flexion and right side-flexion, followed by right side-flexion and flexion
- Extension and right side-flexion, followed by right side-flexion and extension
- Extension and left side-flexion, followed by left side-flexion and extension

Motions that involve flexion and side-flexion away from the symptoms invoke a stretch to the structures on the side of the symptoms, whereas motions that involve extension and side-flexion toward the side of the symptoms produce a compression of the structures on the side of the symptoms.[61–63] An example of a stretching pattern would be pain on the right side of the spine that is increased with a flexion followed by a left side-flexion movement, or a left side-flexion motion followed by a flexion movement. A compression pattern would involve pain on the right side of the spine that is increased with a movement involving either extension followed by right side-flexion, or right side-flexion followed by extension.

The combined motions mentioned thus far, and the reproduction of symptoms, could be said to follow a logical and predictable pattern. Indeed, there are recognized patterns that can be used to aid in the correct diagnosis of a patient, and these are detailed in the relevant chapters.

However, there are situations where non-logical patterns are found. An example of a non-logical pattern would be pain on the right side of the spine which is increased with a flexion and right side-flexion combination, but decreased with an extension and right side-flexion combination. The movements just described involve a combination of stretching and compression movements. These non-logical patterns typically indicate that more than one structure is involved.[60–62] Of course, they could also indicate to the clinician that the patient does not have a musculoskeletal impairment.

HYPOMOBILITY, HYPERMOBILITY, AND INSTABILITY

A normal joint has a specific amount of motion available to it, which is based on a number of factors such as the patient's age and sex, as well as the health of the joint. If a joint moves less than one would expect it to, it is described as *hypomobile*; if it moves further than one would expect, it is deemed *hypermobile*; and if it moves so excessively that it becomes pathologic, it is deemed *unstable*. Clearly the clinician needs to identify whether the joint is moving a normal or abnormal amount, and treat it accordingly.

Active range of motion of a joint is traditionally used to test the amount of angular motion available at the joint. Any reduced range will be in either a capsular or a noncapsular pattern, depending on the cause. Because angular motion is directly proportional to linear motion, a loss of angular motion can result in a loss of the linear motion (glide).

If, upon checking the range of motion of a joint, the clinician finds it to be restricted, he or she must determine whether the loss of range is occurring:

● At the joint surfaces, and is thus a linear motion restriction.
● In a structure that surrounds the joint, such as a myofascial[64] or periarticular structure, and is thus a true angular motion restriction.

If the motion is found to be reduced, the joint glide needs to be assessed, so a passive articular motion (PAM) test in the extremities, and passive physiologic articular intervertebral motion (PPAIVM) test in the spine, is performed.

Myofascial restrictions are recognized by a reduction in the passive physiologic range in the presence of a normal accessory or linear glide. Most muscles that cause hypomobility are hypertonic rather than structurally shortened.[65] Structural shortening results from post-traumatic adhesions and scarring, or from adaptive shortening as a result of postural habits. A recommended way to determine the presence of structural shortening is to try to reduce the muscle tone by the nonrepetitive stretches of Janda or Sahrmann.[65] Phasic eye exercises, hold-relax, muscle belly pressure techniques, and brief oscillatory spinal traction are all theorized to decrease tone.[65] If these techniques fail, then traditional stretching techniques are advocated.

Hypertonicity may also be produced by a segmental facilitation.[66] This phenomenon is discussed in Chapter 4 and 12. Vestibular dysfunction has also been implicated in increasing the tone of muscles, reducing head motion, and increasing tone in the trunk and limbs, although the exact mechanism is unknown.[67,68]

Hypermobility is defined as excessive angular motion at a joint. The hypermobile joint retains its stability and functions normally under physiologic loads. In the lumbar spine, a patient with segmental hypermobility typically reports that sustained positions cause discomfort, and that activity eases the pain to some degree. Examination of the lumbar spine reveals that the patient has difficulties moving from flexion to extension, and there is a late onset of resistance with the end feel. An excess of motion in one direction produces a deficit of motion in another direction.

Generalized hypermobility is a nonprogressive and often nonpathologic, syndrome that is characterized by a laxity of connective tissue, ligaments, and muscles resulting in:

● Decreased muscle tone
● Decreased strength
● Increased ROM

Although there is no agreed upon conservative intervention for this syndrome, the clinician needs to be aware of its existence to prevent unnecessary stretching of already lax tissues and to incorporate a prolonged strengthening and sensory motor program to help provide muscular stability. The most useful tests to determine the presence of this syndrome are:

● *Head rotation.* The patient is placed in a sitting position and is asked to perform head rotation. At the end of the available active range of motion, the clinician performs passive over-pressure. The normal range is approximately 80 degrees to each side.
● *High arm cross.* The patient is positioned sitting or standing, and is asked to put his or her arm around the neck from the front to the opposite side. Normally the fingers should reach the spinous process of the

cervical spine while the elbows almost reach the median plane of the body.

- *Touching of the hands behind the neck.* The patient is positioned sitting or standing and is asked to bring both hands together behind the back. Normally the tips of fingers touch without any decrease in the thoracic kyphosis.
- *Crossing of the arms behind the neck.* The patient is positioned sitting or standing and is asked to put his or her arms across the neck with the fingers extended in the direction of the shoulder blades. Normally the fingers reach the spines of the scapula.
- *Extension of the elbows.* The patient is positioned sitting, arms in front, with both elbows and lower arms touching and in maximal elbow flexion. The patient is asked to keep both arms together as he or she extends them at the elbows. Normally, approximately 110 degrees of extension should be achieved before separation of the arms occurs.
- *Hyperextension of the thumb.* Passive extension of the thumb is performed by the clinician. The normal range is up to 20 degrees in the interphalangeal joint and 0 degrees in the metacarpophalangeal (MCP).
- *Fingers in the mouth.* The normal number is about $2^1/_2$ to 3 fingers in the mouth.

Instability is defined as an excessive degree of linear motion (accessory glide) that is nonreversible. Degeneration or degradation of a joint produces a decrease in the angular motion in the form of a capsular pattern, and an increase in the accessory motion, because the degeneration produces cartilage thinning and allows the bone ends to move closer together, thereby slackening off the capsule and surrounding ligaments. Articular instability leads to abnormal patterns of coupled and translational movements, whereas ligamentous instability can lead to multiple planes of aberrant joint motion.[70]

For an instability to be classed as a functional instability, it must interfere with function, and there are a number of criteria to indicate such interference, including:[65,71-73]

- Long term, nonacute low back pain
- Early morning stiffness
- Short-term episodic pain
- A history of ineffective treatments
- Posterior creases
- Full range but abnormal movement, which may include angulation, hinging, deviation, using the thighs to walk up on recovery from flexion, and wiggling
- Apprehension
- A ledge deformity on palpation
- Minimal provocation
- Incomplete recovery from trauma

- A feeling of instability, or giving way
- Consistent clunking or clicking noises
- Inconsistent function and dysfunction
- Hypermobility on segmental testing
- Instability of segmental testing

Ligamentous stability tests utilize a nonphysiological motion/stress in the position of maximal tautness of the joint. For example the anterior talofibular ligament of the ankle is positioned in plantar flexion, tautened with inversion, and then stressed with abduction—a nonphysiologic motion for the ankle.

Articular instability is tested by placing the joint in its close-packed position. In this position, there should be no ability to distract the bone ends or angulate/glide one surface on another except in the presence of articular instability.

SPINAL LOCKING[70,74]

The structure and function of the vertebral column dictate that the therapeutic approach to the spine has to differ from that of the extremity joints in two respects:

1. Because the vertebral column consists of many articulating segments, movements are complex and usually involve several segments, resulting in restrictions that may be complex. For instance, if a single segment is restricted, the adjacent segments may assume part of its normal tasks in executing movement. Thus, hypomobility and forced hypermobility may both exist in a relatively short section of the spine.
2. Because the spinal cord runs along the channel formed by the vertebral column, damage to, or excessive movement of, the column is potentially hazardous to the central nervous system. It is extremely important that the manual clinician have a working knowledge of the combined motions that occur throughout the spine in any given position of flexion or extension.

The movement pattern of the spine delineates the movements attainable by the unrestricted, normal spine. It should not, and normally cannot, be exceeded without injury.

In order to safely and specifically evaluate or treat a spinal segment, the other segments that may be affected by the mobilization must be protected by locking them in such a manner that they are not stressed during the intervention. In addition, once the joints above and below the segment to be treated are locked, they can then be used as a lever to facilitate the treatment technique. There are essentially two main methods of locking: (1) congruent, and (2) incongruent.

Congruent or ligamentous locking involves taking the joint to its full range, using the normal coupling of side-flexion and rotation, to tighten the ligaments and capsule to stabilize the joint. The disadvantage with this type of locking is that the ligaments and capsule take the brunt of the mobilization force and, if the joint is hypermobile in that direction, further damage may ensue. This form of locking has been advocated in cases of articular instability.

Incongruent or articular locking takes the joint to its full range while deliberately employing incongruent rotation and side-flexion to essentially jam the joint surfaces on each other, and so lock the joint, without tautening the capsule or ligaments. Incongruent locking tends to produce a much firmer lock and the potential of overstretching the capsule and ligaments is minimized. It has been promoted as the locking method of choice in cases of ligamentous instability. However, the presence of articular instability obviates this locking method.

In fact, it is difficult to be sure which type of locking is being done at any given series of spinal joints. As previously mentioned, the research into coupled movements in the lower lumbar spine has upset most of the theories on side-flexion and rotation coupling, and there is no reason to suppose that any other area of the spine is any more predictable. While in theory, the use of an incongruent lock in the presence of a ligamentous instability, and the use of a congruent lock in the presence of an articular instability, appears to be reasonable, the lack of consensus as to the coupling, makes it almost impossible to determine which is occurring at any given time. It is probably better to avoid the direction of the instability or hypermobility as these can, with a fair degree of confidence, be detected.

For example, if the L4-5 segment is to be treated and the L3-4 segment is hypermobile into extension and left rotation, then it must be locked into flexion and right rotation. If an anterior instability exists at L5 to S1, then the segment should be locked with nonsequential flexion; that is, the sacrum is extended under L5, thereby flexing the segment, but applying a posterior force while doing so, and avoiding the anterior shear force at the segment.

A further consideration when locking is the intervention technique that will be applied. If the intervention is neurophysiologically based, where grades I or II oscillations are to be employed, the joint must be left in its neutral position, while the remainder of the spine is locked around it. If, on the other hand, mechanical considerations predominate and a grade IV+ or a prolonged stretch are to be used, then the joint should be positioned at its motion barrier, either as part of the locking technique, or separately, after the locking has occurred.

END FEELS[70]

An end feel was defined by Cyriax[75] as the sensation of tissue resistance that is felt by the clinician's hands at the extreme of the possible range during passive ROM testing of a joint. The first resistance that is met on passively moving a joint is muscle. If this is not stretched sufficiently, the underlying end feel cannot be felt. Over the years, Cyriax's original list has been modified and added to, and what is presented here are the common end feels that the clinician can encounter.

Normal End Feels

Bony
A. Produced by bone-to-bone approximation.

B. Characteristics: Abrupt and unyielding, with the impression that further forcing will break something.

C. Examples:
   1. Normal: Elbow extension.
   2. Abnormal: Cervical rotation (may indicate osteophyte).

Elastic
A. Produced by the muscle-tendon unit. May occur with adaptive shortening.

B. Characteristics: Stretch with elastic recoil and exhibits constant-length phenomenon. Further forcing feels as if it will snap something.

C. Examples:
   1. Normal: Wrist flexion with finger flexion, the straight leg raise, and ankle dorsiflexion with the knee extended.
   2. Abnormal: Decreased dorsiflexion of the ankle with the knee flexed.

Soft Tissue Interposition
A. Produced by the contact of two muscle bulks on either side of a flexing joint where the joint range exceeds other restraints.

B. Characteristics: A very forgiving end feel that gives the impression that further normal motion is possible if enough force could be applied.

C. Examples:
   1. Normal: Knee flexion, elbow flexion in extremely muscular subjects.
   2. Abnormal: Elbow flexion in the obese subject.

Capsular

A. Produced by capsule or ligaments.

B. Characteristics:
1. Various degrees of stretch without elasticity. Stretch ability is dependent on thickness of the tissue.
2. Strong capsular or extracapsular ligaments produce a hard capsular end feel whereas a thin capsule produces a softer one.
3. The impression given to the clinician is, if further force is applied something will tear.

C. Examples:
1. Normal: Wrist flexion (soft), elbow flexion in supination (medium), and knee extension (hard).
2. Abnormal: Inappropriate stretch ability for a specific joint. If too hard, may indicate a hypomobility caused by arthrosis; if too soft, a hypermobility.

Abnormal End Feels

Springy

A. Produced by the articular surface rebounding from an intra-articular meniscus or disc. The impression is that if forced further, something will collapse.

B. Characteristics: A rebound sensation, as if pushing off from a Sorbo rubber pad.

C. Examples:
1. Normal: Axial compression of the cervical spine.
2. Abnormal: Knee flexion or extension with a displaced meniscus.

Boggy

A. Produced by viscous fluid (blood) within a joint.

B. Characteristics: A "squishy" sensation as the joint is moved toward its end range. Further forcing feels as if it will burst the joint.

C. Examples:
1. Normal: None.
2. Abnormal: Hemarthrosis at the knee.

Spasm

A. Produced by reflex and reactive muscle contraction in response to irritation of the nociceptor, predominantly in articular structures and muscle. Forcing it further feels as if nothing will give.

B. Characteristics:
1. An abrupt and "twangy" end to movement that is unyielding while the structure is being threatened, but disappears when the threat is removed (kicks back).

2. With joint inflammation, it occurs early in the range, especially toward the close-packed position to prevent further stress.
3. With an irritable joint hypermobility, it occurs at the end of what should be normal range as it prevents excessive motion from further stimulating the nociceptor.
4. Spasm in grade II muscle tears becomes apparent as the muscle is passively lengthened and is accompanied by a painful weakness of that muscle.

Note: Muscle guarding is not a true end feel as it involves a co-contraction.

C. Examples:
1. Normal: None.
2. Abnormal: Significant traumatic arthritis, recent traumatic hypermobility, grade II muscle tears.

Empty

A. Produced solely by pain. Frequently caused by serious and severe pathologic changes that do not affect the joint or muscle and so do not produce spasm. Demonstration of this end feel is, with the exception of acute subdeltoid bursitis, evidence of serious pathology. Further forcing simply increases the pain to unacceptable levels.

B. Characteristics: The limitation of motion has no tissue resistance component, and the resistance is from the patient being unable to tolerate further motion because of severe pain. Although, by definition, an end feel is something the clinician must feel, the empty end feel is very difficult to obtain, even with the most compliant patient.

C. Examples:
1. Normal: None.
2. Abnormal: Acute subdeltoid bursitis, sign of the buttock.

Facilitation

A. Not truly an end feel because facilitated hypertonicity does not restrict motion. It can, however, be perceived near the end range.

B. Characteristics: A light resistance, as from a constant light muscle contraction, throughout the latter half of the range that does not prevent the end of range being reached. The resistance is unaffected by the rate of movement.

C. Examples:
1. Normal: None.
2. Abnormal: Spinal facilitation at any level.

Biomechanical

A. Speculated to be produced by a pathomechanical incongruity at the articular surface level.

B. Characteristics: An abrupt, hard end feel at one extreme of range. Further forcing feels as if something will tear and break simultaneously.

C. Examples:
1. Normal: Any incongruent movement such as flexion of the first MCP joint in medial rotation.
2. Abnormal: Articular subluxation.

TISSUE LOADING

The term *load* describes the type of force applied to the tissue in question and may be tensile, compressive, bending, torsional, or perpendicular, or a combination. Each of these loads produces a certain type of stress within the tissue and tends to produce motion. In addition, each of these types of load tends to produce a certain type of failure if it exceeds the tolerance of the tissue. For example, excessive compressive loading may result in burst vertebral fractures or vertical disc prolapses; bending forces may produce a tension fracture on the convex side of the bone, and compression fracture on the concave. If more than one type of load is applied at any given time, failure is more likely than if an equal single load is applied.

Stiffness, the resistance of a structure to deformation is the force required to produce a unit of deformation. The stiffer the structure, the steeper will be the slope of its stress/strain curve. In collagen fibers, the greater the density of the chemical bonds between the fibers or between the fibers and their surrounding matrix, the greater the stiffness. Collagen fibers at rest are buckled particularly in the larger collagenous structures such as the joint capsule and its ligaments—that is, there are multifiber folds present, owing to its relaxed state. When a force that lengthens the fiber is initially applied, these folds are affected first and, as they unfold, the slack is taken up. This slack is the tissue's crimp.

Once the crimp has been taken out, increasing amounts of force are required to break the chemical bonds between the molecules and the fibrils. If the stress is sufficient, it will break these bonds, and, if enough of these bonds are broken, the tissue fails and is no longer capable of resisting the force. At this point, very little extra force is required to tear the tissue. On average, collagen fibers are able to sustain a 4% increase in elongation (strain) before microscopic damage occurs. If the force is continued beyond the stage that microscopic damage occurs, macro failure, and finally, a complete rupture will occur.

Creep is the time-dependent deformation that occurs as a result of a constantly applied force after the initial lengthening due to crimp has ceased. Clinically, creep is of relevance because prolonged postures can produce it and,

if the tissue does not recover sufficiently before a subsequent stress is applied, failure may occur.

Hysteresis is the difference in the behavior of a tissue when it is being loaded versus unloaded. The deformation of the tissue occurs to a greater extent over a different time period than its recovery. That is, the tissue remains deformed and takes longer to recover its prestress length than it did to become deformed. This is because of a decrease in back pressure, the breaking of bonds, and their subsequent inability to contribute to the recovery of the tissue.

The difference between the resting length and the length immediately after the load has been removed is called the *set*. The more bonds that are broken, the greater is the amount of hysteresis and set. Gradually, providing the chemical bonds remain intact, the collagen and proteoglycans will recover their original alignment but, if the bonds are broken, full recovery cannot occur until they are re-formed. If healing occurs in the set position, permanent elongation may result.

Stress is the force per unit area that is generated by an externally applied force within a tissue. Two types of force are produced within the musculoskeletal system: shear and normal. *Shear stress* is produced by perpendicular forces applied to a tissue that is not able to freely move linearly or angularly. *Normal stress* is generated by nonperpendicular forces such as tension, compression, or bending. Most loads are combined and so tend to produce a combination of normal and shear forces. Stress is expressed as a quotient of the applied force by the area under that force.

CONJUNCT, CONGRUENT, AND ADJUNCT ROTATION

Try this: Stand with your arms by your side, palms facing inward, thumbs extended. Notice that the thumb is pointing forward. Flex one arm 90 degrees at the shoulder so that the thumb is pointing up. From this position, horizontally extend your arm so that the thumb remains pointing up but your arm is in a position of 90 degrees of glenohumeral abduction. From this position, without rotating your arm, return the arm to your side and note that your thumb is now pointing away from your thigh. Referring to the start position, and using the thumb as the reference, it can be seen that the arm has undergone an external rotation of 90 degrees. But where and when did the rotation take place? Undoubtedly, it occurred during the three separate straight plane motions that etched a triangle in space. What you have just witnessed is an example of a conjunct rotation—a rotation that occurs as a result of joint surface shapes, and the effect of inert tissues rather than contractile tissues. It is this rotation that causes the joint capsule to twist when moving toward the close-packed position. An adjunct rotation is any other rotation that occurs with a motion. Conjunct rotations only occur in joints that can internally or externally rotate, but the rotation is only under volitional control in joints with 3 degrees of freedom, not in those with only 2. Although most clinicians think they can name all of the joints that can internally and externally rotate, many would be surprised to learn that almost all joints are capable of achieving these rotations. Consider elbow flexion and extension. While fully flexing and extending your elbow several times, watch the pisiform bone. If you watch carefully, you will notice that the pisiform, and the forearm, move in a direction of pronation during flexion and supination during extension of the elbow. The elbow, which is considered to be a hinge joint with 2 degrees of freedom, does not allow volitional control of this rotation. In fact, all hinge joints do not allow volitional control of the rotation that occurs during flexion and extension. This fact becomes extremely significant when the clinician is restoring the loss of motion in any ovoid joint except the glenohumeral and hip joint. It is no longer sufficient to restore motion using straight plane techniques; a knowledge of the conjunct rotations occurring at each joint is imperative if the clinician is to give the highest level of care.

Try this: Stand with your arms by your side, palms facing inward. Flex your elbow to 90 degrees. Now try to internally rotate your shoulder while simultaneously pronating your forearm. That was easy. Next, try to internally rotate your shoulder while simultaneously supinating your forearm. Although not impossible, it is not something that can be performed without some degree of thought. The former motion, a habitual one, involved a congruent rotation; the latter, an incongruent rotation. Congruent rotations, involved in all habitual motions, should be considered in muscle re-education protocols.

CONCAVE AND CONVEX JOINT SURFACES

Put simply, a joint is a junction between two or more bone ends. The vast majority of these bone ends have surfaces that are either concave or convex in shape, or a combination of both.[76,77] When a bone moves relative to another bone, one of two types of movement can occur between the joint surfaces. A roll occurs if points on the moving surface make contact on the opposing surface at the same intervals (Fig. 3–1). A slide occurs if only one point on the moving surface makes contact with varying points on the opposing surface (Fig. 3–1). In reality, these two movements occur simultaneously with most movements. Although the roll of a joint always occurs in the same direction as the swing of a bone, the shape of the end of the bone that is moving determines the direction of the joint glide, or slide, that occurs at the joint surface when the joint moves.

If the bone end presents a convexity to its joint partner, the glide (accessory motion) occurs in the opposite direction to the bone movement (angular motion)[76] (Fig. 3–2A). To give a clinical example, the talocrural joint is the junction between the bone end, or joint surface, of the talus and the bone end of the tibia and fibula. The bone end

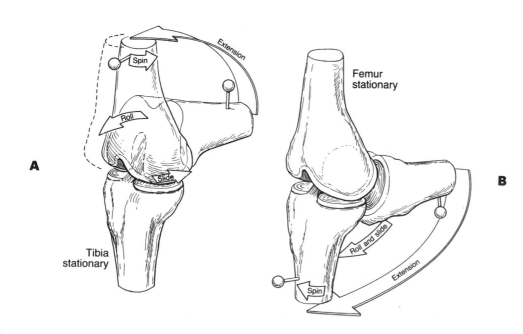

FIGURE 3–1 Joint movements. **A.** Roll and slide occurring with knee extension with a stationary tibia. **B.** Roll and slide occurring with knee extension with a stationary femur.

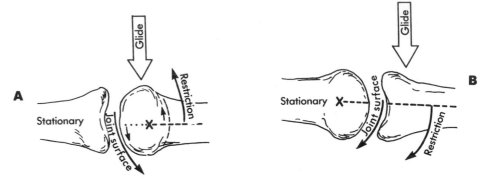

FIGURE 3–2 Gliding motions. **A.** Glides of the convex segment should be in the direction opposite to the restriction. **B.** Glides of the concave segment should be in the direction of the restriction.

of the talus is convex, whereas the bone ends of the tibia and fibula are concave. To restore dorsiflexion, the clinician needs to mobilize the talus on the stabilized crura in a posterior direction. Using the principles concerning conjunct rotation, the clinician also applies an external rotation to the mobilization direction. Conversely, to restore plantar flexion, an anterior glide with an internal rotation is used.

If the bone end presents a concavity to its joint partner, the glide (accessory motion) occurs in the same direction to the bone movement (angular motion)[76] (see Fig. 3–2B). To give a clinical example, the tibiofemoral joint is the junction between the bone or joint surface of the tibia and the bone end of the femur. The bone end of the tibia is concave, whereas the bone ends of the femur— the femoral condyles—are convex. To restore knee flexion, the clinician needs to mobilize the tibia on the stabilized femur in a posterior direction to restore flexion. Using the principles concerning conjunct rotation, the clinician also applies an internal rotation to the mobilization direction.

As a general rule, if the concave-on-convex glide is restricted, there is a contracture of the trailing portion of the capsule, whereas if the convex-on-concave glide is restricted, there is an inability of the moving surface to glide into the contracted portion of the capsule. This, of course, is not always the case, but it serves as a useful guideline.

The Maitland grading system, based on amplitude of motion, is followed throughout this book.[78] In this system, the range of motion is defined as the available range, not the full range, and is usually in one direction only (Fig. 3–3). Each joint has an anatomic limit (AL), which is determined by the configuration of the joint surfaces and the surrounding soft tissues. The point of limitation (PL) is the point in the range that is short of the anatomic limit and is reduced by either pain or tissue resistance.

The joint mobilization techniques, which are used to improve the joint glides of a joint, are usually of a small amplitude, incorporating an oscillatory component. Maitland has described five types of oscillations, each of which falls within the available range of motion that exists at the joint—a point somewhere between the beginning point and the anatomic limit (see Fig. 3–3).

- *Grade I:* Low amplitude and performed at, or near, the beginning of the range.
- *Grade II:* High amplitude and performed through a greater range of motion, but still does not reach the end of available motion and so does not stretch the limiting tissue.
- *Grade III:* High amplitude and performed to the end of the range.

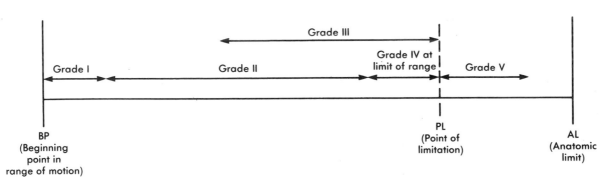

FIGURE 3–3 Maitland's five grades of motion. PL = point of limitation; AL = anatomic limit.

- *Grade IV:* Low amplitude and performed in the range that exceeds the restricted range
- *Grade V:* Low amplitude and high velocity performed at the end of available range

Although the relationship that exists between the five grades in terms of their positions within the range of motion is always constant, the point of limitation shifts further to the left as the severity of the motion limitation increases. The direction of the glide incorporated is determined by the convex–concave rule described earlier, and the joint to be mobilized is placed in its loose-packed position. If mobilizing in the appropriate direction according to the convex–concave rule appears to exacerbate the patient's symptoms, the clinician should apply the technique in the opposite direction until the patient can tolerate the appropriate direction.[79] Refer to Chapter 12 for more details on joint mobilizations.

CAPSULAR AND NONCAPSULAR PATTERNS OF RESTRICTION

A capsular pattern is a characteristic pattern of restriction adopted by those synovial joints controlled by muscles in response to an arthritis of that joint.[75] This pattern is the result of a total joint reaction resulting in muscle spasm, contracture of the joint capsule, or osteophyte formation, or a combination. Each joint has its own characteristic pattern although some have the same type of pattern. The presence of the capsular pattern does not indicate to the clinician the type of joint involvement, but it does serve to help the clinician determine if the underlying cause for a loss in range is the result of joint arthritis.

Noncapsular patterns occur when there is a loss of range in a synovial joint controlled by muscles that does not correspond to the capsular pattern for that joint. Causes for this include a ligamentous adhesion, an internal derangement (loose fragment within the joint), or an extra-articular impairment such as an inflamed sciatic nerve limiting a straight leg raise.

REVIEW QUESTIONS

1. With a convex bone surface, moving on a concave bone surface, in which direction does the bone shaft move relative to the direction of the glide?
2. What are the 10 types of end feel?
3. List some of the pathologic processes that can cause a capsular pattern?
4. List some of the causes of a noncapsular pattern?
5. The deformation that occurs after the crimp has ceased is called what?
6. What is a common cause of creep seen in the clinic?
7. What is the name given to the difference in behavior of a tissue when being loaded and unloaded?
8. What is a definition of the term *set*?
9. Which end feel is always normal?
10. Which end feels are always abnormal?
11. Which end feels can have both normal and abnormal findings?
12. A boggy end feel indicates the presence of what in the joint?
13. What would be an example of an abnormal elastic end feel?
14. What could cause an abnormal bony end feel in the cervical region?
15. What is a biomechanical end feel speculated to be produced by?

ANSWERS

1. Opposite to the glide.
2. Bony, spasm, capsular, springy, empty, soft tissue approximation, facilitation, elastic, boggy, biomechanical.
3. Arthritis, prolonged immobilization, acute trauma, effusion.
4. Internal derangement, adhesion, or muscle tightness.
5. Creep.
6. Prolonged postures.
7. Hysteresis.
8. The difference between the resting length and the length immediately after removal of the load.
9. Soft tissue approximation (except with obese individuals).
10. Boggy (painless emptiness to the feel), facilitation (near end range hypertonicity that is unaffected by the speed of passive range of motion), and empty.
11. All of them except facilitation and empty.
12. Blood or fluid.
13. No change in range of motion when comparing dorsiflexion of the ankle with the knee flexed versus with the knee extended. The range of motion of ankle dorsiflexion should improve with the knee flexed.
14. The presence of an osteophyte.
15. A pathomechanical incongruity at the articular surfaces.

REFERENCES

1. MacConaill MA, Basmajian JV. *Muscles and Movements: A Basis for Human Kinesiology.* Baltimore, Md: Williams & Wilkins, 1969.

2. Pope MH, Lehmann TR, Frymoyer JW. Structure and function of the lumbar spine. In: Pope MH, Frymoyer JW, Andersson G, eds. *Occupational Low Back Pain*. New York, NY: Praeger, 1984.

3. White AA, Panjabi MM. *Clinical Biomechanics of the Spine*. Philadelphia, Pa: JB Lippincott, 1978.

4. Alexander MJL. Biomechanical aspects of lumbar spine injuries in athletes: A review. Can J Appl Sports Sci 1985;10:1–20.

5. Rolander SD. Motion of the lumbar spine with special reference to the stabilizing effect of posterior fusion. Acta Orthop Scand 1966;(suppl 90).

6. Troup JDG, Hood CA, Chapman AE: Measurements of the sagittal mobility of the lumbar spine and hips. Ann Phys Med 1967;9:308–321.

7. Farfan HF. Muscular mechanism of the lumbar spine and the position of power and efficiency. Orthop Clin North Am 1975;6:135–144.

8. Grieve GP. *Common Vertebral Joint Problems*. New York, NY: Churchill Livingstone, 1981.

9. White AA, Panjabi MM. The basic kinematics of the human spine: A review of past and current knowledge. Spine 1978;3:16.

10. Krag MH. Three-dimensional flexibility measurements of preload human vertebral motion segments, PhD dissertation Yale University School of Medicine, 1975.

11. White AA. Analysis of the mechanics of the thoracic spine in man. Acta Orthop Scand (suppl) 1969;127:8–105.

12. Farfan HF. *Mechanical Disorders of the Low Back*. Philadelphia, Pa: Lea & Febiger, 1973.

13. Panjabi MM, Brand RA, White AA. Mechanical properties of the human thoracic spine: As shown by three-dimensional load displacement curves. J Bone Joint Surg 1976;58A:642.

14. Panjabi MM, Summers DJ, Pelker RR, Videman T, Friedlaender, GE, Southwick WO: Three-dimensional load displacement curves due to forces on the cervical spine. J Orthop Res 1986;4:152.

15. Panjabi MM, Krag MH, White AA, Southwick WO. Effects of preload on load displacement curves of the lumbar spine. Orthop Clin North Am 1977;88:181.

16. Panjabi MM, Yamamoto I, Oxland TR, Crisco JJ. How does posture affect the coupling in the lumbar spine? Spine 1989;14:1002.

17. Aiderink GJ. The sacroiliac joint: Review of anatomy, mechanics and function. J Orthop Sports Phys Ther 1991;13:71.

18. Lee D. *The Pelvic Girdle: An Approach to the Examination and Treatment of the Lumbo-Pelvic-Hip Region*. 2nd ed. New York, NY: Churchill Livingstone, 1999.

19. Grieve GP. The sacroiliac joint. Physiotherapy 1976;62:384–400.

20. Kirkaldy-Willis WH, Hill RJ. A more precise diagnosis for low back pain. Spine 1979;4:102–109.

21. Wang M, Bryant JT, Dumas GA. A new in vitro measurement technique for small three-dimensional joint motion and its application to the sacroiliac joint. Med Eng Physics 1996;18:495–501.

22. Ross J. Is the sacroiliac joint mobile and how should it be treated? Br J Sports Med 2000;34:226.

23. van der Wurff P, Meyne W, Hagmeijer RH. Clinical tests of the sacroiliac joint. Manual Therapy 2000;5:89–96.

24. Sturesson B, Uden A, Vleeming A. A radiostereometric analysis of movements of the sacroiliac joints during the standing hip flexion test. Spine 2000;25:364–368.

25. Miller JAA, Schultz AB, Andersson GBJ. Load-displacement behaviour of sacroiliac joints. J Orthop Res 1987;5:92–101.

26. Vleeming A. The sacroiliac joint [thesis]. Rotterdam Holland: Erasmus University, 1990.

27. Vleeming A, Van Wingerden JP, Dijkstra PF, Stoeckart R, Snijders CJ, Stijnen T. Mobility in the sacroiliac joints in the elderly: A kinematic and radiological study. Clin Biomech 1992;7:170–176.

28. Egund N, Olsson TH, Schmid H, Selvik G. Movements in the sacroiliac joints demonstrated with roentgen stereophotogrammetry. Acta Radiol Diagn 1978;19:833–846.

29. Sturesson B, Selvik G, Udén A. Movements of the sacroiliac joints: A roentgen stereophotogrammetric analysis. Spine 1989;14:162–165.

30. Sturesson B, Udén A, Önsten I. Can an external frame fixation reduce the movements of the sacroiliac joint? A radiostereometric analysis. Acta Orthop Scand 1999;70:42–46.

31. Tullberg T, Blomberg S, Branth B, Johnsson R. Manipulation does not alter the position of the sacroiliac joint. Spine 1998;23:1124–1129.

32. Kissling RO, Jacob HAC. The mobility of the sacroiliac joint in healthy subjects. In: *The Integrated Function of the Lumbar Spine and Sacroiliac Joints*. San Diego, Calif: Second Interdisciplinary World Congress on Low Back Pain, 1995:411–422.

33. Kissling RO, Brunner CH, Jacob HAC. Zur Beweglichkeit der Iliosacralgelnke in vitro. Z Orthop 1990;128:282–288.

34. Smidt GL, McQuade K, Wei S-H, Barakatt E. Sacroiliac kinematics for reciprocal straddle positions. Spine 1995;20:1047–1054.

35. Smidt GL. Interinnominate range of motion. Movement, stability and low back pain. New York, NY: Churchill Livingstone, 1997.

36. Smidt GL, Wei S-H, McQuade K, Barakatt E, Tiansheng S, Stanford W. Sacroiliac motion for extreme hip positions. Spine 1997;22:2073–2082.

37. Borenstein D, Wiesel SW. *Low Back Pain: Medical Diagnosis and Comprehensive Management*. Philadelphia, Pa: WB Saunders, 1989:60–78.

38. Bourdillon JF, Day EA. *Spinal Manipulation*. London, England: Heinemann Medical Books, 1987:100–117.

39. Cipriano JJ. *Photographic Manual of Regional Orthopaedic and Neurological Tests*. Baltimore, Md: Williams & Wilkins, 1991:75–82.

40. Cox JM. *Low Back Pain: Mechanism, Diagnosis, Treatment*. Baltimore, Md: Williams & Wilkins, 1985:123–124;313–320.

41. Greenman PE. *Principles of Manual Medicine*. Baltimore, Md: Williams & Wilkins, 1989:225–270.

42. Kirkaldy-Willis WH. *Managing Low Back Pain*. New York, NY: Churchill Livingstone, 1988:135–142.

43. Magee DJ. *Orthopedic Physical Assessment*. Philadelphia, Pa: WB Saunders, 1987:224–231.

44. Palmer ML, Epler ME. *Clinical Assessment Procedures in Physical Therapy*. Philadelphia, Pa: JB Lippincott, 1990.

45. Saunders HD. *Evaluation, Treatment and Prevention of Musculoskeletal Disorders*. Bloomington, Ill: Educational Opportunities, 1985.

46. Scully R, Barnes ML. *Physical Therapy*. Philadelphia, Pa: JB Lippincott, 1989:453–462.

47. Levangie PK. The association between static pelvic asymmetry and low back pain. Spine 1999;24:1234–1242.

48. Dunn EJ, Bryan DM, Nugent JT, et al. Pyogenic infections of the sacro-iliac joint. Clin Orthop 1976;118:113–117.

49. Fowler C. Muscle energy techniques for pelvic dysfunction. In: Grieve GP, ed. *Modern Manual Therapy of the Vertebral Column*. Edinburgh, Scotland: Churchill Livingstone, 1986:805–814.

50. LaBan MM, Meerschaert JR, Taylor RS, et al. Symphyseal and sacroiliac joint pain associated with pubic symphysis instability. Arch Phys Med Rehabil 1978;59:470–472.

51. Bernard TN, Kirkaldy-Willis WH. Recognizing specific characteristics of nonspecific low back pain. Clin Orthop 1987;217:266–280.

52. Cibulka MT. The treatment of the sacroiliac joint component to low back pain: A case report. Phys Ther 1992;72:917–922.

53. Vleeming A, Stoeckart R, Snijders CJ. The sacrotuberous ligament: A conceptual approach to its dynamic role in stabilizing the sacroiliac joint. Clin Biomech 1989;4:201–203.

54. Dunn EJ, Bryan DM, Nugent JT, et al. Pyogenic infections of the sacro-iliac joint. Clin Orthop 1976;118:113–117.

55. Cibulka MT. Sinacore DR. Cromer GS. Delitto A. Unilateral hip rotation range of motion asymmetry in patients with sacroiliac joint regional pain. Spine 1998; 23:1009–1115.

56. Potter NA, Rothstein JM. Intertester reliability for selected clinical tests of the sacroiliac joint. Phys Ther 1985;65;1671.

57. Fryette HH. *The Principles of Osteopathic Technique*. Carmel, Calif: Academy of Applied Osteopathy, 1954.

58. Mitchell FL, Moran PS, Pruzzo NA: *An Evaluation and Treatment Manual of Osteopathic Muscle Energy Procedures*. Mitchell, Moran and Pruzzo Associates, Manchester, MO, 1979.

59. Lee D. *Manual Therapy for the Thorax—A Biomechanical Approach*. Delta, BC, Canada: DOPC, 1994.

60. Brown L. An introduction to the treatment and examination of the spine by combined movements. Physiotherapy 1988;74:347–353.

61. Edwards BC. Combined movements of the lumbar spine: Examination and significance. Aust J Physiother 1979;25:147–152.

62. Edwards BC. Combined movements of the lumbar spine: Examination and treatment. In: Grieve GP, ed. *Modern Manual Therapy of the Vertebral Column*. Edinburgh, Scotland: Churchill Livingstone, 1986:561–566.

63. Brown L. An introduction to the treatment and examination of the spine by combined movements. Physiotherapy 1988;74:347–353.

64. Greenman PE. *Principles of Manual Medicine*. Baltimore, Md: Williams & Wilkins, 1989.

65. Meadows JTS. The principles of the Canadian approach to the lumbar dysfunction patient. In: *Management of Lumbar Spine Dysfunction*. APTA Independent Home Study Course, Orthopedic Section, APTA, Inc. 1999.

66. Patterson MM. A model mechanism for spinal segmental facilitation. J Am Osteopath Assoc 1976;76:62–72.

67. Chester JB Jr. Whiplash, postural control and the inner ear. Spine 1991;16:716.

68. Herdman S, ed. *Vestibular Rehabilitation*. Philadelphia, Pa: FA Davis; 1994.

69. Muhlemann D. Hypermobility as a common cause for chronic back pain. Ann Swiss Chiro Assoc (in press).

70. Meadows J, Pettman E. *Manual Therapy: NAIOMT Level II and III Course Notes*. Denver, Colo: Course notes, 1995.

71. Meadows JTS. *Differential Diagnosis in Orthopedic Physical Therapy: A Case Study Approach*. New York, NY: McGraw-Hill, 1999.

72. Grieve GP. Lumbar instability. Physiotherapy 1982; 68:2.

73. Schneider G. Lumbar instability. In: Boyling JD, Palastanga N, eds. *Grieve's Modern Manual Therapy*. 2nd ed. Edinburgh, Scotland: Churchill Livingstone, 1994.

74. Evjenth O, Hamberg J. *Muscle Stretching in Manual Therapy; A Clinical Manual. Vol 1: The Extremities; Vol 2: The Spinal Column and the TMJ.* Alfta, Sweden: Alfta rehab Forlag, 1980.

75. Cyriax J. *Textbook of Orthopedic Medicine.* vol 1, 8th ed. London, England: Balliere Tindall and Cassell, 1982.

76. Kaltenborn F. *Mobilization of the Spinal Column.* Wellington, New Zealand: New Zealand University Press, 1970.

77. Warwick R, Williams P, eds. *Gray's Anatomy.* 35th ed. Philadelphia, Pa: WB Saunders, 1973.

78. Maitland GD. *Vertebral Manipulation.* 5th ed. London, England: Butterworths, 1986.

79. Wadsworth C. *Manual Examination and Treatment of the Spine and Extremities.* Baltimore, Md: Williams & Wilkins, 1988.

80. Grieve GP. *Common Vertebral Joint Problems,* 2nd ed. New York, NY: Churchill Livingstone, 1988.

CHAPTER FOUR

THE NERVOUS SYSTEM AND ITS TRANSMISSION OF PAIN

Chapter Objectives

At the completion of this chapter, the reader will be able to:

1. Classify the various types of neurons.
2. Describe how nerve impulses are transmitted.
3. Understand how muscle spindles and Golgi tendon organs function.
4. Discuss the various spinal pathways pertinent to the manual clinician and the information they convey.
5. Describe the categorization, receptors, transmission, sources, distribution patterns, and modulation of pain.
6. Describe the characteristics of each of the neural impairments.
7. Understand the principles behind the clinical applications that modulate pain.

CLASSIFICATION OF NEURONS[1]

Each part of the nervous system is characterized by the size, shape, and arrangement of its smallest units, the neurons. Although some neurons may have many similar characteristics, their differences allow them to be classified according to type.

Cell bodies of neurons are usually found in groups. A group of such cell bodies in the central nervous system (CNS) are called *nuclei* (singular: nucleus). The cell bodies of the CNS are unencapsulated, and multitudes of these neuronal cell bodies, and neuroglia, largely contribute to the gray matter of the brain and spinal cord. The counterparts of these cell bodies, located in the peripheral nervous system (PNS), and generally encapsulated, are called *ganglia* (singular: ganglion).

When neurons are arranged into long fibers, they are called *axons*. In the CNS, bundles of axons carrying information or commands of one type are called *tracts*, and these tracts form the white matter of the CNS. In the PNS, bundles of axons bringing information to the CNS from peripheral structures, and conducting motor commands are called *nerves*.

The basic neuronal unit consists of a cell body, and one or more processes called *dendrites*. Neurons without processes or with only one can be classified as apolar and unipolar. Bipolar neurons, those neurons limited to two processes, are usually formed from one dendrite and one axon, occasionally, from two dendrites. Multipolar neurons are distinguished by one axon and two or more dendrites, and are the most common neurons in the nervous system. Golgi I neurons are multipolar cells whose axons extend considerable distances to their target cells, and are thus found throughout the nervous system. The anterior horn cell of the spinal cord is an example.

Neurons can be sensory or motor, or serve as an interneuron.

- Sensory neurons conduct information (touch, pain, etc.) from receptors to the brain and spinal cord. Sensory neurons are the afferent component of the spinal and cranial nerves, and their cell bodies largely constitute the posterior root of the spinal nerve and the cranial ganglia.
- Motor neurons conduct impulses from the brain and spinal cord to muscles, producing a contraction of muscle fibers. Motor neurons are the efferent component of spinal and cranial nerves, and are referred to as *lower motor neurons*.
- Interneurons are entirely contained within the CNS, and have no direct contact with peripheral structures. From the manual therapist's perspective, the most important group of interneurons, whose axons descend and terminate on motor neurons in the brain stem and spinal cord, are called upper motor neurons. The function of interneurons is to modify, coordinate,

integrate, facilitate, and inhibit sensory and motor output.

NERVE IMPULSES[1]

Nerve impulses travel both along axons, and from cell to cell. This traveling, or transmission, is called *synaptic transmission,* and the sites of this transmission are called *synapses.* The terminal branch of an incoming nerve axon, called the *presynaptic cell,* connects with the target cell, or postsynaptic cell, and the distance between these two cells at a synapse is called the *synaptic cleft.*

Transmission of Nerve Impulses[1]

Transmissions can be electrical, but more often, transmission occurs through the release of a neurotransmitter. The sequence of events in chemical transmission is as follows.

1. The impulse arrives at the terminal branch of the incoming axon and depolarizes the presynaptic membrane. This depolarization opens Ca^{2+} channels in the presynaptic membrane, and Ca^{2+} flows down its gradient from outside the cell, where its concentration is high, to inside, where it is very low.
2. The raised concentration of intracellular Ca^{2+} promotes the fusion of vesicles with the presynaptic membrane. This process releases neurotransmitters that had been stored within the vesicles into the synaptic cleft.
3. The neurotransmitter particles diffuse across the synaptic cleft and bind to proteins called *receptors* on the postsynaptic membranes.
4. The transmitter-receptor complex promotes the opening of specific postsynaptic ion channels.
5. Ions flow through the open channels and, if excitatory channels are opened, the postsynaptic membrane is depolarized. The resulting membrane potential generated across the postsynaptic membrane is called an *excitatory postsynaptic potential* (EPSP). This depolarization (EPSP) stimulates other voltage-activated channels adjacent to the synaptic region. If enough of these channels are activated, the postsynaptic cell membrane becomes excited, and the impulse is disseminated out from the synaptic region, over the surface of the postsynaptic cell membrane by the same electrical mechanism that brought the impulse into the synapse on the presynaptic axon.
6. If the open channels are inhibitory, the postsynaptic membrane hyperpolarizes. Now the membrane potential generated across the postsynaptic membrane is

called an *inhibitory postsynaptic potential* (IPSP), because the hyperpolarization spreads to some extent to the adjacent voltage-activated channels, inhibiting them from responding to a stimulus from any other source.

Synapses are not alike. Those that occur at neuromuscular junctions, between nerve and skeletal muscle, use acetylcholine as a neurotransmitter and are always excitatory. Those that occur in visceral organs (i.e., autonomic synapses) use either norepinephrine or acetylcholine and may be either excitatory or inhibitory. Finally, the synapses that occur between neuron and neuron in the CNS are the most varied, and use a multitude of neurotransmitters.

Axons vary in diameter as well as length. The larger the diameter, the faster the conduction of nerve impulses. The speed of conduction depends on how far away the electrical effects of the excitatory impulse reach. The farther they reach, the quicker the distant regions become excited. These electrical effects are propagated by charge movement (i.e., electrical current) inside the axon as well as out, and the narrower the axon, the more resistant it becomes to these movements. As a result, the electrical impulse created in a narrow axon is confined to regions close by, and the velocity of conduction is small.

Rapid reflexes require fast impulses. Invertebrates acquire rapid responses by using very large nerve axons. However, their behavior is uncomplicated, and they do not require very many of these nerves. Because vertebrates have complex behavior, and require many more axons, large axons would be cumbersome and create a storage problem. The problem is solved by using myelin sheaths to achieve rapid conduction velocities along narrow axons. These white, fatty, myelin sheaths are not continuous but are broken at intervals called *nodes of Ranvier.* The nodes of Ranvier are about 1 to 2 mm apart, and they are the only place that the bare axon membrane is exposed to the external solution. A neighboring node becomes depolarized, and the impulse jumps from node to node in a process called *saltatory conduction.*

The transmission of nerves occurs along groups of axons called *tracts* or *pathways.* Spinal pathways are ascending, in which case they carry information to the brain; descending, in which case they transmit instructions from the brain and CNS; or mixed. Three of the more important ascending pathways to the manual clinician include the spinothalamic tract, which conveys information about pain and temperature (Table 4–1); the dorsal medial lemniscus tract, which conveys information about well-localized touch, movement, and position (Table 4–2); and the spinocerebellar tract, which conveys information about proprioception (Table 4–3).

TABLE 4–1 THE SPINOTHALAMIC TRACT

- Helps mediate the sensations of pain, cold, warmth, and touch from receptors throughout the body (except the face) to the brain.[34–37]
- Laterally projecting spinothalamic neurons are more likely to be situated in laminae I and V.
- Medially projecting cells are more likely to be situated in the deep dorsal horn and in the ventral horn.
- Most of the cells project to the contralateral thalamus, although a small fraction projects ipsilaterally.[4]
- Spinothalamic axons in the anterior-lateral quadrant of the spinal cord are arranged somatotopically—at cervical levels, spinothalamic axons representing the lower extremity and caudal body are placed more laterally, and those representing the upper extremity and rostral body, more anterior-medially.[38,39]
- Most of the neurons show their best responses when the skin is stimulated mechanically at a noxious intensity. However, many spinothalamic tract cells also respond, although less effectively, to innocuous mechanical stimuli, and some respond best to innocuous mechanical stimuli.[40]
- A large fraction of spinothalamic tract cells also responds to a noxious heating of the skin,[41] whereas others respond to stimulation of the receptors in muscle,[42] joints, or viscera.[43]
- Spinothalamic tract cells can be inhibited effectively by repetitive electrical stimulation of peripheral nerves,[44] with the inhibition outlasting the stimulation by 20–30 minutes.
- Some inhibition can be evoked by stimulation of the large myelinated axons of a peripheral nerve, but the inhibition is much more powerful if small myelinated or unmyelinated afferents are included in the volleys.[45] The best inhibition is produced by stimulation of a peripheral nerve in the same limb as the excitatory receptive field, but some inhibition occurs when nerves in other limbs are stimulated. A similar inhibition results when high-intensity stimuli are applied to the skin with a clinical transcutaneous electrical nerve stimulator (TENS unit) in place of direct stimulation of a peripheral nerve.[46]
- As the spinothalamic tract ascends, it migrates from a lateral position to a posterior-lateral position. In the midbrain, the tract lies adjacent to the medial lemniscus. The axons of the secondary neurons terminate in one of a number of centers in the thalamus.

STRETCH RECEPTORS[1]

Special receptors are needed in muscles, tendons, ligaments, and joints to provide information about muscle and joint movements and their positions. Information about joint position is called *proprioception*. There are four types of mechanoreceptors in muscle, of which two are commonly cited. These two encapsulated proprioceptors, called *muscle spindles* and *Golgi organs*, are activated by the stretching of the muscles and tendons, respectively, within which they are located. Impulses from these receptors reach the CNS (via the spinal nerves or cranial nerves), resulting in the coordination of muscle activity during movement.

TABLE 4–2 THE DORSAL MEDIAL LEMNISCUS TRACT

- Conveys impulses concerned with well-localized touch, and with the sense of movement and position (kinesthesis).
- Important in moment-to-moment (temporal) and point-to-point (spatial) discrimination.
- Makes it possible for you to put a key in a door lock without light or to visualize the position of any part of your body without looking.
- Lesions to the tract from destructive tumors, hemorrhage, scar tissue, swelling, infections, direct trauma, and so on, abolish or diminish tactile sensations and movement or position sense.
- The cell bodies of the primary neurons in the dorsal column pathway are in the spinal ganglion. The peripheral processes of these neurons begin at receptors in the joint capsule, muscles, and skin (tactile and pressure receptors).

Muscle Spindle

These spindles are numerous in the muscles of the limbs and especially the small muscles of the hands and feet, and are located throughout the belly of each muscle. They lie parallel to the surrounding skeletal muscle fibers and are attached at each of their ends to the fascial envelope of the adjacent skeletal muscle. Within each spindle there are 2 to 12 long, slender, specialized skeletal muscle fibers called *intrafusal fibers* (intra-, "within"; fusal, "fusiform, slender").[2] The central portion of the intrafusal fiber, containing only sensory receptors, is devoid of actin or myosin, and so is incapable of contracting and contributing to the movement of bones around joints. Intrafusal fibers are smaller than extrafusal muscle fibers, and put tension on the spindle only.

Intrafusal fibers are of two types: nuclear bag fibers and nuclear chain fibers. Nuclear bag fibers extend beyond the capsule ends, and tighten relatively slowly. Nuclear chain fibers each contain a single row or chain of nuclei, and are each attached at their ends to the bag fibers.

Muscle spindles are supplied by axons of both sensory and motor neurons.

A. The sensory axons are of two kinds: large myelinated fibers that come into the spindle and terminate around the nuclear bag and chain fibers with wraparound or annulospiral endings; and smaller myelinated axons (group II or class A secondary muscle spindle afferents) that terminate primarily around nuclear chain fibers with flowerspray endings.[2] The sensory endings of these

TABLE 4–3 THE SPINOCEREBELLAR TRACT

- Conducts impulses related to the position and movement of muscles to the cerebellum. This information enables the cerebellum to add smoothness and precision to patterns of movement initiated in the cerebral hemispheres.
- Spinocerebellar impulses, by definition, never reach the cerebrum directly and, therefore, have no conscious representation.
- Four tracts constitute the spinocerebellar pathway: posterior spinocerebellar and cuneocerebellar, and anterior and rostral spinocerebellar tracts.
- The posterior spinocerebellar tract conveys muscle spindle– or tendon organ–related impulses from the lower half of the body (below the level of the T6 spinal cord segment); the cuneocerebellar tract is concerned with such impulses from the body above T6. The "grain" of information carried in these two tracts is fine, often involving single muscle cells or portions of a muscle-tendon complex. A much broader representation is carried by the individual fibers of the anterior and rostral spinocerebellar tracts.
- The axons conducting impulses from muscle spindles, tendon organs, and skin in the lower half of the body are large type Ia, Ib, and type II fibers, the cell bodies of which are in the spinal ganglia of spinal nerves T6 and below.
- Primary neurons below L3 send their central processes into the posterior columns. These processes then bend and ascend in the columns to the L3 level. From L3 to T6, incoming central processes and those in the posterior columns project to the medial part of lamina VII, where there is a well-demarcated column of cells, called Clarke's column. Largely limited to the thoracic cord, Clarke's column can be seen from segments L3 to C8 of the cord. Here the central processes of the primary neurons synapse with secondary neurons, the axons of which are directed to the lateral funiculi as the posterior spinocerebellar tracts.

---

axons are stimulated in two ways:

1. Lengthening or stretching of the entire muscle, producing a stretch or elongation of the intrafusal fibers. They are not sensitive to extrafusal muscle contraction.
2. Stimulation of the intrafusal fibers by the γ afferent system resulting in a stretching of the central portion.

B. The motor axons to muscle spindles are specialized, relatively small, myelinated efferents (classified A-γ efferents). γ Efferents cause the contraction of intrafusal fibers in response to involuntary commands from the CNS, resulting in a resetting of afferent nerve-ending sensitivity to extrafusal muscle and muscle spindle stretch.[2]

A major functional role of the muscle spindle is to produce a smooth contraction and relaxation of muscle and, thereby, eliminate any jerkiness during movement. Over 30% of all motor nerve fibers entering the muscle, are γ efferent rather than α motor fibers. These γ neurons are stimulated simultaneously with the α neurons. This is called coactivation and causes simultaneous contraction of both the intra- and extrafusal fibers and no stimulation of the sensory fibers of the spindle. This keeps the muscle spindle from opposing the contraction or relaxation of the muscle.

In addition, if the relative degree of contraction between the two sets of muscle fibers is not equal, such as during a contraction under heavy load, where the intrafusal shortening is greater than the extrafusal, the extra stretch in the intrafusal fibers would elicit a stretch reflex that would, in turn, cause extra excitation of the extrafusal. This mechanism would provide a number of advantages:

- The muscle spindle rather than the brain would provide most of the nervous energy in muscle contraction against heavy load.

- It would make the length of the contraction less load sensitive, as it would control the desired length of the muscle under almost any load.
- It would compensate for muscle fatigue as any failure of the muscle in its contraction would cause an extra muscle spindle reflex that would excite the extrafusal fibers.

Clinical exploitation of the stretch reflex includes the so-called deep tendon reflex (ankle jerk, etc.) and clonus.[2]

Golgi Tendon Organ

Golgi organs are encapsulated receptors found in tendons. The capsules of these receptors are tightly layered cellular sheets. The receptors consist of twisted braids of small collagen fibers, called *fibrils*, intertwined with group Ib afferents.[2] It is believed that tension on the tendon during muscle lengthening or shortening stretches the twisted fibrils, tightening them and deforming the entrapped axons sufficiently to generate an action potential.

In the state of contraction, extrafusal muscle fibers are stimulated to shorten by the alpha (α) motor neurons (α efferent axon). Muscle contraction puts the tendon under tension and moves the bone. In this situation, the contraction of the extrafusal fibers takes the tension off the resident muscle spindle. This action removes the stimulus for activation of the afferent endings around the intrafusal fibers, and the afferent axons of the spindle do not fire. The neurotendinous organ within the tendon is stretched, however, and it fires impulses along the tendon afferent axon to the spinal cord.

If a muscle is stretched and then contracted, the conditions are no different from the preceding situation. During the stretch phase, the spindle is tensed, and the afferent endings begin to fire. Once the α efferent axon fires, however, the extrafusal fibers contract, taking the tension off the muscle spindle, and the afferent endings do not fire. The neurotendinous organ is stimulated in both cases, as the tendon is tensed in stretch and in contraction.

In a static stretch of the extrafusal muscle, the muscle spindle is put under stretch, and both primary and secondary endings fire. The secondary afferent axons have an increased rate of firing over the primary (annulospiral) afferents during sustained stretch, suggesting that the nuclear chain fibers are more sensitive to changes in length than in the rate of change in lengthening (stretching). In static stretch, the neurotendinous organ fires as before, but there is no activity in the efferent axons.

During varying degrees of lengthening or dynamic stretch, the primary afferents fire at a faster rate than the secondary axons; in fact, the rate of firing of the secondary axons does not change significantly during variations in muscle stretch. This suggests that the nuclear bag fibers are more sensitive to changes in the rate of stretch (velocity, acceleration) than the nuclear chain fibers, which seem sensitive only to the lengthening itself.

It is important that the CNS have the capacity to alter the sensitivity of the spindles in the face of changing lengths of extrafusal muscle fibers, so as to have a continual, updated input on the position and activity of the body musculature. It does so through the gamma (γ) efferent system of neurons. As the spindle is stretched, the afferent endings fire, and the CNS is informed of the stretch via the primary and secondary afferent axons, as well as by the tendon afferent axon. In succeeding stretches and contractions, the γ efferents fire and stimulate contraction of the intrafusal fibers, tensing up the spindle and enhancing its sensitivity to changing conditions. Although γ efferents fire during muscle stretching, it is probable that they also fire during contractions, making possible a continuum of muscle-state information to the CNS throughout a spectrum of muscle activity.

PAIN SYSTEM

Our knowledge of the pain system has greatly improved over the past few years with discoveries that have increased our understanding of the role of nociceptors and the processing of nociceptive information in the CNS. Furthermore, new findings have illuminated our knowledge about descending pathways that modulate nociceptive activity. It would appear from these findings that:

- Pain sensation normally results from the activity of nociceptors, and not from overactivation of other kinds of receptors.[3]

- There are distinct sensory channels for different qualities of pain.[4]
- Pain can result from activation of central nociceptive pathways without involving peripheral nociceptors; for example, in cases of central pain that may follow damage to the CNS.[5]

Pain is felt by everyone. No longer considered just a sensation and a symptom of many diseases, pain is an emotional experience that is highly individualized and extremely difficult to evaluate. It is, thus, very important that the clinician have an understanding of the mechanisms involved with pain perception, because a knowledge of its transmission, referral patterns, and control is essential for intervention planning.

The purpose of pain is to serve as a protective mechanism—to make the subject aware of a situation's potential for producing tissue damage, and to provoke a response from the subject that results in minimizing the damage.

Pain can be categorized according to its speed of transmission or its source.

Speed

Slow or sclerotomic pain travels via unmyelinated C fibers and is a deep, aching, burning, or throbbing type of sensation. This type of pain is caused by the stimulation of any innervated tissue, and can last for prolonged periods.

Fast or dermatomal pain occurs within a tenth of a second of the stimulus application. Whereas slow, or sclerotomic, pain takes a second or more and continues to increase over a relatively protracted period, fast, or dermatomal, pain, travels over small, myelinated A-delta (δ) fibers; tends to be sharp, such as when a pin is stuck into the skin; and is usually not felt when deeper tissues are stimulated.

Source

Pain may be referred from a wide variety of sources, including both visceral and somatic structures. The severity of the pain, and the distance of referral away from the involved source, is directly proportional to the strength of the stimulus. A given stimulus may or may not result in pain, and it is possible to have pain behavior in the absence of nociception. The determination as to whether or not referred pain is diffuse or localized appears to depend more on the depth of the involved structure than on its type.[6] Superficial structures give rise to well-localized dermatomal pain, whereas deep structures give rise to pain that is more difficult to localize.

Pain that is of a chronic nature is easier to localize than pain that is acute. Pain is usually referred distally to the involved structure.

Pressure on the spinal cord as well as the dura mater produces extrasegmental pain.

A study by Kellgren and associates,[7] involving the injection of saline into various structures, found that the structures most sensitive to noxious stimulation are the periosteum and the joint capsule. Subchondral bone, tendons, and ligaments were found to be moderately pain sensitive; and muscle and cortical bone were less sensitive.

The quality of the pain sensation depends on the tissue innervated by the nociceptors being stimulated; for example, stimulation of the cutaneous A-δ nociceptors leads to pricking pain,[8] whereas stimulation of the cutaneous C nociceptors results in burning or dull pain.[9] Activation of nociceptors in muscle nerves by electrical stimulation produces aching pain.[10] Electrical stimulation of visceral nerves at low intensities results in vague sensations of fullness and nausea, but higher intensities cause a sensation of pain.[11]

Motivational-affective circuits can also mimic pain states, most notably in patients with anxiety, neurotic depression, or hysteria.[12]

Pain Receptors

A major discovery in the 1980s indicated that many nociceptors, possibly most, are inactive and rather unresponsive under normal circumstances.[6] This observation was first made in recordings from the nerves supplying the knee joint[13,14] and led to the description of these afferents as "silent" or "sleeping" nociceptors.[6] However, it appeared that inflammation could cause the sensitization of these nerve fibers, after which they "awoke," by developing spontaneous discharges, and became much more sensitive to peripheral stimulation.[15] Silent nociceptors have now been described not only in joint nerves, but also in cutaneous and visceral nerves.[16] Sensitization of nociceptors appears to depend on the activation of "second-messenger" systems by the action of inflammatory mediators released in the damaged tissue, such as bradykinin (BK), prostaglandins, serotonin, and histamine.[17,6]

These tissue pain receptors appear to exist as free nerve endings or in plexi. They are found extensively in the skin, periosteum, arterial walls, the outer layers of the annulus fibrosis, joint capsules, and ligaments.[6] They are less widespread in the viscera. Most pain receptors are sensitive to varying types of stimuli, but some are responsive to only one type.

Pain receptors, unlike other receptors, are nonadapting in nature; that is, they will continue to fire for as long as the stimulus is applied. Painful responses to inflammation or injury can be classified as either hyperalgesia or allodynia.

- *Hyperalgesia* is a term used to describe an abnormal or increased response to a previously noxious stimuli.[18] Hyperalgesia can be further divided into primary and secondary hyperalgesia. Primary hyperalgesia is believed to be a consequence of the sensitization of nociceptors during the process of inflammation.[19] Whereas primary hyperalgesia refers to an increase response to peripheral noxious stimuli in the area of the injury, secondary hyperalgesia is felt at a site remote from the original injury.[20,21]
- *Allodynia* is a term used to describe a painful response to a previously innocuous stimuli, such as the brushing or stroking of the skin.[18]

The activity of nociceptors can be affected not only by adequate stimuli—such as strong mechanical, thermal, or chemical stimuli—but also by chemical actions on the surface membrane receptors of their axons.[6]

Pain Transmission[6,22,4]

Tissue degeneration leads to an excitation of the nerve endings. This, in turn, produces afferent sympathetic impulses to the sympathetic chain. The central pathways for processing nociceptive information begin at the level of the spinal cord (and medullary) dorsal horn. Interneuronal networks in the dorsal horn not only are responsible for the transmission of nociceptive information to neurons that project to the brain, but also help modulate that information, passing it on to other spinal cord neurons, including the flexor motoneurons and the nociceptive projection neurons. For example, certain patterns of stimulation have the effect of both enhancing reflex actions and increasing the speed of nociceptive transmissions. Other inputs result in the inhibition of projection neurons. The common free nerve endings have two distinct pathways into the CNS that correspond to the two different types of pain.

The fast, or dermatomal, pain signals are transmitted in the peripheral nerves by small myelinated A fibers at velocities between 6 and 30 m (20 and 98 ft) per second, whereas the slow, or sclerotomal, pain is transmitted in even, small, and unmyelinated nerves at much slower velocities between 0.5 and 2 m (1.6 and 6.6 ft) per second. The fast pain impulse is an emergency signal telling the subject that there is a threat present and provoking an almost instantaneous and often reflexive response. This is often followed a second or more later by a duller pain that tells of either tissue damage or continuing stimulation.

On entering the dorsal horn of the spinal cord, the pain signals from both visceral and somatic tissues ascend or descend one to three segments in the tract of Lissauer (dorsolateral fasciculus) before entering the gray matter of the dorsal horn.[22] They then relay with cells in the substantia gelatinosa (laminae II and III), and some proceed to synapse ipsilaterally in the dorsal funicular gray matter (lamina V) and are transmitted upward in one of two pathways:

1. The fast pain fibers terminate in laminae I and V of the dorsal horn. Here they excite neurons (internuncial neurons, segmental motor neurons, and flexor reflex afferents) that send long fibers to the opposite side of the cord and then upward to the brain in the lateral division of the anterior-lateral sensory pathway (lateral spinothalamic tract) (see Table 4–1).

2. The slow signals of the C fibers terminate in laminae II and III of the dorsal horn. Most of the signal then passes through another short fiber neuron to terminate in lamina V. Here the neuron gives off a long axon, most of which joins with the fast signal axons to cross the spinal cord, and continue on upward in the brain in the same spinal tract.

About 75% to 90% of all pain fibers terminate in the reticular formation of the medulla, pons, and mesencephalon. From here, other neurons transmit the signal to the thalamus, hypothalamus (pituitary), limbic system, and the cerebral cortex. A small number of fast fibers are passed directly to the thalamus, and then to the cerebral cortex, bypassing the brain stem. It is believed that these signals are important for recognizing and localizing pain, but not for analyzing it. Of the slow signals, none, or at least very few, avoid the reticular system. Because most of the fast, and all of the slow, pain signals go through the reticular formation, they can have wide-ranging and potent effects on almost the entire nervous system, because the reticular formation is the autonomic system's center and transmits activating signals into all parts of the brain. Signals that pass through this system can only localize to gross body areas and are, therefore, of little use in pain localization; however, they are more important in interpreting and producing an awareness of ongoing destructive processes. The fast and slow pain fibers remain undifferentiated from each other in the spinothalamic tract, with the fast pain fibers having a larger diameter, and a correspondingly faster transmission rate (see Table 4–1).

Lamina V is the area for convergence, summation, and projection. This lamina has the most complex responsiveness of all of the posterior laminae. Almost all nociceptive and mechanoreceptive impulses eventually reach this lamina. A few of the fast pain signals bypass this lamina and go directly to higher centers. The response of the cells in lamina V depends largely on the intensity of the stimulus. High-intensity stimulation leads to facilitation of the cell and relatively easy transmission across the cord to the other side and, from here, upward. More gentle stimulation inhibits this transmission. This inhibition is, according to theory, the result of pre- and postsynaptic effects produced by the cells of laminae II and III. In addition, where the impulses originate also determines whether facilitation occurs, or not. Successive impulses from the nociceptive system, have a "wind-up" effect so that further impulses that occur for longer durations facilitate transmission. If the signal arises from the A-beta (β) fibers, a quiet period follows each discharge and so tends to inhibit transmission. The effect of pain signals at lamina V tends to facilitate transmission upward, the greater the intensity of stimulation. However, milder intensities, and mild to moderate input from the mechanoreceptor, tend to inhibit lamina V as far as pain transmission is concerned. Thus, the net effect at lamina V will determine whether or not the pain signal is relayed upwards. Thus, the pain signal is prevented from progressing if mild mechanoreceptor dominates, but if the pain input dominates, the transmission of the pain signal occurs.

Sources of Pain

Referred
This is basically a misrepresentation of pain and generally follows the main innervating segment's embryologic derivation, although in more severe pain, several segments may be involved.

Tissue Ischemia
Tissue ischemia is a source of very intense pain. This pain intensity is greater, and occurs faster, if the ischemic tissues are functioning and demand a greater blood supply, or if the metabolic rate of the tissue is high. It was once believed that the pain was caused by a buildup of lactic acid, but as ischemic pain can also occur in the skin where lactic acid is not a significant factor, this theory lost favor. It is now believed that the ischemia causes actual tissue damage, and the pain is a result of the release of those chemicals associated with the damage.

TABLE 4–4 SIGNS AND SYMPTOMS ASSOCIATED WITH NERVE ROOT IRRITATION

DORSAL	VENTRAL	SYMPATHETIC
Neurogenic	Myogenic	Autonomic nervous system (ANS) reactions: sweating, nausea
Sharp, electric-like	Dull, achy, boring	ANS reactions: sweating, nausea
Superficial	Deep	ANS reactions: sweating, nausea
Distal paresthesia (hyperesthesia)	Tenderness of specific points	ANS reactions: sweating, nausea
Fairly well localized	Moderately well localized	ANS reactions: sweating, nausea
Dermatomal distribution	Myotomal/ sclerotomal distribution; increased reflexes	ANS reactions: sweating, nausea

Excessive Physical Deformation

Excessive physical deformation is a source of pain. The stimulation from the deformation can be sudden, as in the pain of a partial tear of a tendon or ligament before the chemicals have been released, or the deformation can be slow and gradual. A good example of this occurs when sitting on one chair with the legs crossed, while resting the feet on another chair, with the knees unsupported, for a prolonged period. No pain is felt initially but after a period of time, an ache occurs in the back of the knees.

With nerve root deformation, the symptoms vary according to which nerve is involved and whether the nerve is compressed or irritated.

Irritated Nerve Root

Refer to Table 4–4.

Compressed Nerve Root

Refer to Table 4–5.

TABLE 4–5 SIGNS AND SYMPTOMS ASSOCIATED WITH NERVE ROOT COMPRESSION

DORSAL	VENTRAL	SYMPATHETIC
Loss of sensation	Weakness/paralysis	Decreased autonomic nervous system reactions
	Decreased reflexes No tenderness	

CENTRAL NERVOUS SYSTEM SIGNS AND SYMPTOMS

Quite obviously, a lesion to the CNS is a major cause for a concern for any clinician, especially because it is out of the practice domain of most. Thus, it is very important that clinicians be able to identify a CNS impairment when it presents itself. Listed below are signs and symptoms that originate from a lesion of the CNS.

- Ataxia
- Spasticity
- Subjective complaints of a multisegmental paresis or paralysis
- Subjective complaints of a multisegmental sensory deficit or paresthesia
- Subjective complaints of a bilateral or quadrilateral paresthesia
- Hyper-reflexia
- Clonus or Babinski reflex
- Nystagmus
- Dysphasia
- Wallenberg's syndrome
- Cranial nerve signs—these include nystagmus, diplopia, and other visual disturbances, and loss of the pupillary reflex

This is by no means an all-inclusive list, and the reader should refer to Chapters 8, 9, and 10 for more information.

Dural Sleeve

Lesions to the dural sleeve produce the following findings:

- Subjective complaints of a localized pain
- Subjective complaints of an extrasegmental radiating pain (in a nondermatomal pattern)
- Restricted dural mobility tests as evidenced during adverse neural tissue testing

Posterior Root Ganglion

Compression of this structure results in the following:

- Subjective complaints of a paresthesia in a dermatomal distribution
- Subjective complaints of a radicular-type pain in a dermatomal distribution
- Subjective complaints of a hypoesthesia in a dermatomal distribution
- Hyporeflexic or areflexic deep tendon reflexes

Posterior Nerve Root

This can occur in the disc impingement syndrome, producing any of the following sensory and reflex changes:

- Subjective complaints of a dermatomal paresthesia
- Subjective complaints of a dermatomal hypoesthesia
- Hyporeflexic or areflexic deep tendon reflexes
- Possible associated dural signs, and nerve root tension signs

Anterior Nerve Root

This can also occur in the classic disc impingement syndrome, producing any of the following motor and reflex changes:

- Segmental paresis (key muscle weakness)
- Hyporeflexic or areflexic deep tendon reflexes
- Possible associated dural and nerve root tension signs

Spinal Nerve

Following a spinal nerve root impairment, the symptoms described by the patient will be paresthesia, occurring first, followed by paresis or cutaneous analgesia. A spinal nerve root impairment leads to pain only if the dural sheath is inflamed; if just the parenchyma is involved, paresthesia results. Both motor and sensory deficits are seen; these are related to the involved segment and can be felt in all, or any part of, the dermatome. A mixture of anterior and posterior nerve root signs is usually present.

Nerve Trunk or Plexus Lesions

A lesion to a nerve trunk or plexus leads to paresthesia and numbness in the distal part of the cutaneous supply. For example, a lesion to the sciatic nerve is felt in the foot. The sensation is usually felt in a vague area rather than in an area of dermatomal distribution. With a trunk or plexus impairment, a loss of motor and sensory function is noted as well as the release phenomenon, which is related to the length of compression. The release phenomenon occurs following compression of a nerve; in this condition, the neurologic signs go from numbness to tingling and are accompanied by some pain as the ischemia to the nerve is released. If the release phenomenon is present, the patient reports increased feelings of paresthesia over the analgesic part of the skin during passive range of motion or stroking of the area. The release

phenomenon is nonpathologic and can occur with a variety of postural positions, such as prolonged sitting on a railing. The railing compresses the sciatic nerve, resulting in paresthesia in the foot upon walking. It is interesting to note that the release phenomena does not occur in the brachial plexus.

Peripheral Nerve (Small Nerve) Lesions

A lesion to a small peripheral sensory nerve leads to pain, paresthesia, and numbness in a clearly defined boundary served by that peripheral nerve.

PAIN MODULATION

Gate Control Theory

Melzack and Wall[23] postulated that interneurons in the substantia gelatinosa act as a "gate" to modulate sensory input. They proposed that the substantia gelatinosa interneuron projected to the second-order neuron of the pain-temperature pathway located in lamina V, which they called the *transmission cell*. It was reasoned that if the substantia gelatinosa interneuron were depolarized, it would inhibit transmission cell firing, and thus decrease further transmission of input ascending in the spinothalamic tract. The degree of modulation appeared to depend on the proportion of input from the large A fibers, and the small C fibers, so that the gate could be closed by either decreasing C-fiber input or by increasing A-fiber input (Fig. 4–1).

Melzack and Wall also believed that the gate could be modified by a descending inhibitory pathway from the brain, or brain stem,[24] suggesting that the CNS apparently plays a part in this modulation in a mechanism called *central biasing* (Fig. 4–1).

The gate control theory was, and is, supported by practical evidence, although the experimental evidence for the theory is lacking. Researchers have identified many clinical pain states that cannot be fully explained by the gate control theory.[25] A problem with this theory is that there is evidence to suggest that the A-β fibers from the mechanoreceptor do not synapse in the substantia gelatinosa. In this case, the modulation at the spinal cord level must occur in lamina V, where there is a simple summation of signals from the pain fibers and the mechanoreceptor fibers. However, severe or prolonged pain tends to have the segment identifying all input as painful, and summation modulation has little if any effect. The likelihood is that our pain perception is much more complicated, and that further research is needed.

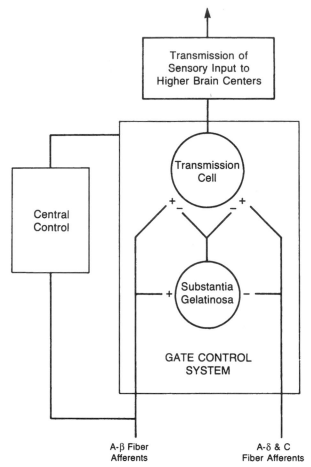

FIGURE 4–1   Modulation of pain by the Gate Control System.

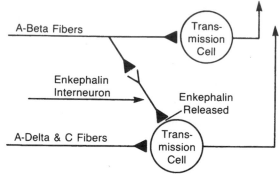

FIGURE 4–2   A schematic representation of the descending analgesia system of the periaquaductal gray, raphe nucleus, pons, and medulla regions.

Chemical

In 1969, Reynolds[26] reported that he found it possible to perform abdominal surgery on rats without chemical anesthesia during stimulation in the periaqueductal gray (PAG) region of the midbrain. The rats did not have motor impairment, and they showed normal responses to innocuous stimuli. Since then, numerous investigations have been made of what became known as the "descending analgesia systems." These pathways have been shown to utilize several different neurotransmitters, including opioids, serotonin, and catecholamines, and the anatomic structures giving rise to them include not only the PAG, but also the locus ceruleus, subceruleus, and Kölliker-Fuse nuclei, the nucleus raphe magnus, and several nuclei of the bulbar reticular formation (Fig. 4–2). In addition, structures at higher levels of the nervous system (including the cerebral cortex) and various limbic structures (including the hypothalamus) contribute to the analgesia pathways. The system is thought to work in the following manner.

The PAG area of the upper pons sends signals to the raphe magnus nucleus in the lower pons and upper medulla. This structure relays the signal down the cord to a pain inhibitory complex located in the dorsal horn of the cord. Stimulation in the lateral column of the PAG evokes a defense response, which consists of avoidance behavior in rats, retraction of the ears or arching of the back in cats, sympathetic activation, vocalization, and sometimes a flight reaction,[27] as well as analgesia. By contrast, stimulation in the ventrolateral PAG results in immobility and sympathoinhibition, as well as analgesia.[28] Therefore, the PAG is believed to be involved in complex behavioral responses to stressful or life-threatening situations, or to promote recuperative behavior after a defense reaction.

The nerve fibers derived from the gray area secrete enkephalin and serotonin, whereas the raphe magnus releases enkephalin only (Fig. 4–3). The fibers terminating in the cord's dorsal horn secrete serotonin, which has been shown to act on another set of cord neurons that, in turn, release enkephalin. This enkephalin is believed to produce presynaptic inhibition of the incoming pain signals to laminae I through V, thereby blocking pain signals at their entry point into the cord.[29] It is further believed that the chemical releases in the upper end of the pathway can inhibit pain signal transmission in the reticular formation and thalamus. The inhibition from this system is effective on both fast and slow pain. The more important morphine-like substances that act in synaptic receptors are:

● β-endorphin, found in the hypothalamus and pituitary gland.
● Met-enkephalin.
● Leu-enkephalin.
● Dynorphin, found only in minute quantities in nervous tissue; it acts as an extremely powerful analgesic.

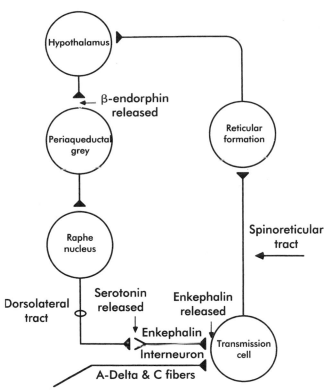

FIGURE 4–3 The nerve fibers derived from the grey area secrete enkephalin and serotonin while the raphe magnus releases enkephalin only.

Neurophysiologic

A negative feedback loop exists in the cortex called the *corticifugal system*.[30] This originates at the termination point of the various sensory pathways. Excessive stimulation of the feedback loop results in a signal being transmitted down from the sensory cortex to the posterior horn of the level from which the input arose. This produces lateral or recurrent inhibition of the cells adjacent to the stimulated cell, thereby preventing the spread of the signal. This is an automatic gain control system to prevent overloading of the sensory system.

CLINICAL IMPLICATIONS

The Facilitated Segment

A *facilitated segment* is a theoretical explanation of a phenomenon seen clinically and is thought to be the result of a breakdown in the nervous system of the body.

The CNS is continuously subject to afferent impulses arising from countless receptors throughout the body.

Within any given segment of the spine, there are a fixed number of sensory and motor neurons. Much like a relay center in a telephone exchange, there are limits to the number of "calls" that can be handled. If the number or amplitude of impulses from the proprioceptors, and nociceptors throughout the body, exceeds the capacity of the normal routing pathway, the electrochemical discharges may begin to affect collateral pathways. This spillover effect may be exerted ipsilaterally, contralaterally, or vertically. The closer to the spine that this phenomenon occurs, the greater the effect it has on the other areas within the body. When these impulses extend beyond their normal sensorimotor pathways, the CNS begins to misinterpret the information because of the effect of an overflow of neurotransmitter substance within the involved segment. For example, afferent impulses intended to register as pain in the gallbladder manifest as shoulder pain, because the phrenic nerve, and portions of the brachial plexus, share common spinal origins.

The resulting overload at the CNS level is referred to as a facilitated segment.

- Chronic irritation of a joint can involve the sympathetic and autonomic pathways and lead to trophic and metabolic changes, which may be the basis for some of the local tissue changes associated with musculoskeletal impairment.
- The excessive motion that occurs at a hypermobile segment can produce a hyperexcitable reaction in terms of the impulses, as it moves beyond the normal ranges it is designed for.

The neuromuscular reflex arc is at the crossroads for several sources of noxious stimuli, including trauma, viscerosomatic reflexes, and emotional distress, as well as the vast proprioceptive system reporting from striated muscle throughout the body. According to Upledger,[31] the facilitated segment is exemplified by the following:

- *Hypersensitivity.* Minimal impulses may produce excessive responses or sensations because of a reduced threshold for stimulation and depolarization at the level of the facilitated segment.
- *Overflow.* Impulses may become nonspecific and spill over to adjacent pathways. Collateral nerve cells, lateral tracts, and vertical tracts may be stimulated and produce symptoms of a widely divergent nature, such as those which occur with referred pain.
- *Autonomic dystrophy.* The sympathetic ganglia become excessively activated, leading to reduced healing and

repair of target cells, reduced immune function, impaired circulation, accelerated aging, and deterioration of peripheral tissues. Digestive and cardiovascular disturbances and visceral parenchymal dystrophy may also develop over time.

Because of the excessive discharge arising from a variety of receptors, the facilitated segment may eventually become a self-perpetuating source of irritation in its own right. An injury of the biceps, for example, produces an increase in high-frequency discharge (increased neural impulses), which is transmitted to the spinal segment at the level of C-5. If the discharge is excessive, other muscles connected to this segment (supraspinatus, teres minor, levator scapula, pectoralis minor, etc.) may receive a certain amount of spillover discharge. This results in an increase in the γ gain to these muscles. Thus several muscles supplied by the same segment may have a generally increased setting of their γ bias (background tone fed to the muscle spindle apparatus), which leads to increased hypertonicity and susceptibility to strain. Other tissues (skin receptors, viscera, and cerebral emotional centers) may also feed into this loop either as primary sources of high-frequency discharge or secondary to the neuromuscularly induced hyperirritability. Another clinical example of a facilitated segment could involve the posterior tibialis which, when facilitated, produces a relative inhibition of the peroneus longus resulting in metatarsalgia, as the peroneus longus is relatively inhibited. Conversely, if the segment that innervates the peroneus longus is facilitated, shin splints can occur, as its antagonist, the tibialis posterior is relatively inhibited.

Positional release and muscle energy therapy appear to have a damping influence on the general level of excitability within the facilitated segment, and they exert an influence in reducing the threshold within the facilitated segment. This may open a window of opportunity for the CNS to normalize the level of neural activity.

Use of Direct Interventions to Control Pain

Pain can be described using many terms. Perhaps the simplest descriptors are "acute" and "chronic."

A. *Acute pain.* This is the pain that usually precipitates a visit to a physician because it has one or more of the following characteristics:[32]
1. It is new and has not been experienced before.
2. It is so severe and disabling.
3. It is continuous or recurs very frequently.
4. The site of the pain may cause alarm (e.g., chest, eye).
5. The associated symptoms may be alarming.

B. *Chronic pain.* This is the pain that is more aggravating than worrying. It typically has the following characteristics:[32]
1. It has been experienced before and has remitted spontaneously, or after simple measures.
2. It is usually mild to moderate in intensity.
3. It is usually of limited duration.
4. The pain site does not cause alarm (e.g., knee, ankle).
5. There are no alarming associated symptoms.

The presence of pain should not always be viewed negatively by the clinician. After all, its presence helps to determine the location of the injury, and its behavior aids the clinician in determining the stage of healing, the prognosis, its source, the degree of patient dysfunction, and its degree of irritability. As discussed in Chapter 12, pain is used as a guide in determining the grade of mobilization to be employed. A number of factors need to be considered by the clinician when planning an intervention:

● Stage of healing (refer to Chapter 2).
● Source. Cyriax[33] devised a sequential scheme of systematic analysis to provide the clinician with a portrait of the joint dysfunction in relation to signs and symptoms. He coined the expression "selective tissue tension tests" and reasoned that if one isolates and then applies tension to a structure, one could make a conclusion as to the integrity of that structure. The intervention should involve techniques geared toward alleviating the stresses from that structure.
● Degree of patient dysfunction. When pain is associated with a loss of function, the major focus of the clinician should be to seek methods to control the pain, and address the strength and flexibility deficits, so that the function can be improved. Obviously the degree of dysfunction can vary between individuals and diagnoses, and even between individuals with the same diagnosis.
● Degree of irritability. An irritable structure is one that produces a sharp increase in pain with the minimal amount of intervention. Irritable structures, which suggest an acute stage of healing or a serious underlying cause, should always be approached with care.

The observation that most nociceptors are normally "sleeping" but "awaken" when they are sensitized (e.g., by inflammation) suggests that the pain of inflammation should be reduced if sensitization is minimized.[6] The traditional approach has been the use of nonsteroidal anti-inflammatory agents, such as aspirin, to block the synthesis of prostaglandins. However, many other substances also contribute to peripheral sensitization, including bradykinin, serotonin, and a variety of cytokines released from immune cells. Presumably, pharmacologic agents directed against the actions of these agents should prove as useful as aspirin, at least under some conditions.[6]

Peripheral nerve damage causes changes in the concentrations of several peptides in the dorsal root ganglia, and in the dorsal horn of the spinal cord, possibly contributing to neuropathic or other pain states.[6]

Our knowledge of the descending endogenous analgesia system remains incomplete.

The gate control theory, utilizing either a decrease in C-fiber input, or an increase in the A-δ fiber input, can be applied in the clinic setting. C-fiber input can be decreased by removing the chemical or physical irritant, through the application of protection, rest, ice, compression, and elevation (PRICE). The application of manual therapy techniques such as joint mobilizations, massage, and transverse frictions is thought to increase A-δ fiber input, thereby "closing the gate" and preventing C-fiber transmission. A-δ fiber input can also be increased through the use of exercise, hot packs, whirlpools, vibrators, or transcutaneous electrical nerve stimulation (TENS). These methods are discussed in more detail in Chapter 12.

REVIEW QUESTIONS

1. Loss of light touch is the result of a lesion of which tract?
   a. Spinothalamic tracts—posterior columns
   b. Spinocerebellar
   c. Corticospinal
   d. Medial lemniscus—posterior columns
2. A nerve impulse travels in which direction?
   a. One direction, dendrites to axon
   b. One direction, axon to dendrites
   c. Either direction
   d. None of the above
3. Sensory or afferent nerve fibers enter the spinal cord through the:
   a. Dorsal roots
   b. Ventral roots
   c. Peripheral nerves
   d. None of the above
4. Efferent nerve fibers leave the spinal cord through the:
   a. Dorsal roots
   b. Ventral roots
   c. Peripheral nerves
   d. None of the above
5. In which lamina(e) is the spinal gating's presynaptic inhibition supposed to occur?

6. What are the two types of anterior motor neurons called, and what are their functions?
7. The presence of nystagmus, dysphasia, dysphagia, or Wallenberg's syndrome indicates a compromise to what?
8. Schwann cells, nodes of Ranvier, and saltatory conduction are associated with which nerve fibers?
9. Are cranial nerves considered part of the CNS or PNS?
10. What is the major function of the muscle spindle?
11. What is the major function of the Golgi tendon organ?

ANSWERS

1. a.
2. a.
3. a.
4. b.
5. Laminae II and III.
6. α—Innervation of large muscle fibers; γ—supply the small intrafusal muscle fibers of the muscle spindle.
7. CNS.
8. Myelinated.
9. CNS.
10. To give information regarding the length of the muscle.
11. To provide information with regard to tension of the muscle.

REFERENCES

1. Diamond MC, Scheibel AB, Elson LM. *The Human Brain Coloring Book*. New York, NY: Harper & Row; 1985.
2. Gordon J, Ghez C. Muscle receptors and spinal reflexes: The stretch reflex. In: Kandel ER, Schwartz JH, Jessel TM, eds. *Principles of Neural Science*, 3rd ed. Norwalk, Conn: Appleton & Lange, 1991:564–580.
3. Wall PD, McMahon SB. Microneurography and its relation to perceived sensation. A critical review. Pain 1985;21:209–229.
4. Willis WD, Coggeshall RE. *Sensory Mechanisms of the Spinal Cord*, 2nd ed. New York, NY: Plenum Press; 1991.
5. Boivie J, Leijon G, Johansson I. Central post-stroke pain—a study of the mechanisms through analyses of the sensory abnormalities. Pain 1989;37:173–185.
6. Willis WD, Westlund KN. Neuroanatomy of the pain system and of the pathways that modulate pain. J Clin Neurophys 1997;14:2–31.
7. Kellgren JH, Samuel EP. The sensitivity and innervation of the articular capsule. J Bone Joint Surg 1950; 32(B):84–92.

8. Konietzny F, Perl ER, Trevino D, Light A, Hensel H. Sensory experiences in man evoked by intraneural electrical stimulation of intact cutaneous afferent fibers. Exp Brain Res 1981;42:219–222.

9. Ochoa J, Torebjörk E. Sensations evoked by intraneural microstimulation of C nociceptor fibres in human skin nerves. J Physiol 1989;415:583–599.

10. Torebjörk HE, Ochoa JL, Schady W. Referred pain from intraneural stimulation of muscle fascicles in the median nerve. Pain 1984;18:145–156.

11. Ness TJ, Gebhart GF. Visceral pain: A review of experimental studies. Pain 1990;41:167–234.

12. Chaturvedi SK. Prevalence of chronic pain in psychiatric patients. Pain 1987;29:231–237.

13. Schaible HG, Schmidt RF. Activation of groups III and IV sensory units in medial articular nerve by local mechanical stimulation of knee joint. J Neurophysiol 1983;49:35–44.

14. Schaible HG, Schmidt RF. Responses of fine medial articular nerve afferents to passive movements of knee joint. J Neurophysiol 1983;49:1118–1126.

15. Schaible HG, Schmidt RF. Effects of an experimental arthritis on the sensory properties of fine articular afferent units. J Neurophysiol 1985;54:1109–1122.

16. Häbler HJ, Jänig W, Koltzenburg M. Activation of unmyelinated afferent fibres by mechanical stimuli and inflammation of the urinary bladder in the cat. J Physiol 1990;425:545–562.

17. Dray A, Bettaney J, Forster P, Perkins MN. Bradykinin-induced stimulation of afferent fibres is mediated through protein kinase C. Neuroscience Lett 1988;91:301–307.

18. Bonica JJ. Clinical importance of hyperalgesia. In: Willis WD, ed. *Hyperalgesia and Allodynia*. New York, NY: Raven Press; 1992:17–43.

19. Meyer RA, Campbell JN. Myelinated nociceptive afferents account for the hyperalgesia that follows a burn to the hand. Science 1981;213:1527–1529.

20. Lewis T. *Pain*. London, England: Macmillan Press; 1942.

21. Hardy JD, Wolff HG, Goodell H, eds. Pain sensations and reactions. New York, NY: Williams & Wilkins, 1952; reprinted by New York: Hafner; 1967.

22. Bonica JJ. Neurophysiological and pathological aspects of acute and chronic pain. Arch Surg 1977;112:750–761.

23. Melzack R, Wall PD. On the nature of cutaneous sensory mechanisms. Brain 1962;85:331–356.

24. Melzack R. The gate theory revisited. In: LeRoy PL, ed. *Current Concepts in the Management of Chronic Pain*. Miami, Fla: Symposia Specialists; 1977.

25. Nathan PW. The gate-control theory of pain—A critical review. Brain 1976;99:123–158.

26. Reynolds DV. Surgery in the rat during electrical analgesia induced by focal brain stimulation. Science 1969;164:444–445.

27. Bandler R, Depaulis A. Midbrain periaqueductal gray control of defensive behavior in the cat and the rat. In: Depaulis A, Bandler R, eds. *The Midbrain Periaqueductal Gray Matter*. New York, NY: Plenum Press; 1991: 175–187.

28. Lovick TA. Inhibitory modulation of the cardiovascular defense response by the ventrolateral periaqueductal grey matter in rats. Exp Brain Res 1992;89:133–139.

29. Mayer DJ, Price DD. Central nervous system mechanisms of analgesia. Pain 1976;2:379–404.

30. Fields HL, Anderson SD. Evidence that raphe-spinal neurons mediate opiate and midbrain stimulation-produced analgesias. Pain 1978;5:333–349.

31. Upledger J, Vredevoogd JD. *Craniosacral Therapy*. Seattle, Wash: Eastland Press; 1983.

32. Wiener SL. *Differential Diagnosis of Acute Pain by Body Region*. New York, NY: McGraw-Hill, 1993:1–4.

33. Cyriax J. *Textbook of Orthopedic Medicine*, vol 1, 8th ed. London, England: Balliere Tindall and Cassell; 1982.

34. Willis WD. *The Pain System*. Basel, Switzerland: Karger; 1985.

35. Spiller WG, Martin E. The treatment of persistent pain of organic origin in the lower part of the body by division of the anterior-lateral column of the spinal cord. JAMA 1912;58:1489–1490.

36. Gowers WR. A case of unilateral gunshot injury to the spinal cord. Trans Clin Lond 1878;11:24–32.

37. Vierck CJ, Greenspan JD, Ritz LA. Long-term changes in purposive and reflexive responses to nociceptive stimulation following anterior-lateral chordotomy. J Neurosci 1990;10:2077–2095.

38. Hyndman OR, Van Epps C. Possibility of differential section of the spinothalamic tract. Arch Surg 1939;38: 1036–1053.

39. Willis WD, Trevino DL, Coulter JD, Maunz RA. Responses of primate spinothalamic tract neurons to natural stimulation of hindlimb. J Neurophysiol 1974;37: 358–372.

40. Ferrington DG, Sorkin LS, Willis WD. Responses of spinothalamic tract cells in the superficial dorsal horn of the primate lumbar spinal cord. J Physiol 1987;388: 681–703.

41. Kenshalo DR, Leonard RB, Chung JM, Willis WD. Responses of primate spinothalamic neurons to graded and to repeated noxious heat stimuli. J Neurophysiol 1979;42:1370–1389.

42. Foreman RD, Schmidt RF, Willis WD. Effects of mechanical and chemical stimulation of fine muscle afferents upon primate spinothalamic tract cells. J Physiol 1979;286:215–231.

43. Milne RJ, Foreman RD, Giesler GJ, Willis WD. Convergence of cutaneous and pelvic visceral nociceptive inputs onto primate spinothalamic neurons. Pain 1981;11:163–183.

44. Chung JM, Fang ZR, Hori Y, Lee KH, Willis WD. Prolonged inhibition of primate spinothalamic tract cells by peripheral nerve stimulation. Pain 1984;19:259–275.

45. Chung JM, Lee KH, Hori Y, Endo K, Willis WD. Factors influencing peripheral nerve stimulation produced inhibition of primate spinothalamic tract cells. Pain 1984;19:277–293.

46. Lee KH, Chung JM, Willis WD. Inhibition of primate spinothalamic tract cells by TENS. J Neurosurg 1985; 62:276–287.

CHAPTER FIVE

THE VERTEBRAL ARTERY

Chapter Objectives

At the completion of this chapter, the reader will be able to:

1. Describe the anatomy of the vertebral artery.
2. Identify the areas of vulnerability in the vertebral artery.
3. List the signs and symptoms that indicate a vertebral artery insufficiency.
4. Perform an examination of the vertebral artery.

OVERVIEW

The first description of a spontaneous occlusion of a vertebral artery was provided by Wallenberg in 1895.[1] Since that time, there have been numerous reports outlining the pathomechanics of vertebral artery compromise.

No other artery in the body has been discussed in as much detail by manual therapists as the vertebral artery. To fully comprehend its significance, a review of its anatomy and function is in order.

The vertebral artery appears at the fourth to fifth week of intrauterine development.[2] An anastomosis of the upper six cervical and posterior-lateral intersegmental arteries forms the posterior costal anastomosis, which, in turn, eventually forms most of the vertebral artery.[2] The vertebral arteries are different from other arteries in the body, in that they run for most of their length within an osteofibrotic channel that has movable segments. However, the vertebral arteries are susceptible to mechanical compression, especially with cervical extension and rotation, because of their anatomic relationship with neighboring bone, muscle, ligaments, and fascia. Anatomically the artery, along its course, can be viewed as four segments: the proximal, transverse, suboccipital, and intracranial portions (Fig. 5–1).[3,4]

Proximal Portion[3,5]

This segment normally originates from the first part of the subclavian artery, although it can originate from the aortic arch. It ascends posteriorly between the longus colli and scalenus anterior, behind the common carotid artery and vertebral vein to enter the foramina transversaria of C6 although its exact direction is dependent on its exact point of origin. Posterior to it are the first rib, the seventh cervical transverse process, the stellate ganglion and the ventral rami of the seventh and eighth cervical spinal nerves.

Although the typical entry point to the cervical spine is at the C6 transverse foramen, other levels of entry between C3 and C7 occur. Tortuosity and kinking of this portion of the artery is more common than it is elsewhere and the artery can also be compressed by the fascia of the scalenovertebral angle.[6]

Transverse Portion[3,5]

The second part of the vertebral artery runs with a large branch of sympathetic nerve fibers from the stellate ganglion, from the point of entry at the spinal column to the transverse foramen of C2 (see Fig. 5–1). Throughout this section of the spinal column, the artery travels anterior to the ventral rami of the cervical spinal nerves (C2–C6), and medial to the uncinate processes, in a canal called the *transverse canal*, which is formed by the bony transverse foramina at each spinal level, and by the overlying ligamentous and muscular structures. Within the canal, the artery is encased in a sheath that is adherent to the periosteum of the transverse processes and uncinate processes which form a protective boundary and restrict motion of the artery.

Tortuosity of this portion of the artery is characterized by looping within the intervertebral foramina to the extent of causing pedicle erosion, and widening of the intervertebral foramen with nerve root compression.[7]

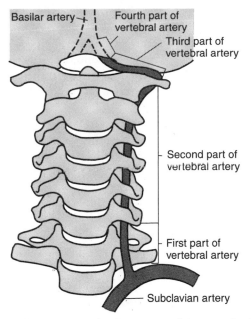

FIGURE 5-1 The four parts of the vertebral artery.

Arthrotic changes at these levels may have important consequences for the blood flow. The artery is susceptible to compression at this portion by osteophytes and other degenerative changes of cervical spondylosis.

Suboccipital Portion[3,5]

This part of the artery extends from its entry into the transverse foramen of C2 to its point of penetration into the foramen magnum (Fig. 5–2). In this portion the vertebral artery has four curves:

1. Within the transverse foramen of C2. This portion lies in a complete bony canal formed by the two curves of the C2 transverse foramen.
2. Between C2 and C1. The second part bends laterally and slightly anteriorly to the transverse foramen of C2. At the atlantoaxial joint, the artery can be compressed by fibers from the inferior oblique capitis, intertransversarius muscle, membrane hypertrophy, or vertebral subluxation. The length of this segment varies with head position, being elongated on the side contralateral to head rotation.
3. In the transverse foramen of C1. In its third part, the suboccipital portion of the vertebral artery curves superiorly within the transverse foramen of C1 in which it is completely enclosed (see Fig. 5–2).
4. Between the posterior arch of the atlas and its entry into the foramen magnum (see Fig. 5–1). On exiting from the transverse foramen of C1, the artery winds posteriorly behind the lateral mass of the superior

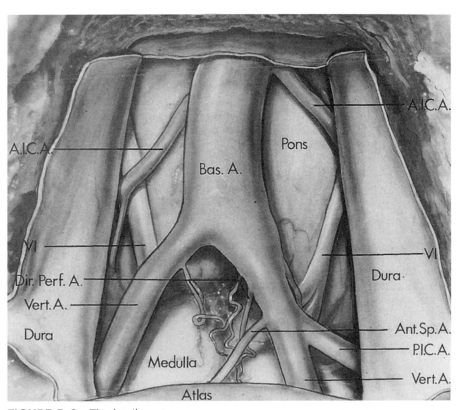

FIGURE 5-2 The basilar artery.

articular process of the atlas in a groove on the superior aspect of the posterior arch of the atlas. The groove extends horizontally from the medial border of the transverse foramen to the medial edge of the posterior ring of the atlas. In the vertebral artery groove, the vertebral artery lies lateral to the spinal canal, posterior to the lateral mass, anterior to the atlanto-occipital membrane, and medial to the rectus capitis lateralis muscle (Fig. 5–2).

Occasionally, this groove is closed to form an arterial canal. As the artery leaves the groove it is surrounded anteriorly by the joint capsules of the atlanto-occipital joints and posteriorly by the superior oblique capitis and rectus capitis posterior major muscles.

After leaving the groove, the artery penetrates the dural sac on the lateral aspect of the foramen magnum by piercing the posterior atlanto-occipital membrane and dura mater (see Fig. 5–1). This upper portion of the extracranial vertebral artery is relatively superficial. Having bone beneath it, and only muscles above, it is vulnerable to direct blunt trauma.[8] Indeed, because of their unique course through four or five transverse foramina, the vertebral arteries are vulnerable to direct traumatic damage which results in a dissection. The pathomechanics behind a vertebral artery dissection have yet to be established, but it would appear there are changes in the arterial wall.

In addition to blunt trauma, the vertebral artery is vulnerable during movement of the head and neck. Although the artery is affected by vertebral motion in the lower cervical region, it is affected even more between C2 and the occipital bone. This is a result both of the osteology and the biomechanics of the upper cervical spine. Because the transverse foramen of C1 is more lateral than that of C2, the artery must incline laterally between the two vertebrae. At this point, the artery is vulnerable to impingement from:

- Abnormal posture.[9]
- Excursion of the C1 transverse mass during rotation. Because a larger amount of axial rotation occurs between C1 and C2, there is a large excursion of the transverse mass of C1 with rotation. The artery is stretched during this process, and the size of the lumen can be reduced. The artery most vulnerable to the rotation is usually the one that is contralateral to the side of the rotation.[10] During head rotation to the right, the left transverse foramen of C1 moves anteriorly and slightly to the right. This movement imparts a marked stretch on the left artery, and it increases the acuteness of the angle formed between its ascending and posterior-medial courses. It has been demonstrated

that kinking and stretching of the contralateral artery can be observed at this site with 30 degrees of head rotation and becomes well marked at 45 degrees.[6] Thus, both stenotic and aneurysmal lesions are most common in the distal segment of the artery, at the level of the first and second cervical vertebra.

Intracranial Portion[3,5]

After entering the skull, the right and left vertebral arteries bend superiorly to meet on or near the midline of the clivus, to form the basilar artery. The basilar artery (Fig. 5–2) serves much of the medulla, pons and cerebellum. The periosteal sheath continues intracranially for about half a centimeter. Unlike the internal carotid artery, which enters the skull through this narrow osseous foramen, the vertebral artery enters the skull through the foramen magnum, which explains why as many as 10 percent of vertebral-artery dissections extend intracranially.[10]

BRANCHES

The vertebral artery gives off both cervical and cranial branches.

A. The cervical branches include spinal and muscular branches.
  1. The spinal branch divides in two.
    a. One branch enters the vertebral canal by the intervertebral foramen, anastomoses with other spinal arteries, and supplies the dural sleeve of the nerve roots, the spinal cord, and its membranes.
    b. The other branch supplies the periosteum, bone, and ligaments of the posterior aspect of the vertebral body.
  2. The muscular branches arise from the vertebral artery as it curves around the lateral mass of the atlas, supply the deep suboccipital muscles, and anastomose with the occipital and cervical arteries.

B. Intracranially, the vertebral artery generates small meningeal branches that supply the bone and dura mater of the cerebellar fossa.

The total blood supply to the brain is carried by four arteries: the two internal carotid arteries, and the two vertebral arteries. In all, the vertebral arteries contribute about 11% of the total cerebral blood flow, the remaining 89% being supplied by the carotid system.[11]

Near the termination of the artery, the anterior spinal artery arises. This branch unites with its opposite number and then descends, receiving reinforcement from the spinal branches of the regional arteries (vertebral, cervical, or posterior intercostal and lumbar arteries). Together these arteries supply the spinal cord and cauda equina.

The posterior spinal arteries commonly arise from the posterior inferior cerebellar artery, which is the largest branch of the vertebral artery, supplying either directly or indirectly, the medulla and the cerebellum and, via the posterior spinal arteries, the dorsal portion of the spinal cord.

The formation of the basilar artery by the union of the two vertebral arteries (see Fig. 5–2) at the lower border of the pons marks the termination of the vertebral artery. The basilar artery and its branches supply the pons, the visual area of the occipital lobe, the membranous labyrinth, the medulla, the temporal lobe, the posterior thalamus, and the cerebellum.

A major change in the structure of the artery occurs as it becomes intracranial. The tunica adventitia and tunica media become thinner, and there is a gross reduction in the number of elastic fibers in these coats.[12] Variations in the elasticity of the vertebral artery occur in the transverse and proximal portions, and it is thought that these are an adaptation to the greater mobility required in these sections of the artery.

General Anomalies

The vertebral artery is subject to variations in the gross anatomy of its general structure. These variations are of particular concern and significance to the manipulating clinician.

By far the most common variant is the side-to-side caliber of the two arteries.[13,14] Asymmetry in the size of the two vertebral arteries is common, with one study finding that only 41% were equal in diameter.[13] Of the remaining subjects, the left vertebral artery was the larger of the two in 36% of the cases, with the right one larger in the remaining 24%.[13,15] Where there is nonequivalency, the larger artery, is termed the *dominant artery* and the smaller, the *minor artery*.

Unilateral occlusion of the vertebral artery by thrombosis or dissection may not lead to clinical signs and symptoms when contralateral flow via the contralateral vertebral artery is sufficient. However, it can be assumed that patients with a unilateral dependence on one artery will be particularly vulnerable if that dependence is on the dominant artery.

VERTEBRAL ARTERY INSUFFICIENCY

The vertebral artery is subject to occlusion from internal and external causes.

Internal Causes[16]

Atherosclerosis and Thrombosis
Atherosclerosis of the extracranial part of the vertebral artery primarily affects the proximal and transverse portions. Castaigne and colleagues[17] investigated 44 patients with vertebrobasilar artery occlusions and found that in 35 of the 44 patients the cause was atherosclerosis.

Another study[13] found that vertebral artery stenosis was about equal to that seen in the cerebral vessels, and that the right side was affected more frequently than the left, a finding coincident with the relative sizes of the two sides. The chief site of occlusion occurred at the origin of the artery, at the angle formed between the subclavian and vertebral arteries. It was also noted that the stenosis occurred more frequently in the smaller of the two arteries, although no possible explanation was given as to the reason for this observation.

Thrombosis can occur at any level of the vertebral artery, but is rarer in the transverse part, and more common in the suboccipital and intracranial parts.

Atherosclerosis has the potential to produce signs and symptoms resulting from ischemia of the tissues supplied by the artery distal to the occlusion.

Fibromuscular Dysplasia (FMD)
This condition is a multifocal, noninflammatory, angiopathy of unknown etiology which commonly affects the renal arteries, but has also been described in the vertebral arteries.

Angiographic changes of fibromuscular dysplasia are found in about 15 percent of patients with a spontaneous dissection of the vertebral artery.[13]

Stanley and associates[18] reporting on 15 patients, described multiple intracranial aneurysms of which seven ruptured, killing the patient. He further found that of 14 vertebral arteries investigated, 6 were fibrodysplastic.

Arteriovenous Fistula
This is an abnormal communication between the extracranial vertebral artery, or one its muscular or radicular branches, and an adjacent vein. It has variable causes, including traumatic dissections or dissecting aneurysms, and may occur spontaneously as a result of existing disease, or as a congenital condition. Most spontaneous arteriovenous fistulas occur at the level of C2-3.

Traumatic causes of atriovenous fistulas include penetrating trauma, such as bullet and knife wounds; and blunt trauma.

External Compression

The vertebral artery is particularly vulnerable to external compression in the portion that courses through the foramina transversaria from C6 to C1.[19] Because of its fixation to the spine in this segment, subluxations of one vertebral body on another may exert undue tension and traction on the artery. Unilateral occlusion of the vertebral artery rarely results in a neurologic deficit because of collateral supply through the contralateral vertebral and posterior inferior cerebellar arteries.[20] However, extracranial compression of the vertebral artery may cause neurologic symptoms, depending on the acuteness of the occlusion and preexisting conditions such as atherosclerosis, and the absence of a contralateral vertebral artery. Signs of vertebral artery insufficiency may manifest as dizziness, speech deficits, dysphagia, diplopia, blurred vision, and tinnitus,[21] whereas vertebral artery occlusion may result in death.[22,23]

The constant feature of nonpenetrating trauma injures to the vertebral artery is hyperextension of the neck, with or without rotation and lateral flexion.[24,25] The most common mechanism of injury to the vertebral artery after nonpenetrating trauma is stretching and tearing of the intima and media in a vessel tethered to bone.[22,26] There are some weaker areas that are subjected to great stresses during anterior-posterior, lateral, or rotatory movements of the head. The vertebral artery is prone to injury at the following sites: (1) its entry point into the transverse foramen of C6; (2) anywhere in the bone canal secondary to fracture-dislocations of the spine, and (3) its course from the foramen of C1 to its entry point into the skull.[27]

Dissection

Spontaneous dissections of the carotid and vertebral arteries affect all age groups, including children, but there is a distinct peak in the fifth decade of life.[28] Although there is no overall sex-based predilection, women are on average about five years younger than men at the time of the dissection.[28] Although spontaneous dissections can occur in arteries throughout the body, they are more likely to occur in the extracranial segments of the vertebral and carotid arteries, and extracranial vertebral artery dissection has been reported with increasing frequency during the last decade.[28,29] The most common clinical findings are brain stem or cerebellar ischemic symptoms preceded by severe neck pain or occipital headache, or both. Occasionally, patients report radicular symptoms.[30]

A headache is often the earliest symptom of carotid artery dissection, and is reportedly present in 60% to 75% of patients.[31] The typical patient with vertebral artery dissection presents with pain in the back of the head or neck which can be bilateral, and ischemic symptoms related to the lateral medulla (Wallenberg's syndrome), thalomus, cerebral hemispheres and cervical spinal cord.

Dissections of the vertebral artery usually arise from a primary tear of the intima. The tear allows blood under arterial pressure to enter the wall of the artery, between the intima and media, and form an intramural hematoma, the so-called false lumen. Subintimal hemorrhage can produce various degrees of stenosis; subadventitial hemorrhage can cause a aneurysmal dilatation. Tearing of the artery is not always related to remarkable trauma and so this aspect may not appear in the history unless the symptoms appear immediately following the injury. The activities that have immediately preceded a spontaneous dissection of the vertebral artery range from boxing, trampolining, athletics, being bitten by a dog, coughing, "bottoms-up" drinking, "head banging" to music, moving furniture, parking a car, roller coaster riding, vomiting, performing yardwork, and nose blowing.

A potential link with common risk factors for vascular disease, such as tobacco use and hypertension, has not been systematically evaluated, but atherosclerosis appears to be distinctly uncommon in patients with a vertebral artery dissection.

Two clinical studies examined vertebral artery injuries after cervical spine trauma. Louw and co-workers[32] studied 12 consecutive patients with facet joint dislocations, and documented vertebral artery occlusions in 9 of 12 patients (75%) using digital subtraction angiography. Willis and associates[33] similarly looked at 26 patients with facet dislocations and angiographically identified vertebral artery injuries in 12 patients (46%).

The vertebral artery can be damaged with road traffic accidents. The mechanism of arterial injury is often not entirely clear and may be multifactorial, although in some cases there appears to be a close association with the head and neck motions produced during the accident. Such motions, particularly when they are sudden, may injure the artery as a result of mechanical stretching.

Postmortem studies[34] have shown that vertebral artery lesions are found in about one-third of fatally injured road traffic accident victims with vertebral atlas injury. In other reports, neurologic deficits or death have followed posterior neck injuries up to 8 days after the accident.[35,36] One report described a case of lethal basilar thrombotic embolus occurring as late as 2 months after a serious whiplash injury.[37] In the time interval between the accident and death, the victim complained of episodic visual disturbances. The authors of this report suggest that anticoagulant therapy be considered, particularly in patients who, after whiplash trauma, develop signs of transient ischemic attacks resulting from posterior cerebral circulation disturbances.[37]

Other Activities Associated with Dissection of the Vertebral Artery Sherman and colleagues[38] described two cases of vertebrobasilar infarction after turning the head while driving an automobile. In both cases, the patients reported a headache and temporary visual loss.

A myriad of sports activities have been implicated in the etiology of vertebrobasilar artery infarction. Nagler[39] described an infarction occurring in an 18-year-old high school student doing a handstand on a set of parallel bars, when the head was thrown back into extension to maintain balance. The patient lost strength in his upper and lower extremities, but denied losing consciousness. Eighteen months after the onset of quadriplegia, the patient was still wheelchair-bound. In the same series of case studies, a 55-year-old man who became concerned about his health and posture decided to begin an exercise regimen. As he performed a series of lumbar extension exercises over the edge of a table, he hyperextended his neck and experienced sudden dizziness with bilateral C-4 and C-5 sensory and motor weakness. Radiographs showed osteoarthritic changes at the C1-2 level, and a myelogram demonstrated an abnormally small foramen magnum.

Even Yoga has been documented as the immediate cause of vertebral artery infarction in two separate cases.[39,40]

Diving has been reported to produce a vertebrobasilar thrombosis following cervical trauma.[41] Although the 42-year-old man was conscious, oriented, and alert when he arrived at the emergency department, he began to complain of paresthesias all over his body 3 hours after admission, and he abruptly became unresponsive, with disconjugate gaze and pinpoint pupils. The patient died 1 week after the initial injury.

Softball, a relatively benign sport, was reported by Goldstein[42] as a cause of vertebral artery dissection in a 31-year-old woman. The patient had a sudden onset of headache, speech slurring, dizziness, and left-sided weakness while playing softball. The patient was found to have irregular narrowing of the left vertebral artery and a smaller than normal right artery.

Chiropractic manipulations have been linked to vertebrobasilar complications.[43] One report estimated that as many as 1 in 20,000 spinal manipulations causes a stroke,[44] whereas Dvorak and Orelli[45] estimated an incidence of 1 in 400,000. Various assumptions obviously had to be made regarding the total number of treatments being performed, so these estimates are speculative. The prevalence of strokes with cervical manipulations is related to the initial symptoms of vertebral artery dissection mimicking those of a musculoskeletal cervical dysfunction. Although cervical manipulations are used with the intention of relieving pain and improving range of motion, and are generally perceived as being safe, they are obviously fraught with danger. Summarizing reported cases of injury following cervical spine manipulation published between 1925 and 1997, di Fabio[46] found 177 cases

of severe injury, mainly arterial dissection or brainstem lesions, of which 18% were fatal.

Whether as a result of manipulative intervention, sudden movement, or spontaneity, the portion of the artery most frequently damaged is the suboccipital part between C1 and C2. Among the possible reasons for this preference is the large range of motion available at the atlanto-axial joint, and the relatively large degree of rotation at the atlanto-occipital joint.[47] If the main restraint to atlanto-axial rotation, the alar ligament, is ruptured, the degree of this movement has been shown to increase by 30%.[48]

A recent history of a respiratory tract infection appears to be a risk factor for spontaneous dissections of the vertebral artery,[49] although an infection with Chlamydia pneumoniae or the associated mechanical factors such as coughing do not appear to be the cause.[49]

Even in the absence of underlying disease or trauma, functional ranges of motion, especially the extremes of rotation and extension, have been shown to compromise the flow of the vertebral artery to almost nonexistence. In a cross-sectional study, 64 symptomatic individuals with well-documented brain stem ischemic events (average age, 70.9 years) and 37 control subjects (average age, 66.3 years) were evaluated using a dynamic MRA technique designed to mimic activities of daily living. Occlusion was noted in all subjects with contralateral neck rotation.[50] The same study demonstrated that the degree of rotation required to compromise the artery could be very small if underlying osteophytosis was present, already preoccluding the artery, and this was compounded if the artery had lost some of its inherent elasticity.

The correlative finding of increased blood flow through the carotid artery during vertebral artery occlusion was made by Stern,[51] who demonstrated that the flow rate in the contralateral carotid artery increased by one-and-half to two times with experimental occlusion of the vertebral artery.[16] These alterations in flow rates, following an occlusion of the parallel artery, serve as an apparent safety mechanism and may explain why more patients are not injured during cervical manipulation.[16]

This view is clinically supported by Nagler,[52] who stated that the risk of vertebrobasilar insufficiency symptomatology from hyperextension movements was increased in the presence of pathologic changes in the artery or the spine.[16]

The Association of Dizziness with Vertebral Artery Compromise   The pathogenesis of dizziness must be considered in the context of the vascular anatomy and physiology of the vestibular system. At the level of the brain stem, the vestibular nuclei are supplied by penetrating and short circumferential arterial branches of the basilar artery.

In turn, the internal auditory artery, arising either directly from the basilar artery or from the anterior inferior cerebellar artery (AICA), supplies the vestibulocochlear nerve, the cochlea, and the labyrinth.[53–55]

Because the labyrinthine branches are small and receive less collateral flow, it is possible that the labyrinth becomes a more prominent target of the effects of atherosclerosis of the vertebrobasilar system.[53,56] In contrast, the cochlea receives collateral flow from branches of the internal carotid artery that supply the adjacent portions of the petrous bone and, thus, may have more protection against vascular insufficiency.[53,56]

Traditionally, the examination of patients with vertigo has been centered on the differentiation between central and peripheral vestibular dysfunction, with vertebrobasilar insufficiency included among the potential causes for centrally mediated vertigo. This approach, however, is clearly inadequate because ischemia may affect both the central and the peripheral portions of the vestibular system. Support for this hypothesis comes from a report by Oas and Baloh[57] of two patients with isolated vertigo lasting several months who later developed extensive infarcts in the territory of the AICA. It was only when widespread infarction occurred that hearing loss and tinnitus were noted by the patients.

The testing for dizziness has been a part of patient screening by manual therapists for many years, being first described by Maitland in 1968.[58] However, other signs and symptoms have now been linked, directly or indirectly, to vertebral artery insufficiency; these include:

- Wallenberg's, Horner's, and similar syndromes
- Bilateral or quadrilateral paresthesia
- Hemiparesthesia
- Ataxia
- Scotoma
- Nystagmus
- Drop attacks
- Periodic loss of consciousness
- Lip anaesthesia
- Hemifacial para/anaesthesia
- Hyperreflexia
- Positive Babinski, Hoffman, or Oppenheimer reflexes
- Clonus
- Dysphasia
- Dysarthria
- Absent auditory reflexes
- Neural hypoacousia diplopia

These signs and symptoms are discussed in relevant chapters of this book.

It should be apparent from the preceding discussion that the vertebral artery is a structure that requires testing if the clinician plans to evaluate or treat the neck.

VERTEBRAL ARTERY EXAMINATION

Prior to any grade 1 to 5 passive mobilization of the cervical spine, maintaining the immediate premobilization position for 30 seconds tests vertebral artery patency. A positive test is one in which any signs or symptoms, especially those mentioned earlier, occur. Following a positive test, the patient must be handled very carefully, and further treatment, particularly manipulation of the cervical spine, should not be delivered. The patient should not, under any circumstance, be allowed to leave the clinic until his or her physician has been contacted, or until the necessary arrangements have been made for safe transport to an appropriate facility. As always, the patient should be educated as to the condition and should be strongly advised to defer from any neck motions that induce either extension, lateral flexion, or rotation of the cervical spine.

Upper Part

The patient is positioned in supine lying, with the head supported over the edge of the table, and the clinician standing at the patient's head, facing the shoulders. With one hand the clinician supports the mid- and lower cervical spine while the other hand supports the occiput.

- Maintaining the lower and the mid-cervical spine in a neutral position, the clinician extends the craniovertebral region, holding this position for 30 seconds, and noting any symptoms or signs produced.
- The clinician adds a compression force through the cranium and holds this force for 30 seconds, noting any symptoms or signs produced.
- The clinician rotates the craniovertebral region to the left, holding this position for 30 seconds, and noting any symptoms or signs produced (Fig. 5–3).

This test is repeated with right rotation of the craniovertebral region.

Lower Part

The patient is positioned in supine lying, with the head resting on the table without a pillow, and the clinician standing at the patient's head, facing the shoulders. With one hand the clinician palpates the cervicothoracic junction while the other hand palpates the cranium and craniovertebral joints.

- The clinician fixes the cervicothoracic junction and craniovertebral region, and extends the mid- and lower cervical spine. This position is held for 30 seconds, and a note is made of any symptoms or signs produced.

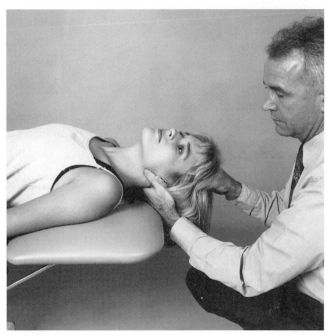

FIGURE 5–3 The vertebral artery test of the upper cervical spine. Note the lack of excessive cervical extension.

● From this maximally extended position, the clinician rotates the mid-cervical spine to the left (Fig. 5–4), and holds this position for 30 seconds, noting any symptoms or signs produced.

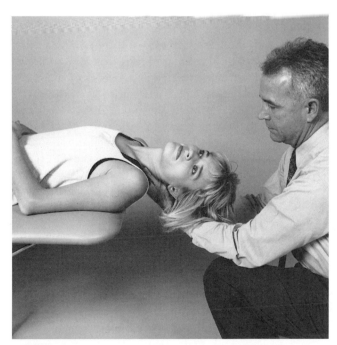

FIGURE 5–4 The vertebral artery test of the lower cervical spine. Note the opened eyes of the patient.

● From this position of extension and left rotation, the clinician applies a traction force through the mid-cervical spine. This position is held for 30 seconds, and a note is made of any symptoms or signs produced.

This test is repeated with the cervical spine extended, with right rotation and traction.

Case Study: The Dizzy Patient[59]

The following case study illustrates the common subjective and objective findings for a vertebrobasilar artery insufficiency.

Subjective

A 62-year-old woman with no history of vertigo or dizziness reported to the clinic for her scheduled therapy session for cervical degenerative joint disease. During the course of conversation, the patient reported experiencing dizziness after a shampoo treatment of her hair at a hairdressing salon. She had visited her hairdresser the previous day and reported severe vertigo, occipital pain, difficulty standing, and a periodic numbness of the right arm and leg. A recent radiograph and MRI of the cervical spine had shown cervical spondylosis and narrowing of C-4, and minor cervical compression at the same level.

Examination

A glove-and-stocking–type hypesthesia was present. Deep tendon reflexes and muscle power were normal. However, disturbances of equilibrium were noted, and nystagmus was present.[60] The patient was referred back to her physician for further testing.

Discussion

MRA showed a blood flow defect in the left vertebral artery at the atlanto-occipital junction. MRI of the brain revealed a few low-intensity areas, which were supplied by the vertebral artery, and testing showed right and left nystagmus.

A diagnosis of vertebrobasilar artery insufficiency with cerebellar infarction caused by neck hyperextension in the hair dressing salon was made. The patient was treated conservatively with rest and medication, and the vertigo improved 1 week after injury, at which time the patient could walk without assistance.

Beauty parlor stroke syndrome was first described by Weintraub[61] in 1992. Since then, various authors have reported similar cases.[62,63] Because this syndrome is not widely recognized, a careful history is necessary in the presence of symptoms such as those described. Such symptoms are often thought to be nonspecific and might be attributed to neurosis, psychogenic headache, or menopause, particularly when imaging studies do not show specific findings. Routine radiography, CT, and MRI studies usually do not help to identify lesions in this syndrome. Special care is therefore necessary to evaluate the clinical findings during examination of the nervous and auditory systems for back lifting or cerebellum dysfunction.

The most likely pathophysiologic mechanism of the beauty parlor stroke syndrome is stenosis of the vertebral artery caused by compression at the atlanto-occipital junction. This stenosis leads to damage of the intima, thrombus formation, stenosis of the artery by fibrosis, or embolism, followed by infarction of the brain stem or cerebellum. The vertebral arteries can also be compressed by the posterior edge of foramen magnum and the first cervical vertebra in cervical extension (approximately 20 degrees) and right rotation (approximately 20 degrees) in cases involving the left vertebral artery, and by left rotation in cases involving the right artery, respectively.[59]

On the other hand, Thiel and colleagues[64] found no occlusion in the vertebral artery blood flow during various head and neck positioning tests on the patient. Williams and Wilson[65] provided a detailed description of vertebrobasilar artery insufficiency almost 40 years ago and indicated that reversible symptoms were related to inefficiency of the basilar system.

Mas and associates[29] described 25 patients with previous transient ischemic attacks. Among these, 18 reported the appearance of symptoms after neck hyperextension. Usually, vertebrobasilar artery insufficiency occurs as a minor attack (temporary vertigo or dizziness), with no clinical or radiologic evidence of neural abnormalities.

Many cases are not caused by occlusion of the basilar artery, but rather by narrowing, structural anomaly, or arterial hypotension. Therefore, a correlation between symptoms and reduced blood flow has been postulated. In the majority of cases, however, symptoms stabilize within 8 months.[63]

Beauty parlor syndrome can be explained not only by this mechanism but also by whiplash injury, dental work, endotracheal intubation, certain radiograph positioning, perimetry, and chiropractic manipulation, which may also produce cervical vertigo.

REVIEW QUESTIONS

1. From which artery does the vertebral artery normally arise?
2. What are the four parts of the vertebral artery and from where do they originate?
3. What is the most common variation in the origin of the vertebral artery?
4. Give one adverse and one beneficial consequence of the second part of the artery beginning much more cranially.
5. List the structures that form the transverse tunnel.
6. Describe the course of the third part of the artery (suboccipital).
7. List the branches generated directly by the vertebral artery.
8. What structures are vascularized by the vertebral artery and its branches?
9. List the anomalies in each of the parts of the vertebral artery and its branches.
10. Which of the cranial nerves is (are) not vascularized by the vertebral artery?
11. Give two types of intrinsic occlusion.
12. Give four causes of extrinsic occlusion.
13. What is a pseudoanuerysm?
14. What is fibromuscular dysplasia with reference to the vertebrobasilar system?
15. How could cervical manipulation adversely affect the vertebrobasilar system?
16. List four anomalies of the vertebral artery that may predispose a patient to vertebrobasilar compromise.
17. What cervical movements have been found to occlude the vertebral artery?

ANSWERS

1. The usual site of origin is from the proximal part of the subclavian artery.
2. The four parts are (1) osteal—arises from the C6 foramen and travels to the transverse tunnel; (2) transverse—arises from the entry of the transverse tunnel and travels cranially through the tunnel to the C2 transverse foramen; (3) suboccipital—arises from the C2 transverse foramen and travels into the foramen magnum; and (4) intracranial—arises from the foramen magnum and travels to the lower border of the pons.
3. Four percent of the left arteries arise from the aorta. The left artery runs vertically and slightly medial and posterior to reach the transverse foramen of the lower cervical spine, although its exact direction is dependent on its exact point of origin (any anomalies result in tortuosity). The typical point of entry is at the C6 transverse foramen, but 10% of the population have entry points from C5 to C7. Also, the postsubclavian artery could have a kink in it.
4. *Adverse:* Abnormalities in entry point are most commonly associated with origin of the artery from the aorta. This causes increased blood pressure in the vertebral artery and may be a factor in vertebral bone erosion, tortuosity of the artery, and widening of the intervertebral foramen with nerve root compression. The artery loses bony protection, is more vulnerable, and is further away from the axis of movement. *Beneficial:* Increased slack occurs in the artery, preventing

compression of the vertebral artery between the transverse and suboccipital portions. The artery may thus avoid impingement from osteophytes; also it is less vulnerable to instability and disc prolapse.

5. The bony transverse foramina at each spinal level, the overlying anterior and posterior intertransverse muscles, the lateral border scaleni and longus anterior colli muscles, the lateral margins of the vertebral bodies, and the superior facets of the apophyseal joints. The transverse tunnel dimensions are proportional to the diameter of the artery. The average diameter is 6 mm, or about 1 to 2 mm greater than the vertebral artery. The vertebral artery is surrounded by a periosteal sheath that is adherent to the boundaries of the canal and affords further protection of the artery.

6. Divided into four parts: (1) Within the transverse foramen of C2, the C2 vertebral foramen has two curves. (2) Between C2 and C1. The second part runs vertically upwards in the transverse foramen of C2 and is covered by the levator scapulae and the inferior capitis muscles. (3) In the transverse foramen of C1. In the third part, the suboccipital portion of the vertebral artery bends backward and medially in the transverse foramen of C1. (4) Between the posterior arch of the atlas and its entry into the foramen magnum. The artery is vulnerable to direct blunt trauma in this portion.

7. *Extracranial branches:* (1) Spinal branch—one branch anastomoses with other spinal arteries to supply the dural sleeve of the nerve roots, the spinal cord, and the meninges of the cord (?) Muscular branch the other branch supplies the periosteum, bone and ligaments of the posterior aspect of the vertebral body.
Intracranial branches: (1) Meningeal branches—occipital meninges.

8. The dural sleeve of the nerve roots; spinal cord; meninges of the cord; atlas and axis bones; periosteum, bone, and ligaments of the posterior aspect of the vertebral bodies; deep suboccipital muscles; occipital meninges; anterior portion of the spinal cord; posterior spinal cord; medulla, cerebellum, pons, and midbrain, as follows: Medulla—CN IX, X, XI, and XII. Pons—CN VI, VII, and VIII. Midbrain—CN III, IV, and V. Thalamus/midbrain—CN II.

9. Variation in diameter of the two vertebral arteries; left artery is usually dominant (larger).

10. Olfactory (CN I).

11. Possible answers are atherosclerosis, embolus or thrombus, pseudoaneurysm, spasm.

12. Possible answers are osteophytosis, instability, subluxation, disc prolapse (C4-6), motion—traction, extension, rotations, or a combination of rotation-extension-traction.

13. There is damage of the tunica intima and tunica media of the arterial wall. The blood flow strips the intima and media away from the adventitia. The pressure causes the adventitia to balloon outward.

14. Stenosis of the vertebral artery associated with normal anatomic variation of the dominant left vertebral artery.

15. Because of the location of the vertebral artery in the transverse tunnel and the sharp directional changes that occur in the third portion of the artery (suboccipital), rotation, extension, and traction can occlude one or both arteries.

16. Hypoplastic artery, atretic artery, direct origin of vertebral artery from aorta, or an absent vertebral artery.

17. Rotation-extension-traction is most stressful, followed by rotation-extension, rotation alone, extension alone, and flexion.

REFERENCES

1. Wallenberg A. Acute bulbaraaffection. Arch Psychiat Nervenkr 1895;27:504–540.

2. Williams PL, Warwick R, eds. *Gray's Anatomy*, 38th ed. Edinburgh, Scotland: Churchill Livingstone; 1995; 91–341.

3. Williams PL, Warwick R, eds. *Gray's Anatomy*, 38th ed. Edinburgh, Scotland: Churchill Livingstone; 1995; 1530–1534.

4. George B, Laurian C. The vertebral artery: Pathology and surgery. New York, NY: Springer-Verlag Wien; 1987:6–22.

5. Thiel HW. Gross morphology and pathoanatomy of the vertebral arteries. J Manipulative Phys Ther 1991; 14:133–141.

6. Hadley LA. Tortuosity and deflection of the vertebral artery. AMR 1958;80:306–312.

7. Anderson RE, Sheally CN. Cervical pedicle erosion and rootlet compression caused by a tortuous vertebral artery. Radiol 1970;96:537–538.

8. Cooper DF. Bone erosion of the cervical vertebrae secondary to tortuosity of the vertebral artery. J Neurosurg 1980;53:106–108.

9. Aspinall W. Clinical testing for cervical mechanical disorders which produce ischemic vertigo. Orthop Sports Phys Ther 1989;11:176–182.

10. Fast A, Zincola DF, Marin EL. Vertebral artery damage complicating cervical manipulation. Spine 1987;12: 840.

11. Hardesty WH, Whitacre WB, Toole JF, et al. Studies on vertebral artery blood flow in man. Surg Gyn Obstet 1963;116:662.

12. Wilkinson IMS. The vertebral artery: Extra and intracranial structure. Arch Neurol 1972;27:393–396.

13. Franke JP, Dimarina V, Pannier M, et al. Les artéres vertébrales. Segments atlanto-axoidiens V3 et intracranien V4 collatérales. Anat Clin 1980;2:229.

14. Cavdar S, Arisan E. Variations in the extracranial origin of the human vertebral artery. Acta Anat 1989;135:236.

15. Newton TH, Potts DG. Radiology of the skull and brain. In: *Angiography*, vol. 2, book 2. St. Louis, Mo: Mosby; 1974.

16. Meadows J. *NAIOMT Course Notes Level II and III.* Denver, Colo:1995.

17. Castaigne P, Lhermitte F, Gautier JC, et al. Arterial occlusions in the vertebro-basilar system. A study of 44 patients with post-mortem data. Brain 1973;96:133–154.

18. Stanley JC, Fry WJ, Seeger JF, Hoffman GL, Gabrielsen TO. Extracranial internal carotid and vertebral artery fibrodysplasia. Arch Surg 1974;109:215–222.

19. Parent A, Harvey L, Touchstone D, Smith E. Lateral cervical spine dislocation and vertebral artery injury. Neurosurgery 1992;31:501–509.

20. Golueke P, Sclafani S, Phillips T. Vertebral artery injury—Diagnosis and management. J Trauma 1987;27:856–865.

21. Kubernick M, Carmody R. Vertebral artery transection from blunt trauma treated by embolization. J Trauma 1984;24:854–856.

22. Auer RN, Krcek J, Butt JC. Delayed symptoms and death after minor head trauma with occult vertebral artery injury. J Neurol Neurosurg Psych 1994;57:500–502.

23. Woolsey RM, Hyung CG. Fatal basilar artery occlusion following cervical spine injury. Paraplegia 1980;17:280–283.

24. Hayes P, Gerlock AJ, Cobb CA. Cervical spine trauma: A cause of vertebral artery injury. J Trauma 1980;20:904–905.

25. Schwarz N, Buchinger W, Gaudernak T, Russe F, Zechner W. Injuries of the cervical spine causing vertebral artery trauma: Case reports. J Trauma 1991;31:127–133.

26. Bose B, Northrup BE, Osterholm JL. Delayed vertebrobasilar insufficiency following cervical spine injury. Spine 1985;10:108–110.

27. Miyachi S, Okamura K, Watanabe N, Inoue N, Nagatani T, Takagi T. Cerebellar stroke due to vertebral artery occlusion after cervical spine trauma: Two case reports. Spine 1994;19:83–89.

28. Hart RG, Easton JD. Dissections. Stroke. 1985;16:925–927.

29. Mas JL, Bousser MG, Hasboun D, Laplane D. Extracranial vertebral artery dissections: a review of 13 cases. Stroke 1987;18:1037–1047.

30. Schievink WI, Mokri B, O'Fallon WM. Recurrent spontaneous cervical artery dissection. N Engl J Med 1994;330:393–397.

31. Biousse V, D'Anglejan J, Touboui P-J, Evrard S, Amarenco P, Bousser M-G. Headache in 67 patients with extracranial internal carotid artery dissection. Cephalalgia 1991;11(suppl 11):232–233.

32. Louw JA, Mafoyane NA, Small B, Nesser CP. Occlusion of the vertebral artery in cervical spine dislocations. J Bone Joint Surg [Br] 1990;72:679–681.

33. Willis B, Greiner F, Orrison W, Benzel E. The incidence of vertebral artery injury after midcervical spine fracture or subluxation. Neurosurgery 1994;34:435–442.

34. Vanezis P. Vertebral artery injuries in road traffic accidents: A post-mortem study. J Forensic Sci Soc 1986;26:281–291.

35. Schmitt HP, Gladisch R. Multiple Frakturen des Atlas mit zweizeitiger todlicher Vertebralisthrombose nach Schleudertrauma der Halswirbelsaule. Archiv Orthop Unfall-Chir 1977;87:235–244.

36. Schneider RC, Schemm GW. Vertebral artery insufficiency in acute and chronic spinal trauma. J Neurosurg 1961;18:348–360.

37. Viktrup L, Knudsen GM, Hansen SH. Delayed onset of fatal basilar thrombotic embolus after whiplash injury. Stroke 1995;26:2194–2196.

38. Sherman DG, Hart RG, Easton JD. Abrupt change in head position and cerebral infarction. Stroke 1981;12:2–6.

39. Nagler W. Vertebral artery obstruction by hyperextension of the neck: Report of three cases. Arch Phys Med Rehabil 1973;54:237–240.

40. Russell WR. Yoga and vertebral artery injuries. BMJ. 1972;1:685–690.

41. Prabhu V, Kizer J, Patil A, Hellbusch L, Taylon C, Leibrock L. Vertebrobasilar thrombosis associated with nonpenetrating cervical spine trauma. Trauma-Inj Infect Crit Care 1996;40:130–137.

42. Goldstein SJ. Dissecting hematoma of the cervical vertebral artery. Case report. J Neurosurg 1982;56:451–454.

43. Huffnagel A, Hammers A, Schonle P-W, Bohm K-D, Leonhardt G. Stroke following chiropractic manipulation of the cervical spine. J Neurol 1999;246:683–688.

44. Vickers A, Zollman C. The manipulative therapies: osteopathy and chiropractic BMJ 1999;319:1176–1179.

45. Dvorak J, von Orelli F. [The frequency of complications after manipulation of the cervical spine (case report and epidemiology) [author's transl]]. [German] Schweiz Rundschau Medizin Praxis 1982;71:64–69.

46. Di Fabio RP. Manipulation of the cervical spine: risks and benefits Phys Ther 1999;79:50–65.

47. Dvorak J, Hayek J, Zehnder R. CT-functional diagnostics of the rotatory instability of the upper cervical spine. Part 2. An evaluation on healthy adults and patients with suspected instability. Spine 1987;12:726–731.

48. Panjabi M, Dvorak J, Crisco J 3d, Oda T, Hilibrand A, Grob D. Flexion, extension, and lateral bending of the upper cervical spine in response to alar ligament transections. J Spinal Disord 1991;4:157–167.

49. Grau AJ, Brandt T, Buggle F, et al. Association of cervical artery dissection with recent infection. Arch Neurol 1999;56:851–856.

50. Weintraub MI, Khoury A. Critical neck position as an independent risk factor for posterior circulation stroke. A magnetic resonance angiographic analysis. J Neuroimag 1995;5:16–22.

51. Stern WE. Circulatory adequacy attendant upon carotid artery occlusion. Arch Neurol 1969;21:455–465.

52. Nagler W. Vertebral artery obstruction by hyperextension of the neck: Report of three cases. Arch Phys Med Rehabil 1973;54:237–240.

53. Grad A, Baloh RW. Vertigo of vascular origin. Clinical and electronystagmographic features in 18 patients. Arch Neurol 1989;46:281–284.

54. Fife TD, Baloh RW, Duckwiler GR. Isolated dizziness in vertebrobasilar insufficiency: Clinical features, angiography, and follow-up. J Stroke Cerebrovasc Dis 1994;4:4–12.

55. Oas JG, Baloh RW. Vertigo and the anterior inferior cerebellar artery syndrome. Neurology 1992;42: 2274–2279.

56. Mazzoni A. Internal auditory artery supply to the petrous bone. Ann Otol Rhinol Laryngol 1974;81: 13–21.

57. Oas JG, Baloh RW. Vertigo and the anterior inferior cerebellar artery syndrome. Neurology 1992;42:2274–2279.

58. Maitland GD. *Vertebral Manipulation*, 2nd ed. London, England: Butterworths; 1968.

59. Endo K, Ichimaru K, Shimura H, Imakiire A. Cervical vertigo after hair shampoo treatment at a hairdressing salon: A case report. Spine 2000;25:632.

60. Sakata E, Ohtsu K, Shimura H, Sakai S, Takahashi K. Transitory, counterolling and pure-rotatory positioning nystagmus caused by cerebellar vermis lesion. Pract Otol 1985;78:2729–2736 [in Japanese with English abstract].

61. Weintraub MI. Beauty parlor strokes syndrome: Report of five cases. JAMA 1993;269:2085–2086.

62. Nakagawa T, Yamane H, Shigeta T, Takashima T, Konishi K, Nakai Y. Evaluation of vertebro-basilar hemodynamics by magnetic resonance angiography. Equilibrium Res 1997;56:360–365.

63. Shimura H, Yuzawa K, Nozue M. Stroke after visit to the hairdresser. Lancet 1997;350:1778.

64. Thiel H, Wallace K, Donat J, Yong-Hing K. Effect of various head and neck position on vertebral blood flow. Clin Biomech 1994;9:105–110.

65. Williams D, Wilson T. The diagnosis of the major and minor syndromes of basilar insufficiency. Brain 1962; 85:741–744.

CHAPTER SIX

THE SPINAL NERVES

Chapter Objectives

At the completion of this chapter, the reader will be able to:

1. Describe the anatomy and distribution of the spinal and peripheral nerves.
2. Describe the components of the brachial and lumbosacral plexus.
3. Recognize the characteristics of a peripheral nerve lesion.
4. List the clinical syndromes associated with impairments to each of the peripheral nerves.

OVERVIEW

Knowledge of the spinal nerves and the peripheral nerves that they serve is essential to the manual clinician, as many apparent "peripheral" dysfunctions, such as tennis elbow, can be caused by a spinal dysfunction. In addition, the manual clinician must be able to discriminate between the sensory changes that follow a spinal nerve lesion, and those that are produced by a peripheral nerve lesion. A muscle weakness can result from disuse, inhibition, or nerve palsy. Weakness from a spinal nerve root lesion differs from that of a peripheral nerve lesion in its distribution. For example a compression of the C7 nerve root can result in a weakness of the elbow extensors and wrist flexors, whereas a radial nerve injury, although also resulting in a weakness of the elbow extensors, produces a weakness of the wrist extensors rather than the wrist flexors.

A total of 31 symmetrically arranged pairs of nerves exit from all levels of the vertebral column, except for those of C1 and C2,[1] each of which is derived from the spinal cord. They are divided topographically into 8 cervical pairs (C1-8), 12 thoracic (T1-12), 5 lumbar (L1-5), 5 sacral (S1-5), and 1 coccygeal (Fig. 6–1). The spinal nerve proper is not within the vertebral canal, and usually occupies the intervertebral foramen. However, the dorsal and ventral roots, which form the spinal nerves, are in the vertebral canal. Nerve roots must penetrate the dura mater before passing through dural sleeves within the intervertebral foramen, that are continuous with the epineurium of the nerves.

Spinal nerves contain several kinds of fibers, as follows:

- Motor fibers originate in large cells in the anterior gray column of the spinal cord. These form the ventral root and pass to the skeletal muscles.
- Sensory fibers originate in unipolar cells in the spinal ganglia and are interposed in the course of the dorsal roots. Peripheral branches of these ganglion cells are distributed to both visceral and somatic structures as mediators of sensory impulses to the central nervous system (CNS). The central branches convey these impulses through dorsal roots into the dorsal gray column and the ascending tracts of the spinal cord.
- Sympathetic fibers, which originate from the thoracic and lumbar cord segments, are distributed throughout the body to the viscera, blood vessels, glands, and smooth muscle.
- Parasympathetic fibers, located in the middle three sacral nerves, pass to the pelvic and lower abdominal viscera.

The spinal nerve roots are thought to have different mechanical properties than a peripheral nerve. There are no connective tissue components (at least they are not developed to the same degree) comparable to the epineurium and perineurium.[2] As a result, the spinal nerve roots are more sensitive to both tension and compression. These roots also are devoid of lymphatics and, thus, are predisposed to prolonged inflammation.

Sensory levels

Hearing, equilibrium
Taste
Pharynx, esophagus
Larynx, trachea
Occipital region (C1, 2)
Neck region (C2, 3, 4)
Shoulder (C4, 5)
Arm {
Axillary (C5, 6)
Radial (C6, 7, 8)
Median (C6, 7, 8)
Ulnar (C8, T1)

Thorax {
Spine of scapula (T3)

Epigastrium {
Inferior angle of scapula (T7)

Abdomen {
Umbilicus (T10)

Gluteal region (T12, L1)
Inguinal region (L1, 2)

Femoral region (L1, 2, 3) {
Anterior
Median
Lateral
Posterior

Crural region (L4, 5) {
Median
Lateral

Scrotum, penis, labia, perineum (S1, 2)
Bladder (S3, 4)
Rectum (S4, 5)
Anus (S5, Co1)

Spinous processes
Spinal nerves
First rib

Medulla oblongata
Cervical plexus
Brachial plexus
Intercostal and thoracic muscles
Abdominal muscles
Lumbar muscles
Lumbar plexus
Sacral plexus
Sacro-coccygeal plexus
Filum terminale

Motor levels

Facial muscles VII
Pharyngeal, palatine muscles X
Laryngeal muscles XI
Tongue muscles XII
Esophagus X
Sternocleidomastoid XI (C1, 2, 3)
Neck muscles (C1, 2, 3)
Trapezius (C3, 4)
Rhomboids (C4, 5)
Diaphragm (C3, 4, 5)
Supra-, infraspinatus (C4, 5, 6)
Arm {
Deltoid, brachioradialis, and biceps (C5, 6)
Serratus anterior (C5, 6, 7)
Pectoralis major (C5, 6, 7, 8)
Teres minor (C4, 5)
Pronators (C6, 7, 8; T1)
Triceps (C6, 7, 8)
Forearm {
Long extensors of carpi and digits (C6, 7, 8)
Latissimus dorsi, teres major (C5, 6, 7, 8)
Long flexors (C7, 8; T1)
Hand {
Thumb extensors (C7, 8)
Interossei, lumbricales, thenar, hypothenar (C8, T1)

Iliopsoas (L1, 2, 3)
Sartorius (L2, 3)
Quadriceps femoris (L2, 3, 4)
Gluteal muscles (L4, 5; S1)
Tensor fasciae latae (L4, 5)
Adductors of femur (L2, 3, 4)
Abductors of femur (L4, 5; S1)
Tibialis anterior (L5)
Gastrocnemius, soleus (L5; S1, 2)
Biceps, semitendinosus, semimembranosus (L4, 5; S1)
Obturator, piriformis, quadratus femoris (L4, 5; S1)
Flexors of the foot, extensors of toes (L5, S1)
Peronei (L5, S1)
Flexors of toes (L5; S1, 2)
Interossei (S1, 2)
Perineal muscles (S3, 4)
Vesicular muscles (S4, 5)
Rectal muscles (S4, 5; Co1)

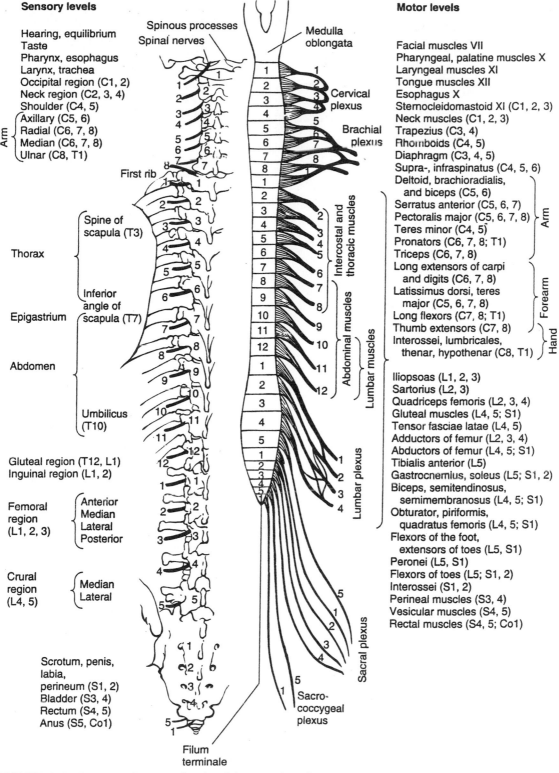

FIGURE 6–1 Motor and sensory levels of the spinal cord.

Meninges and Related Spaces

The meninges and related spaces are important to both the nutrition and protection of the spinal cord. The three meningeal layers (dura mater, arachnoid, pia mater) anchor the spinal cord and create spaces, one of which contains the cerebrospinal fluid, which provides a cushion for the spinal cord. The meninges also form barriers that resist the entrance of a variety of noxious organisms.

The dura mater (Latin, "tough mother") is the outermost and strongest of the layers, composed of tough fibrous connective tissue. It runs from the interior of the cranium through the foramen magnum, and surrounds the spinal cord throughout its distribution from the cranium to the coccyx at the second sacral level (S2).[3] It is also attached to the posterior surfaces of C2 and C3.[4]

The dura forms a vertical sac (dural sac) around the spinal cord, and its short lateral projections blend with the epineurium of the spinal nerves. The dura is separated from the bones and ligaments that form the walls of the vertebral canal by an epidural space. This space contains the internal venous (Baton's) plexus, embedded in epidural fat.[3] The internal venous plexus is a valveless system of veins that interconnects the body cavities and the cranial cavity, and can provide the means by which metastatic disease can spread from the viscera (i.e., from the lungs to the vertebral canal or cranial cavity).[3] This space also contains branches of the radicular arteries.

The pia mater is the deepest of the layers, and is intimately related to the outer surface of the spinal cord and nerve roots. It is firmly attached to the surfaces of both, and follows the contours intimately. It covers the nerve roots and blends with the connective tissue investments of the spinal nerve. The pia is the vascular layer and conveys the blood vessels that supply the spinal cord.[3] The inner pia mater and intermediate arachnoid are interconnected by variable numbers of trabeculae.

The pia mater has a series of lateral specializations, the denticulate (dentate) ligaments, which anchor the spinal cord to the dura mater.[3] These ligaments, which derive their name from their tooth-like appearance, extend the whole length of the spinal cord, serving an important tethering function.

A specialization of the pia mater, the filum terminale, anchors the spinal cord inferiorly from the tip of the conus medullaris. A cord of pia and dura, called the *coccygeal ligament*, attaches to the coccyx and anchors the spinal cord and dural sac inferiorly. This inferior anchor ensures that tensile forces applied to the spinal cord are distributed through its entire length.

The arachnoid is a thin and delicate nonvascular layer, coextensive with the dura mater and the pia mater. Even though the arachnoid and pia mater are interconnected by trabeculae, there is a space between them called the *subarachnoid space*, that contains the cerebrospinal fluid that is also found within the ventricles of the brain, and the central canal of the spinal cord. It is the supposed rhythmic flow of this cerebrospinal fluid which is used by craniosacral therapists to explain the rationale behind their techniques (refer to Chapter 12).

Because the arachnoid is held against the dura mater by the cerebrospinal fluid, an accumulation of material, including blood, inflammatory or infectious material, can create a subdural space.[3]

Definitions

- *Sclerotome:* An area of segmental innervation of bone.
- *Myotome:* The group of muscles supplied from a single spinal segment. Very few muscles fall into this category, as most are supplied from two or more segmental levels.
- *Dermatome:* The cutaneous area supplied by a single posterior root and its ganglion through the intermediation of one or more peripheral nerves. For every spinal segment, there is a corresponding dermatome (except C1). Refer to Chapter 10.
- *Doubly innervated muscles:* Some muscles are innervated by two peripheral nerves. Examples of such muscles include: Pectoralis major, subscapularis, adductor magnus, flexor digitorum profundus, biceps femoris.

CERVICAL NERVES

The eight pairs of cervical nerves are derived from cord segments between the level of the foramen magnum and the middle of the seventh cervical vertebra. The spinal nerves from C3 to C7, exiting from the intervertebral foramen, divide into a larger ventral ramus and a smaller dorsal ramus. The ventral ramus of the cervical spinal nerve courses on the transverse process in an anterior-lateral direction to form the cervical plexus and brachial plexus. The dorsal ramus of the spinal nerve runs posteriorly around the superior articular process, supplying the facet joint, ligaments, deep muscles, and skin of the posterior aspect of the neck.[3]

Each nerve joins with a gray communicating ramus from the sympathetic trunk. It also sends a small recurrent meningeal branch back into the spinal canal to supply the dura with sensory and vasomotor innervation, and branches into anterior and posterior primary divisions, which are mixed nerves that pass to their respective peripheral distributions. The motor branches carry a few sensory fibers that convey proprioceptive impulses from the neck muscles.

Daniels and colleagues[5] and Pech and associates[6] studied magnetic resonance imaging (MRI) and computed tomography (CT) of the cervical intervertebral foramens and found that the cervical nerve root is located in the lower part of the interpedicular foramen and occupies the major inferior part of the intertransverse foramen.

Posterior Primary Divisions

C1 (suboccipital nerve) is the only branch of the first posterior primary divisions; it is a motor nerve to the muscles of the suboccipital triangle, with very few sensory fibers.

Anterior Primary Divisions

The anterior primary divisions of the first four cervical nerves (C1-4) collectively form the cervical plexus (Fig. 6–2). Those of the second four nerves (C5-8), together with the first thoracic nerve, form the brachial plexus.

Cervical Plexus (C1-4)

Sensory Branches
- The small occipital nerve (C2, 3) supplies the skin of the lateral occipital portion of the scalp, the upper median part of the auricle, and the area over the mastoid process.
- The great auricular nerve (C2, 3) supplies sensation to the ear and face over the ascending ramus of the mandible. The nerve lies on or just below the deep layer of the investing fascia of the neck, arises from the anterior rami of the second and third cervical nerves, and emerges from behind the sternomastoid muscle, before ascending on it to cross over the parotid gland.
- The cervical cutaneous nerve (cutaneous coli) (C2, 3) supplies the skin over the anterior portion of the neck.
- Supraclavicular branches (C3, 4) supply the skin over the clavicle and the upper deltoid and pectoral regions, as low as the third rib.

Communicating Branches
The ansa cervicalis nerve (see Fig. 6–2) is formed by the junction of two main nerve roots derived entirely from ventral cervical rami. A loop is formed at the point of their anastomosis, and sensory fibers are carried to the dura of the posterior fossa of the skull via the recurrent meningeal branch of the hypoglossal nerve.

Muscular Branches
Communication with the hypoglossal nerve from C1-2 carries motor fibers to the geniohyoid and thyrohyoid muscles, and to the sternohyoid and sternothyroid muscles by way of the superior root of the ansa cervicalis (see Fig. 6–2). The nerve to the thyrohyoid branches from the hypoglossal nerve, and runs obliquely across the hyoid bone to innervate the thyrohyoid. The nerve to the superior belly of the omohyoid branches from the superior root (see Fig. 6–2), and enters the muscle at a level between the thyroid notch and a horizontal plane 2 cm inferior to the notch. The nerves to the sternohyoid and sternothyroid share a common trunk, which branches from the loop (Fig. 6–2). The nerve to the inferior belly of the omohyoid also branches from the loop (Fig. 6–2). The loop is most frequently located just deep to the site where the superior belly (or tendon) of the omohyoid muscle crosses the internal jugular vein. There is a branch to the sternocleidomastoid muscle from C2, and branches to the trapezius muscles (C3-4) via the subtrapezial plexus. Smaller branches to the adjacent vertebral musculature supply the rectus capitis lateralis and rectus capitis anterior (C1), the longus capitis (C2, 4) and longus coli (C1-4), the scalenus medius (C3, 4) and scalenus anterior (C4), and the levator scapulae (C3-5).

The phrenic nerve (C3-5) passes obliquely over the scalenus anterior muscle and between the subclavian artery and vein to enter the thorax behind the sternoclavicular joint, where it descends vertically through the superior and middle mediastinum to the diaphragm (see Fig. 6–2). Motor branches supply the diaphragm. Sensory branches supply the pericardium, the diaphragm, and part of the costal and mediastinal pleurae. The phrenic nerve is the largest branch of the cervical plexus and plays an important role in respiration.

Lesions of the First Four Cervical Nerves
Phrenic nerve involvement has been described in several neuropathies, including critical illness, polyneuropathy, Guillain-Barré syndrome, brachial neuritis, and hereditary motor and sensory neuropathy type 1.[7,8] The symptoms depend largely on the degree of involvement, and whether one, or both of the nerves are involved. Thus, the following can occur:

- Unilateral paralysis of the diaphragm, which causes few or no symptoms except with heavy exertion.
- Bilateral paralysis of the diaphragm, which is characterized by dyspnea on the slightest exertion; and difficulty in coughing and sneezing.
- Phrenic neuralgia, resulting from neck tumors, aortic aneurysm, and pericardial or other mediastinal infections, which is characterized by pain near the free border of the ribs, beneath the clavicle, and deep in the neck.

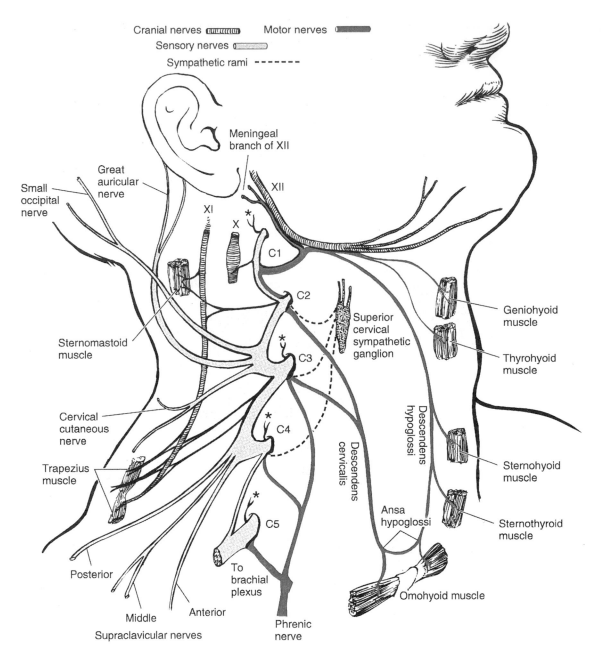

FIGURE 6–2 The cervical plexus.

Rigidity of the neck can occur with neuralgia, and with other irritative lesions of the meninges, such as meningitis.[9]

As early as the fifth century BC the seriousness of infectious meningitis was recognized.[10] In the 20th century, the annual incidence of bacterial meningitis ranged from approximately 3 per 100,000 population in the United States,[11] to 500 per 100,000 in the "meningitis belt" of Africa.[12]

The brain is protected from infection by the skull, the pia, arachnoid, and dural meninges covering its surface, and the blood–brain barrier. When any of these defenses are broached by a pathogen, infection of the meninges and subarachnoid space can occur, resulting in meningitis.[13] Predisposing factors for the development of community-acquired meningitis include preexisting diabetes mellitus, otitis media, pneumonia, sinusitis, and alcohol abuse.[14]

The clinical features of meningitis are a reflection of the underlying pathophysiologic processes.[9] Systemic infection generates nonspecific findings such as fever, myalgia, and rash. Once the blood–brain barrier is breached, an inflammatory response within the cerebrospinal fluid occurs. The resultant meningeal inflammation and irritation elicit a protective reflex to prevent stretching of the inflamed and hypersensitive nerve roots, which is detectable clinically as neck stiffness or Kernig or Brudzinski signs.[15,16] The meningeal inflammation may also cause headache and cranial nerve palsies.[17] If the inflammatory process progresses to cerebral vasculitis or causes cerebral edema and elevated intracranial pressure, alterations in mental status, headache, vomiting, seizures, and cranial nerve palsies may ensue.[13]

Despite classic descriptions of meningeal signs and sweeping statements about its clinical presentation, the signs and symptoms of meningitis have been inadequately studied.[9] Based on the limited studies, the following should be remembered during the assessment:[9]

● The absence of all 3 signs of the classic triad of fever, neck stiffness, and an altered mental status virtually eliminates a diagnosis of meningitis. Fever is the most sensitive of the classic triad of signs of meningitis, and occurs in a majority of patients, with neck stiffness the next most sensitive sign. Alterations in mental status also have a relatively high sensitivity, indicating that normal mental status helps to exclude meningitis in low-risk patients. Changes in mental status are more common in bacterial than viral meningitis.

● Among the signs of meningeal irritation, Kernig and Brudzinski signs appear to have low sensitivity but high specificity.

BRACHIAL PLEXUS

The brachial plexus arises from the anterior primary divisions of the fifth cervical through the first thoracic nerve roots, with occasional contributions from the fourth cervical and second thoracic roots (Fig. 6–3). The roots of the plexus, which consist of C5 and C6, join to form the upper trunk; C7 becomes the middle trunk; and C8 and T1 join to form the lower trunks. Each of the trunks divide into anterior and posterior divisions and then form cords. The anterior divisions of the upper and middle trunk form the lateral cord; the anterior division of the lower trunk forms the medial cord; and all three posterior divisions unite to form the posterior cord. The three cords (named for their relationship to the axillary artery) split to form the main branches of the plexus. These branches give rise to the peripheral

nerves: musculocutaneous (lateral cord), axillary and radial (posterior cord), ulnar (medial cord), and median (medial and lateral cords).[18] Numerous smaller nerves arise from the roots, trunks, and cords of the plexus, as follows:

A. From the Roots
1. A small branch passes to the phrenic nerve from C5.
2. The dorsal scapular nerve (C5). The origin of the dorsal scapular nerve frequently shares a common trunk with the long thoracic nerve (see Fig. 6–3), and passes through the scalenus medius anterior-internally and posterior-laterally with the presence of some tendinous tissues. Leaving the long thoracic nerve, it often gives branches to the shoulder and the subaxillary region before the branches join the long thoracic nerve again. The dorsal scapular nerve supplies the rhomboids and levator scapulae.
3. The long thoracic nerve (C5-7). The long thoracic nerve is purely a motor nerve that originates from the ventral rami of the fifth, sixth, and seventh cervical roots (see Fig. 6–3). It is the sole innervation to the serratus anterior muscle. The fifth and sixth cervical roots, along with the dorsal scapular nerve, pass through the scalenus medius muscle, whereas the seventh cervical root passes anterior to it.[19] The nerve then travels beneath the brachial plexus and clavicle to pass over the first rib. From there, it descends along the lateral aspect of the chest wall, where it innervates the serratus anterior muscle. The nerve extends as far inferior as the eighth or ninth rib. Its long, relatively superficial course makes it susceptible to injury. Pathomechanics postulated to cause injury to the long thoracic nerve include entrapment of the fifth and sixth cervical roots as they pass through the scalenus medius muscle, compression of the nerve during traction to the upper extremity by the undersurface of the scapula as the nerve crosses over the second rib, and compression and traction to the nerve by the inferior angle of the scapula during general anesthesia or passive abduction of the arm.[20–23]

The serratus anterior, along with the levator scapulae, trapezius, and rhomboids, is a scapular rotator. It takes its origin from the first through ninth ribs. The muscle is composed of three functional components.[24,25] The upper component originates from the first and second ribs and inserts on the superior angle of the scapula. The middle component arises from the second, third, and fourth ribs, and inserts along the anterior aspect of the medial scapular border. The lower component is the largest and most

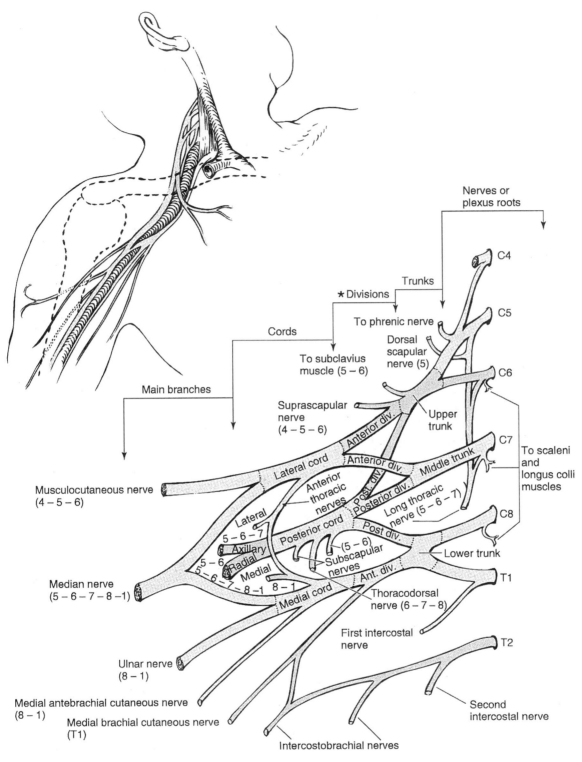

Nerves or plexus roots

Trunks

★ Divisions

To phrenic nerve

Cords

To subclavius muscle (5 – 6)

Dorsal scapular nerve (5)

Main branches

Suprascapular nerve (4 – 5 – 6)

Anterior div.

Upper trunk

C4

C5

C6

C7

To scaleni and longus colli muscles

Musculocutaneous nerve (4 – 5 – 6)

Lateral cord

Anterior div.

Middle trunk

Anterior thoracic nerves

Post. div.

Posterior div.

Long thoracic nerve (5 – 6 – 7)

Lateral 5 – 6 – 7

Axillary 5 – 6

Radial 5 – 6 – 7 – 8 –1

Posterior cord

Post. div.

(5 – 6)

Subscapular nerves

C8

Lower trunk

Median nerve (5 – 6 – 7 – 8 –1)

Medial 8 –1

Medial cord

Ant. div.

Thoracodorsal nerve (6 – 7 – 8)

T1

First intercostal nerve

Ulnar nerve (8 – 1)

Medial antebrachial cutaneous nerve (8 – 1)

Medial brachial cutaneous nerve (T1)

Intercostobrachial nerves

T2

Second intercostal nerve

★ Splitting of the plexus into anterior and posterior divisions is one of the most significant features in the redistribution of nerve fibers, because it is here that fibers supplying the flexor and extensor groups of muscles of the upper extremity are separated. Similar splitting is noted in the lumbar and sacral plexuses for the supply of muscles of the lower extremity.

FIGURE 6–3 The brachial plexus.

powerful, originating from the fifth through ninth ribs, and converging to insert on the inferior angle of the scapula.

The main function of the serratus anterior is to protract and upwardly rotate the scapula.[26,27] In synergy with the trapezius, the serratus anterior acts to provide a strong, mobile base of support to position the glenoid optimally for maximum efficiency of the upper extremity.[28,29] This action causes the entire shoulder to be brought forward, as in fencing. The serratus anterior is more active in forward flexion than pure abduction, as abduction requires some retraction of the scapula.[25] Without upward rotation and protraction of the scapula by the serratus anterior, full glenohumeral elevation is not possible. In patients with complete paralysis of the serratus anterior, Gregg and colleagues[28] reported that abduction is limited to 110 degrees.

An injury to the long thoracic nerve causes scapular winging, as the scapula assumes a position of medial translation and upward rotation of the inferior angle.[30] The medial border of the scapula becomes prominent as the dysfunctional serratus anterior no longer is able to hold the scapula against the thoracic cage. The greater the degree of muscle impairment, the greater the displacement or winging.[31] The deformity is accentuated as the patient elevates the arm into forward flexion against resistance. Resisted shoulder protraction also accentuates the winging.

4. Smaller branches extend to the scaleni and longus coli muscles from C6 to C8.
5. The first intercostal nerve extends from T1.

B. From the Trunks

1. A nerve extends to the subclavius muscle (C5-6) from the upper trunk or fifth root. The subclavius muscle acts mainly on the stability of the sternoclavicular joint, with more or less intensity according to the degree of the clavicular interaction with the movements of the peripheral parts of the superior limb, and seems to act as a substitute for the ligaments of the sternoclavicular joint.[32]
2. The suprascapular nerve originates from the upper trunk of the brachial plexus formed by the roots of C5 and C6 (see Fig. 6–3) at Erb's point. The nerve travels downward and laterally, behind the brachial plexus and parallel to the omohyoid muscle beneath the trapezius, to the superior edge of the scapula, through the suprascapular notch. The roof of the suprascapular notch is formed by the transverse scapular ligament. The notch may assume various shapes such as the letter "U" or may be deep and narrow or shallow and

wide. Rengachary and associates[33] describes six types of notches, depending on their configuration and enclosure. The suprascapular artery and vein initially run with the nerve and then run above the transverse suprascapular ligament over the notch. After passing through the notch, the nerve supplies the suprascapular muscle and provides articular branches to the glenohumeral and acromioclavicular joints, providing sensory and sympathetic fibers to two-thirds of the shoulder capsule, and to the glenohumeral and acromioclavicular joints. The nerve then turns around the lateral edge of the scapular spine to innervate the infraspinatus. There are no skin sensory branches.

C. From the Cords

1. The medial and lateral pectoral nerves extend from the medial and lateral cords, respectively (see Fig. 6–3), and are usually united by a loop. They supply the pectoralis major and pectoralis minor muscles. The pectoralis major muscle has dual innervation.[34] The lateral pectoral nerve (C5-7) is actually more medial in the muscle; it travels with the thoracoacromial vessels and innervates the clavicular and sternal heads. The medial pectoral nerve (C8 to T1) shares a course with the lateral thoracic vessels and provides innervation to the sternal and costal heads.[35] The main trunk of these nerves can be found near the origin of the muscle's vascular supply.
2. The three subscapular nerves from the posterior cord consist of:
   a. The upper subscapular nerve (C5-6) to the subscapularis muscle (see Fig. 6–3).
   b. The thoracodorsal nerve, or middle subscapular nerve, which arises from the posterior cord of the brachial plexus with its motor fiber contributions from C6, C7, and C8 (see Fig. 6–3). It courses along the posterior-lateral chest wall, along the surface of the serratus anterior, and deep to the subscapularis, giving rise to branches that supply the latissimus dorsi. The latissimus dorsi originates from the lumbar aponeurosis at the spines of the T6-12 and L1-5 vertebrae, the supraspinous ligament, the iliac crest, and the lower four ribs, and inserts on the inferior aspect of the intertubular groove of the humerus. It acts as an extensor, adductor, and powerful internal rotator of the shoulder, and also assists in scapular depression, retraction, and downward rotation.[36]
   c. The lower subscapular nerve (C5-6) to the teres major and part of the subscapularis muscle (see Fig. 6–3)

3. Sensory branches of the medial cord (C8 to T1) comprise the medial antebrachial cutaneous nerve to the medial surface of the forearm and the medial brachial cutaneous nerve to the medial surface of the arm (see Fig. 6–3). Several anatomic studies on the medial antebrachial cutaneous nerve trunk have been performed, showing variable derivation of the medial antebrachial cutaneous sensory fibers. In 1918, Kerr[37] reported that the medial antebrachial cutaneous nerve trunk branched from the medial cord in 82% of patients. It received contributions from the C8 and T1 segments in 97% of individuals, and from T1 alone in only 4 of 167 individuals. Wichman,[38] in the same year, reported 51 patients in whom the medial antebrachial cutaneous nerve trunk was derived from C8 and T1 fibers, and 38 patients in whom it was derived from T1 fibers alone.

Brachial Plexus Lesions

The rate of occurrence of brachial plexus injuries in the North American population is presently unknown. By using the Mayo Clinic records, an overall annual incidence rate of 1.64 cases per 100,000 population for idiopathic brachial plexus neuropathy was identified.[39] Unfortunately, this type of data collection has not been performed for patients with traumatic brachial plexus injuries. The pathomorphologic spectrum of traumatic brachial plexus impairments most often includes combinations of various types of injuries: compression of spinal nerves, traction injuries of spinal roots and nerves, and avulsions of spinal roots. If the rootlets are traumatically disconnected from the spinal cord, they normally exit the intradural space; in rare cases, however, they also may remain within the dural space.

Brachial plexus injuries are most commonly seen in children, and are usually caused by birth injuries. Obstetric brachial plexus palsy is quite different from adult brachial plexus injury, and needs a different analysis. Although the mechanisms resulting in plexus injury in both are similar (i.e., traction), in obstetric brachial plexus palsy the traction force is less in energy velocity. Stretch (neurapraxia or axonotmesis) and incomplete rupture are more common in obstetric brachial plexus palsy than complete rupture or avulsion, which is often seen in adult brachial plexus injury. Often, there is paresis (incomplete paralysis) rather than flaccid paralysis (complete paralysis) in obstetric brachial plexus palsy. Even when there is complete rupture, the gaps are short and regeneration is still possible, whereas in adult brachial plexus injury the gaps are long and the scars are dense, which makes regeneration impossible.

Obstetrical brachial plexus palsy is classified into upper (involving C5, C6, and usually C7 roots), lower (predominantly C8 and T1), and total (C5, C6, C7, C8, and sometimes T1) plexus palsies.[40,41] Upper brachial plexus palsy, although described first by Duchenne,[42] bears the name Erb's palsy.[43] Lower brachial plexus palsy is extremely rare in birth injuries[44] and is referred to as Klumpke's palsy.[45] Most cases of obstetric brachial plexus palsy are of Erb's palsy, and the lesion is always supraclavicular.

The infant with Erb's palsy typically shows the classic "waiter's tip" posture of the paralyzed limb.[46,47] The arm lies internally rotated at the side of the chest, the elbow extended (paralysis of C5, C6) or slightly flexed (paralysis of C5, C6, C7), the forearm pronated, and the wrist and fingers flexed. This posture occurs because of paralysis and atrophy of the deltoid, biceps, brachialis, and brachioradialis muscles, and hence the surgical results in patients with Erb's palsy traditionally have been expressed in terms of recovery of shoulder abduction and external rotation, elbow flexion and extension, forearm supination, and extension of the wrist, fingers, and thumb.[48]

Klumpke's paralysis is characterized by paralysis and atrophy of the small hand muscles and flexors of the wrist ("claw hand"). Prognosis of this type is more favorable. If the sympathetic rami of T1 are involved, Horner's syndrome may be present.

Peripheral Nerves

The large peripheral nerves are enclosed in three layers of tissue of differing character. From the inside outward, these are the endoneurium, perineurium, and epineurium.[49] Nerve fibers embedded in endoneurium form a funiculus surrounded by perineurium, a thin but strong sheath of connective tissue. The nerve bundles are embedded in a loose areolar connective tissue framework called the *epineurium*. The epineurium that extends between the fascicles is termed the *inner* or *interfascicular epineurium*, whereas that surrounding the entire nerve trunk is called the *epifascicular epineurium*.[50] The connective tissue outside the epineurium is referred to as the *adventitia of the nerve* or *epineural tissue*.[50] Although the epineurium is continuous with the surrounding connective tissue, its attachment is loose, so that nerve trunks are relatively mobile except where tethered by entering vessels or exiting nerve branches.[51]

There are basically three types of peripheral nerves that are affected by a neuropathy: sensory, motor, and mixed.

Sensory Nerves

Sensory nerves carry afferents from a portion of the skin. They also carry efferents to the skin structures. When a sensory nerve is involved, the pain occurs in the area of its distribution. This pain can be sharp, burning, or accompanied with paresthesia. Commonly affected sensory nerves are the lateral femoral cutaneous nerve, the saphenous nerve, and the interdigital nerves.

Motor Nerves

The motor nerves carry efferents to muscles, and return sensation from muscles, joints, and associated ligamentous structures. Pain produced as the result of a motor nerve involvement is not well localized, because it encompasses a wider region. This pain may be sharp and severe, or a dull ache. The muscle is usually tender to palpation, and there may be atrophy. Examples include the ulnar nerve, the suprascapular nerve, and the dorsal scapular nerve.

Mixed Nerves

A mixed nerve is a combination of skin, sensory, and motor fibers to one trunk. Involvement of a mixed nerve presents with a combination of sensory and motor findings. Some examples of mixed nerves are the median nerve, the ulnar nerve at the elbow or as it enters the tunnel of Guyon, the peroneal nerve at the knee, and the ilioinguinal nerve.

Any nerve that innervates a muscle also mediates the sensation from the joint on which that muscle acts. In nerve entrapments the primary concern is axonocachexia, which is a narrowing of the axon at the site of compression and distal to it, with a subsequent reduction in the conduction speed across the site of compression as well as along the entire distal portion of the nerve. Conduction velocity for motor and sensory nerve fibers is generally decreased significantly, and the latency is prolonged. The usual causes of nerve entrapment are swelling and compression during muscle contraction, tight fascia, osteochondroma, ganglia, lipomas and other benign neoplasms, and bony protuberances.

The diagnosis of peripheral nerve impairments depends on a careful history and physical examination.

Musculocutaneous Nerve (C5-6)

The musculocutaneous nerve is the terminal branch of the lateral cord, which in turn is derived from the anterior division of the upper and middle trunks of the fifth through seventh cervical nerve roots.[52,53] It arises from the lateral cord of the brachial plexus at the level of the insertion of the pectoralis minor.[53,54] The nerve proceeds caudally and laterally, giving one or more branches to the coracobrachialis, before penetrating this muscle 3 to 8 cm below the coracoid process.[53,55] It then courses through and supplies the biceps brachii and brachialis muscles, before emerging between the biceps brachii and the brachioradialis muscles 2 to 5 cm above the elbow (Fig. 6–4). At this level, it is called the

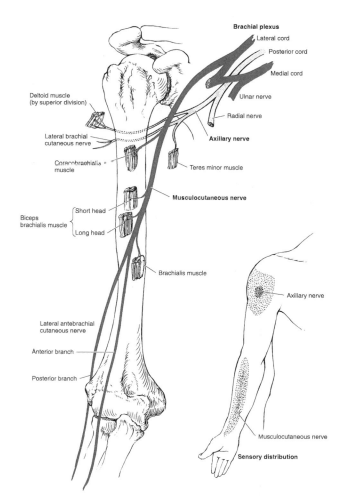

FIGURE 6–4 Musculocutaneous (C5, 6) and axillary (C5, 6) nerves.

lateral antebrachial cutaneous nerve, which then divides into anterior and posterior divisions to innervate the anterior-lateral aspect of the forearm[53] (see Fig. 6–4).

Atraumatic, isolated musculocutaneous neuropathies are rare. Reported cases have been associated with positioning during general anesthesia[56] and peripheral nerve tumors.[57] Several cases have been attributed to strenuous upper extremity exercise without apparent underlying disease.[58–61] These activities included weight lifting,[58] football throwing,[61] rowing,[60] and carrying heavy textile rolls on the shoulder with the arm curled over the roll.[59] Mechanisms proposed for these exercise-related cases include entrapment within the coracobrachialis,[58–60] as well as traction between a proximal fixation point at the coracobrachialis and a distal fixation point at the deep fascia at the elbow.[53] Because the musculocutaneous nerve does not penetrate the coracobrachialis muscle in some anatomic variants,[53] coracobrachialis entrapment may not account for all of the exercise-related cases.

The brachialis is a pure elbow flexor, whereas the biceps brachii is an elbow flexor and supinator of the forearm.[53,62] With complete loss of motor function of these two muscles, functional elbow flexion strength can still be obtained with contraction of the brachioradialis and pronator teres.[63,64] The extensor carpi radialis longus, flexor carpi ulnaris, flexor carpi radialis, and palmaris longus may also assist with flexing the elbow.[65] The brachioradialis has a better mechanical advantage when the elbow is flexed to 90 degrees and is more active when the forearm is in the pronated or neutral position.[62,65] The pronator teres can produce full elbow flexion, but this is accompanied by forearm pronation.[64,66] Thus, with a complete musculocutaneous nerve palsy, full antigravity elbow flexion can still be obtained and is strongest with the elbow flexed at 90 degrees and the forearm pronated.

An isolated injury to the proximal musculocutaneous nerve should not result in weakness of all shoulder motions. The coracobrachialis and long and short heads of the biceps brachii all cross the shoulder joint. They are active with shoulder flexion and abduction,[62,65,67,68] and slightly active with shoulder adduction,[65,68] and internal rotation.[68] These muscles also help stabilize the shoulder joint,[53] and maintain the static position of the arm.[67] Therefore, it is probable that with complete paralysis of these muscles, slight weakness of all shoulder motions would occur.

Thus, the clinical features of musculocutaneous involvement include the weaknesses described previously, loss of biceps jerk, muscle atrophy, and loss of sensation to the anterior-lateral surface of the forearm.

Axillary Nerve (C5-6)

The axillary nerve is the last nerve of the posterior cord of the brachial plexus before the latter becomes the radial nerve (see Fig. 6–4). The axillary nerve arises as one of the terminal branches of the posterior cord of the brachial plexus, with its neural origin in the fifth and sixth cervical nerve roots. The axillary nerve crosses the anterior-inferior aspect of the subscapularis muscle, where it then crosses posteriorly through the quadrilateral space and divides into two major trunks. The posterior trunk gives a branch to the teres minor muscle and the posterior deltoid muscle, before terminating as the superior lateral brachial cutaneous nerve (see Fig. 6–4). The anterior trunk continues, giving branches to supply the middle and anterior deltoid muscle, while traveling on the deep subfascial surface and within the deltoid muscle. The axillary nerve is susceptible to injury at several sites, including the origin of the nerve from the posterior cord, the anterior-inferior aspect of the subscapularis muscle and shoulder capsule, the quadrilateral space, and within the subfascial surface of the deltoid muscle.

A deltoid paralysis causes an inability to protract or retract the arm, or raise it to the horizontal position. After some time, supplementary movements may partially take over these functions. Teres minor paralysis causes weakness of external rotation. Sensation is lost over the deltoid prominence.

Radial Nerve (C6-8, T1)

The radial nerve is the largest branch of the brachial plexus. Originating at the lower border of the pectoralis minor as the direct continuation of the posterior cord, it derives fibers of the last three cervical and first thoracic segments of the spinal cord. During its descent in the arm, it accompanies the profunda artery behind, and around, the humerus and in the musculospiral groove. It pierces the lateral intermuscular septum and reaches the lower anterior side of the forearm, where its terminal branches arise (Fig. 6–5). This nerve is frequently entrapped at its bifurcation in the region of the elbow, where the common radial nerve becomes the sensory branch and a deep or posterior interosseous

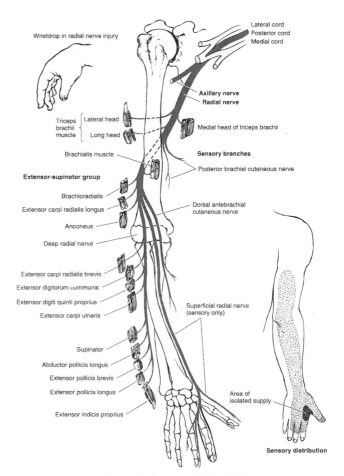

FIGURE 6–5 The radial nerve (C6-8; T1).

branch. The radial nerve crosses the elbow immediately anterior to the radial head, just beneath the heads of the extensor origin of the extensor carpi radialis brevis, then divides. The deep branch runs through the body of the supinator muscle to gain the posterior aspect of the forearm. In this relationship, it is therefore subject to the fibrous edge of the extensor carpi radialis brevis, and some fibers over the radial head. When it enters the fibrous slit in the supinator, or arcade of Frohse, the deep branch is often trapped.[69] A neuropathy of the superficial branch causes pain and alteration in the sensation of its distribution, and therefore it appears to be stemming from the first carpometacarpal joint or the tendons of the anatomical snuff box, or both, and is often confused with de Quervain's disease. When the deep branch is involved, it innervates the group of muscles that extend the wrist and the fingers, and weakness can occur. There is pain in the elbow region, and this is often confused with tennis elbow. A very significant test is to extend the third digit against resistance while the elbow is maintained in extension. This reproduces the elbow pain caused by entrapment of the posterior interosseous nerve.

The radial nerve in the arm supplies the triceps, anconeus, and the upper portion of the extensor-supinator group of forearm muscles. In the forearm, the muscles are supplied by the posterior interosseous nerve, which innervates all muscles of the six extensor compartments of the wrist, with the exception of the second compartment, namely the extensor carpi radialis brevis (ECRB) and extensor carpi radialis longus (ECRL).

The skin areas supplied by the radial nerve, include the posterior brachial cutaneous nerve, to the dorsal aspect of the arm; the posterior antebrachial cutaneous nerve, to the dorsal surface of the forearm; and the superficial radial nerve, to the dorsal aspect of the radial half of the hand. The isolated area of supply is a small patch of skin over the dorsum of the first interosseous space (see Fig. 6–5).

The radial nerve is the most commonly injured peripheral nerve. Because of the radial nerve's spiral course across the back of the mid-shaft of the humerus, and its relatively fixed position in the distal arm as it penetrates the lateral intermuscular septum, it is the most frequently injured nerve associated with fractures of the humerus. Radial nerve injuries usually involve a contusion or a mild stretch, and full recovery can generally be expected.

Conditions that may produce nontraumatic paralysis of the posterior interosseous nerve include compression by the fibrous edge of the entrance[70] or exit[71] of the supinator; benign tumors or tumorous conditions, including a lipoma[72,73] or a ganglion;[74] fibrous adhesions;[75] rheumatoid arthritis;[76,77] neuralgic amyotrophy;[78] constriction of the nerve;[79,80] delayed paralysis resulting from a Monteggia fracture[81] or unreduced anterior dislocation of

the radial head;[82] chronic minor repetitive motion at work;[83,84] and entrapment by the arcade of Frohse.[85]

The major disability associated with radial nerve injury is a weak wrist and fingers. The hand grip is weakened as a result of poor stabilization of the wrist and finger joints, and the patient demonstrates an inability to extend the thumb, proximal phalanges, wrist, and elbow. Pronation of the hand and adduction of the thumb is also affected, and the wrist and fingers adopt a position termed *wrist drop*. The triceps, radial, and periosteal-radial reflexes are absent, but the sensory loss is often slight, owing to overlapping innervation.

The site of the impairment can often be determined by the clinical findings.

- If the impairment occurs at a point below the triceps innervation, the strength of the triceps is intact.
- If the impairment occurs at a point below the brachioradialis branch, some supination will be retained.
- If the impairment occurs at a point in the forearm, the branches to the small muscle groups, extensors of the thumb, extensors of the index finger, extensors of the other fingers, and extensor carpi ulnaris, may be affected.
- If the impairment occurs at a point on the dorsum of the wrist, only sensory loss on the hand will be affected.

Median Nerve (C5 to T1)

The trunk derives its fibers from the lower three (sometimes four) cervical and the first thoracic segments of the spinal cord. Although it has no branches in the upper arm, the trunk descends along the course of the brachial artery and passes onto the volar side of the forearm, where it gives off muscular branches, including the anterior interosseous nerve. It then enters the hand, where it terminates with both muscular and cutaneous branches (Fig. 6–6). The sensory branches of the median nerve supply the skin of the palmar aspect of the thumb and the lateral 2½ fingers and the distal ends of the same fingers (see Fig. 6–6).

The anterior interosseous nerve arises from the posterior aspect of the median nerve, 5 cm distal to the medial humeral epicondyle, and passes with the main trunk of the median nerve between the two heads of the pronator teres.[86] It continues along the volar aspect of the flexor digitorum profundus and then passes between the flexor digitorum profundus and the flexor pollicis longus, running in close apposition to the interosseous membrane, to enter the pronator quadratus.[86] It provides motor innervation to flexor pollicis longus, the medial part of flexor digitorum profundus, involving the index and sometimes the middle finger, and to the pronator quadratus. It also sends sensory fibers to the distal radioulnar, radiocarpal, intercarpal, and

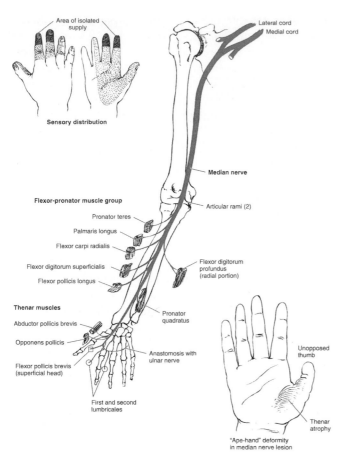

FIGURE 6–6   The median nerve (C6–8; T1).

carpometacarpal joints.[87] Variations in the distribution of the nerve have been noted; it may supply all or none of the flexor digitorum profundus and part of the flexor digitorum superficialis.[88,89]

The congenital abnormality of the distal portion of the humerus that may cause a nerve entrapment is the supratrochlear spur or supracondylar process of the distal anterior-medial surface of the humerus. When this process is present, a fibrous band usually runs from the tip of the spur to the medial epicondylar area. This is the ligament of Struthers, which encloses a foramen through which the nerve travels above the elbow in association with the brachial artery.[90] The important discriminating factor between this syndrome and the pronator syndrome is the fact that, in a pronator syndrome, the innervation of the pronator teres is spared.

Several factors appear to play a part in the production of a paralysis of the anterior interosseous nerve. The anterior interosseous nerve syndrome is a compressive neuropathy of the anterior interosseous nerve characterized by partial or total paralysis of the flexor pollicis longus, the flexor digitorum to the index finger, and the pronator quadratus, with no loss of sensation.[91] Located near the site of origin of the motor branch, which arises from the median nerve 5 to

8 cm distal to the level of the lateral epicondyle, it is vulnerable to injury or compression by the following means:

- A tendinous origin of the deep pronator teres
- A tendinous origin of the flexor superficialis to the long finger
- A thrombosis of crossing ulnar collateral vessels
- An accessory muscle and tendon from the flexor superficialis to the flexor pollicis longus (Zantzer's muscle)
- An aberrant radial artery
- A tendinous origin of a variant muscle, the palmaris profundus
- An enlarged bicipital bursa encroaching on the median nerve near the region of the origin of the anterior interosseous nerve

The patient with this syndrome usually presents with a history of pain in the proximal forearm that lasts for several hours, followed by paresis or total paralysis of the flexor pollicis longus, and the flexor profundus of the index and long finger. The pronator quadratus is also usually paralyzed. The hand that presents with an anterior interosseous paralysis has a typical appearance with a characteristic disturbance of pinch. Additional variations can occur with the anterior interosseous nerve syndrome. A Martin-Gruber anastomosis, a communication between the median and ulnar nerves, was found by Hirasawa[92] in 10.5% of forearms and by Thomson[93] in 15%. It has been reported[91] that half of these communications arise from the anterior interosseous nerve. It is possible that a palsy of the anterior interosseous nerve can lead to weakness or paralysis of the muscles of the hand normally supplied by the ulnar nerve.[91]

The anterior interosseous nerve can also be entrapped as it passes through the pronator teres muscle. The importance of this situation is that it is a mixed nerve, and the sensory involvement will include the radial side of the palm and the palmar aspect of the first, second, third, and half of the fourth digit. Motor loss is reflected in the patient's inability to pronate the wrist, partial loss of flexion of the fingers, and loss of opposition of the thumb.

The clinical features of a median nerve impairment, depending on the level of injury include:[94]

- Paralysis of the flexor-pronator muscles of the forearm, all of the superficial volar muscles except the flexor carpi ulnaris, and all of the deep volar muscles except the ulnar half of the flexor digitorum profundus, and the thenar muscles that lie superficial to the tendon of the flexor pollicis longus.
- In the forearm, pronation that is weak or lost and is supplemented by flexing the forearm and holding the elbow out.

- At the wrist, weak flexion and abduction; the hand inclining to the ulnar side.
- In the hand, an "ape-hand" deformity—an inability to oppose or flex the thumb or abduct it in its own plane; weakened grip, especially in thumb and index finger, with a tendency for these digits to become hyperextended, and the thumb adducted; inability to flex the distal phalanx of the thumb and index finger (never supplemented), tested by having the patient clasp the hands as in prayer or attempt to make a fist. Flexion of the middle finger is weakened.
- Loss of sensation to a variable degree over the cutaneous distribution of the median nerve, most constantly over the distal phalanges of the first two fingers. Pain is present in many median nerve impairments.
- Atrophy of the thenar eminence, which is seen early. Atrophy of the flexor-pronator groups of muscles in the forearm is seen after a few months.
- Skin of the palm that is frequently dry, cold, discolored, chapped, and at times keratotic.

Carpal Tunnel Syndrome

Carpal tunnel syndrome is an important cause of pain and functional impairment of the hand as a result of compression of the median nerve at the wrist. Affected patients report numbness, tingling, and pain in the hand, which often worsens at night, or after use of the hand. The pain may radiate proximally into the forearm and arm. A study of the syndrome in Rochester, Minnesota, that examined medical records, included symptoms compatible with the syndrome, and excluded other illnesses, calculated an incidence of 125 per 100,000 population for the period 1976 through 1980.[95] A survey of physicians in California estimated that 515 of every 100,000 patients sought medical attention for carpal tunnel syndrome in 1988; the syndrome in half of these patients was thought to be occupational in origin.[96] In the Netherlands, 8% of a random sample of 715 persons awoke with nocturnal paresthesias of the hand, and one-third of the subjects were subsequently shown to have carpal tunnel syndrome, for a prevalence of 220 per 100,000.[97]

Examination in the early stages often reveals no abnormality. With more severe nerve compression, the patient will have sensory loss over some or all of the digits innervated by the median nerve (thumb, index finger, middle finger, and ring finger) and weakness of thumb abduction.[98]

Clinical assessment includes Phalen's test (appearance or worsening of paresthesia with maximal passive wrist flexion for 1 minute), and Tinel's sign (paresthesia in the median territory elicited by gentle tapping over the carpal tunnel).[98] Tinel's sign has a sensitivity of 60% and a specificity of 67%; the corresponding values for Phalen's test are 75% and 47%.[99,100] There have been scattered attempts to improve the sensitivity of the sensory examination.[101] In a clinical setting, an assessment of strength, sensory loss, and pain is sufficient to monitor the progress of the syndrome.

Electrodiagnostic testing is particularly useful for differential diagnosis. Radiculopathy resulting from disease of the cervical spine, diffuse peripheral neuropathy, or proximal median neuropathy can pose clinical questions that electrodiagnostic testing can settle.[98]

The diagnosis of carpal tunnel syndrome is most reliably made by an experienced clinician[102] after a review of the patient's history and a physical examination. Cervical radiculopathy may be identified by the occurrence of proximal radiation of pain above the shoulder, paresthesias with coughing or sneezing, or a pattern of motor or sensory disturbances outside of the territory of the median nerve.[98] Ulnar neuropathy must be considered because no more than half the patients with carpal tunnel syndrome can reliably report the location of their paresthesias.[103] Thoracic outlet syndrome is occasionally a concern. Transient cerebral ischemia, not a rare occurrence, can be recognized by the absence of pain during an episode of numbness.

Overuse syndrome (cumulative trauma syndrome) is a common diagnostic problem in occupational settings. Since 1989, these disorders have accounted for more than 50% of all occupational illnesses in the United States.[104]

Ulnar Nerve (C8, T1)

The ulnar nerve is the largest branch of the medial cord of the brachial plexus. It arises from the medial cord of the brachial plexus and contains fibers from the C8 and T1 nerve roots, although C7 may contribute some fibers (Fig. 6–7). The ulnar nerve continues along the anterior compartment of the arm, and it passes through the medial intermuscular septum at the level of the coracobrachialis insertion. As the ulnar nerve passes to the posterior compartment of the arm, it courses through the arcade of Struthers, which is a potential site for its compression. This fascial structure arises to 8 to 10 cm proximal to the medial epicondyle and extends from the medial head of the triceps to the medial intermuscular septum.[105]

At the level of the elbow, the ulnar nerve passes posterior to the medial epicondyle, where it enters the cubital tunnel. This fibro-osseous canal is made up of the medial epicondyle anteriorly and the elbow joint and medial collateral ligament medially. The roof of the tunnel is formed by an aponeurosis, which extends from the medial epicondyle to the olecranon and arises from the origin of the two heads of the flexor carpi ulnaris.[106] This aponeurosis has been given various names, including the arcuate ligament, Osborne's band, the

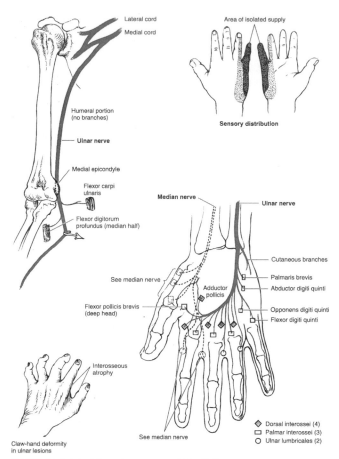

Lateral cord
Medial cord

Humeral portion
(no branches)

Ulnar nerve

Medial epicondyle

Flexor carpi
ulnaris

Flexor digitorum
profundus (median half)

Area of isolated supply

Sensory distribution

Median nerve

Ulnar nerve

See median nerve

Flexor pollicis brevis
(deep head)

Adductor
pollicis

Cutaneous branches

Palmaris brevis

Abductor digiti quinti

Opponens digiti quinti

Flexor digiti quinti

Interosseous
atrophy

See median nerve

◇ Dorsal interossei (4)
□ Palmar interossei (3)
○ Ulnar lumbricales (2)

Claw-hand deformity
in ulnar lesions

FIGURE 6–7 The ulnar nerve (C8, T1).

cubital tunnel retinaculum, and the triangular liga-ment.[105,107,108] The ulnar nerve passes between the two heads of the flexor carpi ulnaris origin and traverses the deep flexor-pronator aponeurosis. This aponeurosis is superficial to the flexor digitorum profundus and deep to the flexor carpi ulnaris and flexor digitorum superficialis muscles.[109,110]

Sunderland[111] described the intraneural topography of the ulnar nerve at various levels of the arm. At the me-dial epicondyle, the sensory fibers to the hand and the mo-tor fibers to the intrinsic muscles are superficial, whereas the motor fibers to flexor carpi ulnaris and flexor digito-rum profundus are deep. This may explain the common finding in cubital tunnel syndrome of sensory loss, weak-ness of the ulnarly innervated intrinsic muscles, but rela-tive sparing of flexor carpi ulnaris and flexor digitorum profundus strength.[106,111]

The ulnar nerve supplies the flexor carpi ulnaris, the ulnar head of the flexor digitorum profundus, and all of the small muscles deep and medial to the long flexor tendon of the thumb, except the first two lumbricales (Fig. 6–7, indi-cated by terminal branches in the hand). Its sensory distri-bution includes the skin of the little finger, and the medial half of the hand and the ring finger (see Fig. 6–7).

As indicated, there are a number of sites, along the nerve's course, at which the ulnar nerve can be compro-mised. It can be trapped in the cubital tunnel, or at the elbow, in the region of the humeral and ulnar edge of the flexor carpi ulnaris. The former entrapment would have sensory changes in the palmar aspect of the fourth and fifth digits, and not in the palm itself. The latter entrap-ment results in disturbed sensation in the fourth and fifth digits, with burning pain in the fingers associated with sen-sory findings in the palm and the fourth and fifth digits.

Normally the ulnar nerve at the elbow is exposed to compression, traction, and frictional forces.[107,112] One cause of ulnar nerve compression is a decrease in canal size. The volume of the cubital tunnel is greatest with the elbow held in extension. As the elbow is brought into full flexion, there is a 55% decrease in canal volume.[106] Several factors have been attributed to this decrease in volume. Vanderpool and colleagues[113] reported that, with each 45-degrees of flexion of the elbow, there was a concomi-tant 5-mm increase in the distance between the ulnar and humeral attachments of the arcuate ligament. At full elbow flexion, there was a 40% elongation of the ligament and a decrease in canal height of approximately 2.5 mm. Bulging of the medial collateral ligament also has been de-scribed as a factor.[113] O'Driscoll and associates[108] reported that the groove on the inferior aspect of the medial epi-condyle was not as deep as the groove posteriorly, and the floor of the canal seems to rise with elbow flexion. These changes lead to an alteration of the cross-sectional area of the cubital tunnel from a rounded surface to a triangular or elliptic surface with elbow flexion.[106]

The clinical features of an ulnar nerve impairment include:[94]

- Claw hand, resulting from unopposed action of the extensor digitorum communis in the fourth and fifth digits.
- An inability to extend the second and distal phalanges of any of the fingers.
- An inability to adduct or abduct the fingers, or to oppose all the fingertips, as in making a cone with the fingers and thumb.
- An inability to adduct the thumb.
- At the wrist, weak flexion and loss of ulnar abduction. The ulnar reflex is lost.
- Atrophy of the interosseous spaces (especially the first) and of the hypothenar eminence.
- Loss of sensation on the ulnar side of the hand, ring finger, and most markedly over the entire little finger.
- Partial lesions may produce only motor weakness or paralysis of a few of the muscles supplied by the ulnar nerve. Lesions low in the forearm or at the wrist spare the deep flexor and the flexor carpi ulnaris.

THORACIC NERVES

Dorsal Rami

The thoracic dorsal rami travel posteriorly, close to the vertebral zygapophysial joints, and divide into medial branches, which supply the short, medially placed back muscles and the skin of the back as far as the mid-scapular line, and into lateral branches, supplying smaller branches to the sacrospinalis muscles.

The medial branches of the upper six thoracic dorsal rami supply the semispinalis thoracis and multifidus, before piercing the rhomboids and trapezius and reaching the skin in close proximity to the vertebral spines, which they occasionally supply.

The lateral branches increase in size the more inferior they are. They penetrate, or pass, the longissimus thoracis to the space between it and the iliocostalis cervicis, supplying both these muscles as well as the levatores costarum. The 12th thoracic lateral branch sends a filament medially along the iliac crest, which then passes down to the anterior gluteal skin.

The recurrent meningeal or sinuvertebral nerve is functionally also a branch of the spinal nerve. This nerve passes back into the vertebral canal through the intervertebral foramen. This nerve supplies the anterior aspect of the dura mater, the outer third of the annular fibers of the intervertebral discs, the vertebral body, and the epidural blood vessel walls, as well as the posterior longitudinal ligament.[114]

Ventral Rami

There are 12 pairs of thoracic ventral rami, and all but the 12th are between the ribs serving as intercostal nerves. The 12th ventral ramus, the subcostal nerve, is located below the last rib. The intercostal nerve has a lateral branch, providing sensory distribution to the skin of the lateral aspect of the trunk, and an anterior branch, supplying the intercostal muscles, parietal pleura, and the skin over the anterior aspect of the thorax and abdomen. All of the intercostal nerves mainly supply the thoracic and abdominal walls, with the upper two nerves also supplying the upper limb. The thoracic ventral rami of T3 to T6 supply only the thoracic wall, whereas the lower five rami supply both the thoracic and abdominal walls. The subcostal nerve supplies both the abdominal wall and the gluteal skin.

Each of the ventral rami is connected with an adjacent sympathetic ganglion by grey and white rami communicantes. The communicating rami are branches of the spinal nerves that transmit sympathetic autonomic fibers to and from the sympathetic chain of ganglia. The fibers pass from spinal nerve to chain ganglia through the white ramus, and the reverse direction through the gray. In the cervical, lower lumbar, and sacral levels, only gray rami are present, and they function to convey fibers from the chain to the spinal nerves. This mechanism ensures that all spinal nerves contain sympathetic fibers.

From each intercostal nerve, a collateral and lateral cutaneous branch leave before the main nerve reaches the costal angle. The intercostobrachial nerve arises from the lateral collateral branch of the second intercostal nerve, piercing the intercostal muscles in the mid-axillary line, traversing the central portion of the axilla, where a posterior axillary branch gives sensation to the posterior axillary fold, and then passing into the upper arm along the posterior-medial border and supplying the skin of this region,[115,116] and connecting with the posterior cutaneous branch of the radial nerve.

The thoracic nerves may be involved in the same types of impairments that affect other peripheral nerves. However, a loss of function of one or even several thoracic nerves is not in itself of great importance, even though impairments of the lower thoracic nerves may produce partial or complete paralysis of the abdominal muscles, and a loss of the abdominal reflexes in the affected quadrants. In unilateral impairments, the umbilicus is usually drawn toward the unaffected side. Upward movement of the umbilicus when the patient tenses the abdomen (as in trying to sit up from a reclining position) is known as Beevor's sign and indicates paralysis of the lower abdominal muscles resulting from a lesion at the level of the 10th thoracic segment. Beevor's sign is a common finding in patients with facioscapulohumeral dystrophy (FSHD) even before functional weakness of abdominal wall muscles is apparent, but is absent in patients with other facioscapulohumeral disorders.[117]

The sensory distribution of the various thoracic cord levels include the anterior aspect of the chest (T1-6), nipple line (T4), upper abdomen (T7-9), umbilicus (T10), and lower abdomen (T11, T12, and L1).

LUMBAR PLEXUS

The lumbar plexus is formed from the ventral nerve roots of the second, third, and fourth lumbar nerves as they lie between the quadratus lumborum muscle and the psoas muscle (Fig. 6–8). In 50% of cases, it receives a contribution from the last thoracic nerve. It then extends anteriorly into the body of the psoas muscle to form the lateral femoral cutaneous, femoral, and obturator nerves.

L1, L2, and L4 divide into upper and lower branches (see Fig. 6–8). The upper branch of L1 forms the iliohypogastric and ilioinguinal nerves. The lower branch of L1 joins the upper branch of L2 to form the genitofemoral nerve (see Fig. 6–8). The lower branch of L4 joins L5 to form the lumbosacral trunk.

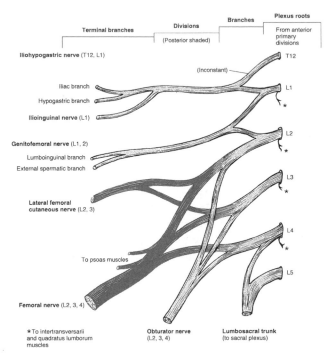

FIGURE 6–8   The lumbar plexus.

- The iliohypogastric nerve (T12, L1) (see Fig. 6–8) emerges from the upper lateral border of the psoas major and passes laterally around the iliac crest between the transversus abdominis and internal oblique muscles, dividing into lateral and anterior cutaneous branches. The iliac (lateral) branch supplies the skin of the upper lateral part of the thigh, whereas the hypogastric (anterior) branch descends anteriorly to supply the skin over the symphysis.
- The ilioinguinal nerve (L1) (see Fig. 6–8), smaller than the iliohypogastric nerve, emerges from the lateral border of the psoas major and follows a course slightly inferior to the iliohypogastric, with which it may anastomose. It pierces the internal oblique, which it supplies, before emerging from the superficial inguinal ring to supply the skin of the upper medial part of the thigh and the root of the penis and scrotum or mons pubis and labium majores. An entrapment of this nerve results in pain in the groin region, usually with radiation down to the proximal inner surface of the thigh, sometimes aggravated by increasing tension on the abdominal wall through standing erect.
- The genitofemoral nerve (L1, 2) (see Fig. 6–8) descends obliquely and anteriorly through the psoas major and emerges from the anterior surface of the psoas, dividing into genital and femoral branches. The genital branch supplies the cremasteric muscle and the skin of the scrotum or labia, and the femoral

branch supplies the skin of the middle upper part of the thigh and the femoral artery.

Collateral muscular branches supply the quadratus lumborum and intertransversarii from L1 and L4 and the psoas muscle from L2 and L3.

The lower branch of L2, all of L3, and the upper branch of L4 split into a smaller anterior and a larger posterior division (see Fig. 6–8). The three anterior divisions unite to form the obturator nerve. The three posterior divisions unite to form the femoral nerve, and the upper two give off smaller branches that form the lateral femoral cutaneous nerve (see Fig. 6–8).

Femoral Nerve (L2-4)

The femoral nerve, the largest branch of the lumbar plexus, arises from the lateral border of the psoas just above the inguinal ligament, and descends beneath this ligament to enter the femoral triangle on the lateral side of the femoral artery, where it divides into terminal branches. Above the inguinal ligament, it supplies the iliopsoas muscle. In the thigh it supplies the sartorius, pectineus, and quadriceps femoris muscles. Its sensory distribution includes the anterior and medial surfaces of the thigh via the anterior femoral cutaneous nerve, and the medial aspect of the knee, the proximal leg, and articular branches to the knee, via the saphenous nerve (Fig. 6–9). Entrapment of the saphenous nerve often results in marked pain at the medial aspect of the knee, which can be confused with an internal derangement of the knee or an anserine bursitis. Confirmation of a saphenous lesion can be made using resisted flexion of the knee, or resisted adduction of the thigh, which should increase the pain or pressure over the saphenous opening in the subsartorial fascia, producing a radiation of the pain.

Although femoral nerve palsy has been reported after acetabular fracture, cardiac catheterization, total hip arthroplasty, or anterior lumbar spinal fusion, and spontaneously in hemophilia,[118–122] an entrapment of the femoral nerve by an iliopsoas hematoma is the most likely cause of the femoral nerve palsy.[118,123] Direct blows to the abdomen or a hyperextension moment at the hip that tears the iliacus muscle may produce iliacus hematomas and subsequent femoral nerve palsy.[124]

Obturator Nerve (L2-4)

The obturator nerve arises from the second, third, and fourth lumbar anterior divisions of the lumbar plexus, emerging from the medial border of the psoas near the brim of the pelvis. Then it passes behind the common iliac vessels, on the lateral side of the hypogastric vessels and

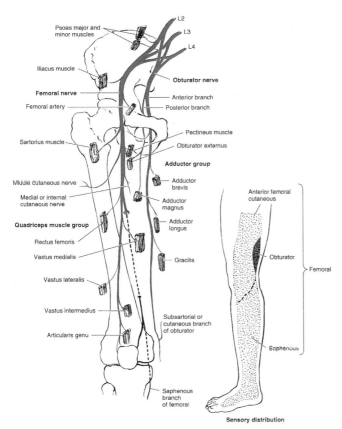

FIGURE 6–9   The femoral (L2-4) and obturator (L2-4) nerves.

ureter, and descends through the obturator canal in the upper part of the obturator foramen to the medial side of the thigh. While in the foramen, the obturator nerve splits into anterior and posterior branches. The anterior division of the obturator nerve gives an articular branch to the hip joint near its origin. It descends anterior to the obturator externus and adductor brevis deep to the pectineus and adductor longus. It supplies muscular branches to the adductors longus, brevis, and the gracilis, and rarely to the pectineus.[125] It divides into numerous named and unnamed branches, including the cutaneous branches to the subsartorial plexus, and directly to a small area of skin on the middle internal part of the thigh, vascular branches to the femoral artery, and communicating branches to the femoral cutaneous and accessory obturator nerves. The posterior division of the obturator nerve pierces the anterior part of the obturator externus, which it supplies, and descends deep to the adductor brevis. It also supplies the adductors magnus and brevis (if it has not received supply from the anterior division) and gives an articular branch to the knee joint (see Fig. 6–9).

The obturator nerve may be affected by the same processes that affect the femoral nerve. Disability is minimal although external rotation and adduction of the thigh are impaired, and crossing of the legs is difficult. The

patient can complain of severe pain, which radiates from the groin down the inner aspect of the thigh (see Fig. 6–9).

Chronic pain in the groin region is a difficult clinical problem to evaluate, and in many cases the cause of the pain is poorly understood. Possible causative clinical syndromes in affected areas include tendinitis, bursitis, osteitis, stress fracture, hernias, conjoint tendon strains, inguinal ligament enthesopathy, and entrapment of the lateral cutaneous nerve of the thigh.[126–128] Compression of the anterior division of the obturator nerve in the thigh has been described recently as one possible cause for adductor region pain, and entrapment of this nerve has been documented by nerve conduction studies.[129] One study indicated that fascia over the nerve contributed to compression of the nerve, or perhaps allowed for the development of a compartment syndrome.[129]

The fascial development, especially with the perivascular condensations around the vessels supplying the adductor mass, constitutes a layer definite enough to create an entrapment of the anterior division of the obturator nerve.[130] This thickening around the vessels becomes more significant in the possible explanation of an entrapment syndrome when the intimate relationship between the nerve branches and the vessels is considered.[130]

Lateral Femoral Cutaneous Nerve

The lateral femoral cutaneous nerve is purely sensory, derived primarily from the second and third lumbar nerve roots, with occasional contributions from the first lumbar nerve root.[131,132] Sympathetic afferent and efferent fibers are also contained within the nerve.[133] The nerve leaves the lumbar plexus and normally appears at the lateral border of the psoas, just proximal to the crest of the ilium; courses laterally across the anterior surface of the iliacus (covered by iliac fascia); and approaches the lateral portion of the inguinal ligament posterior to the deep circumflex iliac artery. The nerve usually crosses beneath the inguinal ligament, just inferior and medial to the anterior superior iliac spine,[134] exiting anteriorly through the fascia lata, several centimeters distal to the inguinal ligament, where it divides into anterior and posterior branches. Ghent[135] described four anatomic variations in the inguinal region, the most common being a split inguinal ligament at the lateral attachment to the anterior superior iliac spine, with the lateral femoral cutaneous nerve running between the fibers. The nerve then splits into anterior and posterior divisions approximately 5 cm below the anterior superior iliac spine and continues distally, dividing into several rami to innervate the skin over the lateral aspect of the thigh[136] (see Fig. 6–9).

Alternately, the nerve may be absent, with a branch from the femoral nerve arising below the inguinal ligament, or it may be replaced by the ilioinguinal nerve.[137]

In 1885, the German surgeon Werner Hager[138] gave the first description of an injury to the lateral femoral cutaneous nerve. This syndrome was described independently by both Bernhardt[139] and Roth[140] in 1895. Roth named the syndrome *meralgia paresthetica* on the basis of the Greek words *meros* (thigh) and *algos* (pain). Numerous causes have been reported,[139,141,142] most of which are associated with either acute or chronic mechanical irritation. Toxic and metabolic disorders, such as diabetes mellitus, alcoholism, and lead poisoning, which have been reported to be causative in several cases, have all been described to increase susceptibility of individual peripheral nerves, including the lateral femoral cutaneous nerve, to mechanical insults.[143,144] This apparent vulnerability of the lateral femoral cutaneous nerve has been investigated by a number of authors[145,146] and has been associated with the unique course of the nerve at its exit from the pelvis. An important factor in development of lateral femoral cutaneous nerve entrapment and subsequent intervention is anatomic variation at the site of passage. Stookey[147] drew attention to the marked angulation of the nerve at the inguinal ligament, postulating that local mechanical factors resulted in chronic nerve damage. Several reports have repeatedly mentioned these anatomic variations, including the unusual mechanism of trauma.[138,148–150]

Symptoms include numbness, tingling, and pain over the outer aspect and front of the thigh, most marked on walking and standing. It is most common in middle-aged men and may occur as the first sign of a lumbar cord tumor.

SACRAL PLEXUS

The lumbosacral trunk (L4, 5) descends into the pelvis, where it enters the formation of the sacral plexus.

The sacral plexus is formed by the ventral rami of the L4-5 and the S1-4 nerves and lies on the posterior wall of the pelvis, anterior to the piriformis, and posterior to the sigmoid colon, ureter, and hypogastric vessels in front. The L4 and L5 nerves join medial to the sacral promontory, becoming the lumbosacral trunk (see Fig. 6–8). The S1-4 nerves converge with the lumbosacral trunk in front of the piriformis muscle, forming the broad triangular band of the sacral plexus (Fig. 6–10). The upper three nerves of the plexus divide into two sets of branches: the medial branches, which are distributed to the multifidi muscles, and the lateral branches, which become the medial cluneal nerves and supply the skin over the medial part of the gluteus maximus. The lower two posterior primary divisions, with the posterior division of the coccygeal nerve, supply the skin over the coccyx.

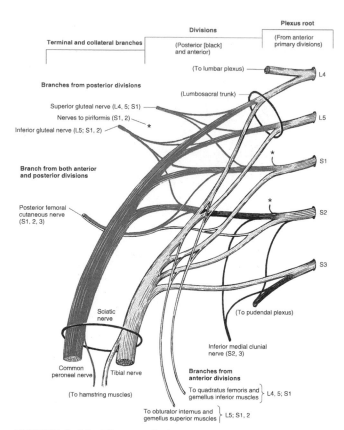

FIGURE 6–10 The sacral plexus.

Sciatic Nerve

The sciatic nerve, the largest nerve in the body, arises from the L4, L5, and S1-3 nerve roots and is considered to be the continuation of the lumbosacral plexus (Fig. 6–11).

The sciatic nerve is composed of independent tibial (medial) and common peroneal (lateral) divisions that usually are united as a single nerve down to the lower portion of the thigh. The tibial division is the larger of the two. Although grossly united, the funicular patterns of the tibial and common peroneal divisions are distinct, and there is no exchange of bundles between them. The common peroneal nerve is formed by the upper four posterior divisions (L4, 5 and S1, 2) of the sacral plexus, and the tibial nerve is formed from all five anterior divisions (L4, 5 and S1, 2, 3).

The sciatic nerve usually enters the gluteal region below the piriformis. In approximately 10% of cases, however, the two divisions exit the pelvis as distinct nerves, being separated by fibers of the piriformis as they pass through the anterior third of the greater sciatic foramen.[151] Also running through the greater sciatic foramen is the superior gluteal artery, the largest branch of the internal iliac artery, and its accompanying vein.

Numerous variations have been described, including cases in which the sciatic nerve passes through the

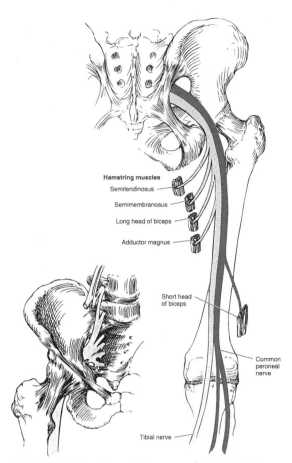

FIGURE 6–11   The sciatic nerve (L4, 5; S1-3).

common peroneal divisions, that showed differences in the relative amounts of nerve tissue (funiculi) and connective tissue within the two divisions. He found that the common peroneal division is composed of fewer and larger funiculi with less connective tissue than the tibial division. It was proposed that nerves with large and tightly packed funiculi are more vulnerable to mechanical injury than those in which the funiculi are smaller and more loosely dispersed in a greater amount of connective tissue. In the latter case, under a deforming force the neural elements are displaced more easily and the mechanical forces can be dissipated to the intervening connective tissue.

Injury to the sciatic nerve may result indirectly from a herniated intervertebral disc (protruded nucleus pulposus) or, more directly, from a hip dislocation, local aneurysm, or direct external trauma of the sciatic notch, the latter of which can be confused with a compressive radiculopathy of the lumbar or sacral nerve root.[152] Some useful clues help distinguish the two conditions:

- Pain from a disc radiculopathy should not significantly change with hip rotation, whereas with a sciatic entrapment by the piriformis, pain is accentuated with hip internal rotation and relieved by external rotation.
- Sensory alteration is present and the distribution is different, in the fact that sciatic neuropathy produces sensory changes on the sole of the foot, whereas the usual disc radiculopathy does not, unless there is a predominant S1 involvement.
- Compressive radiculopathy below the L4 level causes palpable atrophy of the gluteal muscles, whereas a sciatic entrapment spares these muscles.
- The sciatic trunk is frequently tender from root compression at the foraminal level, whereas it is not normally tender in a sciatic nerve entrapment.[153]

Individual case reports of bone and soft-tissue tumors along the course of the sciatic nerve have been described as a rare cause of sciatica.[154,155] The early diagnosis of a tumor as the underlying pathology is crucial because early resection, in addition to producing symptomatic relief and preventing further neurologic damage and unnecessary spine surgeries, may have an impact on patients' survival. A retrospective study[156] of 32 patients who had been treated for pain along the course of the sciatic nerve, and who were subsequently found to have a tumor along the extraspinal course of the sciatic nerve, found that despite the wide variation in histologic diagnosis and anatomic location of these tumors, all 32 patients had a similar and specific pain pattern. At the initial examination, all patients reported pain at least 1 month in duration that was

piriformis, and cases in which the tibial division passes below the piriformis while the common peroneal passes above or through the muscle. It seems that the tibial division always enters the gluteal region below the piriformis, and the variability is in the course of the common peroneal division. The sciatic nerve descends between the greater trochanter of the femur and the ischial tuberosity along the posterior surface of the thigh to the popliteal space, where it usually terminates by dividing into the tibial and common peroneal nerves (Fig. 6–11). Innervation for the short head of the biceps comes from the common peroneal division, the only muscle innervated by this division above the knee. Rami from the tibial trunk pass to the semitendinosus and semimembranosus muscles, the long head of the biceps, and the adductor magnus muscle.

In most reports of sciatic nerve injury, regardless of the cause, the common peroneal division is involved more frequently and often suffers a greater degree of damage than the tibial division, and its susceptibility to injury seems to be related to several anatomic features.

Sunderland[2] performed an investigation of the cross-sectional area of the sciatic trunk, and of the tibial and

unrelated to trauma. All patients described an insidious onset of pain. Although some patients initially had only intermittent pain, all developed pain that was constant, progressive, and unresponsive to change in position or bed rest. Twenty-five patients described significant night pain. The study also commented on the fact that the ability of a patient to locate a sciatic pain to an extraspinal point should be considered an alarming sign.[156]

The roots of the superior gluteal nerve (L4, L5, S1) arise within the pelvis from the sacral plexus (see Fig. 6–10), and enter the buttock through the greater sciatic foramen, above the piriformis. The nerve runs laterally between gluteus medius and gluteus minimus. It is in this region that it is at risk during surgery on the hip.[157] It supplies both gluteus medius and gluteus minimus before terminating in the tensor fascia lata, which it also supplies.

The inferior gluteal nerve (L5 and S1, 2) passes below the piriformis muscle, through the greater sciatic foramen, and travels to the gluteus maximus muscle (see Fig. 6–10). Nerves to the piriformis consist of short, smaller branches from S1 and S2.

The medial branch of the superior cluneal nerve (see Fig. 6–10) passes superficially over the iliac crest and is covered by two layers of dense fibrous fascia. When the medial branch of the superior cluneal nerve passes through the fascia against the posterior iliac crest and the osteofibrous tunnel consisting of the two layers of the fascia and the superior rim of the iliac crest, the possibility of irritation or trauma to the nerve is increased, and this may be a site of nerve compression or constriction.[158] Tenderness of the posterior iliac crest may be found in iliolumbar syndrome, facet syndrome, or disc diseases.[159–161] The iliolumbar syndrome is thought to correspond to the insertion of the iliolumbar ligament.[162] However, because the iliolumbar ligament insertion is always located on the ventral aspect of the posterior iliac crest,[161–163] and shielded by the iliac crest, its insertion is inaccessible to palpation. Consequently, the area over the iliac crest, located 7 to 8 cm from the midline, may not correspond to the iliolumbar ligament attachment. The facet syndrome has been described as pain from a cutaneous dorsal ramus, originating from the thoracolumbar junction, rather than from the iliac insertion of the iliolumbar ligament. The clinical picture frequently may be confused by the finding of radiologic abnormalities at the lumbosacral region, to which the cause of the low back pain is erroneously attributed. However, disc and lower lumbar facet joint disease do not account for all cases of low back pain. When pain and deep tenderness are located at the level of the iliac crest at a point 7 to 8 cm lateral to midline, it may correspond to the cutaneous emergence of the posterior rami (superior cluneal nerve) crossing over the posterior iliac crest.

The posterior femoral cutaneous nerve constitutes a collateral branch, with roots from both anterior and posterior divisions of S1-2 and the anterior divisions of S2-3. Perineal branches pass to the skin of the upper medial aspect of the thigh and the skin of the scrotum or labium majores. The sciatic nerve is by far the most common nerve accidentally injured during intramuscular injection. Despite its close proximity to the sciatic nerve, however, injury to the posterior femoral cutaneous nerve is apparently quite rare. Collateral branches from the anterior divisions extend to the quadratus femoris and gemellus inferior muscles (from L4, 5 and S1) and to the obturator internus and gemellus superior muscles (from L5 and S1, 2) (see Fig. 6–10).

Tibial Nerve

The tibial nerve (L4, 5 and S1-3) is formed by all five of the anterior divisions of the sacral plexus, thus receiving fibers from the lower two lumbar and the upper three sacral cord segments (Fig. 6–12). The tibial nerve forms the largest component of the sciatic nerve in the thigh, and runs parallel and slightly lateral to the midline. Inferiorly, it begins its own course in the upper part of the popliteal space and descends vertically through this space, passing between the heads of the gastrocnemius muscle, to the dorsum of the leg, and to the posterior-medial aspect of the ankle, from which

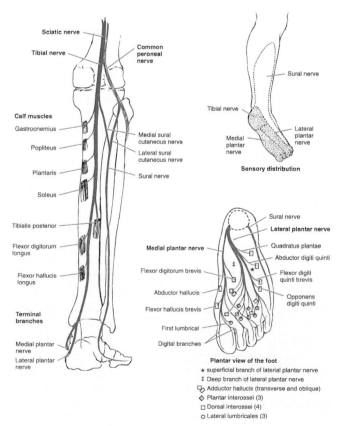

FIGURE 6–12 The tibial nerve (L4, 5; S1-3).

point its terminal branches, the medial and lateral plantar nerves, continue into the foot (see Fig. 6–12). The portion of the tibial trunk below the popliteal space was formerly called the posterior tibial nerve; the portion within the space was called the internal popliteal nerve.

The tibial nerve supplies the gastrocnemius, plantaris, soleus, popliteus, tibialis posterior, flexor digitorum longus pedis, and flexor hallucis longus muscles. Articular branches pass to the knee and ankle joints (see Fig. 6–12).

In the distal leg, the tibial nerve lies on the posterior surface of the tibia. It lies lateral to the posterior tibial vessels, and it supplies articular branches to the ankle joint. As it passes beneath the flexor retinaculum, it gives medial calcanean branches to the skin of the heel, then divides into the medial and lateral plantar nerves (see Fig. 6–12). These nerves supply sensation to the sole of the foot and toes, articular branches to the foot joints, and muscular branches to the small muscles of the foot.[164]

- The medial plantar nerve (comparable to the median nerve in the hand) supplies the flexor digitorum brevis, abductor halluces, flexor halluces brevis, and first lumbrical muscles; and sensory branches to the medial side of the sole, the plantar surfaces of the medial 3½ toes, and the ungual phalanges of the same toes (see Fig. 6–12).
- The lateral plantar nerve (comparable to the ulnar nerve in the arm and hand) supplies the small muscles of the foot, except those innervated by the medial plantar nerve; and sensory branches to the lateral portions of the sole, the plantar surface of the lateral 1½ toes, and the distal phalanges of these toes (see Fig. 6–12). The interdigital nerves are most commonly entrapped between the second and third, and the third and fourth web spaces. This occurs as a result of forced hyperextension of the toes, causing mechanical irritation of the nerve, by the intermetatarsal ligaments, eventually resulting in an interdigital neuroma. These patients are often incorrectly diagnosed as having metatarsalgia. The medial and lateral plantar nerves can be entrapped just distal to the tarsal tunnel and cause painful situations in the plantar aspect of the feet and toes. The usual clinical picture is a patient with pronated feet and burning pain on the plantar surface of the foot and toes that worsens at night or upon arising in the morning.
- The medial sural cutaneous nerve (see Fig. 6–12), joins the lateral sural cutaneous nerve from the common peroneal to form the sural nerve (external saphenous), which supplies the skin of the posterior-lateral part of the leg and the lateral side of the foot.

Tarsal tunnel syndrome is a compressive neuropathy of the posterior tibial nerve or one of its branches. This relatively rare syndrome was first described by Keck[165] and Lam[166] in two separate reports in 1962. The nerve often is entrapped as it courses through the tarsal tunnel, passing under the deep fascia, the flexor retinaculum, and within the abductor hallucis muscle. The etiology is multifactorial and may be posttraumatic, neoplastic, or inflammatory.[167–169] The diagnosis is based on history and clinical examination. The typical patient reports a poorly localized burning sensation or pain and paresthesia at the medial plantar surface of the foot. Discomfort is worse after activity and typically is accentuated during the end of a working day. Some patients have cramps in the longitudinal foot arch. Resting pain is reported infrequently. Tinel's sign, at the medial malleolus just above the margin of the flexor retinaculum, is often positive, sometimes with pain that radiates distally toward the midsole, along the posterior branch of the nerve.

Common Peroneal Nerve

The common peroneal nerve (L4, 5 and S1, 2) is formed by a fusion of the upper four posterior divisions of the sacral plexus and thus derives its fibers from the lower two lumbar and the upper two sacral cord segments (Fig. 6–13). In the thigh, it is a component of the sciatic nerve as far as the upper part of the popliteal space.

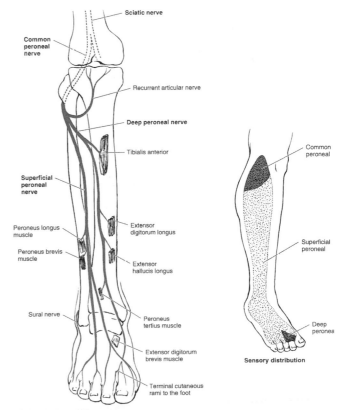

FIGURE 6–13   The common peroneal nerve (L4, 5; S1-2).

Sensory branches are given off in the popliteal space and include the superior and inferior articular branches to the knee joint, and the lateral sural cutaneous nerve, which joins the medial calcaneal nerve (from the tibial nerve) to form the sural nerve, supplying the skin of the lower dorsal aspect of the leg, the external malleolus, and the lateral side of the foot and fifth toe (see Fig. 6–13).

At the apex of the popliteal fossa, the sciatic nerve divides into the tibial and common peroneal nerves, and the common peroneal begins its independent course, descending along the posterior border of the biceps femoris, diagonally across the dorsum of the knee joint to the upper external portion of the leg near the head of the fibula. The nerve curves around the lateral aspect of the fibula toward the anterior aspect of the bone, before passing deep to the two heads of the peroneus longus muscle, where it divides into three terminal rami.

The three terminal branches are the recurrent articular, and the superficial and deep peroneal nerves.

1. The recurrent articular nerve accompanies the anterior tibial recurrent artery, supplying the tibiofibular and knee joints, and a twig to the tibialis anterior muscle.
2. The superficial peroneal nerve arises deep to the peroneus longus (see Fig. 6–13). It then passes forward and downward between the peronei and the extensor digitorum longus muscles, to supply the peroneus longus and brevis muscles, and sensory distribution to the lower front of the leg, to the dorsum of the foot, part of the big toe, and adjacent sides of the second to fifth toes up to the second phalanges. When this nerve is entrapped, it causes pain over the lateral distal aspect of the leg and ankle that is often confused with a disc herniation, with involvement of the L5 nerve root.
3. The deep peroneal nerve passes anterior and lateral to the tibialis anterior muscle, between the peroneus longus and the extensor digitorum longus muscles, to the front of the interosseous membrane and supplies the tibialis anterior, extensor digitorum longus, extensor hallucis longus, and peroneus tertius muscles (see Fig. 6–13). Terminal branches extend to the skin of the adjacent sides of the first two toes, the extensor digitorum brevis muscle, and the adjacent joints (see Fig. 6–13). When the deep peroneal nerve is entrapped, the patient complains of pain in the great toe that can be confused with a post-traumatic, sympathetic dystrophy.

Compared with the tibial division, the common peroneal division is relatively tethered at the sciatic notch and the neck of the fibula, and may, therefore, be less able to tolerate or distribute tension, such as in acute stretching,

because of a near miss from a high-velocity projectile or because of changes in limb position or length. Finally, the more lateral position of the nerve in the gluteal region may make it more susceptible to direct injury.[170] When the common peroneal nerve is entrapped (and it is very vulnerable, especially at the fibula neck), it can be confused with a herniated disc syndrome, tendonitis of the popliteus tendon, and an internal derangement of the knee. The pain is on the lateral surface of the knee and leg, going into the foot itself.

Lateral knee pain is a common problem among patients seeking medical attention, and entrapment of the common peroneal nerve is frequently overlooked in the differential diagnostic considerations, especially in the absence of trauma or the presence of a palpable mass at the neck of the fibula. There is a wide differential diagnosis for peroneal neuropathy that includes mononeuritis, idiopathic peroneal palsy, intrinsic and extrinsic nerve tumors, and extraneural compression by a synovial cyst, ganglion cyst, soft tissue tumor, osseous mass, or a large fabella.[171] Traumatic injury of the nerve may occur secondary to a fracture, dislocation, surgical procedure, application of skeletal traction, or a tight cast.[171]

The pudendal and coccygeal plexuses are the most caudal portions of the lumbosacral plexus and supply nerves to the perineal structures (Fig. 6–14).

A. The pudendal plexus supplies the coccygeus, levator ani, and sphincter ani externus muscles. The pudendal nerve is a mixed nerve, and a lesion that affects it or its ascending pathways can result in voiding and erectile dysfunction.[172] A lesion in the afferent pathways of the pudendal nerve is often suspected clinically by suggestive patient histories, including organic neurologic disease or neurologic

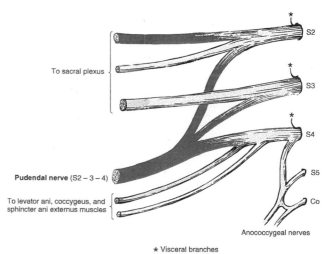

* Visceral branches

FIGURE 6–14 The pudendal and coccygeal plexuses.

trauma. Lesions are also suspected when a neurologic examination to assess the function of sacral segments S2, S3, and S4 is abnormal. The pudendal nerve divides into:

1. The inferior hemorrhoidal nerves to the external anal sphincter and adjacent skin.
2. The perineal nerve.
3. The dorsal nerve of the penis.

B. The nerves of the coccygeal plexus are the small sensory anococcygeal nerves derived from the last three segments (S4, 5, C). They pierce the sacrotuberous ligament and supply the skin in the region of the coccyx.

DOUBLE CRUSH INJURIES

The theory that many entrapment neuropathies result from "double crush" along the peripheral nerve fibers was proposed by Upton and McComas in 1973, who hypothesized that two focal lesions along the same axon could be related in that one could encourage the development of the other because of "serial constraints of axoplasmic flow": the axoplasmic flow is partially reduced at the proximal site of injury, and then further reduced at the distal compression site, to the point that it drops below the safety margin, and denervation results.[173] They assumed that this may occur even though the proximal lesion, while symptomatic, was not clinically severe. Thus, a cervical radiculopathy, manifesting as little more than neck pain and stiffness, could still precipitate a distal focal entrapment neuropathy. For this mechanism of nerve injury—serial compromise of axonal transport along the same nerve fiber, causing a subclinical lesion at the distal site to become symptomatic—they proposed the term *double-crush syndrome*. In their study, Upton and McComas was postulated that the double-crush syndrome was responsible for the high incidence of dual lesions encountered; of 115 patients with either carpal tunnel syndrome or ulnar neuropathy along the elbow segment, or both, there was evidence of a cervical root lesion in 81 (70%).[173]

The double-crush hypothesis has been used to explain a great number of coexisting proximal and distal nerve impairments, and has been expanded to include triple-crush, quadruple-crush, and multiple-crush syndromes, as well as the reversed double-crush syndrome.[174–176] Despite its acceptance, however, the double-crush hypothesis has raised a number of questions that raise doubts as to its existence in the many clinical situations.

The experimental studies done on the double-crush hypothesis have shown that successive lesions along a peripheral nerve can summate.[177–179] However, no published experimental studies to date have shown that dual lesions along nerve fibers cause magnified damage, nor have any studies demonstrated that the segment of nerve distal to a focal lesion is, in the double-crush syndrome context, particularly susceptible to an additional focal insult.[180] What has been proved is that consecutive focal lesions along a nerve may have an additive effect. It is also interesting to note that with most of the experimental models the second lesion has been manifested as focal slowing, presumably secondary to demyelination, yet the double-crush syndrome hypothesis requires that the distal lesion result in axonal loss.[173]

Case Study: Right Sacral and Gluteal Pain[181]

Subjective

A 30-year-old man presented with complaints of pain in the right sacral and gluteal region that increased with walking or sitting, and decreased with lying supine. The pain had started a few months ago following a fall onto the right buttock area and had progressively worsened. An x-ray had shown nothing abnormal.

Examination

Observation revealed nothing remarkable except a slightly increased lordosis. A modified scan was performed. Active forward flexion reproduced the sacral and gluteal pain, but all of the other motions were negative. An increase in radicular pain with forward flexion warranted a neurologic examination, which revealed the following:

- A positive Lasegue sign at about 25 degrees
- Normal deep tendon reflexes as compared to the contralateral side
- No sensory loss in dermatomes
- No strength loss in lumbar "myotomes"
- Irritability upon palpation of the greater sciatic foramen (the region between the greater trochanter and the posterior superior iliac spine)
- Palpable tenderness and swelling over the region of the piriformis muscle
- Increased pain with internal rotation of the hip when combined with hip flexion and knee extension
- A positive Gowers-Bonnet test (hip flexion, knee flexion, and internal rotation)

Discussion[182]

Multiple etiologies have been proposed to explain the compression or irritation of the sciatic nerve that occurs with the piriformis syndrome. Yeoman[183] emphasized the anatomic relationship of the sciatic nerve and the piriformis and was the first to link sacroiliac disease with piriformis muscle spasm. In 1937, Freiberg[185] described two findings on physical examination that were consistent with sciatic pain referable to the piriformis muscle: Lasegue's sign (pain in the vicinity of the greater sciatic notch with extension of the knee and the hip flexed to 90 degrees, and tenderness to palpation of the greater sciatic notch) and Freiberg's sign (pain with passive internal rotation of the hip). In 1938, Beaton and Anson[186] identified certain anomalies of the piriformis muscle and theorized that sciatica could be secondary to an altered relationship between the piriformis muscle and the sciatic nerve. Pace and Nagle[187] later described a diagnostic maneuver that is now referred to as Pace's sign: pain and weakness in association with resisted abduction and external rotation of the affected thigh.

Robinson[188] has been credited with introducing the term *piriformis syndrome* and outlining its six classic findings:

1. A history of trauma to the sacroiliac and gluteal regions
2. Pain in the region of the sacroiliac joint, greater sciatic notch, and piriformis muscle that usually extends down the limb and causes difficulty with walking
3. Acute exacerbation of pain caused by stooping or lifting (and moderate relief of pain by traction on the affected extremity with the patient in the supine position)
4. A palpable sausage-shaped mass, tender to palpation, over the piriformis muscle on the affected side
5. A positive Lasegue's sign
6. Gluteal atrophy, depending on the duration of the condition.

A flexion contracture at the hip increases the lumbar lordosis, and increased tension in the pelvifemoral muscles develops as these muscles try to stabilize the pelvis and spine in the new position. The involved muscles hypertrophy to handle the tension, but there is no corresponding increase in the size of the bony foramens. With neural tissue being the least tolerant to compression of the neurovascular bundle, neurologic signs of sciatic compression develop earlier than vascular signs.[189]

Trauma, direct or indirect, to the sacroiliac or gluteal region can lead to piriformis syndrome[187] and is a result of hematoma formation and subsequent scarring between the sciatic nerve and the short external rotators. Local anatomic anomalies may contribute to the likelihood that symptoms will develop. In patients who have this condition, movement of the hip may cause radicular pain that is much like the nerve-root pain associated with lumbar disc disease.[182] These patients typically present with a history of gluteal trauma, symptoms of pain in the buttock and intolerance to sitting, tenderness to palpation of the greater sciatic notch, and pain with flexion, adduction, and internal rotation of the hip.

Intervention

This syndrome usually responds well to a conservative course of intervention including:

- A home program of prolonged piriformis stretching[190]
- Corticosteroid and anesthetic injections, and anti-inflammatory medication to alleviate muscle spasm[188]

REVIEW QUESTIONS

1. Injury to the radial nerve in the spiral groove would result in:
   a. Weakness of elbow flexion
   b. Difficulty initiating glenhumeral abduction
   c. An inability to control rotation during abduction
   d. A decreased ability to hold the humeral head in its socket
   e. All of the above
2. A patient with a musculocutaneous nerve injury is still able to flex the elbow. The major muscle causing this elbow flexion is the:
   a. Brachioradialis
   b. Flexor carpi ulnaris
   c. Pronator quadratus
   d. Extensor carpi ulnaris
   e. Pectoralis major
3. Which of the following muscles is *not* innervated by the median nerve?
   a. Abductor pollicis brevis
   b. Flexor pollicis longus
   c. Medial heads of flexor digitorum profundus
   d. Superficial head of flexor pollicis brevis
   e. Pronator quadratus
4. The nerve that innervates the first lumbrical muscle in the hand is the:
   a. Median nerve
   b. Ulnar nerve
   c. Radial nerve
   d. Anterior interosseus nerve
   e. Lateral cutaneous nerve of the hand
5. After a nerve injury, regeneration occurs proximally first and then progresses distally at a rate of about 1 mm per day. Following a radial nerve injury in the axilla, which muscle would be the *last* to recover?
   a. Long head of the triceps
   b. Anconeus
   c. Extensor indicis
   d. Extensor digiti minimi
   e. Supinator

6. A patient complains of a burning sensation in the anterior-lateral aspect of the thigh. Dysfunction of which nerve could lead to these symptoms?
   a. Lateral femoral cutaneous
   b. Femoral
   c. Obturator
   d. Genitofemoral
   e. Ilioinguinal

7. The sciatic nerve consists of two divisions (medial and lateral) which eventually separate into distinct nerves. The medial and lateral divisions, respectively, form the:
   a. Femoral and obturator nerves
   b. Obturator and femoral nerves
   c. Common peroneal and tibial nerves
   d. Tibial and common peroneal nerves
   e. Obturator and tibial nerves

8. The saphenous nerve supplies cutaneous sensation to the medial aspect of the leg. From which nerve does the saphenous nerve arise?
   a. Obturator
   b. Peroneal
   c. Sciatic
   d. Femoral
   e. Saphenous, arising as a direct branch from the sacral plexus

9. The tibial nerve passes into the foot, where it divides into its terminal branches. What route does the tibial nerve follow to enter the foot?
   a. It passes along the dorsal aspect of the ankle, then into the foot
   b. It passes anterior to the lateral malleolus
   c. It passes under the flexor retinaculum and posterior to the lateral malleolus
   d. It passes anterior to the medial malleolus
   e. It passes under the flexor retinaculum and posterior to the lateral malleolus

10. Injury to the deep branch of the peroneal nerve would result in a sensory deficit to which of the following locations?
    a. Medial side of the foot
    b. Lateral side of the foot
    c. Lateral 1½ toes
    d. Medial border of the sole of the foot
    e. Adjacent dorsal surfaces of the first and second toes

11. A brachial plexus injury involving the superior portion of the plexus produces winging of the scapula. Weakness of which of the following muscles would produce the winging observed?
    a. Long head of the triceps
    b. Supraspinatus
    c. Deltoid
    d. Pectoralis major
    e. Serratus anterior

12. The anterior interosseus branch of the median nerve innervates which muscles?
    a. Flexor pollicis longus
    b. Pronator teres
    c. Pronator quadratus
    d. Both a and c
    e. All of the above

13. The lumbar plexus is occasionally injured at the point where it passes through a muscle. The muscle causing the compression is the:
    a. Gluteus maximus
    b. Gluteus medius
    c. Quadratus lumborum
    d. Obturator externus
    e. Psoas major

14. The axillary nerve can occasionally be injured where it passes through a muscle. Which muscle would this be?
    a. Pronator teres
    b. Supinator
    c. Deltoid
    d. Coracobrachialis
    e. Biceps

Directions: Match each of the numbered words or phrases below with the lettered item most closely associated with it. Each item may be used once, more than once, or not at all.

15. Pectineus
16. Gluteus medius
17. Gluteus maximus
18. Tensor fasciae lata
19. Long head of the biceps femoris
20. Short head of the biceps femoris
    a. Innervated by the tibial division of the sciatic nerve
    b. Innervated by the common peroneal division of the sciatic nerve
    c. Innervated by the inferior gluteal nerve
    d. Innervated by the superior gluteal nerve
    e. Innervated by the femoral nerve

Directions: Match each of the numbered words or phrases below with the lettered item most closely associated with it. Each item may be used once, more than once, or not at all.

21. Nerve primarily responsible for knee extension
22. Nerve primarily responsible for ankle plantar flexion
23. Nerve primarily responsible for knee flexion
24. Nerve primarily responsible for ankle dorsiflexion
    a. Sciatic nerve
    b. Peroneal nerve
    c. Femoral nerve
    d. Tibial nerve
    e. Obturator nerve

25. A muscle innervated by the superficial branch of the peroneal nerve is the:
    a. Peroneus longus
    b. Peroneus tertius

c. Peroneus brevis

d. Tibialis anterior

26. Which statement(s) about the brachial plexus is (are) true?

a. The brachial plexus is formed from the posterior rami of nerves C5 to T1

b. The cords of the brachial plexus are named with respect to their anatomic position around the axillary artery

c. The muscles innervated by the posterior portion of the brachial plexus are primarily flexors

d. The nerve to the rhomboid muscles arises from C5 before C5 helps to form the upper trunk

27. Muscles that participate in upward shrugging of the shoulder include the:

a. Rhomboid major

b. Levator scapula

c. Rhomboid minor

d. Trapezius

e. All of the above

28. Anatomic variation can occur in the structure of the lumbosacral plexus. Which of the following is (are) true?

a. A prefixed plexus is one in which the L1 nerve root is incorporated into the lumbar plexus

b. A prefixed plexus is one in which the L4 nerve root is incorporated into the sacral plexus rather than into the lumbar plexus

c. A postfixed plexus is one in which the S3 nerve root is incorporated into the sacral plexus

d. A postfixed plexus one in which the L4 nerve root and part of the L5 nerve root are incorporated into the lumbar plexus

29. Injury to the obturator nerve would cause:

a. Sensory loss on the medial aspect of the thigh

b. Sensory loss on the medial aspect of the leg

c. Weakness of thigh adduction

d. A decrease in the amplitude of the knee-jerk reflex

30. Compression of the medial plantar nerve at the medial malleolus would give rise to:

a. Decreased sensation along the medial side of the sole of the foot

b. Weakness of the abductor hallucis muscle

c. Weakness of the flexor digitorum brevis muscle

d. Weakness of the adductor hallucis muscle

31. A herniated disc between C6 and C7 would impinge on which nerve root level?

32. The cutaneous branch of the femoral nerve that supplies the L4 dermatome innervation is called what?

33. A loss of dorsiflexion strength is the result of a lesion to which nerve?

34. What would you suspect if a patient reports persistent paresthesia with occasional burning pain in the area of the L2-3 dermatomes of the thigh, and hip flexion is strong and pain free?

Directions: Which muscles are innervated by:

35. Deep peroneal nerve

36. Tibial nerve

Which areas are covered by the following dermatomes?

37. C5

38. C6

39. C7

40. C8

41. T1

42. L1

43. L3

44. L5

45. S1

46. S2-3

47. S4-5

48. Which two nerves are formed from the lumbar plexus?

49. Which six nerves are formed from the sacral plexus?

Directions: Which muscles are innervated by the following nerves? Give their nerve root levels.

50. Femoral

51. Obturator

52. Superior gluteal

53. Inferior gluteal

54. Sciatic

55. Superficial peroneal

Directions: What is the generally accepted nerve root of the following?

56. Teres major

57. Biceps, brachialis, brachioradialis

58. Coracobrachialis

59. Triceps

60. Supinator

61. Subscapular

62. Which muscle(s) does the thoracodorsal nerve innervate and what is its root?

63. Which two muscles are innervated by the axillary nerve and what is its root?

64. The lateral and medial pectoral nerves innervate which muscles?

65. The posterior cord serves which two nerves?

66. The lateral cord serves which two nerves?

67. The medial cord serves which two nerves?

68. The divisions from which two trunks form the lateral cord?

69. What is the order of nomenclature for the brachial plexus?

70. What root level is the long thoracic and which muscle(s) does it innervate?

71. What root level is the dorsal scapular and which muscle(s) does it innervate?

Directions: What is the root level and which muscle(s) are innervated by the following?

72. Suprascapular

73. Musculocutaneous

74. Median

75. True or False: With a ligament of Struthers compression, the pronator teres is compromised.

76. True or False: The anterior interosseus nerve innervates strictly sensory distribution.

77. After passing through the pronator teres heads, what does the medial nerve split into?

78. Which three structures form the Guyon canal?

79. What passes through the Guyon canal?

80. Using manual muscle testing, how could you differentiate between cubital tunnel syndrome and a Guyon canal lesion?

81. Klumpke's palsy involves which *trunk* of the brachial plexus?

82. Erb's palsy involves which trunk?

83. How can you differentiate a spinal accessory and a long thoracic impairment?

84. Which nerve innervates the lateral antebrachial cutaneous?

85. Injury to the lateral cord of the brachial plexus would most likely involve damage to the which nerve?

86. The hip adductor muscles are innervated by which nerve(s)?
  a. Obturator and sciatic
  b. Sciatic
  c. Obturator
  d. Femoral

87. Which muscle does not have dual nerve innervation?
  a. Flexor digitorum profundus
  b. Flexor carpi ulnaris
  c. Flexor pollicis brevis
  d. Lumbricales

88. The anterior tibialis muscle is innervated by which nerve?
  a. Lateral plantar
  b. Superficial peroneal
  c. Tibial
  d. Deep peroneal

89. The flexor digitorum profundus is innervated by which nerve(s)?
  a. Ulnar
  b. Median
  c. Median, ulnar
  d. Median, radial

90. The peroneus longus muscle is innervated by which nerve?
  a. Deep peroneal
  b. Superficial peroneal
  c. Common peroneal
  d. Medial plantar

91. The second and third digits in the hand are innervated by which nerve?
  a. Ulnar nerve
  b. Median nerve
  c. Radial nerve
  d. Ulnar, median

92. The deep head of the flexor brevis is innervated by which nerve?
  a. Median
  b. Radial
  c. Radial, ulnar
  d. Ulnar

93. Which nerve arises from the posterior cord of the brachial plexus?
  a. Axillary, radial
  b. Ulnar, median
  c. Musculocutaneous
  d. None of the above

94. The hip adductor muscle group is innervated by several nerves. Which nerves innervate these muscles?
  a. Femoral, tibial
  b. Femoral, superior gluteal
  c. Femoral, obturator, tibial
  d. Obturator, tibial, superior gluteal

ANSWERS

  1. d.
  2. a.
  3. c.
  4. a.
  5. c.
  6. a.
  7. d.
  8. d.
  9. c.
  10. e.
  11. e.
  12. d.
  13. e.
  14. d.
  15. e.
  16. d.
  17. c.
  18. d.
  19. a.
  20. b.
  21. c.
  22. d.
  23. a.
  24. b.
  25. b.
  26. c.

27. e.
28. c.
29. b.
30. a.
31. C7.
32. Saphenous.
33. Common peroneal.
34. Compression of lateral cutaneous nerve of thigh.
35. Tibialis anterior (L4, 5), extensor digitorum longus (L4-S1), extensor hallucis longus (L4-S1), and extensor digitorum brevis (L4-S1).
36. Tibialis posterior and triceps surae (L5-S2), flexor digitorum longus (L5-S2), flexor hallucis longus (L5-S2), flexor digitorum brevis (L5-S1), flexor hallucis longus (L5-S2), and the foot intrinsics (S1-S2).
37. The deltoid area and thin strip down middle of the anterior surface of the arm.
38. Lateral aspect of arm, forearm, thumb, and forefinger.
39. Center line down the dorsal aspect of arm, forearm, and hand, and second and third digits (and middle palm).
40. Medial aspect of arm, forearm, and hand.
41. A thin strip down the anterior surface of the arm, and the axilla area.
42. Iliac crests, and anterior superior iliac spine (ASIS).
43. Medial condyle of femur.
44. Great toe and dorsal surface of second toe.
45. Lateral malleolus.
46. Pubic area.
47. Perianal region.
48. Femoral (L1-4), and obturator (L2-4).
49. Superior and inferior gluteal (L4-S2), sciatic (L4-S2), deep peroneal (L4-5), superior peroneal (L5-S1), tibial (L5-S2), and pudendal (S2-4).
50. Iliopsoas (L1-3), sartorius (L2-3), quadriceps femoris (L2-4), and pectineus (L2,3).
51. Pectineus (L2-3), adductor longus (L2, 3), adductor brevis (L2-4), adductor magnus (L3, 4), gracilis (L2-4), and obturator externus.
52. Gluteus medius and minimus (L4-S2), tensor fascia latae (TFL) (L4,5), and piriformis (S1-2).
53. Gluteus maximus (L4-S2).
54. Biceps femoris (L4-S2), semitendinosus, and membranosus (L4-S1).
55. The peronei (L5-S1).
56. C5-7.
57. C5-6.
58. C6-7.
59. C6-T1.
60. C5-7.
61. C5-7.
62. Latissimus dorsi (C6-8).
63. Deltoid and teres minor (C5-6).
64. Pectoralis major (C5, 6) and minor (C7-T1), respectively.

65. Axillary and radial.
66. Musculocutaneous and median.
67. Ulnar and median.
68. Anterior divisions of the upper-middle trunk (the anterior division of lower trunk forms the medial cord).
69. Trunks, divisions, cords, peripheral nerve.
70. C5-7: serratus anterior.
71. C4-5: rhomboids and levator scapula.
72. C(4), 5(6): supraspinatus and infraspinatus.
73. C5, 6: coracobrachialis, biceps, brachialis (2).
74. C5-T1: arm pronators flexor digitorum profundus second and third, flexor digitorum superficialis, lumbricales 1 and 2, Abductor pollices brevis (APB), Opponens pollices (OP), flexor pollicis longus, flexor pollicis brevis (superior), Flexor carpi radialis (FCR), and palmaris longus.
75. True.
76. False.
77. Anterior interosseus, and a mixed nerve.
78. Volar ligament, hook of hamate, pisiform.
79. Ulnar nerve and artery.
80. Cubital tunnel syndrome produces weakness of the flexor digitorum profundus.
81. Lower.
82. Upper.
83. By observing the winging of the scapula. If the winging occurs with glenohumeral abduction, the accessory nerve is at fault. If the winging occurs in forward flexion and protraction of the shoulder, the long thoracic nerve is at fault.
84. Musculocutaneous.
85. Musculocutaneous.
86. a.
87. b.
88. d.
89. c.
90. b.
91. b.
92. d.
93. a.
94. d.

REFERENCES

1. Bogduk N. Innervation and pain patterns of the cervical spine. In: Grant R, ed. *Physical Therapy of the Cervical and Thoracic Spine.* New York, NY: Churchill Livingstone; 1988.
2. Sunderland S. *Nerves and Nerve Injuries,* 2nd ed. Edinburgh, Scotland: Churchill Livingstone; 1978.
3. Pratt N. *Anatomy of the Cervical Spine. APTA Orthopedic Section, Physical Therapy Home Study Course 96-1;* 1996.

4. Sunderland S. Anatomical perivertebral influences on the intervertebral foramen. In: Goldstein M, ed. *The Research Status of Spinal Manipulative Therapy.* HEW Publication No. (NIH) 76-998. Bethesda, Md: 1975.

5. Daniels DL, Hyde JS, Kneeland JB, et al. The cervical nerves and foramina: Local-coil MRI imaging. AJNR 1986;7:129–133.

6. Pech P, Daniels DL, Williams AL, Haughton VM. The cervical neural foramina: Correlation of microtomy and CT anatomy. Radiology 1985;155:143–146.

7. Carter GT, Kilmer DD, Bonekat HW, Lieberman JS, Fowler WM. Evaluation of phrenic nerve and pulmonary function in hereditary motor and sensory neuropathy type 1. Muscle Nerve 1992;15:459–466.

8. Bolton CF. Clinical neurophysiology of the respiratory system. Muscle Nerve 1993;16:809–818.

9. Attia J, Hatala R, Cook DJ, Wong JG. Does this adult patient have acute meningitis? JAMA 1999;282:175–181.

10. Sprengell C. *The Aphorisms of Hippocrates, and the Sentences of Celsus,* 2nd ed. London, England: R Wilkin; 1735.

11. Tunkel AR, Scheld WM. Pathogenesis and pathophysiology of bacterial meningitis. Clin Microbiol Rev 1993;6:118–136.

12. Scheld WM. Meningococcal diseases. In: Warren KS, Mahmoud AAF, eds. *Tropical and Geographical Medicine,* 2nd ed. New York, NY: McGraw-Hill; 1990:798–814.

13. Lindsay KW, Bone I, Callander R. *Neurology and Neurosurgery Illustrated.* New York, NY: Churchill Livingstone; 1991.

14. Durand ML, Calderwood SB, Weber DJ, et al. Acute bacterial meningitis in adults: A review of 493 episodes. N Engl J Med 1993;328:21–28.

15. Brody IA, Wilkins RH. The signs of Kernig and Brudzinski. Arch Neurol 1969;21:215–218.

16. O'Connell JEA. The clinical signs of meningeal irritation. Brain 1946;69:9–21.

17. Harvey AM, Johns RJ, McKusick VA, Owens AH, Ross RS, eds. *The Principles and Practice of Medicine,* 22nd ed. Norwalk, Conn: Appleton & Lange; 1988.

18. Jenkins DB. *Hollinshead's Functional Anatomy of the Limbs and Back,* 7th ed. Philadelphia, Pa: WB Saunders; 1998.

19. Dumestre G. Long thoracic nerve palsy. J Manual Manip Ther 1995;3:44–49.

20. Gozna ER, Harris WR. Traumatic winging of the scapula. J Bone Joint Surg 1979;61A:1230–1233.

21. Kauppila LI. The long thoracic nerve: Possible mechanisms of injury based on autopsy study. J Shoulder Elbow Surg 1993;2:244–248.

22. Kauppila LI, Vastamaki M. Iatrogenic serratus anterior paralysis: Long-term outcome in 26 patients. Chest 1996;109:31–34.

23. Sunderland S. *Nerves and Nerve Injuries.* London, England: Churchill Livingstone; 1978.

24. White SM, Witten CM. Long thoracic nerve palsy in a professional ballet dancer. Am J Sports Med 1993; 21:626–629.

25. Jobe CM. Gross anatomy of the shoulder. In: Rockwood CA Jr, Matsen FA III (eds). *The Shoulder,* 2nd ed. Philadelphia, Pa: WB Saunders; 1998:34–98.

26. Connor PM, Yamaguchi K, Manifold SG, et al. Split pectoralis major transfer for serratus anterior palsy. Clin Orthop 1997;341:134–142.

27. Schultz JS, Leonard JA. Long thoracic neuropathy from athletic activity. Arch Phys Med Rehabil 1992; 73:87–90.

28. Gregg JR, Labosky D, Harty M, et al. Serratus anterior paralysis in the young athlete. J Bone Joint Surg 1979;61A:825–832.

29. Kendall FP, McCreary EK, Provance PG. *Muscle Testing and Function,* 4th ed. Baltimore, Md: Williams & Wilkins; 1993:284–287.

30. Kuhn JE, Plancher KD, Hawkins RJ. Scapular winging. J Am Acad Orthop Surg 1995;3:319–325.

31. Post M. Orthopaedic management of neuromuscular disorders. In: Post M, Bigliani LU, Flatow EL, Pollock RG, eds. *The Shoulder: Operative Technique.* Baltimore, Md: Williams & Wilkins; 1998:201–234.

32. Rcis FP, de Camargo AM, Vitti M, de Carvalho CA. Electromyographic study of the subclavius muscle. Acta Anatomica 1979;105:284–290.

33. Rengachary SS, Burr D, Lucas S, Hassanein KM, Mohn MP, Matzke H. Suprascapular entrapment neuropathy: a clinical, anatomical, and comparative study. Part 2: anatomical study. Neurosurgery 1979; 5(4):447–451.

34. Hoffman GW, Elliott LF. The anatomy of the pectoral nerves and its significance to the general and plastic surgeon. Ann Surg 1987;205:504.

35. Strauch B, Yu HL. *Atlas of Microvascular Surgery: Anatomy and Operative Approaches.* New York, NY: Thieme; 1993:390–391.

36. Perry J. Muscle control of the shoulder. In: Rowe C, ed. *The Shoulder.* New York, NY: Churchill Livingstone, 1988:17–34.

37. Kerr A. The brachial plexus of nerves in man, the variations in its formation and branches. Am J Anat 1918;23:285–376.

38. Wichman R. Die Rückenmarksnerven und ihre Segmentbezüge. In: Kerr A. The brachial plexus of nerves in man, the variations in its formation and branches. Am J Anat 1918;23:285–376.

39. Beghi E, Kurland LT, Mulder DW, Nicolosi A. Brachial plexus neuropathy in the population of Rochester, Minnesota, 1970–1981. Ann Neurol 1985;18:320–323.

40. Terzis JK, Liberson WT, Levine R. Obstetric brachial plexus palsy. Hand Clin 1986;2:773.

41. Terzis JK, Liberson WT, Levine R. Our experience in obstetrical brachial plexus palsy. In: Terzis JK, ed. *Microreconstruction of Nerve Injuries*. Philadelphia, Pa: WB Saunders; 1987:513.

42. Duchenne GBA. *De l'Électrisation localisée et de son application à la pathologie et à la thérapeutique par courants induits et par courants galvaniques interrompus et continus*, 3rd ed. Paris, France: Librairie JB Baillière et fils, 1872.

43. Erb W. Uber eine eigenthümliche Localisation von Lahmungen im plexus brachialis. Naturhist-Med Ver Heidelberg Verh 1874;2:130.

44. Al-Qattan MM, Clarke HM, Curtis CG. Klumpke's birth palsy: Does it really exist? J Hand Surg 1995;20B:19.

45. Klumpke A. Contribution à l'étude des paralysies radiculaires du plexus brachial. Rev Med 1885;5:739.

46. Brown KLB. Review of obstetrical palsies: Nonoperative treatment. Clin Plast Surg 1984;11:181.

47. Brown KLB. Review of obstetrical palsies: Nonoperative treatment. In: Terzis JK, ed. *Microreconstruction of Nerve Injuries*. Philadelphia, Pa: WB Saunders; 1987:499.

48. Gilbert A, Tassin J-L. Obstetrical palsy: A clinical, pathologic, and surgical review. In: Terzis JK, ed. *Microreconstruction of Nerve Injuries*. Philadelphia, Pa: WB Saunders; 1987:529.

49. Fawcett DW. The nervous tissue. In: Fawcett DW, ed. *Bloom and Fawcett: A Textbook of Histology*. New York, NY: Chapman & Hall; 1984:336–339.

50. Millesi H, Terzis JK. Nomenclature in peripheral nerve surgery. In: Terzis JK, ed. *Microreconstruction of Nerve Injuries*. Philadelphia, Pa: WB Saunders; 1987:3–13.

51. Thomas PK, Olsson Y. Microscopic anatomy and function of the connective tissue components of peripheral nerve. In: Dyck PJ, Thomas PK, Lambert EH, Bunge R, eds. *Peripheral Neuropathy*. Philadelphia, Pa: WB Saunders; 1984:97–120.

52. Delagi EF, Perotto A. Arm. In: Delagi EF, Perotto A, eds. *Anatomic Guide for the Electromyographer*, 2nd ed. Springfield, Ill: Charles C Thomas; 1981:66–71.

53. Sunderland S. The musculocutaneous nerve. In: Sunderland S, ed. *Nerves and Nerve Injuries*, 2nd ed. Edinburgh, Scotland: Churchill Livingstone; 1978:796–801.

54. de Moura WG Jr. Surgical anatomy of the musculocutaneous nerve: A photographic essay. J Reconstr Microsurg 1985;1:291–297.

55. Flatlow EL, Bigliani LU, April EW. An anatomic study of the musculocutaneous nerve and its relationship to the coracoid process. Clin Orthop 1989;244:166–171.

56. Dundore DE, DeLisa JA. Musculocutaneous nerve palsy: An isolated complication of surgery. Arch Phys Med Rehabil 1979;60:130–133.

57. Lusk MD, Kline DG, Garcia CA. Tumors of the brachial plexus. Neurosurgery 1987;21:439–453.

58. Braddom RL, Wolfe C. Musculocutaneous nerve injury after heavy exercise. Arch Phys Med Rehabil 1978;59:290–293.

59. Sander HW, Quinto CM, Elinzano H, Chokroverty S. Carpet carrier's palsy: Musculocutaneous neuropathy. Neurology 1997;48:1731–1732.

60. Mastaglia FL. Musculocutaneous neuropathy after strenuous physical activity. Med J Aust 1986;145:153–154.

61. Kim SM, Goodrich JA. Isolated musculocutaneous nerve palsy: a case report. Arch Phys Med Rehabil 1984;65:735–736.

62. Basmajian JV, Latif A. Integrated actions and functions of the chief flexors of the elbow. J Bone Joint Surg Am 1957;39:1106–1118.

63. Jones FW. Voluntary muscular movements in cases of nerve lesions. J Anat 1919;54:41–57.

64. Sunderland S: Voluntary movements and the deceptive action of muscles in peripheral nerve lesions. Aust N Z J Surg 1944;13:160–183.

65. Kendall FP, McCreary EK, Provance PG. Upper extremity and shoulder girdle strength tests. In: Kendall FP, McCreary EK, Provance PG, eds. *Muscles: Testing and Function*, 4th ed. Baltimore, Md: Williams & Wilkins; 1993:253–269.

66. Bartosh RA, Dugdale TW, Nielen R. Isolated musculocutaneous nerve injury complicating closed fracture of the clavicle: A case report. Am J Sports Med 1992;20:356–359.

67. Bierman W, Yamshon LJ. Electromyography in kinesiologic evaluations. Arch Phys Med Rehabil 1948;29:206–211.

68. Townsend H, Jobe FW, Pink M, Perry J. Electromyographic analysis of the glenohumeral muscles during a baseball rehabilitation program. Am J Sports Med 1991;19:264–272.

69. Drye C, Zachazewski JE. Peripheral nerve injuries. In: Zachazewski JE, Magee DJ, Quillen WS, eds. *Athletic Injuries and Rehabilitation*. Philadelphia, Pa: WB Saunders; 1996:441–463.

70. Capener N. The vulnerability of the posterior interosseous nerve of the forearm: A case report and an anatomical study. J Bone Joint Surg [Br] 1966;48-B:770–773.

71. Spinner M. *Injuries to the Major Branches of Peripheral Nerves of the Forearm*, 2nd ed. Philadelphia, Pa: WB Saunders; 1978.

72. Moon N, Marmor L. Periosteal lipoma of the proximal part of the radius: A clinical entity with frequent

medial-nerve injury. J Bone Joint Surg 1991;16:230–235.

73. Richmond DA. Lipoma causing posterior interosseous nerve lesion. J Bone Joint Surg [Br] 1953;35-B:83.

74. Bowen TL, Stone KH. Posterior interosseous nerve paralysis caused by a ganglion at the elbow. J Bone Joint Surg [Br] 1966;48-B:774–776.

75. Sharrard WJW. Posterior interosseous neuritis. J Bone Joint Surg [Br] 1966;48-B:777–780.

76. Marmor L, Lawrence JF, Dubois EL. Posterior interosseous nerve palsy due to rheumatoid arthritis. J Bone Joint Surg [Am] 1967;49-A:381–383.

77. White SH, Goodfellow JW, Mowat A. Posterior interosseous nerve palsy in rheumatoid arthritis. J Bone Joint Surg [Br] 1988;70-B:468–471.

78. Furusawa S, Hara T, Maehiro S, Shiba M, Kondo T. Neuralgic amyotrophy. Seikeigeka 1969;20:1286–1290.

79. Hashizume H, Inoue H, Nagashima K, Hamaya K. Posterior interosseous nerve paralysis related to focal radial nerve constriction secondary to vasculitis. J Hand Surg [Br] 1993;18-B:757–760.

80. Kotani H, Miki T, Senzoku F, Nakagawa Y, Ueo T. Posterior interosseous nerve paralysis with multiple constrictions. J Hand Surg [Am] 1995;20:15–17.

81. Lichter RL, Jacobsen T. Tardy palsy of the posterior interosseous nerve with a Monteggia fracture. J Bone Joint Surg [Am] 1975;57-A:124–125.

82. Hashizume H, Nishida K, Yamamoto K, Hirooka T, Inoue H. Delayed posterior interosseous nerve palsy. J Hand Surg [Br] 1995;20:655–657.

83. Maffulli N, Maffulli F. Transient entrapment neuropathy of the posterior interosseous nerve in violin players. J Neurol Neurosurg Psychiatry 1991;54:65–67.

84. Weinberger LM. Non-traumatic paralysis of the dorsal interosseous nerve. Surg Gynec Obstet 1939;69:358–363.

85. Kopell HP, Thompson WAL. Peripheral entrapment neuropathies. Baltimore, Md: Williams & Wilkins; 1963.

86. Hollinshead WH. Anatomy for Surgeons, 3rd ed, vol 3. Philadelphia, Pa: Harper & Row; 1982:409.

87. Stern PJ, Kutz JE. An unusual variant of the anterior interosseous nerve syndrome: A case report and review of the literature. J Hand Surg 1980;5:32–34.

88. Hope PG. Anterior interosseous nerve palsy following internal fixation of the proximal radius. J Bone Joint Surg 1988;70-B:280–282.

89. Sunderland S. Nerves and Nerve Injuries, 2nd ed. Edinburgh, Scotland: Churchill Livingstone; 1978.

90. Gunther SF, DiPasquale D, Martin R. Struthers' ligament and associated median nerve variations in a cadaveric specimen. Yale J Biol Med 1993;66:203–208.

91. Maeda K, Miura T, Komada T, Chiba A. Anterior interosseous nerve paralysis: Report of 13 cases and review of Japanese literatures. Hand 1977;9:165–171.

92. Hirasawa K. Plexus brachialis und die Nerven der oberen Extremitat. Anat Inst Kaiserlichen Universitat Kyoto Series A 1931;2:135–140.

93. Thomson A. Third annual report of the Committee of Collective Investigation of the Anatomical Society of Great Britain and Ireland for the year 1891–1892. J Anat Physiol 1893;27:192–194.

94. Chusid JG. Correlative Neuroanatomy & Functional Neurology, 19th ed. Norwalk, Conn: Appleton-Century-Crofts; 1985:144–148.

95. Stevens JC, Sun S, Beard CM, O'Fallon WM, Kurband LT. Carpal tunnel syndrome in Rochester, Minnesota, 1961 to 1980. Neurology 1988;38:134–138.

96. Occupational disease surveillance: Carpal tunnel syndrome. MMWR Morb Mortal Wkly Rep 1989;38:485–489.

97. de Krom MCTFM, Knipschild PG, Kester ADM, Thijs CT, Boekkooi PF, Spaans F. Carpal tunnel syndrome: Prevalence in the general population. J Clin Epidemiol 1992;45:373–376.

98. D'Arcy CA, McGee S. Does this patient have carpal tunnel syndrome? JAMA 2000;283:3110–3117.

99. Stewart JD, Eisen A. Tinel's sign and the carpal tunnel syndrome. BMJ 1978;2:1125–1126.

100. Gellman H, Gelberman RH, Tan AM, Botte MJ. Carpal tunnel syndrome: An evaluation of the provocative diagnostic tests. J Bone Joint Surg [Am] 1986;68:735–737.

101. Rosenbaum RB, Ochoa JL. Carpal Tunnel Syndrome and Other Disorders of the Median Nerve. Boston, Mass: Butterworth-Heinemann; 1993.

102. Katz JN, Larson MG, Sabra A, et al. The carpal tunnel syndrome: Diagnostic utility of the history and physical examination findings. Ann Intern Med 1990;112:321–327.

103. Loong SC. The carpal tunnel syndrome: A clinical and electrophysiological study of 250 patients. Proc Aust Assoc Neurol 1977;14:51–65.

104. Rempel DM, Harrison RJ, Barnhart S. Work-related cumulative trauma disorders of the upper extremity. JAMA 1992;267:838–842.

105. Khoo D, Carmichael SW, Spinner RJ. Ulnar nerve anatomy and compression. Orthop Clin North Am 1996;27:317–338.

106. Apfelberg DB, Larson SJ. Dynamic anatomy of the ulnar nerve at the elbow. Plast Reconstr Surg 1973;51:76–81.

107. Idler RS. General principles of patient evaluation and nonoperative management of cubital syndrome. Hand Clin 1996;12:397–403.

108. O'Driscoll SW, Horii E, Carmichael SE, et al. The cubital tunnel and ulnar neuropathy. J Bone Joint Surg 1991;73B:613–617.

109. Amadio PC, Beckenbaugh RD. Entrapment of the ulnar nerve by the deep flexor-pronator aponeurosis. J Hand Surg 1986;11A:83–87.

110. Hirasawa Y, Sawamura H, Sakakida K. Entrapment neuropathy due to bilateral epitrochlearis muscles: A case report. J Hand Surg 1979;4:181–184.

111. Sunderland S. The ulnar nerve. Anatomical features. In: *Nerves and Nerve Injuries*. Edinburgh, Scotland: E & S Livingstone; 1968:816–828.

112. Lundborg G. Surgical treatment for ulnar nerve entrapment at the elbow. J Hand Surg 1992;17B:245–247.

113. Vanderpool DW, Chalmers J, Lamb DW, Whiston TB. Peripheral compression lesions of the ulnar nerve. J Bone Joint Surg 1968;50B:792–803.

114. Mannheimer JS, Lampe GN. Electrode placement sites and their relationship. In: Mannheimer JS, Lampe GN, eds. *Clinical Transcutaneous Electrical Nerve Stimulation*. Philadelphia, Pa: FA Davis; 1984.

115. Williams PL, ed. *Gray's Anatomy*, 38th ed. New York, NY: Churchill Livingstone; 1995.

116. McMinn RMH, ed. *Last's Anatomy: Regional and Applied*, 9th ed. New York, NY: Churchill Livingstone; 1994.

117. Awerbuch GI, Nigro MA, Wishnow R. Beevor's sign and facioscapulohumeral dystrophy. Arch Neurol 1990;47:1208–1209.

118. Warfel BS, Marini SG, Lachmann EA, Nagler W. Delayed femoral nerve palsy following femoral vessel catheterization. Arch Phys Med Rehabil 1993;74:1211–1215.

119. Hardy SL. Femoral nerve palsy associated with an associated posterior wall transverse acetabular fracture. J Orthop Trauma 1997;11:40–42.

120. Papastefanou SL, Stevens K, Mulholland RC. Femoral nerve palsy: An unusual complication of anterior lumbar interbody fusion. Spine 1994;19:2842–2844.

121. Weale AE, Newman P, Ferguson IT, Bannister GC. Nerve injury after posterior and direct lateral approaches for hip replacement. A clinical and electrophysiological study. J Bone Joint Surg [Br] 1996;78:899–902.

122. Goodfellow J, Fearn CBD'A, Matthews JM. Iliacus haematoma: A common complication of haemophilia. J Bone Joint Surg [Br] 1967;49:748–756.

123. Sreeram S, Lumsden AB, Miller JS, et al. Retroperitoneal hematoma following femoral arterial catheterization: A serious and often fatal complication. Am Surg 1993;59:94–98.

124. Fealy S, Paletta GA Jr. Femoral nerve palsy secondary to traumatic iliacus muscle hematoma: Course after nonoperative management. J Trauma-Injury Infect Crit Care 1999;47:1150–1152.

125. Gray H. Neurology. In: Williams P, Warwick R, eds. *Gray's Anatomy*, 36th ed. London, England: Churchill Livingstone; 1990:1108.

126. Ashby EC. Chronic obscure groin pain is commonly caused by enthesopathy: "Tennis elbow" of the groin. Br J Surg 1994;81:1632–1634.

127. Martens MA, Hansen L, Mulier JC. Adductor tendinitis and musculus rectus abdominis tendonopathy. Am J Sports Med 1987;15:353–356.

128. Zimmerman G. Groin pain in athletes. Aust Fam Physician 1988;17:1046–1052.

129. Bradshaw C, McCrory P, Bell S, Bruckner P. Obturator neuropathy: A cause of chronic groin pain in athletes. Am J Sports Med 1997;25:402–408.

130. Harvey G, Bell S. Obturator neuropathy. An anatomic perspective. Clin Orthop Rel Res 1999;363:203–211.

131. Ecker AD, Woltman HW. Meralgia paresthetica: A report of one hundred and fifty cases. JAMA 1938;110:1650–1652.

132. Keegan JJ, Holyoke EA. Meralgia paresthetica: An anatomical and surgical study. J Neurosurg 1962;19:341–345.

133. Reichert FL. Meralgia paresthetica: A form of causalgia relieved by interruption of the sympathetic fibers. Surg Clin North Am 1933;13:1443.

134. Edelson JG, Nathan H. Meralgia paresthetica. Clin Orthop 1977;122:255–262.

135. Ghent WR. Further studies in meralgia paresthetica. Can Med Assn J 1961;85:871–875.

136. Seddon HJ. *Surgical Disorders of Peripheral Nerves*, 2nd ed. Edinburgh, Scotland: Churchill Livingstone; 1975:124.

137. Sunderland S. Traumatized nerves, roots and ganglia: Musculoskeletal factors and neuropathological consequences. In: Knorr IM, Huntwork EH, eds. *The Neurobiologic Mechanisms in Manipulative Therapy*, vol. 11. New York, NY: Plenum Press; 1978:137–166.

138. Hager W. Neuralgia femoris. Resection des Nerv. cutan. femoris anterior externus. Heilung Dtsch Med Wochenschr 1885;11:218.

139. Bernhardt M. Ueber isolirt im Gebiete des Nervus cutaneus femoris externus vorkommende parasthesien. Neurol Centralbl 1895;14:242–244.

140. Roth VK. Meralgia paraesthetica. Med Obozr Mosk 1895;43:678.

141. Nathan H. Gangliform enlargement of the lateral cutaneous nerve of the thigh: Its significance on the understanding of meralgia paresthetica. J Neurosurg 1960;17:843.

142. Stookey B. Meralgia paraesthetica: Etiology and surgical treatment. JAMA 1928;90:1705.

143. Dellon AL, Mackinnon SE, Seiler WA IV. Susceptibility of the diabetic nerve to chronic compression. Ann Plast Surg 1988;20:117.

144. Asbury AK. Focal and multifocal neuropathies of diabetes. In: Dyck PJ, Thomas PK, Winegrad AI, Porte D, eds. *Diabetic Neuropathy.* Philadelphia, Pa: WB Saunders; 1987:45–55.

145. Macnicol MF, Thompson WJ. Idiopathic meralgia paresthetica. Clin Orthop 1990;254:270.

146. Lee FC. An osteoplastic neurolysis operation for the cure of meralgia paresthetica. Ann Surg 1941;113:85.

147. Stookey B. Meralgia paraesthetica: Etiology and surgical treatment. JAMA 1928;90:1705.

148. Ecker AD, Woltman HW. Meralgia paraesthetica: A report of one hundred and fifty cases. JAMA 1938;110:1650–1652.

149. Massey EW, O'Brian JT. Mononeuropathy in diabetes mellitus. Postgrad Med 1979;65:128.

150. Nahabedian MY, Dellon AL. Meralgia paresthetica: Etiology, diagnosis and outcome of surgical decompression. Ann Plast Surg 1995;35:590.

151. Netter FH. Lumbar, sacral, and coccygeal plexuses. In: *Nervous System,* pt I. (The CIBA collection of medical illustrations; vol. 1) West Caldwell, NJ: Ciba, 1991:122–123.

152. Sogaard I. Sciatic nerve entrapment: Case report. J Neurosurg 1983;58:275–276.

153. Robinson DR. Pyriformis syndrome in relation to sciatic pain. Am J Surg 1947;73:355–358.

154. Benyahya E, Etaouil N, Janani S, et al. Sciatica as the first manifestation of leiomyosarcoma of the buttock. Rev Rheum 1997;64:135–137.

155. Lamki N, Hutton L, Wall WJ, Rorabeck CH. Computed tomography in pelvic liposarcoma: A case report. J Comput Tomogr 1984;8:249–251.

156. Bickels J, Kahanovitz N, Rubert CK, et al. Extraspinal bone and soft-tissue tumors as a cause of sciatica. Clinical diagnosis and recommendations: Analysis of 32 cases. Spine 1999;24:1611–1616.

157. Kenny P, O'Brien CP, Synnott K, Walsh MG. Damage to the superior gluteal nerve after two different approaches to the hip. J Bone Joint Surg [Br] 1999;81:979–981.

158. Lu J, Ebraheim NA, Huntoon M, Heck BE, Yeasting RA. Anatomic considerations of superior cluneal nerve at posterior iliac crest region. Clin Orthop Rel Res 1998;347:224–228.

159. Garvey TA, Marks MR, Wiesel SW. A prospective, randomized, double-blind evaluation of trigger point injection therapy for low-back pain. Spine 1989;14:962–964.

160. Luk KDK, Ho HC, Leong JCY. The iliolumbar ligament: A study of its anatomy, development and clinical significance. J Bone Joint Surg 1986;68B:197–200.

161. Maigne JY, Maigne R. Trigger point of the posterior iliac crest: Painful iliolumbar ligament insertion or cutaneous dorsal ramus pain? An anatomic study. Arch Phys Med Rehabil 1991;72:734–737.

162. Basadonna PT, Gasparini D, Rucco V. Iliolumbar ligament insertions: In vivo anatomic study. Spine 1996;21:2313–2316.

163. Cooper JW. Cluneal nerve injury and chronic postsurgical neuritis [abstract]. J Bone Joint Surg 1967;49A:199.

164. Neurology. In: Williams PL, Warwick R, Dyson M, Bannister LH, eds. *Gray's Anatomy.* 37th ed. London, England: Churchill Livingstone; 1989:1145–1148.

165. Keck C. The tarsal tunnel syndrome. J Bone Joint Surg 1962;44A:180–182.

166. Lam S. A tarsal tunnel syndrome. Lancet 1962;2:1354–1355.

167. DiStefano V, Sack J, Whittaker R, Nixon J. Tarsal tunnel syndrome: Review of the literature and two case reports. Clin Orthop 1972;88:76–79.

168. Edwards W, Lincoln C, Bassett F, Goldner J. The tarsal tunnel syndrome: Diagnosis and treatment. JAMA 1969;207:716–720.

169. Radin E. Tarsal tunnel syndrome. Clin Orthop 1983;181:167–170.

170. Schmalzried TP, Amstutz HC, Dorey FJ. Nerve palsy associated with total hip replacement. J Bone J Surg 1991;73A:1074–1080.

171. Resnick D. *Diagnosis of Bone and Joint Disorders,* 3rd ed. Philadelphia, Pa: WB Saunders; 1995:2773–2777,3400.

172. Ohsawa K, Nishida T, Kurohmaru M, Hayashi Y. Distribution pattern of pudendal nerve plexus for the phallus retractor muscles in the cock. Okajimas Folia Anat Jpn 1991;67:439–441.

173. Upton RM, McComas AJ. The double crush in nerve entrapment syndromes. Lancet 1973;2:359–362.

174. Dahlin LB, Lundborg G. The neurone and its response to peripheral nerve compression. J Hand Surg [Br] 1990;15:5–10.

175. Narakas AO. The role of thoracic outlet syndrome in double crush syndrome. Ann Chir Main Memb Super 1990;9:331–340.

176. Wood VE, Biondi J. Double-crush nerve compression in thoracic-outlet syndrome. J Bone Joint Surg [Am] 1990;72A:85–88.

177. Dellon Al, Mackinnon SE. Chronic nerve compression model for the double crush hypothesis. Ann Plast Surg [Br] 1991;26:259–264.

178. Nemoto K, Matsumoto N, Tazaki K-I, Horiuchi Y, Uchinshi K-I, Mori Y. An experimental study on the "double crush" hypothesis. J Hand Surg [Br] 1987;12A:552–559.

179. Seiler WA, Schelgel R, Mackinnon S, Dellon AL. Double crush syndrome: Experimental model in the rat. Surg Forum 1983;34:596–598.

180. Swensen RS. The "double crush" syndrome. Neurol Chronicle 1994;4:1–6.

181. Pećina MM, Krmpotić-Nemanić J, Markiewitz AD. *Tunnel Syndromes: Peripheral Nerve Compression Syndromes,* 2nd ed. Boca Raton, Fla: CRC Press;1996.

182. Benson ER, Schutzer SF. Posttraumatic piriformis syndrome: Diagnosis and results of operative treatment. J Bone Joint Surg [Am] 1999;81:941–949.

183. Yeoman W. The relation of arthritis of the sacro-iliac joint to sciatica, with an analysis of 100 cases. Lancet 1928;2:1119–1122.

184. Levin PH. JAMA 1924;82:965.

185. Freiberg AH. Sciatic pain and its relief by operations on muscle and fascia. Arch Surg 1937;34:337–350.

186. Beaton LE, Anson BJ. The sciatic nerve and the piriformis muscle: their interrelation a possible cause of coccygodynia. J Bone Joint Surg 1938;20:686–688.

187. Pace JB, Nagle D. Piriformis syndrome. Western J Med 1976;124:435–439.

188. Robinson DR. Pyriformis syndrome in relation to sciatic pain. Am J Surg 1947;73:355–358.

189. Pećina M. Contribution to the etiological explanation of the piriformis syndrome. Acta Anat 1979; 105(2):181–187.

190. Barton PM. Piriformis syndrome: a rationale approach to management. Pain 1991;47(3):345–352.

CHAPTER SEVEN

THE INTERVERTEBRAL DISC

Chapter Objectives

At the completion of this chapter, the reader will be able to:

1. List the various components of the intervertebral disc.
2. Describe the chemical makeup and function of each of the intervertebral components.
3. Define the similarities and differences of the disc in each spinal area.
4. Describe the pathologic processes involved with disc degeneration and disc degradation.
5. Describe the differences between a protrusion, an extrusion, and a sequestration.
6. Identify the various forces that act on the disc and how the disc responds.
7. List the characteristics of a disc impairment at each segmental level.
8. Use various strategies to treat disc impairments.

OVERVIEW

Phylogenically, the intervertebral disc is a relatively new structure, which evolved to handle the twin problems of weight bearing and motion. The presence of a disc, not only allows free motion in any direction, up to the point that the disc itself is stretched, but also allows for a significant increase in the weight bearing capabilities of the spine.

The intervertebral disc is composed of three parts, the anulus, the vertebral end plate and the nucleus pulposus (Fig. 7–1). The nucleus pulposus sits in, or near, the center of the disc, lying slightly more posteriorly than anteriorly, and surrounded by an anulus fibrosis. Although the nucleus pulposus and anulus fibrosis are quite distinct entities, except in youth, no clear boundary exists between the anulus and the peripheral parts of the nucleus pulposus that merge together. The two vertebral end plates are the third component of the intervertebral disc. Each vertebral end plate consists of a layer of cartilage, which covers the top or bottom aspects of the disc, separating the disc from the adjacent vertebral body.

The intervertebral disc forms a symphysis or amphiarthrosis between two adjacent vertebrae, functioning to:

- Increase the potential range of motion between vertebrae.
- Maintain contiguity between the vertebral bodies.
- Attenuate and transfer vertebral loading.

Anulus Fibrosis

The anulus fibrosis consists of approximately 10 to 12 (often as many as 15 to 25) concentric sheets[1] of collagen tissue, whose fibers are oriented at about 65 degrees from vertical. The fibers of each successive sheet or lamella maintain the same inclination of 65 degrees, but in the opposite direction to the preceding lamella, resulting in every second sheet having the same orientation. Only 50% of the fibers work at any given time. The number of layers decreases with age, but the remaining layers get thicker. Incomplete lamellae, ones that do not pass around the circumference of the disc, seem to be more frequent in the middle portions of the anulus.[2] There are three types of orientation for the lamella, all of which involve a blending of the sheets into junctions (two sheets become one, or three sheets blend into one).

Each lamella is thicker anteriorly than posteriorly, leading to the disc being thinner posteriorly than anteriorly. The lamellae are also thicker toward the center of the disc.[3] In addition, the shape of the posterior aspect of the anulus is concave, and this results in a tighter packing of the collagen in this area than anteriorly, resulting in the posterior aspect of the anulus being thinner than the other aspects.[4]

Consequently, the posterior part of the anulus has thin but stronger fibers, and it is capable of withstanding

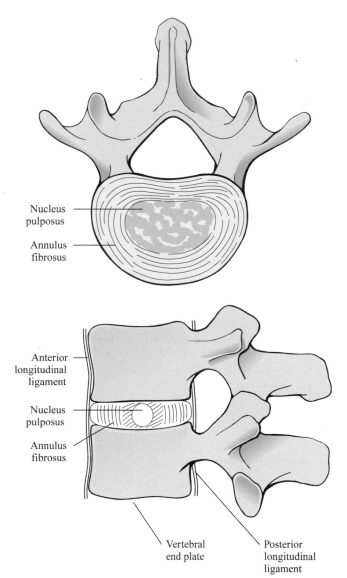

Nucleus
pulposus

Annulus
fibrosus

Anterior
longitudinal
ligament

Nucleus
pulposus

Annulus
fibrosus

Vertebral
end plate

Posterior
longitudinal
ligament

FIGURE 7–1 Intervertebral disc—lateral and superior view.

the tension applied to this area during flexion activities and postures that occur more frequently than with extension.[5]

The intervertebral joint operates as an osmotic system. Fluid flow is caused by pressure changes on the disc. Increased load causes fluid to be expelled, whereas low pressure allows the disc to suck in fluid from the surrounding tissues. Two main anatomic and biomechanical properties make the posterior aspect of the disc vulnerable. These are:

1. The posterior part of the nuclear annular boundary receives less nutrition.
2. The posterior longitudinal ligament affords only weak reinforcement.

This is unfortunate because all of the nociceptive tissues responsible for backache and sciatica emerge from just beyond the posterior aspect of the disc. Clinically, if the anulus is damaged, subjective complaints of pain increase with sustained traction as this leads to further breakdown of the anulus.

Only the most peripheral annular fibers receive a blood supply, and this comes from the metaphyseal arteries that anastomose on the outer surface of the anulus. Nutrition of the disc comes via a diffusion of nutrients from the anastomosis over the anulus and from the arterial plexi underlying the end plate. Almost the entire anulus is permeable to the nutrients, in contrast to only the center portions of the end plate. In addition, there is some evidence that a mechanical pump action also aids nutrition. This is one of the proposed mechanisms attributed to the success of repeated motions in the McKenzie exercise protocols for the spine.

Vertebral End Plates

Each vertebral end plate is a layer of cartilage about 0.6 to 1 mm thick[6] that covers the area on the vertebral body. Peripherally, the end plate abuts and attaches to the ring apophysis. Over about 10% of the surface of the end plate, the subchondral bone of the centrum is deficient and, at these points, the bone marrow is in direct contact with the end plate, thereby augmenting the nutrition of the disc and end plate. Because the adult disc has no blood supply, it relies on diffusion for nutrition.[7]

The two end plates of each disc, therefore, cover the nucleus pulposus in its entirety, but fail to cover the entire extent of the anulus fibrosis. The collagen of the inner lamellae of the anulus enters the end plate and swings centrally within it.[8] By tracing these fibers along their entire length, it can be seen that the nucleus pulposus is enclosed around all aspects by a sphere of collagen fibers, more or less like a capsule.[5]

Because of the attachment of the anulus fibrosis to the vertebral end plates on the periphery, the end plates arc strongly bound to the intervertebral disc. In contrast, the vertebral end plates are only weakly attached to the vertebral bodies.[9] Thus, the end plates are regarded as constituents of the intervertebral disc, rather than as a part of the vertebral body.[10]

At birth, the end plate is part of the vertebral body growth plate, but by the 20th year, it has been separated from the body by a subchondral plate. During this time, the plate is bilaminar, with a growth zone and an articular area. Gradually, the growth zone becomes thinner and disappears so that, by the end of this period, it leaves only a thickened articular plate. The end plate in younger subjects consists of hyaline and fibrocartilage, with hyaline dominating toward the vertebral body and fibrocartilage nearer the nucleus.[5] Between 20 and 65 years, the end plate thins and the vascular foramina in the subchondral bone become occluded, resulting in decreased nutrition to the disc. In old age, the plate consists entirely of fibrocartilage, formed by the collagen of the inner lamellae of the anulus. At the same time, the underlying bone becomes weaker, and the end plate gradually bows into the vertebral body, becoming more vulnerable centrally, where it may fracture into the centrum.[5] The presence of damage to a vertebral body end plate reduces the pressure in the nucleus of adjacent disc by up to 57%, and doubles the size of "stress peaks" in the posterior anulus.[11] Other structural changes in the disc that increase the space available for the nucleus, such as radial fissures or posterior disc prolapse, have a similar effect.[12]

Clinical findings for an isolated vertebral end plate fracture are an increase in pain with manual traction or compression, as well as the typical signs and symptoms of an inflammatory reaction. No neurologic signs are typically present, and the intervention usually involves bed rest in the acute stage.

Nucleus Pulposus

The intervertebral discs of a healthy young adult contain a nucleus pulposus that is composed of a semifluid mass of mucoid material (with the consistency more or less of toothpaste).[5] In the second and third decades, the nucleus is clear, firm, and gelatinous, but subsequently it becomes drier as the water content decreases with age. At birth, the water content of the nucleus is about 80% of the nucleus. In the elderly, the water content is about 68%. Most of this water content change occurs in childhood and adolescence, with only about 6% occurring in adulthood.[13]

Within the structural framework of the intervertebral disc, collagen plays a pivotal role. It is well established that in normal intervertebral discs, seven collagen types occur (i.e., types I, II, III, V, VI, IX, and XI[14-18]). Their proportion, however, varies between the different structures. There is an inverse "gradient" of collagen types I and II from the outer anulus fibrosus to the nucleus pulposus.[19] Accordingly, the anulus fibrosus contains more collagen type I (fibrous) than type II (elastic), whereas the nucleus pulposus is composed mainly of collagen type II. Besides these major collagens, the so-called minor collagen types, mainly types III, V, VI, IX, and XI, have a particular role in the organization of the collagen fibrils and are, therefore, essential for disc biomechanics, despite their low percentage within the disc tissue.

The biomechanical makeup of the nucleus is similar to that of the anulus except that the nucleus has higher content of water (70% to 90%)[20] whereas the anulus, at 60% to 70% of water,[21] has a higher concentration of collagen (50% to 60% of the dry weight) and proteoglycans (20%).

The cartilage cells are located primarily near the end plates and are responsible for the synthesis of the nuclear collagen and proteoglycans. The water provides the fluid properties of the nucleus, and the collagen and proteoglycans, its viscosity.

ALTERATIONS IN DISC STRUCTURE

Although the intervertebral disc appears destined for tissue regression and destruction, it remains unclear why similar age-related changes remain asymptomatic in one individual and may cause severe low back pain in others, although the basic changes that influence the responses of the disc to aging are biochemical. In early adulthood, the proteoglycan content of the dry weight of the nucleus is about 65%; by 60 years, this has dropped to 30%.[22] In addition, the proteoglycan content also changes, with a decrease in the concentration of chondroitin sulphate. As the keratin sulphate level remains constant, this decrease results in a relative rise in the keratin sulphate level. Chondroitin sulphate is the major substance that binds water to the proteoglycans, and its loss results in a decreased water content in the nucleus. However, most of the water loss occurs early in life, so the mechanism is thought to be more subtle than this alone, and may concern the collagen content levels in the nucleus.

There is, with age, an increase in the collagen content[23] of both the nucleus and anulus and also a change in the type of collagen present. The elastic collagen of the nucleus becomes more fibrous, whereas the type 1 collagen of the anulus becomes more elastic.[23] Eventually, they come to resemble each other. In addition, the concentration of noncollagenous proteins increases in the nucleus. These changes in the makeup of the collagen alter the biomechanical properties of the disc, making it less resilient and perhaps leading to changes from microtrauma. It is thought that the altered relationships between the proteoglycans and the collagen protein may be responsible for the early life alteration in the water content of the disc.[23]

In general, with age, the disc becomes drier, stiffer, less deformable, and less able to recover from creep, a process that can be delayed through a course of regular stretching. Although an individual becomes shorter in height throughout late adult life, the cause of this height change has always been attributed to the alteration in disc height that occurs with aging as a result of the aforementioned biomechanical changes. More recently, it has been demonstrated that the disc actually increases its height with age by about 10% between the ages of 20 and 70 years, and that the loss of height with age occurs because of erosion of the end plate of the disc.[24]

As the disc becomes more fibrous, the distinction between the anulus and nucleus is minimized. The handling of the compressive load becomes compromised, and more weight is taken by the anulus. This function, for which it is not designed, causes a separation of the lamellae and the formation of cavities within it.[23]

Between 2 and 7 years of age, the lumbar disc is a biconcave structure interposed by the convex surfaces of the centra, but in later childhood, all of the surfaces reverse their shape. As childhood progresses, the thickness of the disc increases, with L4 increasing 3 to 10 mm between birth and 12 years of age.[5] Up to the age of 8 years, the cartilaginous end plates are penetrated by blood vessels passing into the peripheral layers of the nucleus and anulus. Thereafter, the disc nutrition is achieved by diffusion through the end plate. The outermost layer of the anulus is attached to the vertebral body by mingling with the periosteal fibers (fibers of Sharpey). The outer two-thirds of the anulus fibrosus are attached firmly to the cartilaginous end plate, but the inner third is more loosely attached.[5]

The proper organization and interactions of the human lumbar intervertebral disc are a fundamental requirement for adequate biomechanical function of the intervertebral discs. Under normal conditions, the central gelatinous nucleus pulposus is contained by the anulus fibrosus, and the longitudinal ligaments provide added stability. Any disturbance of the balance of these tissue structures leads invariably to tissue destruction and functional impairment,[25–27] and may result in low back pain.

Embryologically, the lower half of the lumbar vertebra and the upper half of the one below it, originate from the same segment.

Degeneration seems to start early in the upper lumbar spine, with end plate fractures and Schmorl's nodes related to the vertical loading of those segments.[23] Autopsy results show that disc degeneration begins at 20 to 25 years of age.[28] One study provided evidence that a family history of operated lumbar disc herniation has a significant implication in lumbar degenerative disc disease, indicating that there may be a genetic factor in the development of lumbar disc herniation as an expression of disc degeneration.[29]

The posterior-lateral aspect of the anulus tends to weaken first and develops clefts and tears. If the inner layers of the posterior anulus tear in the presence of the nucleus pulposus, which is still capable of bulging into the space left by the tear, the symptoms of disc disease are likely to be experienced. The size of the tear will determine the outcome.

- *Protrusion or herniation.* The nuclear material bulges outward through the tear to strain, but not escape from, the outer anulus or the posterior longitudinal ligament (Fig. 7–2). This usually results in a deep,

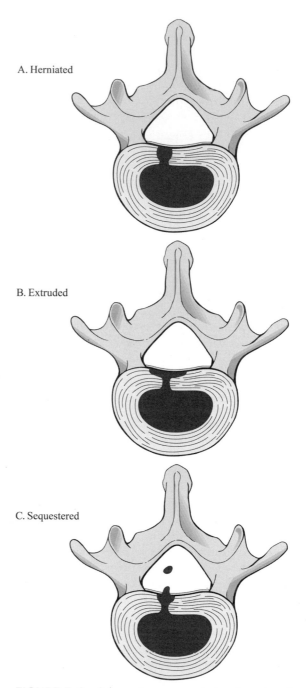

A. Herniated

B. Extruded

C. Sequestered

FIGURE 7–2   Schematic representation for a herniated, extruded, and sequestered intervertebral disc.

somatic type of pain that is localized. Because the nucleus is still contained, the patient is likely to feel more pain in the morning after the nucleus has imbibed more fluid, resulting in added volume and a subsequent increase in pressure on pain-sensitive structures. Recent attention has been given to the internal disruption of the nucleus, termed the *contained herniation*,[30] in which the nucleus becomes inflamed and invaginates itself between the anular layers. Compression of the disc during sitting and bending increases the pain, as the nociceptive structures within the anulus are further irritated. There is usually no or minimal leg pain and no or minimal limitation in the straight leg raise.

- *Prolapse or extrusion.* The nuclear material remains attached to the disc but escapes the anulus or the posterior longitudinal ligament to bulge externally into the intervertebral, or neural, canal (see Fig. 7–2).
- *Sequestration.* The migrating nuclear material escapes contact with the disc entirely and is a free fragment in the intervertebral canal (see Fig. 7–2).

Prolapses and sequestrations impinge on nerve tissue. Central prolapses, although fairly rare, may produce upper motor neuron impairments if they occur in the cervical spine, and bowel, or bladder impairments if they occur in the lumbar spine. As part of its unnatural history, the disc may travel through each stage of herniation sequentially, producing symptoms that range from backache to bilateral sciatica.

The effects of a disc impairment depend on its size, position, and segmental level. A substantial compression of the root affects the nerve fibers, producing paresthesia and interference with conduction. Mixter and Barr[31] suggested that tissue of the intervertebral disc protrudes into the spinal canal, compressing and therefore irritating the nerve root and causing sciatic pain. Although this concept is widely accepted, the mechanical compression of the nerve root itself does not explain sciatic pain and radiculopathy.[32,33] The operative finding that mechanically compressed nerve roots become tender[32,34,35] and results of recent histologic and biochemical studies on herniated lumbar disc tissue led to the notion of inflammatory-induced sciatic pain.

Low back pain with or without radiculopathy is a significant clinical problem, but the cause of low back pain and the exact pathophysiology of lumbar pain and sciatica often remain unclear. In patients with sciatic pain from disc herniation, radiographic examinations such as myelograms, computed tomographic (CT) scans, and magnetic resonance imaging (MRI) scans demonstrate nerve root compression by a herniated disc. However, approximately 20% to 30% of individuals without any history of sciatic pain have abnormal findings in radiographic examinations.[36,37] Recent models of lumbar radiculopathy suggest that the mechanisms underlying thermal hyperalgesia are probably caused, in part, by a local chemical irritant, an autoimmune reaction from exposure to disc tissues, an increased concentration of lactic acid, or a lower pH around the nerve roots.[38]

Inflammation certainly could play some part in the pathophysiology of discogenic lumbar radiculopathy.

Investigators have repeatedly demonstrated inflammatory cells, proinflammatory enzyme phospholipase A2, immunoglobulins, and various inflammatory mediators in herniated disc tissues.[38–44,52,53] Several investigators have hypothesized that the adult nucleus pulposus is somehow concealed from the immune system, and that the exposure of nuclear disc material to the circulatory system provokes an autoimmune reaction. Some credibility is given to this with the identification of antibodies to nucleus pulposus in patients' sera and in animal models.[45,54–57] It is also thought that neovascularization in herniated disc tissue could promote the formation of granulation tissue[46–48] and, in association with blood vessels, deposits of immunoglobulins have been reported.[49,50]

A recent experimental study in dogs placed the nucleus pulposus adjacent to the nerve root without mechanical compression. After 1 week, new blood vessels and infiltration of inflammatory cells, including lymphocytes and macrophages, were observed in the transplanted nucleus pulposus.[62]

Presence of inflammation in disc herniations could explain the clinical findings of improvement in radicular pain following the administration of corticosteroid or nonsteroidal anti-inflammatory agents.[51,60,61]

However, the occurrence of inflammatory cells has not so far been related to the duration of radicular pain symptoms.

Degeneration

Degenerative changes are the body's attempts at self-healing. If part of this healing involves the stabilization of an unstable joint, the joint can be immobilized by muscle spasms, or by increasing the surface area of the joint.[63]

The biology of intervertebral disc degeneration is not well understood. As alluded to, it is known that the matrix of the nucleus pulposus is rich in proteoglycans, whereas the anulus fibrosus is predominantly collagenous.[8] The proteoglycan content of the disc declines with age, a process that, at least partly, reflects decreased synthesis of these macromolecules by the disc cells.[26,64] Although the reasons for this decline are unknown, any reduction in proteoglycan content could have severe consequences for the disc's ability to resist mechanical loads.

The clinical syndromes associated with degenerative disc disease include:[65–69]

- Idiopathic low back pain
- Cervical and lumbar radiculopathy
- Cervical myelopathy
- Lumbar stenosis
- Spondylosis
- Osteoarthritis
- Herniated disc (degenerative disc disease)

TABLE 7–1 PHASES OF DEGENERATION[70]

PHASE	ZYGAPOPHYSIAL JOINTS	THREE-JOINT COMPLEX	INTERVERTEBRAL DISC
Early dysfunction	Synovitis and effusion Early cartilage destruction Painful facet syndrome	Minor pathologic changes	Circumferential tears in anulus Possible herniation secondary to radial tears
Intermediate instability	Perifacetal osteophyte formation Traction spurs Capsular laxity	Possible permanent changes of instability Spondylolisthesis Retrolisthesis[309]	Internal disruption Lateral or central nerve entrapment[310]
Final stabilization	Fibrosis of posterior joints and capsule Osteophyte formation on posterior vertebral body Central canal stenosis if osteophyte is large enough Circumferential osteophytes around the disc space, which can produce lateral or central stenosis		Loss of disc material

Kirkaldy-Willis[70] proposed a system to describe the spectrum of degeneration involving three phases or levels. The three phases (Table 7–1) are defined as early dysfunction, intermediate instability, and final stabilization.

- *Early dysfunction.* Characterized by minor pathologic changes, resulting in abnormal function of the posterior elements and disc. Disc herniations most commonly occur at the end of this phase but may occur during the final stabilization phase.
- *Intermediate instability.* Characterized by laxity of the posterior joint capsule and anulus.
- *Final stabilization.* Characterized by fibrosis of the posterior joints and capsule, loss of disc material, and the formation of osteophytes.[71] Osteophyte formation around the three-joint complex increases the load-bearing surface, and decreases the amount of motion, producing a stiffer and thus less painful motion segment.

Clinical experience has shown that it is possible for the three-joint complex to go through all of these phases with little symptomology.

Disc degeneration appears to involve structural disruption of the anulus fibrosus and cell-mediated changes throughout the disc and subchondral bone.[72] Disruption of the anulus is associated with back pain,[73] although some other degenerative changes in discs, such as dehydration of the nucleus pulposus, may simply be signs of aging. All skeletal tissues adapt to increased mechanical demands, but they may not always adapt quickly enough. People who suddenly change to a physically demanding occupation may subject their skeletons to increased repetitive loading, causing fatigue damage to accumulate rapidly. In the spine,

exercise-induced strengthening of the back muscles would exacerbate the problem, because most spinal compressive loading comes from back-muscle tension.[74] The ability of spinal tissues to strengthen in response to increased muscle forces may be restricted by health and age, so that fatigue damage would accumulate most rapidly in sedentary middle-aged people who suddenly become active.

Disc Degradation

This is a more aggressive process than that of the degenerative age changes (Table 7–2), and although the macroscopic changes are similar to age degeneration, it is a more accelerated process, involving a loss of disc height.

An increase in the hydrostatic pressure in both the nucleus pulposus and anulus fibrosus, and an increase in the hoop stress in the anulus layers balance an axial compressive force applied to the intervertebral disc.[5] The geometric consequences of a compressive force are a reduction in

TABLE 7–2 COMPARISON OF DEGENERATION AND DEGRADATION OF THE DISC

DEGENERATION	DEGRADATION
Changes occur to the biochemistry in early adulthood and middle age	Vasculogenic degradation of the nucleus
Circumferential clefting and tearing of the anulus	Circumferential and radial tearing of the anulus
No migration of nucleus	Nucleus migrates through the radial fissures
Undisplaced	Nucleus herniates through the anulus
The disc maintains or increases height	The disc is reabsorbed

disc height and a bulging of the anulus fibrosus. The extent of the bulging and the magnitude of the stress in the anulus layers depend on the applied compressive force, the disc height, and the cross-sectional area of the disc. Variations in disc height can be divided into two categories: primary disc height variations and secondary disc height changes.

- Primary disc height variations are related to intrinsic individual factors such as body height, gender, age, disc level, and geographic region.[75-78]
- Secondary disc height changes are associated with extrinsic factors such as degeneration, abnormality, or clinical management. Surgical procedures such as nucleotomy, discectomy, and chemonucleolysis cause a decrease in disc height, resulting from the removal of a portion of the nucleus pulposus or damage to the water-binding capacity of the extracellular matrix.[79-82] In addition, diurnal changes in disc height occur, caused by fluid exchange and creep deformation. These height changes are estimated to be about 0.68 mm on average for each intervertebral disc[83] or about 1.5 mm for each lumbar disc.[84]

With variations in disc height, one would expect changes in mechanical behavior of the disc, and it is speculated that repeated torsional trauma leads to posterior or posterior-lateral radial fissuring. An important result to emerge from a recent study is that axial displacement, posterior-lateral disc bulge, and tensile stress in the peripheral anulus fibers are a function of axial compressive force and disc height.[85] Under the same axial force, discs with a higher height-to-area ratio generated higher values of axial displacement, disc bulge, and tensile stress on the peripheral anulus fibers.

It should also be apparent that the unequal load distribution in asymmetric joints is a major predisposing factor in radial tearing of the anulus fibrosis, as the superior vertebra tends to rotate to the more coronal joint, producing a routine torsional effect in a constant direction with sagittal movements.

It is recognized that the adult intervertebral disc is avascular by young adulthood; after this time, nutrients are presumed to reach disc cells mainly by diffusion.[86-88] When a pathway to the periphery is opened for the nucleus, further stresses can force it to migrate through the tear. However, normal, even aged, nuclear material cannot be made to herniate through an annular defect, and it is believed that some mechanism must degrade the nucleus to allow it to migrate peripherally.[5] The appearance of nuclear material in the vertebral canal accelerates the autoimmune reaction as more of the avascular nucleus is exposed to the body's circulation. This process has been demonstrated both in vitro and in vivo by the presence of inflammatory products and increased levels of immunoglobulins.[89,90]

Nuclear material migration may be asymptomatic. It can be argued that the presence of free nerve endings in the outer part of the anulus could indicate a nociceptive ability in the disc, and anything disturbing these endings may then be considered to be potentially painful. There is, however, no direct evidence to prove that this is, in fact, the case.

Disc cell density is known to decrease with aging and degeneration,[91] and it is probable that apoptotic cell death (programmed cell death) is a major contributing factor to this decline. Apoptosis is essential during many stages of normal development and homeostasis, and it is now known from numerous studies that apoptosis may be triggered by a variety of exogenous or environmental stimuli.[92,93]

Actions of the Disc During Stress

The disc is a dynamic structure that responds to stresses applied from vertebral movement or the application of a static load. The major stresses that must be withstood are axial compression, shearing, bending, and twisting, either singly or in combination. Intervertebral discs are able to distribute compressive stress evenly between adjacent vertebrae because the nucleus pulposus and inner anulus act like a pressurized fluid, in which the pressure does not vary with location or direction.[11,94]

Axial Compression

It has been demonstrated experimentally that the anulus, even without the nucleus, can withstand the same vertical forces that an intact disc can for short periods,[95] providing the lamellae do not buckle. However, if the compression is prolonged or if the lamellae are not held together by the proteoglycan gel, the sheets buckle and the system collapses on itself.

Therefore, the nucleus is absolutely essential to the disc in the application of prolonged or repeated axial loading. The nucleus, being a ball of gel, is deformable but relatively incompressible; therefore, when a load is applied to it vertically, it tends to bulge around its equator and apply a radial pressure to the anulus.[5] This peripheral pressure increases the tension on the collagen fibers, which resist it until a balance is reached, when the radial pressure is matched by the collagen tension.

The loaded nucleus also tends to apply pressure against the end plates, but the end plates and the underlying vertebral bodies resist this pressure. When both of these mechanisms are balanced, the nucleus cannot deform any further. This equilibrium achieves two things:

1. Pressure is transferred from one end plate to another, so relieving the load on the anulus.

2. The nucleus braces the anulus and prevents it from buckling under the sustained axial load.

Axial compression, or spinal loading occurs in weight bearing, whether in standing or sitting. These forces also occur when the disc is damaged, which leads to excessive rotation and excessive lateral shearing. The amount of resistance to this compression is shared by the various structures of the intervertebral disc. During static, slow loading:

- The nuclear pressure rises, absorbing and transmitting the compression forces.
- The end plate, which is inherently weak, bows away from the disc and toward the vertebra[96] but the load is evenly distributed over its surface.[97] Fractures occur in the center with overload. The resistance of the end plate is dependent on the strength of the bone beneath and the blood capacity of the vertebral body.
- The anterior longitudinal ligament offers resistance if the spine is in its normal lordosis. The lumbar lordosis while standing is about 50% greater than when seated.[98]
- The anulus fibrosis bulges radially,[99] delaying and graduating the forces.
- The vertebral body absorbs and transmits the compression forces.
- The inferior articular process can impact on the lamina below during strong lordosis.

During axial compression of the intervertebral disc:

A. Water is squeezed out of disc.

B. Water loss is 5% to 11%.[100]
   1. Creep occurs rapidly (1.5 mm in the first 2 to 10 minutes),[101] then more slowly, at 1 mm per hour.[102]
   2. The creep plateaus at 90 minutes.[103]
   3. Over a 16-hour day, a 10% loss in disc height occurs.
   4. A person's height is restored with unloading. The best unloading position is the supine-with-knees-up posture (more effective than the extended supine posture).[104]

C. Compression increases the intradiscal pressure (but this effect varies with posture and activity).

The ability of the disc to act as a hydrostatic "cushion" depends on the high water content of the tissues and, in particular, on the volume of the nucleus pulposus. As alluded to, the nucleus acts like a sealed hydraulic system in which the fluid pressure rises substantially when volume is increased (by fluid injection[105]) and falls when volume is decreased (by surgical excision[106]). By a similar mechanism, age-related degenerative changes that reduce the water content of the nucleus pulposus by 15% to 20%,[107] cause a 30% fall in the nucleus pressure.[108] In effect, the load is being transferred from the nucleus to the anulus. The posterior anulus is affected most because it is the narrowest part of the disc, and the least able to sustain large compressive strains.[109]

As the nuclear material is intrinsically cohesive under normal conditions, the material will not herniate through the anulus. However, if the anulus is defective, and the nuclear material is altered, it becomes expressible and erodes the anulus along radial fissures. Under compression, the end plate is the weakest part of the disc mechanism, being able to withstand about nine times less stress than the anulus.[110] Axial loading over the surface of the end plate occurs evenly. However, failure of this structure occurs over the nucleus. It is reasonable to assume, therefore, that this central part of the end plate is weaker than the periphery. It is thought that this results from a selective absorption of the horizontal trabeculae. The clinical sign of this internal disc disruption is pain at rest, aggravated by activities that stress the disc; neurologic signs are absent and imaging studies are normal.

In life, structural disruption in the discs is often accompanied by cell-mediated degenerative changes. However, it is not necessary to postulate two independent processes because evidence is mounting that structural changes cause the biologic changes. Before the age of 40 years, up to 55% of the compressive load through the centrum is taken by the cancellous bone,[111] the remainder, by cortical. After this age, horizontal trabeculae are absorbed in the center of the vertebral body, thereby weakening the part of the centrum overlying the nucleus. This results in only about 35% of the axial stress being taken by the cancellous bone, with the greater proportion now going through cortical bone. Because cortical bone fails with a smaller degree of deformation than cancellous bone—2% compared with 9.5%—compressive failure occurs much more readily.

Another possible consequence of stress concentrations is pain. High stresses and stress gradients might elicit pain from nociceptive endings in the outer anulus,[112] because this region of the disc appears to be sensitive to mechanical stimulation.[113] Alternatively, stress peaks in the disc might elicit pain from adjacent vertebrae by deforming the relatively weak vertebral body endplate. Pain originating from either of these mechanisms would be expected to increase during the course of a day, especially in an individual who had spent a considerable amount of time with the lumbar spine flexed, so that disc creep would have been unchecked by the apophysial joints. This could explain why prolonged automobile driving is so closely associated with back pain and disc prolapse.[114]

Distraction

Symmetric distraction of the spine is a rare force and, as a consequence, the disc is less resistant to distraction that it is to compression.[115] Although asymmetric distraction occurs constantly with spinal movement (side-flexion causes ipsilateral compression, and contralateral distraction), symmetric distraction—in which all points of the one vertebral body are moved an equal distance away from its adjacent body—occurs only during vertical suspension or therapeutic traction. The anulus appears to bear the principal responsibility for restricting distraction, with the oblique orientation of the collagen fibers becoming more vertical as the traction force is applied.

A cadaveric study[116] demonstrated an initial average lengthening of 7.5 mm under 9 kg of traction (9 mm in younger subjects, 5.5 mm in the middle aged, and 7.5 mm in the elderly). A creep of 1.5 mm followed this during the next 30 minutes, and a set of 2.5 mm, reducing to 0.5 mm with release. There was greater elongation of the healthy spine (11 to 12 mm) and lesser elongation of the degenerative spine (3 to 5 mm). The creep was more rapid in the young, and there was no set in this age group. Forty percent of the lengthening was a result of straightening of the lordosis, with only 0.9 mm of segmental separation, and 0.1 mm of segmental set.

Torsion

During torsion, the collagen fibers of the anulus that are orientated in the same direction as the twist are stretched and resist the torsional force, whereas the others remain relaxed. As a result, only half of the anulus is able to share the stress of twisting. It may be partly for this reason, and because the maximum range of rotation for an intervertebral disc without incurring an injury is 3 degrees,[117] that torsion is one of the most common methods for injuring the disc. Macroscopic failure of the disc has been found to occur at 12 degrees of rotation.[118]

Shear

This is the movement of one vertebral body across the surface of its neighbor. Shear can occur in any plane. In forward sliding, the anulus fibers, which are angled forward on the lateral aspects of the disc, predominantly resist the movement, because they lie parallel to the movement. Those angled posteriorly are relaxed during forward shearing, but tensed during backward shearing. The anterior and posterior fibers make some contribution, but this is much less than that of the lateral fibers. The effect of these fibers is seen mainly during lateral shearing, again with those orientated in the direction of the shear, undergoing tension. As with torsion, only half of the fibers can contribute to the resistance and, as with torsion, shear forces are potentially very disruptive to the disc.

Bending

This motion can occur in any direction, producing both a rocking motion, and a translation shearing effect on the disc. The rocking motion results in deformation of the nucleus, and ipsilateral compression and contralateral tension of the anulus. The nucleus is compressed, the anulus buckles in the direction of the rock,[119] and there is a tendency for the anulus to be stretched in the opposite direction, while the pressure on the posterior aspect of the nucleus is relieved. Although the deformation can occur in a healthy disc, displacement of the nucleus is prevented by the anulus that encapsulates it. The anulus buckles at its compressed aspect because it is not braced by the nucleus, which is exerting that effect on the anular fibers at the opposite side of the disc.

DISC IMPAIRMENTS

Pain Production[50,51]

Nerve root fiber irritation is responsible for paresthesia, pain, and decreased conductivity. At the L1 and L2 levels, the nerves exit the intervertebral foramen above the disc. From L2 downward, the nerves leave the dura slightly more proximally than the foramen through which they pass, thus having an increasingly oblique direction, and an increasing length within the spinal canal. The L3 nerve root travels behind the inferior aspect of the vertebral body and the L3 disc. The L4 nerve root crosses the whole vertebral body to leave the spinal canal at the upper aspect of the L4 disc. The L5 nerve root emerges at the inferior aspect of the fourth lumbar disc, and crosses the fifth vertebral body to exit at the upper aspect of the L5 disc (Fig. 7–3). Several consequences of this anatomic relationship are discussed.

First Lumbar

Rarely encountered (0.3%), palsy here may be caused by a neoplasm. Disc impairments are often secondary to lower level fusions.

- *Pain:* Genital and groin area, outer buttock, and trochanter
- *Dural signs:* Neck flexion, slump
- *Articular signs:* Lumbar flexion most affected depending on size, extension also (see above)
- *Conduction signs:* Motor—none; sensory—hypoesthesias just below the medial half of the inguinal ligament; reflex—untestable
- *Differential diagnosis:* Neoplasm

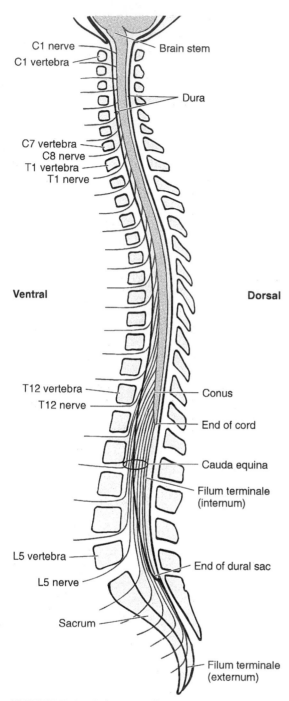

FIGURE 7–3 Schematic illustration of the relationships between the spinal cord, spinal nerves, and vertebral column (lateral view).

Second Lumbar

Rarely (less than 2%) encountered, a neoplasm here or at L1 may cause a palsy. Disc impairments are often secondary to lower level fusions.

- *Pain:* Upper lumbar, anterior thigh to knee
- *Dural signs:* Neck flexion

- *Articular signs:* Lumbar flexion is most affected, depending on size; extension is affected also (see earlier discussion)
- *Conduction signs:* Motor—hip flexion weak; sensory—anterior thigh; reflex—untestable
- *Differential diagnosis:* Upper lumbar or femoral neoplasm, meralgia paresthetica, claudication

Third Lumbar Root

Disc impairment at this level is uncommonly (4% to 8%) encountered.

- *Pain:* Mid-lumbar, upper buttock, whole anterior thigh and knee, medial knee to just above the ankle
- *Dural signs:* Prone knee flexion, occasionally a positive straight leg raise (SLR)
- *Articular signs:* Major motion loss of extension
- *Conduction signs:* Motor—slight weakness of psoas, grosser loss of quadriceps; sensory—hypoesthesia of inner knee and lower leg; reflex—knee jerk absent or reduced
- *Differential diagnosis:* Hip or knee arthritis, loose body, femur neoplasm, claudication, long saphenous neuritis

Fourth Lumbar Root

About 40% of disc impairments affect this level, about an equal amount as those that effect the L5 root. A disc protrusion can irritate the fourth or fifth root, or with a larger protrusion, both roots.

- *Pain:* Mid-lumbar or iliac crest, inner buttock, outer thigh and leg, over the foot to the great toe.
- *Dural signs:* SLR, bilateral and crossed SLR, and neck flexion (see Chapter 10)
- *Articular signs:* Marked deviation is common, as is gross limitation of flexion on one side
- *Conduction signs:* Motor—weak dorsiflexion; sensory—hypoesthesia of the outer lower leg and great toe; reflex—tibialis posterior and anterior
- *Differential diagnosis:* Spondylolisthesis, claudication

Fifth Lumbar Root

This root is equally affected with the fourth root and frequently compressed by the fourth as well as the fifth disc. A disc protrusion can irritate the fifth root, the first sacral root, or both.

- *Pain:* Sacroiliac area, lower buttock, lateral thigh and leg, inner three toes, and medial sole of foot
- *Dural signs:* Unilateral SLR, neck flexion
- *Articular signs:* May deviate during flexion; otherwise, as expected for size

- *Conduction signs:* Motor—weakness of peroneal, extensor hallucis, and hip abductor muscles; sensory—hypoesthesia of the outer leg and inner three toes and medial sole; reflex—peroneus longus, extensor hallucis
- *Differential diagnosis:* Peroneal neuritis, claudication, and loose body or meniscal derangement at the knee, with subsequent pressure on the tibial nerve

Fourth Sacral Root

Impairment here is always a concern because a permanent palsy may lead to incontinence and impotence.

- *Pain:* Lower sacral, peroneal, and genital areas; saddle area paresthesia
- *Dural signs:* None, or neck flexion
- *Articular signs:* May or may not have gross limitation of all movements
- *Conduction signs:* Motor—bladder, bowel, or genital dysfunction, alone or in combination; sensory—none; reflex—anal wink reduced
- *Differential diagnosis:* Genital and bladder dysfunctions, but always assume a root palsy; neural deficits cannot be detected in S3 impairments as it is the S4 nerve root that serves the saddle area (it is not possible to test the mobility of the S3 and S4 roots because they do not reach the lower limb)

Adherent Root

An adherent root is evidenced by prolonged sciatica on trunk flexion in the younger patient, protracted limitation of trunk flexion, and unilateral SLR. The intervention is careful stretching. This diagnosis should be made only after careful rejection of other, more common, conditions.

As mentioned previously, there are number of proposed mechanisms for the pain produced by a disc herniation. These include:

- Irritation of the free nerve endings in the outer anulus[112]
- Pain from the autoimmune reaction
- Direct irritation of the dura
- Contact inflammation of the dura from an autoimmune reaction
- Direct irritation of an already damaged nerve root
- Ischemia of the dura or root, caused by pressure from the disc on the vascular tissues of the segment
- Compression of the dura, or root, by edema caused by an inflammatory reaction
- Direct irritation of the nociceptors of the posterior longitudinal ligament

Types of Disc Herniations[50,51]

Disc herniations vary in size and position, and there are a number of different types.

A. Small posterolateral protrusion:
Onset: Slow, following sustained flexion or no apparent cause
Observation: Nothing extraordinary
Dural signs: Negative
Conduction signs: Negative or facilitated
Articular signs: Flexion is limited and painful; ipsilateral posterior quadrant (extension and side-flexion) is limited
Intervention: Bed rest, analgesics

B. Large posterior-lateral prolapse:
Onset: Within hours of sustained flexion or occurring suddenly
Observation: Kyphotic or deviated, or both
Dural signs: Positive SLR, positive coughing, sneezing
Conduction signs: Ranges from negative findings to a full palsy
Articular signs: Severely painful and limited flexion; ipsilateral posterior quadrant (extension and side-flexion) is limited
Intervention: Rest, analgesics, traction, manipulation, surgery

There are two categories for the posterior-lateral prolapse, primary or secondary, each with their own characteristics.

Primary Posterolateral Prolapse

The protrusion compresses the nerve root but not the dura. These protrusions are lateral to the canal. This is the disc protrusion of the young (15- to 30-year-olds). Typical signs and symptoms are as follows:

- Onset occurs in the leg rather than in the back (the major differentiating feature)
- Unilateral leg pain (often only in the calf)
- Good range of motion in the lumbar spine, but pain reproduced on flexion during which deviation may occur
- Positive slump test and SLR—dural signs are positive unilaterally, but conduction signs are usually negative

The recommended intervention for these individuals is: (1) sustained traction for 20 to 30 minutes at 50 to 60 pounds, checking progress with slump findings; (2) epidural injection, which gives an anti-inflammatory affect by bathing the dura; (3) surgery.

Secondary Posterior-Lateral Prolapse

This type initiates as a central protrusion on the dura (causing back pain for 2 to 4 weeks, before shifting laterally and causing leg pain). Typical signs and symptoms are as follows:

● Characterized by an onset of back pain, then leg pain
● Pain in the back or leg, or both
● Depending on the size of the protrusion, it may produce conduction signs unilaterally
● Unilateral dural signs

The recommended intervention for these individuals is intermittent traction.

Other types of protrusions include the following:

A. Large posterior-lateral extrusion:
Onset: Within hours of sustained flexion or occurring suddenly
Observation: Kyphotic or deviated, or both
Dural signs: Positive SLR
Conduction signs: Range from negative findings to a full palsy
Articular signs: Severely painful and limited flexion; ipsilateral posterior quadrant (extension and side-flexion) is limited
Intervention: Rest, analgesics, traction, manipulation, surgery

B. Massive posterior extrusion:
Onset: Slow or sudden
Observation: Kyphotic
Dural signs: SLR may be positive bilaterally or negative
Conduction signs: Cauda equina and S4 signs and symptoms
Articular signs: Possibility of severe limitation in all ranges
Intervention: Rest, analgesics, surgery

C. Anterior protrusion in the elderly (Mushroom phenomenon): Has essentially the same features as stenosis, and may, in fact, be stenosis rather than a disc impairment

D. Anterior prolapse in the adolescent (osteochondritis): May or may not be symptomatic, and if so, usually only results in a vague backache

E. Vertical prolapse (Schmorl's node): Often asymptomatic and an incidental finding on x-ray. A Schmorl's node is the herniation of disc substance through the cartilaginous plate of the intervertebral disc into the body of the adjacent vertebra[120] (Fig. 7–4). The chronic Schmorl's node has been reported to be the most common impairment of the intervertebral discs, indeed, of the whole spine.[26] Theories proposed to explain the pathogenesis of Schmorl's nodes include origins that are:

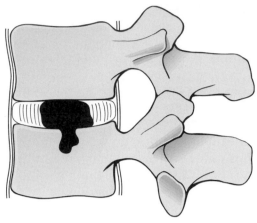

FIGURE 7–4 Lumbar degenerative joint disease and Schmorl's node.

1. Developmental, in which embryonic defects such as ossification gaps, vascular channels, and notochord extrusion defects form points of weakness where Schmorl's nodes may occur.[8,121]
2. Degenerative, in which the aging process produces sites of weakness in the cartilaginous endplate, resulting in Schmorl's nodes formation.[26,122]
3. Pathologic, in which diseases weaken the intervertebral disc or vertebral bodies, or both.[123,124]
4. Traumatic, in which acute and chronic trauma destroy the cartilaginous end plates, resulting in disc herniation. Although most spine physicians accept that Schmorl's nodes occur as a result of trauma, no studies have shown a direct causal relation between a traumatic episode and the formation of an acute Schmorl's node.

F. Traumatic back pain related to a specific incident and accompanied by muscle spasm, referred pain, but a negative SLR, usually indicates one of the following:
1. Tear of the outer anulus fibers
2. End plate fracture
3. Capsular ligament tear
4. Interspinous ligament tear
5. Muscle tear
6. Fluid ingestion (if there is no referred pain)[125]
These patients usually respond to bed rest and analgesics.

G. High lumbar disc protrusions[126]

Although a herniated disc most commonly originates from the L4-5 or L5-S1 level,[127] 1% to 11% of herniated discs originate from the L1-2, L2-3, or L3-4 level.[128–131] Reduced motion and stress at the upper lumbar spine and the protective influence of the posterior longitudinal ligament may account for the disparity.[131,132]

Clinical Considerations

Much confusion still exists in regard to the diagnosis and proper management of the high lumbar (L2-4) disc. "Sciatica" is a dated term to describe pain in the lower back and hip that radiates down the back of the thigh and into the lower leg, usually caused by a herniated lumbar disc.[133]

Clinicians who treat low back pain that radiates into the leg are often under the misconception that the pain is secondary to a herniated disc, and that it must always radiate down the back of the leg. In fact, the high lumbar radiculopathy does not radiate pain down the back of the leg, but often causes an insidious onset of pain in the groin or anterior thigh, which is often relieved in a flexed position and worsened on standing.

Several plausible diagnoses for anterior thigh pain must be eliminated before a high lumbar radiculopathy can be confirmed:

- Degenerative hip joint
- Avascular necrosis of the hip[134]
- Muscle strain
- Stress fracture
- Isolated femoral nerve injury—although uncommon, it is more common in a younger, athletic population[135–137]
- Diabetic amyotrophy—also relatively uncommon, but it can occasionally be the presenting symptom of uncontrolled diabetes mellitus[138]

The most important aspect of the examination of low back pain with possible nerve root herniation is the history and physical examination. The patient often describes back and leg pain, with the leg pain often involving below-the-knee symptoms. For patients with herniated discs, the accuracy of the medical history can be extremely valuable. Typically, true radiculopathy produces pain radiating below the knee, usually to the foot or ankle, and is often associated with some numbness or paresthesias. Coughing, sneezing, or a Valsalva maneuver often aggravates the pain. Sciatica is such a sensitive finding (95%) that its absence almost rules out a clinically important disc herniation, although it is only 88% specific for herniation. In contrast, the sensitivity of pseudo-claudication in detecting spinal stenosis is 60%, whereas the combination of pseudoclaudication and age greater than 50 years has a sensitivity of 90% (specificity, 70%).[139]

A physical examination that reveals nerve root tension signs further suggests true radiculopathy. For the sciatic nerve, this generally means straight leg raising. For the femoral nerve, however, this means the femoral nerve stretch test (flexing the knee with the patient prone). The SLR test is moderately sensitive, but relatively nonspecific, in the diagnosis of a herniated disc. Crossed straight leg raising occurs when straight leg raising on a patient's healthy leg elicits pain in the leg with sciatica.[140] This test is less sensitive but substantially more specific than the ipsilateral SLR.[139] Thus, this test affirms the diagnosis, whereas ipsilateral straight leg raising is more effective in ruling out the diagnosis. (Refer to Chapter 10)

The reverse SLR test, or femoral nerve stretch test, is probably the single best screening test to evaluate for a high lumbar radiculopathy. It has been shown to be positive in 84% to 95% of patients with high lumbar discs,[127,145,146] although the test may be falsely positive in the presence of a tight iliopsoas or rectus femoris or any pathology in or about the hip joint and, therefore, should be performed bilaterally. (Refer to Chapter 10)

Ninety-eight percent of all disc herniations occur at the L4-5 or L5-S1 levels,[141] although, in the older population there is a relative increased risk of a prolapse at the L3-4 and L2-3 levels.[142] Herniations occur in a predictable manner:

- The disc bulges against the dura and the posterior longitudinal ligament, producing a dull, poorly localized pain in the back and sacroiliac region. Bilateral low back pain probably results from an irritation of the connecting branch of the sinuvertebral nerve, which joins the right and left portions of that nerve[143]
- The disc bulges posterior-laterally against the nerve root, resulting in sharp, lancinating pain. If the disc ruptures, the fluid of the nucleus pulposus comes into contact with the vascular system, which sets up a chain reaction of inflammation and back and/or leg pain.

As a general rule, the presence of leg pain indicates a larger protrusion than does back pain alone.[144] Reflex testing is usually normal in high lumbar involvement, and both strength and reflexes may be influenced by the presence of pain.

The natural history of sciatica and disc herniation is not quite as favorable as for simple low back pain, but it is still excellent, with approximately 50% of patients recovering in the first 2 weeks, and 70% recovering in 6 weeks.[147] Both Hakelius and Weber treated patients with sciatica nonoperatively with very good results. Thirty-eight percent of Hakelius' patients improved in the first month, 53% in the second, and 78% in the third.[148,149] In Weber's series, 25% of patients admitted with documented disc herniation improved after a 2-week hospital stay.[150] However, 25% remained significantly symptomatic and were surgically treated. The remaining 126 patients in that study were randomized to nonsurgical and surgical intervention. At 1 year, good results were found in 90% of surgically treated patients compared with 60% in the conservative group. In the nonsurgical group, 17 patients had undergone surgery because of intolerable pain. At 4- and 10-year follow-up, the results were similar in the two groups. At 10 years, return of muscle function was the same regardless of intervention, as was sensory function, which remained abnormal in 35%.

The McKenzie program can be valuable to the overall intervention strategy, and if centralization of pain occurs, a good response to physical therapy can be anticipated. (Refer to Chapter 11)[151,152] A comprehensive examination of the patient is performed in the neutral, flexed, and extended positions for the presence of the centralization phenomenon. The same maneuvers are repeated with the trunk in the neutral position, shifted toward the side of pathology, and away from pathology. The goal is to reduce the radiating pain and to centralize it. Once this centralizing position is identified, the patient is instructed to perform these maneuvers repetitively throughout the day.[153] In addition, the patient is instructed in a spinal stabilization program in which neutral zone mechanics are practiced in various positions to decrease stress to the lumbosacral spine. The intervention program is only as good as the concomitant home exercise program, and the clinician must continually monitor the home exercise program, evaluating the patient's knowledge of the exercises and upgrading the program when appropriate.

CERVICAL DISC

The morphology and biochemistry of the lumbar intervertebral discs have been studied extensively, and several insights have emerged regarding the pathology of mechanical disorders of the lumbar disc. However, when considering cervical intervertebral discs, most authors have been content with extrapolating data from the lumbar spine, even though it is clear that the pathology affecting the cervical intervertebral disc is different from that affecting the lumbar disc.

Differences in the Cervical Disc

A small number of studies have indicated that the structure of the cervical discs,[154–156] and their development, is distinctly different from that of the lumbar discs. The nucleus at birth constitutes no more than 25% of the entire disc, not 50% as in lumbar discs.[157] With aging, the nucleus pulposus rapidly undergoes fibrosis such that, by the third decade, barely any nuclear material is distinguishable.[158] In the cervical spine, the nucleus pulposus sits in, or near, the center of the disc, lying slightly more posteriorly than anteriorly. Although the nucleus pulposus and anulus fibrosis are quite distinct entities, as in the young lumbar spine, there is no clear boundary between the anulus, and the peripheral parts of the nucleus pulposus merge with the deeper parts of the anulus fibrosis. The nucleus pulposus of the cervical spine is a semifluid mass

of mucoid material composed of relatively few collagen fibers. The proteoglycan component of the cervical nucleus pulposus makes the nucleus highly hydrophilic, resulting in a water content of approximately 80%.[20] As in the lumbar spine the disc functions as a closed but dynamic system, distributing the changes in pressure equally to all components of the container (i.e., the end plates and the anulus, and across the surface of the vertebral body).

The cervical discs form an anterior weight-bearing link between each of the mobile cervical segments. The disc height-to-body height ratio is greatest (2:5) in the cervical spine, therefore allowing the greatest possible range of motion. There are six cervical discs, the first of which occurs between C2 and C3. A normally functioning disc is extremely important to permit the normal biomechanics of the spine to occur, and to maintain sufficient space between the vertebral segments. Unlike the lumbar and thoracic intervertebral discs, degeneration of the cervical disc appears to be a natural consequence of aging, producing predictable changes in cervical function and movement patterns. In addition, the configuration and functional demands of the lower cervical vertebrae are significantly different from those of the lumbar region, so some variations in the discs should be expected.[159]

The cervical anulus fibrosus does not consist of obliquely oriented concentric lamellae of collagen fibers that uniformly surround the nucleus pulposus, as it does in the lumbar spine.[159] Rather, the cervical anulus is crescent shaped, being thick anteriorly but tapering in thickness laterally as it approaches the uncovertebral region.

The cervical discs are rendered different from the lumbar discs by certain key features:[159]

- Anteriorly, the cervical anulus consists of interwoven alar fibers, whereas posteriorly, the anulus lacks any oblique fibers and consists exclusively of vertically orientated fibers.
- Essentially, the cervical anulus has the structure of a dense, anterior interosseous ligament with few fibers to contain the nucleus pulposus posteriorly. That is the role of the overlying posterior longitudinal ligament.
- In no region of the cervical anulus fibrosus do successive lamellae exhibit alternating orientations. In fact, only in the anterior portion of the anulus, where obliquely orientated fibers upward and medially interweave with one another, does a cruciate pattern occur. This weave, regarded in x-ray crystallography studies[160] as alternating layers, is not produced by alternate lamellae.
- Posterior-laterally, the nucleus is contained only by the alar fibers of the posterior longitudinal ligament, under or through which the nuclear material must pass if it is to herniate.

- The vertical orientation of the posterior anulus of cervical discs is similar to that of the thoracic discs.[161]
- The absence of an anulus over the uncovertebral region. In this region, collagen fibers are torn by 15 years,[162] or as early as 9[163] or 7 years,[164] leaving clefts that progressively extend across the back of the disc.[162] Rather than an incidental age change, this disruption has been interpreted either as enabling[165] or resulting from[166] rotatory movements of the cervical vertebrae.
- Axial rotation of a typical cervical vertebra occurs around an oblique axis perpendicular to the plane of its facets.[166]

Considering the structure of the cervical anulus, the possibilities that emerge for mechanisms of discogenic pain are strain or tears of the anterior anulus, particularly after hyperextension trauma, and strain of the alar portions of the posterior longitudinal ligament when stretched by a bulging disc.[159,167]

The cervical spine is vulnerable to the same impairments as those of the lumbar spine, and any weakness in the surrounding structures results in either a bulge or rupture. A rupture through the cartilage plate results in a Schmorl's node; whereas a rupture of the anulus can produce a disc herniation.

The cartilaginous joint, formed by the union between two vertebral bodies and the intervertebral disc, permits some motion, although the motion is much less than that found in most synovial joints. The role of the disc is unique because it holds the bodies together while simultaneously pushing them apart. The disc is preloaded, its internal pressure exceeding atmospheric pressure, and it exerts a force on the surrounding vertebra. This is true even when a person is recumbent and the vertebral column is unloaded.

Considering the anatomic proportions, it is evident that cervical discogenic disease can have an impact on neural structures in the bony spinal canal. The available space occupied by the spinal cord and nerve roots is determined primarily by the diameter of the bony spinal canal. Degenerative processes such as cervical spondylosis and disc herniation are the most common diseases that threaten the spinal cord and nerve roots.

In the lumbar disc, a prolapse is common. In the cervical spine, a straightforward prolapse is uncommon, and degenerative changes are reported to occur typically in the form of end plate sclerosis, disintegration and collapse of the disc, bulging anulus fibrosus, development of osteophytes from the margins of the vertebral body, uncovertebral or zygapophysial joints, and narrowing of the intervertebral foramina or spinal canal by chondroosseous spurs.[168–170] A cervical disc herniation is not a miniature version of lumbar disc herniation. It is, unlike lumbar disc herniation,[171,172] extremely rare under 30 years of age.[173,174] The disc spaces concerned frequently remain normal in height on plain radiographic films.[173] These characteristics may be based on the pathomechanisms peculiar to cervical disc herniation.

Asymptomatic cervical disc herniation is often found in magnetic resonance images for other diseases.[175] The anterior-posterior diameter of the cervical spinal canal tends to be narrower in patients with herniation resulting in myelopathy.[173,176] That is, patients with wide canals might be nonmyelopathic even with the same degree of herniation.

Abnormalities in the osseous and the fibroelastic boundaries of the bony cervical spinal canal affect the availability of space for spinal cord and nerve roots. In 1937, Lindgren[185] was the first to stress the importance of the sagittal diameter of the bony cervical spinal canal. In 1954, Verbiest[186] defined "developmental stenosis" as a narrowing of the bony spinal canal caused by an inadequate development of the vertebral arch. Although this stenosis often remains asymptomatic for a long time, it can become a major influence in the production of radiculomyelopathic compressive disturbances when other conditions such as spondylosis, discal hernia, and trauma become superimposed. One study concluded that the relation between the sagittal diameter of the bony spinal canal and the sagittal diameter of the hernia determines the severity of neurologic symptoms after soft cervical disc herniation.[187] As the resulting space for neural structures becomes smaller, the risk of developing motor disturbances of medullary or radicular origin increases. The "developmental sagittal diameter" of the bony cervical spinal canal is, therefore, a reliable parameter for estimating the risk of developing medullary or radicular compression by an intraspinal space-occupying process.[188,189]

Patients with cervical disc herniations often report a history of neck pain for days to weeks before the onset of their arm pain. As time passes, radicular symptoms may develop. The annual incidence of cervical herniated nucleus pulposus with radiculopathy was 5.5 per 100,000 in Rochester, Minnesota.[177] The age range of peak incidence for cervical herniated nucleus pulposus was 45 to 54 years, and incidence was only slightly less common in the 35- to 44-year-old group. C5-6 was the most commonly affected level, followed by C6-7 and C4-5.

In a large U.S. population survey, the combined prevalence of C5-6 and C6-7 herniated nucleus pulposi accounted for 75% of cervical disc herniations.[180] Of these disc herniations, 23% were attributed to a motor vehicle accident. It is likely that many of these radiographic findings were present before the injury; Boden and colleagues[181] reported the incidence of cervical disc protrusions in the asymptomatic population to be 10% to 15%, depending on age.

Cervical discs may become painful as part of the degenerative cascade, from repetitive microtrauma, or from an excessive single load. Depending on the size and location of the impairment, pain from the disc injury may result from inflammation[178,179] or compression of local nervous or vascular tissue.

Cigarette smoking and frequent lifting have been shown to be associated with a higher risk of herniated nucleus pulposus.

When herniations occur, there are two distinct types:

1. *Soft.* These are small, well-contained herniations that push through the radial tears in the anulus. In a soft hernia, part of the nucleus pulposus is pushed through the ruptured anulus fibrosus, forming an anatomically well-defined mass beneath the posterior longitudinal ligament. In some cases, there is also rupture of the posterior longitudinal ligament, causing sequestration of a herniated fragment in the spinal canal. Soft disc herniations are much more common in younger patients who have not yet experienced cervical spondylotic changes.[182–184]

2. *Hard.* These are large herniations or fragmentations of nucleus material, usually in a posterior direction, into the wide spinal canal and can prove to be very problematic. A disc protrusion tends to affect the motor nerve, whereas a degeneration of the zygapophysial joint can lead to an impingement on the sensory nerve.

Cervical intervertebral discs with herniation usually remain normal in height, or change only slightly without abnormality in the Luschka joints.[173] Sclerosis and formation of osteophytes in the Luschka joints accompany narrowed discs in spondylosis. These facts indicate that the Luschka joints bear a part of the axial load to the intervertebral disc. Accordingly, disc degeneration may play a more important role than trauma in the production of herniation in the cervical spine, and it is not unusual for a patient to awake with a cervical disc herniation, misinterpreting it as a "crick" in the neck. The indication that degeneration plays a greater role in cervical disc herniations may explain why cervical disc herniation is extremely rare in those younger than 30 years of age and why the mean age of onset is around 50 years.[173,174]

Cervical disc degeneration occurs in a predictable fashion. The nucleus pulposus and anulus fibrosus form small cysts[190,191] and fissures as the first disruptive changes after the death of chondrocytes and the separation of fibers or fiber bundles. Subsequently, they extend and join together to form horizontal and vertical clefts. Pritzker[192] compared the nucleus pulposus and the cartilaginous end plate to synovial fluid and articular cartilage of a diarthroidal joint from the anatomic and functional aspects. From the aspect of degeneration, a disc with a horizontal cleft could be likened to the osteoarthritic joint. Shearing stress to the disc by translational motion may lead to fibrillation of the matrix as in osteoarthritic joint cartilage. Some of the vertical clefts extend to the cartilaginous end plate, and portions of the cartilaginous end plate may be torn off. Regarding the modes of lumbar disc herniation, Yasuma and associates[191] described the degenerative process of the matrix and concluded that most herniations are protrusions of the nucleus pulposus before the age of 60 years, whereas after that age, prolapse of the anulus fibrosus predominates. Eckert and Decker[193] and Taylor and Akeson,[194] however, found cartilaginous end plate in 60% of herniated masses, and in approximately 50% of sequestrated fragments, respectively. Harada and Nakahara[195] found that fragments of cartilaginous end plate with anulus fibrosus more often herniate than nucleus pulposus alone in those more than 30 years of age, especially in the elderly more than 60 years of age.

Frykholm[196] in 1951 advocated the classification of cervical disc herniation into nuclear herniation and anular protrusion as in lumbar disc herniation. Mixter and Barr[197] reported that herniated tissue consisted of anular fiber, whereas Peet and Echols[198] reported herniation masses contained nucleus pulposus. Bucy and co-workers[199] noted that the protruded tissue was fibrocartilage.

In the cervical region, the discs are named after the vertebra above (the C4 disc lies between C4 and C5). Cervical roots exit horizontally. The cervical nerves C1-7 exit above the vertebra of the same number (C1 exits above the C1 vertebra). There is no disc at C1 or C2. At the C2-7 levels, the disc, if it protrudes, will hit the nerve root number above. The C8 nerve root exits below the C7 vertebra.

A C3 nerve impingement is very rare as there is no disc at the C2 level. A dura mater impairment (any level), or a trigeminal impairment should be suspected.

C4 nerve impingements as a result of a C3 disc herniation are also uncommon. Findings include no paresthesia, but pain reported in the C4 dermatome distribution (top of the shoulder and anterior chest).

A C5 nerve root injury is often the result of an osteophyte, or a traction injury, and not a C4 disc protrusion. If pain is present, it is felt in a C5 dermatome, but often the clinician finds painless weakness and a decreased deep tendon reflex in the biceps and brachioradialis.

A C6 nerve impingement is often as a result of a C5 disc protrusion or an osteophyte. Findings include a decreased biceps deep tendon reflex.

C7 nerve root irritation, a common impairment, is likely the result of a C6 disc protrusion.

The C7 disc impinges the C8 nerve root. Clinical findings include weakness of the extensor pollicis longus and brevis, the ulna deviators, thumb adductors, finger extensors, and the abductor indices.

The T1 nerve root is rarely impinged by a disc and is often related to a serious pathology, such as a Pancoast's tumor. With T1 involvement, the clinician often sees atrophy of the hand intrinsics.

More recently, postmortem studies have found that after whiplash injuries, ligamentous injuries are extremely common in the cervical spine but that herniation of the nucleus pulposus is rare.[200–203] The impairments found in the cervical spine included bruising and hemorrhage of the uncinate region, so-called rim lesions or transections of the anterior anulus fibrosus, and avulsions of the vertebral endplate.[200–203]

The disc's capacity to self-repair is limited by the fact that only the peripheral aspects of the anulus receive blood, and a small amount at that. As in the lumbar spine, both the nucleus pulposus and anulus fibrosus undergo age-related changes that are evident chemically and morphologically. However, they are evident to a much greater extent in the nucleus pulposus than in the anulus fibrosus. Oda and colleagues[158] studied the histologic changes that occur with age. They described significant changes in the composition of the nucleus: fibrocartilage and dense fibrous tissue replace the cellular and very fine fibrillar composition of the neonate by the end of the second decade.

Clinical Findings[167,204,205]

Upper trunk brachial plexus disorders can be confused with a C5 or C6 radiculopathy. The etiology is unknown but usually presents first with severe pain that resolves and then is followed by weakness and subsequent atrophy.[206–208] There generally is an absence of neck symptoms, and the Spurling test is negative. Electrodiagnostic studies and MRI are helpful in establishing the diagnosis.

Peripheral nerve entrapment within the upper limb may also be confused with a cervical radiculopathy. This includes entrapment or compression of suprascapular, median, and ulnar nerves. A suprascapular neuropathy can be confused with a C5 or C6 radiculopathy but would spare the deltoid and biceps muscles. C6 and C7 radiculopathies are most likely to be confused with median neuropathies, whereas C8 radiculopathy must be differentiated from ulnar neuropathies and thoracic outlet syndrome.

The seventh (C7, 60%) and sixth (C6, 25%) cervical nerve roots are the most commonly affected.[210–212] There is limited information regarding the true incidence of cervical radiculopathy in sports. One study found increased cervical disc disease from diving and weight lifting.[213] Golfers were found to have a statistically insignificant increase in cervical disc disease. Other factors associated with increased risk include heavy manual labor, requiring lifting of more than 25 lb, smoking, and driving or operating vibrating equipment.[215]

It is important to obtain a detailed history to establish a diagnosis of a cervical radiculopathy and to rule out other causes of the complaints. The examiner should first determine the main complaint (i.e., pain, numbness, weakness) and location of symptoms. Anatomic pain drawings can be helpful by supplying the clinician with an outline of the pain pattern. Activities and head positions that increase or decrease symptoms help in making the diagnosis, as well as in guiding the intervention. The position of the head and neck at the time of injury should also be noted. Prior episodes of similar symptoms or localized neck pain are important for diagnosis.

The typical patient presents with an insidious onset of neck and arm discomfort, which ranges from a dull ache to severe burning. The pattern of radiation is variable and may include referred pain to the scapular, or down the upper extremity in a pattern related to the involved nerve root, depending on the nerve root that is involved. Acute disc herniations or sudden narrowing of the neural foramen may also occur from injuries involving cervical extension, side-flexion, or rotation and axial loading.[226–228] This is a common mechanism for "burner" or "stinger" injuries which result from an injury caused by either traction or compressive forces to the upper trunk of the brachial plexus or upper cervical nerve roots.[216–225] Patients with these types of injury usually complain of increased pain with neck positions that place the brachial plexus on stretch: side-flexion, or rotation away from the symptomatic side.

Typically, the patient with cervical radiculopathy has a head list away from the side of injury to avoid further impingement of the nerve root.

Active range of motion is typically limited into cervical extension, rotation toward the side of the lesion, and side-flexion in either direction, and the patient is usually unwilling to attempt these motions, or sustain these positions.

On palpation, tenderness is usually noted at the site of injury and along the ipsilateral cervical paraspinals. There may also be muscle tenderness along muscles where the symptoms are referred as described above, as well as associated hypertonicity or spasm.

Manual muscle testing can detect subtle weakness in a myotomal, or key muscle, distribution. Weakness of shoulder abduction suggests C5 pathology, elbow flexion and wrist extension weakness suggests a C6 radiculopathy, weakness of elbow extension and wrist flexion would occur with a C7 radiculopathy, and weakness of thumb extension and ulnar deviation of the wrist would be seen in C8 radiculopathies.[229]

On sensory examination, a dermatomal pattern of diminished, or loss, of sensation is typically reported. In addition, there may be reports of hyperesthesia to light touch and pin-prick examination.[214,230]

Deep tendon reflexes are useful tests to determine the level of involvement. As reflexes can vary from individual to individual and yet be considered normal,[231] the clinician must look for asymmetry in the reflexes when comparing one extremity to the other. The biceps brachii reflex occurs at the C5-6 level. The brachioradialis is another C5-6 reflex. The triceps reflex tests the C7-8 nerve roots. The pronator reflex can be helpful in differentiating C6 and C7 nerve root problems. If it is abnormal in conjunction with an abnormal triceps reflex, then the level of involvement is more likely to be C7. This reflex is performed by tapping the volar aspect of the forearm, with the forearm in a neutral position and the elbow flexed.[231,232]

Provocative tests for cervical radiculopathy include the Spurling test. This test is performed by extending or flexing the neck, rotating the head and then applying downward pressure on the head.[207,233,234] (Refer to Chapter 10) The Spurling test has been found to be very specific, but not sensitive in diagnosing acute radiculopathy.[207,235]

Gentle manual cervical distraction can also be used as a diagnostic tool. A positive response is indicated by a reduction of neck or limb symptoms with the distraction. (Refer to Chapter 10)

Little is known about the natural history of cervical radiculopathy or controlled randomized studies comparing operative versus nonoperative intervention.[207,236] The pathogenesis of radiculopathy occurs from the inflammatory process initiated by nerve root compression, resulting in nerve root swelling.[214,224,237] A study of patients under local anesthesia found that compression of a nerve root produced limb pain, whereas pressure on the disc produced pain in the neck and the medial border of the scapula.[214,238] Intradiscal injection and electrical stimulation of the disc has also suggested that neck pain is referred by a damaged outer anulus.[214,239] Muscle spasms of the neck have also been found after electrical stimulation of the disc. In addition to the resolution of inflammation, the reabsorption of extruded disc material itself probably occurs in the cervical herniated nucleus pulposus as it does in the lumbar disc herniated nucleus pulposus.[240–242] The outcome data support the concept that an extruded disc actually may have a more favorable nonoperative prognosis than contained disc pathology. Conceptually, this is consistent with the premise that a contained disc pathology represents a distinct clinical entity pathophysiologically different than nuclear extrusion.

Nonsurgical management consists of rest, a cervical collar, oral corticosteroid "dose-packs," nonsteroidal anti-inflammatory drugs, and nonspecific modalities.[243–245]

Oral steroids have been found to be clinically useful in reducing the associated inflammation, although there are no controlled studies to support the use of oral steroids in the treatment of cervical radiculopathy.[207,226] The beneficial effect of corticosteroids may occur as a result of the anti-inflammatory properties of these drugs. If the inflammatory response can be controlled pharmacologically, the neural elements will adapt to the deformation caused by the disc material to which they were initially intolerant.

A small percentage of patients with cervical herniated nucleus pulposus do require surgery for radiculopathy. There are not adequate data currently in the medical literature to allow a comparison of nonsurgical treatment methods with surgical treatment for patients with cervical herniated nucleus pulposus (CHNP) and radiculopathy.[240,241,249] There are limited published reports of patients with cervical herniated nucleus pulposus treated nonsurgically.[241,250] Lees and Turner[251] have reported that if the symptoms of cervical spondylitic radiculopathy are persistent, the prognosis is considered guarded based on their observational study. However, the majority can be treated successfully with a carefully applied and progressive nonoperative program.

Typically, the decision to proceed with surgical intervention is made when a patient has significant extremity or myotomal weakness, severe pain, or pain that persists beyond an arbitrary "conservative" intervention period of 2 to 8 weeks.[245,252,253] For nonvalidated reasons, cervical disc extrusions have been frequently considered a definite indication for surgery.[244,252]

THORACIC INTERVERTEBRAL DISC[254]

Thoracic discs have been poorly researched. They are narrower and flatter than those in the cervical and lumbar spine. Disc size gradually increases from superior to inferior. The disc height-to-body height ratio is 1:5, making it the smallest ratio in the spine. The nucleus is rather small in the thorax relative to the rest of the spine, is more centrally located within the anulus, and has a lower capacity to swell.[255] Therefore, protrusions are usually of the annular type, and a true nuclear protrusion is very rare in this region.

In contrast to the cervical and lumbar regions, where the spinal canal is triangular to oval in cross-section, with a large lateral excursion to the nerve roots, the mid-thoracic spinal canal is small and circular, becoming triangular at the upper and lower levels. At the levels of T4 through to T9, the canal is at its narrowest. The spinal canal is also restricted in its size by the pedicles, remaining within the confines of the vertebra, unlike they do in the cervical spine. This would tend to predispose the spinal cord to compression more than in the cervical spine, were it not for the smaller cord size and more oval shape of the thoracic canal. However, this is an area of poor vascular supply, receiving its blood from only one radicular artery, which renders the thoracic spinal cord extremely vulnerable to damage by extradural masses or by an overzealous manipulation.

Symptomatic thoracic disc herniations are rare, and their clinical manifestations differ widely from those of cervical and lumbar disc herniations.[256] In a review of 280 patients, Arce and Dohrmann[256] found that thoracic disc herniation constitutes 0.25% to 0.75% of all disc herniations. Most prolapsed thoracic discs show degenerative change. The duration of symptoms of thoracic disc herniation is longer than 6 months in 70% of patients. Its clinical appearance varies, and its diagnosis is often delayed.[257] Midline back pain and compressive myelopathy symptoms progressing over months or years are the predominant clinical features.[256,258] By the time of diagnosis, 70% of patients had signs of spinal cord compression, and isolated root pain occurred in only 9% of patients. Unusual features of thoracic disc herniation include Lhermitte's symptom, precipitated by rotation of the thoracic spine,[259] neurogenic claudication with positionally dependent weakness,[260] flaccid paraplegia,[261] and chronic abdominal pain mimicking chronic pancreatitis.[262] These soft neurologic symptoms and signs indicate a thoracic spine impairment rather than a lumbar disc disease. Pain radiating to the buttock, which suggested lumbosacral root compression, have also been reported in some cases with lower thoracic disc herniation.[263] One patient who experienced a clinical manifestation of lumbosacral radiculopathy, without any sign of thoracic cord or root, was found to have a lower thoracic disc herniation. How a herniated disc at low thoracic level could appear to be lumbosacral radiculopathy is best explained by the anatomic arrangement of the spinal cord and vertebral bodies. In adults, the conus medullaris ends between the 12th thoracic and second lumbar vertebrae, and the lumbar enlargement of the spinal cord usually locates at the lower thoracic level. Therefore, a lower thoracic disc herniation could compress the lumbosacral spinal nerves after their exit from the lumbar enlargement of the spinal cord, producing symptoms of compressive lumbosacral radiculopathy. Thus, a herniation at an already tight canal may produce bilateral symptoms and sphincter disturbance, as in patients with a conus medullaris impairment.[264]

SPINAL NERVE ROOT EXITS

The angle at which the spinal nerve root exits the vertebral column varies according to level. In the cervical region, and the upper to mid-thoracic regions, the roots exit horizontally.

In the thoracic region, a nerve root can only generally be compressed by its corresponding disc. However, the more caudal in the spine, the more oblique the nerve root

exits. And as a consequence, the lowest thoracic nerve roots can be compressed by disc impairments of two consecutive levels (the T12 root can be compressed by the 11th or 12th disc in the thoracic region).

In the lumbar region, the L3 nerve root travels behind the inferior aspect of the vertebral body and the L3 disc. The L4 nerve root crosses the whole vertebral body to leave the spinal canal at the upper aspect of the L4 disc. The L5 nerve root emerges at the inferior aspect at the fourth lumbar disc and crosses the fifth vertebral body to exit at the upper aspect of the L5 disc. Consequently, the following can occur:

- At L4, a disc protrusion can pinch the fourth root, the fifth root, or with a larger protrusion, both roots.
- At L5, a disc can compress the fifth root, first sacral root, or both.
- Root L5 can be compressed by an L4 or an L5 disc.

Because of the L1 and L2 levels, the nerves exit the intervertebral foramen above the disc. An impingement here is very rare.

IMAGING STUDIES[167]

Plain Radiographs

X-rays of the spine are usually the first diagnostic test ordered in patients presenting with back and limb symptoms, and they are very helpful in providing a gross assessment of the severity of degenerative changes, and detecting the presence of fractures and subluxations in patients with a history of trauma.[214] In patients with cervical trauma, the physician will often order lateral, anterior-posterior, and oblique views, together with an open-mouth view. The open-mouth view helps the physician to rule out injury to the atlanto-axial joint. The atlantodens interval (ADI) is the distance from the posterior aspect of the anterior C1 arch and the odontoid process. This should be less than 3 mm in the adult and less than 4 mm in children.[266] An increase in the ADI suggests atlanto-axial instability.

A recommendation for flexion and extension views should be made to the patient's physician if the clinician suspects the presence of an instability. Greater than 2 mm of motion occurring at any segment with flexion or extension suggests instability.

Problems exist with both specificity and sensitivity of plain radiographs and comparison studies on plain x-rays and cadaver dissections have found a 67% correlation between disc space narrowing and presence of disc degeneration.[267] However, x-rays identified only 57% of large posterior osteophytes and only 32% of the abnormalities of the apophyseal joints found on dissection. It is also worth remembering that degenerative changes occur in asymptomatic subjects. Radiographic evidence of degenerative changes on x-rays have been found in 35% of asymptomatic subjects by the age of 40 and up to 83% by the age of 60.[268] As with any diagnostic study, the findings on x-ray must be correlated with the history and physical examination.

Computed Tomography (CT)

CT can be helpful in the assessment of acute injury. The accuracy of CT imaging of the cervical spine ranges from 72% to 91% in the diagnosis of disc herniation, but approaches 96% when CT is combined with myelography.[209,269–271] CT of the spine provides superior anatomic imaging of the osseous structures of the spine and good resolution for disc herniation.[272] However, its sensitivity for detecting disc herniation when used without myelography is inferior to that of MRI.[273]

CT with myelography is felt to best assess and localize spinal cord compression and underlying atrophy.[274] It can also determine the functional reserve of the spinal canal in evaluating patients with possible cervical stenosis.[275]

Magnetic Resonance Imaging

MRI has demonstrated excellent sensitivity in the diagnosis of lumbar disc herniations and is considered the imaging study of choice for root impingement.[273] This is tempered, however, by the prevalence of abnormal findings in asymptomatic subjects[276] and, therefore, its use is reserved for selected patients. It can, however, detect ligament and disc disruption, which cannot be demonstrated by other imaging studies.[277–278] The entire spinal cord, nerve roots, and axial skeleton can be visualized.

The major indicator for an immediate MRI of the spine may include patients with a large prolapse, progressive neurologic deficits, or cauda equina syndrome, and those with symptoms and a known history or high risk of malignancy or infection.

ELECTRODIAGNOSIS

Electrodiagnostic studies play an important role in identifying physiologic abnormalities of the nerve root and in ruling out other neurologic causes for the patient's complaints such as peripheral neuropathy and motor neuron disease, radiculopathy,[207,280] and have been shown to correlate well with findings at the time of surgery and with myelography.[207,281,282]

There are two parts to the electromyogram (EMG): nerve conduction studies and needle electrode examination.

Nerve conduction studies are performed by placing surface electrodes over a muscle belly or sensory area and stimulating the nerve, supplying either the muscle or sensory area from fixed points along the nerve. From this, the amplitude, distal latency, and conduction velocity can be measured. The amplitude reflects the number of intact axons, whereas the distal latency and conduction velocity is more of a reflection of the degree of myelination.[167,207,283,284] The timing of the examination is important, because positive sharp waves and fibrillation potentials will first occur 18 to 21 days after the onset of a radiculopathy.[167,207,285] It is, therefore, best to delay this study until 3 weeks after the injury so that the results can be as precise as possible.

The primary use of electromyography is to confirm nerve root impairment when the diagnosis is uncertain or to distinguish a radiculopathy from other impairments that are unclear on physical examination.[167,207,286,287]

INTERVENTION

Various protocols for disc impairments throughout the spine have been proposed over the years. All of them have involved one or combinations of the following measures.

Patient Education

It is very important that patients understand the likely cause of their pain. Their education should include a review of the basic anatomy and biomechanics of the spine and the plan of care which should include a description of recommended therapeutic exercises, postural education, biomechanics of the spine in activities of daily living, and simple methods to reduce symptoms should be reviewed.[288] The more education the patient receives increases the likelihood that they will become active participants in their rehabilitative process, and that they will develop a lifelong commitment to preventing future episodes of spine pain. Over time, the patients learn that all pain is not harmful and that some pain is a natural consequence of the healing process.

Although most of the education occurs early in the rehabilitative process, the clinician's goal should be to ensure that the patient becomes independent with their maintenance exercise program, and that they can refine the exercises as needed as the healing progresses.

The patient should be advised to avoid sitting, bending, and lifting. If sitting is necessary, the lumbar and cervical lordosis should be maintained.[289] The patient should initially sleep in whatever position is comfortable, progressing to the fetal position. The patient should avoid standing with both knees in extension. If prolonged standing is necessary, the patient should raise one foot onto a low stool or other object. In addition the patient should avoid vacuuming, making beds, raking leaves, and any activity involving trunk rotation while in a flexed position.

Manual Therapy

Although manipulations have been advocated for disc herniations, particularly in the lumbar spine, the success rate is not very high, whereas the risk of exacerbation is. Although several studies have demonstrated the efficacy of manipulation and soft tissue mobilization in the intervention of acute low back pain, some have not found this approach to be effective.[290,291] The studies[292,293] that have compared manipulative therapy with other interventions such as medications and sham therapy concluded that short-term manipulative interventions may afford a temporary decrease in pain and increase in function.[288] The initial manipulation technique should be performed once a week in conjunction with the exercise program, and patient-activated interventions (or muscle energy) can be done up to 2 to 3 times per week in conjunction with an active exercise program.[288] If the patient has not improved after three to four treatments, manipulation should be discontinued, and the patient should be reassessed.[288]

The various manual techniques for each of the types of disc lesions are described in the case studies that follow. The manual techniques should be incorporated into the initial intervention of acute pain to facilitate the patient's active exercise program.

Manual shift corrections seem to work well for lumbar protrusions, but are less successful for the prolapsed and extruded discs, owing to the fact that the attempts to correct often result in spasm and reproduction of the patient's symptoms. McKenzie[294] theorizes that because of a prolonged flexed lumbar posture or lifting and walking with the lumbar spine flexed, or both, the nucleus pulposus migrates posteriorly or posterior-laterally. Mechanical correction of the lateral shift usually causes an increase in pain. Ideally, the increase in pain should be noted centrally and not peripherally. An increase in peripheral pain indicates the need to discontinue the correction, because this increase is the result of further irritation to the nerve root.

Therapeutic Exercises

Improvement in aerobic fitness can increase blood flow and oxygenation to all tissues, including the muscles, bones, and ligaments of the spine. Aerobic exercise may also decrease the psychological effect of low back pain by improving mood, decreasing depression, and increasing pain tolerance.[295]

Theoretically, aerobic exercise may help to improve the body's ability to break down scar tissue via tissue plasminogen activator.[296] One study[297] reviewed the available literature on the role of aerobic training and cardiovascular conditioning and noted that it is unclear whether low back pain reduces fitness or whether reduced fitness promotes low back pain. Furthermore, the authors noted that physically fit persons have less low back pain, and they believe that aerobic exercise is "reasonable" as a part of a rehabilitation program.[297]

The clinician should select a series of pain-free exercises if possible. Theoretically, these exercises should provide some relief through an increase in the large-fiber input. The exercises progress to exercises that regain strength. Once full pain-free range of flexion and extension is gained, the patient is encouraged to progress to isometric flexion exercises.

The most important exercise of all is walking. Dynamic stabilization exercises may be used concomitantly to provide dynamic muscular control and protect the patient from biomechanical stresses, including tension, compression, torsion, and shear. Spinal stabilization exercises provide this by emphasizing the synergistic activation or coactivation of the trunk and spinal musculature in a 'neutral spine' position. A progressive challenge is provided through movement of the upper and lower extremities in various planes while the patient is in therapy and, later, during work and activities of daily living.[288] The overall goals of this comprehensive exercise program are to reduce pain, develop the muscular support of the trunk and spine, and diminish stress to the intervertebral disc and other static stabilizers of the spine.[298]

Traction: Mechanical or Manual

Manual or mechanical traction is used to regain normal range of motion. During mechanical traction, electrical stimulation is recommended over the paraspinal muscles to aid in the muscle pumping of the edema.

Traction has long been a preferred method for treating lumbar and cervical disc problems. In the lumbar spine, approximately $1\frac{1}{2}$ times a patient's body weight is needed to develop distraction of the vertebral bodies and, thus, requires a fair amount of strength if performed manually.

Traction is time consuming, is a difficult procedure in the lumbar spine if done manually, and is difficult to tolerate if done mechanically. Vertebral axial decompression, a newer method to cause distraction, probably represents a higher-tech version of traction, although there is no evidence in the current peer-reviewed literature to support this type of intervention.[288] No significant difference in outcome has been demonstrated with traction versus sham traction, with greater morbidity in the traction group.[288,299]

Generally speaking, traction appears to yield better results if at least one of the lumbar motions is full and pain free. However, a one-session trial of short duration is worthwhile if all of the motions are restricted.

Traction is indicated for the following conditions:

- Nuclear disc protrusions
- Indeterminate protrusions
- Primary and secondary lumbar disc impairments
- Backache together with a long-standing limitation of bilateral straight leg raising
- Pain with fourth sacral reference

Lumbar traction is contraindicated in the following conditions:

- Acute lumbago
- Abdominal surgery
- Respiratory or cardiac insufficiency
- Respiratory irritation
- Painful reactions
- A large protrusion
- Altered mental state; this includes the inability of the patient to relax
- Instability of lumbar segments; although intermittent traction with no more than about 40 to 50 lbs can be successful, sustained traction should be avoided

Therapeutic Modalities and Physical Agents

Modalities should always be considered an adjunct to an active intervention program in the management of acute neck or back pain, and should never be used as the sole method of intervention. The clinician should be aware of all indications and contraindications for a prescribed modality and have a clear understanding of each modality and its level of tissue penetration.[288] (see Chapter 12).

A program that is modality intensive rather than exercise based is not helpful to the patient and results in a poor functional outcome.[300] If possible, patients should be instructed in the use of simple modalities in conjunction with their home exercise program.[288]

Modified Rest

This is always an option, especially in acute cases, because most symptoms result from a chemical irritation. Complete rest in the intervention of acute neck and back pain is controversial.

Although there may be some beneficial effects via pain modulation and reduction of intradiscal pressure, bed rest has many detrimental effects on bone, connective tissue, muscle, and cardiovascular fitness.[288] The proactive approach emphasizes activity modification rather than bed rest and immobilization.[288] For severe radicular symptoms, limited bed rest in conjunction with standing and weight bearing, as tolerated, can be used.[288] The patient can often relate a position of comfort to the clinician and if this position does not appear to produce pain during or afterward, it should be encouraged. For low back symptoms, the use of pillows to support the legs while lying should be demonstrated.

In the acutely painful stage when the lumbar deviation cannot be corrected because of pain, the initial resting position for the first 48 hours should be in flexed supine lying with the hips in about 90 degrees of flexion and the legs supported with pillows.[301] The patient is progressed to supine lying with one pillow under the knees and, eventually, to prone lying (30 to 60 minutes at a time) to counteract the amount of flexion and sitting during the day.

Case Studies

It is recommended that the reader review the material in Chapter 10 before proceeding with these case studies.

Case Study: Low Neck Pain

Subjective

A 35-year-old woman presented at the clinic with what she described as a "crick" in her neck upon arising from bed a few mornings ago. The patient described experiencing pain in the lower part of the neck that radiated into the right shoulder and arm, and anteriorly and posteriorly over the upper right chest area. The patient also reported a tingling sensation over the radial aspect of the right forearm, the hand, and the fingers. The pain was reported to be aggravated by coughing, sneezing, and straining. The pain was lessened by maintaining the upright position and when ambulating.

Questions
1. What is the working hypothesis?
2. Does this presentation or history warrant a scan? Why?
3. Pain that is aggravated by coughing, sneezing, and straining usually indicates what kind of diagnosis?
4. Tingling sensations are usually in response to an impairment of which system?

Examination

Observation of the patient revealed that the cervical lordosis was reduced and that her head was held in neutral flexion and deviation to the left. Although all indications pointed to a working hypothesis of a herniated disc in the cervical region, the insidious onset, although not uncommon for the aforementioned pathology, deemed it necessary to perform a scan. In addition, the scan can be used to confirm the hypothesis while ruling out the more serious causes for these symptoms. The scan revealed the following:

- Marked limitation of active and passive cervical motion, with a spasm end feel with right rotation, right side-flexion, and extension.
- Gentle compression through the patient's head reproduced the pain. There was no need to perform the Spurling test.
- Palpable tenderness was elicited over the right aspect of the C6-7 segment.
- Hypoesthesia in the seventh cervical dermatome
- Hyporeflexive triceps deep tendon reflexes
- Weakness of the C7 key muscles

Questions
1. Did the scan confirm the working hypothesis?
2. Given the findings from the scan, what is the diagnosis, or is further testing warranted in the form of a biomechanical examination?

Evaluation[302]
The findings from the scan alone indicated that the patient had a rupture of the sixth cervical disc with compression of the seventh cervical nerve, so there was no real need at this time to proceed with a biomechanical examination.

It is, however, important to rule out other possible causes of neck and limb symptoms prior to establishing a diagnosis of radiculopathy. The differential diagnosis includes musculoskeletal disorders, among them, rotator cuff tendinitis or tears, subacromial bursitis, bicipital tendinitis, and lateral epicondylitis.

Questions
1. Having confirmed the diagnosis, what intervention is needed?
2. In order of priority, and based on the stages of healing, what are the goals of the intervention?

Intervention
Although a less common entity than lumbar disc herniation, cervical intervertebral disc herniation is more frequently managed on a case-by-case basis. The initial intervention should be directed at reducing pain and inflammation, and can begin with local icing, in conjunction with the nonsteroidal anti-inflammatories prescribed by the physician. Manual or mechanical traction can be tried in an attempt to temporarily remove the compression from the nerve.

Specific Manual Traction at C6-7 The patient is positioned sitting, and the clinician stands to the side of the patient, with the hips and knees slightly flexed. Using a lumbrical grip of the index finger and thumb of the dorsal hand, the clinician palpates the laminae and transverse processes of C7. The rest of this hand is used to support the patient's lower cervical spine. The ulnar border of the fifth finger of the ventral hand is applied to the laminae and inferior articular processes of C6. The rest of this hand supports the cranium and the upper cervical spine. An incongruent lock of the cranial segment is accomplished by applying side-flexion and rotation at the C5-6 joint complex, leaving the craniovertebral joints in a neutral position (Fig. 7–5). C7 is fixed, and a vertical traction force of grade I is applied to the C6-7 joint complex.

Mechanical Cervical Traction Mechanical cervical traction can be used to treat both zygapophysial joint impairments and cervical disc herniations.

- Zygapophysial joint impairments: The patient's cervical spine is positioned in about 15 degrees of extension, not flexion, as flexion causes a binding when a pull is exerted.
- Intervertebral foramen narrowing: The typical presentation for this type of patient is a combination of

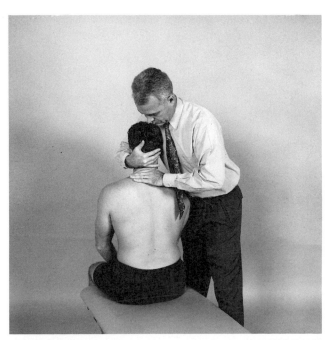

FIGURE 7–5 Patient and clinician position for specific traction at C6-7.

sensory and motor changes. *Anterior foramen* (motor symptoms) opened more in flexion (30 degrees); *posterior foramen* (sensory) opened more in 0 degrees or 30 degrees of flexion.

Manipulative Technique for Cervical Nerve Root Impingement at C6-7 (When Traction Has Failed)   The patient is positioned supine, with the clinician at the head of the table. The clinician supports the patient's head in the hands and contact is made with the upper bone of the segment to be mobilized (C6), using the metacarpophalangeal joint of the index finger of the right hand. The patient's neck is fully flexed up from below, beyond the upper bone (C6) before being unflexed (extended) so that the segment to be mobilized (C6-7), is in neutral—thereby utilizing a ligamentous lock of the neck below the caudal bone of the segment in question. Locking from above then takes place. While the clinician maintains contact with the right hand on C6, he or she moves to the right side of the patient and cradles the patient's head with the left arm and forearm, wrapping around the left side of the patient's face and grasping the chin. Noncongruent locking from above is achieved with right side-flexion and then slight left rotation down to the point where motion is felt to occur by the right hand (C6) (Fig. 7–6). Distraction of the C6-7 segment is manually applied by the clinician, and then a distractive impulse is superimposed on the traction force using the right hand.

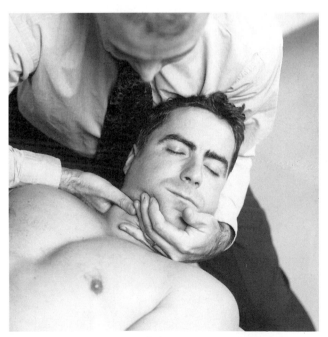

FIGURE 7–6   Patient and clinician position for thrust technique at C6-7.

Modalities such as electrical stimulation have also been found helpful in uncontrolled studies.[226] They appear to be helpful in reducing the associated muscle pain and spasm often found with cervical problems but should be limited to the initial pain-control phase of the intervention.

Once there is control of pain and inflammation, the patient's therapy should be progressed to restore full range of motion and flexibility of the neck and shoulder girdle muscles. Various soft tissue mobilization techniques can be helpful to stretch the noncontractile elements of soft tissues.[226,303] Patients should be instructed on proper stretching technique that they can do 1 to 2 times per day. Gentle, prolonged stretching is recommended. This is best done after a warm-up activity such as using an exercise bike.

As range of motion and flexibility improve, cervical muscle strengthening should begin with isometric strengthening in a single plane and include flexion, extension, side-flexion and rotation. In addition, the scapular stabilizing muscles, including the trapezius, rhomboids, serratus anterior, and the latissimus dorsi, should be strengthened.[167] Strength training can progress to manual resistance cervical stabilization exercises in various planes. All exercises should be performed without pain, although some degree of postexercise soreness can be expected. Isolated strengthening of weakened muscle secondary to the radiculopathy is important before beginning more complex activities involving multiple muscles.[167] In the initial phases of the intervention, the clinician should monitor the patients response to exercise closely, and should only progress the patient as tolerance allows. Closed kinetic chain activities can also be very helpful in rehabilitating weak shoulder girdle muscles.[167]

It is important throughout the rehabilitation process for patients to maintain their level of cardiovascular fitness as much as possible, so aerobic conditioning should be started as early as healing permits to prevent deconditioning. These exercises also serve as a great warm-up prior to a stretching program.[167]

Management need not be overly aggressive in exercise. Continued efforts must be made to progressively reduce the patient's pain and advance physical function through exercise.[249] However, aggressive measures at pain and inflammation control probably help a patient to progress while suffering considerably less pain and enabling him or her to return to work.

Case Study: Low Back and Leg Pain

Subjective

A 32-year-old man presented with complaints of severe pain in the lower back and radiating into the right buttock, posterior thigh, calf, and lateral foot and two toes. The pain in the back started about 2 weeks ago after sitting for a period of a few hours, and was initially relieved by rest. Over the next few days the pain gradually got worse. He reported the pain to be aggravated with bending at the waist and sitting, and lessened with right-side-lying with the hips and knees flexed. Difficulty with assuming an erect posture after lying down or sitting was also reported. Further questioning revealed that the patient had a history of minor back pain but was otherwise in good health and had no reports of bowel or bladder impairment.

Questions
1. What is the working hypothesis at this stage?
2. Does this presentation and history warrant a scan? Why or why not?
3. Low back pain that is aggravated by bending at the waist and sitting, usually indicates what kind of diagnosis?
4. Radiation of pain in the described distribution is usually in response to an impairment of which structure?

Examination
The patient was a slightly obese man who had preferred to stand in the waiting room. His standing posture revealed a flexed hip and knee on the right side when weight bearing, moderate kyphosis and a rotoscoliosis with right convexity of the lumbar spine, and shoulder girdle retraction. Because of the reports of a relatively insidious onset of symptoms and the report of leg pain, a lumbar scan was performed with the following findings:

- The patient demonstrated a marked restriction of lumbar motion.
- Active range of motion revealed a significant restriction of trunk flexion at about 35 degrees from the kyphotic start position, which reproduced the posterior leg pain. The patient attempted to compensate during the trunk flexion by bending at the hips and knees.
- The patient was unable to perform extension or right side-flexion because of a sharp increase in the radiation of pain into the right buttock and posterior thigh.
- Left side-flexion was limited by 25%, producing a slight ache in the right side of the low back.
- Compression testing reproduced the back, right buttock, and posterior thigh pain, and posterior-anterior pressure applied at the L4 and L5 segments provoked a spasm end feel.
- The right SLR reproduced the radiating pain into the posterior right leg, and a hamstring spasm at 15 degrees. The application of passive ankle dorsiflexion increased the patient's symptoms. The left SLR was

limited by spasm at 60 degrees, producing right low back, right buttock, and posterior thigh pain. The addition of neck flexion or dorsiflexion to the left SLR had no effect on the symptoms. The slump test was deferred as it was felt that no additional information would be achieved at the expense of aggravating the patient's condition.
- The prone knee-flexion test was negative on both sides.
- The ipsilateral and contralateral kinetic tests for the sacroiliac joint were positive on both sides. (Refer to Chapter 17)
- Key muscle testing revealed fatigable weakness of the right ankle plantar flexors and evertors.
- Sensory testing revealed some pin-prick loss over the lateral border of the right foot and toe and over the skin of the posterolateral right calf.
- Deep tendon reflexes were decreased at the right ankle, but the spinal cord tests were unremarkable. Palpation revealed tenderness over the paravertebral area on the right side.

Questions
1. Did the scan confirm the working hypothesis? How?
2. Given the findings from the scan, what is the diagnosis, or is further testing warranted in the form of a biomechanical examination? What information would further testing reveal?
3. A positive SLR at 15 degrees with muscle spasm indicates what type of herniation?
4. Why was the prone knee-flexion test negative?

At the end of the scan, a provisional diagnosis of a disc prolapse could be made, so the performance of the biomechanical part of the examination was unnecessary. If performed, the biomechanical examination would have revealed further evidence of the diagnosis, as both the passive physiological intervertebral motion (PPIVM) and passive physiological articular intervertebral motion (PPAIVM) tests would be limited owing to spasms, stiffness, and pain.

Assessment
The findings for this patient indicate the presence of a prolapse, or extrusion of the fifth lumbar disc, with an isolated compression of the first sacral spinal nerve. The patient was referred back to his physician, who then ordered an MRI that confirmed the diagnosis. The patient returned to the clinic for treatment.

Questions
1. Having confirmed the diagnosis, what intervention should be performed?

2. In order of priority, and based on the stages of healing, what will be the goals of the intervention?

Intervention

The treatment of a disc impairment obviously depends on the size of the impairment. This patient presented with either a disc prolapse or extrusion and, therefore, caution is needed as the progression to a cauda equina syndrome is a possibility. The intervention for this patient included:

● Manual shift correction
● Patient education
● Specific manual traction
● The McKenzie exercise approach.[304] The McKenzie program is initiated only after a comprehensive assessment in which the positions that centralize pain are determined.[305]
● A unilateral extension protocol, consisting of manual therapy, electric stimulation, and exercises to close down the segment on the disc and force it anteriorly
● Initiation of a walking program

Specific lumbar traction (refer to Chapter 13) afforded the patient some relief. The patient was advised on a period of modified rest for 48 hours. When the patient returned, a series of short-duration (8 minutes), sustained mechanical traction sessions were initiated with the patient in supine 90-90 at 60% of body weight.[306] The patient was instructed on gentle active range of motion exercises of unilateral heel slides and pelvic rotations to be performed without increasing peripheral signs and symptoms. After a few sessions, the patient progressed to prone traction, posterior pelvic tilts, and the McKenzie program.[307]

Case Study: Severe Low Back Pain[308]

Subjective

A 49-year-old woman presented to the clinic with a 1-week history of severe low back pain. The patient experienced an acute onset of severe lumbar shooting pain that radiated immediately into the left buttock and the lateral aspect of the left leg and left foot. The pain was exacerbated by movement, sneezing, or coughing, and was lessened by resting. Paresthesia and numbness were present over the lateral aspect of the left leg and foot and the dorsum of the left foot, and mild pain in the right leg. In addition, the patient mentioned urinary urgency. The patient's history showed that she had a history of intermittent low back pain for the past year. There was no history of back trauma. The patient had the results of a conventional CT myelogram of the lumbosacral spine with her, which were normal.

Questions
1. Given the classic symptoms, what would be the working hypothesis at this stage?
2. Does this presentation and history warrant a scan? Why or why not?
3. Should the fact that there was no trauma concern the clinician?

Examination

Given the history and described symptoms and the strong possibility that the patient was presenting with a disc herniation, a lumbar scan was performed to confirm the diagnosis. It elicited the following results:

● Symptoms were reproduced with end range flexion and thoracic rotation to the left. All other motions were normal.
● There was decreased muscle strength (4/5) in the foot dorsiflexors, plantar flexors, gluteus maximus, anterior tibialis, and gastrocnemius muscles on the left side.
● There was reduced sensation to pin-prick at the L5 and S1 dermatomes.
● The ankle jerk was reduced on the left side, and plantar responses were flexor bilaterally.
● Stretching of the sciatic nerve by an SLR test to 15 degrees reproduced the low back pain that sometimes radiated into the left leg. A crossed SLR test produced negative results.

Questions
1. Having apparently confirmed the diagnosis, what intervention is appropriate?
2. In order of priority, and based on the stages of healing, list the various goals of the intervention?
3. What should the clinician tell the patient about the intervention?
4. Estimate this patient's prognosis.
5. What modalities could be used in the intervention of this patient?
6. What exercises should be prescribed?

Evaluation

The patient's clinical presentation, including an acute low back pain radiating down the weak leg through the L5-S1 dermatomes, positive SLR, and sensory and motor impairments of the corresponding roots, strongly indicated acute lumbar disc disease, although the subjective report of urinary urgency suggests cavda equina involvement. The initial diagnosis was a lumbar disc herniation with L5-S1 root compression.

Intervention was initiated, but the patient failed to respond and was referred back to her physician for further testing.

An MRI study of the thoracolumbar spine showed a bulging disc and posterior osteophytes at T11-12, with encroachment of the underlying spinal canal and compression on the underlying cord. There was no evidence of L5 or S1 root compression at the exiting intervertebral foramens. One month later, a surgical procedure was performed to remove the bulging disc and osteophytes at T11-12. Following the surgery, the patient's sensory and motor deficits, and her urinary urgency completely resolved, and the low back pain was much diminished.

REVIEW QUESTIONS

1. Which of the two processes is the more aggressive, degeneration or degradation?
2. What are the three components of the intervertebral disc?
3. Give three functions of the disc
4. Does the water content of the disc increase or decrease with age?
5. Does the collagen content in the disc increase or decrease with age?
6. Does the height of the disc increase or decrease with age?
7. At what age range is disc degeneration thought to begin?
8. List seven signs or symptoms characteristic of a posterior-lateral disc herniation.
9. Which area of the anulus tends to weaken first?
10. True or false: When the nuclear material remains attached to the disc but escapes the anulus or the posterior longitudinal ligament to bulge externally into the intervertebral, it is termed a *protrusion* or *herniation*.
11. List four clinical syndromes that are associated with disc degenerative disease.
12. Name the three phases of disc generation proposed by Kirkaldy-Willis.
13. Which of the three phases of Kirkaldy-Willis is characterized by fibrosis of the posterior joints and capsule, loss of disc material, and the formation of osteophytes?
14. Which nerve supplies the intervertebral disc?
15. What are the patterns of paresthesia with compression of the following: (a) spinal nerve, (b) spinal cord, and (c) spinothalamic tract.
16. List five signs and symptoms of spinal cord compression.
17. List three causes of spinal cord compromise.
18. List six signs of cauda equina syndrome.
19. List three causes of cauda equina syndrome.
20. What is a Schmorl's node?

21. In a large U.S. population survey, the combined prevalence of which two segmental levels accounted for 75% of cervical disc herniations?
22. A C7 nerve root impairment is likely the result of the protrusion of which disc?
23. Of the three spinal regions, cervical, thoracic, and lumbar, which region has the least number of intervertebral disc herniations?

ANSWERS

1. Degradation.
2. Nucleus pulposus, end plate, and anulus fibrosis.
3. It increases the potential range of motion between vertebrae; maintains contiguity between the vertebral bodies; attenuates and transfers vertebral loading.
4. Decrease.
5. Increase.
6. Increase.
7. Between 20 and 25 years.
8. Key muscle weakness at a specific level; paresthesia in dermatomal distribution; decreased deep tendon reflexes; positive SLR in 30- to 60-degree range; pain with lumbar flexion and opposite side-flexion; limited lumbar range of motion with flexion and ipsilateral extension quadrant; positive bowstring test(s).
9. Posterior-lateral.
10. False. It is a prolapse or extrusion.
11. Possible answers include idiopathic low back pain, cervical and lumbar radiculopathy, cervical myelopathy, lumbar stenosis, spondylosis, osteoarthritis, and herniated disc (degenerative disc disease).
12. The three phases are defined as early dysfunction, intermediate instability, and final stabilization.
13. The final, stabilization phase.
14. Sinuvertebral nerve.
15. (a) Spinal nerve—dermatomal single segment loss; (b) spinal cord—multisegmental dermatomal loss below the level of the lesion; (c) spinothalamic tract—loss of pain and temperature sense below the level of the lesion.
16. Spasticity, multisegmental paresis or paralysis, clonus, Babinski, and hyper-reflexia.
17. Traumatic damage, ischemia, pathology (disease, cancer).
18. Hypotonicity, incontinence, normal extensor and plantar response, marked atrophy, coarse fasiculations with time, multisegmental radicular symptoms.
19. Possible answers include major posterior disc protrusion, tumor, fracture–dislocation, and significant spondylolisthesis.
20. A vertical disc prolapse.

21. C5-6 and C6-7.
22. The C6 disc.
23. Thoracic.

REFERENCES

1. Taylor JR. The development and adult structure of lumbar intervertebral discs. J Man Med 1990;5: 43–47.
2. Tsuji H, Hirano N, Ohshima H, Ishihara H, Terahata N, Motoe T. Structural variation of the anterior and posterior anulus fibrosus in the development of the human lumbar intervertebral disc: A risk factor for intervertebral disc rupture. Spine 1993;18: 204–210.
3. Marchand F, Ahmed AM. Investigation of the laminate structure of lumbar disc anulus fibrosus. Spine 1990;15:402–410.
4. Armstrong JR. *Lumbar Disc Lesions*, 3 ed. Edinburgh, Scotland: Churchill Livingstone; 1965:13.
5. Bogduk N, Twomey LT. *Clinical Anatomy of the Lumbar Spine and Sacrum*, 3d ed. Edinburgh, Scotland: Churchill Livingstone; 1997:2–53,81–152,171,176.
6. Eyring EJ. The biochemistry and physiology of the intervertebral disc. Clin Orthop 1969;67:16–28.
7. Nachemson AL. The lumbar spine: An orthopedic challenge. Spine 1976;1:59–71.
8. Coventry MB, Ghormley RK, Kernohan JW. The intervertebral disc: Its microscopic anatomy and pathology. Part I. Anatomy, development and physiology. J Bone Joint Surg 1945;27:105–112.
9. Inoue H. Three dimensional architecture of lumbar intervertebral discs. Spine 1981;6:138–146.
10. Coventry MB. Anatomy of the intervertebral disk. Clin Orthop 1969;67:9–17.
11. Adams MA, McNally DS, Wagstaff J, Goodship AE. Abnormal stress concentrations in lumbar intervertebral discs following damage to the vertebral body: A cause of disc failure. Eur Spine J 1993;1:214–221.
12. Adams MA, Dolan P. Which comes first: Disc degeneration or mechanical failure? Proceedings of the Spine Society of Australia, Cairns, November 1996.
13. Naylor A. The biophysical and biomechanical aspects of intervertebral disc herniation and degeneration. Ann R Coll Surg 1962;31:91–114.
14. Beard HK, Ryvar R, Brown R, Muir H. Immunochemical localization of collagen types and proteoglycan in pig intervertebral discs. Immunology 1980;41:491–501.
15. Beard HK, Roberts S, O'Brien JP. Immunofluorescent staining for collagen and proteoglycan in normal and scoliotic intervertebral discs. J Bone Joint Surg [Br] 1981;63B:529–534.
16. Roberts S, Menage J, Duance V, Wotton S, Ayad S. Collagen types around the cells of the intervertebral disc and cartilage end plate: An immunolocalization study. Spine 1991;16:1030–1038.
17. Roberts S, Ayad S, Menage PJ. Immunolocalization of type VI collagen in the intervertebral disc. Ann Rheumatol Dis 1991;50:787–791.
18. Roberts S, Menage J, Duance V, Wotton SF. Type III collagen in the intervertebral disc. Histochem J 1991;23:503–508.
19. Ghosh P, Bushell GR, Taylor TFK, Akeson WH. Collagens, elastins and noncollagenous protein of the intervertebral disc. Clin Orthop 1977;129:124–132.
20. Gower WE, Pedrini V. Age related variation in protein polysaccharides from human nucleus pulposus, annulus fibrosus and costal cartilage. J Bone Joint Surg 1969;51A:1154–1162.
21. Schmorl G, Junghanns H. *The Human Spine in Health and Disease*, 2nd Amer ed. New York, NY: Grune & Stratton; 1971:18.
22. Happey T, Pearson CH, Palframan J, et al. Proteoglycans and glycoproteins associated with collagen in the human intervertebral disc. Z Klin Chem 1971;9:79.
23. Farfan HF. *Mechanical Disorders of the Low Back.* Philadelphia, Pa: Lea & Febiger; 1973.
24. Roberts N, Gratin C, Whitehouse GH. MRI analysis of lumbar intervertebral disc height in young and older populations. J MRI 1997;7:880–886.
25. Buckwalter JA. Spine update: Ageing and degeneration of the human intervertebral disc. Spine 1995;20:1307–1314.
26. Coventry MB, Ghormley RK, Kernohan JW. The intervertebral disc: Its microscopic anatomy and pathology. Part II. Changes in the intervertebral disc concomittant with age. J Bone Joint Surg 1945;27A: 233–237.
27. Fraser RD, Osti OL, Vernon-Roberts B. Intervertebral disc degeneration. Eur Spine J 1993;1:205–213.
28. Kelsey JL, White AA. Epidemiology and impact of low back pain. Spine 1980;5:133–142.
29. Matsui H, Kanamori M, Ishihara H, Yudoh K, Naruse Y, Tsuji H. Familial predisposition for lumbar degenerative disc disease. A case-control study. Spine 1998; 23:1029–1034.
30. Jonsson B, Stromqvist B. Clinical appearance of contained and non-contained lumbar disc herniation. J Spinal Disord 1996;9:32.
31. Mixter WJ, Barr JS. Rupture of the intervertebral disc with involvement of the spinal canal. N Engl J Med 1934;211:210–215.
32. Howe JF, Loeser JD, Calvin WH. Mechanosensitivity of dorsal root ganglia and chronically injured axons: A physiological basis for the radicular pain of nerve root compression. Pain 1977;3:25–41.

33. Rydevik B, Garfin SR. Spinal nerve root compression. In: Szabo RM, ed. *Nerve Compression Syndromes, Diagnosis and Treatment*. Thorofare, NJ: Slack; 1989: 247–261.

34. Brown MD. The source of low back pain and sciatica. Semin Arthritis Rheum 1989;18(Suppl):67–72.

35. Smyth MJ, Wright V. Sciatica and the intervertebral disc. An experimental study. J Bone Joint Surg [Am] 1958;40:1401–1418.

36. Boden S, Davis DO, Dina TS, Patronas NJ, Wiesel SW. Abnormal magnetic resonance scans of the lumbar spine in asymptomatic subjects. J Bone Joint Surg [Am] 1990;72:403–408.

37. Hiselberger WE, Witten RM. Abnormal myelograms in asymptomatic patients. J Neurosurg 1968;28: 204–206.

38. Weinstein JN, Gordon SL. *Low Back Pain: A Scientific and Clinical Overview*. Rosemont, Ill: American Academy of Orthopedic Surgeons; 1996.

39. Gronblad M, Virri J, Tolonen J, et al. A controlled immuno-histochemical study of inflammatory cells in disc herniation tissue. Spine 1994;19:2744–2751.

40. Kang JD, Georgescu HI, McIntyre-Larkin L, Stefanovic-Racic M, Donaldson WF, Evans CH. Herniated lumbar intervertebral discs spontaneously produce matrix metalloproteinases, nitric oxide, interleukin-6, and prostaglandin E2. Spine 1996;21: 271–277.

41. Doita M, Kanatani T, Harada T, Mizino K. Immuno-histologic study of the ruptured intervertebral disc of the lumbar spine. Spine 1996;21:235–241.

42. Gronblad M, Virri J, et al. A controlled biochemical and immunohistochemical study of human synovial-type (group II) phospholipase A2 and inflammatory cells in macroscopically normal, degenerated, and herniated human lumbar disc tissues. Spine 1996;22: 1–8.

43. Habtemariam A, Virri J, Gronblad M, et al. Inflammatory cells in experimental disc herniation. Presented at the annual meeting of the International Society for the Study of the Lumbar Spine, Singapore, June 2–6, 1997.

44. Hampton D, Laros G, McCarron R, Franks D. Healing potential of the anulus fibrosus. Spine 1989;14: 398–401.

45. Bobechko WP, Hirsch C. Autoimmune response to nucleus pulposus in the rabbit. J Bone Joint Surg [Br] 1965;47:574–580.

46. Tolonen J, Gronblad M, Virri J, Seitsalo S, Karaharju E. Basic fibroblast growth factor immunoreactivity in blood vessels and cells of disc herniations. Spine 1995;20:271–276.

47. Virri J, Gronblad M, Savikko J, et al. Prevalence, morphology and topography of blood vessels in herniated disc tissue: A comparative immunocytochemical study. Spine 1996;21:1856–1863.

48. Yasuma T, Kouichi A, Yamauchi Y. The histology of lumbar intervertebral disc herniation: The significance of small blood vessels in the extruded tissue. Spine 1993;18:1761–1765.

49. Habtemariam A, Gronblad M, Virri J, Seitsalo S, Ruuskanen M, Karaharju E. Immunocytochemical localization of immunoglobulins in disc herniations. Spine 1996;16:1864–1869.

50. Meadows J. NAIOMT course notes Level II and III Derver, Colo: 1995.

51. Cyriax J. Textbook of Orthopedic Medicine 8th Ed. London. Baillière Tindal, 1982.

52. Marshall LL, Trethewie ER, Curtain CC. Chemical radiculitis: A clinical, physiological and immunological study. Clin Orthop 1977;129:61–67.

53. McCarron RF, Wimpee MW, Hudkins PG, Laros GS. The inflammatory effect of nucleus pulposus: A possible element in the pathogenesis of low back pain. Spine 1987;12:760–764.

54. Gertzbein SD, Tile M, Gross A, Falk R. Autoimmunity in degenerative disc disease of the lumbar spine. Orthop Clin North Am 1975;6:67–73.

55. Gertzbein SD. Degenerative disc disease of the lumbar spine: Immunological implication. Clin Orthop 1977;129:68–71.

56. Pennington JB, McCarron F, Laros GS. Identification of IgG in the canine intervertebral disc. Spine 1988;13:909–912.

57. Takenaka Y, Kahan A, Amor B. Experimental autoimmune spondylodiscitis in rats. J Rheumatol 1980,13:397–400.

58. Gronblad M, Virri J, Tolonen J, et al. A controlled immunohistochemical study of inflammatory cells in disc herniation tissue. Spine 1994;24:2744–2751.

59. Virri J, Sikk S, Gronblad M, et al. Concomitant immunocytochemical study of macrophage cells and blood vessels in herniated disc tissue. Eur Spine J 1994;3:336–341.

60. Dilke TFW, Burry JC, Grahame R. Extradural corticoid injection in management of lumbar nerve root compression. BMJ 1973;2:635–637.

61. Green LN. Dexamethasone for lumbar radiculopathy. J Neurol Neurosurg Psychiatry 1975;38:1211–1217.

62. Shizu N, Yoshizawa H, Kobayashi S, Nakai S. Effects of disc tissue on the nerve root. Presented at the annual meeting of the International Society for the Study of the Lumbar Spine, Singapore, June 2–6, 1997.

63. Dupuis PR. The natural history of degenerative changes in the lumbar spine. In: Watkins RG, Collis JS, eds. *Principles and Techniques in Spine Surgery*. Rockville, Md: Aspen Publications; 1987:1–4.

64. Adams P, Muir H. Qualitative changes with age of proteoglycans of human lumbar discs. Ann Rheum Dis 1976;35:289–296.

65. Adams MA, Hutton WC. Gradual disc prolapse. Spine 1985;10:524–531.

66. Arnold JG Jr. The clinical manifestation of spondylochondrosis (spondylosis) of the cervical spine. Ann Surg 1955;141:872–889.

67. Bohlman HH, Emery SE. The pathophysiology of cervical spondylosis and myelopathy. Spine 1988;13:843–846.

68. Frymoyer JW, Donaghy RM. The ruptured intervertebral disc: Follow-up report on the first case fifty years after recognition of the syndrome and its surgical significance. J Bone Joint Surg 1985;67A:1113–1116.

69. Park WM, McCall IW, O'Brien JP, et al. Fissuring of the posterior annulus fibrosus in the lumbar spine. Br J Radiol 1979;52:382–387.

70. Kirkaldy-Willis WH. The three phases of the spectrum of degenerative disease. In: Kirkaldy-Willis WH, ed. *Managing Low Back Pain.* New York, NY: Churchill Livingstone; 1983:75–90.

71. Wedge JH. The natural history of spinal degeneration. In Kirkaldy-Willis WH, ed. *Managing Low Back Pain.* New York, NY: Churchill Livingstone; 1983:3–8.

72. Adams MA, McNally DS, Dolan P. Stress distributions inside intervertebral discs: The effects of age and degeneration. Bone Joint Surg 1996;78:965–972.

73. Moneta GB, Videman T, Kaivanto K, et al. Reported pain during lumbar discography as a function of annular ruptures and disc degeneration. Spine 1994;19:1968–1974.

74. Dolan P, Earley M, Adams MA. Bending and compressive stresses acting on the lumbar spine during lifting activities. J Biomech 1994;27:1237–1248.

75. Fang D, Cheung KMC, Ruan D, Chan FL. Computed tomographic osteometry of the Asian lumbar spine. J Spinal Disord 1994;7:307–316.

76. Farfan HF, Huberdeau RM, Dubow HI. Lumbar intervertebral disc degeneration: The influence of geometrical features on the pattern of disc degeneration—A post mortem study. J Bone Joint Surg [Br] 1972;54:492–510.

77. Meschan I. *An Atlas of Anatomy Basic to Radiology.* Philadelphia, Pa: WB Saunders; 1975:521–556.

78. Rolander SD. Motion of the lumbar spine with special reference to the stabilizing effect of posterior fusion. An experimental study on autopsy specimens. Acta Orthop Scand 1966;90(Suppl):1–144.

79. Anderson BJG, Schultz A, Nathan A, Irstam L. Roentgenographic measurement of lumbar intervertebral disc height. Spine 1981;6:154–158.

80. Bradford DS, Cooper KM, Oegema TR. Chymopapain, chemonucleolysis, and nucleus pulposus regeneration. J Bone Joint Surg [Am] 1983;65:1220–1231.

81. Brinckmann P, Grootenboer H. Change of disc height, radial disc bulge, and intradiscal pressure from discectomy. An in vitro investigation on human lumbar discs. Spine 1991;16:641–646.

82. Konings JG, Williams JB, Deutman R. The effects of chemonucleolysis as demonstrated by computerized tomography. J Bone Joint Surg [Br] 1984;66:417–421.

83. De Puky P. The physiological oscillation of the length of the body. Acta Orthop Scand 1935;6:338–347.

84. Adams MA, Dolan P, Hutton WC, Porter RW. Diurnal variations in the stresses on the lumbar spine. Spine 1987;12:130–137.

85. Lu YM, Hutton WC, Gharpuray VM. Can variations in intervertebral disc height affect the mechanical function of the disc? Spine 1996;21:2208–2216; discussion: 2217.

86. Crock HV, Goldwasser M, Yoshizawa H. Vascular anatomy related to the intervertebral disc. In: Ghosh P, ed. *The Biology of the Intervertebral Disc,* vol. I. Boca Raton, Fla: CRC Press; 1988:109–133.

87. Eyre D, Benya P, Buckwalter J, et al. Basic science perspectives. In: Frymoyer JW, Gordon SL, eds. *New Perspectives on Low Back Pain.* Park Ridge, Ill: American Academy of Orthopaedic Surgeons; 1988:147–214.

88. Maroudas A. Nutrition and metabolism of the intervertebral disc. In: Ghosh P, ed. *The Biology of the Intervertebral Disc,* vol II. Boca Raton, Fla: CRC Press; 1988:1–37.

89. Bobechko WP, Hirsch C. Autoimmune response to nucleus pulposus in the rabbit. J Bone Joint Surg [Br] 1965;47:574–580.

90. Marshall LL, Trethewie ER, Curtain CC. Chemical radiculitis: A clinical, physiological and immunological study. Clin Orthop 1977;129:61–67.

91. Buckwalter JA. Aging and degeneration of the human intervertebral disc. Spine 1995;20:1307–1314.

92. Fabregat I, Sánchez A, Alvarez AM, Nakamura T, Benito M. Epidermal growth factor, but not hepatocyte growth factor, suppresses the apoptosis induced by transforming growth factor-beta in fetal hepatocytes in primary culture. FEBS Lett 1996;384:14–18.

93. Uren AG, Vaux DL. Molecular and clinical aspects of apoptosis. Pharmacol Ther 1996;72:37–50.

94. Adams MA, McNally DM, Chinn H, Dolan P. Posture and the compressive strength of the lumbar spine. International Society of Biomechanics Award Paper. Clin Biomech 1994;9:5–14.

95. Markolf KL, Morris JM. The structural components of the intervertebral disc. J Bone Joint Surg 1974;56A:675–687.

96. Brinkmann P, Frobin W, Hierholzer E, Horst M. Deformation of the vertebral end-plate under axial loading of the spine. Spine 1983;8:851–856.

97. Horst M, Brinkmann P. Measurement of the distribution of axial stress on the end plate of the vertebral body. Spine 1981;6:217–232.

98. Lord MJ, Small JM, Dinsay JM, Watkins RG. Lumbar lordosis: Effects of sitting and standing. Spine 1997;22:2571–2574.

99. Adams MA, Dolan P. Recent advances in lumbar spinal mechanics and their clinical significance. Clin Biomech 1995;10:3–19.

100. Kraemer J, Kolditz D, Gowin R. Water and electrolyte content of human intervertebral discs under variable load. Spine 1985;10:69–71.

101. Kazarian LE. Dynamic response characteristics of the human lumbar vertebral column. Acta Orthop Scandinav Supp 1972;146:1–86.

102. Markolf KL, Morris JM. The structural components of the intervertebral disc. J Bone Joint Surg 1974;56A: 675–687.

103. Kazarian LE. Creep characteristics of the human spinal column. Orthop Clin North Am 1975;6:3–18.

104. Tyrell AJ, Reilly T, Troup JDG. Circadian variation in stature and the effects of spinal loading. Spine 1985;10:161–164.

105. Andersson GBJ, Schultz AB. Effects of fluid injection on mechanical properties of intervertebral discs. J Biomech 1979;12:453–458.

106. Brinckmann P, Grootenboer H. Change of disc height, radial disc bulge and intradiscal pressure from discectomy: An in-vitro investigation on human lumbar discs. Spine 1991;16:641–646.

107. Adams MA, Hutton WC. The effect of posture on the fluid content of lumbar intervertebral discs. Spine 1983;8:665–671.

108. Nachemson A. Disc pressure measurements. Spine 1981;6:93–97.

109. Adams MA, McMillan DW, Green TP, Dolan P. Sustained loading generates stress concentrations in lumbar intervertebral discs. Spine 1996;21:434–438.

110. Hickey DS, Hukins DWL. Relation between the structure of the annulus fibrosus and the function and failure of the intervertebral disc. Spine 1980;5: 100–116.

111. Yoganandan N, Myklebust JB, Wilson CR, Cusick JF, Sances A. Functional biomechanics of the thoracolumbar vertebral cortex. Clin Biomech 1988;3: 11–18.

112. Bogduk N, Twomey LT. *Clinical Anatomy of the Lumbar Spine.* Edinburgh, Scotland: Churchill Livingstone; 1991.

113. Kuslich SD, Ulstrom CL, Michael CJ. The tissue origin of low back pain and sciatica. Orthop Clin North Am 1991;22:181–187.

114. Kelsey JL, Hardy RJ. Driving of motor vehicles as a risk factor for acute herniated lumbar intervertebral disc. Am J Epidemiol 1975;102:63–73.

115. Markolf KL. Deformation of the thoracolumbar intervertebral joints in response to external loads. J Bone Joint Surg 1972;54A:511–533.

116. Twomey L. Sustained lumbar traction. An experimental study of long spine segments. Spine 1985;10: 146–149.

117. Hickey DS, Hukins DWL. Relation between the structure of the annulus fibrosus and the function and failure of the intervertebral disc. Spine 1980;5: 100–116.

118. Farfan HF, Cossette JW, Robertson GH, Wells RV, Kraus H. The effects of torsion on the lumbar intervertebral joints: The role of torsion in the production of disc degeneration. J Bone Joint Surg 1970;52A: 468–497.

119. Shah JS. Structure, morphology and mechanics of the lumbar spine. In: Jayson MIV, ed. *The Lumbar Spine and Backache,* 2nd ed. London, England: Pitman; 1980:359–405.

120. Schmorl G, Junghanns H. *The Human Spine in Health and Disease.* New York, NY: Grune & Stratton; 1971.

121. Moore KL. *The Developing Human: Clinically Orientated Embryology.* Philadelphia, Pa: WB Saunders; 1988.

122. Hilton RC, Ball J, Benn RT. Vertebral end plate lesions (Schmorl's nodes) in the dorsolumbar spine. Ann Rheum Dis 1976;35:127–132.

123. Keyes DC, Compere EL. The normal and pathological physiology of the nucleus pulposus of the intervertebral disc. J Bone Joint Surg 1932;14:897–938.

124. Yasuma T, Saito S, Kihara K. Schmorl's nodes: Correlation of x-ray and histological findings in postmortem specimens. Acta Pathol Japonica 1988;38: 723–733.

125. Charnley J. Acute lumbago and sciatica. Br Med J 1955;1:344.

126. Nadler SF, Campagnolo DI, Tomaio AC, Stitik TP. High lumbar disc: diagnostic and treatment dilemma. Am J Phys Med Rehab 1998;77:538–544.

127. Porchet F, Frankhauser H, de Tribolet N. Extreme lateral lumbar disc herniation: A clinical presentaion of 178 patients. Acta Neurochir (Wien) 1994;127: 203–209.

128. Bosacco SJ, Berman AT, Raisis LW, Zamarin RI. High lumbar disc herniation. Orthopedics 1989;12:275–278.

129. Fontanesi G, Tartaglia I, Cavazzuti A, Giancecchi F. Prolapsed intervertebral disc at the upper lumbar level. Ital J Orthop Traumatol 1987;13:501–507.

130. Usher BW Jr, Friedman RJ. Steroid-induced osteonecrosis of the humeral head. Orthopedics 1995; 18:47–51.

131. Hsu K, Zucherman J, Shea W, et al. High lumbar disc degeneration: Incidence and etiology. Spine 1990;15: 679–682.

132. Cailliet R. *Low Back Pain Syndrome.* Philadelphia, Pa: FA Davis; 1988:14.

133. Sciatica. *Dorland's Medical Dictionary,* 27th ed. Philadelphia, Pa: WB Saunders; 1988:1494.

134. Halland AM, Klemp P, Botes D, Van Heerden BB, Loxton A, Scher AT. Avascular necrosis of the hip in systemic lupus erythematosus: The role of MRI. Br J Rheumatol 1993;32:972–976.

135. Cooper KL. Insufficiency stress fractures. Curr Probl Diagn Radiol 1994;23:29–68.

136. Weber M, Hasler P, Gerber H. Insufficiency fractures of the sacrum. Spine 1993;18:2507–2512.

137. Sammarco GJ, Stephens MM: Neuropraxia of the femoral nerve in a modern dancer. Am J Sports Med 1991;19:413–414.

138. Naftulin S, Fast A, Thomas M. Diabetic lumbar radiculopathy: Sciatica without disc herniation. Spine 1993;18:2419–2422.

139. Deyo R. Understanding the accuracy of diagnostic tests. In: Weinstein J, Rydevik B, Sonntag V, eds. *Essentials of the Spine.* Philadelphia, Pa: Raven Press; 1995:55–70.

140. Deyo R, Rainville J, Kent D. What can the history and physical examination tell us about low back pain? JAMA 1992;268:760–765.

141. Spangfort EV. The lumbar disc herniation: A computer aided analysis of 2,504 operations. Acta Orthop Scand Suppl 1972;142:1–95.

142. Frymoyer JW. Back pain and sciatica. N Engl J Med 1988;318:291–300.

143. Finneson BE. *Low Back Pain.* Philadelphia, Pa: JB Lippincott; 1980.

144. McKenzie RA. *The Lumbar Spine: Mechanical Diagnosis and Therapy.* Waikanae, New Zealand: Spinal Publications Ltd; 1981.

145. Christodoulides AN. Ipsilateral sciatica on the femoral nerve stretch test is pathognomonic of an L4/5 disc protrusion. J Bone Joint Surg Br 1989;71:88–89.

146. Abdullah AF, Wolber PG, Warfield JR, Gunadi IK: Surgical management of extreme lateral lumbar disc herniations. Neurosurgery 1988;22:648–653.

147. Weinstein JN. A 45-year-old man with low back pain and a numb left foot. JAMA 1998;280:730–736.

148. Hakelius A. Prognosis in sciatica. Acta Orthop Scand. 1970;129:1–76.

149. Saal JA, Saal JS. Nonoperative treatment of herniated lumbar intervertebral disc with radiculopathy. Spine 1989;14:431–437.

150. Weber H. Lumbar disc herniation. Spine 1983;8: 131–140.

151. Stankovic R, Johnell O. Conservative management of acute low back pain. A prospective randomized trial: McKenzie method of treatment versus patient education in "mini back school." Spine 1990;15:120–123.

152. Donelson R. The McKenzie approach to evaluating and treating low back pain. Orthop Rev 1990;19: 681–686.

153. Saal JS, Franson R, Dobrow RC, Saal JA, White AH, Goldthwaite N. High levels of phopholipase A2 activity in lumbar disc herniation. Spine 1990;15: 674–678.

154. Ecklin U. Die Altersveranderungen der Halswirbelsaule. Berlin, Germany: Springer; 1960.

155. Taylor JR. Growth and development of the human intervertebral disc (Thesis). University of Edinburgh, 1974.

156. Tondury G. *Entwicklungsgeschichte und Fehlbildungen der Halswirbelsaule.* Stuttgart, Germany: Hippokrates; 1958.

157. Taylor JR. Regional variation in the development and position of the notochordal segments of the human nucleus pulposus. J Anat 1971;110:131–132.

158. Oda J, Tanaka H, Tsuzuki N. Intervertebral disc changes with aging of human cervical vertebra: From neonate to the eighties. Spine 1988;13:1205–1211.

159. Mercer SB, Bogduk N. The ligaments and anulus fibrosus of human adult cervical intervertebral discs. Spine 1999;24:619–626.

160. Pooni JS, Hukins DWL, Harris PF, Hilton RC, Davies KE. Comparison of the structure of human intervertebral discs in the cervical, thoracic, and lumbar regions of the spine. Surg Radiol Anat 1986;8:175–182.

161. Zaki W. Aspect morphologique et fonctionnel de l' anulus fibrosus du disque intervertebrale de la colonne dorsale. Arch Anat Path 1973;21:401–403.

162. Hirsch C. Some morphological changes in the cervical spine during ageing. In: Hirsch C, Zotterman Y, eds. *Cervical Pain.* Oxford, England: Pergamon; 1971.

163. Tondury G. The behavior of the cervical discs during life. In: Hirsch C, Zotterman Y, eds. *Cervical Pain.* Oxford, England: Pergamon; 1971.

164. Hirsch C, Schajowicz F, Galante J. Structural changes in the cervical spine: A study on autopsy specimens in different age groups. Acta Orthop Scand 1967; Suppl 109.

165. Bogduk N. Biomechanics of the cervical spine. In: Grant R, ed. *Physical Therapy of the Cervical and Thoracic Spine,* 2nd ed. New York, NY: Churchill Livingstone; 1994:27–45.

166. Penning L. Differences in anatomy, motion, development, and ageing of the upper and lower cervical disk segments. Clin Biomech 1988;3:37–47.

167. Malanga GA. The diagnosis and treatment of cervical radiculopathy. Medicine and Science in Sports and Exercise 1997;29(7 suppl): S236–245.

168. Brooker AEW, Barter RW. Cervical spondylosis: A clinical study with comparative radiology. Brain 1965;88:925–936.
169. Goodman BW. Neck pain. Prim Care 1988;15:689–707.
170. Gore DR, Sepic SB, Gardner GM, Murray MP. Neck pain: A long-term follow-up of 205 patients. Spine 1987;12:1–5.
171. Kirita Y. Intervertebral disc herniation. Seikeigeka 1961;12:65–87. In Japanese.
172. Spangfort EV. The lumbar disc herniation. Acta Orthop Scand Suppl 1972;142:1–95.
173. Kokubun S. Cervical disc herniation. Rinsho Seikei Geka 1989;24:289–297. In Japanese.
174. O'Laoire SA, Thomas DGT. Spinal cord compression due to prolapse of cervical intervertebral disc (herniation of nucleus pulposus): Treatment in 26 cases by discectomy without interbody bone graft. J Neurosurg 1983;59:847–853.
175. Teresi LM, Lufkin RB, Reicher MA, et al. Asymptomatic degenerative disk disease and spondylosis of the cervical spine: MR imaging. Radiology 1987;164:83–88.
176. Lourie H, Shende MC, Stewart DH Jr. The syndrome of central cervical soft disk herniation. JAMA 1973;226:302–305.
177. Kondo K, Molgaard C, Kurland L, et al. Protruded intervertebral cervical disc. Minn Med 1981;64:751–753.
178. Franson R, Saal J. Human disc phospholipase A2 in inflammatory. Spine 1992;17(suppl 6):S129–132.
179. Saal J, Franson R, Dobrow R, et al. High levels of inflammatory phospholipase A2 activity in lumbar disc herniations. Spine 1990;15:674–678.
180. Kelsey J, Githens P, Walter S, et al. An epidemiological study of acute prolapsed cervical intervertebral disc. J Bone Joint Surg [Am] 1984;66:907–914.
181. Boden SD, McCowin PR, Davis DO, Dina TS, Mark AS, Wiesel SW. Abnormal magnetic resonance scans of the cervical spine in asymptomatic subjects: A prospective investigation. J Bone Joint Surg [Am] 1990;72:1178–1184.
182. Aldrich F. Posterolateral microdiscectomy for cervical monoradiculopathy caused by posterolateral soft cervical disc sequestration. J Neurosurg 1990;72:370–377.
183. De Graaff R. *Cervicale spondylogene myelopathie*. Utrecht: Proefschrift; 1982.
184. Espersen JO, Buhl M, Eriksen EF, et al. Treatment of cervical disc disease using Cloward's technique: I. General results, effect of different operative methods, and complications in 1,106 patients. Acta Neurochir 1984;70:97–114.
185. Lindgren E. Über Skelettveränderungen bei Rückenmarkstumoren. Nevenartz 1937;10:240–248.
186. Verbiest H. Moderne overwegingen over compressio medullae. Ned Tijdschr Geneeskd 1954;98:2972–2982.
187. Debois V, Herz R, Berghmans D, Hermans B, Herregodts P. Soft cervical disc herniation: Influence of cervical spinal canal measurements on development of neurologic symptoms. Spine 24:(19):1996–2002,1999.
188. Burrows HE. The sagittal diameter of the spinal canal in cervical spondylosis. Clin Radiol 1963;17:77–86.
189. Edwards WC, La Rocca SH. The developmental segmental sagittal diameter of the cervical spinal canal in patients with cervical spondylosis. Spine 1983;8:20–27.
190. Motoe T. Studies on topographic architecture of the annulus fibrosus in the developmental and degenerative process of the lumbar intervertebral disc in man. J Jpn Orthop Assoc 1986;60:495–509. In Japanese.
191. Yasuma T, Koh S, Okamura T, Yamauchi Y. Histological changes in aging lumbar intervertebral discs: Their role in protrusions and prolapses. J Bone Joint Surg [Am] 1990;72:220–229.
192. Pritzker KPH. Aging and degeneration in the lumbar intervertebral disc. Orthop Clin North Am 1977;8:65–77.
193. Eckert C, Decker A. Pathological studies of intervertebral discs. J Bone Joint Surg 1947;29:447–454.
194. Taylor TKF, Akeson WH. Intervertebral disc prolapse: A review of morphologic and biochemical knowledge concerning the nature of prolapse. Clin Orthop 1971;76:54–79.
195. Harada Y, Nakahara S. A pathologic study of lumbar disc herniation in the elderly. Spine 1989;14:1020–1024.
196. Frykholm R. Lower cervical vertebrae and intervertebral discs: Surgical anatomy and pathology. Acta Chir Scand 1951;101:345–359.
197. Mixter WJ, Barr JS. Rupture of the intervertebral disc with involvement of the spinal canal. N Engl J Med 1934;211:210–215.
198. Peet MM, Echols DH. Herniation of the nucleus pulposus: A cause of compression of the spinal cord. Arch Neurol Psychiatry 1934;32:924–932.
199. Bucy PC, Heimburger RF, Oberhill HR. Compression of the cervical spinal cord by herniated intervertebral discs. J Neurosurg 1948;10:471–492.
200. Jonsson H, Cesarini K, Sahlstedt B, Rauschning W. Findings and outcome in whiplash-type neck distortions. Spine 1994;19:2733–2743.
201. Jonsson H, Bring G, Rauschning W, Sahlstedt B. 1991 Hidden cervical spine injuries in traffic accident

victims with skull fractures. J Spinal Disord 1991;4: 251–263.

202. Rauschning W, McAfee PC, Jonsson H. Pathoanatomical and surgical findings in cervical spinal injuries. J Spinal Disord 1989;2:213–222.

203. Twomey LT, Taylor JR. The whiplash syndrome: Pathology and physical treatment. J Man Manip Ther 1993;1:26–29.

204. Kokubun S, Sakurai M, Tanaka Y. Cartilaginous endplate in cervical disc herniation. Spine 1996;21: 190–195.

205. Saal JS, Saal JA, Yurth EF. Nonoperative management of herniated cervical intervertebral disc with radiculopathy. Spine 1996;21:1877–1883.

206. Dyck PJ, et al, eds. *Peripheral Neuropathy*, 2nd ed. Philadelphia, Pa: WB Saunders; 1984;1392–1393.

207. Ellenberg MR, et al. Cervical radiculopathy. Arch Phys Med Rehabil 1994;75:342–352.

208. Favero KJ, et al. Neuralgic amyotrophy. J Bone Joint Surg [Br] 1987;69:195–198.

209. Ahlgren BD, et al. Cervical radiculopathy. Orthop Clin North Am 1996;27:253–262.

210. Murphey F, Simmons JC, Brunson B. Ruptured cervical discs, 1939–1972. Clin Neurosurg 1973;20:9.

211. Radhakrishnan, K., et al. Epidemiology of cervical radiculopathy: a population-based study from Rochester, Minnesota, 1976–1990. Brain 1994;117: 325–335.

212. Ward R. Myofascial release concepts. In: Nyberg, N. Basmajian J. V. (eds). Rational Manual Therapies. Baltimore, Md Williams & Wilkins, 1993:223–241.

213. Leblhuber F, Reisecker F, Boehm-Jurkovic H, et al. Diagnostic value of different electrophysiologic tests in cervical disc prolapse. Neurology 1988;38: 1879–1881.

214. Schutter H. Intervertebral disc disorders. In: *Clinical Neurology*, vol. 3. Philadelphia, Pa: Lippincott-Raven; 1995:chap 41.

215. Kelsey JL, et al. An epidemiological study of acute prolapsed cervical intervertebral disc. J Bone Joint Surg [Am] 1984;66:907.

216. Barnes R. Traction injuries to the brachial plexus in adults. J Bone Joint Surg [Br] 1949;31:10–16.

217. Clancy WG. Brachial plexus and upper extremity peripheral nerve injuries. In: Tong JS, ed. *Athletic Injuries to the Head Neck and Face*. Philadelphia, Pa: Lea & Febiger; 1982:215–222.

218. Clancy WG, Brand RL, Bergfeld JA. Upper trunk brachial plexus injuries in contact sports. Am J Sports Med 1977;5:209–216.

219. Markey K, Di Benedetto M, Curl W. Upper trunk brachial plexopathy: The stinger syndrome. Am J Sports Med 1993;21:650–655.

220. Speer KP, Bassett FH. The prolonged burner syndrome. Am J Sports Med 1990;18:591–594.

221. Di Benedetto M, Markey K. Electrodiagnosis localization of traumatic upper trunk brachial plexopathy. Arch Phys Med Rehabil 1984;65:15–17.

222. Poindexter DP, Johnson EW. Football shoulder and neck injury: A study of the stinger. Arch Phys Med Rehabil 1984;65:601–602.

223. Wilbourn AJ, Hershman EB, Bergfeld JA. Brachial plexopathies in athletes: The EMG findings. Muscle Nerve 1986;9(5 suppl):254.

224. Robertson W, Eichman P, Clancy W. Upper trunk brachial plexopathy in football players. JAMA 1979; 241:1480–1482.

225. Rockett FX. Observation on the burner: Traumatic cervical radiculopathy. Clin Orthop Rel Res 1992;164: 18–19.

226. Cole AJ, Farrell JP, Stratton SA. Cervical spine athletic injuries. Phys Med Rehabil Clin North Am 1994;5:37–68.

227. Gamburd RC. Sports related cervical injuries. In: *The Cervical and Lumbar Spine: State of the Art' 91*. San Francisco, Calif: San Francisco Spine Institute; March 24, 1991.

228. Marks MR, et al. Cervical spine injuries and their neurologic implications. Clin Sports Med 1990;9: 263–278.

229. Magee DL. *Orthopedic Physical Assessment*, 2nd ed. Philadelphia, Pa: WB Saunders; 1992:48–50.

230. Frykholm R. Cervical nerve root compression resulting from disc degeneration and root-sleeve fibrosis. Acta Chiropract Scand Suppl 1951;160:1.

231. Braddom RL. Management of common cervical pain syndromes, In: De Lisa JA, ed. *Rehabilitation Medicine: Principles and Practice*, 2nd ed. Philadelphia, Pa: JB Lippincott; 1993:1038.

232. Malanga GA, Campagnolo DI. Clarification of the pronator reflex. Am J Phys Med Rehabil 1994;73: 338–340.

233. Spurling RG, Scoville WB. Lateral rupture of the cervical intercerebral discs. A common cause of shoulder and arm pain. Surg Gynecol Obstet 1944;78:350–358.

234. Jahnke RW, Hart BL. Cervical stenosis, spondylosis, and herniated disc disease. Radiol Clin North Am 1991;29:777–791.

235. Viikari-Juntura E, et al. Validity of clinical tests in the diagnosis of root compression in cervical disk disease. Spine 1989;14:253–257.

236. Reiners K, Toyka KV. Management of cervical radiculopathy. Eur Neurol 1995;35:313–316.

237. Farfan HF, Kirkaldy-Willis WH. The present status of spinal fusion in the treatment of lumbar intervertebral joint disorders. Clin Orthop 1981;158:198.

238. Murphey F, Simmons JC. Ruptured cervical disc: Experience with 250 cases. Am Surg 1966;32:83.

239. Cloward RB. The clinical significance of the sinuvertebral nerve of the cervical spine in relation to the cervical disk syndrome. J Neurol Neurosurg Psychiatry 1960;23:321.

240. Krieger AJ, Maniker AH. MRI-documented regression of a herniated cervical nucleus pulposus: A case report. Surg Neurol 1992;37:457–459.

241. Maigne JY, Deligne L. Computed tomographic follow-up study of 21 cases of nonoperatively treated cervical intervertebral soft disc herniation. Spine 1994;19:189–191.

242. Saal JA, Saal JS, Herzog R. The natural history of lumbar intervertebral disc extrusions treated nonoperatively. Spine 1990;15:683–686.

243. Gore DR, Sepic SB. Anterior cervical fusion for degenerated or protruded discs. A review of one hundred forty-six patients. Spine 1984;9:667–671.

244. Grisoli F, Graziani N, Fabrizi AP, et al. Anterior discectomy without fusion for treatment of cervical lateral soft disc extrusion: A follow-up of 120 cases. Neurosurgery 1989;24:853–859.

245. Lans M, Pignatti G. Anterior surgery for treatment of soft cervical HNP. Chir Degli Org di Mov 1992;77:101–109.

246. Rowlingson JC, Kirschenbaum LP. Epidural analgesic techniques in the management of cervical pain. Anesth Analg 1986;65:938–942.

247. Schulman J. Treatment of neck pain with cervical epidural steroid injection. Reg Anesth 1986;11:92–94.

248. Warfield CA, Biber MP, Crews DA, et al. Epidural steroid injection as a treatment for cervical radiculitis. Clin J Pain 1988;4:201–204.

249. Sweeney TB, Prentice C, Saal JA, Saal JS. Cervicothoracic muscular stabilization techniques. In: Saal JA, ed. *Physical Medicine and Rehabilitation, State of the Art Reviews: Neck and Back Pain*, vol. 4. Philadelphia, Pa: Hanley & Belfus; 1990:335–359.

250. Kumano K, Umeyama T. Cervical disc injuries in athletes. Arch Orthop Trauma Surg 1986;105:223–226.

251. Lees F, Turner J. Natural history and prognosis of cervical spondylosis. BMJ 1963;2:2607–2620.

252. Aldrich F. Posterolateral microdiscectomy for cervical monoradiculopathy caused by posterolateral soft cervical disc sequestration. J Neurosurg 1990;72:370–377.

253. Lunsford LD, Bissonette DB, Jannetta PJ, et al. Anterior surgery for cervical disc disease. Part I: Treatment of lateral cervical disc herniation. J Neurosurg 1980;53:1–11.

254. Lyu RK, Chang HS, Tang LM, Chen ST. Thoracic disc herniation mimicking acute lumbar disc disease. Spine 1999;24:416–418.

255. Beadle OA. The intervertebral discs. His Majesty's Stationery Office, London, 1931. In White AA. Analysis of the mechanics of the thoracic spine in man. Acta Orthop Scand (suppl 127), 1969.

256. Arce CA, Dohrmann GJ. Thoracic disc herniation: Improved diagnosis with computed tomographic scanning and a review of the literature. Surg Neurol 1985;23:356–361.

257. Maiman DJ, Larson SJ, Luck E, El-Ghatit A. Lateral extracavitary approach to the spine for thoracic disc herniation: Report of 23 cases. Neurosurgery 1984;14:178–182.

258. El-Kalliny M, Tew JM Jr, van Loveren H, Dunsker S. Surgical approaches to thoracic disc herniations. Acta Neurochir (Wien) 1991;111:22–32.

259. Jamieson DRS, Ballantyne JP. Unique presentation of a prolapsed thoracic disk: Lhermitte's symptom in a golf player. Neurology 1995;45:1219–1221.

260. Morgenlander JC, Massey EW. Neurogenic claudication with positionally weakness from a thoracic disk herniation. Neurology 1989;39:1133–1134.

261. Hamilton MG, Thomas HG. Intradural herniation of a thoracic disc presenting as flaccid paraplegia: Case report. Neurosurgery 1990;27:482–484.

262. Whitcomb DC, Martin SP, Schoen RE, Jho HD. Chronic abdominal pain caused by thoracic disc herniation. Am J Gastroenterol 1995;90:835–837.

263. Albrand OW, Corkill G. Thoracic disc herniation: Treatment and prognosis. Spine 1979;4:41–46.

264. Byrne TN, Waxman SG. *Spinal Cord Compression: Diagnosis and Principles of Management*. Philadelphia, Pa: FA Davis; 1990.

265. Thomas M, Bell GB. Radiologic examination and imaging of the spine. In: Nicholas JA, Hershman EB, eds. *The Lower Extremity and Spine*, 2nd ed. St Louis, Mo: Mosby-Year Book; 19–:1096–1097, 1102.

266. Fielding JW, Fietti VG, Mardam-Bey TH. Athletic injuries to the antlantoaxial articulation. Am J Sports Med 1978;6:226.

267. Friedenberg ZB, Edeiken J, Spencer HN, Tolentino SC. Degenerative changes in the cervical spine. J Bone Joint Surg [Am] 1959;41:1:61–70.

268. Gore DR, Sepic SB, Gardner GM. Roentgenographic findings of the cervical spine in asymptomatic people. Spine 1986;11:521–524.

269. Jahnke RW, Hart BL. Cervical stenosis, spondylosis, and herniated disc disease. Radiol Clin North Am 1991;29:777–791.

270. Landman JA, Hoffman JC, et al. Value of computed tomographic myelography in the recognition of

cervical herniated disc. Am J Neuroradiol 1988;5: 391–394.

271. Modic MT, Ross JS, Masaryk TJ. Imaging of degenerative disease of the cervical spine. Clin Orthop 1989;239:109–120.

272. Thornbury JR, Fryback DG, Turski PA, et al. Disk-caused nerve compression in patients with acute low-back pain: Diagnosis with MR, CT myelography, and plain CT [published correction appears in Radiology. 1993;187:880]. Radiology 1993;186:731–738.

273. Forristall RM, Marsh HO, Pay NT. Magnetic resonance imaging and contrast CT of the lumbar spine: Comparison of diagnostic methods and correlation with surgical findings. Spine 1988;13:1049–1054.

274. Jackson RP, Cain JE, Dacobs RR, et al. The neuroradiographic diagnosis of lumbar herniated pulposus: II. A comparison of computed topography, myelography, CT-myelography and magnetic resonance imaging. Spine 1989;14:1362.

275. Cantu RC. Functional cervical spinal stenosis: A contraindication to participation in contact sport. Med Sci Sports Exerc 1993;25:316–317.

276. Boden SD, Davis DO, Dina TS, Patronas NJ, Wiesel SW. Abnormal magnetic-resonance scans of the lumbar spine in asymptomatic subjects: A prospective investigation. J Bone Joint Surg [Am] 1990;72:403–408.

277. Emery SE, et al. Magnetic resonance imaging of posttraumatic spinal ligament injury. J Spinal Disord 1989;2:229.

278. Harris JH, Yeakley JW. Hyperextension-dislocation of the cervical spine: Ligament injuries demonstrated by magnetic resonance imaging. J Bone Joint Surg [Br] 1992;74:567.

279. Thomas M, Bell GB. Radiologic examination and imaging of the spine. In: Nicholas JA, Hershman EB, eds. The Lower Extremity and Spine, 2nd ed. St Louis, Mo: Mosby-Year Book; 19–:1096–1097,1102.

280. Wilbourn AJ, Aminoff MJ. The electrophysiologic examination in patients with radiculopathies. AAEE Minimonograph 32. Muscle Nerve 1988;11:1099–1114.

281. Herring SA, Weinstein SM. Electrodiagnosis in sports medicine. Phys Med Rehabil State Art Rev 1989;3: 809–822.

282. Marinacci AA. A correlation between operative findings in cervical herniated disc with electromyograms and opaque myelograms. Electromyography 1966;6: 5–20.

283. Eisen A, Aminoff MJ. Somatosensory evoked potentials. In: Aminoff MJ, ed. Electrodiagnosis in Clinical Neurology, 2nd ed. New York, NY: Churchill Livingstone; 1986:535–573.

284. Leblhuber F, Reisecker F, Boehm-Jurkovic H, et al. Diagnostic value of different electrophysiologic tests in cervical disc prolapse. Neurology 1988;38:1879–1881.

285. Johnson EW, ed. Practical Electromyography, 2nd ed. Baltimore, Md: Williams & Wilkins: 1988:229–245.

286. Bergfeld JA, Hershman E, Wilbourne A. Brachial plexus injury in sports: A five-year follow-up. Orthop Trans 1988;12:743–744.

287. Speer KP, Bassett FH. The prolonged burner syndrome. Am J Sports Med 1990;18:591–594.

288. Malanga GA, Nadler SF. Nonoperative treatment of low back pain [review]. Mayo Clin Proc 1999;74: 1135–1148.

289. Lord MJ, Small JM, Dinsay JM, Watkins RG Lumbar lordosis: Effects of sitting and standing. Spine 1997;22:2571–2574.

290. Anderson R, Meeker WC, Wirick BE, Mootz RD, Kirk DH, Adams A. A meta-analysis of clinical trials of spinal manipulation. J Manip Physiol Ther 1992;15: 181–194.

291. Koes BW, Assendelft WJ, van der Heijden GJ, Bouter LM. Spinal manipulation for low back pain: An updated systematic review of randomized clinical trials. Spine 1996;21:2860–2871.

292. DiFabio RP. Clinical assessment of manipulation and mobilization of the lumbar spine: A critical review of the literature. Phys Ther 1986;66:51–54.

293. Haldeman S. Spinal manipulative therapy as a status report. Clin Orthop 1983;179:62–70.

294. McKenzie RA. The Lumbar Spine: Mechanical Diagnosis and Therapy. Waikanae, New Zealand:Spinal Publications Ltd, 1981.

295. Anshel MH, Russell KG. Effect of aerobic and strength training on pain tolerance, pain appraisal and mood of unfit males as a function of pain location. J Sports Sci 1994;12:535–547.

296. Szymanski LM, Pate RR. Effects of exercise intensity, duration, and time of day on fibrinolytic activity in physically active men. Med Sci Sports Exerc 1994; 26:1102–1108.

297. Casazza BA, Young JL, Herring SA. The role of exercise in the prevention and management of acute low back pain. Occup Med. 1998;13:47–60.

298. Saal JA. Dynamic muscular stabilization in the nonoperative treatment of lumbar pain syndromes. Orthop Rev 1990;19:691–700.

299. Beurskens AJ, de Vet HC, Koke AJ, et al. Efficacy of traction for nonspecific low back pain: 12-week and 6-month results of a randomized clinical trial. Spine 1997;22:2756–2762.

300. Jette DU, Jette AM. Physical therapy and health outcomes in patients with spinal impairments [published correction appears in Phys Ther 1997;77:113]. Phys Ther 76:930–941,1996.

301. Deyo RA, Diehl AK, Rosenthal M. How many days of bed rest for acute low back pain? A randomized clinical trial. N Engl J Med. 1986;315:1064–1070.

302. Malanga GA. The diagnosis and treatment of cervical radiculopathy. Med Sci Sports Exercise 1997;29 (7 suppl):S236–245.

303. Ward R. Myofascial release concepts. In: Nyberg, N. Basmajian J. V. (eds). Rational Manual Therapies. Baltimore, Md Williams & Wilkins, 1993:223–241.

304. McKenzie RA. Manual correction of sciatic scoliosis. N Z Med J 1972;76:194–199.

305. Donelson R, Silva G, Murphy K. Centralization phenomenon: Its usefulness in evaluating and treating referred pain. Spine 1990;15:211–213.

306. Frymoyer JW. Back pain and sciatica. N Engl J Med 1988;318:291–300.

307. Vanharanta H, Videman T, Mooney V. McKenzie exercise, back track and back school in lumbar syndrome [abstract]. Orthop Trans 1986;10:533.

308. Lyu RK, Chang HS, Tang LM, Chen ST. Thoracic disc herniation mimicking acute lumbar disc disease. Spine 1999;24:416–418.

309. Dupuis PR, Yong-Ling K, Cassidy JD, et al. Radiologic diagnosis of degenerative lumbar spinal instability. Spine 1985;10:262–276.

310. Van Akkerveeken PF, O'Brien JP, Park W. Experimentally induced hypermobility in the lumbar spine. Spine 1979;4:236–241.

CHAPTER EIGHT

DIFFERENTIAL DIAGNOSIS— SYSTEMS REVIEW

Chapter Objectives

At the completion of this chapter, the reader will be able to:

1. Describe the characteristics of musculoskeletal pain.
2. Identify the signs and symptoms of nonmusculoskeletal pain.
3. Describe the categories of musculoskeletal pain.
4. List the five types of spondylolisthesis.
5. Understand the motives and manifestations of the malingering patient.
6. Perform tests to identify nonorganic signs.

OVERVIEW

The systems review is the part of the examination that identifies possible health problems that require consultation with, or referral to, another health care provider.[1]

MUSCULOSKELETAL PAIN

Pain is the most common reason for a patient to seek intervention. When a patient requests help for pain, the physician makes a determination as to the cause, labeling it as musculoskeletal or nonmusculoskeletal, and decides on a course of intervention to provide relief for the patient. If the pain is musculoskeletal in nature, the physician may prescribe physical therapy.

It is important to assume that all reports of insidious pain by the patient are serious in nature until proven otherwise with a thorough assessment.[2] MacNab[3] originally devised the following categories of spinal pain:

1. Viscerogenic
2. Vasculogenic
3. Neurogenic
4. Psychogenic
5. Spondylogenic

Viscerogenic Pain

The pain in this category can be referred from any viscera. Visceral pain differs from superficial pain in that highly localized damage to an organ may produce no pain at all or, at worst, nonacute pain. However, an impairment that causes a diffuse nociceptor response may cause extremely severe pain. The viscera tend to have only pain, and no other sensory, nerve endings. The stimuli that can produce visceral pain include chemical damage, ischemia, spasm of smooth muscle, and distension. All visceral pain from the abdominal or thoracic cavities is transmitted through small C fibers within the sympathetic nervous system, resulting in the slow type of pain. The referral of visceral pain is thought to be produced when the nociceptive fibers from the viscera synapse in the spinal cord with some of the same neurons that receive pain from the skin. When the visceral nociceptors are stimulated, some are transmitted by the same neurons that conduct skin nociception, and so take on the characteristics of those impulses, appearing to arise from the skin.

Pain arising from problems in the peritoneum, pleura, or pericardium differs from that of other visceral impairments. These parietal walls are supplied extensively with both fast and slow pain fibers, which have their fibers in spinal, rather than sympathetic nerves. These structures can, therefore, produce the sharp pain of superficial impairments.

Visceral pain has five important clinical characteristics:

1. It is not evoked from all viscera. (Organs such as the kidney, most solid viscera, and lung parenchyma are not sensitive to pain.)

2. It is not always linked to visceral injury. (Cutting the intestine causes no pain and is an example of visceral injury with no attendant pain, whereas stretching the bladder is painful and is an example of pain with no injury.)
3. It is diffuse and poorly localized.
4. It is referred to other locations.
5. It is accompanied by motor and autonomic reflexes, such as the nausea, vomiting, and lower-back muscle tension that occurs in renal colic.

The fact that visceral pain cannot be evoked from all viscera, and that it is not always linked to visceral injury, has led to the notion that some viscera lack afferent innervation. It is postulated that these features are owing to the functional properties of the peripheral receptors of the nerves that innervate certain visceral organs, and to the fact that many viscera are innervated by receptors that do not evoke conscious perception and, thus, are not sensory receptors in the strict sense.

Visceral pain tends to be diffuse because of the organization of visceral nociceptive pathways in the central nervous system, particularly the absence of a separate visceral sensory pathway, and the low proportion of visceral afferent nerve fibers, compared with those of somatic origin.

Head[5] provided the following potential areas of cutaneous referral from various viscera:

- *Heart:* T1-5—Under the sternum, base of the neck, over the shoulders, over the pectorals and down one or both arms (left greater than right)
- *Bronchi and lung:* T2-4
- *Esophagus:* T5-6—Pharynx, lower neck, arms, midline of the chest from the upper to the lower sternum
- *Gastric:* T6-10—Lower thoracic to upper abdomen
- *Gall bladder:* T7-9—Upper abdomen, lower scapular and thoracolumbar
- *Pancreas:* Upper lumbar or upper abdomen
- *Kidneys:* T10-L1—Upper lumbar, occasionally anterior abdomen about 2 inches lateral to the umbilicus
- *Urinary bladder:* T11-12—Lower abdomen or low lumbar
- *Uterus:* Lower abdomen or low lumbar

Although it might appear to be difficult to differentiate the source of somatic versus visceral pain, it is worth remembering that if the patient's pain or symptoms are not altered with movement, a visceral source should be suspected, and ruled out, before proceeding. For example, pain that is related to eating probably has a gastric source but must still be confirmed by the examination. Pain that appears to be unrelated to rest, or activity, could also be an acute musculoskeletal dysfunction.

In general, the greater the degree of pain radiation, the greater the chance that the problem is acute or that it is occurring from a proximal structure. Eliciting the date of the mechanism will clarify the cause. However, having the ability to apply the selective stresses through a specific structure, described in other chapters, allows the clinician to isolate the cause, and rule out other possibilities. Visceral back pain is not very often confused with pain originating in the spine, because other specific signs and symptoms are present to localize the problem correctly. For example, although pain in the low back region can be referred by the kidneys, pelvic organs, peritoneal area, and liver, the musculoskeletal examination would result in normal ranges of motion, with little if any pain. If a movement is found to aggravate the visceral pain, it does not follow a musculoskeletal pattern of motion restriction. For example, an inflamed liver, might be aggravated by side-flexion of the trunk to the right, but no other motion. Low back pain of a mechanical spondylitic origin is normally relieved by rest, whereas impairments in solid or hollow viscera are not relieved in this way and are unrelated to the level of activity.[6,7] Visceral impairments tend to cause other problems that turn the clinician's attention away from the spine, as the pain is often associated with symptoms such as blood in the stool, fever, or night chills. Visceral back pain is more likely to result from visceral disease in the abdomen and pelvis than from intrathoracic disease.[8]

A. Kidney or urologic disorders, such as acute pyelonephritis, may cause bilateral aching flank pain and costovertebral area tenderness. However, a distinction can often be made between these conditions and a musculoskeletal lesion due to the accompanying signs of fever, chills and vomiting, as well as a history of irritative bladder symptoms or urinary tract infections.

B. Bladder calculi (bladder stones) may produce dull suprapubic discomfort, with sharper pain precipitated by jarring or exercise. Frequency, urgency and dysuria such as diminished stream and hesitation.

The pain from the stone is typically increased as the stone passes from the bladder to the urethra.

Bladder stones are usually secondary to chronic obstruction, prostatic disease, urethral stricture, or the chronic use of catheters. Gout and hyperuricemia (excess uric acid in the blood) have also been implicated.[9]

C. A renal stone traversing the ureter may give rise to a constant severe pain in the left lumbar and left iliac area. Direct iliac area tenderness may be present. The urine usually contains erythrocytes or is grossly bloody.[9]

D. Patients with a history of urinary frequency, dysuria, or hematuria may have an irritation of the bladder and urethra, with low back pain as the chief complaint.[4] Further questioning may elicit additional urologic symptoms, such as urinary frequency, urinary urgency, dysuria, or hematuria.

E. Prostatitis or prostate cancer can cause low back, and sciatic pain. Dysuria accompanied by frequency, suprapubic and perineal pain, fever, chills and general malaise are common findings, as well as changes in bowel function. Men from the fifth decade on are most commonly affected.[4]

F. A pancreatic carcinoma can cause severe and persistent back pain.

G. Gynecologic disorders have the potential to cause mid-pelvic or low back discomfort. These disorders encompass:
1. Tubal pregnancy
2. Ovarian cysts
3. Uterine fibroids or myoma
4. Endometritis
5. Pelvic inflammatory disease (PID)
6. Septic abortion

Gynecologic disorders are most common in 20- to 45-year-old women, who present with sharp, bilateral, pain in the lower quadrants.[4] If such a gynecologic disorder is suspected, the patient should be referred back to their physician so that a careful pelvic examination can be performed to help rule out a more serious cause for the pain. The clinician is encouraged to ask appropriate questions to determine the need for a gynecologic examination, especially in the absence of objective musculoskeletal findings.[4]

The patient may reveal iliac and hypogastric pain that can be referred as a result of a sexually transmitted disease, ectopic pregnancy, use of an intrauterine device (IUD), dysuria, ovarian abscess, or tubal pregnancy.

Tumors may involve the sacral plexus or its branches, causing severe, burning pain in a sciatic distribution.[9]

Associated symptoms of gynecologic disorders include:

- Amenorrhea, irregular menses, history of menstrual disturbances
- Tender breasts
- Tenderness in the broad ligaments bilaterally
- Nausea, vomiting
- Chronic constipation (with laxative and enema dependency) or diarrhea
- Fever, night sweats, chills
- History of vaginal discharge
- Late menstrual periods with persistent bleeding
- Irregular, longer, or heavier menstrual periods
- Pain on defecation
- Spotting, or frank vaginal bleeding
- Crampy pain and tenderness

Vasculogenic Pain

The location of vasculogenic pain depends on the location of the vascular pathology.[10] Pain that is vasculogenic in origin tends to occur as a result of venous congestion or arterial deprivation to the musculoskeletal areas, and is often worsened by activity, as with intermittent claudication or thromboangiitis obliterans (Buerger's disease). Some conditions, however, can be improved with activity, such as a disc impairment, which tends to worsen with sustained positions, but improves with exercise. The symptoms of vasculogenic back pain may be mistaken for those of a wide variety of disorders. Conversely, the diagnosed presence of vascular impairment of a minor degree may direct attention away from a primary disorder that originates elsewhere.[4] Such disorders include low back pain of musculoskeletal origin, nerve root compression, or arthritis of the low back or hip.[10]

A. Peripheral vascular disease with claudication can be confused with neurogenic claudication and spinal stenosis.[4] The major difference in the clinical features is the response of pain to rest, and the position of the spine. Peripheral vascular disease pain is not relieved by trunk flexion, or aggravated with sustained trunk extension (Table 8–1). Because vascular and neurogenic claudication occur in approximately the same age group, vascular studies and myelography may be necessary to help determine the source.[10]

B. Gradual obstruction of the aortic bifurcation produces:[4]
1. Bilateral buttock and leg pain
2. Weakness, fatigue and atrophy of the lower extremities
3. Absent femoral pulses
4. Color and temperature changes in the lower extremities
5. Pain that is often aggravated with lumbar extension
6. A pulsing sensation in the abdomen (abdominal aortic aneurysm). Additional symptoms can include back pain. Suspicion for an abdominal aortic aneurysm should be raised with male patients aged 60 or above who have a past medical history of coronary disease and whose peripheral pulses are diminished or absent[9]

C. Involvement of the femoral artery along its course, or at the femoral-popliteal junction, produces thigh and calf pain, and absent pulses below the femoral pulse.[4] Obstruction of the popliteal artery or its branches produces pain in the calf, ankle, or foot.[4]

TABLE 8-1 DIFFERENTIATING THE CAUSES OF CLAUDICATION[4]

VASCULAR CLAUDICATION	NEUROGENIC CLAUDICATION	SPINAL STENOSIS
Pain* is usually bilateral	Pain is usually bilateral, but may be unilateral	Usually bilateral pain
Occurs in the calf (foot, thigh, hip, or buttocks)	Occurs in back, buttocks, thighs, calves, feet	Occurs in back, buttocks, thighs, calves, feet
Pain occurs consistently in all spinal positions	Pain is decreased in spinal flexion, increased in spinal extension	Pain is decreased in spinal flexion, increased in spinal extension
Pain is brought on by physical exertion (e.g., walking)	Pain is increased with walking	Pain is increased with walking
Pain is relieved promptly by rest (1–5 min)	Pain is decreased by recumbency	Pain is relieved with prolonged rest (may persist hours after resting)
Pain is increased by walking uphill		Pain is decreased when walking uphill*
No burning or dysesthesia	Burning and dysesthesia from the back to the buttocks and leg(s)	Burning and a numbness are present in lower extremities
Decreased or absent pulses in lower extremities	Normal pulses	Normal pulses
Color and skin changes in feet; cold, numb, dry, or scaly skin; poor nail and hair growth	Good skin nutrition	Good skin nutrition
Affects those aged 40 to over 60	Affects those aged 40 to over 60	Peaks in the seventh decade; affects men primarily

*Pain associated with vascular claudication may also be described as an "aching," a "cramping," or a "tired" feeling.

D. A superior gluteal artery claudication can produce buttock pain, which is aggravated by walking and relieved with standing still.

E. Problems during pregnancy can occur when the fetus lies on the lateral cutaneous nerve of the thigh, producing meralgia paresthetica, or on the pelvic veins, resulting in an increase in venous pressure and low back pain.

Although spinal stenosis is not a vasculogenic cause of back pain, it is included in this category to assist the reader in comparing back pain and symptoms with a vasculogenic, as opposed to a neurogenic, cause.

A narrowing of the spinal canal, nerve root canals, or intervertebral foramina results in spinal stenosis. The canal tends to be narrow at the lumbosacral junction, and any combination of degenerative changes, such as disc protrusion or osteophyte formation, can reduce the space needed for the spinal cord and its nerve roots.[8]

There exists a third, widely unknown type of intermittent claudication that causes leg pain with any muscular effort similar to the vascular type.[11] In this condition, the pain is mostly localized to the pelvis. The pain is followed by paresthesia and a diminishing of the tendon reflexes, with possible motor weakness. This special type of intermittent claudication is usually associated with stenosis of the pelvic arteries, including the internal iliac arteries.

The blood supply of the lumbosacral plexus usually derives from branches of the internal iliac artery (iliolumbar artery, superior and inferior gluteal artery, lateral sacral artery), and the deep iliac circumflex artery.[12] Acute ischemic impairments of the lumbosacral plexus are caused by high-grade stenoses and occlusion of the iliac arteries or of the distal abdominal aorta. The internal iliac artery plays the predominant part. However, the most frequent cause of such acute ischemic impairments of the lumbosacral plexus is surgery of the aortic bifurcation and the pelvic arteries, or radiation therapy.[13] Finally intra-arterial injections of cytostatic agents into the iliac arteries or accidental intra-arterial injections of vasotoxic agents into the gluteal arteries[14] may result in persistent ischemic plexopathy. Distinct from those persisting plexopathies with acute onset, there is only an intermittent ischemic plexopathy during walking, with relapsing pain and sensomotoric deficits.

Reduced perfusion within the area of the internal iliac artery can result in a temporary ischemic impairment of the lumbosacral plexus that appears only during muscular activity of the legs. The neurophysiologic finding of temporal dispersion of lumbar motor evoked potentials after exertion proves the involvement of the peripheral nerve, and excludes ischemia of the lower spinal cord or conus medullaris.

Although peripheral nerves have a high tolerance for ischemia because they have a double blood supply,[15] the peripheral nerve has a significantly increased energy metabolism during activity[16] and a low capability of autoregulation of the blood supply.[17] Therefore, it must be assumed that, during inactivity, the perfusion of the plexus is still sufficient. However, during activity of those leg muscles supplied by branches of the external iliac arteries, a steal-phenomenon appears to occur that privileges the leg muscles over the pelvic organs. Thus, localized pelvic pain results, followed by paresthesia and sensomotoric deficits in the area of the lumbosacral plexus. After a rest of a few minutes, the symptoms resolve completely.

The neurologic examination of the inactive patient usually discloses no abnormality; however, the clinical diagnosis of this type of intermittent claudication resulting from exercise-induced ischemia of the lumbosacral plexus is based mainly on two specific features:

- Firstly, as in the more frequent type of intermittent claudication caused by arterial occlusive disease of the legs, the symptoms appear in correlation with the degree of muscle activity. In early stages of the disease, symptoms occur only when walking uphill or riding a bicycle. This allows a distinction from the intermittent claudication caused by spinal stenosis, in which symptoms predominantly appear when walking downhill. In addition, patients with spinal stenosis can ride a bicycle for a long distance without developing symptoms, because of the kyphosis of the lumbar spine and subsequent widening of the lumbar canal.
- Secondly, in addition to pain, progressive sensomotoric deficits in the area of the lumbosacral plexus occur during exertion. This cannot be seen in patients with peripheral arterial occlusive disease. Moreover, the localization of the pain in the buttock differs from the latter condition.

Neurogenic Pain

Neoplasms of the cord, dura and cauda equina, can mimic spondylogenic pain.[3] Neurogenic pain is usually the result of a space-occupying lesion. The space-occupying lesion can be the result of a normal reaction to trauma (e.g., relatively benign), or the result of something more insidious, or of something as nonthreatening as a gravid uterus. The following findings should be of great concern to the clinician:

- An insidious onset of severe pain with no specific mechanism of injury
- Neurologic symptoms from more than two lumbar levels, or more than one cervical level
- Pain at night that awakens the patient from a deep sleep, usually at the same time every night. The pain is unremitting and is not relieved with movement. Night pain of this nature is believed to be associated with the relative decrease in core temperature that occurs during the night, and the subsequent response of the hypothalamus. Because tumors are avascular and anoxic, their temperature is not regulated by blood flow, and tumors appear colder to the body's internal monitoring system, controlled by the hypothalamus. This difference in temperature is interpreted erroneously by the hypothalamus, and symptoms of pain are provoked.
- Painless weakness on resistive testing without root pain

Other examples of a neurogenic cause of pain are:

- A thalamic tumor producing causalgic leg pain[3]
- An irritation of the arachnoid space producing back pain[3]
- A nerve root irritation secondary to a diabetic neuropathy, producing a clinical picture that is indistinguishable from sciatica. This similarity may lead to long and serious delays in diagnosis.[7] Such a situation may require persistence on the part of the clinician and patient in requesting further medical follow-up.
- A nerve root impingement. The assessment and intervention of this condition is discussed in more detail in Chapter 7.
- A peripheral nerve entrapment. These entrapments and their findings are discussed in more detail in Chapter 6.

Psychogenic Pain

Emotional overtones are common with low back and neck pain. A dysfunctional central nervous system, grief, or medications, as well as fear of reinjury, can inhibit the central biasing system. Psychogenic back pain can be observed in the hysterical or extremely anxious patient that leads to an increase in the person's perception of pain. Anxiety leads to an increase in muscle tension, more anxiety, and muscle spasm.[4] These patients often demonstrate full active range of motion with few objective findings to match the subjective complaints of a serious pathology.

The term *nonorganic* is used to define pain exhibited by patients suffering from depression, emotional disturbance, or anxiety states.[18] It is extremely difficult to assess a patient who has pain that is nonorganic in origin, and whose symptoms are exacerbated or prolonged by psychological factors.

In addition to this patient type, there is the patient who is involved in litigation. This type can be subdivided into patients with a legitimate injury and cause for litigation who genuinely want to improve, and patients who are merely motivated by the lure of a litigation settlement and who have no intention of showing signs of improvement until their case is settled. Unfortunately, the latter group, aptly named "happy cripples," display exaggerated complaints of pain, tenderness, and suffering that are not unlike those of the nonorganic patient. However, in this group, it is the potential for financial gain that produces behaviors that can mimic those of psychogenic dysfunction (objective findings not matching subjective complaints).

Malingering[19]

Any patient involved in litigation, whether as the result of a motor vehicle accident, work injury, or other accident, has the potential for malingering. *Malingering* is defined as the intentional production of false symptoms or the gross exaggeration of symptoms that truly exist. These symptoms may be physical or psychological but have in common the conscious intention of achieving a certain goal.[20] Malingering is synonymous with faking, lying, or fraud, and it represents a frequently unrecognized medical diagnosis. Malingerers, when identified, are commonly mismanaged, and are a source of frustration for the clinician.

When a clinician engages a patient, it is assumed that both work together to treat a pathologic condition that is causing the patient harm or in some way decreasing the optimal function of the patient. This assumption is not true in the case of the diagnosis of malingering.

Malingering can be differentiated into "pure" versus "partial." Pure malingering occurs when there is a claim of a disease or the false production of symptoms that do not exist; partial malingering occurs when the symptoms exist, but are exaggerated in intensity.[21]

Identifying the source of secondary gain associated with malingering is critical to establishing the diagnosis. Typically, secondary gain is related to the situation in which malingering is presenting.

Such deception often causes a significant, negative response from the clinician. It is most important, therefore, that the clinician address suspected deception in a structured, unemotional manner. It should be recollected that malingering can be deemed to have a nonpathologic, adaptive function under certain circumstances. It is the obligation of the clinician to interact in a problem-oriented, constructive, and helpful fashion with the malingering patient. The diagnosis of malingering should be made based on the observation of signs and symptoms during the examination, and the clinician should avoid introducing a negative connotation in the documentation or a negative emotional response of the clinician.

Regardless of the criterion utilized to justify a suspicion of malingering, the diagnosis requires an attempt to confirm this suspicion. This attempt can be achieved by two methods: observation and inference. The observational method can be further divided into two subcategories:

1. Controlled-environment observation
2. Covert "real-world" surveillance

An example of controlled environment observation would be clinical observations of behaviors on an inpatient unit, in a partial hospitalization program, or in a multidisciplinary pain intervention program. An example of covert, real-world surveillance would be videotaping the claimant in their natural environment.

Unfortunately malingerers and nonmalingerers are often grouped together because of similarities in the assessment findings. With very few exceptions, patients in significant pain look and feel miserable, move extremely slowly, and present with consistent findings during the examination. Inconsistent findings in the presence of severe pain could, of course, indicate a serious pathologic process of a nonmusculoskeletal origin. It cannot be stressed enough that all patients should be given the benefit of the doubt until the clinician, with a high degree of confidence, can rule out an organic cause for the pain. As research by MacNab[22] has shown, serious injury can result from low-speed impacts in motor vehicle accidents (20 miles per hour), and other studies have demonstrated that neck fractures do not show up on x-rays, or are missed when they do, for about 6 weeks after the injury.[23,24]

Various tests and observations have been devised to help differentiate between the organic and nonorganic types of back pain, and they are outlined here:

A. *Distraction test.*[25] This test involves checking a positive finding elicited during the examination on the distracted patient. For example, if a patient is unable to perform a seated trunk flexion maneuver, the same patient can be observed when asked to remove the shoes. If marked improvement is noted, the patient's response is inconsistent.

B. *Simulation tests.* A series of tests that should be comfortable to perform. If pain is reported, a nonorganic origin should be suspected.
    1. *Hip and shoulder rotation.*[26] With the patient positioned standing, the clinician passively rotates the patient's hips or shoulders while the feet are kept on the ground.
    2. *Axial loading.*[26] The clinician applies an axial load through the standing patient's head.
    3. *Burn's test.*[18] The patient is asked to kneel on a stool and is then asked to bend over and try to touch the floor. Most patients will at least attempt the task. Patients with nonorganic pain often refuse on the grounds that it will cause too much pain, or overbalance them on the chair.
    4. Overreaction during the examination, such as disproportionate verbalization, muscle tension, tremors, and tenderness.[27]

There are a number of clinical signs and symptoms that serve to alert the clinician to the possibility of a malingerer:[4]

- Subjective complaints of paresthesia in a stocking-glove distribution
- Reflexes inconsistent with the presenting problem
- Cogwheel motion of muscles during strength testing for weakness
- The inability of the patient to complete a straight leg raising test in the supine position, but having no difficulty performing the equivalent range in a seated position
- The straight leg raising test in the supine position reproduces symptoms with plantar flexion instead of dorsiflexion

Whatever the reasoning or motivation behind pain of a nonorganic origin, the success rate from the clinician's viewpoint will be low, and so it is well worth recognizing these individuals from the outset.

Spondylogenic Pain

Severe pathologic processes involving the vertebra, such as infections, neoplasms, and metabolic disorders, frequently present as back pain. Spondylogenic pain, produced by bone impairments, is relatively limited in nature and quality, although the conditions producing these symptoms are numerous, making this the largest group.[4] The age of the patient, character of the pain, history of unexplained weight loss, presence of a fever, and bone tenderness are helpful to the clinician in making the correct diagnosis.[4]

A. Osseous impairments
  1. Infective
    a. Pyogenic osteomyelitis: This usually results from PID but can be the result of surgery or poor dental hygiene.
    b. Tuberculous vertebral osteomyelitis: Produced by tuberculosis bacteria, which spread from the lungs, or urinary tract. The most frequent site of vertebral involvement is the vertebral body of the upper lumbar and lower thoracic regions. This condition can be a cause of low back pain in diabetics, drug addicts, alcoholics, patients who take corticosteroid drugs, and otherwise debilitated patients.[4] The most constant clinical finding is backache with marked tenderness over the spinous process of the involved vertebrae, gross spinal rigidity due to paravertebral muscle spasms, fever, sweats, anorexia, weight loss, and easy fatiguability. All spinal motions, and jarring, intensify the pain.[3]

c. Miscellaneous infections: These include fungal (e.g., mycotic osteomyelitis), parasitic (e.g., hydatid disease) or syphilitic (e.g., Charcot arthropathy of the thoracolumbar junction) infections.[3]
  2. Neoplastic: Tumors can be either benign or malignant. The benign form tends to occur more often in the under-30 age group.[3]
    a. Benign
      (1) Osteoid osteoma: A benign, blood-filled tumor of cortical bone found in the spine that may not present with the characteristic history of night pain relieved by aspirin.[4] A hamstring spasm with a marked limitation of the straight leg raise are characteristic findings with this lesion.[3]
      (2) Osteoblastoma: This tumor has a marked predilection for the spine.[3]
    b. Malignant: Malignant tumors can be primary or secondary, and are more common in the under-40 age group.[3]
      (1) Primary
        (a) Multiple myeloma: The most common malignant primary bone tumor of the spine. Early in its course it can easily be overlooked as the cause of back pain. The complaints may be nonspecific, but a general feeling of malaise is usually an indication for a medical referral.
        (b) Chordoma: A slowly developing, locally invasive and destructive tumor.
      (2) Secondary: Secondary cancer from the breast, thyroid, lung, kidney, and prostate can present as back pain.[3] The first suggestion of a malignant disease lies in the history, which is not of pain varying with exertion, but of a steady aggravation, irrespective of activity.[4] The distinguishing feature is one of an unrelenting, intense, and progressive nature to the pain.[7] Severe weakness without pain is very suggestive of spinal metastasis.[4] Gross muscle weakness with a full range of straight leg raising, is also suggestive of spinal metastasis.[6]

Neoplasms, whether primary or secondary, may interfere with the sympathetic nerves of the autonomic nervous system, resulting in thermal changes in the extremities.[4] For example, the foot on the affected side may be warmer to the touch than the foot on the unaffected side.

It is more difficult to detect a sacral neoplasm than a lower lumbar metastasis, because the spinal joints retain a full and painless range of movement, whereas a patient with the former condition complains of sacral pain or coccygodynia (painful coccyx), only. Paresis of the gross muscles of one, or both feet, in the absence of root pain, suggests a tumor. Back pain resulting from degenerative joint disease is seldom, if ever, unrelenting and usually responds to bed rest. The patient's past medical history regarding previous cancer must be obtained. The clinician should keep in mind that removal of a breast due to primary cancer may seem so remote from the present symptoms that the patient may not volunteer this information.[7]

3. Metabolic[28]

   a. Osteoporosis and osteomalacia: The problem in the diagnosis of osteoporosis is that there are no preceding symptoms before a fracture occurs. Osteoporosis, a decrease in the mass of bone, can result in compression fractures, although a recent meta-analysis of 11 separate study populations and over 2000 fractures concluded that bone mineral density "cannot identify individuals who will have a fracture."[29] The reader is referred to Chapter 2 for more details about osteoporosis and osteomalacia.

   b. Paget's disease: Paget's disease (osteitis deformans) is a metabolic bone disorder characterized by slowly progressive enlargement and deformity of multiple bones associated with unexplained acceleration of both deposition and resorption of bone.[4] The disorder causes the bones to become sponge-like, weakened, and deformed. The bones most commonly involved are those of the pelvis, lumbar spine, and sacrum. Although this disorder is often asymptomatic, when symptoms occur, they do so insidiously and may include deep, aching bone pain, nocturnal pain, joint stiffness, fatigue, headache, dizziness, increased temperature over the long bones, and periosteal tenderness.

4. Traumatic

   a. Fractures of the transverse processes have the potential to produce low-grade back pain, which can interfere with leisure activities and may remain undetected. These fractures typically result from gross muscular violence, often from a resisted rotation strain.

   b. Fractures of the neural arch.

   c. Dislocations.

   d. A wedge compression fracture of the vertebral body is often produced by damage to the related posterior joints, and can result in prolonged back pain.

   e. End plate fractures result from a compression force applied to the spine, and they set up a chain of processes that results in changes to the disc. (See Chapter 7)

   (1) The initial injury with an end plate fracture may be pain-free as the end plate is not well innervated. However, as the nucleus is exposed to body's immune system for the first time, it is not recognized and elicits an immune response in the vertebral body's spongiosa.

   (2) The degradation of the nucleus results in a progressive loss of its water-binding capacity, resulting in a decreased ability to take load, putting more load on the anulus. The continued loading of the anulus results in the formation of vertebral body osteophytes and load sharing through the zygapophysial joints, with resulting osteophytosis.

   (3) Over time, the degradation may extend peripherally along radial fissures in the anulus, resulting in internal disc disruption.

   (4) The patient may complain of pain at rest or pain with activity, but demonstrates no external signs of disc bulge, herniation, or loss of height with most imaging studies; x-rays, computed tomography (CT), and myelography are normal. CT discography and magnetic resonance imaging (MRI) show the injury. It is thus important to test the ability of the spinal segment to tolerate a compression force. (Refer to Chapter 10)

B. Spondylogenic impairments

   1. Osseous

   a. Spondylosis: Defined as degeneration of the intervertebral disc.

   b. Spondylolysis: The result of traumatic, congenital, or hereditary damage to one of the pars interarticularis, resulting in the characteristic x-ray resembling the side view of a "Scotty dog." Spondylolysis causes no significant change in lifestyle, except for the very athletic. It tends to be common in weight lifters, wrestlers, rowers and fast-bowlers in cricket.

   c. Spondylolisthesis: There are five main types.[30,31]

   (1) Type I, isthmic: An anatomic defect of the pars interarticularis.

   (2) Type II, congenital: The posterior elements are structurally inadequate because of developmental abnormalities.

   (3) Type III, degenerative: The facets and their supporting ligamentous structures are deficient and a listhesis or slippage results. There is no defect of the pars interarticularis. The condition, related to trauma and aging, is potentially progressive.

   (4) Type IV, elongated pedicles: Often considered a variant of the isthmic type. The neural arch is elongated, placing the facets more posteriorly.

(5) Type V, destructive disease: Secondary to metabolic, malignant, or infectious diseases.

Whatever the cause, spondylolisthesis involves an anterior slippage of one vertebra over another and is graded according to severity.[30] Grade I corresponds to a 25% slippage (3/8 inch) and is usually the point at which intervention is sought. (See Chapter 13)

Patients with this condition feel an increase of symptoms when the lumbar lordosis is increased, as this slackens the posterior longitudinal ligament system, which works to prevent anterior slippage once the primary restraints (facets and discs) are no longer available. The incidence for true spondylolisthesis is zero at birth, but it increases with age up to adulthood, and rarely increases during the next decades. Although the etiology is unclear, in Eskimos the incidence is considerably higher, and it increases in this population up to 40 years of age.[32,33]

   d. Spina bifida, and other congenital abnormalities.
   e. Scheuermann's disease (juvenile vertebral osteochondritis).
   f. Sacroiliac: Injuries to the sacroiliac joint can result from:
     (1) Trauma.
     (2) Pregnancy, resulting in increased laxity of the ligaments.
     (3) Disease: Rheumatic diseases, such as ankylosing spondylitis, Reiter's syndrome, psoriatic arthritis, or arthritis associated with chronic inflammatory bowel disease, may present with back and sacroiliac joint pain. In addition to back pain, rheumatic diseases usually include a constellation of associated signs and symptoms, such as fever, skin lesions, anorexia, and weight loss, to alert the clinician to the presence of a systemic disease.

C. Soft tissue
   1. Myofascial sprains or strains.
   2. Fibrositis, myofascial pain syndrome, Travell trigger points.
   3. Kissing spines: An approximation of the spinous processes indicative of a ligamentous sprain or instability; also known as a "sprung back."
   4. Disc degeneration.
   5. Disc herniation.
   6. Nerve root entrapments or dural adhesions.
   7. Stenosis, central or lateral recess, producing a lateral or central narrowing of the intervertebral foramen as a result of a disc impairment, osteophyte formation, degeneration, or calcification.

   8. Facilitated segment.
   9. Postural back pain.

Pain Related to Specific Regions

Cervical Pain

A number of conditions can cause cervical pain and include meningitis, subarachnoid hemorrhage, cervical disc degeneration and/or herniation, epidural abscess, lyme disease, retropharyngeal abscess, torticollis, vertebral artery dissection, and cervical cord tumors. Tracheobronchial pain can be referred to sites in the neck or anterior chest at the same levels as the points of irritation in the air passages.[4] This irritation may be caused by inflammatory lesions, irritating foreign materials, or cancerous tumors.[34]

Tumors of the cervical cord may be primary, metastatic, extramedullary, or intramedullary. Pain of insidious onset, with or without neurologic signs and symptoms (e.g., progressive leg weakness, bladder paralysis, and sensory loss), may occur.[4]

Thoracic Pain

Systemic origins of musculoskeletal pain in the thoracic spine (Table 8–2) are usually accompanied by constitutional symptoms affecting the whole body, along with other associated symptoms that the patient may not relate to the back pain and, therefore, may fail to mention to the clinician.[4] Perhaps the most common sources of nonmusculoskeletal chest pain are the heart and lungs. An acute myocardial infarction can produce mild to severe

TABLE 8–2 SYSTEMIC CAUSES OF THORACIC PAIN[4]

SYSTEMIC ORIGIN	LOCATION
Gallbladder disease	Midback between scapulae
Acute cholecystitis	Right subscapular area
Peptic ulcer, stomach or duodenal ulcers	5th–10th thoracic vertebrae
Pleuropulmonary disorders	
Basilar pneumonia	Right upper back
Empyema	Scapula
Pleurisy	Scapula
Spontaneous pneumothorax	Ipsilateral scapula
Pancreatic carcinoma	Middle thoracic or lumbar spine
Acute pyelonephritis	Costovertebral angle (posteriorly)
Esophagitis	Midback between scapulae
Myocardial infarction	Midthoracic spine
Biliary colic	Right upper back; midback between scapulae; right interscapular or subscapular areas

sub-sternal pain, that may radiate to one or both breasts, the shoulders, the jaw, the neck, and one or both arms. The pain is described as a heaviness, a weight, a viselike pain and may be accompanied with sweating, nausea and weakness. The duration of the discomfort can vary from 15 min to 24 hours, and is not relieved by antacids, a change in position, or rest.

Other causes of thoracic pain include esophagitis, acute coronary insufficiency, angina, dural inflammation pericarditis, herpes zoster, and costochondritis.

When screening the patient through the subjective history, the clinician should remember that symptoms of pleural, intercostal and costal origin all increase on coughing or deep inspiration.[4]

Peptic Ulcer   Although the pain of a peptic ulcer typically occurs in the left hypochondrium, it occasionally occurs in the back between the eighth and tenth thoracic vertebrae. Perforated duodenal ulcers may refer pain to the left upper quadrant or right shoulder. Patients with this disorder prefer to avoid all movement. If the ulcer is not perforated, relief can be obtained by antacids. The patient usually describes periodic symptoms, relief with antacids, and the relationship of pain to eating. For example, the patient may have relief from pain after eating only to find that the pain returns and increases 1 to 2 hours after eating when the stomach is emptied.[4]

Pancreatic Carcinoma   The most frequent symptom of a pancreatic carcinoma is upper abdominal/thoracic pain. It begins over a period of minutes as a knife-like or steady, dull pain, radiating from the epigastrium into the back, and left shoulder. Anorexia, nausea, and vomiting usually accompany the pain, and there may be postural dizziness and weakness, and gastrointestinal difficulties unrelated to meals. This disease is predominantly found in men (3:1) and occurs in the sixth and seventh decades.

Acute Cholecystitis   Acute cholecystitis (gallbladder infection) may occur in association with pancreatitis causing diffuse upper abdominal pain and tenderness. Associated symptoms include muscle guarding, jaundice, chills and fever.

Biliary Colic   A bile duct obstruction may be caused by various disorders. The pain of biliary colic begins suddenly and builds in intensity over a period of seconds or minutes. It is usually constant and is referred to the right posterior upper quadrant, with pain in the right shoulder. There may be back pain between the scapulae, with referred pain to the right side in the interscapular or subscapular area.[4]

Acute Pyelonephritis   Acute pyelonephritis, an inflammation of the kidney and renal pelvis, presents with aching pain at one or several costovertebral areas, posteriorly, with radiation to the pelvic crest or groin possible.[4] The patient may describe febrile chills, frequent urination, hematuria, and shoulder pain (if the diaphragm is irritated).[4]

Mediastinal Tumors   Mediastinal tumors may refer pain to the thoracic spine, but the pain is disproportionate to any musculoskeletal problem.[4] Tumors occur most often in the thoracic spine because of its length, the proximity to the mediastinum, and the proximity to direct metastatic extension from lymph nodes involved with lymphoma, breast, or lung cancer.[4]

Esophagitis   Severe esophagitis, a condition common in alcoholics, may refer pain to the thoracic spine. This referred pain is always accompanied by epigastric pain and heartburn.[4]

Myocardial Infarction   A myocardial infarction, or heart attack, results from ischemia of the heart muscle. As with any pain associated with ischemia, the pain is severe and is often accompanied by a crushing sensation which is usually located across the chest. Despite associated signs of a cold sweat, and weak blood pressure, the most common symptom in this condition is one of denial by the patient.

Pneumothorax[4]   Patients presenting with a pneumothorax develop acute pleuritic chest pain localized to the side of the pneumothorax. This pain may be referred to the ipsilateral scapula or shoulder, across the chest, or over the abdomen. Associated symptoms may include dyspnea, cough, hemoptysis (blood in sputum), tachycardia (increased heart rate), tachypnea (rapid respirations), and cyanosis (blue lips and skin due to a lack of oxygen). The patient may have severe pain in the upper and lateral thoracic wall, which is aggravated by any movement and by the cough and dyspnea that accompany it.[34] The patient may be most comfortable sitting in an upright position.

Lumbar Pain

Metastatic Lesions   Metastatic lesions affecting the lumbar spine occur most commonly from the ovary, breast, kidney, lung, or prostate gland.[4] Cancer of the prostate which can metastasize to other areas in the body is the second most common site of cancer among men, and is often diagnosed when the man seeks medical assistance because of symptoms of urinary obstruction or sciatica, the latter resulting from a metastasis to the bones of the pelvis, lumbar spine, or femur.[4]

Case Study: Low Back and Buttock Pain

Subjective

A 30-year-old woman presented with a history of periodic and vague right lower back and buttock pain. The patient also complained of right heel pain, but she was unsure if the two were related. The latest episode had lasted longer than the previous ones and had been progressively worsening, and the patient had sought medical advice. The pain was described as worse in the morning, improving with activity, but worsening after sitting in one position for a long period. Coughing also appeared to worsen the pain. No imaging studies had been performed.

Examination

Observation of the patient revealed a decrease in lordosis but was otherwise unremarkable. Owing to the insidious nature of the low back pain, a lumbar scan was performed with the following results:

- Diminished lumbar spine motion in all planes but especially side-flexion to the right because of pain. Flexion produced a slight deviation toward the right.
- Hypertonus of the lumbar paraspinals.
- Pain was elicited at the end of the straight leg raise, but no dural tension signs were present.
- Positive anterior SI joint distraction test.
- Positive Gaenslen's torsion test.[35]
- Rib expansion of only 2 cm was noted on inspiration.
- Positive manubrium test.

Although not part of the typical lumbar scan, the last three special tests were performed on the basis of suspicion regarding the patient's diagnosis.

Discussion

The patient demonstrated a number of the classic signs for ankylosing spondylitis and was referred back to her physician for further testing. Her lumbar spine x-rays were unremarkable, but her laboratory tests found an increased erythrocyte sedimentation rate and slight anemia, and she was HLA-B27–positive. The patient was referred to physical therapy.

The spondyloarthropathies are a group of inflammatory arthritic conditions that share certain clinical and laboratory features:[36]

- An inflammatory arthritis of the back that manifests with pain associated with stiffness in the buttocks and back
- The absence of a rheumatoid factor, hence the distinction of the group as "seronegative" spondyloarthropathies

- Arthritis that tends to be asymmetric and most commonly involves the lower extremities
- Inflammation, often at the insertion of tendons into bone (enthesitis), accompanied by certain extra-articular features, including skin and mucous membrane impairments, bowel complaints, eye involvement, and aortic root dilation.
- The familial aggregation, which occurs within each condition and among the entities within the group
- An association with HLA-B27, which has also been documented in the diseases included in this group. Almost 30 years have passed since the initial reports in 1972 of the association of HLA-B27 with ankylosing spondylitis,[37,38] which was soon followed by similar associations in Reiter's syndrome,[39,40] psoriatic spondylitis,[41] and the spondylitis of inflammatory bowel disease.[42] The association of HLA-B27 with the seronegative spondyloarthropathies has remained one of the best examples of a disease association with a hereditary marker.

Ankylosing Spondylitis Ankylosing spondylitis (Bekhterew's or Marie Strümple disease) is a chronic rheumatoid disorder that is usually progressive, resulting in a full ankylosing of the sacroiliac joints, although the course can also be mild, particularly in women.[36,43] The patient is usually between 15 and 40 years of age, and the condition affects 1 to 3 per 1000 people. Although men are affected more often than women, mild courses of ankylosing spondylitis are more common in the latter.[44] Patients with ankylosing spondylitis who lack HLA-B27 comprise approximately 5% to 10% of the total patient population, and tend to have clinical differences from HLA-B27–positive patients. Inflammatory eye or cardiac disease is nearly absent in these individuals.[45]

The most characteristic feature of the back pain associated with ankylosing spondylitis is pain at night.[46] Patients often awaken in the early morning (between 2 and 5 AM) with back pain and stiffness, and usually either take a shower or exercise before returning to sleep.[44] In time, the disorder progresses to involve the whole spine and results in spinal deformities, including flattening of the lumbar lordosis, kyphosis of the thoracic spine, and hyperextension of the cervical spine. These, in turn, result in flexion contractures of the hips and knees with significant morbidity and disability.[44] Men generally have the more severe form, which affects the spine, whereas in women, the peripheral joints are more often affected. There is a 10% to 20% risk that the offspring of patients with the disease will later develop it.

Although signs of this disease are also common in the thoracic region, the sacroiliac joints are commonly the initial site of inflammation. Backache in ankylosing spondylitis is typically intermittent and comes and goes irrespective of exertion or rest.[44] The disease includes involvement of the anterior longitudinal ligament and ossification of the disc, the thoracic zygapophysial joint joints, the costovertebral joints, and the manubrial sternal joint, which is affected in 50% of all cases, producing painful forced inspiration, making the checking of chest expansion measurements a required test in this region.

Peripheral arthritis is uncommon in ankylosing spondylitis, but when it occurs, it is usually late in the course of the arthritis.[47] Peripheral arthritis developing early in the course of the disease is a predictor of disease progression.[48] The arthritis usually presents in the lower extremities in an asymmetric distribution.[44] Involvement of the "axial" joints, including shoulders and hips, is more common than involvement of more distal joints.[49] In the shoulder, there may be a unique lesion of erosion at the insertion of the rotator cuff.

The disease in women may not be as severe as it is in men, and it may present with neck pain and, on occasion breast pain, in the absence of the typical lower back pain of sacroiliitis.[50] This may account for the fact that the disease in women is often diagnosed at a later age than in men.[51]

Longitudinal studies in patients with ankylosing spondylitis reveal that deformities and disability occur within the first 10 years of disease.[48] Most of the loss of function occurs during the first 10 years, and correlates significantly with the occurrence of peripheral arthritis, radiographic changes in the spine, and the development of "bamboo" spine.

The following findings are suggestive of spondylitis.[50]

- General malaise
- Weight loss
- Positive family history
- Eye disorders such as iritis and iridocyclitis
- Colitis
- Peripheral arthritides
- Heel pain

Inspection usually shows a flat lumbar spine and gross limitation of side-flexion in both directions. Mobility loss tends to be bilateral and symmetric. There is loss of spinal elongation on flexion (Shober's test) and, often, a history of lower limb peripheral involvement (20% to 30% of patients), such as arthritis, plantar fasciitis, or Achilles tendinitis. The patient may relate a history of costochondritis and, with examination, rib springing may give a hard end feel. Basal rib expansion is often decreased. The glides of the costotransverse joints, and distraction of the sternoclavicular joints, are decreased and the lumbar spine exhibits a capsular pattern.

As the disease progresses, the pain and stiffness can spread up the entire spine, pulling it into forward flexion, so that the patient adopts the typical "stooped-over" position. The patient gazes downward, the entire back is rounded, the hips and knees are semiflexed, and the arms cannot be raised beyond a limited amount at the shoulders.[53] Radicular pain occurs, the sacroiliac joints develop tenderness, and chest expansion is restricted because of disease of the costovertebral joints.

Although radiologic evidence of sacroiliitis is accepted as being obligatory for the diagnosis of ankylosing spondylitis, the clinical signs may predate radiologic abnormalities by months or even years. When the signs begin to show on x-ray, they demonstrate erosions with subsequent ankylosis of the joints. The New York criteria[54] describe the sacroiliac involvement according to four grades: grade 1 is suspicious; grade 2 shows erosions and sclerosis; grade 3 shows erosions, sclerosis, and early ankylosis; and grade 4 reflects total ankylosis. The following findings with x-ray are characteristic, depending on the region:

- Sacroiliac joint: Early, patchy osteoporosis develops, and the joint margins become ill-defined. Subchondral erosions develop and, when multiple, produce a "rosary" effect. Initially, the increasing bone density is patchy before becoming widespread and obliterating the joints.[55]
- Lumbar spine: The early radiologic sign is the Romanus lesion,[55] which reflects an erosion at the disc margin. Squaring of the vertebra then results, followed by the development of the syndesmophyte, as a result of ossification of the outer layer of the nucleus fibrosus of the intervertebral disc. The anterior concavity of each body is lost, and the normal lordosis is straightened. Paravertebral ossification gradually develops beneath the anterior longitudinal ligament at each level, resulting eventually in the typical "bamboo" spine appearance.
- In the late stages of the disease, total ankylosis of the spine occurs, with ossification of the longitudinal ligaments.

Intervention

An exercise program is particularly important for these patients to maintain functional spinal outcomes.[56] The goal of exercise therapy is to maintain the mobility of the spine and involved joints for as long as possible, and to prevent the spine from stiffening in an unacceptable kyphotic position. A strict regimen of daily exercises, which include positioning and extension exercises, breathing exercises, and exercises for the peripheral joints, must be followed. Several times a day, patients should lie prone for 5 minutes, and they should be encouraged to sleep on a hard mattress and avoid the side-lying position. Swimming is the best form of routine exercise.

REFERENCES

1. Guide to physical therapist practice. Phys Ther (Suppl) 1997;77:1163–1650.
2. Grieve GP: The masqueraders. In: Boyling JD, Palastanga N, eds. *Grieve's Modern Manual Therapy,* 2nd ed. Edinburgh, Scotland: Churchill Livingstone; 1994.
3. McNab I. *Backache.* Baltimore, Md: Williams & Wilkins; 1978.
4. Goodman CC, Snyder TE. *Differential Diagnosis in Physical Therapy,* 2nd ed. Philadelphia, Pa: WB Saunders; 1995.
5. Head H. *Studies in Neurology.* London, England: Oxford Medical; 1920:653.
6. Cyriax J. *Textbook of Orthopedic Medicine,* vol 1, 8th ed. London, England: Balliere Tindall and Cassell; 1982.
7. Wedge JH. Differential diagnosis of low back pain. In: Kirkaldy-Willis WH, ed. *Managing Low Back Pain.* New York, NY: Churchill Livingstone; 1983:129–143.
8. Hall A. Back pain. In: Blacklow RS, ed. *MacBryde's Signs and Symptoms,* 6th ed. Philadelphia, Pa: JB Lippincott; 1983:195–221.
9. D'Ambrosia R. *Musculoskeletal Disorders: Regional Examination and Differential Diagnosis,* 2nd ed. Philadelphia, Pa: JB Lippincott; 1986.
10. Zohn DA, Mennel J. *Musculoskeletal Pain: Principles of Physical Diagnosis and Physical Treatment,* 2nd ed. Boston, Mass: Little, Brown; 1988.
11. Wohlgemuth WA, Rottach KG, Stoehr M. Intermittent claudication due to ischaemia of the lumbosacral plexus. J Neurol Neurosurg Psychiatry 1999;67:793–795.
12. Day MH. The blood supply of the lumbar and sacral plexuses in the human foetus. J Anat 1964;98:104–116.
13. Wohlgemuth WA, Rottach K, Stoehr M. Radiogene Amyotrophie: Cauda equina Läsion als Strahlenspätfolge. Nervenarzt 1998;69:1061–1065.
14. Stoehr M, Dichgans J, Dörstelmann D. Ischaemic neuropathy of the lumbosacral plexus following intragluteal injection. J Neurol Neurosurg Psychiatry 1980;43:489–494.
15. Roberts JT. The effect of occlusive arterial diseases of the extremities on the blood supply of nerves. Experimental and clinical studies on the role of the vasa nervorum. Am Heart J 1948;35:369–392.
16. Low PA, Ward KK, Schmelzer JD, et al. Ischemic conduction failure and energy metabolism in experimental diabetic neuropathy. Am J Physiol 1985;248:457–462.
17. Low PA, Tuck RR. Effects of changes of blood pressure, respiratory acidosis and blood flow in sciatic nerve of the rat. J Physiol (Lond) 1984;347:513–524.
18. Corrigan B, Maitland GD. *Practical Orthopaedic Medicine.* Boston, Mass: Butterworth; 1985.
19. LoPiccolo CJ, Goodkin K, Baldewicz TT. Current issues in the diagnosis and management of malingering. Ann Med 1999;31:166–174.
20. American Psychiatric Association. *Diagnostic and Statistical Manual of Mental Disorders,* 4th ed. Washington, DC: American Psychiatric Association; 1994.
21. Resnick PJ. Malingering. *Review Course in Forensic Psychiatry.* Bloomfield, CT: American Academy of Psychiatry and the Law; Oct 1993.
22. MacNab I. Acceleration injuries of the cervical spine. J Bone Joint Surg [Am] 1964;46:1797.
23. Dalinka MK, et al. The radiographic evaluation of spinal trauma. Emerg Med Clin North Am 1985;3:475.
24. Reid DC, et al: Etiology and clinical course of missed spinal fractures. J Trauma 1987;27:980.
25. Kenna O, Murtagh A. The physical examination of the back. Aust Fam Physician 1985;14:1244–1256.
26. Waddell G, Main CJ, Morris EW, et al. Chronic low back pain, psychological distress and illness behavior. Spine 1984;9:209–213.
27. Waddell G, McCulloch JA, Kummel EG, et al: Nonorganic physical signs in low back pain. Spine 1980;5:117–125.
28. Wilkin TJ. Changing perceptions in osteoporosis BMJ. 1999;318:862–864.
29. Marshall D, Johnell O, Wedel H. Meta-analysis of how well measures of bone mineral density predict occurrence of osteoporotic fractures. BMJ 1996;312:1254–1259.
30. Bradford DS, Hu SS. Spondylolysis and spondylolisthesis. In: Weinstein SL, ed. *The Pediatric Spine.* New York, NY: Raven; 1994.
31. Cailliet R. *Low Back Pain Syndrome,* 4th ed. Philadelphia, Pa: FA Davis; 1991:276–277.
32. Stewart TD. The age incidence of neural arch defects in Alaskan natives, considered from the standpoint of etiology. J Bone Joint Surg 1953;35A:937.
33. Stewart TD. The incidence of separate neural arch in the lumbar vertebrae of Eskimos. Am J Phys Anthropol 1931;16:51.
34. Bauwens DB, Paine R. Thoracic pain. In: Blacklow RS, ed. *MacBryde's Signs and Symptoms,* 6th ed. Philadelphia, Pa: JB Lippincott; 1983:139–164.
35. Hoppenfeld S. *Physical Examination of the Spine and Extremities.* New York, NY: Appleton-Century-Crofts;1976.
36. Gladman DD. Clinical aspects of the spondyloarthropathies. Am J Med Sci 1998;316:234–238.

37. Schlosstein L, Terasaki PI, Bluestone R, Pearson CM. High association of an HL-A antigen, W27, with ankylosing spondylitis. N Engl J Med 1972;288:704–706.

38. Brewerton DA, Hart FD, Nichols A, Caffrey M, James DCO, Sturrock RD. Ankylosing spondylitis and HL-A27. Lancet 1973;1:904–907.

39. McClusky OE, Lordon RE, Arnett FC Jr. HL-A 27 in Reiter's syndrome and psoriatic arthritis: A genetic factor in disease susceptibility and expression. J Rheumatol 1974;1:263–268.

40. Brewerton DA, Nicholls A, Oates JK, James DCO. Reiter's disease and HLA-27. Lancet 1973;2:996–998.

41. Metzger AL, Morris RI, Bluestone R, Terasaki PI. HL-A W27 in psoriatic arthropathy. Arthritis Rheum 1975; 18:111–115.

42. Dekker-Saeys BJ, Meuwissen SGM, Van Den Berg-Loonen EM, DeHaas WHD, Meijers KAF, Tytgat GNJ. Clinical characteristics and results of histocompatibility typing (HLA B27) in 50 patients with both ankylosing spondylitis and inflammatory bowel disease. Ann Rheum Dis 1978;37:36–41.

43. Wright V, Moll JMH. *Seronegative Polyarthritis.* North Holland; 1976.

44. Haslock I. Ankylosing spondylitis. Baillieres Clin Rheumatol 1993;7:99.

45. Khan MA, Kushner I, Braun WE. Comparison of clinical features of HLA-B27 positive and negative patients with ankylosing spondylitis. Arthritis Rheum 1977;60: 909–912.

46. Gran JT. An epidemiologic survey of the signs and symptoms of ankylosing spondylitis. Clin Rheumatol 1985;4:161–169.

47. Cohen MD, Ginsurg WW. Late onset peripheral joint disease in ankylosing spondylitis. Arthritis Rheum 1983;186–190.

48. Carrett S, Graham D, Little H, Rubenstein J, Rosen P. The natural disease course of ankylosing spondylitis. Arthritis Rheum 1993;26:186–190.

49. Gladman DD. Clinical aspects of the spondyloarthropathies. Am J Med Sci 1998;316:234–238.

50. Gladman DD, Brubacher B, Buskila D, Langevitz P, Farewell VT. Differences in the expression of spondyloarthropathy: A comparison between ankylosing spondylitis and psoriatic arthritis: genetic and gender effects. Clin Invest Med 1993;16:1–7.

51. Rubin LA, Amos CI, Wade JA, et al. Investigating the genetic basis for ankylosing spondylitis: Linkage studies with the major histocompatibility complex region. Arthritis Rheum 1994;37:1212–1220.

52. Winkel D, Aufdemkampe G, Meijer OG, Phelps V. *Diagnosis and Treatment of the Spine: Nonoperative Orthopaedic Medicine and Manual Therapy.* Aspen; 1996: 119.

53. Turek SL. *Orthopaedics: Principles and Their Application,* vol 2, 4th ed. Philadelphia, Pa: JB Lippincott; 1984: 1570–1575.

54. Bennett PH, Burch TA. The epidemiological diagnosis of ankylosing spondylitis. In: Bennet PH, Wood PHN, eds. *Proceedings of the 3rd International Symposium of Population Studies of the Rheumatic Diseases.* Amsterdam, Holland: Exerpta Medica; 1966:305–313.

55. Resnick D, Niyawama C. Ankylosing spondylitis. In: Resnick D, ed. *Diagnosis of Bone and Joint Disorders,* 3rd ed. Philadelphia, Pa: WB Saunders; 1994:1008–1074.

56. Kraag G, Stokes B, Groh J, Helewa A, Goldsmith CH. The effects of comprehensive home physiotherapy and supervision on patients with ankylosing spondylitis: An 8-month follow-up. J Rheumatol 1994;21: 261–263.

CHAPTER NINE

THE SUBJECTIVE EXAMINATION

Chapter Objectives

At the completion of this chapter, the reader will be able to:

1. Perform a detailed subjective examination.
2. Describe the purpose of the subjective examination.
3. List the mandatory questions for each spinal area.
4. Understand the relevance of additional questions pertaining to each joint.
5. Discuss the importance of the past medical history.
6. Recognize the importance of a thorough subjective examination in aiding the clinician to screen for patients with a medical diagnosis.

OVERVIEW

The examination of the patient consists of two parts of equal importance, the subjective examination (history) and the objective examination (systems review, and tests and measures). The tests and measures are further subdivided into the scanning examination and the biomechanical examination. Usually the subjective examination precedes the objective examination, but they can, and often do, occur concurrently.

THE SUBJECTIVE EXAMINATION

The subjective part of the examination, or patient history, is the cornerstone of every examination, for it is only the patient who can describe the symptoms and, more often than not, give the clinician the information needed to formulate a hypothesis. However, the right questions must be asked, and a correct interpretation must be made by the clinician from the responses. The general purpose of the subjective examination is to:

A. Develop a working relationship and establish lines of communication with the patient.

B. Assist with the planning of the objective examination.

C. Elicit reports of potentially dangerous symptoms.

D. Determine the mechanism of injury, and the severity.

E. Determine the irritability and nature of the symptoms.

F. Assist with the generation of a working pathologic hypothesis.

G. Establish a baseline for intervention and examination.

H. Elicit information on the history and past history of the current condition.

I. Elicit information on:[1]
   1. Past medical and surgical history
   2. General demographics (age, primary language, race and ethnicity, sex)
   3. Social history
   4. Medications
   5. Family history
   6. Other tests and measures (imaging studies, laboratory tests, etc.)
   7. Occupation and employment
   8. Growth and development
   9. Living environment
   10. Functional status and activity level
   11. General health status
   12. Social habits

J. Ask joint-specific questions.

Past Medical History

A complete medical history of the patient should be taken to give the clinician an idea as to the general health of the patient. The patient can fill out a medical history form, such as the one in Table 9–1, upon arrival for the

TABLE 9–1 SAMPLE MEDICAL HISTORY QUESTIONNAIRE

GENERAL MEDICAL HISTORY

General Information:

_____ Date: _____

Last Name   First Name

The information requested may be needed if you have a medical emergency

_____ _____ Relationship:_____

Person to be notified in emergency   Phone

Are you currently working?   (Y)   (N)   Type of work:_____

If not, why? _____

General Medical History:

Please check (✓) if you have been treated for:

( ) Heart Problems
( ) Fainting or Dizziness
( ) Shortness of Breath
( ) Calf Pain with Exercise
( ) Severe Headaches
( ) Recent Accident
( ) Head Trauma/Concussion
( ) Muscular Weakness
( ) Cancer
( ) Joint Dislocation(s)
( ) Broken Bone
( ) Difficulty Sleeping
( ) Frequent Falls
( ) Unexplained Weight Loss
( ) Tremors
( ) High Blood Pressure (Hypertension)
( ) Kidney Disease
( ) Liver Disease
( ) Weakness or Fatigue
( ) Hernias
( ) Blurred Vision
( ) Bowel/Bladder Problems
( ) Night Pain (while sleeping)
( ) Nervous or Emotional Problems
( ) Any Infectious Disease (TB, AIDS, hepatitis)
( ) Tingling, Numbness, or Loss of Feeling? If yes, where? _____
( ) Constant Pain or Pressure During Activity

( ) Difficulty Swallowing
( ) A Wound That Does Not Heal
( ) Unusual Skin Coloration
( ) Lung Disease/Problems
( ) Arthritis
( ) Swollen and Painful Joints
( ) Irregular Heart Beats
( ) Stomach Pains or Ulcers
( ) Pain with Cough or Sneeze
( ) Back or Neck Injuries
( ) Diabetes
( ) Stroke(s)
( ) Balance Problems
( ) Muscular Pain with Activity
( ) Swollen Ankles or Legs
( ) Jaw Problems
( ) Circulatory Problems
( ) Epilepsy/Seizures/Convulsions
( ) Chest Pain or Pressure at Rest
( ) Allergies (latex, medication, food)
( ) Constant Pain Unrelieved by Rest
( ) Pregnancy

Do you use tobacco? (Y)   or   (N)   If yes, how much? _____ _____
Are you presently taking any medications or drugs? (Y)   or   (N)
If yes, what are you taking them for? _____ _____

1. Pain
On a scale of 0 to 10, with 0 being no pain and 10 being the worst pain imaginable, give yourself a score for your _current level_ of pain _____

2. Simple Movements (moving your involved region)
On a scale of 0 to 10 with 0 being normal movement of your involved region and 10 being unable to move your involved region at all, give yourself a score for your _current ability_ to perform simple movements with your involved region _____

3. Function (getting out of a bed or a chair, driving, getting dressed, etc.)

(Continued)

TABLE 9–1   (Continued)

On a scale of 0 to 10 with 0 being able to perform all of your normal daily activities and 10 being that you are unable to perform any of your normal daily activities, give yourself a score for your *current ability* to perform your activities of daily living _____

Please list any major surgery or hospitalization:
Hospital: _____   Approx Date:_____   _____
Reasons: _____

Hospital: _____   Approx Date:_____
Reasons: _____

Have you recently had an X-ray, MRI, or CT scan for your condition? (Y)   or   (N)
Facility:_____   Approx Date:_____
Findings:_____

Please mention any additional problems or symptoms you feel are important:

_____

_____

Have you been evaluated and/or treated by another physician, physical therapist, chiropractor, osteopath, or health care practitioner for this condition?   (Y)   or   (N)   If yes, please circle which one.

I, the undersigned, state that I have answered this form to the best of my knowledge.

Patient's Signature _____   Date: _____

first treatment session. The form serves to alert the clinician about any potential serious signs and symptoms that the patient may be experiencing, and the responses to these questions should be clarified, as necessary, with more detailed questions.[2]

General questions about medical history can give the examiner some useful information. Although this can potentially open the flood gates to a wealth of unwanted information, the skilled clinician uses the technique of asking the correct ratio of open-ended and closed-ended questions to elicit the pertinent information. Open-ended questions encourage longer answers, whereas close-ended questions demand "yes" and "no" answers. Direct questions need to be asked, as the patient may fail to relate information that he or she considers to be unimportant.

Joint-Specific Questions[3]

Related to the Thoracic Region

Thoracic pain can be referred from any of the structures that comprise the thoracic cage, or from the structures encased by the cage. As indicated in Chapter 8, visceral causes of thoracic pain must always be considered. The patient should be asked about any history of:

A. Cord signs, especially bilateral or hemiparesthesia (Table 9–2).
1. The cord signs may be caused by compression of the spinal cord by a space-occupying lesion, or the result of ischemia. The spinal canal in this region is relatively narrow compared with the width of the spinal cord,

and the blood supply to the cord is very tenuous in this region. Posterior disc herniations or osteophytic encroachments can compress the spinal cord.
2. Seventy percent of spinal metastases affect the thoracic spine.[4] The ribs are a common site of metastasis from the breast.
3. If a rib impairment is present, the patient may have noticed a reduction in shoulder movement, because of the pulling action of the attached muscles, or pain with breathing.

B. Pain with a deep breath, cough, or sneeze.
1. Pain felt on deep respiration could be caused by either the movement of the ribs and spine, or from the lining of the lungs, or from cardiac ischemia. A quick screen to help differentiate between the two involves having the patient breathe deeply while the

TABLE 9–2   CAUSES OF PARESTHESIA

PARESTHESIA LOCATION	PROBABLE CAUSE
Lip (perioral)	Vertebral artery occlusion
Bilateral lower or bilateral upper extremities	Central protrusion of disc impinging on the spine
All extremities simultaneously	Spinal cord compression
One-half of the body	Cerebral hemisphere
Segmental (in a dermatomal pattern)	Disc or nerve root
Glove-stocking distribution	Diabetes mellitus neuropathy, lead or mercury poisoning
Half of face and opposite half of body	Brain-stem impairment

thoracic spine is placed in various positions (refer to Chapter 16).

2. A patient who reports thoracic pain associated with coughing should be referred back to the physician, because pain of a pleural origin is very difficult to rule out, even with a very thorough musculoskeletal examination.

C. Severity. Anterior chest wall pain should alert the clinician to the possibility of a heart attack. However, heart attacks often occur with a myriad of symptoms, including arm pain and jaw pain. If the symptoms are reported to be increased with exertion or emotional stress, the patient should be referred back to the physician.

Related to the Lumbar Region

Most low back pain is not induced with trauma. The fact that a herniated disc is more common here than in the cervical spine is thought not only to be the result of the stresses incurred by the lumbar spine, but also of their differing modes of degeneration (refer to Chapter 7).[5] Large lumbar disc protrusions have the potential to produce cauda equina compressions. The patient should be asked about any history of:

A. Bladder or bowel impairment.[3]
   1. Usually the result of S4 nerve root compression but can result from prostate cancer. The typical problems reported include:
      a. Problems with starting and stopping the flow of urine.
      b. Incontinence. This indicates a complete impairment.
      c. Retention. The patient feels like "going," but cannot. This may be the result of a facilitation of the sphincter nerve.
      d. Various degrees of incontinence, indicating compromise to any combination of the L5-S1, S2-4 nerve roots.

B. Saddle paresthesia or anesthesia (Table 9–2). This is the classic symptom of cauda equina pressure. Lesions of the spinal cord or conus medullaris produce the upper motor neuron symptoms of a neurogenic bladder.[6] Cauda equina impairments are also typically associated with severe low back pain and bilateral sciatica.

C. Pain with cough or sneeze. This usually has a discogenic or dural cause and is produced as the result of an increase in intra-abdominal pressure associated with these two actions.

D. Night pain not related to movement. Twenty percent of spinal metastasises occur in the lumbar spine. The question of pain at night, which is not related to movement,

should be asked with all patients who report an insidious onset of pain. Although an acute injury should be expected to hurt at night, and at rest, other pain of a musculoskeletal origin should improve with rest.

E. Effects on the symptoms during standing, sitting, and walking.
   1. Although a spinal stenosis can be caused by disc herniation, and spondylolisthesis at any age, it is usually found in the older population, owing to the effects of degeneration. In both central and lateral stenosis, the symptoms are increased with extension postures, or activities that produce an increase in lumbar lordosis.
   2. Pain resulting from intermittent claudication is also reproduced with walking, or any other exertional activity that involves the lower extremities such as cycling.
   3. Seated postures tend to exacerbate the symptoms of a lumbar disc herniation.
   4. The symptoms of spondylolisthesis, like stenosis, are exacerbated with extension postures or activities, including sitting erect (refer to Chapters 8 and 13).

Related to the Cervical Region

Inquire about a history of:

A. Dizziness, drop attacks, or nausea. Although most causes of dizziness are benign in origin, no assumptions should be made. Traumatic dizziness may be the result of:
   1. Damage to the vestibular system.
   2. Damage to the vertebrobasilar system.
   3. Damage to the upper cervical joints.

B. Rheumatoid diseases. One study[7] showed that 30% of patients with rheumatoid arthritis have neck pain, and about 30% have an anterior or vertical instability of the atlanto-axial segment.

C. Cord signs associated with neck position or movements. Obviously, any evidence of serious pathology should preclude further examination. The patient's neck should be stabilized in a hard collar, and the patient should be transported to the emergency department.

D. Radicular pain or paresthesia with, or without, coughing. Any radicular symptoms that do not follow a segmental distribution may indicate an underlying, and serious, pathology.

E. History of trauma. The most common cause of trauma to the neck is a hyperextension injury, such as occurs in rear-end collisions. The injury is far worse if the head is rotated or extended at the point of impact.[8] An immediate onset of severe pain following a whiplash is indicative of profound damage to the musculoskeletal system, whereas a gradual onset is the more likely scenario with an inflammation.

The primary focus of the subjective examination is to question the patient as to the reason he or she is seeking an intervention. More often than not, pain is the reason that a patient seeks help, so it is well worth spending some time questioning the patient about his or her pain.

Nature of Symptoms

To assess the relevance of the patient's responses during the examination, further questioning from the examiner is needed to find out as much information as possible about the nature and behavior of the patient's symptoms.

Type

Are the symptoms solely related to the pain, or are there other symptoms that accompany the pain, such as tingling, numbness, weakness, stiffness, dizziness, increased sweating, bowel and bladder changes, and so on.

A common definition of acute pain is "the normal, predicted physiological response to an adverse chemical, thermal or mechanical stimulus . . . associated with surgery, trauma and acute illness."[9] Yet patients' attitudes, beliefs, and personalities also strongly affect their immediate experience of acute pain.

Somatic pain has an aching quality, and typically originates from local or distal tissues of the musculoskeletal system. This type of pain, unlike neurogenic pain, can vary in intensity from mild to severe. It is thought that spinothalamic neurons that convey nociceptive input from the skin may also respond to noxious visceral stimuli, and that such viscero-somatic convergence provides a neural substrate for the phenomenon of cutaneous referral of visceral pain.[10]

Visceral pain[11–13] is typically described by the clinician as referred pain. Although the precise mechanisms of visceral pain differ between the different organs and organ systems, there seem to be two common principles that apply to all visceral pain. The first principle is that the neurologic mechanisms of visceral pain differ from those involved in somatic pain; therefore, findings in somatic pain research cannot necessarily be extrapolated to visceral pain. The second principle is that the perception and psychological processing of visceral pain also differ from that of somatic pain. To learn more about visceral pain, the reader is referred to Chapter 8.

Neurogenic pain is typically described by the clinician as radicular pain, and by the patient as sharp, or shooting. In broad terms, pain may be classified as nociceptive or as neurogenic. Although neurogenic pain arises from neural injury, the mechanisms of neurogenic pain are complex and incompletely understood, making it imperative to objectively demonstrate and quantify a physiologic disruption in sensory function that may be the cause of pain. The role of somatosensory cortex has been recently emphasized in the genesis of neurogenic pain.[14]

Radicular pain, a form of neurogenic pain, was once thought to be solely the result of nerve root compression. However, it is now clear that this type of pain can only occur if the nerve root is irritated, rather than merely compressed, or if there is ischemia of the nerve root as a result of edema.[15,16]

Radicular pain should not be confused with radiating pain, in which there is an increase in pain intensity that results in a spreading of the pain, usually distally.

Areas and Definition of Symptoms

With an acute injury (within the first 24 to 48 hours following the trauma), the area of pain surrounds the injury site—everything hurts. As the injury begins to heal, the area of subjective pain becomes more localized, giving the examiner a clearer idea as to the structure at fault.

Intensity

Is it sufficient to prevent sleep or to wake the patient at night? What effect on the pain do activities of daily living (ADLs), work, sex, and so forth, have on the pain? Does the patient exhibit a socially withdrawn pattern of behavior that should be a cause for concern. Is the pain constant, which suggests the presence of a chemical irritation. An inability to reproduce the constant pain with a specific motion is not a good sign. Is the pain continuous? Although one might expect constant and continuous pain to have the same interpretation, continuous pain is pain that is perpetual, but that varies in intensity, indicating the involvement of both a chemical and a mechanical source. This type of pain gives the clinician a good perspective on the irritability of a structure, the stage of healing, or the severity of the injury. As mentioned previously, pain of a nonacute derivation that is not alleviated with rest should alert the examiner.

Behavior of Symptoms

A. The patient should be questioned about how the pain behaves over a 24-hour period. The questions need to be specific:[17]
   1. On waking. If the pain is noticeable after sleeping soundly, the patient's sleeping posture or the bed itself may be the cause.

2. On rising. If the patient has a disc impairment or an arthritic joint, stiffness and pain in the morning is a common complaint.
3. Traveling to work. How does the patient travel to work and for how long?
4. At work. Is the patient sedentary or active?
5. Relaxing in evening. What kind of chair or position does the patient relax in?
6. Initially going to bed. How long does it take for the pain to subside? Does it subside?
7. During sleep. Is the patient able to fall asleep naturally or does he or she use medication or alcohol, both of which can interfere with the body's normal mechanism to change position if it is painful.

B. Specific aggravating activities or postures. If no activities or postures are reported to aggravate the symptoms, the clinician needs to probe for more information. The examiner needs to find out about activities such as walking, bending, sleeping position, prolonged standing, and sitting. When the patient sits, does he or she sit upright or slouched. Sitting or standing upright increases lordosis and can be a source of aggravation for patients with an anterior instability, spondylolisthesis, stenosis, or a zygapophysial joint irritation. Sitting slouched typically aggravates a lumbar disc.

C. Specific relieving factors. This is *very* important to ascertain, because the patient can often provide the clinician with an intervention plan based on the answers to these questions. If neither activity nor rest relieves the symptoms, the cause may be systemic.

D. Relationship of symptoms to nonmechanical events.
1. Eating: Pain that increases with eating may suggest gastrointestinal involvement.
2. Stress: An increase in overall muscle tension prevents muscles from resting.
3. Cyclical events (e.g., menstruation).

Consider the following patient example. If the tests used during this example are unfamiliar to you, do not be concerned; they will be explained in detail later in the book.

Case Study[18]

Subjective
A 32-year-old healthy looking man with no past health problems of significance complains of pain in the right upper lumbar region. The pain is sharp and stabbing and radiates downward and around the groin to the scrotum and upper medial thigh about 2 inches below the hip. The pain has been present since waking this morning and comes and goes, but is never absent for more than 10 to 15 minutes at a time. The onset and offset of pain is not related to activity or postures. The patient ran a marathon 2 days ago. The patient saw his physician who prescribed Tylenol and Naprosyn and physical therapy. The patient was in no pain at the time of the examination.

Examination
The patient is of medium build and healthy, with no excess weight. No evidence of postural deformities or deficits, bruising, muscle deficits, or atrophy in the trunk or legs, was noted. Neither were there any congenital abnormalities.

Spinal Scan Examination A full range of pain-free movements was elicited with normal end feel. There were no neurologic deficits. Compression and traction tests were pain free. The straight leg raise (SLR) tests were 90 degrees bilaterally, and the prone knee-flexion tests produced full range; neither produced pain. The slump test was negative. Posterior-anterior pressures were a little tender over T12 and L1, with some increased resistance to movement from hypertonicity. The patient was asked to jump up and down on the painful leg. This provoked the pain, which lasted 10 minutes, but the sacroiliac (SI) stress tests did not reproduce the pain.

Biomechanical Examination Passive physiologic intervertebral movement (PPIVM) tests at T12-L1 demonstrate some hypomobility into flexion and left side flexion. Passive physiologic articular intervertebral movement (PPAIVM) tests were negative. The right L5-S1 joint was hypermobile into extension and there was mild instability into right rotation at L5-S1. The right hip was hypomobile into extension.

Examination and Intervention Although the pain appeared to be related to running the marathon, it occurred some time later. If the patient had torn a muscle or had done significant damage to a spinal segment, the pain would have been experienced much earlier. Pain-modulating systems are generally not so effective that they can abolish pain for 2 days. It is possible that the patient may have sustained a low-level injury that was subclinical, and then some minor provocation imposed on the injury made it symptomatic. However, the pain was not typical musculoskeletal pain. Some patients do complain of stabbing pain, but it is an unusual descriptor. The pain was unpredictable and not related to physical stresses or their relief, except when asked to jump up and down on the painful leg. This did set up the pain, which lasted 10 minutes and could suggest sacroiliitis—if the SI stress tests had reproduced the pain, which they did not.

These findings tend to argue against a mechanical cause. The pain was not constant nor even continuous, reducing the likelihood of it being inflammatory in nature. The pain radiated from the flank to the groin, suggesting that whatever tissue was causing the symptoms, its derivation was somewhere between T12 and L2. The scrotal component in the absence of sciatica (S4) would support higher levels rather than lower.

Thus far, the patient appears to be presenting with a nonmechanical, noninflammatory condition arising from a tissue derived from the thoracolumbar high lumbar area. This by itself should be enough for the clinician to refer the patient back to his physician. One other test that would help confirm this decision is heavy, dull percussion over the kidney. This reproduced the patient's pain.

Provisional differential diagnosis: Viscerogenic pain—renal colic caused by kidney stones. The low lumbar and hip impairments were coincidental and had nothing to do with the patient's complaints.

History of Present Condition

At the end of the last section of questions, the examiner must have ascertained whether or not the symptoms are related to biomechanical stresses. The next series of questions examines the natural history of the condition.

A. Onset. When? How? Time factor—A sudden onset (i.e., within 4 hours) indicates an acute impairment such as a tear, whereas immediate pain and "locking" indicates a facet, disc, or meniscoid impairment.
   1. Rapid swelling is an indication of bleeding into the joint.
   2. A gradual increase of symptoms over time indicates that the condition is worsening.
   3. An insidious onset needs to be investigated fully.

B. Does the mechanism or severity of the described injury account for the symptoms? Clinical evidence would suggest that most cervical injuries from a motor vehicle accident will be found in the 20- to 60-year-old age range. This may be the result of the younger population having a high degree of flexibility, which reduces the chances of a serious injury. In the older population, a loss of flexibility and an increase in stability, secondary to ossification and fibrosis, results in a decreased incidence of motor vehicle accident injuries. More back injuries seem to occur as a result of taking something out of a car trunk than putting it in, and this may be secondary to the hysteresis of the tissues following the prolonged driving position. It is no secret that most injuries are predisposed secondary to unhealthy tissue.

C. Previous history.
   1. Initial onset of symptoms.
   2. Successive onsets—Frequency, ease of onset, duration of episodes.
   3. Previous intervention and results.

Case Study: Dizzy Patient[19]

This case study, although extreme in its clinical presentation, serves to illustrate the manifestation of serious signs and symptoms.

Subjective

A 41-year-old woman who had undergone several surgical interventions of the cervical spine reported experiencing vertigo, nausea, and oscillopsia while cooking. Further questioning revealed that these symptoms were related to neck flexion. Other symptoms included diplopia, left facial and tongue numbness, swallowing difficulties, and balance problems with gait impairment. Five years ago, after neck surgery, she had reported neck pain and paresthesia in all four limbs, and a C3-4 disc protrusion, surgically managed, relieved her symptoms. Four years later, she was admitted to the hospital with neck pain and deformity of the cervical spine. She underwent further surgery, and her pain and neck deformity improved. She had done well for 10 months until experiencing her current symptoms.

Questions

1. List all of the reported symptoms that are of concern to the clinician.
2. Explain the possible causes for these symptoms, giving both benign and nonbenign causes.

Examination

Results of the patient's general physical examination were remarkable for a severe cervical kyphosis with severely limited range of movement. Flexion could be accomplished using en bloc movements of the neck. However, extension and lateral rotation were limited to only a few degrees. The left arm and left foot were colder than the right, and were slightly cyanotic. On neurologic examination, the patient was oriented and cooperative. Cranial nerve testing (Table 9–3) revealed the following:

● Prominent bilateral rotatory nystagmus, which was evident at rest, became more pronounced on left lateral and downward gaze.
● The left corneal reflex was absent.
● Palatal sensation and gag reflex were absent.
● Speech was hypophonic.

TABLE 9–3 CRANIAL NERVE TESTING

CRANIAL NERVE	TEST
I Olfactory	Smell (usually not tested)
II Optic	Light reaction
	Accommodation
	Confrontation
III Oculomotor	Fixation
IV Trochlear	Fixation
V Trigeminal	Facial sensation
	Jaw reflex
VI Abducens	Fixation
VII Facial	Smile, frown
VIII Vestibulocochlear	Lie down, sit up
	Side tilt
	Caloric
	Finger rustle
	Humming
	Weber's test
	Rhine's test
IX Glossopharyngeal	Gag reflex (usually not tested)
X Vagal	Gag reflex (usually not tested)
XI Accessory	Sternomastoid and trapezius strength
	Trapezius reflex
XII Hypoglossal	Tongue protrusion

On motor examination, normal tone and strength were found in all muscle groups with the exception of the hand intrinsics (3/5 on the left and 4/5 on the right). Sensory examination showed diffuse bilateral hypalgesia below the neck, which was more pronounced on the left side and markedly worse on both hands. Positional and vibratory sensations were intact. Tendon reflexes were normal bilaterally without clonus or Babinski sign. The patient's gait was wide based, and she could not walk in tandem.

Questions
1. Given these findings on the physical examination, would you proceed with a biomechanical examination? Why and why not?
2. Why do you think the tendon reflexes were normal, and the clonus and Babinski signs were absent?
3. What could explain the hand intrinsic weakness?

The patient was referred back to her physician for imaging studies. A dynamic flexion–extension radiography of the cervical spine demonstrated no gross osseous instability.

Cervical magnetic resonance imaging (MRI) scans obtained in flexion and extension showed the residual C3 vertebral body clearly protruding into the canal. While in extension, it only abutted the spinal cord. During neck flexion, however, the C3 remnant became compressive, with the spinal cord placed in traction. This dynamic spinal cord compression was believed to be the cause of the patient's symptoms.

Discussion
The close anatomic and functional relation between the upper spinal cord and lower brain stem makes these structures prone to concomitant involvement by different pathologic processes that affect the occipitocervical region. The etiologies of these processes include congenital malformations, inflammatory or arthritic diseases, and neoplastic impairments, among others.[20]

Pathophysiologic mechanisms are related to either impairment of blood supply or direct mechanical compression of the neural structures.

The clinical picture varies depending on the compressed structures and may include cervical pain, occipital pain, torticollis, radiculopathy, myelopathy, or symptoms and signs related to impairment of the brain stem, or lower cranial nerves, including nausea, vomiting, dizziness, blurred vision, nystagmus, dysarthria, swallowing disturbances, loss of consciousness, and Lhermittes sign.

In this patient, some of the symptoms, such as vertigo and nystagmus, may be explained by either cervical or brain stem impairment. However, vertigo of cervical vertebral origin typically is associated with cervical hyperlordosis and lack of mobility of the first three vertebral segments.[24] The patient reported here demonstrated a kyphotic deformity of the neck and had neither proprioceptive deficits nor vascular compromise. In addition, she experienced swallowing disturbances and oscillopsia, which indicate brain stem rather than spinal involvement.

REVIEW QUESTIONS

1. What are two characteristics of brain stem impairment?
2. What are the purposes for performing a subjective examination?
3. Name three ill-effects that a patient might experience from taking non-steroidal antiinflammatory drugs (NSAIDs).
4. The manual techniques of manipulation and transverse friction massage are contraindicated for patients prescribed which medications?
5. What are the four topics that must be discussed in the mandatory questions for the thoracic region?
6. What are the four topics that must be discussed in the mandatory questions for the lumbar region?
7. List four topics that are mandatory when questioning a patient about cervical spine pathology.
8. List four conditions that tend to worsen if the lumbar lordosis is increased.

ANSWERS

1. Unilateral facial symptoms accompanied by contralateral body symptoms.

2. (1) Develop a working relationship and establish lines of communication with the patient; (2) assist with the planning of the examination; (3) elicit reports of potentially dangerous symptoms; (4) determine the mechanism of injury, and the severity; (5) determine the irritability and nature of the symptoms; (6) assist with the generation of a working pathologic hypothesis; (7) establish a baseline for intervention and examination; (8) elicit information on any relevant previous history, other medical conditions, and medications.

3. Possible answers include peptic ulceration, impaired renal function, fluid retention, photodermatitis, hyperkalemia, central nervous system effects, and impaired liver function.

4. Anticoagulants.

5. Cord signs; pain with deep breath; pain changes with cough or sneeze; and night pain.

6. Bowel and bladder impairment; saddle paresthesia; pain with cough or sneeze; and night pain.

7. Possible answers include history of dizziness; nausea or drop attacks; rheumatoid arthritis; medications, especially steroids; and spinal cord signs.

8. Anterior instability, spondylolisthesis, stenosis, and zygapophysial joint irritation.

REFERENCES

1. Rothstein J, ed. Guide to physical therapist practice. Phys Ther (Suppl) 1997;77:1163–1650.

2. Stith JS, Sahrmann SA, Dixon KK, Norton BJ. Curriculum to prepare diagnosticians in physical therapy. J Phys Ther Educ 1995;9:46–53.

3. Meadows J, Pettman E, Fowler C. *Manual Therapy: NAIOMT Level II and III Course Notes.* Denver; 1995.

4. Roth P. Neurological problems and emergencies. In: Cameron RB, ed. *Practical Oncology.* Norwalk, Conn: Appleton & Lange; 1994.

5. Twomey LT, Taylor JR. Joints of the middle and lower cervical spine: Age changes and pathology. Man Ther Assoc Austr Conf, Adelaide, 1989.

6. Gomella L, Stephanelli J. Malignancies of the prostate. In Cameron RB, ed. *Practical Oncology.* Norwalk, Conn: Appleton & Lange; 1994.

7. Sherk HH. Atlantoaxial instability and acquired basilar invagination in rheumatoid arthritis. Orthop Clin North Am 1978;9:1053.

8. Sturzzenegger M, et al. The effect of accident mechanisms and initial findings on the long-term course of whip-lash injury. J Neurol 1995;242:443.

9. Federation of State Medical Boards of the United States. *Model Guidelines for the Use of Controlled Substances for the Treatment of Pain.* Euless, Tex: FSMB; 1998.

10. Milne RJ, Foreman RD, Giesler GJ Jr, Willis WD. Convergence of cutaneous and pelvic visceral nociceptive inputs onto primate spinothalamic neurons. Pain 1981;11:163–183.

11. Cervero F, Laird JM. Visceral pain. Lancet 1999;353: 2145–2148.

12. Cervero F. Visceral pain. In: Dubner R, Gebhart GF, Bond MR, eds. *Proceedings of the Vth World Congress on Pain.* Amsterdam, Holland: Elsevier; 1988:216–226.

13. Cervero F, Morrison JFB. Visceral sensation. Progr Brain Res 1986;67:1–324.

14. Canavero S, Pagni CA, Castellano G, et al. The role of cortex in central pain syndromes: Preliminary results of a long-term technetium-99 hexamethylpropyleneamineoxime single photon emission computed tomography study. Neurosurgery 1993;32:185–191.

15. Smyth MJ, Wright V. Sciatica and the intervertebral disc. An experimental study. J Bone Joint Surg 1958;40:1401–1418.

16. Groves MD, McCutcheon IE, Ginsberg LE, Kyritsis AP. Radicular pain can be a symptom of elevated intracranial pressure. Neurology 1999;52:1093–1095.

17. Meadows JTS. *Manual Therapy: Biomechanical Assessment and Treatment, Advanced Technique.* Lecture and video supplemental manual, Swodeam Consulling, Calgary, AB, 1995.

18. Meadows JTS. Available: http://swodeam.com/mto. html: 1999.

19. Rosenberg WS, Salame KS, Shumrick KV, Tew JM Jr. Compression of the upper cervical spinal cord causing symptoms of brainstem compromise. A case report. Spine 1998;23:1497–1500.

20. Menezes AH. Craniocervical abnormalities. Neurosurg Consult 1990;1:1–7.

21. Murase S, Ohe N, Nokura, et al: Vertebral artery injury following mild neck trauma: Report of two cases. No Shinkei Geka 1994;22:671–676.

22. Deen HG Jr, McGirr SJ. Vertebral artery injury associated with cervical spine fracture. Spine 1992;17: 230–234.

23. Sherman MR, Smialek JE, Zane WE. Pathogenesis of vertebral artery occlusion following cervical spine manipulation. Arch Pathol Lab Med 1987;111:851–853.

24. Biesinger E. Vertigo caused by disorders of the cervical vertebral column: Diagnosis and treatment. Adv Otorhinolaryngol 1988;39:44–51.

25. Weinstein SM, Cantu RC. Cerebral stroke in a semipro football player: A case report. Med Sci Sports Exerc 1991;23:1119–1121.

26. Schneider RC. Vascular insufficiency and differential distortion of brain and cord caused by cervicomedullary football injuries. J Neurosurg 1970;33: 363–375.

CHAPTER TEN

THE SCANNING EXAMINATION

Chapter Objectives

At the completion of this chapter, the reader will be able to:

1. Describe the significance of patient observation.
2. Perform neurologic tests to assess the integrity of the sensory and motor systems of the body and recognize the difference between upper motor neuron and lower motor neuron impairments.
3. Describe the differences between contractile and noncontractile tissues and understand the principles of strength testing in the scanning examination.
4. Describe the significance of deep tendon reflexes and the pathologic reflexes.
5. Understand the principles of dural tension and the various tests that examine the dural structures.
6. List the seven "signs of the buttock."
7. Perform a detailed lumbosacral, cervical, and thoracic scanning examination.
8. List the signs and symptoms for cervical, thoracic, and lumbar disc impairments.
9. Describe the indications and contraindications for proceeding beyond the scanning examination.

OVERVIEW

As the flow diagram shown in Figure 10–1 illustrates, the scan traditionally follows the subjective history component of the examination. The scan is not always an essential part of the examination, and it is only used if the examiner has heard or seen anything during the observation and subjective history that might indicate the presence of serious pathology, such as an insidious onset or radiculopathy.

Two scans are commonly recognized: the upper scan and the lower scan. Both of these are discussed, in addition to a less common scan, the thoracic scan.

A scan may be performed for a number of reasons:

- To help confirm the physician's diagnosis
- To help rule out any serious pathology
- To assess the patient's neurologic status
- To assess the status of the contractile and inert tissues
- To focus the examination to a specific area of the body
- To generate a working hypothesis

The scan (Fig. 10–2) is a combination of screening tests and a selective tissue tension examination which consist of a comprehensive clinical examination of the musculoskeletal system that will, if positive, confirm a medical diagnosis rather than a biomechanical one.[1] Designed by Cyriax,[2] the scan is based on sound anatomic and pathologic principles, and although two studies[3,4] questioned the validity of some aspects of the selective tissue tension examination, no definitive conclusions were drawn from these studies. The scarcity of research to refute the work of Cyriax would suggest that the principles of the scanning examination are sound, and that its use be continued.

For each joint or region of joints, the examination has, in common, active, passive, and resisted testing. The scanning examination should be carried out until the clinician is confident that no serious pathology is present, and it is routinely carried out unless there is some good reason for postponing it, such as recent trauma when a modified differential diagnostic examination is used.[1]

As much as any clinical examination can, the scanning examination attempts to generate a working hypothesis as to the patient's diagnosis. It can yield a diagnosis by generating a number of signs and symptoms that, taken together, form a pattern distinct enough to base an effective intervention on. Such diagnoses that the scan can elicit include the possibility of:

A. Visceral referral

B. Neoplastic disease

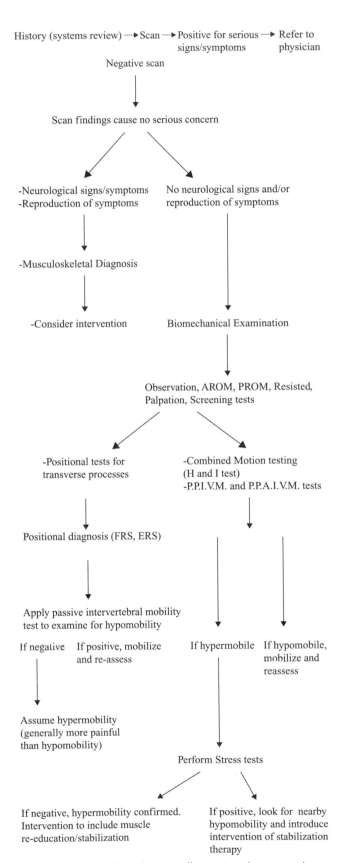

FIGURE 10–1 Flow diagram illustrating the general examination sequence for the spine.

C. Fracture

D. Ligament tears

E. Muscle tears

F. Tendonitis

G. Arthritis

H. Disc impairment (protrusion, prolapse, or extrusion)

I. Postural deficits

J. Ankylosing spondylitis

K. Spinal stenosis

L. Spondylolisthesis

If a working diagnosis can be made, the scanning examination is considered positive, and the clinician can take some immediate action. This will include such things as referring the patient to the physician for further consideration, rest, exercises, modalities, traction, postural correction, and so on.

If, however, the scan does not afford a diagnosis, the clinician is required to obtain further information from the biomechanical examination, which generates a statement about the movement status of the joint, or joints, in question. (Refer to Chapter 11)

OBSERVATION

Much can be learned from a thorough observation. The focus of the observation during a scan differs from that of the biomechanical examination. During the scanning examination, the clinician is observing for any signs or symptoms that would be suggestive of a nonmusculoskeletal condition or serious pathology. The clinician not only needs to be able to recognize these, but also needs to have an understanding about the underlying pathology.

The clinician should look or listen for indications of:

● *Nystagmus.* Nystagmus has many forms and causes. The pathologic nature of positional nystagmus as a sign of vestibular disease has long been recognized.[5,6] The most common form is benign paroxysmal positional nystagmus, which results from a labyrinthine lesion.[7]

● *Dysphasia.* This is defined as a problem with vocabulary. Dysphasia is caused by a cerebral lesion in the speech areas of the frontal or temporal lobes. The temporal lobe receives its blood supply to a large extent from the temporal branch of the cortical artery of the vertebrobasilar system and may become ischemic periodically, producing an inappropriate use of words.

● *Dizziness.* Although most causes of dizziness are relatively benign, dizziness may signal a more serious problem,

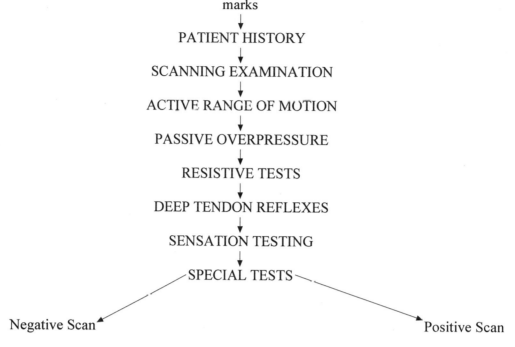

INITIAL OBSERVATION
This involves everything from the initial entry of the patient including their gait, demeanor, standing and sitting postures, obvious deformities and postural defects, scars, radiation burns, creases, and birth marks
↓
PATIENT HISTORY
↓
SCANNING EXAMINATION
↓
ACTIVE RANGE OF MOTION
↓
PASSIVE OVERPRESSURE
↓
RESISTIVE TESTS
↓
DEEP TENDON REFLEXES
↓
SENSATION TESTING
↓
SPECIAL TESTS

Negative Scan

If, at the end of the scan, the clinician has determined that the patient's condition is appropriate for physical therapy, but has not determined the diagnosis to treat the patient, the clinician will need to perform a Biomechanical Examination.

Positive Scan

Results in a Medical Diagnosis

1. Specific interventions can now be given if the diagnosis is one that will benefit from physical therapy (traction, frictions, rest, and specific exercises)

2. Return patient to a physician for more tests if signs/symptoms are a cause for concern

FIGURE 10–2   Flow diagram illustrating the sequence of the scanning examination.

such as damage to the vertebral artery, especially if the patient reports having had immediate post-traumatic dizziness. The clinician must ascertain whether the symptoms result from vertigo, nausea, giddiness, unsteadiness, fainting, or some other cause. Vertigo requires that the patient's physician be informed, as it is a definite pathologic entity that needs to be investigated more fully. However, it is not, of itself, a contraindication to the continuation of the examination.

● *Paresthesia.* The seriousness of the paresthesia depends on its distribution. Complaints of paresthesia can be the result of a benign impingement of a peripheral nerve, but the reasons for its presence can vary in severity and seriousness (Table 10–1).

● *Wallenberg's syndrome.* This is the result of a lateral medullary infarction (LMI).[8] Classically, sensory dysfunction in LMI is characterized by selective involvement of the spinothalamic sensory modalities, with dissociated distribution (ipsilateral trigeminal and contralateral hemibody and limbs).[9] However, various patterns of sensory disturbance have been observed in LMI that include contralateral or bilateral trigeminal sensory impairment, restricted sensory involvement, and a concomitant deficit of lemniscal sensations.[10,11]

TABLE 10–1 CAUSES OF PARESTHESIA[1]

PARESTHESIA LOCATION	PROBABLE CAUSE
Lip (perioral)	Vertebral artery occlusion
Bilateral lower or bilateral upper extremities	Central protrusion of disc impinging on the spine
All extremities simultaneously	Spinal cord compression
One-half of the body	Cerebral hemisphere
Segmental (in a dermatomal pattern)	Disc or nerve root
Glove-and-stocking distribution	Diabetes mellitus neuropathy, lead or mercury poisoning
Half of face and opposite half of body	Brain stem impairment

- *Ataxia.* Ataxia is often most marked in the extremities. In the lower extremities it is characterized by the so-called drunken-sailor gait pattern, in which the patient veers from one side to the other, with a tendency to fall toward the side of the lesion. Ataxia of the upper extremities is characterized by a loss of accuracy in the reaching for, or placing of, objects. Although ataxia can have a number of causes, it generally suggests central nervous system disturbance, specifically a cerebellar disorder, or a lesion of the posterior columns.[12–14]

- *Spasticity.*[15–17] Immediately following any trauma causing tetraplegia or paraplegia, the spinal cord experiences spinal shock, resulting in the loss of reflexes innervated by the portion of the cord below the site of the lesion. The direct result of this spinal shock is that the muscles innervated by the traumatized portion of the cord and the portion below the lesion, as well as the bladder, become flaccid. Spinal shock, which wears off between 24 hours and 3 months after injury, can be replaced by spasticity in some, or all, of these muscles. Spasticity occurs because the reflex arc to the muscle remains anatomically intact despite the loss of cerebral innervation and control via the long tracts. During spinal shock, the arc does not function, but as the spine recovers from the shock, the reflex arc begins to function without the inhibitory or regulatory impulses from the brain, creating local spasticity and clonus.

- *Drop attack.* This is described as a loss of balance resulting in a fall but no loss of consciousness. It is never a good or benign sign and is the consequence of a loss of lower extremity control. The patient, usually elderly, falls forward, with the precipitating factor being extension of the head. Recovery is immediate. Causes include (1) a vestibular system impairment,[18] (2) neoplastic and other impairments of the cerebellum,[19] (3) vertebrobasilar compromise,[20,21] (4) sudden spinal cord compression, (5) third ventricle cysts, (6) epilepsy, and (7) type 1 Chiari malformation.[22]

- *Wernicke's encephalopathy.* Impairment, typically localized in the dorsal part of the midbrain,[23] produces the classic triad of Wernicke's encephalopathy: abnormal mental state, ophthalmoplegia, and gait ataxia.[24]

- *Vertical diplopia.*[25] Descriptions of "double vision" by the patient should alert the clinician to this condition. Patients with vertical diplopia complain of seeing two images, one atop or diagonally displaced from the other.

- *Dysphonia.* This condition presents as a hoarseness of the voice. If it occurs post-traumatically the causes can include (1) damage to the larynx, especially if pain is reported; and (2) damage to nerve supply of vocal chords (vagal/vagal accessory). Usually no pain is reported. Painless dysphonia is a common symptom of Wallenberg's syndrome.[8]

- *Hemianopia.* This is defined as a loss in half of the visual field and is always bilateral. A visual field defect describes sensory loss restricted to the visual field and arises from damage to the primary visual pathways linking optic tract and striate cortex.

- *Ptosis.* Ptosis is a pathologic depression of the superior eyelid such that it covers part of the pupil because of a palsy of the levator palpabrae and Muller's muscles.

- *Miosis.* This is defined as the inability to dilate the pupil (damage to sympathetic ganglia). It is one of the symptoms of Horner's syndrome.

- *Horner's syndrome.*[26] This syndrome is caused by interference of the cervicothoracic sympathetic outflow resulting from a lesion to (1) reticular formation, (2) descending sympathetic, or (3) oculomotor nerve caused by a sympathetic paralysis. The other clinical signs of Horner's syndrome are ptosis, enophthalamus, facial reddening, and anhydrosis. If Horner's syndrome is identified, the patient should immediately be returned or referred to a physician for further examination and not treated again until the cause is found to be relatively benign.

- *Dysarthria.* Dysarthria is an undiagnosed change in articulation. Dominant or nondominant hemispheric ischemia, as well as brain-stem and cerebellar impairments, may result in altered articulation.

NEUROLOGIC TESTS

Cyriax divided the neuromusculoskeletal system into neurologic, contractile, and noncontractile (or inert) tissues.[2]

The neurologic tissues comprise those tissues that are involved in nerve conduction, and the neurologic tests of the scan evaluate the transmission capability of the nervous system. Although the passive stretching of the dura is not technically a neurologic test, it is included under the neurologic tests as it is more closely related to the nervous system than the musculoskeletal system.

The evaluation of the transmission capability of the nervous system is performed to detect the presence of either upper motor neuron (UMN) impairment or lower motor neuron (LMN) impairment.

● UMN impairment. This is also known as a central palsy and presents with muscle hypertonicity and a hyper-reflexive deep tendon reflex (DTR) in a nonsegmental distribution. Motor and sensory loss can also be a feature, depending on the location and extent of the injury.

● LMN impairment. This is also known as a peripheral palsy and presents with muscle atrophy and hypotonus, in addition to a diminished DTR of the areas served by a spinal nerve root, or a peripheral nerve.

The differing symptoms are the result of injuries to different parts of the nervous system. LMN impairment involves damage to a neurologic structure distal to the anterior horn cell, whereas UMN impairment involves damage to a neurologic structure proximal to the anterior horn cell, namely the spinal cord or central nervous system, or both.

The other types of tissue, contractile and noncontractile/inert, are a little misleading in their nomenclature. Contractile tissues include the muscle belly, tendon, tenoperiosteal junction, submuscular/tendinous bursa, and bone. Noncontractile tissue includes the joint capsule, ligaments, bursa, articular surfaces of the joint, and synovium, dura, bone, and fascia. Bone, and the bursae, are placed in each of the subdivisions because of their close proximity to contractile tissue, and their capacity to be compressed or stretched during movement. By definition, a contractile tissue is a tissue involved with a muscle contraction and one that can be tested using an isolated muscle contraction. However, contractile tissues such as tendons, which have no ability to contract, could be classified as inert, because whereas they are strongly affected by the contraction of their respective muscle bellies, they are also affected if passively stretched. Conversely, inert tissues, which also have no ability to contract, can be compressed, and therefore affected, during a contraction.

Contractile tissues are most easily affected by isometric testing, whereas inert tissues are mainly affected by passive movement and ligament stress tests. As a general rule, if active and passive motions are limited or painful in the same direction, the lesion is in the inert tissue, whereas if the active and passive motions are limited or painful in the opposite direction, the lesion is in the contractile tissue.[2]

The scan consists of the following components (Fig. 10–2), which test a wide variety of pain-provoking structures:

Components	Tested
Active	Range of motion (ROM), willingness to move, integrity of contractile and inert tissues, pattern of restriction (capsular, or noncapsular), quality of motion, symptom reproduction
Passive	Integrity of inert and contractile tissues, ROM, end feel, sensitivity
Resisted	Integrity of contractile tissues (strength, sensitivity)
Stress	Integrity of inert tissues (ligamentous or disc stability)
Dural	Dural mobility
Neurologic	Nerve conduction
Dermatome	Afferent (sensation)
Myotome	Efferent (strength, fatigability)
Reflexes	Afferent–efferent and central nervous systems

Information about the patient's willingness to move and the status of the inert and contractile tissues could be obtained without a full scan; however, it is the ability to gain information about the integrity of the "myotome" for which the scan is critical. The tests that comprise the scan examine strength, fatigability, sensation, DTRs, and the inhibition of those and other reflexes by the central nervous system. The term *myotome* in this context is incorrect, as a true myotome is a muscle, or group of muscles, innervated exclusively from a segment. *Key muscle* is a better, more accurate term, as the muscles tested in the scan are the most representative of the supply from a particular segment.

In addition to the basic components of the scan, several other tests that are nonroutine are used when indicated. These special tests for each area are dependent on the special needs and structure of each joint. In the spine, the special tests consist of dermatome, reflex testing, and directional stress tests. Directional stressing includes posterior-anterior pressures, and anterior, posterior, and rotational stressing. Other special tests are carried out if there is some indication that they would by helpful in arriving at a diagnosis. These include vascular tests, repeated movement testing, and palpation for tenderness.

Manual Muscle Testing

Manual muscle testing is traditionally used by the clinician to assess the strength of the patient, and much information can be gleaned from the tests, including:

● The amount of force the muscle is capable of producing and whether the amount of force produced varies with the joint angle

- Whether any pain or weakness is produced with the contraction
- The endurance of the muscle, and how much substitution occurs during the tested movement.

Force

The force a muscle is capable of exerting depends on its length. For each muscle cell, there is an optimum length or range of lengths at which the contractile force is strongest. Thus, the significance of the findings in resisted testing depends on the position of the muscle and the force applied:

1. A strong positive finding: — Minimal resistance applied in the rest position for the muscle

2. A moderately positive finding: — Maximal resistance applied in the rest position for the muscle

   Minimal resistance applied in a lengthened position for the muscle

3. A weakly positive finding: — Maximal resistance applied in a lengthened position for the muscle

Pain or Weakness

Key muscle testing in the scan is used to differentiate between a weakness resulting from inactivity or disuse and one occurring as a result of nerve palsy or a grade III-IV muscle or tendon tear. Key muscle testing reveals one of four findings[2]:

1. A strong and pain-free contraction: — Normal finding

2. A strong but painful contraction: — Indicating a bursitis, tendonitis, or grade I muscle tear

3. A weak but pain free contraction: — Indicating a grade III-IV muscle tear, palsy, disuse, inhibition, or facilitation

4. A weak and painful contraction: — Indicating a hyperacute arthritis, fracture, grade II muscle tear, or neoplasm

Note: The latter two both indicate the possibility of serious pathology.

Endurance

To be a valid test, strength testing must elicit a maximum contraction of the muscle being tested. Three strategies ensure this:

1. Placing the muscle to be tested in a shortened position. This puts the muscle in an ineffective physiologic position and has the effect of increasing motor neuron activity.

2. Having the patient perform an eccentric muscle contraction by using the command "Don't let me move you." As the tension at each cross-bridge and the number of active cross-bridges is greater during an eccentric contraction, the maximum eccentric muscle tension developed is greater with an eccentric contraction than with a concentric one. (Refer to Chapter 2)

3. Breaking the contraction. It is important to break the patient's muscle contraction to ensure that the patient is making a maximal effort and that the full power of the muscle is being tested.

Weakness as a result of palsy has a distinct fatigability, and the muscle demonstrates poor endurance, maintaining a maximum muscle contraction for about 2 to 3 seconds before complete failure occurs. This is based on the theories behind muscle recruitment wherein a normal muscle, while performing a maximum contraction, uses only a portion of its motor units, keeping the remainder in reserve to help maintain the contraction. A palsied muscle, with fewer functioning motor units, has very few, if any, in reserve.

If a muscle appears to be weaker than normal, further investigation is required:

- The test is repeated a few times. Muscle weakness resulting from disuse is consistently weak and should not get weaker with several repeated contractions.
- Another muscle that shares the same innervation is tested. Knowledge of both spinal nerve and peripheral nerve innervation aids the clinician in determining which muscle to select. (Refer to Chapter 6)

Substitutions by other muscle groups during testing indicates the presence of weakness. It does not, however, tell the clinician the cause of the weakness.

As always, these tests cannot be evaluated in isolation but have to be integrated into a total clinical profile of the patient before the clinician can come to any conclusion about the patient's condition.

Sensory Testing

Sensory testing during the scan is performed throughout the dermatomal areas (Fig. 10–3). As a degree of overlap exists with the segmental innervation of the skin,[27] it is important to test the full area of the dermatome because the area of greater sensitivity changes. The area of sensitivity, or autogenous area, is a small region of the dermatome with no overlap. It is the only area within a dermatome that is supplied exclusively by a single segmental

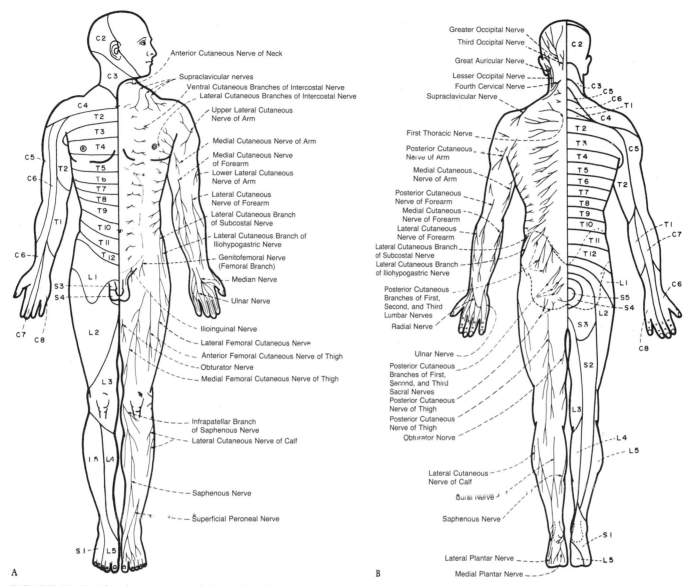

FIGURE 10–3 The dermatomes of the body. *(Reproduced, with permission from Wilkins RH (editor): Neurosurgery, 2e. McGraw-Hill, 1996)*

level. Because there is so much overlap in the dermatome, spinal nerve root compression usually results in hypoesthesia rather than anesthesia within the majority of the dermatome, but in anesthesia or near-anesthesia in the autogenous area of the dermatome. Paresthesia is a symptom of direct involvement of the nerve root. Further irritation and destruction of the neural fibers interfere with conduction, resulting in a motor or sensory deficit, or both. It is, therefore, possible for a nerve root compression to cause pure motor paresis, a pure sensory deficit, or both, depending on which aspect of the nerve root is compressed. If pressure is exerted from above the nerve root, sensory impairment may result, whereas compression from below

can induce motor paresis. There are two components to the dermatome tests:

1. *Light touch.* This tests for hypoesthesia throughout the dermatome and should be performed using the edge of a soft tissue paper so that just the hair follicles are stimulated.
2. *Pin-prick.* This tests for near-anesthesia in the autogemous, no-overlap area and is tested with the pointed end of a paper clip, or by using a disposable pinwheel.

With both tests, it is important to ask the patient to close the eyes. In terms of sensation loss, light touch is the most sensitive, and it is the first to be affected with palsy. If the light touch test is positive, the areas of reduced sensation are mapped out for the autogenous area, and then the pin-prick test is performed to map out the whole of the autogenous area. If everything is perceived as sharp by the patient, then it could indicate:

- The presence of a denervation hypersensitivity (patient is numb to light touch in that area)
- The presence of a hypermobile segment, producing a hyperesthesia in that area (facilitated segment), demonstrating intact light touch sensations and a very painful sharp/dull response. With a facilitated or hypermobile segment, an increased sympathetic response is often noted, with the area involved appearing cold and clammy throughout a dermatomal distribution. A blanching of the skin appears along the path of the finger that is rubbed down the back. (Refer to Chap. 4)

A decreased sympathetic response is often noted with nerve palsy, with the area involved looking pink, shiny, and glasslike throughout a dermatomal distribution. In addition, if a finger is rubbed down a patient's back, a welt will appear along the path of the finger.

Testing temperature sensation is not a necessary part of the scan, as the impulses for temperature sensation travel together with pain sensation in the lateral spinothalamic tract (refer to Chapter 4). However, the testing of skin temperature can help the clinician to differentiate between a venous insufficiency and an arterial insufficiency. With venous insufficiency, an increase in skin temperature is noted in the area of occlusion, and it also appears bluish in color. Pitting edema, especially around the ankles, sacrum, and hands, may also be present. However, if pitting edema is present and the skin temperature is normal, the lymphatic system maybe at fault. With arterial insufficiency, a decrease in skin temperature is noted in the area of occlusion and the area appears whiter. The area is also extremely painful.

A more thorough examination of the various components of the sensory system can be performed if the clinician feels it is warranted. A brief summary is given below.

A. Sensory evaluation[28]
  1. Temperature
     a. Origin: lateral spinothalamic tract
     b. Test: a cold and warm test tube is applied to the patient's skin.
  2. Pressure
     a. Origin: spinothalamic tract
     b. Test: firm pressure is applied to the patient's muscle belly.

  3. Vibration
     a. Origin: dorsal column/medial lemniscal
     b. Test: a vibrating tuning fork is placed on malleoli, patellae, epicondyles, vertebral spinous processes, and iliac crest.
  4. Position sense (proprioception)
     a. Origin: dorsal column/medial lemniscal
     b. Test: the patient is tested for the ability to perceive passive movements of the extremities, especially the distal portions. Proprioception refers to awareness of the position of joints at rest. While the extremity or joint under examination is held in a static position by the clinician, the patient is asked to describe the position verbally or duplicate the position with the opposite extremity.
  5. Movement sense (proprioception–kinesthesia)
     a. Origin: dorsal column/medial lemniscal
     b. Test: the patient is asked to indicate verbally the direction of movement while the extremity is in motion. The clinician must grip the patient's extremity over neutral borders.
  6. Stereognosis
     a. Origin: dorsal column/medial lemniscal
     b. Test: the patient is asked to recognize, through touch alone, a variety of small objects such as comb, coins, pencils, and safety pins.
  7. Graphesthesia
     a. Origin: dorsal column/medial lemniscal
     b. Test: the patient is asked to recognize letters, numbers, or designs traced on the skin.
  8. Two-point discrimination
     a. Origin: dorsal column/medial lemniscal
     b. Test: a measure is taken of the smallest distance between two stimuli that can still be perceived by the patient as two distinct stimuli.
  9. Equilibrium reactions: the patient's ability to maintain balance in response to alterations in the body's center of gravity and base of support is tested.
  10. Protective reactions: the patient's ability to stabilize and support the body in response to a displacing stimulus in which the center of gravity exceeds the base of support is tested (e.g., extension of arms to protect against a fall).

B. Tonal abnormality evaluation[28]
  1. Spasticity: increased resistance to sudden passive stretch
     a. Clasped knife phenomenon: produces a sudden letting go by the patient
     b. Clonus: an exaggeration of the stretch reflex
  2. Rigidity: a resistance is increased to all motions, rendering body parts stiff and immovable.

a. Decorticate: upper extremities are held in flexion and the lower extremities in extension.

b. Decerebrate: upper and lower extremities are held in extension.

c. Cogwheel phenomenon: a ratchet-like response to passive movement characterized by an alternate giving and increased resistance to movement

d. Leadpipe: constant rigidity; a common finding in patients with Parkinson's disease

C. Cranial nerve testing (refer to Table 9–3)

Deep Tendon Reflexes

These tests utilize the muscle spindle to determine the state of both the afferent and efferent peripheral nervous systems, and the ability of the central nervous system to inhibit the reflex. A reflex is a programmed unit of behavior in which a certain type of stimulus from a receptor automatically leads to the response of an effector. Many spinal cord and brain stem mechanisms involved in control of somatic and visceral activities are essentially reflexive. The circuitry that generates these patterns varies greatly in complexity, depending on the nature of the reflex.

The myotatic, or deep tendon, reflex (Fig. 10–4) is one of the simplest known, depending on just two neurons and one synapse,[29,30] and influenced by cortical and subcortical input. The tap of the reflex hammer on the tendon of the quadriceps femoris muscle as it crosses the knee joint causes a brief stretch of the tendon and muscle belly where the Golgi tendon organ and muscle spindle are stimulated (Figs. 10–5 and 10–6). Whenever a muscle is stretched, the intrafusal fibers are stretched with the extrafusal.[29,30] The sensory receptors of the spindle are excited and fire, causing a reflex contraction of the muscle so as to take the stretch off the spindle (see Fig. 10–6). The subsequent volley of impulses reaches the spinal cord over the large peripheral and central processes of the sensory neurons[29,30] (see Fig. 10–5). Although some impulses may head up the cord via ascending branches, the majority reach the synapses with the ipsilateral motor neurons of the anterior horn controlling the muscle that has been lengthened. Impulses are conducted along the axons of these motor neurons to the neuromuscular junctions, exciting the effectors (quadriceps femoris muscle), and producing a brief, weak contraction, which results in a momentary straightening of the leg ("knee jerk").[29,30] The stretch reflex can be divided into two parts:

1. The dynamic stretch reflex, wherein the primary endings and type Ia fibers are excited by a rapid change in length (see Fig. 10–6). The speed of conduction along the type Ia fibers and the monosynaptic connection in the cord ensure that a very rapid contraction of the

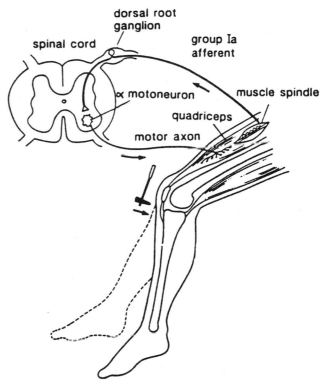

FIGURE 10–4 A schematic representation of the reflex arc. *(Reproduced, with permission from Haldeman S (editor): Principals and Practice of Chiropractic, 2e. Appleton & Lange, 1992)*

muscle occurs to control the sudden and potentially dangerous stretch of the muscle. The dynamic stretch reflex is over within a fraction of a second, but a secondary static reflex continues from the secondary afferent nerve fibers.

2. As long as a stretch is applied to the muscle, both the primary and secondary endings in the nuclear chain continue to be stimulated causing prolonged muscle

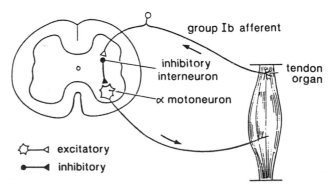

FIGURE 10–5 Reflex pathway of the Golgi tendon organ. *(Reproduced, with permission from Haldeman S (editor): Principals and Practice of Chiropractic, 2e. Appleton & Lange, 1992)*

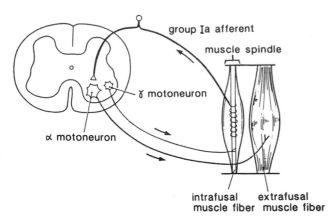

FIGURE 10–6 Role of the gamma motor neuron. *(Reproduced, with permission from Haldeman S (editor): Principals and Practice of Chiropractic, 2e. Appleton & Lange, 1992)*

contraction for as long as the excessive length of the muscle is maintained, thereby affording a mechanism for prolonged opposition to prolonged stretch.

When a load is suddenly taken off a contracting muscle, shortening of the intrafusal fibers reverses both the dynamic and static stretch reflexes, causing both sudden and prolonged inhibition of the muscle so that rebound does not occur.

The absence of a reflex signifies an interruption of the reflex arc. A hyperactive reflex denotes a release from cortical inhibitory influences.

Any muscle that possesses a tendon is capable of producing a DTR. Five grades exist for the manual clinician:

0	Areflexia (no reflex)
1+	Hyporeflexia
2+	Normal
3+	Brisk or hyperactive
4+	Markedly hyperactive or hyperreflexic

Each of these categories can occur as a generalized, or local, phenomenon.

The causes of generalized hyporeflexia run the gamut from neurologic disease, chromosomal metabolic conditions, and hypothyroidism to schizophrenia and anxiety.[31]

Nongeneralized hyporeflexia can result from peripheral neuropathy, spinal nerve root compression and cauda equina syndrome or the patient's physiologic makeup. It is thus important to test more than one reflex, and to evaluate the information gleaned from the examination, before reaching a conclusion as to the relevance of the findings. Hyporeflexia, if not generalized to the whole body, indicates an LMN or sensory paresis, which may be segmental (root), multisegmental (cauda equina), or nonsegmental (peripheral nerve).

True neurologic hyperreflexia contains a clonic component and is suggestive of central nervous system impairment such as brain stem or cerebral impairment, spinal cord compression, or a neurologic disease, any of which are out of the scope of a manual clinician. As with hyporeflexia, the clinician should assess more than one reflex before coming to a conclusion about a hyperreflexia, and can confirm the presence of a UMN with the presence of the pathologic reflexes such as a Babinski, Hoffman, and Oppenheim.

A brisk reflex is a normal finding provided that it is not masking a hyperreflexia caused by an incorrect testing technique. Unlike hyperreflexia, a brisk reflex does not have a clonic component to it.

Pathologic Reflex Testing

Babinski

In 1896, 6 years after taking his new position at the Hôpital de la Pitié, Babinski described the sign that bears his name.[32] Two years later, a full account of the diagnostic significance of the toe phenomenon ("phénomène des orteils"), regarded as a pathognomonic sign of pyramidal dysfunction,[33] was presented. In 1903, Babinski added to the original description the "signe de l'éventail," or fanning of the outer toes, often part of the reflex.[34,35] As Babinski observed, the pyramidal tracts are not well developed in infants, and these signs, which are abnormal past the age of 3 years, are usually present.

In this test, the clinician applies noxious stimuli to the sole of the patient's foot by running a pointed object along the plantar aspect.[36] A positive test, demonstrated by extension of the big toe and splaying (abduction) of the other toes, is indicative of a UMN impairment.

Oppenheim

In the Oppenheim test, the clinician applies noxious stimuli to the crest of the patient's tibia by running a fingernail along the crest. A positive test, demonstrated by the Babinski sign, is indicative of a UMN impairment.

Clonus

To test for clonus, the clinician passively applies a sudden dorsiflexion of the patient's ankle and the stretch is maintained during the test. The examiner notes a gradual increase in tone and then the transient occurrence of ankle clonus. In some patients there is a more sustained clonus, and in others there is only a very short-lived finding. During the testing, the patient should not flex the neck as this can often increase the number of beats. A positive test, demonstrated by four or five reflex twitches of the plantar flexors (two or three twitches are considered normal), is indicative of a UMN impairment.

Neuromeningeal Mobility Tests

The neuromeningeal mobility tests apply a mechanical and compressive stress to the neurologic tissues.[37] The tests assess for the presence of any abnormalities of the dura, both centrally and peripherally, by employing a sequential and progressive stretch to the dura until the patient's symptoms are reproduced. Theoretically, if the dura is scarred or inflamed, a lack of extensibility with stretching occurs. Breig's tissue-borrowing phenomenon offers a plausible explanation for the neuromeningeal tests.[38] He observed that tension produced in a lumbosacral nerve root results in displacement of the neighboring dura, nerve roots, and the lumbosacral plexus toward the site of tension.[38–41] In effect, a borrowing of the resting slack in neighboring meningeal tissues occurs as neural structures are pulled toward the site of increased tension. This results in a decrease in the available slack and potential mobility of the neural tissues throughout the region.[38,39,41–44] This stretching and displacement of the lumbosacral nerve roots and sacral plexus reduces the available caudal mobility of the sciatic nerve.[38–44] As a result of these sites of tension, the neurologic tissues move in different directions, depending on where the stress is applied and in which order it is applied.[44] Tension sites are found at the segmental levels of C6, T6, and L4, and at the elbow, the shoulder, and the knee.

The more common neuromeningeal mobility tests include the straight-leg raise and the slump test, but each has their own variations.

Straight Leg Raise Test

The straight leg raise (SLR) test is recognized as the first neural tissue tension test to appear in the literature,[45] although it was first described by Lasègue more than a hundred years ago.[46] During SLR testing, the patient is positioned supine, and the leg is elevated with the knee extended. The patient gives no assistance to the leg raise so that the results are not altered due to the anterior tilting of the pelvis by a contraction of the psoas major. It is also important to ensure that the patient does not raise the head off the bed during testing, thereby introducing tension to the dura.

The SLR places a tensile stress on the sciatic nerve and exerts a caudal traction on the lumbosacral nerve roots from L4 to S2.[44,45,47–49] Examination of the SLR test requires that the ROM measured is compared with the contralateral side and expected norms.[2,44,45,50,51] Although the SLR is considered to be a reasonably good clinical test of the sciatic nerve, it has no diagnostic significance on its own and must always be interpreted in association with other clinical findings.

Confounding the SLR test are the nonneural structures, such as lumbar zygapophysial joints, muscles, and connective tissue, which can limit leg elevation and provoke patient discomfort during testing.[44,45,50–52]

The sciatic nerve arises from the L4, L5, S1, S2, and S3 nerve roots, and passes out of the pelvis through the greater sciatic foramen, down the back of the thigh to its lower third, where it divides into the tibial and common peroneal nerves (refer to Chapter 6). *Sciatica* is defined as pain along the course of the sciatic nerve or its branches, and is most commonly caused by a herniated disc or by spinal stenosis. Characteristically, patients report gluteal pain radiating down the posterior thigh and leg, paresthesia in the calf or foot, and varying degrees of motor weakness.

Extraspinal Entrapment[53] Extraspinal entrapment of the sciatic nerve (i.e., along its course within the pelvis or the lower extremity) is infrequent and difficult to diagnose because its symptoms are similar to those of the more frequent causes of sciatica.[54,55] Sciatic nerve compression has been reported secondary to piriformis entrapment (refer to the discussion of bowstring tests later in this chapter, and to Chap. 6), heterotopic ossification around the hip,[56] misplaced intramuscular injections, myofascial bands in the distal thigh,[57] and myositis ossificans of the biceps femoris muscle.[58] Additional causes include post-traumatic or anticoagulant-induced extraneural hematomas[59] and compartment syndrome of the posterior thigh.[60] Entrapment sciatic neuropathy complicating total hip arthroplasty has been described secondary to escaped cement, subfascial hematoma, and nerve impingement during trochanteric wiring.[61]

When the SLR is severely limited, it is considered diagnostic for a disc herniation.[62] It should be remembered that:

- The patient must have at least 70 degrees of available hip flexion range to make this test valid.
- The SLR produces a posterior shear and some degree of rotation in the lumbar spine, a region not well suited to shearing or rotational forces. Thus, it may be necessary to differentiate between a physical irritant to the dura and a chemical one. With a physical irritant, the patient's pain occurs at the same point in the range each time it is tested. However, with a chemical irritation, the available range improves in time as the inflammation heals.

Performing the Test The patient is positioned supine, with no pillow under the head, and each leg is tested individually. To ensure that there is no undue stress on the dura, the tested leg is placed in slight medial rotation and adduction of the hip, and extension of the knee. The clinician, holding the patient's ankle, flexes the hip until the patient complains of pain or tightness in the posterior thigh.[41] At this point, the clinician reduces the amount of hip flexion slightly until the patient reports no pain or tightness.

During leg elevation, the L4-5 and S1-2 nerve roots are tracked downward and forward, pulling the dura mater caudally, laterally, and forward. During this maneuver, tension in the sciatic nerve and its continuations occurs in a sequential manner, firstly developing in the greater sciatic foramen, then over the ala of the sacrum, next in the area where the nerve crosses over the pedicle, and finally in the intervertebral foramen.

Anatomic changes at the anterior wall, such as a disc protrusion bulging dorsally in the canal, have the potential to compress the dura. Owing to the downward and anterior direction of the nerve root and the relative fixation of the dural investment at the anterior wall, a downward movement of the nerve always involves an anterior displacement that pulls the root against the posterior-lateral aspect of the disc and vertebra.

In addition, any space-occupying lesions situated at the anterior wall of the vertebral canal at the fourth and fifth lumbar, and first and second sacral segments, may interfere with the dura mater or nerve root structures, or both.

The patient is then asked to flex the neck so the chin is on the chest, or the clinician may dorsiflex the patient's foot (Bragard's test),[63] or medially rotate the patient's hip. Flexing the cervical spine, dorsiflexing the ankle (Fig. 10–7), and medially rotating the hip during the SLR test increases tension exerted on the spinal cord, spinal dura, and

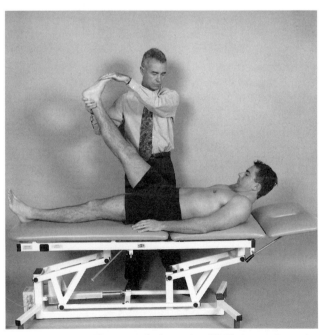

FIGURE 10–7 The straight leg raise (SLR) test with neck flexion superimposed.

lumbosacral nerve roots, and serve as "sensitizers" for the test.[38–40,43,44,64–66] Research conducted by Breig[64] and others[39,40,42,65–68] found that flexing the cervical spine during SLR testing lengthens the spinal cord and dura,[39,40,42,65–68] pulling the lumbosacral nerve roots cranially.[39,40,42,65] This may provoke radicular symptoms without stressing non-neural tissues in the lower extremity.[40,64,69–71]

If the cervical flexion, performed at the point where the SLR is positive, increases or decreases the pain, then the problem almost certainly lies within the neuromeningeal system, the restriction of the nerve root mobility indicating an anterior compression of the root. If, by adding cervical flexion, the patient's symptoms remain unchanged or are alleviated, this would indicate:

● The presence of a medially located disc protrusion.
● The presence of dural scarring or fibrosis resulting from a previous injury to the dura (up to 2 or more years earlier). This results in a painless loss in range of the SLR. Paresthesia may be provoked.
● An injury to the hamstring muscle complex as flexing the neck increases the stretch on the dura but has no effect on the length of the hamstrings.
● A crack fracture of a pedicle. This can often mimic a disc protrusion, or extrusion, with physical testing.

Thus, the dura can be pulled from below, during the SLR, or from above, during neck flexion. An increase of lumbar pain during neck flexion or SLR will therefore implicate the dura mater as the source. Dural signs are extremely important in distinguishing a lesion in which the anterior part of the dura mater is involved (disc displacements) from possible impairments at the posterior wall (zygapophysial joints and ligaments).

It is generally agreed that the first 30 degrees of the SLR serves to take up the slack or crimp in the sciatic nerve and its continuations. Thus, pain in the 0 to 30-degree range may indicate the presence of:

● An acute spondylolisthesis
● A tumor of the buttock
● A gluteal abscess
● A very large disc protrusion or extrusion[72]
● An acute inflammation of the dura
● A malingering patient

The sign of the buttock should always be suspected if pain is reproduced in this range.

Between 30 and 70 degrees, the spinal nerves, their dural sleeves, and the roots of the L4, L5, S1, and S2 segments are stretched, with an excursion of 2 to 6 mm.[73] After 70 degrees, these structures undergo further tension, but other structures are also involved. These structures include the hamstrings, the gluteus maximus, and the hip, lumbar, and sacroiliac joints. An SLR test is positive if:

1. The range is limited by spasm to less than 70 degrees.
2. Flexing the knee allows a greater range of hip flexion to occur.
3. The pain reproduced is neurologic in nature, indicating that the dura is inflamed, which usually occurs 24 hours after the protrusion or extrusion. This should be accompanied by other signs and symptoms, such as pain with coughing, tying of shoe laces, and so on, but not necessarily any muscle weakness.

Positive findings throughout the whole range indicate a muscle or contractile impairment.

Negative findings throughout the whole range may indicate a massive protrusion, and may be accompanied by:

● Ischemic root atrophy, resulting in a complete loss of sensitivity of the dural sheath
● A discontinuation of reflex hamstring contractions, which usually occurs to protect the nerve root, allowing the SLR to return to full range

Cross Straight Leg Sign

The cross SLR sign, or well-leg raising test of Fajersztajn[45] is a phenomenon that can be associated with the SLR test, whereby a lifting of the asymptomatic leg produces pain in the symptomatic leg. There are three recognized types:

1. An SLR producing pain in the contralateral leg, but not when the contralateral leg is raised
2. An SLR producing pain in both legs
3. An SLR producing pain in the contralateral leg, and a contralateral SLR also producing pain. For example, if the pain is felt in the right leg, the SLR of the right leg produces pain in the left leg, and the SLR of the left leg produces pain in the right leg

There are many theories as to the cause and significance of the crossover sign, including sacroiliac joint involvement. It is possible that the neuromeninges are pulled caudally, resulting in a compression of the dural sleeve against a large or medially displaced disc herniation. The crossover sign is thought to be more significant than the SLR test in terms of its diagnostic powers to indicate the presence of a large disc protrusion.[74]

Bilateral Straight Leg Raise

Once the unilateral SLR test is completed, the clinician should test both legs simultaneously (Fig. 10–8). One of the limitations of the unilateral SLR is that it may not highlight the presence of a central disc protrusion, especially a

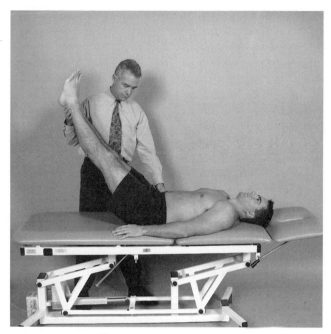

FIGURE 10–8 The bilateral SLR test.

soft disc protrusion. By performing a bilateral SLR and incorporating both neck flexion and dorsiflexion, central protrusions can be detected.

Because a central protrusion can mimic a stenosis, a method of differentiation is needed. The easiest way to do this is to position the patient in a seated flexion position. A stenotic patient will feel better when put in this position. The clinician can also differentiate between a posterior-lateral disc bulge, spinal stenosis and intermittent claudication by using the bicycle test of van Gelderen.[75] The patient is positioned on a stationary bike and asked to pedal against resistance. The patient with stenosis tolerates the seated or flexed position well. The patient with intermittent claudication of the lower extremities experiences a worsening of symptoms with time in whatever spinal position is assumed. The symptoms of a patient with intermittent cauda equina compression worsen with an increase in lumbar lordosis. The patient with a disc herniation initially fairs well in the flexed position, but quickly worsens.

Slump Test

Despite the development of refinements to the SLR test, the test is inadequate in detecting neural tension in some cases.[49,70,71,76,77] A neural tension test performed in a sitting position is necessary to simulate the extremes of spinal motion seen during symptom-provoking activities, such as slouched sitting or entering and exiting a car.[40,70,71,76,77]

The slump test, popularized by Maitland,[77] is a combination of other neuromeningeal tests, namely the seated SLR, neck flexion, and lumbar slumping. In the slump test, the patient is seated in full flexion of the thoracic and lumbar regions of the spine.[78] Sensitizing maneuvers are then systematically applied and released to the cervical spine and lower extremities, while the tester maintains the patient's trunk position. The slump test assesses the excursion of neural tissues within the vertebral canal and intervertebral foramen,[71] detecting impairments to neural tissue mobility from a number of sources identified by Macnab[79] and Fahrni.[80] Maitland asserted that the slump test enables the tester to detect adverse nerve root tension caused by spinal stenosis, extraforaminal lateral disc herniation, disc sequestration, nerve root adhesions, and vertebral impingement.[71,76]

A number of studies[38,43,64,67] have demonstrated the effects of trunk and head position on neural structures within the vertebral canal and intervertebral foramen during slump testing, finding that full spinal flexion, or flexion of the cervical, thoracic, and lumbar regions of the spine, produces lengthening of the vertebral canal. This elongation of the vertebral canal stretches the spinal dura and transmits tension to the spinal cord, lumbosacral nerve root sleeves, and nerve roots.[38,39,42,43,67,81] During full spinal flexion, the cauda equina becomes taut and the lumbosacral nerve roots and root sleeves are pulled into contact with the pedicle of the superior vertebra.[38,39,49,67]

When extension of the cervical spine is introduced, the dura and the nerve roots slacken as the vertebral canal begins to shorten.[38,39,42,49,67,81,82] Extending the thoracic and lumbar spine increases the slack in the neural tissues as the vertebral canal continues to shorten.[38,39,49,67,81,82]

Because the slump test is a combination of other tests, a choice as to its use needs to be made. Either the SLR, or its various adjunct tests, should be performed or the slump test should be used.[1]

The only advantage that the slump test has over the SLR test is that it increases the compression forces through the disc and will, therefore, highlight the presence of dural adhesions better.[1] Depending on the text source, there are a wide variety of progressive steps to the slump test in terms of when the lumbar kyphosis stage is introduced. Although the specific order to use is controversial, it is important that the clinician consistently uses the same sequence with each patient.

As soon as symptoms are reproduced during these tests, they should be terminated. It is worth remembering that during a dural tension test, the dura itself does not move, it is merely stressed; hence the name for the tests. One method is described here.

The patient is positioned sitting with the hands behind the back, and a slight arch in the back (Fig. 10–9), which helps ensure that the lumbar spine is maintained in neutral. This position should be followed by a slump of the lumbar and thoracic spine as the clinician maintains the patient's

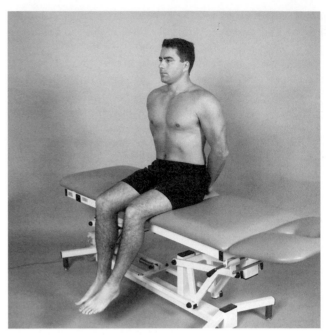

FIGURE 10–9 The start position of the slump test.

neck in neutral (Fig. 10–10). This maneuver has the effect of tightening the entire dura, including the thorax dura. If the test is still negative, the patient is asked to flex the neck by first applying a chin tuck and then placing the chin on the chest, and then to straighten the knee as much as possible. The test is repeated using the other leg and then with both legs at the same time. If the patient is unable to

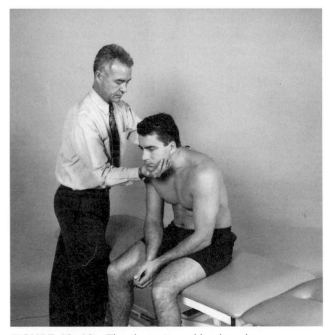

FIGURE 10–10 The thoracic and lumbar slump.

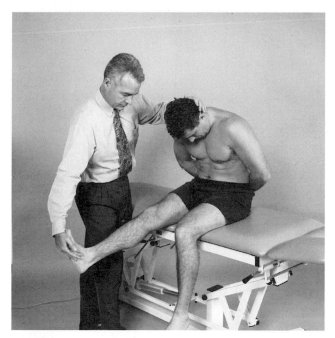

FIGURE 10–11 The full slump test.

straighten the knee because of a reproduction of pain, he or she is asked to actively extend the neck. If, following the neck extension, the patient is able to straighten the knee further, the test can be considered positive.

If symptoms have yet to occur, active dorsiflexion is added (Fig. 10–11). Passive overpressure can be applied to each of these moves. If the patient experiences positive symptoms with the leg extension, the knee is slightly flexed and the dorsiflexion is reapplied passively in an attempt to reproduce the symptoms. Throughout the entire slump test, each time a positive response is reached, the last movement applied is reduced slightly to take the stress off the dura, and tension is applied from the opposite end of the dura. The test should also be done in reverse (as a positive response can be obtained in one direction but not the other) and can be made more objective by numbering each of the motions; for example: (1) thoracic kyphosis, (2) lumbar kyphosis, (3) neck flexion/chin tuck, (4) knee flexion at 90 degrees, (5) knee flexion at 60 degrees, (6) knee flexion at 30 degrees, and (7) knee flexion at 0 degrees (full knee extension). The important numbers for symptom reproduction are 3 through 5.

For a neuromeningeal test to be positive, it must reproduce the patient's symptoms, and the sensitizing tests must increase or decrease those symptoms. The tests themselves often cause pain, but the clinician must be able to differentiate this from dural pain. For example, in the slump test a nonpathologic response includes pain, or discomfort, in the area of T8-9.

The adverse neural tension tests are not a part of every scan but are used if a dural adhesion or irritation is suspected. The examination of neural adhesions is by no means an exact science, but the principles are based on sound anatomic theory. Knowledge of the course of each of the peripheral nerves is essential to put adequate tension through each of them. Because the sinuvertebral nerve innervates the dural sleeve, the pain, experienced as a result of an inflamed dura, is felt by the patient at multisegmental levels and is described as having an achelike quality. If the patient experiences sharp or stabbing pain during the test, a more serious underlying condition should be suspected.

If pain is reproduced with the slump, but not with an SLR, there could be a number of reasons:

● Presence of a soft protrusion, particularly a central soft protrusion. Soft central protrusions need loading through weight bearing, and are often negative in a non–weight-bearing position.
● Presence of an acute spondylolisthesis
● Presence of a posterior instability
● Presence of a malingering patient

The following findings are strongly predictive for a disc herniation[72,74,83]:

● Severely limited SLR
● Crossover SLR
● Severely restricted and painful trunk movements

Bowstring Tests

A positive bowstring test is a strong indicator for surgery, but it need only be performed if the SLR is positive with the addition of dorsiflexion. Bowstring tests will not detect a chronically irritated dura, as insufficient stretch is imparted on the dura during the test, but the tests can help the clinician to differentiate between a lesion to the tibial or common peroneal branch of the sciatic nerve.

Tibial Nerve Test

The roots of the tibial nerve exit from L4 to S2 and travel down the middle of the posterior thigh between the femoral condyles and down the back and middle of the calf, entering the foot under the medial malleolus of the ankle. The nerve is, therefore, put on stretch with the addition of dorsiflexion to the SLR. Once the point of irritation has been reached, the clinician places the patient's leg over one shoulder. The patient's knee is gently flexed until the symptoms fade. The clinician places a thumb behind the patient's knee, between the femoral condyles, and presses into the popliteal fossa, thereby deforming the tibial nerve. If the symptoms are brought on by this maneuver, the bowstring test is positive.

Common Peroneal Test

Typically, the roots of the common peroneal nerve exit from L5 to S2 and travel with the tibial branch to the posterior distal thigh region. It then wraps itself around the fibular head and has strong attachments to the tendon of the biceps femoris. Because the nerve is usually well attached, attempts to stretch it with plantar flexion and inversion may not reproduce the symptoms, whereas the bowstring test will. The procedure is similar to that of the tibial version of the test, except that after the knee is slightly flexed, the clinician pulls the biceps femoris tendon, at the fibular head, medially and laterally. If this maneuver reproduces the symptoms, it is a positive test.

It is possible to have a positive SLR test accompanied by a negative bowstring test, and there are three possible explanations for this:

1. As mentioned previously, the inflammation to the dura is chronic, rather than acute; more stretch is applied to the dura during an SLR than with the bowstring tests
2. *Lateral stenosis.* A loss of disc height will lead to instability of the segment as this loss of height makes the ligaments slack and causes the facets to telescope, which produces lateral stenosis.
3. *Piriformis syndrome.* The sciatic nerve usually travels below the piriformis. In about 15% of the population, the tibial part of the sciatic nerve passes through either the belly of the piriformis muscle, or the piriformis has two muscle bellies, and the nerve passes between the two bellies. Consequently, contraction or tightness of the muscle will produce radicular symptoms. By the time the tibial nerve reaches the piriformis, it is a peripheral nerve and, therefore, compression of it should produce no pain, only numbness and tingling throughout the tibial distribution, unless there is a neuritis resulting from a bacterial infection or from friction.

Piriformis pain can also be caused by:

*   A chronic piriformis spasm, resulting from a facilitated segment in the lumbar spine that causes hypertonicity in the piriformis and chronic irritation to the nerve.
*   A lesion to the piriformis muscle belly. This can be diagnosed by testing the strength of the gluteus medius and minimus. The superior gluteal nerve, which exits from the sciatic nerve before it reaches the piriformis, innervates these muscles. The muscles below the piriformis that are innervated by the sciatic nerve are then tested. Weakness of these in the presence of strong glutei is a positive sign of piriformis syndrome.

Piriformis involvement can also be ruled out using a modified SLR. The piriformis is placed on slack by externally rotating the hip during the SLR. The range obtained is compared with that obtained from an SLR with the hip in internal rotation. If the piriformis is involved, more range will be obtained with the hip in external rotation, which places the piriformis on slack.

A modification to the SLR tests can also be used to help rule out radicular symptoms resulting from stenosis. The SLR is taken to the point of symptom reproduction, and then a longitudinal traction force is applied through the leg by the clinician. This imparts a distraction force on the lumbar spine and alleviates the symptoms if stenosis if present, but aggravates the symptoms if the dura is irritated.

Further modifications can be incorporated to place stress through different branches of the sciatic and common peroneal nerves by adjusting the ankle and foot position:

1. Dorsiflexion, foot eversion, and toe extension:	Stresses the tibial branch
2. Dorsiflexion and inversion:	Stresses the sural nerve
3. Plantar flexion and inversion:	Stresses the common peroneal (deep and superficial)

Prone Knee Bending Test

The prone knee bending test stretches the femoral nerve using hip extension and knee flexion to stretch the nerve termination in the quadriceps muscle, and has been used to indicate the presence of upper lumbar disc herniations,[84] especially when hip extension is added.[85] The femoral nerve travels anteriorly to both the hip and the knee (as does the rectus femoris). Therefore, the nerve roots are stretched with a combination of knee flexion and hip extension. Some clinicians recommend performing a prone knee bend test prior to executing a sacroiliac upslip correction, because there is a small potential of avulsing the L2-3 nerve roots with this maneuver.

The lateral femoral cutaneous nerve also travels anterior to the thigh and can be stressed with the hip extension component of this maneuver. Neuropathy of this nerve is usually associated only with hypoesthesia, but in some patients it may cause pain and dysesthesia in the anterior-lateral aspect of the thigh.[86] In many patients, the cause of the neuropathy is not found,[87] but compression along the long course of the nerve is the main cause. The compression may be at the level of the roots, such as by disc hernia[88] or by tumor in the second lumbar vertebra,[89] but it

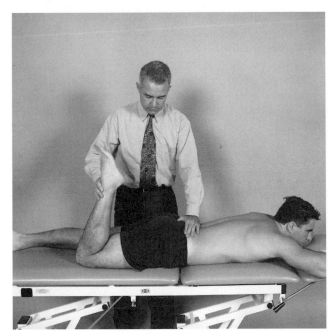

FIGURE 10–12   The prone knee bending test.

also may be compressed along the retroperitoneal course by a space-occupying lesion such as a tumor.[90] Abnormal posture, tight-fitting braces or corsets, and thigh injuries are other common causes of injury to the nerve.[91] A recent study found an injury to the lateral femoral cutaneous nerve to be a common complication during spinal surgery, occurring in 20% of these patients.[93]

The patient is positioned in prone lying, and the clinician stabilizes the ischium to prevent an anterior rotation of the pelvis. The patient's knee is then flexed as far as possible (Fig. 10–12). If no pain is reproduced thus far, the hip is extended while the knee flexion is maintained. The zone where the dura is stretched is 80 to 100 degrees of knee flexion. Knee flexion greater than 100 degrees introduces both a rectus femoris stretch and lumbar spine motion into the findings.

The test is positive if there is a reproduction of unilateral pain in the lumbar area, buttock, and/or posterior thigh, which would indicate an L2, L3, or L4 nerve root impairment, but acute L4-S1 disc protrusions can also produce positive findings.[93] As with the SLR test, neck flexion or extension (Fig. 10–12) can be added.[94] This test can also be positive with patients who have undergone a cardiac grafting procedure.

Sign of the Buttock[2]

This syndrome is described here because its underlying pathologies occur in the lower quadrant and because it can be assessed as part of the SLR test. The "sign of the

buttock" is not a single sign, as the name would suggest, but rather a collection of signs indicating a serious pathology present posterior to the axis of flexion and extension in the hip. Among the causes of the syndrome are osteomyelitis, infectious sacroiliitis, and fracture of the sacrum/pelvis, septic bursitis, ischiorectal abscess, gluteal hematoma, gluteal tumor, and rheumatic bursitis. The patient lies supine and the clinician performs a passive unilateral SLR. If there is a unilateral restriction, the clinician flexes the knee and notes whether the hip flexion increases. If the restriction was caused by the lumbar spine or hamstrings, hip flexion increases. If the hip flexion does not increase when the knee is flexed, it is a positive sign of the buttock test. If the sign of the buttock is encountered, the patient must be immediately referred back to the physician for further investigation. The sign of the buttock typically includes almost all of the following:

- Limited SLR
- Limited hip flexion
- Limited trunk flexion
- Noncapsular pattern of hip restriction
- Painful and weak hip extension
- Gluteal swelling
- Empty end feel on flexion

SCANS

Suggested Sequence of the Lumbar and Sacroiliac Scan

Chronic low back pain is among the most common musculoskeletal disorders and is the single most common disorder associated with disability, with the costs estimated to be at least 50 billion dollars per year in the United States alone.[95,96] There are a number of warning signs to watch for during a lumbar examination:

- Pain in the upper lumbar region. This suggests the possibility of aortic thrombosis, neoplasm, dental caries, ankylosing spondylitis, or visceral disease.
- Sign of the buttock. The first indication is usually a discrepancy noted between trunk flexion and the SLR.
- Signs of interference with conduction of more than one nerve root.
- Bilateral nerve root palsy.
- Complete paralysis.
- A significantly warmer foot on the affected side.[2] The warmer foot results from interference with the sympathetic nerves at the upper lumbar levels.
- Glove and sock neuropathy. This finding could indicate lead or mercury poisoning, or both.

History

PATIENT STANDING

Observation
The observation should be performed with the patient standing and then seated.

Posture Good posture is a subjective finding based on what the clinician believes to be correct and should not be of a major concern to the clinician at this stage of the examination. The subject of posture, more pertinent to the biomechanical examination, is discussed later in Chapter 11.

Scoliosis The clinician should note any abnormal spinal curvature. Structural changes in the lumbar region associated with pain are fairly common. One of the most common is scoliosis.

Scoliosis can be found in four forms: static, sciatic, idiopathic, and psychogenic. With static scoliosis, a leg length difference is the source of the scoliosis. Sciatic scoliosis is caused by painful disorders in the lower lumbar spine. The extent of a scoliosis should be noted if it is thought to be significant, and an attempt should be made to manually correct it to ascertain whether this can be done painlessly. A compensatory shift or scoliosis is often easy and painless to correct.

Lateral Shift The sight of a patient with a pelvic shift or list is a common one. The shift is thought to result from the body finding a position of comfort and protection due to:

- An irritation of a zygapophysial joint
- An irritation of a spinal nerve and/or its dural sleeve, due to a disc herniation[97] and the resulting muscle spasm[98]

It is theorized that this protective spasm is created by the quadratus lumborum muscle and, occasionally, the iliacus muscle. The direction of the list, although still controversial, is believed to result from the relative position of the disc herniation to the spinal nerve. Theoretically, a contralateral list occurs when the spinal nerve/dura is compressed on its lateral aspect, whereas an ipsilateral list occurs when the compression is on its medial aspect.[99]

The technique to correct a lateral shift is described in Chapter 13.

Lordosis Is the lordosis excessive or reduced? An increase in lumbar lordosis is usually as the result of:

- Short, tight, and weak erector spinae
- Stretched, slack, and weak abdominals

- Short and strong psoas muscles, especially if associated with an anterior pelvic tilt, or a flexion deformity of the hip joint

A flattened back may indicate that the patient has either lumbar spinal stenosis, or a lateral recessed stenosis. An excessive lordosis may indicate that the patient has a spondylolisthesis.

Kyphosis Is the lumbar spine kyphotic? Kyphosis of the lumbar spine may indicate damage to the supraspinous ligament complex.

Atrophy If atrophy is present, does it follow a segmental or nonsegmental pattern?

Creases Creases in the posterior aspect of the trunk may indicate areas of hypermobility or instability. A very low abdominal crease may indicate a spondylolisthesis.

Deformity, Birthmarks, and Hairy Patches These are all evidence of congenital deficits of the integumentary system and can indicate underlying anomalies in the systems derived from the same embryological segments.[100] A hairy patch or tuft, typically located at the base of the lumbar spine, may indicate a spina bifida occulta or diastematomyelia.[101]

Bony Landmarks The anterior superior iliac spines, medial malleoli, and lateral malleoli should all be level with their counterparts on the opposite side.

Active Range of Motion
Normal active motion involves fully functional contractile and inert tissues, and optimal neurologic function. While standing, the patient performs flexion, extension, and side-flexion to both sides (Fig. 10–13A, B, C and D). At the end of each motion, a gentle overpressure is applied to assess the end feel. At the end of the side-flexion motion, which tends to be less irritating than other movements, overpressure is applied on the shoulder opposite to the side-flexion to avoid any unnecessary compression (Fig. 10–13C and D). Although some clinicians feel that overpressure should not be applied in the presence of pain, most, if not all, of the end feels that suggest acute or serious pathology are to be found in the painful range, including spasm and the empty end feel.

The clinician should consider having the patient remain at the end range for 10 to 20 seconds if sustained positions were reported to increase the symptoms in the subjective history; likewise, if repetitive or combined motions have been reported. McKenzie[102] advocates the use

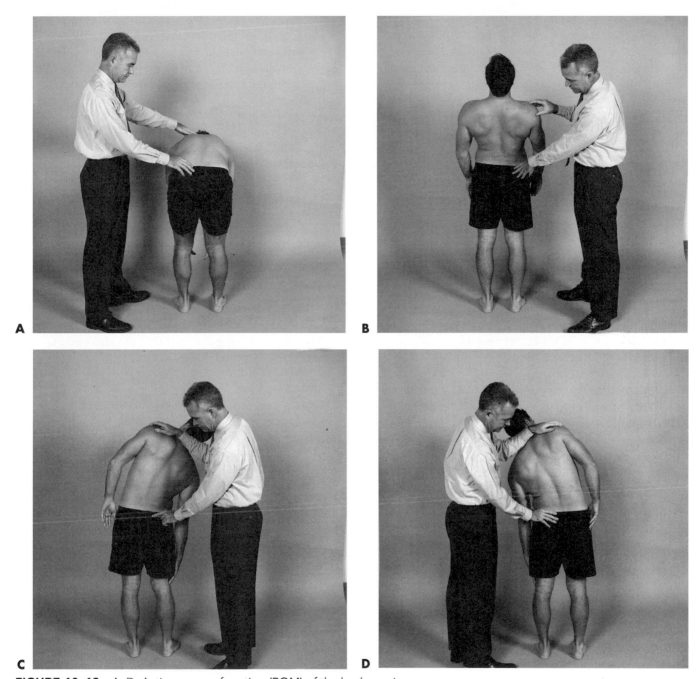

FIGURE 10–13 A–D. Active range of motion (ROM) of the lumbar spine.

of repeated active movements, especially flexion and extension.

The amount of range available depends on a number of factors, including age and stage of healing, and even in so-called normal spines there is a great deal of variability. Some individuals are able to touch their toes with only hip or thoracic motion. However, the focus of the scan is not with actual ranges, but the quality of the

motion, the symptoms the motions provoke, and the end feel—it is the biomechanical examination that assesses the ranges in more depth. An apparently normal range could indicate normalcy, hypermobility, or instability. Restricted range will be in either a capsular or noncapsular pattern.

As mentioned earlier in this chapter, the various components of the range of motion and strength tests examine different aspects:

Components	Tests (Tissues and Other)
Active	ROM, willingness to move, contractile and inert tissues, pattern of restriction, quality of motion, symptom reproduction
Passive	Inert and contractile tissues, ROM, end feel, sensitivity
Resisted	Contractile (strength, sensitivity)

A good view of the spine is essential so that the examiner can focus on the following areas.

- The curve of the spine in flexion, extension, and side-flexion, which should be smooth. An angulation occurring during extension could indicate an area of instability. In side-flexion, an angulation indicates an area of hypomobility, the point at which it curves, representing the first segment capable of side-flexion, not the hypomobile segment.
- Creases in the lumbar spine area during extension, which could indicate an area of rotational instability or hypermobility if unilateral, or an anterior instability and extension hypermobility, if bilateral and symmetric.
- Deviations during or at the end of range. Trunk deviation during flexion is believed to be associated with a disc herniation, with the direction of the deviation determined by the relative position of the compression on the nerve, as previously discussed. Deviations during flexion may also result from neuromeningeal adhesions, hypomobile segment(s) on the contralateral side, hypermobile segment(s) on the ipsilateral side, a structural scoliosis, or a shortened leg on the ipsilateral side.[1]
- Failure to recover motion smoothly, which is indicative of an instability. This typically occurs at the end point of flexion as the patient begins to return to the erect stance and has to extend by walking the hands up the thighs or using a series of jerking motions.
- The provocation of symptoms. Are the symptoms neurologic or nonneurologic, and how far does the distribution of pain extend? If there is lower extremity pain, does it travel below the knee? Leg pain provoked by any motion other than flexion is not a good prognostic sign[2]; neither is posterior leg pain, reproduced with extension, rotation, or side-flexion, possibly indicating a significant prolapse or extrusion.
- Gross limitation of both side-flexions, possibly indicating ankylosing spondylitis.
- End feel. It is the end feel that indicates to the clinician the cause of the motion restriction. It must be remembered that the significant end feels, such as

spasm and empty, are associated with pain, so the overpressure needs to be performed gently. However, if radicular pain is reproduced with active ROM, it would seem pointless to inflict overpressure further into the range. Nonradicular pain that occurs at the end of full range may indicate a hypermobility.

Standing Up on the Toes
The patient raises both heels off the ground. The key muscles tested during this maneuver are the plantar flexors (S1-2). These are difficult muscles to fatigue, so the patient should perform 10 heel raises unilaterally with his or her arms resting on the clinician's shoulders. In addition to observing for fatigability, the clinician should also look for Trendelenburg's sign, which could indicate a hip impairment (coxa vara), or a gluteus medius weakness secondary to a superior gluteal nerve palsy.

Unilateral Squat while Supported
The patient performs unilateral squats while supported. The key muscles being tested during this maneuver are the quadriceps (L3-4).

Heel Walking
The patient walks toward, or away from, the clinician while weight bearing through the heels. The key muscles being tested during this maneuver are the dorsiflexors (L4).

PATIENT SEATED

Active Range of Motion
The patient, keeping the knees together, twists at the waist to each side, and overpressure is applied at the end of range (Fig. 10–14). The clinician should perform this maneuver from in front of, and behind, the patient.

Seated Lumbar Flexion
The flexion component of this test is a good way to scan for rotoscoliosis.

Key Muscle Tests
- *Knee extension (L3).* If the mini-squat maneuver was not used in the standing section, this is another opportunity to test the fatigability of the quadriceps. At this level, the L3 nerve root is not commonly compressed by a disc, but it is a common site for a metastasis. The clinician positions the patient's knee in 25 to 35 degrees of flexion and then applies a resisted flexion force at the midshaft of the tibia (Fig. 10–15). Both sides are tested for comparison.
- *Hip flexion (L1-2).* With palsy, the patient is unable to raise the thigh off the table. Palsy at this level should

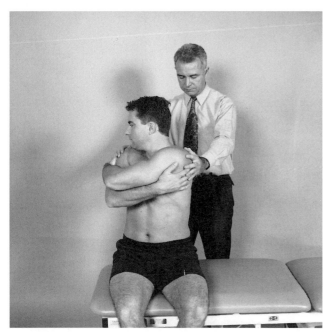

FIGURE 10–14 Active lumbar rotation with overpressure applied by the clinician.

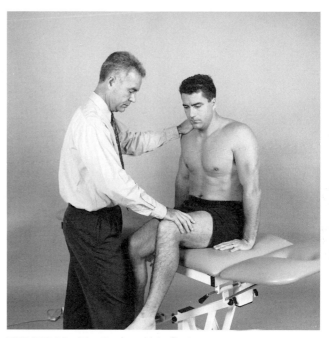

FIGURE 10–16 Resisted hip flexion.

serve as a red flag, as disc protrusions here are rare, but this is also a common site for metastasis. The patient's hip is actively raised off the treatment table. The clinician then applies a resisted force proximal to the knee, into hip extension (Fig. 10–16), while ensuring that the heel of the patient's foot is not contacting the examining table. Both sides are tested for comparison.

A combined L3-4 palsy is extremely rare. Because L2 disc impairments are also extremely rare, an L2 palsy always suggests a nondiscogenic impairment. A bilateral palsy at this level is rarely the result of a disc impairment; more likely it is the result of a space-occupying structure such as a neoplasm.

Slump Test (L4-S2)
(See earlier discussion.)

PATIENT SUPINE

McKenzie advocates the testing of lumbar flexion motion in the supine as well as standing positions.[102] In the standing position, flexion occurs from above downward, so pain at the end of the range indicates that L5-S1 is affected. When the patient is in the supine position, lifting both knees to the chest (Fig. 10–17), causes flexion to occur from below upward, so that pain at the beginning of movement indicates that L5-S1 is affected.

Key Muscle Tests
The testing of these levels is very important as 90% of all lumbar disc impairments occur at the levels of L4-5. Serious impairments should be suspected if total loss of power from these muscles is present, because it is

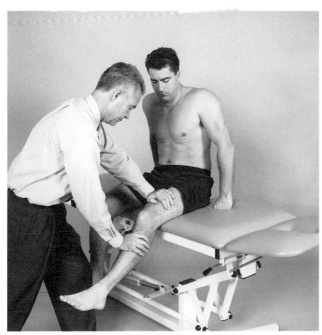

FIGURE 10–15 Resisted knee extension.

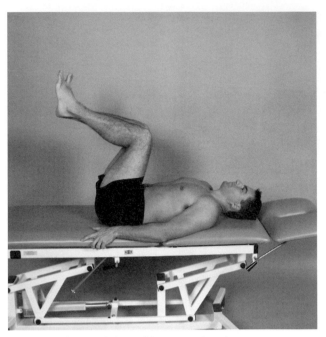

FIGURE 10–17   Bilateral knees to the chest.

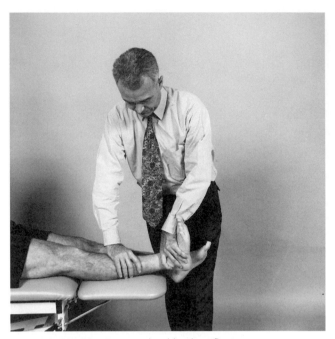

FIGURE 10–18   Resisted ankle dorsiflexion.

extremely unlikely for a disc impairment to cause a complete palsy.[1]

- *Ankle dorsiflexion (L4).* The patient is asked to place the feet at 0 degrees of plantar and dorsiflexion relative to the leg. A resisted force is applied to the dorsum of each foot by the clinician (Fig. 10–18) and a comparison is made.
- *Great toe extension (L5).* The patient is asked to hold both big toes in a neutral position, and the clinician applies resistance to the nails of both toes and compares the two sides.
- *Ankle eversion (L5-S1).* The patient is asked to place the feet at 0 degrees of plantar and dorsiflexion relative to the leg. A resisted force is applied by the clinician to move each foot into inversion, and a comparison is made.

Straight Leg Raise Test
(See earlier discussion.)

Bowstring Tests
(See earlier discussion.)

Compression Test (Modified Farfan Test)[103]
The patient is supine. The clinician flexes the patient's hips and knees to the point where the pelvis starts to posteriorly rotate (Fig. 10–19). The clinician then squeezes the patient's thighs against the chest and exerts a cranially directed pressure against the patient's feet or buttocks, and applies an

axial compression force to the patient's spine. Farfan's original version of this test had the patient positioned supine with the hips flexed to 45 degrees and the feet on the bed. The clinician then placed a hand over the patient's sacrum and attempted to push the patient up the bed.

The test is positive if pain is produced. There are two scenarios for the pain production. The pain can occur

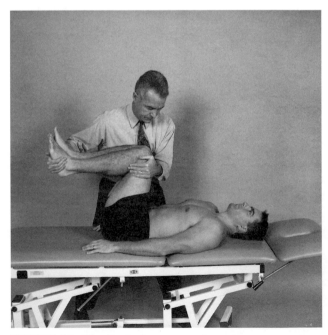

FIGURE 10–19   Farfan's compression text.

before the posterior rotation of the pelvis, or during the axial loading. If it occurs before, the following pathologies may be present:

- Anterior spondylolisthesis
- Muscle tear
- Acute instability
- Malingering patient

If the pain is reproduced with the axial loading, there is the possibility of an end-plate fracture or acute disc herniation. If a disc herniation is present, the pain should increase if the clinician taps the ischial tuberosities with the heel of the palm.

Anterior Sacroiliac Joint Stress Test

The anterior stress test, also called the gapping test, is performed with the patient supine. The clinician stands to one side of the patient and, crossing his or her arms, places the palms of the hands on the patient's anterior superior iliac spines (Fig. 10–20). The crossing of the arms ensures that the direction of the applied force is lateral, thereby gapping the anterior aspect of the sacroiliac joint. The stress is maintained for 7 to 10 seconds, or until an end feel is felt. The procedure stresses the ventral ligament and compresses the posterior aspect of the joint. A positive test is one in which the patient's groin or sacroiliac joint pain is reproduced either anteriorly, posteriorly, unilaterally, or bilaterally.[104]

This test and its posterior counterpart (see later discussion) are believed to be sensitive for arthritis or ventral ligament tears, and they are commonly positive in ankylosing spondylitis.[1]

FABER (Flexion, abduction, external rotation) Positional Test

The patient lies supine. The clinician places the foot of the test leg on top of the knee of the opposite leg (Fig. 10 21). The clinician then slowly lowers the test leg into abduction, in the direction toward the examining table. A positive test occurs when the test leg remains above the opposite straight leg, which may indicate a problem affecting the hip joint. However, because the lumbar spine and sacroiliac joint are involved in this maneuver, pathologies of those joints cannot be ruled out without selective stabilization of the pelvis. Placing the sole of the test leg foot against the medial aspect of the opposite thigh and then lowering the test leg toward the examining table can modify the FABER test for the patient with knee pathology.

FADE Positional Test

The set up for the flexion, adduction, extension (FADE) test is similar to that of the FABER test, except that the start position involves moving the patient's hip into flexion and adduction (Fig. 10–22). From that position, the clinician moves the patient's hip into extension and slight abduction. The FADE test assesses the integrity of the hip joint.

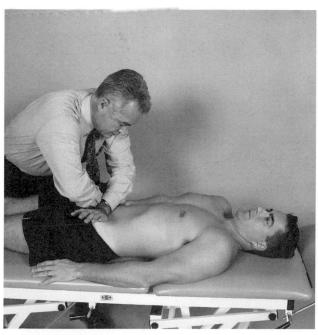

FIGURE 10–20   Gapping of the anterior sacroiliac joint.

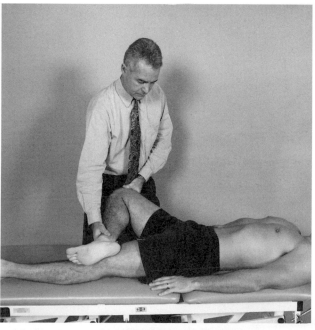

FIGURE 10–21   The FABER test.

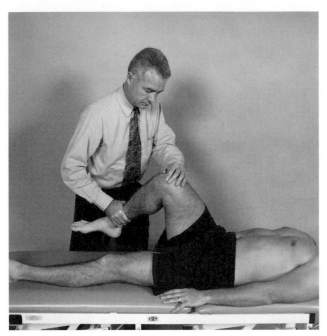

FIGURE 10–22 The start position for the FADE test.

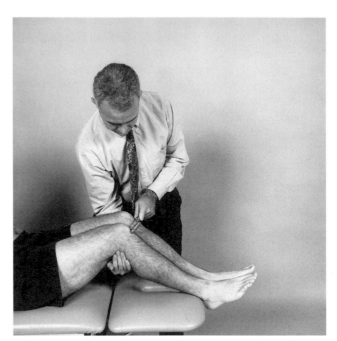

FIGURE 10–23 A variation of the patient position for the patella reflex.

Deep Tendon Reflexes

The reflexes should be assessed and graded accordingly. The clinician should note any differences between the two sides.

0	No deep tendon reflex present (Areflexia)
1+	Diminished (Hyporeflexia)
2+	Normal
3+	Brisk or hyperactive
4+	Markedly hyperactive or hyperreflexic

The DTRs are tested with a reflex hammer, with the patient relaxed.

- *Patella reflex (L3).* The patient is positioned supine so that the hip is abducted and externally rotated and the knee is flexed to about 30 degrees. Alternatively, both knees can be supported in flexion (Fig. 10–23).
- *Achilles reflex (S1-2).* The patient should be positioned so that the ankle is at 90 degrees or slightly dorsiflexed (Fig. 10–24).

Ankle and knee jerks sometimes disappear earlier than muscle power or skin sensitivity. A loss of the ankle jerk is permanent in about half of the cases, whereas the knee jerk often recovers.

As mentioned previously, DTRs can be performed on any muscle that contains a spindle. Other examples include:

- Adductor magnus reflex (L3), on the distal-medial aspect of the thigh over its insertion

- Posterior tibialis reflex (L4), on the proximal aspect of the foot arch
- Anterior tibialis reflex (L4), on the anterior aspect of the midshin
- Peroneal reflex (L4), on the lateral aspect of the leg
- Extensor digitorum brevis reflex (L5), on its muscle belly on the dorsum of the foot

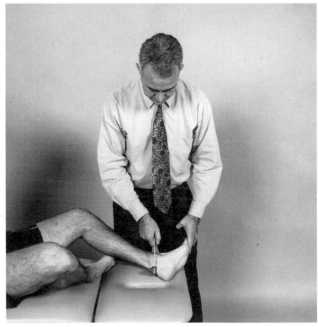

FIGURE 10–24 The Achilles reflex.

- Medial hamstrings reflex (L5-S1), on the medial aspect of knee
- Lateral hamstrings reflex (S1-2), which can be difficult to find. The clinician places a thumb over the tendon and taps the thumbnail to elicit the reflex.

Pathologic Reflexes
(See earlier discussion.)

Sensory Testing
The clinician checks the dermatome patterns of the nerve roots as well as the peripheral sensory distribution of the peripheral nerves. Dermatomes vary considerably between individuals.

PATIENT SIDE LYING

Posterior Sacroiliac Joint Stress Test
The posterior stress test, also called the compression test, is performed with the patient in the side lying position. The clinician, standing behind the patient, applies a downward force on the side of the patient's uppermost innominate using both hands (Fig. 10–25). The procedure creates a medial force that tends to gap the posterior aspect of the joint while compressing its anterior aspect. The reproduction of pain over one or both of the sacroiliac joints is considered positive. The dorsal ligament is accessible just below the posterior inferior iliac spine and should be palpated for tenderness.[105]

Key Muscle Test
Hip abduction (L5 and superior gluteal).

PATIENT PRONE LYING

Key Muscle Tests
- *Hip extension (L5-S1).* This test is only performed if the patient is unable to perform plantar flexion in standing or resisted ankle eversion. The patient's knee is flexed to 90 degrees and the thigh is lifted slightly off the examining table by the clinician, while the other leg is stabilized. A downward force is applied to the patient's posterior thigh while the clinician ensures that the patient's thigh is not in contact with the table. Both sides are tested for comparison. The S1 nerve root is commonly injured with hip surgery.
- *Knee extension (L3-L4).* This is the position preferred by many clinicians for testing knee extension, provided the patient has no knee pathologies. The patient's leg is positioned in about 90 degrees of knee flexion, taking care to do this passively. The clinician rests the superior aspect of his or her shoulder against the dorsum of the patient's ankle, and a superior force is applied while the clinician grips the edges of the examining table (Fig. 10–26). Both sides are tested for comparison.
- *Knee flexion (L5 and S1-2).* The patient's knee is flexed and an extension isometric force is applied just above the ankle (Fig. 10–27). Both sides are tested for comparison.

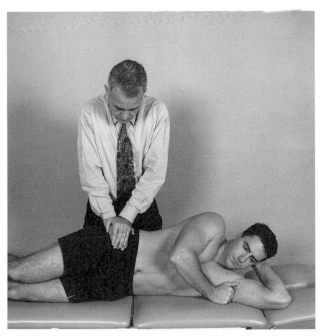

FIGURE 10–25 Gapping of the posterior sacroiliac joint.

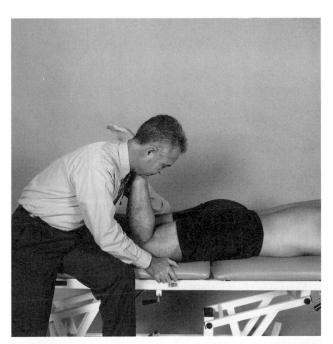

FIGURE 10–26 Resisted knee extension in prone position.

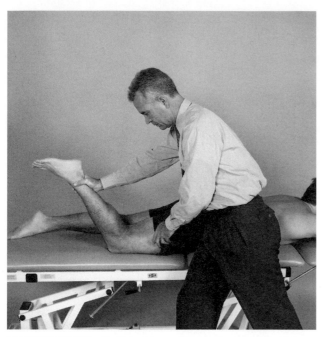

FIGURE 10–27 Resisted knee flexion in prone position.

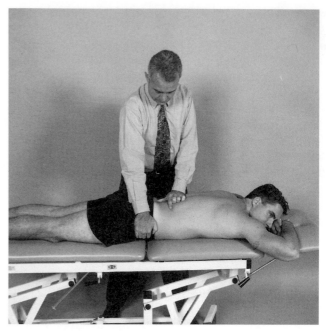

FIGURE 10–28 Farfan's torsion test.

An S2 palsy produces atrophy of the buttock. The patient is asked to contract the buttock muscles while the clinician pushes into the buttocks with a closed fist. Failure by the patient to hold the tightness could be indicative of an S2 impairment.

Farfan's Torsion Stress Test[1,103]

The intent of this test is to deform the pars articularis and compress the facets on one side, while distracting them on the opposite side. A positive finding is the reproduction of pain. The patient is prone and the clinician stabilizes the spinous process of T12. The clinician reaches over the patient and grasps the anterior superior iliac spine. The anterior superior iliac spine is then pulled directly backward, resulting in a torsional force and a pure axial rotation to the lumbar spine (Fig. 10–28). A rotation to the left of the lumbar spine produces a gapping of the left zygapophysial joints and a compression of the right zygapophysial joints. The test is then repeated on the other side. Bearing in mind that the lumbar spine is only capable of 3 to 4 degrees of axial rotation, this test has the ability to highlight the presence of a rotational instability. The test also provokes pain from the following pathologies:

● Neural arch fracture; the patient typically complains of pain with both tests
● Unilateral subchondral fracture of the zygapophysial joint
● Very large disc protrusion

If the test is positive, the clinician needs to check each level. The clinician stabilizes the spinous process of L5 and repeats the test. Moving cranially, each level is similarly tested. The testing is stopped at the first level where pain is reproduced, as findings at higher levels will also be painful and, therefore, inconclusive. The test can also be performed in reverse by lifting the patient's shoulder from the bed. For example, lifting the right shoulder of the patient induces right rotation at the lumbar spine. The findings from the reverse test should be consistent with the standard test; that is, pain reproduced with the same direction of rotation.

Posterior-Anterior Pressures

Posterior-anterior pressures over the vertebra via pressure on the spinous processes of each lumbar vertebra are a form of stress test, although not very specific. For example, pressure over L3 produces an anterior shear at L3-4 but a posterior shear of L4-5. In addition, L2 extends and L4 flexes, both resulting in an extension of L2-3 and L3-4.

However, as a screen it has its uses, serving to help detect the presence of excessive motion or spasm, or both. The clinician applies the posterior-anterior force in a slow and gentle fashion, using the thumb of one hand while monitoring the paravertebrals with the other hand (Fig. 10–29). Modifications of this test can be performed; for example, applying the force over one transverse process produces a rotational force and will help to check the multifidus.

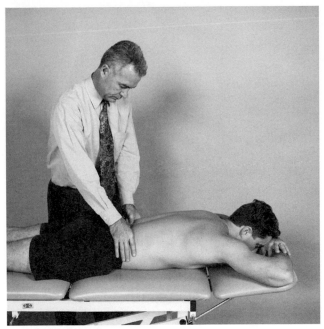

FIGURE 10–29 Posterior-anterior pressures over the lumbar spine.

Prone Knee Bending Test
(See earlier discussion.)

Suggested Sequence of the Cervical Scan

Warning signs in the cervical region (in addition to those serious signs already mentioned) include:

- Unexplained weight loss
- Involvement of two or three nerve roots
- Gradual increase in pain
- Expanding pain
- Spasm with passive ROM of the neck
- Visual disturbances
- Painful and weak resistive testing
- Hoarseness
- Limited scapular elevation
- Horner's syndrome
- T1 palsy (weakness and atrophy of hand intrinsics); the first sign of amyotrophic lateral sclerosis
- Arm pain in a patient who is less than 35 years old, or in any patient for more than 6 months
- Side-flexion away from the painful side that causes pain (if this is the only motion that causes pain)

In this region:

- The uncovertebral joint is the main threat to the vertebral artery
- The zygapophysial joint is the main threat to the nerve root

As with the lumbar scan, the basic sequence of testing is geared to patient convenience, to prevent unnecessary movement of the patient. However, the clinician will also decide the order of the testing based on the observation and subjective examination. Thus, testing of the vertebral artery and the transverse ligament should be considered if the observation and subjective examination reveal any of the signs and symptoms that have been linked, directly or indirectly, to vertebral artery insufficiency. These include:

- Wallenberg's, Horner's, and similar syndromes
- Bilateral or quadrilateral paresthesia
- Hemiparesthesia
- Ataxia
- Scotoma
- Nystagmus
- Drop attacks
- Periodic loss of consciousness
- Lip anesthesia
- Hemifacial para/anesthesia
- Hyperreflexia
- Babinski, Hoffman, and Oppenheimer signs
- Clonus
- Dysphasia
- Dysarthria
- Absent auditory reflexes
- Neural hypoacousia diplopia

History
The cervical spine is an area with a high potential for serious injury, which makes this an area of the body that needs to be approached with caution. As with the other scans, the subjective history is extremely important. Many of the symptoms that occur in an upper limb have their origins in the neck. Unless there is a history of definite trauma to a peripheral joint, a scanning examination must be done to rule out problems with the neck. The patient can report bizarre symptoms, and these need to be heeded until the clinician can rule out serious pathology. The history must include questions that will elicit any symptoms that might suggest a central nervous system condition, or a vascular compromise to the brain. In addition to those already mentioned for this region, the following questions, made specific to the cervical spine must be asked:

A. History of trauma. When was the trauma and what was the mechanism? Were there neurologic symptoms? If there were, this could indicate more severe damage.[106]

B. Presence of dizziness, nausea, or visual disturbances

C. Lhermitte's symptom, or "phenomenon." This is an electric shock–like subjective sensation that radiates down the spinal column into the upper or lower limbs when flexing the neck. It can also be precipitated by extending the head, coughing, sneezing, or bending forward or by moving the limbs.[107] It was described in detail by Lhermitte,[108] who insisted that demyelination was the underlying pathology. Lhermitte's symptom and abnormalities in the posterior part of the cervical spinal cord on magnetic resonance imaging (MRI) are strongly associated. Smith and McDonald[109] postulated that there is an increased mechanosensitivity to traction on the cervical cord of injured axons located within the dorsal columns, causing transient activity of normally silent sensory units as well as increasing the firing rate of spontaneously active units. Although a herniated disc is an anteriorly placed lesion, and the spinothalamic tract is usually more affected than the posterior columns, flexion of the neck will produce stretching of the posterior aspects of the cord but not the anterior part at the site of the impairment, and this may explain this particular symptom.

1. Multisegmental paresthesia (cord symptoms)
2. Does the patient have headaches? If so, where? What is their frequency and intensity? Does a position alter the headache? If the patient reports relief of pain and referred symptoms with the placement of the hand or arm of the affected side on top of the head, this is Bakody's sign and is indicative of an impairment in the C4 or C5 area.[110]
3. Does the patient have trouble with walking or balance? Positive responses may indicate a cervical myelopathy or a systemic neurologic impairment.[111]

PATIENT SEATED

Observation

The clinician should look for gross deformities such as:

- Torticollis
- Sprengel's deformity, an embryologic condition giving the patient the appearance of having no neck, secondary to a high-riding scapula
- Scars (particularly long, transverse scars indicative of cervical surgery)
- Scoliosis
- Muscle atrophy or hypertrophy
- Swelling
- Stance
- Gait

- Bone deformities
- Autonomic skin changes
- Birthmarks
- Posture
- Cervical rib, indicated by a higher trapezius.

The clinician should observe the position of the patient's head. If it is shifted to one side, it could be indicative of a disc protrusion. If it is deviated, acute arthritis might be present. Does the patient change posture often, indicating a degree of discomfort?

The clinician should look for asymmetries when the patient is unaware of being observed. A major driving force to give the appearance of symmetry exists in people, examples of which occur when people look into a mirror or when they know they are being observed. During the observation portion of the examination, the clinician looks for subtleties and attempts to determine the origin of any asymmetries seen.

Side View

- Is the forehead vertical, as in a normal individual?
- Is a forward head posture present? The amount of compression occurring at the L5-S1 disc doubles for every inch beyond the correct position and can lead to recurrent disc protrusions. A forward head posture produces a change in head position and a change in the bite biomechanics. Most forward head postures are the result of a thoracic hypomobility. In normal individuals, the tip of the chin is perpendicularly in line with the manubrium.

If in doubt, the clinician should measure the distance the chin protrudes anteriorly, or measure the distance from the apex of the thoracic kyphosis to the deepest point in the cervical lordosis.[112]

Is the patient able to reduce the degree of forward head posture?

Front View

- Is the head in midline or is there evidence of torticollis? A cervical disc protrusion at C3-4 or C4-5 produces a horizontal side shift of the head while the patient maintains eye level
- Are the eyes level? Are their depths and sizes equal?
- Is the nasal bone observable between the eyelids, and does it continue down symmetrically? Are there any obvious nostril defects?
- Does the mouth have any tilts or upturns? The presence of dry and cracked lips indicates a mouth breather. Are the teeth or tongue visible, which also indicates mouth breathing? Mouth breathing encourages a forward head posture. Is there an

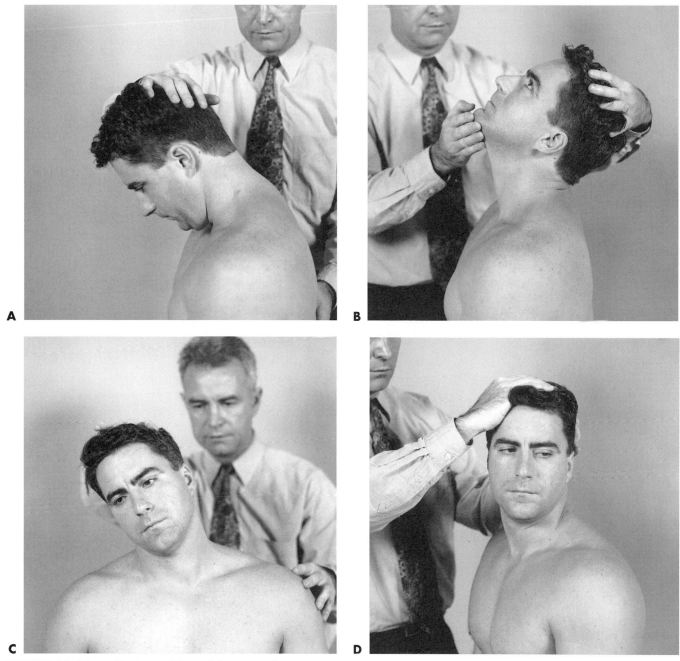

FIGURE 10–30   A–D. Active ROM of the cervical spine.

overbite? Overbites push the head of the mandible up and back.

● Are the shoulders level? The shoulder on the dominant side is usually higher. Is there any atrophy of the deltoid, suggesting an axillary nerve palsy?

Active Range of Motion

The patient performs the six cardinal motions: flexion, extension, both side-flexions, and both rotations

(Fig. 10–30A to D). Each of the motions is tested with a gentle overpressure, applied at the end of range if the active range appears to be full and pain free, although, with the exception of rotation, the weight of the head usually provides sufficient overpressure. As previously mentioned, it is necessary to apply overpressure even in the presence of pain, in order to get an end feel. If the application of overpressure produces pain, the presence of an acute muscle spasm is possible. Caution must be taken when using overpressure in the direction of rotation, especially if the rotation is combined with ipsilateral side-flexion and extension.[113] The clinician should evaluate the following:

- Quality
- End feel
- Symptoms provoked
- Willingness of the patient to move
- Patterns of restriction

The available ROM in the cervical spine is a combination of many factors, including the shape and orientation of the zygapophysial joints and the degree of muscle flexibility. As with other joints in the body, the available ROM typically decreases with age, the only exception being the rotation available at C1-2, which may increase.[114] It is possible to assess both the upper and mid-to lower cervical segments by modifying the active ROM tests, and by asking the patient to resist at the end of range once the end feel has been assessed:

- *Short neck flexion.* The clinician instructs the patient to place his or her chin on the Adam's apple. If this maneuver produces tingling in the feet, it is highly indicative of a C0-1 or C1-2 instability, or both, resulting from a dens fracture or a laxity of the transverse ligament. If the patient reports a pulling sensation, the cervicothoracic junction may be at fault. The C1 "myotome" can be tested in this position by testing the short neck *extensors*. The clinician attempts to gently push the patient's chin towards the Adam's apple while the patient resists. The short neck extensors are innervated by the spinal accessory. Positive findings with this test are nausea or rigidity, which may indicate a dens fracture or a tumor.
- *Mid-low cervical flexion.* The clinician instructs the patient to place his or her chin on the chest while keeping the teeth together. If this produces tingling in the feet, it could indicate a cervical myelopathy or scarring of the dura.
- *Short neck extension.* The clinician instructs the patient to look upward by only lifting the chin. The patient extends the head on the neck, and the clinician attempts to lift the occiput in the direction of the ceiling. If this produces tingling in the feet, it may indicate a "buckling" of the ligamentum flavum, producing pressure on the spinal cord. A loss of balance or a drop attack strongly suggest a compromise of the vertebrobasilar system. The C1 "myotome" can also be tested in this position by testing the short neck *flexors*. The clinician attempts to lift the patient's chin toward the ceiling while the patient resists. The short neck flexors are in-

nervated by the spinal accessory nerve. Positive findings with this test are nausea or rigidity, which may indicate a dens fracture, or a tumor.

- *Long neck extension.* The clinician instructs the patient to "look up to the ceiling." From this position, the clinician gently pushes the patient's chin posteriorly and assesses the end feel.
- *Side-flexion.* Active side-flexion is typically the first motion to demonstrate problems of the cervical spine. Most of the side-flexion occurs between C0-1 and between C1-2. The clinician should note the rotation that accompanies this motion. Resisted side-flexion tests the C3 "myotome."
- *Rotation.* Resisted rotation tests the C2 "myotome."

The clinician should consider having the patient remain at the end range for 10 to 20 seconds if sustained positions were reported in the subjective history to increase the symptoms; likewise, if repetitive or combined motions have been reported. The use of distraction and compression can be employed following the motion tests.

Distraction Test

Distraction is applied in the neutral position first (Fig. 10–31), and then in cervical flexion and extension.

- Distraction in extension produces a distraction of the zygapophysial joint surfaces and a compression of the disc.

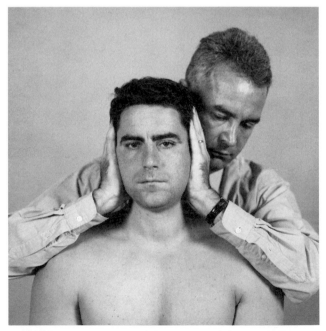

FIGURE 10–31 General distraction of the cervical structures.

- Distraction in flexion increases the compression of the zygapophysial joint surfaces and distracts the disc.

A reproduction of pain with distraction suggests:

- A tear of a spinal ligament
- A tear or inflammation of the annulus fibrosis
- An irritated dura

Other signs and symptoms may present themselves during distraction. These include a loss of consciousness, lower extremity paresthesia, or a drop attack.[1]

Compression Test

Compression of the spine (Fig. 10–32) gives an indication of vertical irritability. A reproduction of pain with compression suggests:

- A disc problem
- An end plate fracture
- A fracture of the vertebral body
- An acute arthritis of the zygapophysial joint

The compression test should be applied in the neutral position first before attempting it in flexion or extension.

Key Muscle Tests

The clinician looks for relative strength and fatigability. These isometric tests are first performed with the muscles in a stretched position. If this proves positive for pain or weakness, the muscles are retested in their shortened position, and are palpated along the suspect muscle and tendon unit. There are numerous smaller muscles throughout this area, so resistance needs to be applied gradually. Pain that occurs with resistance, accompanied by pain at the opposite end of passive range, indicates a muscle impairment. Alternates are given for each "myotome":

- *Levator scapulae (C4).* The clinician places a thumb on the superior aspect of the medial border of the patient's scapula and then tries to push the border in the direction of the ipsilateral iliac crest while the patient resists.
- *Diaphragm (C4).* The patient takes a deep breath while the clinician stabilizes the patient's ribs, trying to prevent the expansion
- *Scapular elevators (C2-4).* The clinician asks the patient to elevate the shoulders about one-half of full elevation. The clinician applies a downward force on both shoulders while the patient resists (Fig. 10–33).
- *Shoulder abduction (C5).* The clinician asks the patient to abduct the arms to about 75 to 80 degrees with the forearms in neutral. The clinician applies a downward force on the humerus while the patient resists (Fig. 10–34).
- *Shoulder external rotation (C5).* The clinician asks the patient to put the arms by the sides, with the elbows flexed to 90 degrees and the forearms in neutral. The clinician applies an inward force to the forearms (Fig. 10–35)

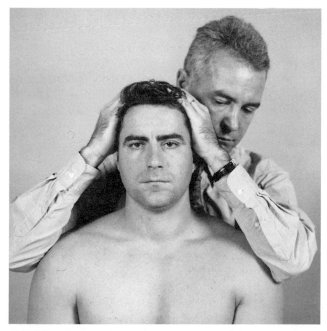

FIGURE 10–32 General compression of the cervical structure.

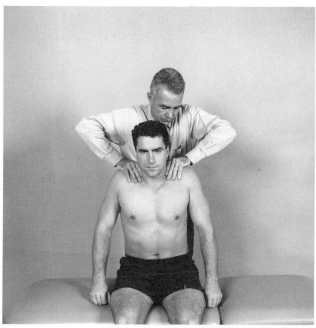

FIGURE 10–33 Resisted shoulder elevation.

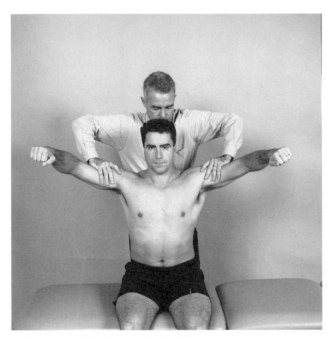

FIGURE 10–34 Resisted shoulder abduction.

- *Elbow flexion (C6).* The clinician asks the patient to put the arms by the sides, with the elbows flexed to 90 degrees and the forearms in neutral. The clinician applies a downward force to the forearms.
- *Wrist extension (C6).* The clinician asks the patient to place the arms by the sides, with the elbows flexed to 90 degrees and the forearms, wrists, and fingers in

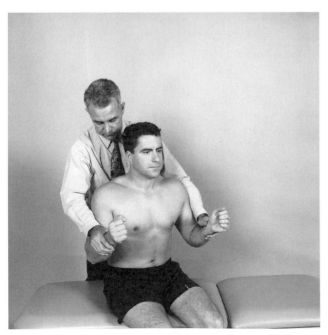

FIGURE 10–35 Resisted shoulder external rotation.

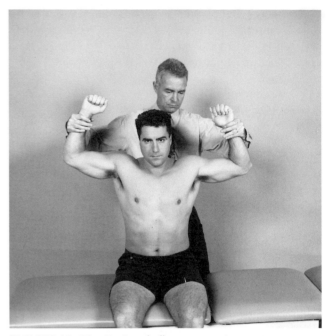

FIGURE 10–36 Resisted elbow extension.

neutral. The clinician applies a downward force to the back of the patient's hands.
- *Shoulder internal rotation (C6).* The clinician asks the patient to put the arms by the sides, with the elbows flexed to 90 degrees and the forearms in neutral. The clinician applies an outward force to the forearms.
- *Elbow extension (C7).* The patient is seated with their shoulders and elbows flexed to about 90 degrees. The clinician stands behind the patient and tests the triceps bilaterally by grasping the patient's forearms and attempting to flex the elbows (Fig. 10–36).
- *Wrist flexion (C7).* The clinician asks the patient to place the arms by the sides, with the elbows flexed to 90 degrees and the forearms, wrists, and fingers in neutral. The clinician applies an upward force to the palm of the patient's hands.
- *Thumb extension (C8).* The patient extends the thumb just short of full ROM. The clinician stabilizes the proximal interphalangeal joint of the thumb with one hand, and applies an isometric force into thumb flexion with the other.
- *Ulnar deviation (C8).* The clinician asks the patient to place the arms by the sides, with the elbows flexed to 90 degrees and the forearms, wrists, and fingers in neutral. The clinician applies a lateral force to the back of the patient's hands
- *Hand intrinsics (T1).* The patient is asked to squeeze a piece of paper between the fingers while the clinician tries to pull it away.

Neuromeningeal Tests

Foraminal Compression (Spurling's Test)[115]   A progression
of three stages is recommended with this test. The first two
stages, compression in neutral (see Fig. 10–32) and then
compression in extension, have already been mentioned.
If no symptoms were provoked in the first two stages, the
Spurling test is performed. Spurling's test involves an axial
compression loading, which is manually applied at the end
of all four quadrants to fully open or close the intervertebral formina and stress the disc. It is only used if the
patient does not report any arm symptoms prior to the
scan; otherwise, compression is applied in neutral only.

- Neck flexion, combined with side-flexion away from
  the pain, tests the integrity of the disc (Fig. 10–37).
- Neck extension, combined with side-flexion toward
  the painful side, tests for foraminal encroachment
  (Fig. 10–38).

Upper Limb Tension Tests   The reader is encouraged to refer to the work of David Butler, from whom these tests are
taken.[41] The upper limb tension tests (ULTTs) are equivalent to the SLR test in the lumbar spine. They are tests
designed to put stress on the neuromeningeal structures of
the upper limb. Each test begins by testing the normal side
first. Normal responses include:

- Deep stretch or ache in the cubital fossa

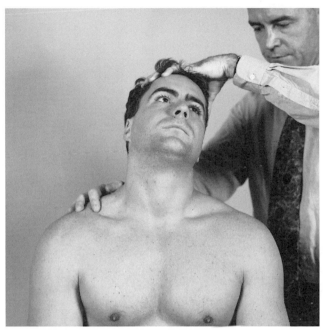

FIGURE 10–38   The Spurling test demonstrating neck
extension and side-flexion toward the painful side.

- Deep stretch or ache into the anterior or radial aspect
  of the forearm and radial aspect of the hand
- Deep stretch in the anterior shoulder area
- Sensation felt down the radial aspect of the forearm
- Sensation felt in the median distribution of the hand

Positive findings include:

- Production of the patient's symptoms
- A sensitizing test in the ipsilateral quadrant that alters
  the symptoms

*ULTT 1—Median Nerve (Anterior Interosseous Bias [(C5-6,
7])*   The patient is supine, with the head unsupported.
The clinician places a hand on top of the patient's shoulder and depresses that shoulder. The patient's arm is
then abducted to about 110 degrees and the elbow
extended to 0 degrees. This is followed by supination of
the forearm and extension of the wrist and fingers. The
patient then side-flexes the head away from the tested
side.

*ULTT 2A—Median Nerve (Musculocutaneous and Axillary
Nerve Bias)*   The patient is supine, head unsupported.
Shoulder depression is applied. The shoulder is then
placed in 10 degrees of abduction. The elbow is extended,
the forearm supinated, and the wrist and thumb extended.
The patient then side-flexes the head away from the tested
side.

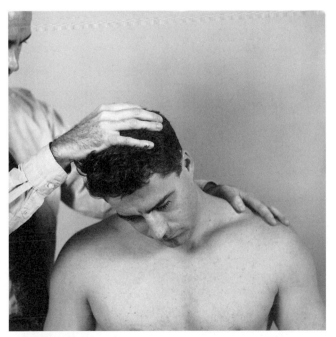

FIGURE 10–37   The Spurling test demonstrating neck
flexion and side-flexion away from the painful side.

ULTT 3—Radial Nerve Bias (C5-T1) The patient is supine, head unsupported. The clinician, facing the patient's feet, supports the patient's arm in about 80 degrees of elbow flexion. The shoulder is in internal rotation and about 10 degrees of abduction. Shoulder depression is applied, followed by full extension of the elbow, pronation of the forearm, wrist and finger flexion, and ulnar deviation. The shoulder is then internally rotated, followed by the patient side-flexing the neck away from the tested side.

ULTT 4—Ulnar Nerve Bias (C8-T1) The patient is supine, head unsupported. The clinician places a hand on top of the patient's shoulder and depresses that shoulder. The patient's arm is then abducted to about 10 degrees with the elbow flexed to 90 degrees. The forearm is supinated, and the wrist and fingers are then extended and radially deviated. The shoulder is externally rotated. The patient side-flexes the neck away from the tested side.

Evans[116] described a modification of the ULTT. The patient is asked to abduct the humerus with the elbows straight, stopping just short of the onset of symptoms. The patient then externally rotates the shoulder just short of symptoms, and the clinician then holds this position. Finally, the patient flexes the elbows so that the hands are placed behind the head. Reproduction of radicular symptoms with elbow flexion is considered positive.

Modifications to these tests allow the clinician to test some of the other peripheral nerves.

Musculocutaneous Nerve The patient is supine, head unsupported. The clinician, facing the patient's feet, supports the patient's arm in about 80 degrees of elbow flexion. The shoulder is in external rotation and about 10 degrees of abduction. Shoulder depression is then applied, followed by glenohumeral extension (the "sensitizer"), elbow extension, and wrist ulnar deviation.

Axillary Nerve Patient is supine, head unsupported. The clinician places a hand on top of the patient's shoulder and depresses that shoulder. The glenohumeral joint is then externally rotated, and the patient side-flexes the head away from the tested side. The shoulder is then abducted to about 40 degrees.

Suprascapular Nerve The patient is supine, head unsupported. The clinician places a hand on top of the patient's shoulder. The patient's arm is then placed into internal rotation and shoulder girdle protraction. Then the arm is moved into horizontal adduction, and the patient side-flexes the head away from the tested side. The clinician now depresses that shoulder.

Sensory (Afferent System) The clinician instructs the patient to say "yes" each time he or she feels something touching the skin. The clinician notes any hypo- or hyperesthesia within the distributions. Light touch of the hair follicles is used throughout the whole dermatome, followed by pin-prick in the area of hypoesthesia. Remember that there is no C1 dermatome! (see Fig. 10–3)

Deep Tendon Reflexes
The following reflexes should be checked for differences between the two sides:

- C4: Levator scapulae
- C4-5: Rhomboids
- C5: Deltoid—the anterior belly on the superior-lateral tip of the shoulder
- C5-6: Brachioradialis
- C5-6: Infraspinatus
- C6: Biceps (Fig. 10–39)
- C6: Wrist extensors
- C7: Triceps (Fig. 10–40)
- C7: Wrist flexors
- C8: Extensor pollices longus and abductor pollices
- T1: Thenar muscles
- T1: Pisiform pressure—the clinician pushes the patient's pisiform bone distally, producing a reflex contraction of the hypothenar muscles

Spinal Cord Reflexes
- Hoffman's sign. This sign is the upper limb equivalent of the Babinski sign. The clinician holds the patient's middle finger and briskly flicks the distal phalanx, thereby applying a noxious stimuli to the nail bed of

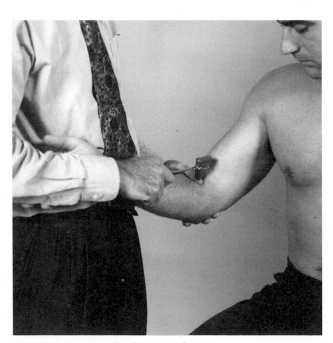

FIGURE 10–39 The biceps reflex.

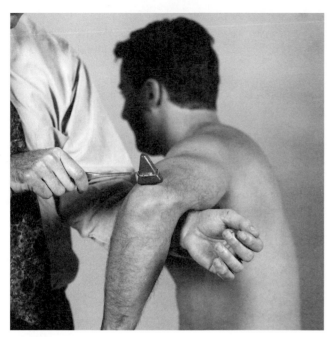

FIGURE 10–40   The triceps reflex.

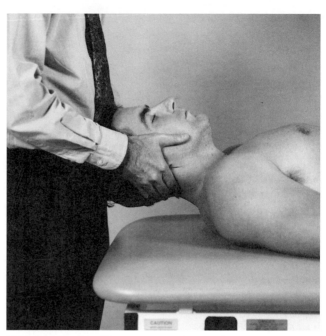

FIGURE 10–41   The transverse ligament stress test.

the middle finger. Denno and Meadows[117] devised a dynamic version of the Hoffman sign, which involves the patient performing repeated flexion and extension of the head before being tested for the Hoffman sign, as previously described.

- Clonus at the wrist (extension) or elbow (pronation/ supination)
- Lower limb tendon reflexes

PATIENT SUPINE AND PRONE

Craniovertebral Ligamentous Stress Tests

Transverse Ligament   This ligament is tested by positioning the patient supine. The clinician locates the anterior arches of C2 by following around the vertebra from the back to the front using the thumbs. The patient is instructed to keep the eyes open. Using the fingers of both hands, the clinician cups the patient's occiput and the C1 segment, and the patient's head is lifted, keeping the head parallel to the ceiling but in slight flexion (Fig. 10–41). The position is held for approximately 15 seconds, and the patient is asked to count backward aloud.

Alar Ligament   A laxity of this ligament is not life threatening, but it can produce symptoms such as headaches. The patient is seated or supine. The patient's neck is placed in slight flexion, and the C2 segment is stabilized with a lumbrical grip by pushing down on its posterior neural arch

with the thumb on the side opposite to the side-flexion (to block the rotation) and the index finger placed over the other posterior neural arch of C2 (to block the side bend of C2). The patient's head is then side-flexed with the neck in flexion (chin tuck), neutral (the ligament will be fairly lax in this position), (Fig. 10–42) and then extension. The end feel is assessed for laxity in all three positions.

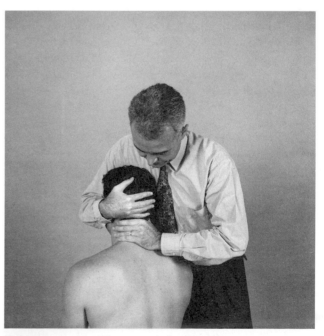

FIGURE 10–42   The seated alar ligament stress test.

Vertebrobasilar Artery

A full description of the tests for the vertebral artery can be found in Chapter 5.

Palpation

The patient should be supine to allow for maximum relaxation of the neck muscles. During palpation of this region, the clinician should note any tenderness, trigger points, muscle spasm, hypertonicity, skin texture changes, and reactivity.

Posterior-Anterior Pressures

Posterior-anterior pressures over the vertebra via pressure on the spinous processes of the cervical vertebrae are a form of stress test, although not very specific. The clinician uses these pressures to test for pain or reactivity of the segment.

Special Tests

The following test may be performed, if indicated:

- Cranial nerve tests
- Specific long tract tests

Suggested Sequence of the Thoracic Scan

Owing to the proximity of the viscera, particularly the heart, serious disease must always be a major consideration in this region. In addition, the pleura, because it is attached to both the ribs and the lungs, reproduces pain when it is stretched, both by breathing as well as by trunk movements, a situation that could lead the clinician to believe that the problem is musculoskeletal. Because of the proximity and vulnerability of the spinal cord in this region, long tract signs (Babinski, clonus, DTR) should be routinely assessed.

The vascularization of the vertebrae in the mid- to lower thoracic spine, is generally through a watershed effect rather than by direct segmental arteries.[1] This leaves the region susceptible to a metastatic invasion.

The thoracolumbar outflow of the autonomic nervous system has its location here and can lead to the presence of facilitated segments, as well as to trophic changes in the skin of the periphery.

Cautions

- Elderly patients with no causal factor
- All bladder diseases
- Cardiac disease
- Osteoporosis
- Juvenile osteochondrosis (Scheuermann's disease) and subsequent Schmorl's nodes
- Night pain, although the pain may just be because the patient has an increased, and fixed, kyphosis and needs a softer bed to accommodate the deformity

History

In the thoracic spine, protection and function of the thoracic viscera take precedence over intersegmental spinal mobility. The thoracic spine is also the area of the spine that is very prone to postural impairments.

In the thoracic region, with the diagnosis of a musculoskeletal disorder, it is important to:

A. Look for muscular and neurologic signs. Thoracic disc herniation does not have a characteristic clinical presentation, and its symptomatology may be confused with other diagnoses. In a review of the literature covering 280 cases of thoracic disk herniation,[118] 23% had sensory symptoms, most commonly numbness, paresthesias, or dysesthesias. (See Chapter 7)

B. Ensure that no visceral signs are present. Serious signs to look for include:
   1. Disturbed coordination accompanied by a spastic gait (UMN impairments to the cord can only occur above L2)
   2. Increased muscle tone, with the affected muscles not limited to one myotome
   3. Hyperreflexia of the patella or Achilles DTRs
   4. Babinski, Oppenheim, and clonus signs present
   5. Lhermitte's symptom. The impairment is usually considered to be in the cervical spinal cord and is associated with demyelination, prolapsed cervical disc, neck trauma, or subacute combined degeneration of the cord. It is rarely a presenting symptom of thoracic cord disease such as compression by metastatic malignant deposits,[119] impairments of the thoracic vertebrae,[120] and thoracic spinal tumor.[121] Because the thoracic cord is immobilized by the denticulate ligaments, flexion produces only limited stretching of the cord, and thus less excursion. This presumably explains why symptoms attributable to flexion are rare in thoracic cord disease.
   6. Occasionally, Brown-Séquard's syndrome is found. It is characterized by ipsilateral flaccid segmental palsy, ipsilateral spastic palsy below the impairment, and ipsilateral anesthesia and loss of proprioception, and loss of appreciation of the vibration of a tuning fork (dysesthesia). Contralateral discrimination of pain sensation and thermoanesthesia may be present and are both noted below the impairment.

If a neurologic impairment is suspected, the clinician must first exclude a neoplastic process, infectious process, or fracture, and then consider a disc protrusion. A nondiscal disorder of the thoracic spine could include a neurofibroma. Some of the signs to help confirm its presence are:

- The patient reports preferring to sleep sitting up.
- The pain, which slowly increases over a period of months, is felt mainly at night and is uninfluenced by activities.
- The patient reports a band-shaped area of numbness that is related to one dermatome.
- The patient reports the presence of a pins-and-needles sensation in one or both feet, or reports any other sign of cord compression.

Disc herniations in this region are considered a rarity[122] and unless they compress the spinal cord, they are difficult to diagnose (refer to Chapter 7). The following landmarks may be helpful to determine which root is impinged.

- If pain is felt around the nipple, the T5 nerve root is likely to be at fault.
- Because the epigastrium belongs to the T7 and T8 segments, pain here arises from the structure of the same origin.

A disc herniation in the thoracic spine can have the following presentation:

- Severe pain, which may be posterior, anterior, or radicular (bilateral or unilateral) and can be so severe that many of these patients are admitted to hospital with a suspected cardiac infarct.
- All movements are severely limited and extremely painful and may or may not reproduce radicular pain.
- Owing to the small caliber of the spinal canal, these impairments often compress the spinal cord.

Tumors of T12 to L2 (typically multiple myeloma) may compress the conus medullaris containing the S3 to S5 nerve roots. This may lead to an impairment of the urinary or anal sphincter, which is sometimes associated with saddle anesthesia. One of the early signs of cauda equina compromise is the inability to urinate while sitting down due to the increased levels of pressure. Any space-occupying lesion, benign or otherwise, provides a threat to the spinal cord. Because of its location, pain in the thoracic region can be referred from just about all of the viscera. Severe chest pain of an abrupt onset should arouse suspicion of:

- Dissecting aneurysm
- Pneumothorax
- Myocardial infarction
- Pulmonary embolism

- Rupture of the esophagus
- Acute thoracic disc protrusion

The thoracic spine is also capable of referring symptoms to distal regions (groin, pubis, and lower abdominal wall).

Signs of ankylosing spondylitis are common in the thoracic region. They include involvement of the anterior longitudinal ligament and ossification of the disc, the thoracic zygapophysial joints, the costovertebral joints, and the manubrial sternal joint, (which is affected in 50% of all cases), producing painful forced inspiration and making chest expansion measurements a requirement in this region. This systemic disease usually affects the sacroiliac joint initially and then appears in the thoracolumbar area. Backache in ankylosing spondylitis is typically intermittent and is not related to exertion or rest. However, the pain and stiffness are greatest in the morning and usually improve with movement. Inspection usually shows a flat lumbar spine, and a gross limitation of side-flexion in both directions is demonstrated.

A similar metabolic disease is diffuse idiopathic skeletal hyperostosis (DISH), in which too much bone is present, giving a "dripped cement/icing" appearance on imaging. In addition, the anterior and posterior longitudinal ligaments become ossified. Other diseases that can affect the thoracic spine include tuberculosis, Paget's disease, pyogenic spondylitis, vertebral melanomas, and ochronosis, a condition thought to result from alkaptonuria and oxidized homogentisic acid, which results in dark pigmentations on the vertebral bodies, cartilage, muscle, and bones as well as the skin of the face and hands. The patient may also experience dark-colored urine.

As mentioned earlier, special attention has to be paid to signs and symptoms of osteoporosis and spinal cord compression in this region. Because of the proximity of the visceral organs, it is important that the clinician determine whether or not the pain the patient is experiencing is musculoskeletal in nature, and be able to rule out visceral causes for the pain (Table 10–2).

PATIENT SITTING

Observation

The patient should be suitably disrobed to expose as much of this region as is necessary. As a quick orientation to the relationship of the bony structures, the clinician should confirm the following:

- The spine of the scapula is level with the spinous process of T3.

TABLE 10–2 SYMPTOMS AND POSSIBLE CONDITIONS ASSOCIATED WITH PAIN IN THE THORACIC REGION[1]

INDICATION	POSSIBLE CONDITION
Severe bilateral root pain in the elderly	Neoplasm (most common areas for metastasis are the lung, breast, prostate, and kidney)
Wedging/compression fracture	Osteoporotic (estrogen deficiency) or neoplastic fracture
Onset-offset of pain unrelated to trunk movements	Ankylosing spondylitis, visceral
Decreased active motion, contralateral side-flexion painful, with both rotations full	Neoplasm
Severe chest wall pain without articular pain	Visceral
Spinal cord signs and symptoms	Cord pressure or ischemia
Pain onset related to eating or diet	Visceral

- The inferior angle of the scapula is in line with the T7-9 spinous processes.
- The medial border of the scapula is parallel with the spinal column and about 5 cm lateral to the spinous processes.

Scoliosis is easy to see in this region, the rib hump occurring on the convex side of the curve. The curve patterns are named according to the level of the apex of the curve. For example, a right thoracic curve has a convexity toward the right, and the apex of the curve is in the thoracic spine. There may be a number of curves spanning the thoracic and lumbar region, and the clinician needs to determine if the scoliosis is:

- Contributing to the patient's pain. Frequently, these curves can be asymptomatic.
- Nonstructural, in which case the patient is able to correct the curves relatively easily, or structural, which may be genetic, congenital, or idiopathic, producing a structural change to the bone and a loss of spinal flexibility. With a structural scoliosis, the vertebral bodies rotate toward the convexity of the curve, producing a distortion.[123] The distortion in the thoracic spine is called a *rib hump*. The rotation of the vertebral bodies causes the spinous processes to deviate toward the concave side.
- The result of poor posture, a nerve root irritation, a leg length discrepancy, atrophy, or a hip contracture.

Varying degrees of kyphosis occur in the thoracic spine. A slight kyphosis is normal. There are, however, a number of kyphotic deformities[124]:

- *Dowager's hump:* a result of postmenopausal osteoporosis, producing anterior wedge fractures in several vertebra of the middle to upper thoracic spine
- *Hump back:* a localized, sharp, posterior angulation called gibbus produced by an anterior wedging of one of two thoracic vertebra caused by a fracture, tumor, or bone disease
- *Round back:* a decreased pelvic inclination (20 degrees) with an excessive kyphosis
- *Flat back:* A decreased pelvic inclination (20 degrees) with a kyphosis and mobile thoracic spine

The clinician should observe the ribs during quiet breathing. Respiratory excursion is measured under the axilla, at the level of the nipple line, and at the 10th rib level. A decreased expansion could be the result of a diaphragm palsy (C4), intercostal weakness, pulmonary (pleura) problems, old age, a rib fracture, a chronic lung condition, or ankylosing spondylitis.

The skin should be examined for scars, suggesting surgery or trauma, and for skin eruptions that might suggest herpes zoster. While examining the skin, the clinician should observe for any discrete muscle atrophy or hypertrophy:

- Rotatores atrophy could suggest a nerve palsy.
- Rotatores hypertonicity could suggest a segmental facilitation.

Lastly, the clinician should look for evidence of deformity.

- *Barrel chest:* a forward- and upward-projecting sternum that increases the anterior-posterior diameter
- *Pigeon chest:* a forward- and downward-projecting sternum that increases the anterior-posterior diameter
- *Funnel chest:* a posterior-projecting sternum secondary to an outgrowth of the ribs[125]

Active Range of Motion

The capsular pattern of the spine appears to be symmetric limitation of rotation and side-flexion, extension loss, and least loss of flexion. This is the case if the clinician is dealing with a symmetric impairment. With an asymmetric impairment, such as trauma, the capsular pattern appears to be an asymmetric limitation of rotation and side-flexion, extension loss, and a lesser loss of flexion.

The patient is seated with the arms crossed. Care must be taken to ensure that the motion occurs in the thoracic spine and not in the lumbar, cervical, or hip joints. It is also important to ensure that all parts of the thoracic spine are

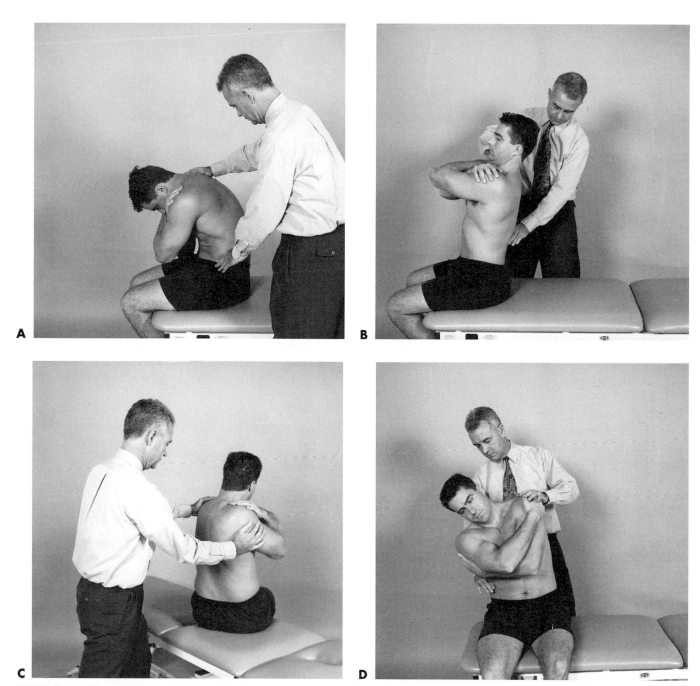

FIGURE 10–43 A–D. Active ROM of the thoracic spine, guided by the clinician.

involved in the ROM testing. Active, passive, and resisted flexion, extension, rotation, and side-flexion are performed (Fig. 10–43). The clinician should look for noncapsular patterns of restriction, pain, or painful weakness (possible fracture or neoplasm). As with the other scans, the clinician is not overly concerned with the actual ranges, but with the quality and the signs and symptoms reproduced. End feels should be noted.

- If the normal elastic end feel of thoracic rotation is replaced by a stiffer one, it may indicate the presence of osteoporosis or ankylosing spondylitis.
- During forward flexion, the nonstructural scoliosis disappears, the structural scoliosis does not.
- If side-flexion is more seriously affected than rotation, neoplastic disease of the viscera or chest wall may be present.[1]

- If, during side-flexion, the ipsilateral paraspinal muscles demonstrate a contracture (Forestier's bowstring sign), ankylosing spondylitis may be present.[116]
- Side-flexion away from the painful side, which is the only painful and limited movement, always indicates a severe extra-articular impairment, such as a pulmonary or abdominal tumor or a spinal neurofibroma. The functional examination normally confirms the patient history.
- A marked restriction of motion in a noncapsular pattern with one or more spasm end feels could indicate a thoracic disc herniation.
- Anterior or lateral pain with resisted thoracic rotation could indicate a muscle tear. Localized pain with resisted testing could indicate a rib fracture.

Costovertebral Expansion

The extremes of respiration should be assessed for their ability to produce pain. Breathing in extends the spine, and breathing out flexes it. Therefore, as part of the examination, breathing should be combined with flexion and extension to help rule out rib involvement. For example, if the patient is in a position of thoracic flexion and breathing in reproduces the pain, there is likely to be a rib impairment.

Neurologic Tests[1]

A neurologic deficit is very difficult to detect in the thoracic spine. Sensation should be tested over the abdomen; the area just below the xiphoid process is innervated by T8, the umbilicus by T10, and the lower abdominal region, level with the anterior superior iliac spines, by T12. Too much overlap exists above T8 to make sensation testing reliable (see Fig. 10–3).

Strength testing is similarly difficult. The resisted isometric tests in this region are merely gross tests and are more likely to detect muscle strains.

A number of tests have been devised to help assess the integrity of the neurologic system. They include:

- *Beevor's sign (T7-12).* The patient lies supine, with the knees bent, feet flat on the bed. The patient is asked to raise the head against resistance, coughs or attempts to sit up with the hands resting behind the head[126] (Fig. 10–44). The clinician observes the umbilicus for motion. It should remain in a straight line. If it deviates diagonally, this suggests a weakness in the diagonally opposite set of three abdominal muscles. If it moves distally, weak upper abdominals are suggested, whereas if it moves proximally, this suggests weak lower abdominals. For example, if the umbilicus moves upward and to the right, the muscles in the lower left quadrant must be weak. The weakness may be caused by a spinal nerve root palsy, in this case the 10th, 11th, and 12th thoracic nerves on the left.[127]

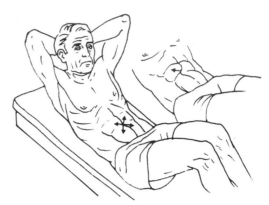

FIGURE 10–44 Beevor's sign. *(Reproduced, with permission from Haldeman S (editor): Principals and Practice of Chiropractic, 2e. Appleton & Lange, 1992)*

- *Slump test.* This is described at length earlier in the chapter in the discussion of the lumbar scan.
- *First thoracic nerve root stretch.* The patient is asked to abduct the arms to 90 degrees and to flex the pronated forearms to 90 degrees. This position should not provoke any symptoms. From this position, the patient fully flexes the elbows and places the hands behind the neck (Fig. 10–45). This maneuver stretches the ulnar nerve and T1 nerve root, and pain into the scapular area produced by this maneuver is indicative of a T1 nerve root irritation.
- *Abdominal cutaneous reflex.* Deep stroking over the abdominal muscles using the handle of a reflex hammer

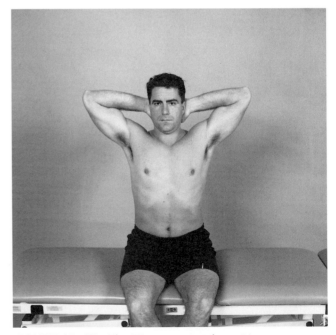

FIGURE 10–45 The T1 nerve stretch position.

tests the abdominal cutaneous reflex. Each quadrant is tested by etching diagonal lines around the patient's umbilicus. The clinician observes for symmetry of skin rippling or umbilicus displacement.

- *Spinal cord reflexes.* These must be tested on all patients with thoracic pain and include lower extremity DTRs, Babinski, and Oppenheim's clonus.

Stress Tests

These are a useful adjunct to the scan. Although they are also performed as part of the biomechanical examination of the thorax, positive findings with these tests can indicate serious conditions.

Axial   Axial compression is induced by the clinician leaning on the patient's shoulders for the upper half of the thoracic spine and via the lumbar spine for the lower half. Reproduction of the symptoms is considered a positive test and may be indicative of a vertical instability; that is, end plate fracture, discal problems, or acute centrum fracture. In the acutely painful patient, a positive test may result from apophyseal joint inflammation.

Traction   Traction for the upper half of the spine is through the shoulder girdle (see Fig. 16–14) and via lumbar traction for the lower half. If the test reproduces the patient's symptoms, an injury of the longitudinal ligaments may be present or, again, in the acutely painful patient, inflammation of the zygapophysial joint.

Anterior-Posterior   The patient is seated with the arms held in front and the elbows flexed while the clinician stands in front of the patient. The clinician reaches around the patient with both arms and stabilizes the transverse processes of the lower vertebra of the segment to be tested. The patient places the pronated forearms on the clinician's chest and then applies light pressure against the clinician's shoulders with his or her forearm, while the clinician palpates for any posterior motion of the caudal vertebra of the segment (Fig. 10–46). If the test reproduces the patient's symptoms, it may be indicative of an anterior or posterior instability, a disc herniation or, again, in the acutely painful patient, inflammation of the apophyseal joint.

CONCLUSION

At the end of the scanning examination, either a medical diagnosis can be made (e.g., disc impairment [protrusion, prolapse, or extrusion], acute arthritis, specific tendonitis or muscle belly tear, spondylolisthesis, or stenosis) or the examination is considered negative. Usually, the scanning examination proves to be negative. A negative scanning

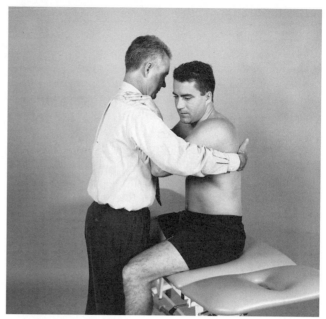

FIGURE 10–46   Posterior stress test of the thoracic and lumbar spine.

examination does not imply that there were no findings but, rather, that the results of examination were insufficient to generate a diagnosis upon which an intervention could be based. In this case, further examination is required. The inability to treat following the scanning examination requires that a biomechanical examination be carried out before any intervention is initiated.

If a diagnosis is rendered from the scan, and there are no serious signs and symptoms, an intervention can be initiated using the guidelines in Table 10–3.

TABLE 10–3   CONDITIONS AND INTERVENTION PROTOCOLS

CONDITIONS	FINDINGS	PROTOCOL
Disc protrusion, prolapse, and extrusion	Severe pain All movements reduced	Gentle manual traction in progressive extension
Anterior-posterior instability	Flexion and extension reduction greater than rotation	Traction or traction manipulation in extension
Arthritis	Hot capsular pattern	PRICE (protection, rest, ice, compression, and elevation)
Subluxation	One direction is restricted	Flexion or extension
Arthrosis	All directions restricted	Flexion or extension

Masqueraders

It was Grieve[128] who coined the term *Masqueraders* to indicate conditions that may not be musculoskeletal in origin, and that may require skilled intervention elsewhere.

Generally speaking, symptoms from a musculoskeletal condition are provoked by certain postures, movements, or activities, and relieved by others. However, this is a generalization and must be viewed as such. We can all recall patients whose symptoms mimicked a musculoskeletal impairment, but who were later diagnosed with a life-threatening condition. It is important that the reader refers to Chapter 9, on the subjective examination, as well as to Chapter 8, on differential diagnosis.

The findings in Table 10–4 should always alert the clinician to a more sinister pathology.

The following case studies serve to highlight some of the conditions that mimic musculoskeletal impairments. Although there are times when these conditions can be benign, more often than not, they are serious.

Case Study: Back and Leg Pain

Subjective

A 55-year-old patient presented with complaints of an insidious onset of severe back and left leg pain. Progressively worsening symptoms of pain over the last few months were followed by left foot drop. An MRI examination was interpreted as mild lumbar spine degenerative disc disease without evidence of nerve root compromise. The patient could report no specific aggravating or relieving activities, but did report pain at night, not related to movement in bed. The patient's past medical history was significant for a renal transplantation approximately 20 years earlier.

Questions

1. What aspects of the subjective history should alert the clinician to the possibility of a serious pathology?
2. What is the significance of night pain, which is unrelated to movement?
3. Does this presentation and history warrant further investigation? Why or why not?

Examination

The patient appeared to be a well-nourished and healthy-looking individual with no obvious postural deformities. Given the insidious nature of his back pain and the history suggesting a nerve root impairment, a scan was performed with the following results:

- Active lumbar ROM, with passive overpressure and resistance, was full and pain free in all directions, although some trunk pain was elicited with end range

TABLE 10–4 EXAMINATION FINDINGS AND THE POSSIBLE CONDITIONS CAUSING THEM[1]

FINDINGS	POSSIBLE CONDITION
Dizziness	Upper cervical impairment, vertebrobasilar ischemia, craniovertebral ligament tear
Quadrilateral paresthesia	Cord compression, vertebrobasilar ischemia
Bilateral upper limb paresthesia	Cord compression, vertebrobasilar ischemia
Hyperreflexia	Cord compression, vertebrobasilar ischemia
Babinski or clonus sign	Cord compression, vertebrobasilar ischemia
Cardinal signs and symptoms	Cord compression, vertebrobasilar ischemia
Consistent swallow on transverse ligament stress tests	Instability, retropharyngeal hematoma, rheumatoid arthritis
Nontraumatic capsular pattern	Rheumatoid arthritis, ankylosing spondylitis, neoplasm
Arm pain lasting >6–9 months	Neoplasm
Persistent root pain <30 years	Neoplasm
Radicular pain with coughing	Neoplasm
Pain worsening after 1 month	Neoplasm
>1 level involved (cervical region)	Neoplasm
Paralysis	Neoplasm or neurologic disease
Trunk and limb paresthesia	Neoplasm
Bilateral root signs and symptoms	Neoplasm
Nontraumatic strong spasm	Neoplasm
Nontraumatic strong pain in the elderly patient	Neoplasm
Signs worse than symptoms	Neoplasm
Radial deviator weakness	Neoplasm
Thumb flexor weakness	Neoplasm
Hand intrinsic weakness or atrophy, or both	Neoplasm, thoracic outlet syndrome, carpal tunnel syndrome
Horner's syndrome	Superior sulcus tumor, breast cancer, cervical ganglion damage, brain stem damage
Empty end feel	Neoplasm
Severe post-traumatic capsular pattern	Fracture
Severe post-traumatic spasm	Fracture
Loss of ROM post-trauma	Fracture
Post-traumatic painful weakness	Fracture

extension. No other positions or activities appeared to change the pain.
- Fatigable muscle weakness, graded at 4/5, was found in the L5-S1 distribution.
- The Achilles tendon reflex on the left was diminished.

Questions
1. Did the scanning examination confirm your working hypothesis? How?
2. What is the significance of the fatigable weakness?
3. What is the significance of having pain that is not reproducible with activities or positions?

The distribution of the patient's symptoms appeared to fit that of a disc herniation at L5-S1, but the clinician returned the patient to his physician for further testing because:

● The clinician was unable to reproduce the pain with movement.

● There were subjective reports of night pain, unrelated to movement

● There were no relieving or aggravating positions or activities.

The results of the physical therapy examination prompted the physician to order a second MRI examination of the lumbosacral spine, and an electromyogram (EMG) study. The MRI uncovered an aneurysm extending posterior-medially, and adjacent to the left lumbosacral nerve plexus. Arteriography verified the aneurysm's origin from the left internal iliac artery. After prompt excision of the aneurysm, the patient reported significant reduction of back and limb pain in the immediate postoperative period. The EMG studies clearly showed severe ongoing denervation changes in distal and proximal limb muscles supplied by L5-S1 root levels on the left side but no significant denervation changes were observed in lumbosacral paraspinal muscles that are typically affected in radiculopathies.[129]

Evaluation[130]
In addition to demonstrating how a visceral source of pain can mimic a musculoskeletal impairment, this case illustrates two other points.

1. The importance of the subjective history.
2. The use of imaging studies to confirm the clinical findings. The initial MRI showed no significant evidence for nerve root compromise in the lumbosacral spine, and yet the subjective history indicated the possibility of nerve root irritation. However, it is not unusual for MRI results to give both false positives or false negatives while clinical findings are more reliable.

Although this patient's symptoms resembled a radiculopathy, and the strength testing did little to refute the hypothesis, there was nothing in the motion tests to confirm the diagnosis. The EMG results clearly indicated that the lumbosacral plexus was the location of the neuropathic process. Because paraspinal muscles are innervated by dorsal rami of spinal nerves that branch immediately after exiting the vertebral foramina, they are subject to active denervation changes in radiculopathies caused by disc or bone disease. Sural sensory nerve action potentials are usually absent in lumbosacral plexopathies (postganglionic impairment), but should not be affected in radiculopathies.[131] In this case, bilateral absence of sural sensory nerve action potentials may be also attributed to polyneuropathy secondary to chronic uremia.

Visceral lumbosacral radiculopathy, although uncommon, is reported to develop secondary to abdominal aortic aneurysms, retroperitoneal abscesses, neoplasms, and hemorrhages.[130,132,133] The importance of recognizing the development of post-transplant pseudoaneurysms cannot be overstated because they are prone to acute rupture, resulting in significant hemorrhage,[134] and they are considered surgical emergencies. A careful EMG analysis in this case was the key to determining that the patient's symptoms were caused by a process affecting the lumbosacral plexus. Electrodiagnostic studies are invaluable tools in localizing processes causing pain and limb weakness and they often help procure an accurate diagnosis.

Case Study: Right Buttock Pain[135]

Subjective
A 55-year-old woman presented for physical therapy with a physician diagnosis of "right lumbosacral radiculitis." The patient had a 10-month history of right buttock pain with radiation to her posterior-lateral right lower limb, which was associated with intermittent numbness and tingling of her distal lower limb and foot. She denied any low back pain and denied any radiation of pain down her left lower limb. Her pain was exacerbated by walking uphill, by lying on her right side, and after exercise. Her pain was not worse with bending or with Valsalva maneuver. Past medical history was significant for chronic low back pain, lymphoma (diagnosed when aged 23 and treated successfully with local radiation to the neck and axillae), status post-meningioma resection, status postbilateral-modified radical mastectomy for carcinoma in-situ, and hypothyroidism. An MRI of the lumbosacral spine revealed multi-level degenerative disc disease from L3-4 through L5-S1, with mild foraminal narrowing bilaterally. There was no evidence of focal herniation or canal stenosis.

Questions
1. What structure(s) could be the cause of these symptoms?
2. Does the history of the symptoms follow a pattern associated with a musculoskeletal disorder? If not, why not?

3. What in the patient's past medical history needs to be noted?
4. What questions would you ask to help rule out a cauda equina impairment?
5. What impairment could cause an increase in these symptoms with walking uphill and lying on the right side?
6. Why would the patient's symptoms increase after exercise?
7. What is your working hypothesis at this stage based on the various diagnoses that could present with leg pain and paresthesia, and the tests you would use to rule out each one.
8. Does this presentation and history warrant a scan? Why or why not?

Examination

This type of history warrants a scan. A lumbar scan examination produced the following results:

● A negative SLR test on the left; but a positive SLR on the right side at approximately 45 degrees, which reproduced right buttock and posterior thigh pain
● Motor and sensory examinations otherwise intact in bilateral lower limbs
● No spinal or paraspinal tenderness or spasm on palpation
● Moderate spasm and tenderness of the right piriformis and gluteus medius muscles, and marked tenderness over the right sciatic notch
● Active ROM of the lumbar spine was full and pain-free in all directions
● Active and passive ROM of the patient's hips were somewhat decreased in internal and external rotation as well as abduction bilaterally

Questions
1. Did the scanning examination confirm your working hypothesis? How?
2. List the examination findings that surprised you, given the subjective history.
3. What do you do now?

The scan findings were inconclusive for a right lumbosacral radiculitis, so a biomechanical examination was performed. The biomechanical examination failed to reproduce the patient's pain and symptoms. After a discussion with the patient's physician, a trial of physical therapy was ordered for symptomatic pain relief. The patient underwent a physical therapy program, which consisted of modalities to her right piriformis and gluteal muscles, stretching exercises, hip ROM exercises, instruction in proper posture and body mechanics, and generalized conditioning exercises. Her symptoms improved somewhat

initially, but then returned to the previous level, and the patient was returned to her physician.

Questions
1. What are some of the problems associated with proceeding to treat this patient?
2. How would you describe this condition to the patient?
3. Based on the findings thus far, and the rationale to provide pain relief, is there anything else you would add to the patient's intervention?
4. Estimate this patient's prognosis.
5. What modalities could you use in the intervention of this patient?
6. Given the lack of progress from the patient, how long would you wait before returning her to the physician?

Evaluation   Because of persistent pain, an MRI of the pelvis was obtained. The MRI examination of the pelvis revealed a markedly enlarged uterus with multiple small myomata within the entire uterus. There was a large pedunculated myoma measuring 6 cm in maximal cross-sectional diameter, which was impinging on the right sciatic foramen at the level of exit of the right sciatic nerve. No other pelvic abnormalities were noted.

The impression at that time was right sciatic neuropathy secondary to uterine myoma. Because of her persistent complaints, the patient was referred for a subtotal abdominal hysterectomy, which was performed without complications. At follow-up, approximately 6 months postoperatively, the patient reported a very rare, mild right buttock pain without any lower limb radiation, which was a significant improvement compared with her preoperative pain.

Discussion

The sciatic nerve arises from the L4 through S2 nerve roots, and maintains a short intrapelvic course, before exiting the pelvis through the greater sciatic foramen.[136] Although impairments of the sciatic nerve outside the pelvis have been well described, impairments within the pelvis are far less common. Intrapelvic endometriosis has been reported to cause cyclic sciatic nerve pain.[137] Intrapelvic tumors such as lipomas have also been reported to result in sciatica.[138] A case of idiopathic internal iliac artery aneurysm has been reported, causing sciatic nerve involvement.[139]

Uterine fibroids, also known as leiomyomas, fibromyomas, fibromas, and myomas, are well circumscribed but nonencapsulated benign uterine tumors. These are mainly composed of smooth muscle but have some fibrous connective tissue components.

Although the exact incidence of fibroids is unknown, they are the most common form of pelvic tumors, and estimations indicate that as many as 25% of women over the age of 35 has a uterine fibroid.

A history of sciatica that is worse with certain positions, is not worse with Valsalva, and is not associated with low back pain, should prompt clinicians to consider a uterine fibroid as a potential cause, especially in women with a history of uterine fibroids. Likewise, failure to respond to an intervention for the more common causes of sciatica, such as herniated intervertebral disc, should initiate a return to the physician for further workup, which may include pelvic ultrasound, computed axial tomography, or MRI.

Case Study: Bilateral Arm and Wrist Weakness[140]

Subjective

A 36-year-old man who sustained a left tibial plateau fracture presented at the clinic with complaints of bilateral arm and wrist weakness, which had progressively worsened over the last month since his discharge from hospital. The patient was ambulating with crutches and non–weight-bearing on the left side. There was no history of cervical trauma. The patient reported no pain in his upper extremities but had noticed a mild and vague numbness in his hands. There had been no preceding viral infection and no proximal migration of the weakness, nor did he have any other areas of weakness. The patient complained of pain in his axillae and commented that his crutches had been rubbing against his axillae.

Questions

1. What structure(s) could be at fault when weakness is the major complaint?
2. Why was the history of no cervical trauma pertinent?
3. Why was the statement about preceding viral infection pertinent?
4. Why was the statement about the proximal migration of the weakness pertinent?
5. What is your working hypothesis at this stage? List the various diagnoses that could present with bilateral arm numbness and the tests you would use to rule out each one.
6. Does this presentation and history warrant a scan? Why or why not?

Examination

Because of the insidious nature of the patient's symptoms and the fact that the symptoms were in a distribution that could indicate a serious condition or neurologic involvement, a scan was performed with the following findings:

- Examination of the upper extremities found the deltoid strength to be 4/5 and the biceps 5/5.
- All radial nerve–innervated muscles from the triceps distally were 1/5 in strength.
- The wrist and finger flexors were rated at 3+/5, and the intrinsic muscles of the hand were 3−/5.
- The patient's reflexes showed absence of the triceps jerk, with preservation of the biceps jerks, which were 2+. The brachioradialis reflexes were intact up to the biceps reflex.
- There was diminished pin-prick and temperature perception in the hands. These findings were present on both sides.
- The patient's axillae showed marked redness, suggestive of chronic irritation and rubbing.
- Cranial nerve function was found to be normal, as was the cervical spine.
- The lower limbs had normal strength, sensation, and reflexes.
- The patient's axillary crutches were found to be too long, with the axillary bar sitting just under the axillary fold when the patient stood erect. The patient's crutch walking technique was assessed and found to be very poor, with the patient putting all his weight on the axillary bars.

Questions

1. Did the scan confirm the working hypothesis? How?
2. List the muscles that could be used to assess the radial nerve.
3. What are the characteristics about a weakness produced by a nerve palsy?
4. Given the findings from the scan, what is the diagnosis, or is further testing warranted in the form of a biomechanical examination? What information would be gained with further testing?

Evaluation/Intervention

A diagnosis of crutch palsy was suspected based on the history and the findings from the scanning examination. The axillary crutches were initially discontinued, and a forearm-bearing walker was substituted. The patient was asked to return in 6 weeks, but to call if the symptoms did not start to improve after 2 weeks. Six weeks later the patient's sensory function was resolved. Examination found normal sensation in all distributions, to all assessment methods, including pin-prick and temperature perception. Examination of muscle function showed full strength in all muscles innervated by the median, ulnar, musculocutaneous, and axillary nerves.

Question

1. Why was the patient not treated on a regular basis in the clinic?

Discussion[140]

Brachial plexus compressive neuropathy following the use of axillary crutches is rare, but well-recognized. There are a number of documented reports in the medical literature[141,142] of compressive neuropathies stemming from the incorrect use of axillary crutches, the so-called crutch palsy. The diagnosis of a crutch palsy is usually made clinically by taking a careful history and performing a physical examination, including watching the patient ambulate using crutches, as well as looking at the axillae for such signs of chronic irritation as hyperpigmentation and skin hypertrophy. A detailed neurologic examination is usually sufficient to determine the cord or terminal branch(es) involved and the level of the involvement.[143]

The incorrect use of axillary crutches, with excessive weight bearing on the axillary bar leads to a sevenfold increase in force on the axilla.[144] Ensuring that correct crutch-walking technique is taught to the patient, and that the crutches are measured correctly, is the best course of action. There are many techniques for determining the correct crutch length for axillary crutches. Bauer and colleagues[145] found that the best calculation of ideal crutch length was either 77% of the patient's height, or the height minus 16 inches (40.6 cm).

Case Study: Intermittent Leg Numbness

Subjective

A 46-year-old man presented to the clinic with a history of sensations that he described as a mixture both of pins and needles and of cotton wool around the second and third toes of his feet. The symptoms developed suddenly while at work and had progressed to intermittent numbness of both legs from the waist down since his last physician visit. The initial sensation settled, but over the following 10 years he suffered momentarily from electric-shock–type sensations radiating down into his legs, more so on the right than the left. In addition, he noticed stiffness in his gait and reduced sensation on passing urine, and an aching sensation had developed in the buttocks. He had a history of infrequent low back pain over a number of years. The patient's physician had given the patient a workup for multiple sclerosis, but the results were negative.

Questions
1. What aspects of the subjective history should alert the clinician to the possibility of a serious pathology?
2. What is the significance of the gait stiffness?
3. What is the significance of the reduced sensation on passing urine?
4. Does this presentation and history warrant a scan? Why or why not?

Examination
Given the history and symptoms of this patient, a thoracic and lumbar scan was performed with the following findings:

- A broad-based gait pattern
- Weakness of hip flexion on the right
- Brisk knee and ankle jerks with clonus on the right
- Positive Lhermitte's sign
- Normal sensory examination, although it appeared that vibration sensation was absent in the left leg
- Absent abdominal reflexes
- Nystagmus on lateral gaze

Questions
1. Did the scanning examination confirm your working hypothesis?
2. List the findings that could indicate the presence of a serious pathology.
3. What is the significance of the Lhermitte's sign?
4. What do you do now?

Evaluation
All of the signs and symptoms of this patient indicate UMN impairment. He was referred back to his physician, at which time an MRI of the thoracic spine showed a thoracic disc prolapse at T9-10 with an osteophyte impinging the theca and just indenting the cord. A computed tomography myelogram showed a large calcified disk prolapse at T9-10 with calcification in the remaining disk space and considerable compression of the spinal cord from right to left.

REVIEW QUESTIONS

1. Give five examples of noncontractile tissue.
2. Give five examples of contractile tissue.
3. If, when assessing the range of motion of a joint, both the active and passive ROM are limited or painful in the same direction, would this implicate a contractile or noncontractile tissue?
4. The finding of a weak and painful response during strength testing of a key muscle would implicate which four diagnoses?
5. List the five signs of Horner's syndrome.
6. Give five anatomic sites where a lesion could cause Horner's syndrome.
7. What are the differences between a drop attack and fainting?
8. Give three possible causes of drop attacks.
9. How would you differentiate the cause if drop attacks were suspected from the medical history?
10. Define dysphagia.
11. List as many serious signs and symptoms as you can remember from your reading of this chapter.
12. Which muscle is involved with ptosis?

13. What are the key muscles for the following nerve roots?
    a. C4
    b. C6
    c. C8
    d. T1
    e. C1-2
14. Resisted hip abduction tests which root level?
15. If, with a positive SLR test, neck flexion eases the symptoms, where is the disc protrusion likely to be in relation to the nerve root—medial or lateral?
16. List the seven signs of the buttock.
17. A patient presents with severe weakness of the deltoid muscle and wrist extensors. Where would the impairment probably be located?
    a. C6 nerve root
    b. C7 nerve root
    c. Middle trunk of brachial plexus
    d. Posterior cord of the brachial plexus
    e. Radial nerve
18. A patient was involved in a motorcycle accident and it is suspected that he may have avulsed his C5 nerve root at its origin. To test this impression, what is the best muscle to check electrophysiologically?
    a. Biceps
    b. Pronator teres
    c. Supraspinatus
    d. Deltoid
    e. Rhomboids
19. A sensory evaluation reveals light touch impairment to the anterior-lateral thigh, lateral calf, and sole of the foot. When recording these findings, the corresponding dermatomes are:
    a. L2, L4, S3
    b. L1, L3, L5
    c. L2, L5, S1
    d. L3, L5, S1
20. The patellar reflex is used to assess which level?
    a. L2-3
    b. S1-2
    c. L2-3-4
    d. L3-4-5
21. The spinal root, C6, can be tested through which reflex?
    a. Levator scapula
    b. Brachioradialis
    c. Triceps
    d. Pectoralis major
22. Manual muscle testing of the finger abductors helps test which spinal level?
    a. T2
    b. C7
    c. T1
    d. C6

23. Which cranial nerve assists with lifting the shoulder?
    a. Glossopharyngeal
    b. Hypoglossal
    c. Vagus
    d. Spinal accessory
24. Which of the following tests for reflex at level C5?
    a. Elbow extension
    b. Triceps
    c. Biceps
    d. Brachioradialis
25. The triceps reflex tests what level?
    a. C5
    b. C6
    c. C7
    d. C8
26. The Achilles tendon reflex is at what level?
    a. L4
    b. L3
    c. S2
    d. S1
27. This syndrome may be seen after a knife type injury to the spinal cord, causing hemisection of the spinal cord?
    a. Marfan's syndrome
    b. Amyotrophic lateral sclerosis
    c. Cerebellar syndrome
    d. Brown-Séquard's syndrome
28. The diaphragm is innervated by what nerve?
    a. Phrenic
    b. Subscapular
    c. C1-2
    d. Accessory
29. A patient has experienced a loss of strength at the L2-3-4 level. What muscle should you test to confirm weakness secondary to L2-3, and L4 injury?
    a. Quadriceps
    b. Extensor hallucis longus
    c. Gluteus medius
    d. Peroneus longus
30. A patient has experienced a loss of strength at the S1 level. What muscle should you test to confirm weakness secondary to S1 injury?
    a. Quadriceps
    b. Peroneus longus
    c. Extensor digitorum longus
    d. Iliopsoas
31. You are performing a respiratory evaluation, including the following tests: respiratory rate, blood pressure, pulse, and measurement of chest expansion. What is a normal measurement of difference between the rest measurement and full expansion over the xiphoid process?
    a. 1/2 inch
    b. 1 inch

    c. 1 1/2 inches

    d. 2 inches

32. Give five possible diagnoses for the finding of a weak and painless response during strength testing of a key muscle.

33. A herniation between the C4 and C5 vertebrae would cause an impingement of which nerve root?

34. A herniation between the T4 and T5 vertebrae would cause an impingement of which nerve root?

35. A herniation between the L4 and L5 vertebrae would cause an impingement of which nerve root?

36. What is the equivalent upper extremity reflex for the lower extremity ankle clonus?

37. Give three reasons for performing a scan.

38. What segmental levels are tested with the DTRs of the medial and lateral hamstrings?

39. What segmental level is tested with the DTRs of the posterior tibialis?

40. What are the two key muscle tests for L5-S1?

41. What is the key muscle test for L3-4?

42. How would you describe the skin of a patient with venous insufficiency?

43. Which of the two, a lateral shift or a deviation, demonstrates a flexion component?

44. Which nerve roots are stressed with an SLR?

45. What is the critical zone in the range for an SLR to suggest a dural impairment?

46. Which root levels are assessed for dural mobility with the prone knee bending test?

47. What is the critical zone in the range for the prone knee bending test to suggest a dural impairment?

48. Describe the area of the body that you would use to test sensation in the following dermatomes:

    a. C1

    b. S1-2

    c. C5

    d. T1

49. When performing an SLR, in which position would you place the foot to stretch the following nerves:

    a. Posterior tibial

    b. Sural

    c. Common peroneal

50. In which direction should the hip be rotated in order to increase tension on the common peroneal nerve during an SLR?

51. Utilizing the information gleaned from the patient history and the dural tension tests, how can the clinician differentiate between a disc protrusion and a dural adhesion?

52. Utilizing the information gleaned from the patient history and the dural tension tests, how can the clinician differentiate between posterior thigh pain from tight hamstrings, and the presence of a dural adhesion?

53. Which components of the neurologic system (peripheral, central, afferent, or efferent) are tested by:

    a. Sustained or repeated isometric contraction

    b. Sensation testing

    c. DTRs

    d. Pathologic reflexes

54. Pin-prick testing within a dermatome is performed to detect what?

55. Light touch testing within a dermatome is performed to detect what?

56. What is the most common cause of a segmental weakness?

57. What is the most common cause of a nonsegmental weakness or virtual paralysis?

58. The finding of a nonfatigable segmental weakness during strength testing could suggest which two causes?

59. DTRs test the muscle spindle reflex, and which components (afferent, efferent, facilitation, inhibition) of the peripheral and central nervous systems?

60. A hyperreflexive DTR has which component associated with the reflex response?

61. What structures are stressed in the SLR?

62. Increased pain with the lumbar torsion test would indicate what types of impairment?

63. Subjective complaints of bilateral sciatica along with a negative SLR test could indicate an impairment to which structure?

64. List three potential causes for a painful weakness of hip flexion?

65. A painless weakness with knee extension strength testing could indicate what diagnosis?

66. With a C6 palsy, which four muscles should the clinician expect to be weak?

67. Apart from the extensibility of the dural sheaths and roots of L2-3, what anatomic structures are tested with the prone knee flexion test?

68. A painful and strong response to resistive testing indicates which diagnoses?

69. With resistive testing, what is the combination of muscle positioning and force that ensures the strongest positive finding?

70. With resistive testing, what is the combination of muscle positioning and force that ensures the least positive finding?

71. Which key muscle is tested for the C8 segmental level?

ANSWERS

1. Possible answers include joint capsule, ligament, bursa, articular surfaces, synovium, bone, cartilage, dura, and fascia.

2. Muscle belly, tendon, tenoperiosteal junction, submuscular/tendinous bursa, bone.

3. Inert (noncontractile).

4. Fracture, metastases, hyperacute arthritis, grade II tear.

5. Ptosis (drooping eyelid), miosis (constriction of the pupil), enophthalmus (recession of the eyeball), facial reddening, anhydrosis (absence of sweating secondary to sympathetic paralysis).

6. Thalamus, reticular formation, descending sympathetic nerve, inferior cervical ganglia, superior cervical ganglia.

7. A drop attack involves a fall without a loss of consciousness, whereas fainting involves a fall with a temporary loss of consciousness.

8. Possible answers include sudden compression of the spinal cord, compromise of the vertebral artery supply, cerebellar disease, vestibular system impairment.

9. Vestibular system tests, vertebral artery tests, transverse ligament test, and coordination tests for cerebellum. Observe for signs of hyperreflexia and pathologic reflexes.

10. Abnormal difficulty with swallowing.

11. Quadrilateral paresthesia, bilateral upper limb paresthesia, hemifacial paresthesia, hemianopia (loss of vision in one-half of the visual field of one or both eyes), diplopia, perioral anesthesia, nystagmus, drop attacks, ataxia, periodic loss of consciousness, dysphasia (lack of coordination in speech and failure to arrange words in an understandable way), hyperreflexia, Babinski response, positive Hoffman or Oppenheimer test, flexor withdrawal.

12. Muller's muscle.

13. a. C4, levator scapula.
b. C6, forearm supinators.
c. C8, ulnar deviators.
d. T1, finger adductors.
e. C1-2, short neck flexors.

14. L5-S1.

15. Medial.

16. a. Limited SLR.
b. Limited hip flexion.
c. Limited trunk flexion.
d. Noncapsular pattern of the hip.
e. Painful and weak hip extension.
f. Gluteal swelling.
g. Empty end feel with hip flexion.

17. d.

18. e.

19. c.

20. c.

21. b.

22. c.

23. d.

24. c.

25. c.

26. d.

27. d.

28. a.

29. a.

30. b.

31. c.

32. Complete rupture of a contractile tissue, a nerve palsy, muscle disuse, muscle inhibition, or muscle facilitation.

33. C5.

34. T4.

35. L4 *and* L5 (because of obliquity of exit). *Note:* L1 and L2 emerge high up in the foramina and therefore escape the protrusion of that level. An L5 protrusion can impinge on L5 and S1 roots.

36. Hoffman.

37. 1. Identify serious pathology
2. Identify patient's neurological status
3. Identify a regional diagnosis

38. Medial—L5; lateral—S1.

39. L4.

40. Foot evertors (peroneals) and knee flexors (hamstrings).

41. Knee extensors (quadriceps).

42. Blue and warm, with pitting edema.

43. Deviation.

44. L4 through S2.

45. 30 to 60 degrees.

46. L2-4.

47. 80 to 100 degrees.

48. a. No dermatome.
b. Heel of the foot.
c. From the shoulder to the wrist on the anterior aspect of the arm and forearm, to the base of the thumb.
d. Medial aspect of the elbow to the wrist.

49. a. Posterior tibial—dorsiflexed and everted.
b. Sural—dorsiflexed and inverted.
c. Common peroneal—Plantar flexed and inverted (with the toes flexed).

50. Internal rotation.

51. A history of trauma and positive dural tension tests would indicate a disc protrusion. A dural adhesion is implicated when a stretch applied simultaneously to both ends of the dura has no effect on the symptoms.

52. The introduction of neck flexion will not affect the length of the hamstrings but will stretch the dura.

53. a. Efferent (myotome/key muscle testing).
b. Afferent.
c. Afferent, efferent, and central nervous system inhibition.
d. Central nervous system inhibition.

54. Hypoesthesia throughout the dermatome.

55. Near-anesthesia in the autonomous area of the dermatome.
56. Nerve root or spinal nerve compression or irritation.
57. Compression or impairment of a peripheral nerve.
58. Incompletely recovered palsy or segmental facilitation.
59. The afferent and efferent components of the peripheral nervous system; the ability of the central nervous system to inhibit the reflex.
60. Clonus (sustainment).
61. Dural sheaths of roots L4-S2, hamstring length, gluteus maximus length, and sacroiliac, lumbar, and hip joints.
62. Arthritis, annular tear (recent), compression fracture of lamina.
63. Cauda equina (compression).
64. Fracture of the lesser trochanter, abdominal neoplasm, metastases at the upper femur.
65. An L3 palsy.
66. Biceps, brachialis, supinator brevis, and extensor carpi radialis.
67. Quadriceps femoris flexibility, anterior capsule of the hip and knee, femoral nerve.
68. Tendonitis, grade I muscle tear, bursitis.
69. Pain produced with minimum force applied to the muscle in its rest position.
70. Pain produced when maximum resistance is applied to a muscle in its stretched position.
71. Extensor pollices longus.

REFERENCES

1. Meadows JTS. *Differential Diagnosis in Orthopedic Physical Therapy: A Case Study Approach.* New York, NY: McGraw-Hill;1999.
2. Cyriax J. *Textbook of Orthopedic Medicine,* vol 1, 8th ed. London, England: Balliere Tindall and Cassell; 1982.
3. Haynes KW. An examination of Cyriax's passive motion tests with patients having osteoarthritis of the knee. Phys Ther 1994;74:697.
4. Franklin ME. Assessment of exercise induced minor lesions: The accuracy of Cyriax's diagnosis by selective tissue tension paradigm. J Orthop Sports Phys Ther 1996;24:122.
5. Barany R. Diagnose von Krankheitserscheinungen im Bereiche des Otolithenapparates. Acta Otolaryngol 1921;2:434–437.
6. Nylen CO. The otoneurological diagnosis of tumours of the brain. Acta Otolaryngol Suppl (Stockh) 1939;33:5–149.
7. Dix MR, Hallpike CS. The pathology, symptomatology and diagnosis of certain common disorders of the vestibular system. Ann Otol Rhinol Laryngol 1952;61:987–1016.
8. Rigueiro-Veloso MT, et al. Wallenberg's syndrome: A review of 25 cases. Rev Neurol 1997;25:1561.
9. Norrving B, Cronqvist S. Lateral medullary infarction: Prognosis in an unselected series. Neurology 1991;41:244–248.
10. Chia L-G, Shen W-C. Wallenberg's lateral medullary syndrome with loss of pain and temperature sensation on the contralateral face: Clinical, MRI and electrophysiological studies. J Neurol 1993;240:462–467.
11. Kim JS, Lee JH, Suh DC, Lee MC. Spectrum of lateral medullary syndrome: Correlation between clinical findings and magnetic resonance imaging in 33 subjects. Stroke 1994;25:1405–1410.
12. Jenkins IH, Frackowiak RSJ. Functional studies of the human cerebellum with positron emission tomography. Rev Neurol 1993;149:647–653.
13. Kim SG, Ugurbil K, Strick PL. Activation of a cerebellar output nucleus during cognitive processing. Science 1994;265:949–951.
14. Molinari M, Leggio MG, Solida A, et al. Cerebellum and procedural learning: evidence from focal cerebellar lesions. Brain 1997;120:1753–1762.
15. Hoppenfeld S. *Orthopedic Neurology—A Diagnostic Guide to Neurological Levels.* Philadelphia, Pa: JB Lippincott; 1977:97–98.
16. Ashby P, McCrea D. Neurophysiology of spinal spasticity. In: Davidoff RA, ed. *Handbook of the Spinal Cord.* New York, NY: Marcel Decker; 1987:119–143.
17. Pierrot-Deseilligny E, Mazieres L. Spinal mechanisms underlying spasticity. In: Delwaide PJ, Young RR, eds. *Clinical Neurophysiology in Spasticity: Contribution to Assessment and Pathophysiology.* Amsterdam, Holland: Elsevier BV; 1985:63–76.
18. Meissner I, Wiebers DO, Swanson JW, O'Fallon WM. The natural history of drop attacks. Neurology 1986;36:1029–1034.
19. Zeiler K, Zeitlhofer J. [Syncopal consciousness disorders and drop attacks from the neurologic viewpoint]. Wiener Klinische Wochenschrift 1988; 100:93–99.
20. Ross Russell RW. *Vascular Disease of the Central Nervous System,* 2d ed. Edinburgh, Scotland: Churchill Livingstone; 1983.
21. Kameyama M. Vertigo and drop attack. With special reference to cerebrovascular disorders and atherosclerosis of the vertebral-basilar system. Geriatrics 1965;20:892–900.
22. Bardella L, Maleci A, Di Lorenzo N. [Drop attack as the only symptom of type 1 Chiari malformation. Illustration by a case]. [Italian] Rivista di Patologia Nervosa e Mentale 1984;105:217–222.
23. Schochet SS Jr. Intoxications and metabolic diseases of the central nervous system. In: Nelson JS,

Parisi JE, Schochet SS Jr, eds. *Principles and Practice of Neuropathology*. St Louis, MO: Mosby; 1993:302–343.

24. Harper CG, Giles M, Finlay-Jones R. Clinical signs in the Wernicke-Korsakoff complex: A retrospective analysis of 131 cases diagnosed at necropsy. J Neurol Neurosurg Psychiatry 1986;49:341–345.

25. Brazis PW, Lee AG. Binocular vertical diplopia. Mayo Clinic Proc 1998;73:55–66.

26. Giles CL, Henderson JW. Horner's syndrome: An analysis of 216 cases. Am J Ophthalmol 1958;46:289–296.

27. Denny-Brown D, et al. The tract of Lissauer in relation to sensory transmission in the dorsal horn of the spinal cord of the macaque. J Comp Neurol 1973;151:175.

28. Meadows JTS. *Manual Therapy: Biomechanical Assessment and Treatment, Advanced Technique*. Lecture and video supplemental manual, Swocleam Consulting Calgary, AB; 1995.

29. Diamond MC, Scheibel AB, Elson LM. *The Human Brain Coloring Book*. New York, NY: Harper & Row; 1985.

30. Meadows JTS, Pettman E. *North American Institute of Orthopedic Manual Therapy*. Course notes, Denver, Swocleam Consulting Calgary, AB; 1996.

31. Adams RD, et al. *Principles of Neurology*, 6th ed, part 2 (CD-ROM version). New York, NY: McGraw-Hill; 1998.

32. Babinski J. Réflexes tendineux & réflexes osseux. Paris, France: Imprimerie Typographique R. Tancrede; 1912.

33. Babinski J. Du phénomène des orteils et de sa valeur sémiologique. Semaine Med 1898;18:321–322.

34. Babinski J. De l'abduction des orteils. Rev Neurol 1903;11:728–729.

35. Babinski J. De l'abduction des orteils (Signe de l'éventail). Rev Neurol 1903;11:1205–1206.

36. Dommisse GF, Grobler L. Arteries and veins of the lumbar nerve roots and cauda equina. Clin Orthop 1976;115:22–29.

37. Shacklock M. Neurodynamics. Physiotherapy 1995;81:9–16.

38. Breig A. *Adverse Mechanical Tension in the Central Nervous System*. Stockholm, Sweden: Almqvist & Wiskell; 1978.

39. Breig A, Marions O. Biomechanics of the lumbosacral nerve roots. Acta Radiol 1963;1:1141–1160.

40. Breig A, Troup JDG. Biomechanical considerations in the straight leg raising test. Spine 1979;4:242–250.

41. Butler DS. *Mobilization of the Nervous System*. Edinburgh, Scotland: Churchill Livingstone; 1991.

42. Reid JD. Effects of flexion-extension. Movements of the head and spine upon the spinal cord and nerve roots. J Neurol Neurosurg Psychiatry 1960;23:214–221.

43. Smith CG. Changes in length and posture of the segments of the spinal cord with changes in posture in the monkey. Radiology 1956;66:259–265.

44. Slater H, Butler DS, Shacklock MD. The dynamic central nervous system: Examination and assessment using tension tests. In: Boyling JD, Palastanga N, eds. *Grieve's Modern Manual Therapy*, 2nd ed. Edinburgh, Scotland: Churchill Livingstone; 1994.

45. Woodhall B, Hayes GJ. The well leg raising test of Fajersztajn in the diagnosis of ruptured lumbar intervertebral disc. J Bone Joint Surg 1950;32A:786–792.

46. Lasègue C. Considérations sur la sciatique. Arch Gen Med Paris 1864;2:258.

47. Fahrni WH. Observations on straight leg raising with special reference to nerve root adhesions. Can J Surg 1966;9:44–48.

48. Goddard MD, Reid JD. Movements induced by straight leg raising in the lumbosacral nerve roots, nerves and plexus, and in the intrapelvic section of the sciatic nerve. J Neurol Neurosurg Psychiatry 1965;28:12–18.

49. Inman VT, Saunders JB. The clinicoanatomical aspects of the lumbosacral region. Radiology 1941;38:669–678.

50. Smith C. Analytical literature review of the passive straight leg raise test. S Afr J Physiother 1989;45:104–107.

51. Urban LM. The straight leg raising test: A review. In: Grieve GP, ed. *Modern Manual Therapy of the Vertebral Column*. Edinburgh, Scotland: Churchill Livingstone; 1986:567–575.

52. Gajdosik RL, Barney FL, Bohannon RW. Effects of ankle dorsiflexion on active and passive unilateral straight leg raising. Phys Ther 1985;65:1478–1482.

53. Bickels J, Kahanovitz N, Rubert CK, et al. Extraspinal bone and soft-tissue tumors as a cause of sciatica. Clinical diagnosis and recommendations: Analysis of 32 cases. Spine 1999;24:1611–1616.

54. Odell RT, Key JA. Lumbar disc syndrome caused by malignant tumors of bone. JAMA 1955;157:213–216.

55. Paulson EC. Neoplasms of the bony pelvis producing the sciatic syndrome. Minn Med 1951;11:1069–1074.

56. Thakkar DH, Porter RW. Heterotopic ossification enveloping the sciatic nerve following posterior fracture-dislocation of the hip: A case report. Injury 1981;13:207–209.

57. Banerjee T, Hall CD. Sciatic entrapment neuropathy. Neurosurgery 1976;45:216–217.

58. Jones BV, Ward MW. Myositis ossificans in the biceps femoris muscles causing sciatic nerve palsy: A case report. J Bone Joint Surg [Br] 1980;62:506–507.

59. Richardson RR, Hahn YS, Siqueira EB. Intraneural hematoma of the sciatic nerve: Case report. J Neurosurg 1978;49:298–300.

60. Zimmerman JE, Afshar F, Friedman W, Miller C. Posterior compartment syndrome of the thigh with a sciatic palsy. J Neurosurg 1977;46:369–372.

61. Johanson NA, Pellicii PM, Tsairis P, Salvati EA. Nerve injury in total hip arthroplasty. Clin Orthop 1983;179:214–222.

62. Harada Y, Nakahara S. A pathologic study of lumbar disc herniation in the elderly. Spine 1989;14:1020.

63. Reilly BM. *Practical Strategies in Outpatient Medicine.* Philadelphia, Pa: WB Saunders; 1984.

64. Breig A. *Biomechanics of the Central Nervous System.* Stockholm, Sweden: Almqvist & Wiskell; 1960.

65. Breig A, El-Nadi FA. Biomechanics of the cervical spinal cord. Acta Radiol 1966;4:602–624.

66. Lew PC, Morrow CJ, Lew MA. The effect of neck and leg flexion and their sequence on the lumbar spinal cord. Spine 1994;19:2421–2424.

67. Louis R. Vertebroradicular and vertebromedullar dynamics. Anat Clin 1981;3:1–11.

68. Troup JDG. Biomechanics of the lumbar spinal canal. Clin Biomech 1986;1:31–43.

69. Butler DS. *Mobilisation of the Nervous System.* Melbourne, Australia: Churchill Livingstone; 1992.

70. Cyriax J. Perineuritis. Br Med J 1942;1:578–580.

71. Maitland GD. Movement of pain sensitive structures in the vertebral canal and intervertebral foramina in a group of physiotherapy students. S Air J Physiother 1980;36:4–12.

72. Vucetic N, Svensson O. Physical signs in lumbar disc herniation. Clin Orthop 1996;333:192.

73. Scham SM, Taylor TKF. Tension signs in lumbar disc prolapse. Clin Orthop 1971;75:195–204.

74. Supic LF, Broom MJ. Sciatic tension signs and lumbar disc herniation. Spine 1994;19:1066.

75. Dyck P, Doyle JB. "Bicycle test" of van Gelderen in diagnosis of intermittent cauda equina compression syndrome. J Neurosurg 1977;46:667–670.

76. Maitland GD. Negative disc exploration: Positive canal signs. Aust J Physiother 1979;25:129–134.

77. Maitland GD. The slump test: Examination and treatment. Aust J Physiother 1985;31:215–219.

78. Maitland GD. *Vertebral Manipulation,* 5th ed. London, England: Butterworth-Heinemann; 1993.

79. Macnab I. Negative disc exploration. J Bone Joint Surg 1971;53A:891–903.

80. Fahrni WH. Observations on straight leg raising with special reference to nerve root adhesions. Can J Surg 1966;9:44–48.

81. Penning L, Wilmink JT. Biomechanics of lumbosacral dural sac. A study of flexion-extension myelography. Spine 1981;6:398–408.

82. White AA, Punjabi MM. *Clinical Biomechanics of the Spine,* 2nd ed. Philadelphia, Pa: JB Lippincott; 1990.

83. Hakelius A, Hindmarsh J. The comparative reliability of preoperative diagnostic methods in lumbar disc surgery. Acta Orthop Scand 1972;43:234.

84. Dyck P. The femoral nerve traction test with lumbar disc protrusions. Surg Neurol 1976;6:136.

85. Estridge MN, et al. The femoral nerve stretching test. J Neurosurg 1982;57:813.

86. Edelson R, Stevens P. Meralgia paresthetica in children. J Bone Joint Surg [Am] 1994;76:993–999.

87. Macricol MF, Thompson WJ. Idiopathic meralgia paresthetica. Clin Orthop 1990;254:270–274.

88. Cedz ME, Larbre JP, Lequin C, Fischer G, Llorca G. Upper lumbar disc herniation. Rev Rheum Engl Ed 1996;63:421–426.

89. Pinkel GJ, Wokke JH. Meralgia paraesthetica as the first symptom of metastatic tumor in the lumbar spine. Clin Neurol Neurosurg 1990;92:365–367.

90. Amoiridis G, Wohrle J, Grunwald I, Przuntek H. Malignant tumor of the psoas, another cause of meralgia paraesthetica. Electromyogr Clin Neurophysiol 1993;33:109–112.

91. Lorei MP, Hershman EB. Peripheral nerve injuries in athletes: Treatment and prevention. Sports Med 1993;16:130–147.

92. Mirovsky Y, Neuwirth M. Injuries to the lateral femoral cutaneous nerve during spine surgery. Spine 2000;25:1266–1269.

93. Christodoulide AN. Ipsilateral sciatica on femoral nerve stretch test is pathognomic of an L4-5 disc protrusion. J Bone Joint Surg 1989;21:1584.

94. Davidson S. Prone knee bend: An investigation into the effect of cervical flexion and extension. Proc Manip Ther Assoc Austr 5th Biennial Conf, Melbourne; 1987:237.

95. Frymoyer JW, Cats-Baril WL. An overview of the incidences and costs of low back pain. Orthop Clin North Am 1991;22:263–271.

96. Twomey LT, Taylor JR. Joints of the middle and lower cervical spine: age changes and pathology. Man Ther Assoc Austr Conf, Adelaide; 1989.

97. Bianco AJ. Low back pain and sciatica. Diagnosis and indications for treatment. J Bone Joint Surg [Am] 1968;50:170.

98. Maigne R. *Diagnosis and Treatment of pain of Vertebral Origin.* Baltimore, Md: Williams & Wilkins; 1996.

99. DePalma AF, Rothman RH. *The Intervertebral Disc.* Philadelphia, Pa: WB Saunders; 1970.

100. Beals RK, et al. Anomalies associated with vertebral malformations. Spine 1993;18:1329.

101. Matson DD, Woods RP, Campbell JB, Ingraham FD. Diastematomyelia (congenital clefts of the spinal cord). Pediatrics 1950;6:98–112.

102. McKenzie RA. *The Lumbar Spine: Mechanical Diagnosis and Therapy.* Waikanae, New Zealand: Spinal Publications Ltd; 1981.

103. Farfan HF. Mechanical disorders of the low back. Philadelphia, Pa: Lea & Febiger; 1973.

104. Lee D. *The Pelvic Girdle.* Edinburgh, Scotland: Churchill Livingstone; 1989.

105. Vleeming A, et al. The function of the long dorsal sacroiliac ligament: Its implication for understanding low back pain. Spine 1996;21:556.

106. Hohl M. Soft tissue injuries of the neck in automobile accidents; factors influencing prognosis. J Bone Joint Surg [Am] 1974;56:1675.

107. Kanchandani R, Howe JG. Lhermitte's sign in multiple sclerosis: A clinical survey and review of the literature. J Neurol Neurosurg Psychiatry 1982;45:308–312.

108. Lhermitte J, Bollak, Nicolas M. Les douleurs a type de decharge electrique consecutives a la flexion cephalique dans la sclerose en plaque. Rev Neurol (Paris) 1924;2:36–52.

109. Smith KJ, McDonald WI. Spontaneous and mechanically evoked activity due to central demyelinating lesion. Nature 1980;286:154–155.

110. Foreman SM, Croft AC. *Whiplash Injuries: The Cervical Acceleration/Deceleration Syndrome.* Baltimore, Md: Williams & Wilkins; 1988.

111. Bradley JP, Tibone JE, Watkins RG. History, physical examination, and diagnostic tests for neck and upper extremity problems. In: Watkins RG, ed. *The Spine in Sports.* St Louis, Mo: Mosby-Year Book; 1996.

112. Rocabado M. *Notes from Advanced Upper Quarter.* Continuing education course. San Francisco, Calif: Rocabado Institute; 1984.

113. Toole J, Tucker SH. Influence of head position upon cervical circulation. Arch Neurol 1960;2:616–623.

114. Dvorak J, Antinnes JA, Panjabi M, Loustalot D, Bonomo M. Age and gender related normal motion of the cervical spine. Spine 1992;17:S393–S398.

115. Spurling RG, Scoville WB. Lateral rupture of the cervical intervertebral disc. Surg Gynec Obstet 1944;78:350–358.

116. Evans RC. *Illustrated Essentials in Orthopedic Physical Assessment.* St Louis, Mo: Mosby-Year Book; 1994.

117. Denno JJ, Meadows GR. Early diagnosis of cervical spondylotic myelopathy: A useful clinical sign. Spine 1991;16:1353–1355.

118. Acre CA, Dohrmann GJ. Thoracic disc herniation: Improved diagnosis with computed tomographic scanning and a review of the literature. Surg Neurol 1985;23:356–361.

119. Ventafridda V, Caraceni A, Martini C, Sbanotto A, De Conno F. On the significance of Lhermitte's sign in oncology. J Neurooncol 1991;10:133–137.

120. Ongerboer de Visser BW. Het teken van Lhermitte bij thoracale wervelaandoeningen. Ned Tijdschr Geneeskd 1980;124:390–392.

121. Broager B. Lhermitte's sign in thoracic spinal tumour. Personal observation. Acta Neurochir (Wien) 1978;106:127–135.

122. Warren MJ. Modern imaging of the spine; the use of computed tomography and magnetic resonance. In: Boyling JD, Palastanga N, eds. *Grieve's Modern Manual Therapy,* 2nd ed. Edinburgh, Scotland: Churchill Livingstone; 1994.

123. Keim HA. *The Adolescent Spine.* New York, NY: Springer-Verlag, 1982.

124. Wiles P, Sweetnam R. *Essentials of Orthopedics.* London, England: JA Churchill; 1965.

125. Sutherland ID. Funnel chest. J Bone Joint Surg [Br] 1958;40:244–251.

126. Post M. *Physical Examination of the Musculoskeletal System.* Chicago, Ill: Year Book Medical Publishers; 1987.

127. Hoppenfeld S. *Orthopedic Neurology: A Diagnostic Guide to Neurological Levels.* Philadelphia, Pa: JB Lippincott; 1977.

128. Grieve GP. The masqueraders. In: Boyling JD, Palastanga N, eds. *Grieve's Modern Manual Therapy,* 2nd ed. Edinburgh, Scotland: Churchill Livingstone; 1994.

129. Chad DA, Bradley DM. Lumbosacral plexopathy. Semin Neurol 1987;7:97.

130. Luzzio CC, Waclawik AJ, Gallagher CL, Knechtle SJ. Iliac artery pseudoaneurysm following renal transplantation presenting as lumbosacral plexopathy. Transplantation 1999;67:1077–1078.

131. Wilbourn AJ. Electrodiagnosis of plexopathies. Neurol Clin 1985;V3:511.

132. Wilberger JE. Lumbosacral radiculopathy secondary to abdominal aortic aneurysms. J Neurosurg 1983;58:965.

133. Kleiner JB, Donaldson WF, Curd JG, Thorne RP. Extraspinal causes of lumbosacral radiculopathy. J Bone Joint Surg 1991;73:817.

134. Donckier V, De Pauw L, Ferreira J, et al. False aneurysm after transplant nephrectomy. Transplantation 1995;60:303.

135. Bodack MP, Cole JC, Nagler W. Sciatic neuropathy secondary to a uterine fibroid: A case report. Am J Phys Med Rehabil 1999;78:157–159.

136. Kimura J. *Electrodiagnosis of Diseases of Nerve and Muscle: Principles and Practice*, 2nd ed. Philadelphia, Pa: FA Davis; 1989:3–24.

137. Salazar-Gruesco E, Roos R. Sciatic endometriosis: A treatable sensorimotor mononeuropathy. Neurology 1980;36:1360–1363.

138. Vanneste JAL, Burzelaar RMJM, Dicke HW. Ischiadic nerve entrapment by an extra- and intrapelvic lipoma: A rare cause of sciatica. Neurology 1980;30: 532–534.

139. Geelen JA, de Graaff R, Biemans RG, Prevo RL, Koch PW. Sciatic nerve compression by an aneurysm of the internal iliac artery. Clin Neurol Neurosurg 1985;87: 219–222.

140. Raikin S, Froimson MI. Bilateral brachial plexus compressive neuropathy (crutch palsy). J Orthop Trauma 1997;11:136–138.

141. Poddar SB, Gitelis S, Heydemann PT, Piasecki P. Bilateral predominant radial nerve crutch palsy: A case report. Clin Orthop 1993;297:245–246.

142. Rudin LN. Bilateral compression of radial nerve (crutch paralysis). Phys Ther 1951;31:229.

143. Subramony SH. Electrophysiological findings in crutch palsy. Electromyogr Clin Neurophysiol 1989; 29:281–285.

144. Ang EJ, Goh JC, Bose K, Toh SL, Choo A. A biofeedback device for patients on axillary crutches. Arch Phys Med Rehabil 1989;70:644–647.

145. Bauer DM, Finch DC, McGough KP, Benson CJ, Finstuen K, Allison SC. A comparative analysis of several crutch-length-estimation techniques. Phys Ther 1991;71:294–300.

146. Rudin LN. Bilateral compression of radial nerve (crutch paralysis). Phys Ther 1951;31:229.

CHAPTER ELEVEN

THE BIOMECHANICAL EXAMINATION

Chapter Objectives

At the completion of this chapter, the reader will be able to:

1. Define the components that comprise the tests and measures for the biomechanical examination.
2. Describe the rationale for biomechanical screening tests.
3. Describe the purpose and components of a biomechanical examination.
4. Outline the significance of the key findings from a biomechanical examination.
5. Develop a working hypothesis.
6. Understand the purpose of muscle function testing and the various grading systems.
7. Define posture and recognize the common postural syndromes.
8. Describe the significance of muscle imbalance in terms of flexibility and strength.
9. Perform a muscle function analysis.
10. Recognize the common muscle imbalance patterns.
11. Initiate an intervention plan for correcting a muscle imbalance.
12. Discuss the various classification systems for examining back pain.

TESTS AND MEASURES[1]

Tests and measures are a component of the overall examination of the patient, which is a component of the episode of care[2] (Fig. 11–1.) According to the *Guide to Physical Therapist Practice*,[2] the purpose of an examination is to identify impairments, functional limitations, disabilities, or changes in physical function and health status resulting from injury, disease, or other causes to establish the diagnosis and the prognosis and to determine the intervention

(see Fig. 11–1). The components that comprise the examination include the systems review, the subjective history, and the scanning examination—each of which is discussed in a separate chapter of this book—and the biomechanical examination is described herein.

BIOMECHANICAL SCREENING TESTS[3]

Screening tests are quick noncomprehensive tests that allow the clinician to identify a joint or group of joints as possibly contributing to the patient's symptoms and requiring more detailed biomechanical testing. Screening tests are not exclusive to the biomechanical examination. In fact, the scanning examination is a screening examination aimed at screening out those patients with serious pathology, neurologic pathology, or a diagnosis that can be identified by the tests contained within it. The scanning examination in Chapter 10 also contains some biomechanical screening tests, examples of which include the FABER and FADE tests, and active, passive, and resisted testing of each joint.

Biomechanical screening tests are especially useful when the remote cause of an impairment is being investigated, because they allow the numerous areas that have to be examined to be provisionally excluded from a more definitive examination. However, it must be constantly remembered that because screening tests are not all inclusive, and that false negatives are common, they must be subordinate to other considerations in the examination of the patient.

In addition to the scanning examination of the spine, the symptomatic area must obviously be assessed. This can be achieved by utilizing upper and lower limb screening/scanning tests. If any of these tests is positive for pain or aberrant motion, a full selective tissue tension and biomechanical examination of that joint must follow. If negative, a search elsewhere in the quadrant usually demonstrates the site of the cause. If it does not, it becomes necessary to

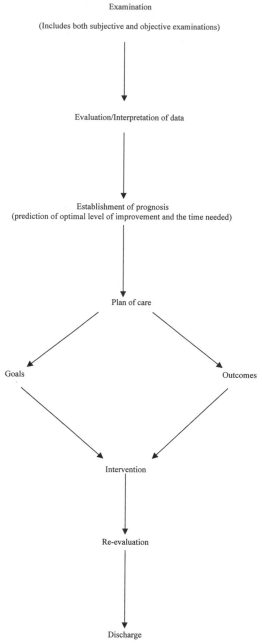

Examination

(Includes both subjective and objective examinations)

Evaluation/Interpretation of data

Establishment of prognosis
(prediction of optimal level of improvement and the time needed)

Plan of care

Goals   Outcomes

Intervention

Re-evaluation

Discharge

FIGURE 11–1 Episode of care.

carry out a comprehensive and definitive scanning and biomechanical examination of every joint in that quadrant. It is only after this proves negative that the clinician can state with some confidence that the pain is not musculoskeletal in origin or, at least, is beyond the clinician's skills to reproduce or demonstrate. Rather than individually examine each of the suspected areas, the screening tests are designed to assess the most likely regions first, thereby expediting the examination process. Specific screening tests are included in each chapter and usually involve:

- Active and passive movements through the full range of each joint, with a maximal isometric contraction performed at each end range.
- Functional motions, such as the squat, to test a group of joints.

BIOMECHANICAL EXAMINATION

Generally speaking, the biomechanical examination is used if the scanning examination does not yield a diagnosis. Following the scanning examination, a number of diagnoses may have been made, either by the subjective history or by the scanning examination, or both. Those diagnoses include, but are not limited to:

A. Visceral pathology

B. Fractures

C. Pathologic space-occupying lesions

D. Neurologic pathology
   1. Treatable
      a. Mechanical nerve root compression (disc, osteophyte, inflammation)
   2. Nontreatable
      a. Mechanical nerve root compression (tumor)
      b. Upper motor neuron impairment
      c. Cauda equina impairment

E. Spondylolisthesis

F. Ankylosing spondylitis

The scan or subjective examination, or both, may also have indicated to the clinician that the patient's condition is in the acute stage of healing. Although this is not a diagnosis in the true sense, it is a diagnosis for the purpose of setting an intervention plan. Patients who are in the acute stage of healing have pain at rest and activity, and all motions of the affected joint are painful, with the exception of gentle passive motion. There may be local muscle guarding, and swelling. The intervention approach for these patients involves the principles of PRICE (protection, rest, ice, compression, and elevation). For further details, the reader is referred to Chapters 2 and 12.

Having ruled out the more serious causes for pain, and the common patterns of the treatable diagnoses listed earlier, the clinician needs to delve deeper and begin examining some of the musculoskeletal reasons for the patient's signs and symptoms, which could include:

- Zygapophysial joint pathology. Although it is difficult to envision a zygapophysial joint impairment without having a disc impairment, it is possible to have a disc impairment without a zygapophysial joint impairment, as the disc is a primary stabilizer.

- Hypomobility, hypermobility, or instability of the three-joint complex
- Bursitis
- Chronic musculotendinous impairment
- Articular impairment
- Capsular impairment
- Ligamentous impairment

Often the scan generates a number of signs and symptoms that, taken together, do not form a pattern distinct enough to base an effective intervention on. Usually, the clinician requires further information in order to proceed. This information is obtained from the tests and measures of the biomechanical examination that inspect, in more detail and with a different focus, the movement status of the joint, or joints, in question.

According to the *Guide to Physical Therapist Practice*,[2] tests and measures for musculoskeletal patterns include the examination of:

- Aerobic capacity and endurance
- Anthropometric characteristics
- Community and work integration
- Ergonomics and body mechanics
- Orthotic, protective, and supportive devices
- Self-care and home management
- Joint integrity and mobility
- Gait
- Posture
- Pain
- Range of motion
- Muscle performance
- Motor function

The main focus in this book is the examination of the following:

- Joint integrity and mobility
- Posture
- Pain
- Range of motion
- Muscle performance
- Motor function

The same principles and, in some cases, the same techniques that were used in the scan are used for the biomechanical examination, the difference being the intention of the examiner. Whereas the aim of the scan is to elicit a medical diagnosis and to help the clinician focus the examination on a specific area of the body, the aim of

TABLE 11–1 REDUCED VERSUS EXCESSIVE JOINT MOTION[1]

REDUCED MOVEMENT		EXCESSIVE MOVEMENT	
ARTICULAR	NONARTICULAR	HYPERMOBILE	UNSTABLE
Subluxed	Myofascial Pericapsular	Irritable Nonirritable	Ligamentous Articular

the biomechanical examination is to elicit a movement diagnosis and to determine:

- Which of the peripheral or spinal joints is impaired
- The presence and type of movement impairment

The biomechanical examination consists of the aforementioned screening tests that help focus on the problem area, specific stress tests to detect an instability, and mobility tests that determine the "motion state" of the joint; that is, is the joint myofascially or pericapsularly hypomobile, subluxed, hypermobile, or ligamentously or articularly unstable[1] (Table 11–1).

A general examination and the principles behind it are described here. The specific examination for each region of the spine, sacroiliac joint, and temporomandibular joint are described in later chapters.

The examination actually begins in the waiting room, when the patient is observed without his or her knowledge. The posture of the patient is recorded, as well as the response to the calling of his or her name.

A more formal observation is then performed with the patient in an appropriate stage of undress. (Refer to Chapter 10)

Active and passive motions are assessed. A joint's active range of motion is determined by its articular design and the inherent tension and resilience in its associated muscular, myofascial, and ligamentous structures. Greenman[5] uses the term *physiologic end barrier* to describe the end point of active joint motion. Full and pain-free ranges suggest normalcy for that movement. The active motions may not reproduce the patient's symptoms, because the patient is able to self-limit, and avoid going into the painful part of the range, having learned from experience the consequences of such a movement. This is particularly true of the patient with a hypermobile or unstable joint. It is efficient to perform the passive motion by applying overpressure at the end of active range. Apprehension from the patient that limits a movement at near or full range suggests instability, whereas apprehension in the early part of the range suggests anxiety due to pain. Resistive tests are performed during this phase of the examination (refer to the later section entitled "Muscle Function Testing").

The next stage in the examination process depends on the clinician's background. For those clinicians heavily influenced by the muscle energy techniques of the osteopaths,[6] position testing is used to determine which segment to focus on. Other clinicians omit the position tests and proceed to the passive physiologic and combined motion tests.

POSITION TESTS[6]

The position tests are screening tests that, like all screening tests, are valuable in focusing the attention of the examiner on one segment, but are not appropriate for making a definitive statement concerning the movement status of the segment. When combined with the results of the passive movement testing, however, they help the clinician to form the working hypothesis.

In consideration of normal anatomic restraints, and viewing the zygapophysial joints as "independent" joints, the superior facet of each joint is capable only of superior or inferior motion.

A. If both facets move symmetrically, this produces the pure motions of the spine.
   1. If both facets move superiorly, the motion produced is termed *flexion.*
   2. If both facets move inferiorly, the motion produced is termed *extension.*

B. If both facets move, but in opposite directions (i.e., one facet moves superiorly while the other moves inferiorly), the motion produced is called a *combined motion.* In the lumbar spine, this motion functionally represents side-flexion.

C. There is a point that may be considered as the "center of segmental rotation," about which all rotation must occur. In the case of a zygapophysial joint impairment (hypermobility or hypomobility), it is presumed that this center of rotation will be altered.

D. In the instance that one apophyseal joint is rendered hypomobile (i.e., the superior facet cannot move to the extreme of superior or inferior motion), then the pure motions of flexion and extension, cannot occur. There will be a relative asymmetric motion of the two superior facets as the end of range of flexion or extension is approached.

E. The structure responsible for the loss of zygapophysial joint motion, whether it be a muscle, disc protrusion, or the apophyseal joint itself, will become the "new" axis of vertebral motion, and will introduce a component of rotation into the segmental motion.

F. Because the zygapophysial joints are more posterior, an obvious rotational change occurring between full flexion and full extension (in the position of a vertebral segment), is indicative of a zygapophysial joint motion impairment. By observing any marked and obvious rotation of a segment occurring between the positions of full flexion and full extension, one may deduce the probable pathologic impairment.

Reasons for this change in rotation, other than movement impairments, include a deformed transverse process, compensatory adaptation, structural scoliosis, and a hemivertebra. An additional weakness of position testing is its insensitivity to symmetric impairments. If a symmetric impairment exists, preventing full motion from occurring, no rotation of the vertebra will result, and the flexion and extension position tests will prove to be negative, giving the false impression of no impairment. Hence, if the position test is negative, the symmetric passive mobility tests need to be performed.

PASSIVE PHYSIOLOGIC TESTS[1]

To determine the segmental mobility, the passive physiologic intervertebral mobility (PPIVM) tests are utilized. The PPIVM tests assess the ability of each segment to move through its normal range of motion while the clinician palpates over each segment in turn. The results give the clinician an idea of the range of motion available and, with some stabilization, allow the clinician to examine the end feel. The end feel is very important in joints that only have very small amounts of normal range, such as those of the spine. A hard, capsular end feel indicates a pericapsular hypomobility, whereas a jammed or pathomechanical end feel indicates a pathomechanical hypomobility. A normal end feel would indicate normal range, whereas an abnormal end feel would suggest abnormal range, either hypomobile or hypermobile. To achieve the end feel, the clinician must supply a sufficient force to assess the elastic limits of the joint, before allowing the joint to spring back to its starting position. Because pain does not generally limit movement in specific and deliberate passive tests, these tests are better for gauging the reality of the limitation based on tissue resistance, rather than patient willingness, and are better at determining the pattern of restriction than the active tests. If pain is reproduced, it is useful to associate the pain with the onset of tissue resistance to gain an appreciation of the acuteness of the problem (Table 11–2).

Once the physiologic range has been assessed, it can be categorized as being normal, excessive, or reduced. A positive finding for a hypomobility would be a reduced

TABLE 11–2 TISSUE RESISTANCE, PAIN, AND MANUAL TREATMENT[1]

BARRIER	END FEEL	TECHNIQUE
Pain	—	None
Pain	Spasm	None
Pain	Capsular	Oscillations
Joint adhesions	Early capsular	Passive articular motion stretch
Muscle adhesions	Early elastic	Passive physiologic motion stretch
Hypertonicity	Facilitation	Hold/relax
Bone	Bony	None

range in a capsular or noncapsular pattern, and a change in the end feel from the expected norm for that joint. The hypomobility can be painful, suggesting an acute sprain of a structure, or painless, suggesting a contracture, or adhesion of the tested structure. Thus, one of three conclusions can be drawn from the PPIVM tests:

1. The joint is determined to be normal. If the PPIVM test of a spinal joint has a normal range and end feel, the joint can usually be considered normal because, in the spine, instability invariably produces a hypermobility. However, in a peripheral joint, it is possible to have a normal range in the presence of articular instability.

2. The motion is determined as being excessive (hypermobile). If the articular restraints are irritable, the range is about normal but is accompanied by a spasm end feel, because a reflex muscle contraction prevents the motion into an abnormal, and painful, range. If nonirritable, the physiologic range is increased and the end feel is softer than the expected capsular one, suggesting a complete tear of the structure under examination. If the motion is determined to be excessive, its stability needs to be assessed.

3. If the motion is determined to be reduced (hypomobile), passive physiologic articular intervertebral mobility (PPAIVM) testing is performed to determine whether the reduced motion is a result of an articular or extra-articular restriction. The PPAIVM tests involve the clinician assessing the joint glides or accessory motions of each joint. Accessory motions are involuntary motions and cannot, for the most part, be controlled by muscular action or position especially if the glides are tested at the end of available range in the spinal joints.[1] Thus, if the joint glide is restricted, the cause is an articular restriction such as the joint surface or capsule. If the glide is normal, then the restriction must be from an extra-articular source such as a periarticular structure or muscle.

DEVELOPING A HYPOTHESIS

Patients often present with a mixture of signs and symptoms that indicate one or more possible problem areas. By adding and subtracting the various findings, the clinician can determine the probable cause of the symptoms and begin developing a working hypothesis on which to base the biomechanical examination. For example if, in the examination of the lumbar spine, the patient demonstrated a limitation of flexion and right side-flexion in the combined motion tests, the L4-5 segment demonstrated a hypomobility during the PPIVM, and the PPAIVM was limited in flexion, the site of the restriction must be the left zygapophysial joint of L4-5. If the end feel is pathomechanical, the left joint is subluxed into extension and cannot flex, whereas if the end feel is hard and capsular, then the left joint is limited into extension by inextensible periarticular tissues. If, however, right side-flexion and flexion are limited, but the PPAIVMs are normal, an extra-articular restriction is present.

Musculoskeletal impairments that have a traumatic origin are often easier to diagnose, especially in the case of macrotrauma. Impairments with an insidious onset, or those that occur as a result of a microtrauma, are more challenging and often more rewarding.

KEY FINDINGS

Once the biomechanical examination is completed, the clinician should have a hypothesis as to what tissue or structure is at fault. A few common impairments make up the majority of those that are seen regularly in the clinic, each of which present with their own key findings:[7]

- *Joint capsule.* Fibrosis of the joint usually occurs with a prolonged immobilization of the joint, which is associated with a chronic, low-grade inflammatory process. Joint motion is limited in a capsular pattern, and there is a capsular end feel at the extremes of movement. If the synovium is inflamed as a result of acute trauma, infection, or arthritis, there is often a spasm end feel, producing pain at the restriction points of motion.
- *Bone.* Fractures and dislocations are best diagnosed through the use of x-rays.
- *Articular cartilage.* Significant degeneration of the articular cartilage presents with crepitus on movement when compression of the joint surfaces is maintained. A fragment of the articular cartilage, referred to as a *loose body,* can become symptomatic, producing a catching or locking sensation to normal movement in a noncapsular pattern.

- *Intra-articular fibrocartilage.* The intra-articular fibrocartilaginous discs and menisci can be torn during trauma, restricting motion in a capsular pattern because of the simultaneous injury to the joint capsule and resultant joint effusion.
- *Ligaments.* Point tenderness, joint effusion, and a history of trauma are all characteristic of a ligament tear. A mild tear presents with a normal, but painful, stress test of the ligament. More severe sprains produce excessive joint mobility accompanied by pain if the ligament remains intact, or no pain if there is a complete rupture of the ligament, in the rare case that no other tissue was involved.
- *Bursa.* A bursa commonly becomes inflamed secondary to chronic irritation or infection. Pain is reproduced when the nearby joint is moved, producing a noncapsular pattern of restriction. A painful arc may exist, and the end feel can be empty if the bursitis is acute.
- *Tendons.* Tendinitis involves microscopic tearing and inflammation of the tendon tissue, commonly resulting from tissue fatigue rather than direct trauma. The key clinical finding is a strong but painful response to resistance of the involved musculotendinous structure. Tenosynovitis is an inflammation of the synovial lining of the tendon sheath, which often produces pain with active motion of the involved tendon within the sheath. Tenovaginitis results from a tendon gliding within a swollen, thickened sheath, producing pain.

Pain that occurs consistently with resistance, at whatever the length of the muscle, may indicate a tear of the muscle belly. Pain with muscle testing may indicate a muscle injury, a joint injury, or a combination of both. Pain with an isometric contraction generally indicates a muscle injury rather than a capsular one.[8] However, to differentiate between a muscle injury and a capsular one, the findings from the isometric test must be combined with the findings of the passive motion and compression tests.[9]

Case Study

A 56-year-old moderately obese woman presents with a prescription that reads "Hip OA, evaluate and treat." The subjective history reveals that the pain is of an insidious onset and that the patient complains of left groin pain. The pain started approximately 3 months ago when the patient started a walking program to lose some weight and has been getting worse. It improves with rest and worsens with activity, especially with walking and stair negotiation. X-rays reveal slight degenerative changes at the hip joint.

Given the age of the patient, the insidious onset and location of pain, the x-ray findings, and the fact that the pain improves with rest, the diagnosis from the physician could be correct. However, any insidious onset should alert the clinician, regardless of the diagnosis, or his or her level of experience. This is a good example of a patient condition that is clearly not life threatening but is unlikely to be diagnosed from the findings of a scan.

As with any examination, a great deal of variety exists as to how it is approached in terms of detail. It is often a good idea to keep the approach simple, only utilizing more complex principles and techniques where needed, and this patient example highlights that approach.

Less intuitive clinicians would proceed with the following tests, with the physician diagnosis in the back of their mind, tainting their judgment:

A. Scan performed:
   1. Slight groin discomfort with lumbar flexion
   2. Slight groin discomfort at 90 degrees of left straight leg raise
   3. Slight groin discomfort with the prone knee bending test if the hip is extended

B. Active, passive, and resisted testing of the hip:
   a. No pain reproduced except with passive hip extension

C. Special tests for the hip performed (the scour test and the FABER (flexion, abduction, external rotation) test):
   a. Both tests reproduce the groin pain

Let us suppose the clinician decides to treat the patient, as per the prescription, for hip osteoarthritis and begins a regime of moist heat pads, hip isometrics, and quadriceps strengthening. Two weeks later, the patient is worse.

In many respects, a clinician could be forgiven for proceeding in the chosen fashion, but basic errors should have indicated that an incorrect conclusion had been made. The most obvious mistake was that there was no capsular pattern at the hip. In fact, the only hip motion that was painful was the one not even mentioned in the capsular pattern. The only other tests on which the clinician based his or her biomechanical diagnosis were the scour test and the FABER test, both of which examine more than just the hip joint. But why did the prone knee bending test reproduce the pain, albeit slightly?

It is to be hoped that, at the 2-week point, having realized that the patient's condition was worsening, the clinician would decide to explore more options. To perform a re-evaluation of the same tests would merely elicit the same findings, except more pronounced, owing to the increased level of irritation that occurred over the intervening 2 weeks.

The easiest course of action would be to make the assumption that the patient is exaggerating her symptoms and that there is some psychological overlay to her condition. Under this assumption it would seem fruitless to change the intervention protocol when the same tests, used to determine the original intervention strategy, are still positive.

It is hoped, though, if the correct diagnosis was not made initially, the clinician would swallow his or her pride and assess the patient in more depth. All clinicians fall into the trap of incorrectly judging the patient, and his or her symptoms, at some point in their careers, usually at the beginning. The good ones do not make a habit of it.

The focus of every examination should be on finding ways to both provoke *and* alleviate the patient's symptoms. In addition to performing the tests already completed, a lumbar and sacroiliac biomechanical examination would be added, with the following results:

- No capsular pattern of left hip noted
- Groin pain also reproduced with lumbar extension
- Slight pain with resisted hip flexion (L1-2), but only when the hip is positioned in extension for the test
- Decreased flexibility of the rectus femoris and hip flexors, more marked on the left
- Left rotation of all of the lumbar segments

As is often the case, a more detailed examination reveals more information, but does not always make the diagnosis easier. The clinician needs to form a mental list of all the structures in the body that can refer pain to the groin, and begin to rule out each one with a series of tests until only one remains. Groin pain is a common finding in patients, and the findings thus far could suggest a number of candidates:

A. Hip osteoarthritis
1. As mentioned, the age of the patient, the insidious onset and location of pain, the x-ray findings, and the fact that the pain improves with rest support this conclusion.
2. A positive scour test and FABER test somewhat support the conclusion.
3. The noncapsular pattern somewhat refutes the conclusion.

B. Pelvic impairment
1. The positive FABER test somewhat supports the conclusion.
2. All of the other sacroiliac tests are negative, which refutes the conclusion.

C. A lumbar or thoracic impairment
1. Pain reproduced with lumbar extension.

2. The positive prone knee bending test somewhat supports the conclusion.
3. The positive FABER test somewhat supports the conclusion.
4. The pain with resisted hip flexion, with the hip in extension, could confirm the conclusion based on the anatomy of the hip flexors.

D. A contractile structure
1. Pain reproduced by resisted hip flexion supports the conclusion.
2. The positive scour test refutes the conclusion.
3. The insidious onset could refute or support the conclusion, depending on whether it was a muscle or tendon impairment.

E. Compression of a structure
1. At this point, the pieces of the puzzle begin to come together. All of the findings thus far could result from the compression of a structure. But which structure? It has to be a structure between the lumbar spine and the hip.

In fact, it is the iliopectineal (iliopsoas) bursa. The patient's pain is the result of a bursitis produced by a tight iliopsoas on the left and the introduction of a walking program. Walking programs typically advocate the "stride" form of gait which, unless there is a good degree of hip joint and muscle flexibility, can induce a lot of stress on the lumbar spine as well as the structures beneath the two joint muscles.

It should be clear from this patient example that the biomechanical examination draws on all of the clinician's resources. The more experienced clinician would now begin to wonder why there is more decreased flexibility of the iliopsoas on the left side.

This case also highlights a problem that many clinicians face, and that is the potential invasion of a patient's intimate areas. Although most clinicians routinely palpate the spine and the extremities if they suspect an impairment, many are reluctant to palpate in the groin or genital areas. It is essential to protect the patient's dignity and modesty at all times; however, the clinician needs to examine *all* potential causes for the pain. A thorough explanation as to the reasons for an examination to these areas must be given to the patient. It is also a wise policy to be accompanied by a member of staff, of the same sex as the patient, if the examination may involve such procedures.

MUSCLE FUNCTION TESTING

Muscle function testing provides the clinician with the following information:[10]

- The strength of individual muscles or muscle groups that form a functional unit
- The presence and extent of a peripheral or spinal nerve impairment
- The nature, range, and quality of simple movement patterns
- The relationship between the strength and the flexibility of a muscle or muscle group

To fully test the integrity of the muscle-tendon unit, a maximum contraction must be performed in the fully lengthened position of that muscle-tendon unit. Although this position fully tests the muscle tendon unit, there are some problems with testing in this manner:

- The joint and its surrounding inert tissues are in a more vulnerable position, and could be the source of the pain.
- As described in Chapter 10, the degree of certainty regarding the findings in resisted testing depends on a combination of the length of the muscle tested, and the force applied. The results of the test reflect the degrees of the severity of the damage to the contractile tissue (Table 11–3). For example, pain reproduced with a minimal contraction in the rest position for the muscle is more strongly suggestive of a contractile lesion than pain reproduced with a maximal contraction in the lengthened position for the muscle.

If the same muscle is tested on the opposite side, using the same testing procedure, the concern about the length of the muscle is removed, as the focus of the test is for comparison with the same muscle on the opposite side.

The examination and grading of muscle strength is covered in a number of texts.[11–13] Although the grading of muscle strength has its role in the clinic, the manual clinician is not overly concerned with giving specific grades to individual muscles or muscle groups, except perhaps to reassure an insurance company that progress is being made. While having the ability to isolate the various muscles is very important,

especially when determining the source of a nerve palsy, specific grading does not give the clinician any information on the ability of the structure to perform functional tasks. Despite attempts to make muscle grading as objective as possible, many variables exist in the testing that make it unreliable. Even if the reliability was improved, the clinician would need to determine what improvement in the patient's function is achieved by increasing the strength of a muscle by half a grade. If the popular methods to grade muscles are analyzed, the frailties and similarities become obvious. Janda[12] uses a 0–5 scale with the following descriptions:

- Grade 5 = N (normal): a normal, very strong muscle with a full range of movement and able to overcome considerable resistance. This does not mean that the muscle is normal in all circumstances (e.g., when at the onset of fatigue or in a state of exhaustion).
- Grade 4 = G (good): a muscle with good strength and a full range of movement, and able to overcome moderate resistance
- Grade 3 = F (fair): a muscle with a complete range of movement against gravity only when resistance is not applied
- Grade 2 = P (poor): a very weak muscle with a complete range of motion only when gravity is eliminated by careful positioning of the patient
- Grade 1 = T (trace): a muscle with evidence of slight contractility but no effective movement
- Grade 0 = a muscle with no evidence of contractility

Sapega[11] uses the descriptions in Table 11–4.

If the muscle strength is less than grade 3, these testing grades are perhaps useful, but it is the grades of 3 and higher that produce the most confusion. Some of the confusion arises from the descriptions of maximal, moderate, and minimal, or considerable, whereby the grading becomes very subjective.

The use of goniometric measurements in the clinic has similar pitfalls, although not through a lack of objectivity. If a patient has 80 degrees of shoulder flexion at the beginning of a session and 90 degrees at the end of the session, it is clear that objective progress has been made, but what effect has the increased range had on the patient's ability to use the arm more effectively?

Some measurement tools are already being employed that address some of these issues.[14–18]

Muscle function testing, therefore, should address the production and control of motion in functional activities. There is general agreement as to the role that the trunk and pelvic musculature play in the normal functioning of the vertebral column, the protection against pain, and the recurrence of low back disorders. As a result, the strengthening of these muscles is advocated in the majority

TABLE 11–3 STRENGTH TESTING RELATED TO JOINT POSITION AND MUSCLE LENGTH

MUSCLE LENGTH	RATIONALE/PURPOSE
Fully lengthened	Muscle in strongest position
	Tightens the inert component of the muscle
	Tests for muscle tears (tendoperiosteal tears) while using minimal force
Mid-range	Tests overall power of muscle
Fully shortened	Muscle in its weakest position
	Used for the detection of palsies, especially if coupled with an eccentric contraction

TABLE 11–4 MUSCLE GRADING

GRADE	VALUE	MOVEMENT
5	Normal (100%)	Complete range of motion against gravity with maximal resistance
4	Good (75%)	Complete range of motion against gravity with some (moderate) resistance
3+	Fair+	Complete range of motion against gravity with minimal resistance
3	Fair (50%)	Complete range of motion against gravity
3−	Fair−	Some but not complete range of motion against gravity
2+	Poor+	Initiates motion against gravity
2	Poor (25%)	Complete range of motion with gravity eliminated
2−	Poor−	Initiates motion if gravity eliminated
1	Trace	Evidence of slight contractility but no joint motion
0	Zero	No contraction palpated

of rehabilitation programs[19–21] even though the effectiveness of these programs has yet to be proven.[22,23]

With the change in emphasis to achieving a coordinated activity between a balanced muscular system, the focus of the examination and intervention of back pain has also changed.

POSTURE

Posture describes the relative positions of different joints at any given moment.[24] Each joint has a direct effect on both its neighboring joint and the joints further away. Individuals have characteristics about their posture that can often define them. Like "good movement," "good posture" is a subjective term based on what the clinician believes to be correct from ideal models. Over the course of time, various definitions have been put forward to describe the attributes of good posture. Any posture that does not satisfy these requirements has thus been considered faulty posture.

Certain factors appear to influence adult posture:

● Heredity and environment[25]
● Disease
● Habit

The focus of therapeutic intervention is to alleviate the symptoms of disease and to play a significant role in educating the patient against misuse of the third influence, habit.

Good Posture

When viewing someone from the side, good posture has traditionally been based on the use of a plumb-line. If the plumb-line passed through the ear lobe; through the bodies of the cervical vertebrae; in line with the tip of the shoulder; through the midline of the thorax; through the bodies of the lumbar vertebrae, slightly posterior to the hip joint; slightly anterior to the axis of the knee joint; and just anterior to the lateral malleolus, the individual was deemed to have good posture.[26] However, the modern concept of good posture views it as the position in which minimum stress is applied to each joint, the maintenance of which requires a minimal amount muscle activity.[27]

Faulty posture is not necessarily poor posture. In general, poor posture refers to the classic stoop-shouldered, flat-chested position that results in a "hollow" back and a pelvis that is tilted well forward. Faulty posture becomes pathologic when an individual can no longer correct the malalignment volitionally, or when musculoskeletal structures become damaged, or when the lifestyle is affected.[27]

The tensile properties of muscle change owing to a number of causes. A muscle can become weak through inhibition, disuse, or as the result of neurologic compromise, whereas a muscle can become shortened and contracted, relative to its resting length, through the habituation of activity or posture. This shortening or contracture can result from a neuromuscular influence, producing hypertonicity, or from connective tissue fibrosis. Shortened and contracted muscles are referred to as "tight" in this text.

A muscle imbalance exists when the resting length of the agonist and the antagonist changes, with one adopting a shorter resting length than normal and the other adopting a longer resting length than normal. Although it is quite normal for muscles to change their lengths frequently during movements, this change in resting length becomes pathologic when it is sustained through habituation, or through a response to pain. This sustained change in muscle length is postulated to influence the information sent by the proprioceptors, the autonomic response, and other reflex activities, and to result in an imbalance between the contractions of the agonist and antagonist.[28] These local changes are theorized to produce a sequence of compensation and adaptation responses in surrounding joints and muscles, causing a variety of syndromes (see later discussion).[29]

SIGNIFICANCE OF MUSCLE IMBALANCE AND ALTERED MOVEMENT PATTERNS[10]

Traditional postural assessment has involved a static analysis of the patient's position in the relaxed state. Over the years, clinicians have begun to evaluate the effects of the soft tissues around the joints, particularly the muscles, which have the potential to pull, and to hold, the skeletal structures.

In the past, muscle testing placed an emphasis on evaluating the ability of a muscle to move in a specified direction against resistance, but did not place much emphasis on the overall quality of the performance. The human motor system is required to perform functions, and adapt to changes in those functions. Most of the motions performed at joints are the result of a combination of muscles working synergistically. For example, hip extension involves a contraction of the hamstrings and the glutei, and the assistance of the adductor magnus, gluteus medius and minimus, abdominals, and erector spinae.[12] If the hip extension strength appears normal, it is difficult for the clinician to determine if all, or only some, of the muscles are working normally. Hip extension is certainly being produced, but the quality of the movement pattern may be poor.

Sahrmann[30] introduced the concept of movement system balance (MSB). According to this concept, the efficient and ideal operation of the movement system is determined by several factors. These include[31]:

- *The maintenance of precise movement of rotating parts.* This is determined by the changing position of the instantaneous axis of rotation (IAR) produced by pathology. Several factors influence the position of the IAR, including the shape and integrity of the joint surfaces, the length and mobility of the soft tissues that cross a joint, and the relative participation of muscles around the joint.
- *Correct muscle length.* Whereas traditionally emphasis has been placed on the assessment of shortened muscles, the MSB theory places more emphasis on identifying lengthened muscles.[30] Muscles maintained in a shortened or lengthened position adapt to their new positions but are initially incapable of producing a maximal contraction.[32] However, after a period of adaptation, the muscle is able to produce maximal tension at this new length, because of the relative changes at the sarcomere level.[30] Although this may appear to be a satisfactory adaptation, a muscle that is lengthened will not be able to generate normal tension if it is subsequently put in a shortened position, especially if this shortened position is produced by the clinician attempting to place the patient's joints in the position of so-called good posture.
- *Correct motor control.* The timing and participation of muscles around a joint are critical in ensuring precise movement.[30]
- *Correct relative stiffness of both contractile and noncontractile tissue.* According to the MSB theory, the body takes the path of least resistance during movement.[30]

- *Correct kinetics.* The MSB theory stresses the importance of observation along both directions of the kinetic chain, and the importance of examining joints proximal to the site of the disorder or symptomology to determine the efficiency and correctness of their function.

Thus, a poor quality of movement results from a muscle imbalance of muscle length and strength, and can have adverse effects. A passively insufficient muscle is activated earlier in movement than a normal muscle. The activity of an inhibited and weakened muscle tends to decrease rather than increase when resisted.[33] If the tight muscle is stretched and its normal length achieved, a spontaneous disinhibition of the previously inhibited muscle occurs, and there is a return to normal responses when the resistance is increased.[33]

Janda noted that the way in which muscles tend to react appears to be fairly consistent for the muscle concerned.[34]

- There is a natural imbalance between the strength of muscle groups controlling the trunk, with extensor strength exceeding flexor strength.[35] Whether this relationship is altered with back pain, has not yet been shown conclusively.
- Trunk muscles are fatigued more easily by a sustained contraction than by repeated isokinetic contractions.[36] In one study, the abdominals were found to fatigue more easily than the back extensors,[36] and in another study under isokinetic study conditions, to fatigue more quickly in the patients with back problems than in control patients.[37]
- Tightness of muscles can influence both static postures and dynamic function. Reduced trunk mobility and decreased extensibility of the hamstrings and iliopsoas are frequently reported in studies of patients with low back pain.[38,39]
- Muscles that span more than one joint have a tendency to become tight.
- Muscles that are prone to tightness are approximately one-third stronger than those prone to inhibition, and this may be because these muscles are readily activated during various movements.[40]
- Typical muscle responses are seen with articular pathologies that are extremely similar to those seen in some structural impairments of the central nervous system[41] (Table 11–5).

There are a number of muscle types. The fatigue resistant fibers (type I) produce the prolonged or slowly repeated contractions used in postural control. The rapidly fatiguing muscle fibers (type IIa) generate high force and are used for specific activities for short periods of time.

TABLE 11–5 FUNCTIONAL DIVISION
OF MUSCLE GROUPS[10]

MUSCLES PRONE TO TIGHTNESS (TYPE I)	MUSCLES PRONE TO WEAKNESS (TYPE II)
Gastrocnemius and soleus	Peronei
Tibialis posterior	Tibialis anterior
Short hip adductors	Vastus medialis and lateralis
Hamstrings	Gluteus maximus, medius, minimus
Rectus femoris	Serratus anterior
Tensor fascia lata	Rhomboids
Erector spinae	Lower portion of trapezius
Quadratus lumborum	Short and deep cervical flexors
Pectoralis major	Upper limb extensors
Upper portion of trapezius	Rectus abdominis
Levator scapulae	
Sternocleidomastoid	
Scalene	
Upper limb flexors	

However, most muscles have a mixture of both fast- and slow-twitch fibers (type IIb) (Table 11–6).

Two mechanisms are thought to provoke muscle imbalances:

1. Acute pain or pathology in the spinal segment(s), which can lead to an alteration in the patient's pattern of motion and which will lead to adverse strain in the lumbar spine, ultimately causing a chain reaction throughout the spine.[42]
2. Impairment of motor control from the central nervous system, which will lead to an overactivity of the muscle.[43] This impairment can also be a result of the influence of stress, fatigue, and pain on the limbic system, which regulates muscle tone.[44]

For this reason, emphasis in the therapeutic programs should be placed on regaining normal length of the muscles using proprioceptive neuromuscular facilitation (PNF) techniques, so that exercises directed toward facilitating

TABLE 11–6 FUNCTIONAL DIVISION OF MUSCLE
FIBER TYPES[10]

TYPE I	TYPE IIa	TYPE IIb
Tonic	Phasic	Phasic
Slow	Fast twitch	Fast twitch
Slow oxidative	Fast glycolytic	Fast oxidative, glycolytic
Red	White	Red
Small neuron	Large neuron	Large neuron
Fatigue resistant	Rapidly fatiguing	Fatigue resistant

and strengthening the weakened muscles and achieving good motor patterns can be successful.

Assessment of Muscle Impairment[10]

The assessment is undertaken in three stages:

1. Examination of standing and seated posture
2. Examination of muscle length
3. Examination of movement patterns

Examination of Standing and Seated Posture
The postural examination gives an overall view of the patient's muscle function, and the clinician should attempt to differentiate between possible provocative causes, such as structural variations, age, altered joint mechanics, muscle imbalances, or residual effects of pathology.

- Does the patient wear high-heeled shoes? This style of footwear has a tendency to increase the lordosis.[46]
- Which hand is dominant? Often the dominant side demonstrates differences to the contralateral side. For example a right-handed individual often has the following characteristics on close inspection: a lower right shoulder, a left spinal scoliosis, the right hip slightly deviated to the right, and the opposite foot slightly more pronated and flattened.[47] A closer inspection would reveal a slight tilt of the eyes to the left, a slight tilt of the jaw to the right, a more anterior right shoulder, an anteriorly rotated right clavicle, an anterior rotation of the right innominate, a left-on-left sacral torsion, and a right knee recurvatum. The findings for a left-handed individual would be the reverse.

Posterior View
- *Upper trapezius.* Tightness of this muscle produces an elevated shoulder and a paravertebral area that is broader and more prominent.
- *Levator scapulae.* Tightness of this muscle results in an elevated scapula and the contour of the neckline appearing as a double line (wave) where the muscle inserts into the scapula. This is described as "gothic" shoulders because it is reminiscent of the form of a gothic church tower.
- *Interscapular area.* This tends to be flattened with weakness. An increase in the distance between the thoracic spinous processes and the medial border of the scapula indicates a rotation of the scapula. A serratus anterior weakness results in an inadequate fixation of the inferior angle to the rib cage, and winging of the scapula.

- *Scapular position*. A downwardly rotated scapula can result from a short levator scapula and rhomboid muscle. A depressed scapula indicates that the upper trapezius muscle is long. The latissimus dorsi and pectoralis major can also depress the scapula. An adducted scapula can result from short rhomboid and trapezius muscles.

- *Spine*. Is a curve apparent? Two terms, *scoliosis* and *rotoscoliosis*, are used to describe curvature of the spine. Scoliosis is the older term and refers to an abnormal side-bending of the spine, but gives no reference to the coupled rotation that also occurs. Rotoscoliosis is a more detailed definition, used to describe the curve of the spine by detailing how each vertebra is rotated and side-flexed in relation to the vertebra below.

  A malalignment of the scapular can produce a rib hump. If the rib hump causes the scapula to wing, the patient should not be encouraged to correct the alignment by sustained contraction of the scapular adductors as this can lead to shoulder and cervical pain.

- *Pelvis*. Does a pelvic asymmetry exist? There appears to be a strong correlation between the position of the pelvis and the forward head.[48] If the pelvic landmarks are asymmetric and the patient has a forward head, the clinician should attempt to correct the forward head. If the attempted correction of the forward head worsens the pelvic asymmetry, the intervention should be aimed at correcting the asymmetry. If the attempted correction of the forward head improves or removes the pelvic position or impairment, the subsequent intervention should be aimed at correcting the forward head.[49] The pelvic crossed syndrome (see later discussion) produces an increase in anterior tilt accompanied by decreased lumbar lordosis. A sacral rotation can be the result of tightness of the piriformis muscle, whereas an innominate rotation can be a result of tightness of the hamstrings, rectus femoris, or iliopsoas muscles.

- *Lateral shift*. This shift might be the result of an acute or chronic lumbar segment pathology[21] or a true leg-length difference.

- Muscle shape and quality of the lower quadrant.
  Glutei. The glutei should be symmetric and well rounded not hanging loosely (as found in the pelvic crossed syndrome, see later discussion).
  Hamstrings. The hamstrings should not predominate when compared with the glutei.
  Hip adductors. Tightness of these muscles is indicated by a distinct bulk in the upper third of the thigh.
  Gastrocnemius/soleus. Tightness of this muscle group is indicated by a prominence of the soleus, particularly on the medial side of the teno-calcaneum.
  Erector spinae. There should be no differences in bulk between both sides and regions of these muscles. A poor sign is a predominance of the thoracolumbar portion, indicating poor stabilization of this area.

- Muscle shape and quality of the upper quadrant *Interscapular muscles*. Loss of bulk in these muscles may indicate tightness in the trapezius and levator scapula.

Anterior View

- *Forward head*. This posture indicates weakness of the deep neck flexors and dominance or tightness of the sternocleidomastoid (SCM).

- *Pectoralis major*. If this muscle is tight or strong, it will be prominent. If an imbalance is present, it will lead to rounded and protracted shoulders and a slight medial rotation of the arm.

- *Sternocleidomastoid*. Normally, its insertion is just visible. If the clavicular insertion is prominent, it indicates tightness. A groove along the SCM is an early sign of weakness of the deep neck flexors. A weakening and atrophy of the deep neck flexors has been proposed as a sign for estimating biologic age.[50]

- *Digastric*. If this muscle is tight, it leads to a straightening of the throat line. Palpation of this muscle can reveal trigger points.

- *Abdomen*. The abdominal wall area should be flat. When the obliques are dominant, a distinct groove is seen on the lateral aspect of the recti.

- *Tensor fascia lata*. The bulk of this muscle should not be distinct. If it is, and there is a groove on the lateral side of the thigh, it usually indicates that the muscle is overused, and both it and the iliotibial band may be tight.

- *Rectus femoris*. If the rectus femoris is involved, the patella will move slightly upwards (and also laterally if there is concurrent tightness of iliotibial band).

Examination of Muscle Length

When considering muscle length, the following muscles are of most importance:

A. *Pectoralis major*. The patient is positioned supine. The clinician passively abducts the patient's arm, with the trunk stabilized, to differentiate between the different bands of the pectoralis major:
   1. Clavicular portion: The patient's arm hangs loosely down over the edge of the table. The clinician moves the patient's shoulder down toward the floor. A slight barrier to the motion is normal; if it is hard, the finding is abnormal.
   2. Sternal portion: While supine on a mat table, the patient abducts the arm fully. The arm should maintain contact with the table throughout the range.

B. *Upper trapezius*. The patient lies supine with the head inclined to the contralateral side. While stabilizing the head, the clinician moves the patient's shoulder girdle distally. A normal finding is free movement with a soft motion barrier. Tightness of this muscle results in a restriction in range of motion, and a hard barrier.

C. *Levator scapulae.* The patient is supine with the hand of the tested side behind the head. The patient's head is inclined toward the contralateral side and then flexed and rotated away from the tested side. The clinician then moves the patient's shoulder girdle distally. If tightness is present, there will be tenderness at the levator insertion, and a restriction of movement.

D. *Pectoralis minor.* The patient is supine with their arms by the sides. The posterior aspect of the shoulder girdle should be resting comfortably on the mat table. If the shoulder girdle is raised off the table, pectoralis minor tightness is present.

E. *Sternocleidomastoid.* (Refer to previous section)

F. *Lumbar erector spinae.*
1. A simple test involves having the seated patient fix the hips by placing his or her hands on the iliac crests and then hunching the lumbar and thoracic spine into kyphosis. This will be hindered if the erector spinae are short, although other factors can affect the results, such as the relative length of the trunk and the thighs. The erector spinae muscles are assessed for hypertonus, especially if an increased lordosis is present.
2. The more comprehensive test involves two parts.
   a. First, the patient is positioned on a mat table with the legs stretched out, keeping the pelvis as vertical as possible. If the pelvis tilts posteriorly in this position, it is a sign of shortened hamstrings. The patient is asked to try to touch his or her forehead on the knees. An adult should achieve a distance of 10 cm or less between the forehead and knees, and should demonstrate an even curve of the spine.
   b. The second part of the test involves the patient sitting over the end of the mat table with the knees flexed. The patient bends forward as far as possible, attempting to move the forehead toward the knees, without moving the pelvis. If the forward bending of the trunk is greater than in the first part of the test, it is usually due to an increased tilt of the pelvis and hamstring shortness.

G. *Hip flexors.*
1. The original Thomas test was designed to test the flexibility of the iliopsoas complex (Fig. 11–2) and involved positioning the patient supine. The clinician flexed one hip and assessed whether the opposite

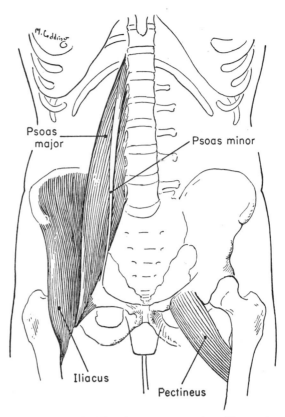

FIGURE 11–2 The iliopsoas complex. (*Reproduced, with permission from Luttgens K, Hamilton N: Kinesiology: Scientific Basis on Human Motion, 9e McGraw-Hill, 1997*)

thigh raised from the bed. If the opposite thigh remained on the bed, the hip flexor length on that side was within normal limits.
2. The test has since been modified to incorporate the assessment of the flexibility of other muscles. The modified technique involves positioning the patient supine with the crease of the buttocks on the edge of the table (Fig. 11–3). The tested leg must hang free over the end of the table and the opposite hip and knee are maintained in flexion to eliminate the lumbar lordosis.
   a. Normal findings on the tested leg are:
      (1) The thigh is horizontal. A flexed hip indicates tightness of the iliopsoas.
      (2) The leg hangs vertically. A diagonal pattern of the leg indicates tightness of the rectus femoris.
   b. To determine which structure is more involved, the application of pressure into the following directions can be applied:
      (1) Hip extension (Fig. 11–3): If less than 10 to 15 degrees is achieved, this indicates a tight iliopsoas. Simultaneous extension of the knee during this maneuver indicates tightness of the rectus femoris.

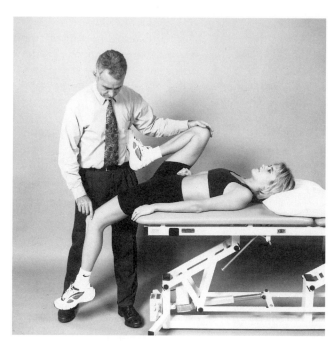

FIGURE 11–3 The modified Thomas test.

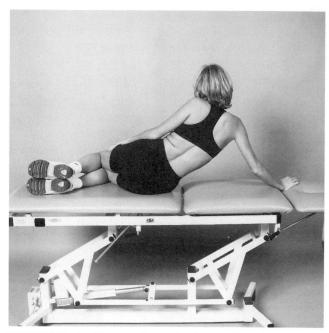

FIGURE 11–4 The quadratus lumborum length test.

(2) Knee flexion: If less than 100 to 105 degrees is available, the rectus femoris is tight.

(3) Hip adduction: If less than 15 to 20 degrees is achieved, the tensor fascia lata and the iliotibial band are tight.

(4) Hip abduction: If less than 15 to 20 degrees is achieved, the short hip adductors are tight.

H. *Hamstrings.* The patient is supine and a towel roll is placed under the lumbar spine. The anterior superior iliac spine (ASIS) is monitored as the straight leg is raised. The hamstrings are considered shortened if the straight leg cannot be raised to an angle of 80 degrees from the horizontal while the other leg is straight.

I. *Quadratus lumborum.* Tightness of the quadratus lumborum can be noted during lumbar side-flexion to the contralateral side in standing, especially if the lumbar spine does not appear to curve. Normal findings would show a smooth, symmetric curve of the spine in both directions, with side bending in standing. A more comprehensive test involves placing the patient in the side-lying position with the hips and knees flexed at about 45 degrees. The patient then pushes up sideways from the table to a point where the pelvis begins to move (Fig. 11–4), while the clinician ensures that the patient's trunk does not flex or rotate during the maneuver.

J. *Piriformis.* An impairment of this muscle would be revealed by a restriction in hip adduction and medial rotation when the hip is flexed. A more reliable test is deep palpation over the greater sciatic foramen. Normal findings would be that the buttock tissue is soft and the piriformis is not palpable. However, signs of tightness would be indicated by a tense muscle belly and acute tenderness over the piriformis.

K. *Short hip adductors.* The patient is positioned supine with the leg to be tested close to the edge of the mat table. The leg not to be tested is abducted 15 to 25 degrees at the hip joint, with the heel over the end of the mat table. Maintaining the tested knee in extension, the clinician passively abducts the tested leg. The normal range is 40 degrees. When the full range is reached, the knee of the tested leg is passively flexed and the leg is abducted further. If the maximum range does not increase when the knee is flexed, the one-joint adductors (pectineus, adductor magnus, adductor longus, adductor brevis) are shortened. If the range does increase with the knee passively flexed, the two-joint adductors (gracilis, biceps femoris, semimebranosus, and semitendinosus) are shortened.

L. *Gastrocnemius/soleus group.* The patient is asked to squat down. If the triceps surae is normal, the patient should be able to place the whole foot on the floor, including the heel, while in the full squatting position. If the soleus is short, the heel will not touch the floor. With the patient supine, if the gastrocnemius is shortened, dorsiflexion of the ankle will be reduced as the knee is extended and increased as the knee is flexed.

Examination of Movement Patterns[10]

These tests are concerned with the coordination, timing, or sequence of activation of the muscles during movement.

A. *Deep neck flexors.* The patient is positioned supine and is requested to slowly raise the head in an arclike motion. With weak deep neck flexors, in the presence of a strong SCM, the jaw juts forward at the beginning of the movement, producing hyperextension of the craniovertebral junction (Fig. 11–5). Clarification can be achieved by resisting the motion with a very slight amount of resistance (2 to 4 g) against the patient's forehead.

B. *Serratus anterior.* The patient is positioned prone and is asked to perform a push-up and then to return to the start position extremely slowly. The clinician checks for the quality of scapula stabilization. If the stabilizers are weak, the scapula on the side of impairment will shift outward and upward, with a resultant winging of the scapula.

C. *Shoulder abduction.* The patient is positioned in sitting with the elbow flexed to control the humeral rotation. The patient is asked to slowly abduct the arm. Three components are evaluated:
1. Abduction at the glenohumeral joint
2. Rotation of the scapula
3. Elevation of the whole shoulder girdle.
   The abduction movement is stopped at the point at which the shoulder begins to elevate. This typically occurs at about 60 degrees of glenohumeral abduction.

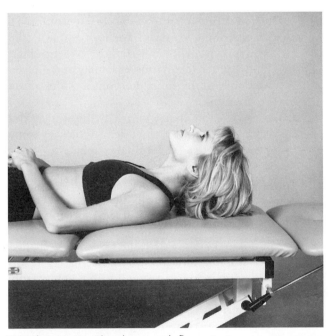

FIGURE 11–5 The deep neck flexor test.

D. *Hip extension (gluteus maximus).* The patient is positioned prone and is asked to extend the hip off the table, keeping the leg straight. For this movement, the hamstrings and the gluteus maximus are the prime movers, with the erector spinae functioning as the stabilizer of the lumbar spine and pelvis. Altered patterning in this test would be demonstrated by:
1. Initial activation of the hamstrings and erector spinae, with a very delayed contraction of the gluteus maximus.
2. The erector spinae initiate the movement with a delayed activity of the gluteus maximus. This would lead to little, if any, extension of the hip joint, as the leg lift would be achieved by an anterior pelvic tilt and a hyperextension of the lumbar spine. This is a very poor movement pattern.

E. *Hip abduction (gluteus medius).* The patient is placed in the side-lying, position, with the uppermost leg straight and the bottom leg slightly bent at the knee and hip. The patient abducts the upper leg from this position. Prime movers for this movement are the gluteus medius and minimus, and the tensor fascia lata. The quadratus lumborum functions as the stabilizer of the pelvis. Altered patterning will demonstrate:
1. Lateral rotation of the leg during the upward movement, indicating an initiation, and dominance, of the movement by the tensor fascia lata, accompanied by a weakness of the gluteus medius and minimus.
2. Full external rotation of the leg during leg lift, indicating a substitution of hip flexion and iliopsoas activity for the true abduction movement.
3. A lateral pelvic tilt at the initiation of movement, indicating that the quadratus lumborum is stabilizing the pelvis and is initiating the movement. This is indicative of a very poor movement pattern.

F. *Trunk curl-up.* This test assesses the patient's ability to sit up from a supine position, and assesses the relationship between the abdominal and iliopsoas muscles. The patient is positioned supine with the hips and knees flexed, both feet flat on the bed (crook-lying position). During the patient's attempt to sit up from the supine position, little flexion of the trunk will be evident if the iliopsoas is dominant, as most of the flexion occurs at the hip. The patient is then asked to perform a sit-up while actively plantar-flexing the ankles, thus removing the effect of the iliopsoas.[51] The patient progressively flexes the spine, starting at the cervical region, until the lumbar region is flexed. As soon as the iliopsoas becomes involved in the motion, the patient's feet will lift from the bed. Normally, the patient should be able to curl up so that the thoracic and lumbar spines are clear of the bed before the feet lift. A patient in excellent condition can complete a full sit-up without the feet lifting from the bed.

Common Postural Syndromes

These syndromes occur via mechanical, neurologic, and neurophysiologic influences, and the speculated causes of these syndromes are based on the sound application of anatomy, biomechanics, and neurologic theory, and are supported by the clinical experience of treating these proposed causes. The syndromes may be caused by the facilitation of a spinal segment, neurologic or neurodevelopmental deficit (palsy), or direct biomechanical impairment, affecting tissues remote from the impaired area. Any, or all, of these can lead to imbalances in the forces acting on the joint capsule, ligament, muscle, fascia and nerve. Some examples of the more common syndromes are described next.

Common Syndromes in the Cervical Region[10,27,52,53] The proximal or shoulder crossed syndrome involves tightness of the levator scapulae, the upper trapezius, pectoralis major and minor, and the SCM, and weakness of the deep neck flexors and lower scapular stabilizers. The syndrome produces elevation and protraction of the shoulder, rotation and abduction of the scapula, together with scapular winging. It also produces a forward head and decreased stability of the glenohumeral joint, which leads to increased muscle activity of the levator scapula and trapezius. The various components and consequences of this syndrome are discussed.

- An asymmetric upper thoracic or, less frequently, a mid-cervical impairment, produces a positional fault that may be compensated for at the C7 level by the C6 or C7 vertebra rotating and side-flexing. If this adjustment closes down a previously asymptomatic stenotic foramen, the spinal nerve root may be compressed, with subsequent neurologic changes. Facilitation of the trigeminal nerve, due to a temporomandibular (TMJ) impairment, can produce suboccipital hypertonus which, if allowed to adaptively shorten, will lead to a craniovertebral hypomobility and symptoms in the spine and upper quadrant. In addition, alteration of the bite plane due to a TMJ impairment may cause the neck to compensate by positioning itself to bring the bite plane back to its normal horizontal orientation. If this occurs on a stenotic segment, it can lead to distal signs and symptoms.

- The forward head produces extension of the craniovertebral joints. A craniovertebral impairment may lead to a rotation or tilting of the head, or both, altering the bite plane and resulting in abnormal forces being generated. Neurophysiologically, craniovertebral impairments can produce trigeminal facilitation,

resulting in hypertonicity of the masticatory muscles and disturbances of joint proprioception.

- Shoulder bursitis, tendonitis, ruptures of the rotator cuff muscles, capsulitis, ligamentous sprains, and calcification are all types of tissue change that can be consequential to an impairment remote from the site of symptoms.[54] Usually, there are local tissue changes, because of the stresses placed on the tissue by the remote impairment. A common cause of many of these syndromes is the forward head posture. In addition to the problems already mentioned, the forward head can produce the impairments described next.

- Hypertonicity of the levator scapulae can produce a facilitation of either the C4 or C5 segment.[55] At rest, this hypertonicity may lead to an overuse syndrome of the supraspinatus tendon as it supports the humeral head on the adducted scapula.

- Protraction of the shoulder girdles limits extension of the upper thoracic spine, which, in turn, limits elevation and abduction of the shoulders. This can lead to a hypermobility or instability of the glenohumeral joint, or both, and to overuse syndromes of the shoulder elevators or abductors. Shoulder protraction can also result in adaptive shortening of the pectoralis minor, which, in turn, alters the motion of the scapula on the chest wall, producing a mechanical impairment of the shoulder, with possible tissue changes and symptoms.[56] Finally, shoulder protraction also causes the humerus to rotate medially and in so doing stretches the posterior glenohumeral joint capsule; in addition, it increases the anterior force at the joint owing to gravity. The former may lead to posterior instability and rotatory hypermobility, and the latter to anterior instability and a biceps tendonitis, as this muscle becomes overused as it tries to stabilize the joint.

- As the zygapophysial joints in the midcervical region incur more weight bearing, owing to the protruding head, marginal osteophytosis may occur. This may result in lateral stenosis (foraminal compression), either facilitating the segment and causing hypertonicity in the early stages, or compromising conduction or axoplasmic flow with resultant hypotonicity. The common levels for this to occur are C5-6 and C6-7. These changes alter scapulothoracic motion, decreasing it with facilitation, and increasing it with a palsy, via the altered muscle tone of the rhomboids (C5), serratus anterior (C7), and pectoralis major (C7-8). When the pectoralis major is hypertonic, the resulting pattern of hypomobility is decreased abduction, lateral rotation, and elevation (the capsular pattern). Hypotonicity, weakness, and reduced coordination of the infraspinatus (C5-6) may destabilize the posterior aspect of the glenohumeral joint.

- Facilitation of the C6 segment may produce an overuse syndrome of the extensor carpi radialis muscles (tennis elbow).
- Facilitation of the C7 or C8 segment may cause a golfer's elbow as the wrist flexor muscles are affected. A C7 facilitation, or palsy, can also alter the neuromuscular coordination of the articularis genu (subanconeus) muscle, leading to olecranon bursitis as the muscle fails to pull the bursa upward during extension. Facilitation of the C8 segment, causing hypertonicity of the abductor and extensor pollicis tendons, may result in De Quervain's syndrome.
- An ulnohumeral impairment, particularly an abducted ulna, may cause a tennis elbow or, less commonly, a golfer's elbow
- An ulnohumeral impairment, particularly an abducted ulna, may cause medial hand paresthesia as a result of an increased carrying angle and subsequent stretching of the ulna nerve. Abduction impairments of the ulna may also produce an apparent radial deviation and extension hypomobility and overstretching of the collateral ligaments.
- Carpal hypomobility may also lead to extensor overuse syndromes at the elbow as the muscles overwork to produce the wrist extension that is limited.

In general, the closer the units are together, the more likely they are to have a pathologic relationship. For example, there is more chance that the head unit will be affected by the shoulder unit than by the hand unit.

Common Syndromes in the Lumbar Region[10,52,57–59] Pathomechanical interaction occurs more readily between certain areas than it does between others in this region (Table 11–7). Some examples of lower quadrant syndromes follow.

- Upper lumbar or thoracolumbar instabilities and hypermobilities can often lead to facilitation of the upper lumbar segments, with resulting psoas hypertonicity. This change leads to reduced hip extension and medial rotation. The loss of full range of motion results in a shortened stride length. Body weight and ground reaction forces, generated by rapid walking, will equalize the stride length by hypermobilizing or destabilizing the lumbosacral junction or the ipsilateral sacroiliac joint. The process is reinforced by the

TABLE 11–7 LOWER QUADRANT SYNDROMES[10,52,57,59,60]

DEFICIT	IMPAIRMENT	EFFECT
Lumbar hyperlordosis	Extension hypermobilities Anterior instabilities	L3 facilitation Retropatellar syndromes L4 facilitation Shin splints Medial foot arch instability L5-S1 facilitation Hamstring injuries Achilles injuries Retropatellar syndromes
Anteriorly rotated pelvis	Hip extension hypomobility	Sacroiliac instability Lumbosacral instability L5-S1 facilitation Hamstring injuries Achilles injuries Retropatellar syndromes
Knee hyperextension	Recurvatum Tibial medial rotation Valgus	Medial collateral sprain Retropatellar syndrome Meniscal injury
Flat foot	Mortice instability Talonavicular instability Calcaneocuboid instability Talocalcaneal instability	Subluxations Plantar cuboid Dorsal navicular Reverted calcaneus Plantar fasciitis Hallux valgus Retropatellar syndrome

mechanical pull of the shortened psoas, and this increases the stress on the upper lumbar spine, increasing facilitation.

- Pelvic crossed syndrome: In this particular syndrome, the erector spinae and the iliopsoas are tight, and the abdominal and gluteus maximus are weak. This syndrome promotes an anterior pelvic tilt, an increased lumbar lordosis, and a slight flexion of the hip. The hamstrings are frequently tight in this syndrome, and this may be a compensatory strategy to lessen the anterior tilt of the pelvis,[60] or because the glutei are weak. The syndrome promotes an increased lumbar lordosis, and a compensatory increase in cervical lordosis. If the hip loses the ability to extend, because of the tight iliopsoas, a compensatory increase in the anterior pelvic tilt needs to occur during gait.
- Layer syndrome: This is an indication of marked impairment of the central nervous system's ability to regulate motor patterns and is thus accompanied by a

deterioration in those patterns. Inherent in this pattern of muscle imbalance is poor muscular stability in the lumbosacral region.

- An L5 palsy alters the function of the peroneus longus, weakening it or causing it to be less coordinated. An impairment of the peroneus longus can also result in metatarsalgia and even second metatarsal stress fracturing as a result of the failure of the first metacarpal to be pulled down to the substrate by the muscle, causing the second metatarsal head to habitually bear weight.

- Facilitation of the L4 segment can lead to hypertonicity and overuse syndromes of the anterior or posterior tibialis, resulting in an anterior or posterior compartment syndrome, or a hypertonicity of the tensor fascia lata, which alters the balance of forces on the patella, resulting in retropatellar syndromes. A palsy of the L4 segment can result in overflattening of the foot, which may lead to instability of the medial arch.

- A palsy or facilitation of the L3 segment may result in altered retropatellar forces, leading to retropatellar pain syndromes. Hypertonicity of the rectus femoris reduces hip extension in the terminal stages of weight bearing during gait and may result in similar problems as those found with a tight psoas. Palsy or facilitation of any of the lumbar segments may predispose the muscle served by that segment to actual damage during exertion, particularly during strong eccentric contractions.

- Extension hypermobility of the knee may result in overflattening of the foot, with resulting medial arch instability. The excessive extension also excessively medially rotates the tibia, increasing the Q angle and altering the forces on the patella.

Intervention

Postural imbalances involve the entire spine, and any corrections should, as well. It is important to remember that postural correction is an intervention, and that prior to any intervention, an appropriate examination must take place. Because postural correction affects every part of the body, a global examination should be undertaken. For the vast majority of people, static postures are a rarity, and dynamic postures are more functional. Thus, it is important that the patient be taught by the clinician to return to the optimal posture between activities, so that they can adopt a good posture without conscious effort.

Therapeutic exercise programs should initially focus on regaining the normal length of a muscle before strengthening the muscle, so that good movement patterns can be achieved.

The intervention of any muscle imbalance is divided into three stages: (1) restorating normal muscle length, (2) strengthening weak or inhibited muscles, and (3) establishing optimal motor patterns to best protect the spine.

Restoration of Normal Muscle Length The activity of selected muscles must be inhibited and, in the inhibitory period, the muscle should be stretched. If the muscle is hypertonic, minimal facilitation and minimal stretch, using muscle energy techniques, can be used. With true muscle shortness, stronger resistance is used to activate the maximum number of motor units, followed by vigorous stretching of the muscle. Stretching should be performed using:

- Low force
- Prolonged duration
- Heat applied to the muscle prior to, and during, stretching
- Postisometric relaxation techniques; reciprocal relaxation is not as effective because of the weakness of the antagonist
- Rapid cooling of the muscle while it is maintained in the stretched position

Strengthening of Inhibited or Weak Muscles Vigorous strengthening should be avoided initially to minimize substitutions by other muscles and to prevent reinforcement of poor patterns of movement.

Establishment of Optimal Motor Patterns to Protect the Spine As an example, a typical intervention protocol for a posture that is having a detrimental effect on the lumbar and thoracic regions, would involve the following actions:

1. The removal of any excessive extension in the midthorax (which has been produced by the increased spinal extensor and diaphragm tone).

2. Correct diaphragmatic breathing is taught. This includes both inspiration and, more importantly, relaxed expiration.

3. Correction of the upper thorax (T1 area) is achieved. The patient is seated. The clinician asks the patient to breathe out while lifting the manubrium and sternum toward the ceiling. This can be encouraged by having the clinician push down on the upper chest over the first and second ribs, while palpating the upper thoracic spinous processes with the other hand during exhalation. The patient may feel pressure between the shoulder blades during this exercise.

4. Posterior pelvic tilting in sitting is taught by having the patient roll onto the tail bone. This begins to help the lower thorax by decreasing the lumbar lordosis. The exercise is, combined with the breathing technique outlined in strategy 2.

Principles

1. Avoid pain during exercise, as this can lead to further inhibition of the muscles.

2. Achieve normal and pain-free movement in the spinal segments.

3. Initially emphasize the normalization of muscle length, differentiating between spasm and structural changes.

USE OF CLASSIFICATION SYSTEMS[61]

The attempt to classify back pain has been the focus of a number of clinicians over recent years. The desire for a classification system probably stems from a degree of frustration that the optimal intervention for patients with acute back and neck pain remains largely enigmatic. In addition, a number of clinical studies have failed to find consistent evidence for improved intervention outcomes with many intervention approaches that rely on exercise, manual therapy, and traction.[62]

One explanation offered for the lack of positive research findings is that patients with "nonspecific" back and neck pain are labeled as a homogeneous group, with all patients equally likely to succeed or fail with any particular intervention.[63,64] Other authors have theorized that patients with back and neck pain actually are a heterogeneous group consisting of several smaller homogeneous subsets.[65–67] Through the use of a classification system, it is proposed that a patient is more likely to respond to a type of intervention unique to that classification, or preferred practice pattern.

To classify patients for an intervention strategy, a number of criteria have been suggested, as outlined next:

A. Pathoanatomy[68,69] This strategy involves using correlations to produce categories. The disadvantage of using pathoanatomy is the difficulty in identifying a relevant pathoanatomic cause for most patients.[70]

B. The presence or absence of sciatica.[71]

C. The duration of the symptoms (acute, subacute, or chronic).[72]

D. Work status.[67]

E. Impairments identified during the physical examination. This approach attempts to link specific interventions with each classification. The system described by McKenzie[21] is reported to be the most commonly used classification system by physical therapists for this purpose.[73] This system uses pain behavior, and its relationship to movements and positions, to determine the appropriate plan of intervention. Each syndrome in the McKenzie classification is broad in terms of pathology, but is specific in terms of clinical behavior, although no attempt is made to be tissue-specific.[74,75] McKenzie uses three syndromes to classify mechanical pain:

1. The *posture syndrome* is proposed to result from over-stretching of normal tissue. The pain, which is of a gradual onset, is dull, local, midline, symmetric, and never referred. Prolonged postures worsen the pain, whereas movement abolishes it. Upon examination, the patient demonstrates no spinal deformity or loss of range, and repeated movements do not produce the symptoms. The onset of symptoms, which is time-dependent (usually occurring after more than 15 minutes), is provoked with sustained end-of-range positions.

2. The *dysfunction syndrome* is proposed to result from an adaptive shortening of soft tissues. The pain, which is intermittent, is local and adjacent to the midline of the spine, and is not referred except in the case of an adherent nerve root when the pain may be felt in the buttock, thigh, or calf. Activities and positions at the end of range worsen the pain, whereas activities that avoid end ranges are better. Upon examination, the patient demonstrates a loss of motion or function, distinguishing this syndrome from the postural syndrome. Repeated movements do not alter the symptoms, and the loss of motion, or function, may be symmetric or asymmetric.

3. The *derangement syndrome* is thought to be produced by a displacement, or alteration in position, of joint structures. The joint structure most commonly involved is the intervertebral disc, and McKenzie divides these disturbances into posterior disc and anterior disc derangements. The posterior derangements are further subdivided into seven derangement categories. Derangements 1 through 6 describe posterior derangements, whereas derangement 7 describes the anterior derangement.

The pain, which is usually of a sudden onset, and associated with paresthesia or numbness, is dull or sharp and can be central, unilateral, symmetric, or asymmetric. Although the pain may be referred into the buttock, thigh, leg, or foot, it varies in both intensity and distribution. Bending, sitting, or sustaining positions worsens a posterior derangement, whereas walking and standing worsen an anterior derangement. Patients with a posterior derangement often feel better with walking and lying, whereas patients with an anterior derangement usually feel better with sitting and other flexed positions. Upon examination, a lateral shift may be noted. There is always a loss of motion and function. Certain motions produce, increase, or peripheralize the symptoms, whereas other motions decrease, abolish, or centralize the symptoms.

Intervention for each of the syndromes is specific, and patients are encouraged to accept responsibility for their intervention and recovery. Although the McKenzie maneuvers are referred to as exercises, most of the procedures are passive self-mobilizations aimed at regaining spinal extension while concurrently maintaining flexion.

Treatment-based Classification System

This system uses information gathered from the physical examination and from patient self-reports of pain (pain scale and pain diagram) and disability (modified Oswestry questionnaire) to classify the patient. The classification then guides the treatment of the patient. The treatment-based classification (TBC) system is designed for patients who are judged to be in the acute stage,[65] with the determination of acuity based on the nature of the patient's symptoms, the degree of disability, and the goals for management, instead of on the elapsed time from injury. Patients in the acute stage are those with higher levels of disability (Oswestry scores generally greater than 30) and substantial patient-reported difficulty with basic daily activities such as sitting, standing, and walking. Management goals are to improve the patient's ability to perform basic daily activities, reduce disability, and permit the patient to advance in his or her rehabilitation. Patients judged to be in the acute stage are assigned to a classification, which guides the initial intervention. Patients judged to be in a more chronic stage are treated with a conditioning program designed to improve strength, flexibility, and conditioning, or with a work-reconditioning program.[65]

Seven classifications are described for patients in the acute stage:[65]

1. Immobilization
2. Lumbar mobilization
3. Sacroiliac mobilization
4. Extension syndrome
5. Flexion syndrome
6. Lateral shift
7. Traction

Each of the classifications is associated with key examination findings and recommended interventions. To facilitate comparisons among classifications, these seven classifications may be collapsed further into four classifications based on similarities in the prescribed interventions:

1. Immobilization
2. Mobilization (either sacroiliac or lumbar)
3. Specific exercise (flexion, extension, or lateral shift correction)
4. Traction

The immobilization classification is purported to identify patients with lumbar segmental instability. Key examination findings are gathered primarily during history-taking and include a history of frequent episodes of symptoms precipitated by minimal perturbations, frequent use of manipulation with short-term relief of symptoms, trauma, or reduced symptoms with the prior use of a corset.[65] Many of these findings have been proposed in the literature to indicate possibly lumbar segmental instability.[76–78] Physical examination findings may include aberrant movements during lumbar flexion (i.e., an "instability catch")[78,79] or generalized ligamentous laxity.[80] Intervention focuses on strengthening exercises for the back extensor and abdominal exercises,[81] as well as stabilization exercises designed to improve dynamic control of the lumbar spine.[82]

The mobilization classification includes patients believed to have indications for either sacroiliac or lumbar region mobilization or manipulation. Sacroiliac region mobilization is indicated by asymmetries of the pelvic landmarks (ASIS, posterior superior iliac spine [PSIS], and iliac crest) with the patient in the standing position and by positive results in three of four tests, as follows: (1) asymmetry of PSIS heights with the patient sitting, (2) the standing flexion test, (3) the prone-knee flexion test, and (4) the supine to long-sitting test. These tests are described in detail elsewhere.[83]

Acute-stage intervention involves a manipulation technique proposed to affect the sacroiliac joint region,[84] muscle energy techniques,[85] and range-of-motion exercises for the lumbosacral spine. Lumbar mobilization is indicated by the presence of (1) unilateral paraspinal pain in the lumbar region and (2) asymmetric amounts of lumbar side-bending range of motion with the patient standing in either an "opening" pattern (limited and painful flexion and side-flexion range of motion to the side opposite the pain) or a "closing" pattern (limited and painful extension and side-flexion range of motion to the same side as the pain). The intervention consists of lumbar mobilization or manipulation techniques[86] and range-of-motion exercises for the lumbosacral spine.

The key examination finding that places patients into a specific exercise classification is the presence of centralization with movement of the lumbar spine.[66] Centralization, which occurs when the patient's pain or paresthesia is abolished or moves from the periphery toward the spine, has been linked to prognosis by other researchers.[87,88] When either lumbar flexion or extension is found to produce centralization, the patient is treated with specific exercises in the direction producing the centralization. Patients also are educated to avoid positions that are found to peripheralize symptoms during examination.

The primary examination findings that lead to a classification of a lateral shift, in which the shoulders are offset from the pelvis in the frontal plane,[66,89,90] are a visible frontal plane deformity and asymmetric side-flexion range of motion when standing. If correction of the deformity produces centralization, the patient is taught specific exercises designed to correct the lateral shift (i.e., pelvic translocation).[66]

The traction classification is reserved for patients with signs and symptoms of nerve root compression who are unable to centralize with any lumbar movements. The acute-stage intervention involves the use of mechanical or autotraction[91] in an attempt to produce centralization.

Although these classifications may have some prognostic value, their ability to direct clinicians to specific interventions that improve outcomes has not been established.[92] The danger of relying on a classification system is that it does not afford patients the benefit of individualized interventions, nor is there any attempt by the clinician to isolate the cause of the problem. In addition, although one study by McKenzie demonstrated a reduction in recurrence through prophylactic advice,[93] most of the classification systems fail to focus sufficiently on prevention.

REVIEW QUESTIONS

1. Using Sapega's 0–5 grading scale, how would you grade a muscle that could complete its range of motion against gravity and with minimal resistance?
2. What position must a muscle be placed in to obtain its strongest contraction?
3. List five diagnoses that should be detected in the biomechanical examination?
4. What is the purpose of the PPIVM test?
5. What is the purpose of the PPAIVM test?
6. What is the purpose of a screening test?

ANSWERS

1. 3+.
2. Fully lengthened.
3. Possible answers include visceral pathology, fracture, pathologic space-occupying impairments, treatable and nontreatable neurologic pathology, spondylolisthesis, and ankylosing spondylitis.
4. To assess the passive physiologic intervertebral mobility of a joint, and its end feel.
5. To determine whether the reduced motion of a joint is a result of an articular or extra-articular impairment by assessing the joint glides or accessory motions of each joint.
6. The purpose of screening tests is to rapidly assess the likelihood that a joint, or group of joints, is impaired and require more detailed biomechanical testing.

REFERENCES

1. Meadows JTS. The principles of the Canadian approach to the lumbar dysfunction patient. In: *Management of Lumbar Spine Dysfunction.* APTA Independent Home Study Course, Orthopedic section APTA, inc.; 1999.
2. Rothstein J, ed. Guide to physical therapist practice. Phys Ther (Suppl) 1997;77:1163–1650.
3. Meadows JTS. *Orthopedic Differential Diagnosis in Physical Therapy.* New York, NY: McGraw-Hill; 1999.
4. Meadows JTS. *Manual Therapy: Biomechanical Assessment and Treatment, Advanced Technique.* Lecture and video supplemental manual, Swodeam Consulting Calgary, Alberta; 1995.
5. Greenman PE. *Principles of Manual Medicine.* Baltimore, Md: Williams & Wilkins; 1989.
6. Mitchell F, Moran PS, Pruzzo NA. *An Evaluation and Treatment Manual of Osteopathic Muscle Energy Procedures,* Manchester, MO; 1979.
7. Hertling D, Kessler RM. *Management of Common Musculoskeletal Disorders,* 2nd ed. Philadelphia, Pa: JB Lippincott; 1983.
8. Cyriax J. *Textbook of Orthopedic Medicine,* vol 1, 8th ed. London, England: Balliere Tindall and Cassell; 1982.
9. Stonebrink RD. *Evaluation and Manipulative Management of Common Musculo-Skeletal Disorders.* Portand, Ore: Western States Chiropractic College; 1990.
10. Jull GA, Janda V. Muscle and motor control in low back pain. In: Twomey LT, Taylor JR, eds. *Physical Therapy of the Low Back: Clinics in Physical Therapy.* New York, NY: Churchill Livingstone; 1987:259–276.
11. Sapega AA. Muscle performance evaluation in orthopedic practice. J Bone Joint Surg [Am] 1990;72: 1562–1574.
12. Janda V. *Muscle Function Testing.* London, England: Butterworths; 1983:2–223.
13. Kendall FP, McCreary EK, Provance PG. *Muscles Testing and Function,* 4th ed. Baltimore, Md: Williams & Wilkins; 1993.
14. Goldstein TS. *Functional Rehabilitation in Orthopedics.* Gaithersburg, Md: Aspen; 1995:19–23.
15. Convery FR, Minteer MA, Amiel D, Connett KL. Polyarticular disability: A functional assessment. Arch Phys Med Rehab 1977;58:498.
16. Rowe CR. *The Shoulder.* Edinburgh, Scotland: Churchill Livingstone; 1988:362.
17. Carroll D. A quantitative test of upper extremity function J Chron Dis 1965;18:482.
18. Potvin AR, Tourtellotte WW, Dailey JS, et al. Simulated activities of daily living examination. Arch Phys Med Rehab 1972;53:478.
19. Nachemson A. Work for all. For those with low back pain as well. Clin Orthop 1982;179:77.

20. Woolbright JL. Exercise protocol for patients with low back pain. J Am Osteopath Assoc 1983;82:919.

21. McKenzie RA. *The Lumbar Spine. Mechanical Diagnosis and Therapy*. Waikanae, New Zealand: Spinal Publications; 1981.

22. Davies JE, Gibson T, Tester L. The value of exercise in the treatment of low back pain. Rheumatol Rehabil 1979;18:243.

23. Jackson CP, Brown MD. Is there a role for exercise in the treatment of low back pain? Clin Orthop 1983;179:39.

24. Godman CC, Snyder TEK. *Differential Diagnosis in Physical Therapy*. Philadelphia, Pa: WB Saunders; 1990:10–13.

25. Darnell MW. A proposed chronology of events for forward head posture. J Craniomandib Prac 1983;1: 49–54.

26. Kisner C, Colby LA. *Therapeutic Exercise: Foundations and Techniques*. Philadelphia, Pa: FA Davis; 1985.

27. Mannheimer JS. Prevention and restoration of abnormal upper quarter posture. In: Gelb H, Gelb M, eds. *Postural Considerations in the Diagnosis and Treatment of Cranio-Cervical-Mandibular and Related Chronic Pain Disorders*. St Louis, Mo: Ishiyaku EuroAmerica; 1991: 93–161.

28. Bailey M, Dick L. Nocioceptive considerations in treating with counterstrain. J Am Osteopath Assoc 1992; 92:334–341.

29. Janda V. In: Grant R, ed. *Physical Therapy of the Cervical and Thoracic Spine*. New York, NY: Churchill Livingstone; 1988.

30. Sahrmann S. *Diagnosis and Treatment of Movement Impairment Syndromes*. St Louis, Mo: Mosby Year Book; 2001.

31. White SG, Sahrmann SA. A movement system balance approach to management of musculoskeletal pain. In: Grant R, ed. *Physical Therapy of the Cervical and Thoracic Spine*, 2nd ed. Clinics in Physical Therapy. New York, NY: Churchill Livingstone; 1988.

32. Tardieu C, Tabary JC, Tardieu G, et al. Adaptation of sarcomere numbers to the length imposed on muscle. In: Guba F, Marechal G, Takacs O, eds. *Mechanism of Muscle Adaptation to Functional Requirements*. Elmsford, NY: Pergamon Press; 1981:99.

33. Janda V. Muscles, motor regulation and back problems. In: Korr IM, ed. *The Neurological Mechanisms in Manipulative Therapy*. New York, NY: Plenum; 1978:27.

34. Janda V. Muscle weakness and inhibition in back pain syndromes. In: Grieve G, ed. *Modern Manual Therapy of the Vertebral Column*. London, England: Churchill Livingstone; 1985.

35. Langrana NA, Lee CK, Alendar H, Maycott CW. Quantitative assessment of back strength using isokinetic testing. Spine 1984;9:287.

36. Hasue M, Fujiwara M, Kikuchi S. A new method of quantitative measurement of abdominal and back muscle strength. Spine 1980;5:143.

37. Suzuki N, Endo S. A quantitative study of trunk muscle strength and fatigability in the low back pain syndrome. Spine 1983;8:69.

38. Triano J, Schultz AB. Correlation of objective measure of trunk motion and muscle function with low back disability ratings. Spine 1987;12:561.

39. Biering-Sorensen F. Physical measurements as risk factors for low back trouble over a one year period. Spine 1984;9:106.

40. Richardson C. The role of knee musculature in high speed oscillatory movements of the knee. Proc IV Biennial Conf Manip Ther Assoc Aust Brisbane 1985; 59.

41. Janda V. Comparison of spastic syndromes of cerebral origin with the distribution of muscular tightness in postural defects. Rehabilitacia Supp 1977; 14–15:87.

42. Horal J. The clinical appearance of low back disorders in the city of Gothenburg, Sweden. Acta Orthop Scand Suppl 1969;118:15.

43. Korr I. Somatic dysfunction, osteopathic manipulative treatment, and the nervous system. J Am Osteopath Assoc 1986;86:109–114.

44. Bannister R. *Brains Clinical Neurology*, 64th ed. London, England: Oxford University Press; 1985.

46. Opila KA, Wagner SS, Schiowitz S, Chen J. Postural alignment in barefoot and high heeled stance. Spine 1988;13:542–547.

47. Kendall FP, McCreary EK. *Muscles: Testing and Function*. Baltimore, Md: Williams & Wilkins; 1983.

48. Brügger A. Die Funktionskrankheiten des Bewegungsapparates. Funktionskrankheiton des Bewegungsapparates. 1986;1:69–129.

49. Silverstolpe L. A pathological erector spinae reflex—a new sign of mechanical pelvic dysfunction. J Manual Med 1989;4:28.

50. Bourliere F. The assessment of biological age in man. WHO, Public Health Papers 37, Geneva; 1979.

51. Janda V. *Muscle Function Testing*. London, England: Butterworths; 1983:163–167.

52. Pettman E. *Level III Course Notes*. Portland, Ore: North American Institute of Orthopedic Manual Therapy; 1990.

53. Troyanovich SJ, Harrison DE, Harrison DD. Structural rehabilitation of the spine and posture: Rationale for treatment beyond the resolution of symptoms. J Manipulative Phys Ther 1998;21:37–50.

54. Peat M, Grahame RE. Electromyographic analysis of soft tissue lesions affecting shoulder function. Am J Phys Med 1977;56:223–240.

55. Eliot DJ. Electromyography of levator scapulae: New findings allow tests of a head stabilization model. J Manipulative Phys Ther 1996;19:19–25.

56. Paine RM, Voight M. The role of the scapula. J Orthop Sports Phys Ther 1993;18:386–391.

57. Kaigle AM, Holm SH, Hansson TH. Experimental instability of the lumbar spine. Spine 1995;20:421–430.

58. Panjabi M, Abumi K, Durenceau J, Oxland T. Spinal stability and intersegmental muscle forces: A biomechanical model. Spine 1989;14:194–200.

59. Panjabi MM, Lyons C, Vasavada A, et al. On the understanding of clinical instability. Spine 1994;19:2642–2650.

60. Lewitt K. *Manipulative Therapy in Rehabilitation of the Motor System.* London, England: Butterworths; 1985.

61. Fritz JM, George S. The use of a classification approach to identify subgroups of patients with acute low back pain. Interrater reliability and short-term treatment outcomes. Spine 2000;25:106–114.

62. van Tulder MW, Koes BW, Bouter LM. Conservative treatment of acute and chronic nonspecific low back pain: A systematic review of randomized controlled trials of the most common interventions. Spine 1997;22:2128–2156.

63. Leboeuf-Yde C, Lauritsen JM, Lauritzen T. Why has the search for causes of low back pain largely been nonconclusive? Spine 1997;22:877–881.

64. Rose SJ. Physical therapy diagnosis: Role and function. Phys Ther 1989;69:535–537.

65. Delitto A, Erhard RE, Bowling RW. A treatment-based classification approach to low back syndrome: Identifying and staging patients for conservative management. Phys Ther 1995;75:470–489.

66. McKenzie RA. *The Lumbar Spine: Mechanical Diagnosis and Therapy.* Waikanae, New Zealand: Spinal Publications Limited; 1981.

67. Spitzer WO. Approach to the problem. In: Scientific approach to the assessment and management of activity-related spinal disorders: A monograph for clinicians. Spine 1987;12(suppl):9–11.

68. Bernard TN, Kirkaldy-Willis WH. Recognizing specific characteristics of nonspecific low back pain. Clin Orthop 1987;217:266–280.

69. Mooney V. The syndromes of low back disease. Orthop Clin North Am 1983;14:505–515.

70. Abenhaim L, Rossignol M, Gobeille D, Bonvalot Y, Fines P, Scott S. The prognostic consequences in the making of the initial medical diagnosis of work-related back injuries. Spine 1995;20:791–795.

71. Bigos S, Bowyer O, Braen G, et al. Acute low back problems in adults. AHCPR Publication 95-0642. Rockville, Md: Agency for Health Care Policy and Research, Public Health Service, US Department of Health and Human Services; 1994.

72. Von Korff M. Studying the natural history of back pain. Spine 1994;19(suppl):S2041–2046.

73. Battie MC, Cherkin DC, Dunn R, Ciol MA, Wheeler KJ. Managing low back pain: Attitudes and treatment preferences of physical therapists. Phys Ther 1994;74:219–226.

74. Stankovic R, Johnell O. Conservative management of acute low back pain. A prospective randomized trial: McKenzie method of treatment versus patient education in "mini back school." Spine 1990;15:120–123.

75. Donelson R. The McKenzie approach to evaluating and treating low back pain. Orthop Rev 1990;19:681–686.

76. Frymoyer JW, Akeson W, Brandt K, Goldenberg D, Spencer D. Clinical perspectives. In: Frymoyer JW, Gordon S, eds. *New Perspectives on Low Back Pain.* Rosemont, Ill: American Academy of Orthopaedic Surgeons; 1989:217–248.

77. Kirkaldy-Willis WH, Farfan HF. Instability of the lumbar spine. Clin Orthop 1982;165:110–123.

78. Pope MH, Frymoyer JW, Krag MH. Diagnosing instability. Clin Orthop 1992;279:60–67.

79. Ogon M, Bender BR, Hooper DM, et al. A dynamic approach to spinal instability: Part II. Hesitation and giving-way during interspinal motion. Spine 1997;22:2859–2866.

80. Beighton PH, Solomon L, Soskolne C. Articular mobility in an African population. Ann Rheum Dis 1973;32:413–418.

81. McGill SM. Low back exercises: Evidence for improving exercise regimens. Phys Ther 1998;78:754–765.

82. O'Sullivan PB, Phyty GD, Twomey LT, Allison GT. Evaluation of specific stabilizing exercise in the treatment of chronic low back pain with radiologic diagnosis of spondylolysis or spondylolisthesis. Spine 1997;22:2959–2967.

83. Cibulka MT, Delitto A, Koldehoff R. Changes in innominate tilt after manipulation of the sacroiliac joint in patients with low back pain. Phys Ther 1988;68:1359–1363.

84. Erhard RE, Delitto A, Cibulka MT. Relative effectiveness of an extension program and a combined program of manipulation and flexion and extension exercises in patients with acute low back syndrome. Phys Ther 1994;74:1093–1100.

85. Mitchell FL, Moran PS, Pruzzo NA. *Evaluation and Treatment Manual of Osteopathic Muscle Energy Procedures.* Valley Park, Mo: Mitchell, Moran, and Pruzzo Associates; 1979.

86. Bourdillon JF, Day EA, Bookout MR. *Spinal Manipulation*, 5th ed. Oxford, England: Butterworth-Heinemann; 1992.

87. Donelson R, Silva G, Murphy K. Centralization phenomena: Its usefulness in evaluating and treating referred pain. Spine 1990;15:211–213.

88. Karas R, McIntosh G, Hall H, Wilson L, Melles T. The relationship between nonorganic signs and centralization of symptoms in the prediction of return to work for patients with low back pain. Phys Ther 1997;77:354–360.

89. Porter RW, Miller CG. Back pain and trunk list. Spine 1986;11:596–600.

90. Tenhula JA, Rose SJ, Delitto A. Association between direction of lateral lumbar shift, movement tests, and side of symptoms in patients with low back pain syndrome. Phys Ther 1990;70:480–486.

91. Natchev E. *A Manual on Autotraction*. Stockholm, Sweden: Folksam Scientific Council; 1984.

92. Bouter LM, van Tulder MW, Koes BW. Methodologic issues in low back pain research in primary care. Spine 1998;23:2014–2020.

93. McKenzie RA. Prophylaxis in recurrent low back pain. NZ Med J 1979;89:22.

CHAPTER TWELVE

DIRECT INTERVENTIONS

Chapter Objectives

At the completion of this chapter, the reader will be able to:

1. Define and describe the components of an intervention.
2. Describe the differences between, and principles behind, joint mobilizations and manipulation.
3. Apply active and passive techniques to a joint in any position using the correct grade, direction, and duration, and explain the mechanical and physiologic effects.
4. List the indications and contraindications for the manual techniques.
5. Understand the concepts behind muscle energy techniques and the effects of a facilitated segment.
6. Understand the principles behind deep transverse friction massage.
7. Understand the principles and rationale of myofascial release, shiatsu, and craniosacral therapy.
8. Describe the various electrotherapeutic modalities and physical agents, including cold, heat, ultrasound, shock-wave, microthermy, iontophoresis, and transcutaneous electrical nerve stimulation (TENS).
9. Describe the therapeutic effects of heat and cold.
10. List the five types of heat transfer.
11. Differentiate between iontophoresis and phonophoresis.
12. Define the similarities and differences between the various types of electrical stimulation.
13. Describe the differences between microthermy and short-wave diathermy.
14. List the various ions that can be used with iontophoresis, and the medications that can be used with phonophoresis.
15. List the indications and contraindications for each of the electrotherapeutic modalities and physical agents.

OVERVIEW

The term *episode of care* is used to describe all of the patient management activities conducted by the clinician from initial contact through discharge.[1] A typical episode of care is outlined in Figure 12–1.

The *Guide to Physical Therapist Practice*[1] defines an intervention as a "purposeful and skilled interaction." Each intervention that the clinician embarks upon should be approached with the intent of reducing pain to a sufficient level that the patient is able to actively participate in a program for strengthening, flexibility, endurance, and postural alignment, and to receive instructions on activities of daily living or work modification, or both.[1]

According to the *Guide to Physical Therapist Practice*, an intervention should encourage the functional independence of the patient, emphasize patient-related instructions, promote a proactive wellness-oriented lifestyle, and facilitate participation of the patient in the plan of care.[1] Three subcategories comprise an intervention:[1]

1. Coordination, communication, and documentation
2. Patient-client–related instruction
3. Direct intervention

This chapter focuses on the subcategory of direct intervention. Examples of direct interventions include manual therapy, therapeutic exercise, and the use of electrotherapeutic modalities and physical agents.

Direct interventions are selected, applied, or modified based on the data from the examination and evaluation, the diagnosis and prognosis, and the anticipated goals and desired outcomes for a particular patient.[1]

From the examination, the clinician needs to determine:

- The site of the impairment and the structure or structures involved.

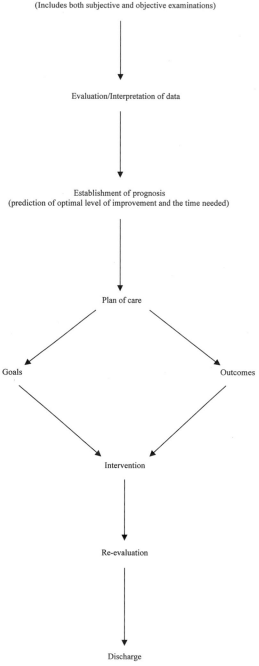

FIGURE 12-1 Episode of care.

TABLE 12-1 THE THREE STAGES OF HEALING

STAGE	GENERAL CHARACTERISTICS
Acute or inflammatory	The area is red, warm, swollen, and painful
	The pain is present without any motion of the involved area
	Usually lasts for 48–72 hours, but can be longer
Subacute or tissue formation	The pain usually occurs with the activity or motion of the involved area
	Usually lasts for 48 hours to 6 weeks[2]
Chronic or remodeling	The pain usually occurs after the activity
	Usually lasts from 3 weeks to 12 months

- The nature and cause of the impairment. Is the impairment a result of macrotrauma, microtrauma, disease, or immobilization?

The scan and biomechanical examinations, described in Chapters 10 and 11, guide the clinician toward a specific diagnosis and a specific plan of care. Once the injured structure has been identified, its stage of healing ascertained, and the reasons as to its presence determined, the clinician can decide which of the direct interventions are the most appropriate.

Pain of a spinal source is a major health problem in western industrialized countries and a major cause of medical expenses, work absenteeism, and disablement.[3] Although the pain is usually the result of a self-limiting and benign disease that tends to improve spontaneously over time,[4] a large variety of direct interventions are available for its management.[5] However, the effectiveness claimed for most of these interventions has not been convincingly demonstrated. This may be, in part, due to inaccurate diagnosis or to incorrect choice or application of the chosen intervention.

MANUAL THERAPY

Manual clinicians are highly competent in the use of specific mobilizations, not only of the spine but also of the peripheral joints.[6] A review of the work by Evjenth,[7] Kaltenborn,[8,9] and Maitland[10] and their use of specific and semispecific techniques illustrates this well. Kaltenborn, who derived much of his approach from the English osteopaths, has done much to promote the field of manual therapy. In association with Evjenth, he helped found the KE system of musculoskeletal management. This system,

- The extent of the pathologic process. How much damage has been inflicted on the structure(s)? This information is often elicited with resistive testing and stress testing as well as subjective reports on the mechanism of injury.
- The stage of healing for the injured structure(s) (Table 12-1).

which emphasizes the testing of intervertebral joint motion to assess the integrity of the joint complex, is used worldwide.[6] The techniques are based on the arthrokinematics of a joint, and introduce the concept of male (convex) and female (concave) joint surfaces. Maitland has made significant contributions in increasing the acceptability of controlled passive movements in the treatment of joint dysfunction.

Manipulations and mobilizations are quite distinct groupings of passive movement. A manipulation involves a high-velocity thrust of small amplitude performed at the limit of available movement to restore joint range. Mobilization involves repetitive passive movement of varying amplitudes of low velocity applied at different parts of the range, depending on the effects desired. Because of the variety of joint reactions over which they can be applied, mobilizations are a powerful group of techniques.

Joint Mobilizations

The techniques of joint mobilization are used to restore the physiologic articular relationship within a joint, and to decrease pain.[11] Additional benefits attributed to joint mobilizations include decreasing muscle guarding, lengthening the tissue around a joint, neuromuscular influences on muscle tone, and increased proprioceptive awareness.[12–14] There are three types:

1. Active, in which the patient exerts the force
2. Passive, in which the clinician exerts the force
3. Combined, in which the clinician and patient work together

To apply joint mobilizations, the components can be utilized in a variety of ways, depending on the method employed.

● *Direct method.* An engagement is made against a barrier in several planes.
● *Indirect method.* Maigne postulated "the concept of painless and opposite motion"[15] whereby disengagement from the barrier occurs and a balance of ligamentous tension is sought.
● *Combined method.* Disengagement is followed by direct retracement.

Joint mobilization techniques are advocated when there is a loss of the accessory motion that occurs at a joint during normal motion, secondary to capsular or ligamentous tightness or adhesions. Manual therapy uses biomechanical principles and should, therefore, only be performed on biomechanical problems. Biomechanical problems worsen in some positions and movements, improve in others, and

usually occur in predictive patterns. If one is not able to identify the behavior of the symptom in a biomechanical fashion, then that patient, at that point in time, is not a candidate for manual therapy.

A number of schools of thought have been put forward to address the concepts of increasing joint range of motion. In addition to Maigne's[15] concept of painless and opposite motion, whereby the direction of a manipulative maneuver is performed in the opposite direction to the motion restriction, Kaltenborn[16] introduced the Nordic program of manual therapy, which utilizes Cyriax's[17] method for evaluation and the specific osteopathic techniques of Mennell[18] for intervention. Further influence from Stoddard,[19] an osteopath, cemented the foundations of the Nordic system of manual therapy. Evjenth,[20] who had joined Kaltenborn's group, brought a greater emphasis on muscle stretching, strengthening, and coordination training. The philosophy of the Nordic system has been to integrate intervention tools from other approaches, and it has incorporated techniques from Rocabado, Kabat, Knott and Voss, McKenzie, and Maitland.[16]

The selection of the manual technique depends on the barrier to movement and the acuteness of the condition (see Table 11–2). Is the barrier to movement pain, muscle, capsule ligament, disturbed mechanics of the joint, or a combination? Muscle is usually the first barrier and is treated with light hold-relax techniques. Often some pain follows this, which is treated with grade III or IV oscillations.[21] As the pain is reduced, the real barrier to movement is approached. If this is periarticular tissue, then grade IV+ rhythmical oscillations are used to stretch the tissue, and if the joint is subluxed, then erratic, jerky grade III+ oscillations are applied.[21]

Whichever technique is employed to increase the range of motion at a joint, a number of further considerations help guide the clinician.

A. The patient and clinician should be relaxed.

B. The position of the joint to be treated must be appropriate for the stage of healing of the joint problem, and the skill of the operator. It is recommended that the resting position of the joint be used with an acute condition, or if the clinician is inexperienced. The resting position in this case refers to the position that the injured joint adopts, rather than the classic resting position for a normal joint. Other positions for starting the mobilization may be used by a skilled clinician in nonacute conditions.

C. One-half of the joint should be stabilized while the other half is mobilized. Both the stabilizing and mobilizing hands should be placed as close to the joint line

TABLE 12–2 COMMONLY COMPOUNDED CHEMICALS FOR IONTOPHORESIS

ION	POLARITY	SOLUTION	PURPOSE/CONDITION
Acetate	Neg	2%–5% acetic acid	Calcium deposits[194]
Atropine sulfate	Pos	0.001%–0.01%	Hyperhidrosis
Calcium	Pos	2% calcium chloride	Myopathy, muscle spasm
Chlorine	Neg	2% sodium chloride	Scar tissue, adhesions
Copper	Pos	2% copper sulfate	Fungus infection
Dexamethasone	Pos	4mg/mL dexamethasone Na-P	Tendonitis, bursitis[195]
Lidocaine	Pos	4% lidocaine	Trigeminal neuralgia[179]
Hyaluronidase	Pos	Wyadase	Edema[198]
Iodine	Neg	Iodex ointment	Adhesions, scar tissue[199]
Magnesium	Pos	2% magnesium sulfate (Epsom salts)	Muscle relaxant,[200] bursitis
Mecholyl	Pos	0.25%	Muscle relaxant
Potassium iodide	Neg	10%	Scar tissue
Salicylate	Neg	2% sodium salicylate	Myalgia, scar tissue
Tap water	Pos/Neg		Hyperhidrosis

Neg = negative; Pos = positive.

as possible. The other parts of the clinician involved in the mobilization should make maximum contact with the patient's body so as to spread the forces over a larger area and reduce pain from contact of bony prominences. The maximum contact also results in more stability and increased confidence from the patient. An alternative technique that produces the desired results must be sought if the contact between opposite sexes is uncomfortable to either the patient or clinician.

D. The direction of the mobilization is almost always parallel or perpendicular to a tangent across adjoining joint surfaces.

E. The mobilization should not move into or through the point of pain.

F. The velocity and amplitude of movement is carefully considered and is based on the goal of the intervention—to restore the joint motion, or to alleviate the pain, or both:
1. Slow stretches are used for large capsular restrictions.
2. Fast oscillations are used for minor restrictions.
3. Maitland's amplitude grades I and II are used solely for pain relief and have no direct mechanical effect on the restricting barrier, but do have a hydrodynamic effect.
4. Maitland's amplitude grades III and IV (or at least III+ and IV+) do stretch the barrier and have a mechanical, as well as a neurophysiologic effect. Grade III and IV have been further subdivided into III+ (++) and IV+ (++), indicating that once the end of the range has been reached, a further stretch to impart a mechanical force to the movement restriction is imparted.[21]

G. One movement is performed at a time, at one joint at a time.

H. Regular reassessment is performed.

I. Reeducation is essential after mobilization or manipulation and will often produce a noticeable reduction in post-treatment soreness. While the joint is maintained in the new range, five to six gentle isometric contractions are asked for from the agonists and antagonists of the motion mobilized.[21]

Mobilizations are indicated when:

- The pain is relieved by rest.
- The pain is relieved by activity.
- The pain is altered by postural changes.
- The pain is provoked by joint motion.

Intensity of the Intervention
Gentle intervention is indicated when the patient has:

- Constant, severe pain
- Extensive radiation
- Pain unrelieved by rest
- Pain that disturbs sleep
- Severe joint irritability (severe pain is easily stirred up, then lasts)
- Range limitation due to pain
- A motion that produces distal pain
- Isometric tests that are all positive
- Pain caused by cough or sneeze
- Severe postural or reactive spasm
- Severe joint range restriction
- Severe latent pain
- A recent neurologic deficit

Vigorous manual intervention is indicated in the receptive patient when he or she has:

- Moderate or mild pain
- A nonirritable condition demonstrated by no sleep disturbance
- Intermittent pain
- Pain relieved by rest
- Minimal radiation of pain
- No static or reactive spasm
- Range limited by resistance of soft tissue
- No recent neurologic deficit
- Radiation not caused by motion
- Negative findings with isometric tests

Indications and Contraindications

Contraindications specific to mobilizations include those that are absolute contraindications, and those that are relative.[22]

A. Absolute:
1. Neoplastic disease
2. Spinal cord or cauda equina involvement
3. Involvement of more than one cervical root or two adjacent roots
4. Tri-level lumbar root signs (rare)
5. Rheumatoid arthritis (cervical spine)
6. Acute inflammatory, infective, or septic arthritis
7. Bone disease
8. Nonmechanical causes (kidney disease)
9. Vertebral artery disease
10. Craniovertebral instability
11. Second lumbar root palsy (uncommon area; therefore, usually a serious pathology)
12. Sign of the buttock
13. Empty end feel
14. Fracture or dislocation
15. Acute rheumatoid episode
16. Psychological pain or marked overlay

B. Relative:
1. Joint effusion or inflammation
2. Acute arthrosis
3. Rheumatoid arthritis
4. Internal derangement
5. Presence of neurologic signs
6. Osteoporosis
7. Spondylolisthesis
8. Hypermobility
9. Pregnancy
10. Dizziness
11. Previous history of neoplastic disease
12. Steroid use
13. Cervical trauma

Manipulation

The term *manipulation* continues to breed controversy among the various schools of manual therapy, which have a long history of internecine and interprofessional rivalry. All of the groups that continue to perform manipulations are the extension of a long line of bone-setters going back to the earliest days of medicine.[23] Two major schools of manipulative therapy have evolved over the years—the chiropractic school and the osteopathic school. The other practitioners of manipulative therapy have had to rely on part or full-time study through sequential course. It is interesting to note that some of the earlier pioneers of manipulative therapy, such as Marlin,[24] Mennel,[25] and Cyriax,[17] were based in physiotherapy departments.

A manipulation is essentially a mobilization with impulse, with the impulse being high velocity and low amplitude in nature. In place of the term *manipulation*, the term *thrust* is often used. The high velocity is used so that the muscles do not have time to contract and prevent the motion. The low amplitude is of paramount importance and ensures that the forces induced to the joint are kept to a minimum.

Indications

As with mobilizations, manipulative techniques can be direct or indirect, with the direct techniques used for locating and addressing the barrier, and the indirect techniques for those cases in which the joint is taken away from the barrier. The detection of abnormalities in joint movement and muscle tension requires trained hands. As manipulation is used to restore joint range, the practicing clinician must have a knowledge of the normal range of motion. Manipulation can be used for the following purposes:[6]

- Releasing minor adhesions
- Altering the position of an intra-articular loose body
- Reducing a displaced articular meniscoid
- Reducing discrete muscle spasm by affecting the input through the gamma (γ) loop system[26]

It should be remembered that although thrust techniques can be used to treat most joint dysfunctions, there are risks associated with their use, especially in the craniovertebral region. The thrust technique should be viewed as another tool at the clinician's disposal and used appropriately.

Mobilizations, or manipulations are unlikely to be of benefit when:

- A neurologic deficit is present.
- There are no local symptoms (negative back pain).
- Lumbar side-flexion is positive to the side of pain (compression pain in extremity)—radiculopathy is present.

- Distal pain is reproduced with spinal range of motion.
- There is a springy end feel.
- There is paresthesia without pain.
- There is a primary posterior-lateral disc protrusion (leg pain, no back pain).

The most difficult aspect of joint mobilizations is the skill of gaining a feel for the appropriate rate, rhythm, and intensity of movement required to administer the intervention. All of the techniques must be adjusted according to the intervention goals and the presentation of the patient's condition.

Muscle Energy Technique

Muscle energy techniques, which utilize the principles of proprioceptive neuromuscular facilitation to increase joint motions, have become very popular in recent years.[27,28] Muscle energy techniques were first developed by Drs. Fred Mitchell Sr.[29] and Jr. and then by Dr. Ed Stiles. Some of these techniques appear in this book in the various chapters devoted to the spine, and what follows is a brief overview to describe the principles on which these techniques are based.

Muscle energy techniques are used when the limit to motion has been determined to be the neuromuscular system. Muscles both produce and control motion. Although it is obvious that muscles produce motion, it is easy to forget that they also resist motion. This resistance to motion is related to muscle tone,[30] a complex neurophysiologic state administered by both cortical and spinal reflexes. Resting muscle tone is modified by the afferent activity from the articular and muscle systems. Afferent input from the type I and II mechanoreceptors located in the superficial and deep aspects of the joint capsule is projected to the γ motor neurons.[31]

According to Korr, an excessive γ motor neuron to the muscle spindle requires less external stretch to fire the primary annulospiral ending, which reflexly fires the extrafusal muscle fiber via the alpha (α) motor neuron.[31] The exaggerated spindle responses are provoked by motions that lengthen the facilitated muscle, creating a restrictive spinal fault. Put simply, the effect of this excitation on the muscle is an increase in resistance to any motion that attempts to lengthen that muscle. Impairment occurs when abnormal or excessive afferent input maintains a state of constant increased excitation at the spinal cord, a state commonly referred to as a *facilitated segment* (refer to Chapter 4). This concept was first proposed by Korr[31] and then integrated with the work of Patterson[32] and Sherrington[33] on spinal reflexes.

The proposed function of muscle energy techniques is to restore the segment to its normal neurophysiologic state. Whereas joint mobilizations are passive techniques in so much as the patient is positioned and instructed to relax while the clinician carries out the technique, muscle energy techniques require the active participation of the patient and can be viewed as a mobilization technique that utilizes muscular facilitation and inhibition.[34] They are likened to proprioceptive neuromuscular facilitation (PNF) techniques,[27] but they employ submaximal rather than maximal contractions.

Muscle energy techniques for joint mobilizations are generally gentle, and the concepts are employed in both the extremities and the spine. The slack of the joint is taken up and the patient is asked to perform a submaximal isometric contraction. The direction of the patient's contraction is precisely controlled, at varying levels of intensity, against a distinctly executed counterforce applied by the clinician.[35] The voluntary control of muscle by the patient is only as efficient as the individual's neuromuscular coordination. Kabat[36] states that "Repeated excitation of a pathway in the central nervous system results in a gradual ease of transmission of nerve impulses through that pathway. This is brought about by a decrease in synaptic resistance and is the basis for the formation of habits and for learning. An impairment in and around a joint produces abnormal motion patterns. These abnormal motion patterns, if repeated often enough, become learned patterns."

The clinician's role is to help retrain normal movement patterns, guiding the patient as to the direction and force applied. A number of techniques can be employed to produce an increase in range due to muscle relaxation. Two types are well recognized and are differentiated by the verbal commands used, and the type of muscle contraction employed by the patient:[37]

Contract-Relax[27]

This technique uses a combination of both concentric or maintained contraction of the antagonist muscle(s), to change the length of a muscle, or muscles when the restriction is one of tightness of the muscle. The agonist muscle is the muscle that contracts to produce a joint motion that is referred to as the *agonist pattern*. The antagonist muscles are the ones that stretch to allow the agonist pattern to occur.

The contract-relax technique is effective in passively moving the body part into the agonist pattern when pain does not accompany, or is not the primary cause of, the restriction in range. In other words, this is the technique of choice when muscle tightness rather than pain is the limit to motion. At the point of limitation of the available range of motion, an isotonic/isometric contraction of the antagonist is performed by the patient against the clinician's resistance by utilizing the antagonist muscle or muscles. The isometric/isotonic contraction is held for up to 5 seconds, after which the patient is instructed to completely relax. The direction of the applied resistance is determined by the neurophysiologic effect desired from the technique. In contrast to hold-relax, the motion gains are greater on two joint muscles using the contract-relax technique in normal subjects.[38]

A contract-relax technique applies the principles of autogenic inhibition.[33] Autogenic inhibition is defined as an inhibition mediated by afferent fibers from a stretched muscle acting on the motor neurons supplying that muscle, thus causing it to relax. Autogenic inhibition appears to function to prevent muscle injury from reflex contractions resulting from an aggressive stretch.[13]

Hold-Relax[27]

This technique involves an isometric contraction of the agonist muscle against resistance. It is an effective technique when pain either accompanies, or is the primary cause of, the restriction in range, or when there is increased tension within the muscle. At the point of limitation of the available range of motion, an isometric contraction of all of the components of the range-limiting, or agonistic, pattern is elicited. The patient is asked to hold the joint in the same position while an isometric contraction is gradually maximized over a period of seconds before the patient is asked to relax. The direction of the applied resistance is determined by the neurophysiologic effect desired from the technique. The shortened muscle is maximally stretched in the immediate postcontraction relaxation phase.

A hold-relax technique relies on the reciprocal inhibition[33] of the antagonist muscle or muscles. Theoretically, a contraction or extended stretch of the agonist muscle must elicit a relaxation, or an inhibition of the antagonist.[39] Similarly, a quick stretch of the antagonist muscle facilitates a contraction of the agonist.

Transverse Friction Massage[40]

While general massage may provide temporary pain relief, probably through the stimulation of the large A-α fibers, as previously discussed, it does not contribute to the long-term relief of pain. Transverse friction massage can be used to provide short-term pain relief, but its main function is to restore the mobility of the various tissues and increase the extensibility of individual structures. Friction massage is mainly indicated for chronic conditions involving muscles, tendons, and ligaments, such as tendinitis and ligament sprains. There are a number of proposed effects of this type of massage, which include traumatic hyperemia and stimulation of mechanoreceptors.

Traumatic Hyperemia

The increased blood flow from the massage reduces pain by removing the products of inflammation, including chemical irritants such as prostaglandin E, potassium, histamine. In addition, the increased blood flow reduces venous congestion and so decreases the hydrostatic pressure, which can cause mechanoreceptor pain.

Mechanical Stimulation

Type I and II mechanoreceptors are stimulated, and so help reduce pain. However, if the frictions are too vigorous, the stimulation of the nociceptors will override the effect of the mechanoreceptors, and so pain will increase.

The movement of the tissue over the underlying bone or tissue helps prevent adhesion formation between the tissue and its neighbors, minimizing cross-linking and enhancing the extensibility of the new tissue. In addition, the transverse nature of the friction assists the orientation of the collagen along the appropriate lines of stress, especially if the structure is stretched immediately after the massage.

Indications

● Acute or subacute partial tears of ligament, tendon, or muscle
● Adhesions in ligament or muscle or between tissues
● Premanipulation

Contraindications

● Hyperacute inflammation
● Recent (within 3 days) hematoma
● Arterial insufficiency
● Patients with bleeding conditions, such as hemophiliacs, and individuals on long-term systemic steroids or anticoagulants
● History of multiple injections of cortisone into the tissue
● Debilitated or open skin
● Patients with compromised skin sensation

Application

The tissue should, whenever possible, be put on a moderate, but not painful stretch. No lubricant is used. Beginning with light pressure, the clinician moves the skin over the site of the impairment back and forth in a direction perpendicular to the normal orientation of its fibers. The patient's skin must move along with the clinician's finger or blistering will occur. Although some degree of discomfort should be expected with transverse friction, the patient's tolerance should be built up gradually over a few minutes. The amplitude should be sufficient to cover all of the affected tissue, and the pressure is dependent on the intensity of the inflammatory process. The rate should be at two to three cycles per second applied in a rhythmic manner. The time length of the frictions is usually gauged by desensitization, which normally occurs within 2 minutes. If the condition is chronic, then frictions continue for some time after this as the mechanical effect on the cross-links and adhesions is required.

The application is condition and patient dependent. For very acute conditions in which the aim is to stimulate the mechanoreceptors, pressure is minimal whereas the amplitude will be as large as tolerated. Most conditions should resolve in six to ten sessions over a 2- or 3-week period.

Intervention Reactions

- *Rapid desensitization.* This occurs if the frictions are given to normal tissues.
- *Expected desensitization.* This occurs if the condition is appropriate and the frictions are correctly applied. Pain relief is present unless further excessive strain is applied.
- *No desensitization.* If desensitization does not occur within 3 minutes: (1) the frictions are being applied incorrectly, or (2) the condition is inappropriate, or (3) the tissue is part of a facilitated segment syndrome.

Myofascial Therapy

In the late 1970s, Stephen Levin, an orthopedic surgeon, introduced a model for the structure of organic tissue that could account for many physical and clinical characteristics. Through a process of systematic examination of the basic physical properties of tissue, he arrived at the conclusion that all organic tissue must be composed of a type of truss (triangular form) and that the essential building block of all tissue must be the tension icosohedron. This model, also referred to as the tensegrity model and the myofascial skeletal truss, has gradually emerged as a viable explanation for the nature of organic tissue.[41a] Recently, this model has been confirmed by electron-microscopic methods and through physical stress extrapolation experiments. This model accounts for the concept of the kinetic chain, which recognizes that impairments transmit tensions throughout the body and that symptoms can be traced back to their source and treated indirectly by aligning fascial lines of force in relation to the primary focus of restriction.

The implications of Levin's model, from a clinical perspective, are that all tissues share certain fundamental characteristics at the molecular and ultrastructural level. The tensegrity model proposes that the body is a functional unit, in that forces applied to it at one point are transmitted uniformly and instantaneously throughout the entire organism.

This model implies that a perceived condition in one area of the body may have its origin in another area and that therapeutic action at the source of the impairment will have an immediate, corrective effect on all secondary areas, including the site of symptom manifestation.

Fringe Manual Therapies

Although the term *fringe* raises images of quackery, it is not the intention of this section to critique the usefulness of the philosophies and techniques discussed. It is true that all of the disciplines within this section have yet to be validated; however, they are included for informational reasons rather than as recommendations.

Shiatsu[41]

Shiatsu is an ancient form of Japanese therapy that involves manual pressure over the body's acupuncture points. Acupuncture, one of the oldest forms of therapy, has its roots in ancient Chinese philosophy. Traditional Chinese medicine is based on a number of philosophical concepts, where manifestation of disease is considered a sign of imbalance between the yin and yang forces in the body. In classical acupuncture theory, it is believed that all disorders are reflected at specific points either on the skin surface or just beneath it. Vital energy circulates throughout the body along the so-called meridians, which have either yin or yang characteristics. A correct choice for needling among the 361 classical acupuncture points located on these meridians is believed to restore the balance in the body.

When manual pressure is applied successfully at these points, the patient is supposed to experience a sensation known as *teh chi*, defined as a subjective feeling of fullness, numbness, tingling, and warmth, with some local soreness and a feeling of distention around the acupuncture point.

In recent decades, new forms of acupressure have developed such as ear (auricular) acupuncture, head (scalp) acupuncture, hand acupuncture, and foot acupressure.[42] Modern acupressurists use not only traditional meridian acupuncture points, but also nonmeridian or extrameridian acupuncture points, which are fixed points not necessarily associated with meridians. Acupressurists also use trigger points, which have no fixed locations and are found by eliciting tenderness at the site of most pain.

It is still not clear what exact mechanisms underlie the action of acupressure. According to traditional Chinese medicine, acupuncture promotes the flow of *qi* (life force energy), thereby balancing the human body system.

Western scientific research has proposed mechanisms for the effect of acupuncture in relieving pain. It has been suggested that acupuncture might act according to principles enunciated by the gate control theory of pain.[43,44] One type of sensory input (low back pain) could be inhibited in the central nervous system by another type of input (pressure). Another theory, diffuse noxious inhibitory control (DNIC), implies that noxious stimulation of heterotopic body areas modulates the pain sensation originating in areas where a subject feels pain. There also is some evidence that acupressure may stimulate the production of endorphins, serotonin, and acetylcholine in the central nervous system, enhancing analgesia.[45,46]

Craniosacral Therapy[47]

Cranial osteopathy and craniosacral therapy are in widespread use today by a number of physical therapists, osteopathic physicians, chiropractors, and other health and wellness providers, both in the United States and abroad,[48,49] and continuing education advertisements under this name are often seen in physical therapy–related publications.[50]

Core to cranial osteopathy is the belief that the cranial vault is a mobile, compliant structure. The originator of this approach is Dr. William G. Sutherland, DO. Within cranial osteopathic circles is the well-known story of a young Dr. Sutherland who, as a medical student at the turn of this century, walked past an exhibit of a disarticulated skull and observed the greater wings of the sphenoid bone. His mind compared these wings to the gill plates of fish, and he wondered if perhaps the skull bones were not mobile and involved in some sort of respiratory process. Twenty years later, this concept of cranial bone motion still nagged at him and he began self-experimenting using a helmet made of leather and thumbscrews. From this initial self-experimentation to later successes in the clinic, the practice of cranial osteopathy was conceived. Based on Dr. Sutherland's theories of cranial bone motion, cranial osteopathy represented a systematic approach to examination and intervention.

More recently, craniosacral therapy has been utilized as a method for evaluating and treating patients. Founded by Dr. John E. Upledger, DO,[50] in the 1970s, craniosacral therapy shares with cranial osteopathy a common theoretical belief in cranial bone motion. Practitioners of craniosacral therapy suggest that periodic fluctuations in cerebrospinal fluid pressure give rise to rhythmic motion of the cranial bones and sacrum. This rhythm is called the craniosacral rhythm. Craniosacral therapists suggest that by applying selective pressure to the cranial bones, they can manipulate the craniosacral rhythm to achieve a therapeutic outcome in their patients.

Little research has been done on cranial bone motion, and agreement about even its existence remains controversial. Though there is more to cranial osteopathic and craniosacral therapy theory than cranial bone motion, without this motion, much of the rationale and many clinical techniques are invalidated.

Irrespective of whether the cranial bones move, the provocation of symptoms from these movements has yet to be proven. The movements that have been measured are very small, and it is difficult to see how these movements can have a widespread influence, if at all. However, being a gentle, hands-on manual therapy, the potential risks of craniosacral therapy can be easily assessed and controlled by judicious application,[47,50] as with many other things we do as therapists. The benefit-to-risk ratio of using craniosacral therapy certainly warrants comparing it with mainstream interventions.

THERAPEUTIC EXERCISE

Therapeutic exercise, including aerobic conditioning, should be the cornerstone of the direct intervention. According to the *Guide to Physical Therapist Practice*:

> Therapeutic exercise includes a broad group of activities intended to improve strength, range of motion (including muscle length), endurance, breathing, balance, coordination, posture, motor function (motor control and motor learning), motor development, or confidence when any of a variety of problems constrains the ability to perform a functional activity. Therapeutic exercise is performed actively, passively, or against resistance. Resistance may be provided manually, by gravity, or through use of a weighted apparatus or of mechanical or electromechanical devices.[1]

Pain does not have to be abolished for the individual to exercise. With decreased pain, however, the individual can exercise and function more easily. Tissues are not consistently reactive throughout the day,[51,52] presenting the challenge that exercises need not only be carefully chosen but that some consideration needs to be given to the time of day when they are performed.

Modalities and agents can also be applied prior to exercise to prepare the muscle and joint for exercise, or after exercise to decrease pain and stiffness, and prevent an increase in swelling.

Purpose

Therapeutic exercises are used early in the rehabilitative process to:[53]

- Prevent or minimize muscle atrophy
- Prevent or minimize excessive scar formation

- Promote fluid movement in the injured area
- Promote activity to minimize fear avoidance behavior
- Restore proper pain-free function

A hierarchy exists for the range of motion and resistive exercises during the subacute (neovascularization) stage of healing to ensure that any progression is done in a safe and controlled fashion. The hierarchy for the range-of-motion exercises is:[53]

1. Passive range of motion
2. Active assisted range of motion
3. Active range of motion

The hierarchy for the resistive exercises is:[53]

1. Single angle, submaximal isometrics performed in the neutral position
2. Multiple angle, submaximal isometrics performed at various angles of the range
3. Multiple angle, maximal isometrics
4. Small arc, submaximal isotonics
5. Full range of motion, submaximal isotonics
6. Functional ranges of motion, submaximal isotonics

Gentle resistance exercises can be introduced very early in the rehabilitative process. Although some delayed-onset muscle soreness can be expected, sharp pain should not be provoked.

Range-of-Motion Exercises

The anticipated goals of range-of-motion exercises are to maintain or increase the mobility of the injured area, and to promote proper healing.

- *Passive range of motion.* By definition, passive range-of-motion exercises are mobilization techniques. The clinician, patient, or patient family member may perform the passive range-of-motion exercises. These exercises are used when the patient is not able, or not supposed to, actively move a segment or segments. All planes of motion of the treated joint are performed through a relatively pain-free range, using the end feel, and stage of healing, as a guide. Passive range-of-motion exercises do not prevent atrophy or increase the strength or endurance of a muscle.
- *Active assisted range of motion.* Once the patient can actively contract the muscles and move a segment with assistance, active assisted exercises are introduced. The clinician provides sufficient assistance to the muscles to aid in the motion desired.

- *Active range of motion.* Once the patient can actively contract the muscles, and move a segment without assistance, active exercises are introduced. All planes of motion should be performed. Active range-of-motion exercises do not maintain or increase strength in the larger muscles of the body.

Exercise Prescriptions

There has been a tendency over the years for clinicians to prescribe exercise programs using the three sets of 10 protocol and to have the patient perform an exercise based on a standard illustration. The exercise segment of the intervention cannot be overemphasized and should, therefore, be as specific as the manual technique used in the clinic. At regular intervals, the clinician should ensure that:

- The patient is being compliant with their exercise program.
- The patient is aware of the rationale behind the home exercise program.
- The patient is performing the exercise program correctly and at the appropriate intensity.
- The patient's exercise program is being updated appropriately.

The therapeutic home exercise program should consist of a series of clear illustrations and accompanying descriptions that give details on the number of repetitions and sets of exercise that must be performed.

- *Repetitions.* This refers to the number of times an exercise is performed. As mentioned, the number 10 is often used. To be as specific as possible, the clinician must teach the patient to exercise to the point of substitution, at which point the exercise is completed. The point of substitution is referred to as the *repetition maximum.*
- *Sets.* This refers to the number of groups of a repetition maximum that are performed during each exercise session. Two to three sets to substitution are recommended.

ELECTROTHERAPEUTIC MODALITIES AND PHYSICAL AGENTS

Electrotherapeutic modalities and physical agents are specific interventions that involve the controlled application of thermal, mechanical, and electromagnetic energy to patients.

- Thermal agents include deep-heating agents, superficial heating agents, and superficial cooling agents.

- Mechanical agents include traction, compression, water, and sound.
- Electromagnetic agents include electromagnetic fields and electrical currents.[54]

Properly harnessed, these agents, or modalities, are powerful adjuncts to an intervention. All of them employ a transfer of energy from a source to a target, but each use different methods to make that transfer.

The electrotherapeutic modalities include biofeedback, electrical muscle stimulation, functional electrical stimulation (FES), neuromuscular electrical stimulation (NMES), transcutaneous electrical nerve stimulation (TENS), and iontophoresis.

The physical agents include athermal modalities (pulsed ultrasound), cryotherapy, deep thermal modalities (ultrasound, short-wave diathermy, microthermy, and phonophoresis), and superficial thermal modalities (hot packs, paraffin baths).

Cryotherapy

The therapeutic application of cold, or cryotherapy, removes heat from the body, producing a decrease in the temperature of body tissues. Cryotherapy is the most commonly used modality for the treatment of acute musculoskeletal injuries.[55–58] The physiologic effects of a local cold application include:

- Decreased blood flow through a reflex vasoconstriction in the cutaneous blood vessels.[59–61] If the tissue temperature reaches 10°C or lower, a cold-induced reflex vasodilation, known as the Hunting reaction is deemed to occur to prevent damage to local tissue caused by cold.[62] However, this reaction may just be a measurement artifact rather than an actual change in blood flow owing to the cold.[63]
- Direct smooth muscle contraction
- Decreased muscle spasm[64,65]
- Decreased cell metabolism[66–68] and cellular activity, which has the potential to decrease inflammation[55,69] through a decrease in the delivery of oxygen and chemical nutrients to the area, an important effect in the acute injury
- Increased tissue viscosity and resistance to movement[69]
- Synaptic inhibition of pain stimuli
- Reduction of nerve conduction velocity

The use of cryotherapy in the intervention of acute musculoskeletal injury has traditionally been based on metabolic inhibition and is described in the secondary injury model.[55,70] In the secondary injury model, the initial

trauma to a tissue is termed *primary injury*, whereas trauma that occurs subsequent to this primary injury is termed *secondary injury*. Secondary injury is thought to result from a period of post-trauma hypoxia (secondary hypoxic injury) and from post-trauma enzymatic activity (secondary enzymatic injury).[55,70] A recent study gave support to the existence of secondary injury in muscle tissue, and the hypothesis that cold can retard secondary injury when used to treat musculoskeletal injuries.[71]

Several methods of applying cryotherapy have been examined in different studies. The use of ice chips in toweling has been shown to be more effective in decreasing skin temperature than ice chips in plastic or cold gel packs.[72] Oosterveld and colleagues[73] demonstrated a significant decrease in the intra-articular knee temperature of normal subjects following a 30-minute ice chip application. Findings from another study[74] would seem to suggest that ice massage and ice bag are equally effective in decreasing intramuscular temperature, and in maintaining the duration of temperature depression, but that ice massage achieves maximal intramuscular temperature decreases sooner than the ice bag. The application of cold to an area is contraindicated in individuals with Raynaud's disease, cold sensitivity, areas with poor circulation or sensation, and over-healing wounds.[75]

Heat

There are five types of heat transfer that can occur with the body.

1. Convection: when a liquid or gas moves past a body part
2. Evaporation: when there is a change in state of a liquid to a gas and a resultant cooling takes place
3. Conversion: when one form of energy is converted into another form
4. Radiation: when there is a transmission and absorption of electromagnetic waves
5. Conduction: when heat is transferred between two objects that are in contact with each other

For a heat application to have a therapeutic effect, the amount of thermal energy transferred to the tissue must be sufficient to stimulate normal function without causing damage to the tissue.[76] Although the human body functions optimally between 36°C and 38°C, an applied temperature of 40°C and 45°C is considered effective for a heat treatment.

The physiologic effects of a local heat application include:

- Dissipation of the heat through selective vasodilation and shunting of blood via reflexes in the microcirculation

- Increased capillary permeability
- Increased cell metabolism and cellular activity, which has the potential to increase the delivery of oxygen and chemical nutrients to the area and decreasing venous stagnation
- Muscle relaxation, probably as a result of a sedative effect on the sensory nerves, decreasing neural excitability and, hence, γ input
- Increased tissue extensibility. This has obvious implications for the application of stretching techniques. The best results are obtained if heat is applied during the stretch, and if the stretch is maintained until cooling occurs after the heat has been removed.

Commercial hot packs or electric heating pads are a conductive type of superficial moist heat. The temperature of the unit is set anywhere between 65°C and 90°C. The moist heat pack causes an increase in the local tissue temperature, reaching its highest point about 8 minutes after the application.[77]

Wet heat produces a greater rise in local tissue temperature compared with dry heat at a similar temperature.[78] However, at higher temperatures, wet heat is not tolerated as well as dry heat.

Moist heat should not be applied to an area with decreased sensation, poor circulation, an open wound, or an acute injury.[75] The application of moist heat to an area of malignancy is also contraindicated because it can increase the temperature of the tumor and increase the rate of growth.[75]

Ultrasound[79]

The selection of a therapeutic heating modality should be based on the desired intervention goals. Superficial heat modalities penetrate tissue up to 1 cm in depth, whereas deep heating modalities penetrate tissue up to 5 cm in depth.[80–82] The most common clinically used deep heating modality to promote tissue healing is ultrasound.[83–85]

Ultrasound treatment involves the use of high-frequency sound waves (greater than 500 kHz) that are generated using the reverse piezoelectric effect to produce thermal and nonthermal effects in tissue.[86] This form of mechanical energy has applications in both diagnosis (see later) and intervention.[87] Therapeutic ultrasound produces thermal and mechanical changes within tissues in the ultrasound field.[87,88] The thermal effects are seen as deep heating in the tissue, whereas the mechanical effects of cavitation and protoplasmic streaming are noted. Cavitation, one of the more controversial effects associated with ultrasound, is the production of gas bubbles in the ultrasonic field that vibrate in resonant frequency with the ultrasound,[89] whereas protoplasmic streaming is the physical movement of protoplasm within the cell.[90–92] The

ultrasound energy must be absorbed by the tissues to produce physiologic changes. Protein-rich hydrophilic tissues, such as muscle, joint capsules, tendons, and extracapsular ligaments, are thought to readily absorb ultrasound energy.[85,93,94] It has been postulated that heating destabilizes intermolecular bonds at the tropocollagen level, thus making dense connective tissue less stiff.[95] However, skin surface contour, the mode of transmission, the dosage (intensity × treatment time), and the ultrasound frequency are the true determinants in the effectiveness of ultrasound treatment.[85,96,97]

Although increasing dense connective tissue extensibility by deep heating seems plausible, the concept has not been studied in vivo. Wessling and associates[98] demonstrated small but statistically significant increases in ankle dorsiflexion with stretching, and with "heat and stretch" (using continuous wattage ultrasound), the increase being greatest with heat and stretch.

The findings from another study suggested that the use of continuous wattage ultrasound made some knee ligaments slightly more extensible, thereby allowing increased joint displacement in the varus/valgus tests and the genu recurvatum tests.[99]

Frequency

Ultrasound frequencies in the megahertz (MHz) region are generally regarded as therapeutically useful.[100,101] At these frequencies, the penetration depth values are such that sufficient energy will reach deeply located tissue and be absorbed and converted there to heat at a suitably high rate.[102] Penetration depth values, and the absorption rate of energy (heat production), are closely related. A low penetration depth is associated with limited transmission of energy, with the rapid absorption of energy, and with a higher heating rate in a relatively limited tissue depth. A high penetration depth is associated with the efficient transmission of energy and with little absorption and, consequently, limited tissue heating. For ultrasound with a frequency of 1 MHz, muscle, ligament, tendon, and bone each have lower penetration depth values than does fat.[100] Consequently, the heating rates in these tissues are higher than in fatty tissue.[103] This feature of conventional ultrasound makes it well suited to the selective intervention of deeply located soft tissues, provided that they are not directly obstructed by intervening bone.[100,101]

Ultrasound machines with frequencies above and below 1 MHz provide therapists with intervention options. For example, ultrasound with a frequency of 3 MHz is used to treat regions where the thickness of tissue overlying bone is relatively small. Penetration depth values are lower at this frequency and, consequently, the rate of energy absorption is greater than for a frequency of 1 MHz. Bradnock[104] argued that therapeutic ultrasound with a frequency of 45 kHz is superior to 1-MHz ultrasound for treating soft tissue impairments, because the ultrasound has an inherently higher penetration depth and would, therefore, (1) allow more effective wave transmission into deep tissue, (2) produce a more even pattern of energy absorption in tissue, and (3) minimize the risk of tissue damage due to local high intensities, which can occur at conventional (MHz) frequencies. However, these claims were not substantiated in a study by Ward and Rohertson,[105] who stated that 45-kHz ultrasound is ineffective as a deep-heating modality and should not be used as an alternative to megahertz-frequency ultrasound units to treat deep soft tissue impairments. They further stated that the 45-kHz frequency may have some value for treating superficial impairments and may require less time to achieve a given temperature elevation.

Effects

Physiologic changes brought about through an ultrasound application are dependent on (1) the extent of temperature rise, (2) the rate at which energy is added to the tissue, and (3) the volume of tissue exposed.[76,84,85,106] Research indicates that tissue temperatures must be elevated to between 40°C and 45°C to achieve therapeutic effects.[107–110] Increasing tissue temperatures too slowly allows cooler blood to dissipate the heat and eliminate the possible therapeutic effects. Increasing temperatures too quickly may cause excessive heat accumulation in the tissues, which may stimulate pain receptors and cause thermal necrosis.[84,106] An average temperature increase of 2.8°C may be produced at a depth of 3 cm in the muscle, and the effects of hyperemia may persist for some 20 to 30 minutes following the intervention session. Increased oxygen uptake accompanies this phenomenon.[111,112]

Pain relief from ultrasound is believed to be related to a washout of pain mediators by increased blood flow, changes in nerve conduction, or alterations in cell membrane permeability that decrease inflammation.[113–116]

Accurate and reliable ultrasound dosage transmission is important for effective intervention. When utilizing modalities such as ultrasound, the device output must be calibrated to deliver appropriate, efficacious, and measurable treatment dosages.[85,106,117] Published reports[117–123] have indicated that the energy output of ultrasound devices significantly differs from manufacturer specification.

After the target area is heated, stretching procedures are begun and, it is hoped, with repeated interventions, normal motion is restored.[124] Some clinicians apply a protocol of continuous ultrasound prior to joint mobilizations with the intent of increasing joint play.

Phonophoresis In addition to applying a thermal effect, therapeutic ultrasound can be used for transdermal delivery of medications through a phenomenon termed *phonophoresis*. Although the terms *phonophoresis* and *iontophoresis* are often used interchangeably, the mechanisms by which each process delivers chemicals to various biologic tissues differ. Iontophoresis, which uses an electrical current to transport ions into the tissues, is discussed at the end of this chapter. Phonophoresis involves the use of acoustic energy to drive whole molecules into the tissues. The medications commonly applied through phonophoresis include cortisol, salicylates, dexamethasone, and analgesics such as lidocaine. The prescribed medication is combined with the ultrasound coupling agent and applied topically to the area to be treated. The ultrasound field is then applied to the area. Both pulsed and continuous ultrasound can be used with phonophoresis.

Other Considerations

Ultrasound can also be used as a diagnostic tool, and has been found to be reliable in the detection of stress fractures.[125] The machine is set to 1 MHz and, using a small transducer with a water-based coupling medium, the clinician slowly moves the transducer over the injured area while gradually increasing the intensity from 0 to 2.0 W/cm². If the patient reports discomfort under the transducer, a stress fracture may be present. A bone scan or radiograph is necessary to confirm the diagnosis.

The application of ultrasound should not occur over the testes, the eyes, the pregnant uterus, and the heart, or in close proximity to cardiac pacemakers, growth plates in children, and areas of malignancy.[75]

There is a need for clinicians to prove the efficacy of different dosages of ultrasound across the therapeutic range, considering different parameters such as pulsing versus continuous beam, intensity, frequency, and probe movement. Each of these different dose parameters should be evaluated with statistically appropriate, and controlled, populations of patients, in order to substantiate results.

Electrical Stimulation

Electrical stimulators are traditionally recognized by their commercial names, and these names have created a great deal of confusion about the terminology. Electrical stimulators should be classified as either direct current (DC), alternating current (AC), or pulsed current.

Electrical stimulation can be a broadly applicable adjunct in the acute, subacute, or chronic phase of rehabilitation for the clinical intervention of neuromuscular and musculoskeletal problems. In the acute phase, it is primarily used for pain and edema reduction. In the subacute and chronic stages, it can be used for pain reduction and neuromuscular reeducation. In muscle reeducation, the individual actively contracts the muscle with the electrical current to obtain a more effective contraction of the muscle.

For the manual therapist, electrical stimulation can be used:

- To create a muscle contraction through nerve or muscle stimulation
- To decrease pain through the stimulation of sensory nerves (see later discussion of TENS)
- To maintain or increase range of motion
- To stimulate tissue healing by creating an electrical field in biologic tissue
- To achieve muscle reeducation or facilitation by both motor and sensory stimulation
- To drive ions into or through the skin (see later discussion of iontophoresis)

By adjusting certain parameters, according to the desired goals of the clinician, the type of electrical stimulation given to the patient can be modified. These parameters include type of current, electrode size and placement, frequency, voltage, intensity, and duration.

Alternating versus Direct Current

Direct current differs from alternating current in that it causes chemical changes. Theoretically, these chemical changes reduce edema by enhancing the movement of charged proteins into the lymphatic channels.[126]

Electrode Size and Placement

Current density (the amount of current flow per cubic area) is highest where the electrodes meet the skin and diminishes as the current penetrates into the deeper tissues.[127] If the electrodes are placed close together, the area of highest current density is relatively superficial, whereas if the electrodes are spaced further apart, the depth of penetration increases.

The relative size of the electrodes used also changes the current density, with the current density being greater under the smaller of the two electrodes, and less under the larger electrode. This is the rationale for using a large dispersive pad that is placed remote from the treatment area, thereby concentrating the current density under the smaller electrode at the site of application.

Frequency

The amount of shortening, and the recovery allowed, of the muscle fiber are a function of the frequency. By adjusting the frequency used to either low or medium, the electrical stimulation has varying affects.

Low-frequency This category includes portable TENS, NMES, and EMS (Electronic muscle stimulators).[128] Low-frequency stimulation is characterized by:

- Stimulus synchronous stimulation
- Faster fatigue
- Lower contraction intensity (30% to 60% of maximal volitional contraction)
- Suitability for smaller, superficial muscles
- Decreased comfort
- The need for accurate placement of electrodes

Medium-Frequency This is also known as Russian stimulation, if time modulated, or interferential stimulation, if amplitude modulated. With the Russian stimulation, the patient is able to tolerate a greater current intensity because of the "burst effect" provided. This is aided by the use of higher frequency currents, which reduce the resistance to current flow, thereby making the treatment more comfortable. The interferential type of stimulation creates an electrical field pattern with a predictable pattern of interference. By using four electrodes in a square pattern, the therapeutic current is applied to the area within the square. The clinician can modify the treatment given by altering the frequency used. A frequency of 20 to 55 pulses per second produces a muscle contraction, 50 to 120 pulses per second produces pain relief, and 1 pulse per second is used for acustim pain relief.[129] The medium-frequency stimulators offer:

- Stimulus asynchronous stimulation
- Slower fatigue
- Higher contraction intensity (80% to 110% of maximal volitional contraction)
- Suitability for all muscle groups
- Greater recruitment capability
- Greater comfort

Voltage

Low-voltage direct current stimulators cause several physiologic changes that are related to polar and vasomotor effects and to the chemical reaction around the positive and negative poles caused by the long duration. An acidic reaction occurs around the positive pole, whereas an alkaline reaction occurs around the negative pole, both of which can cause severe skin reactions.[130] Low-voltage stimulation is indicated when an increased blood flow to the area is desired.[130]

A high-voltage stimulator is not a galvanic stimulator and should be considered as a monophasic pulsed TENS unit, with a very short phase duration, and a very high peak current amplitude. It delivers a monophasic, twin peak waveform.[131] Because of the short duration of the twin peak wave, high voltages with high peak current but low average current can be achieved. These characteristics provide for patient comfort and safety in application, and they can be used with both small and large electrodes. In addition, in contrast to low-voltage direct current devices, thermal and galvanic effects are minimized.[128,132,133] High-voltage stimulators have been applied clinically to reduce or eliminate muscle spasm and soft tissue edema, as well as for muscle reeducation (non-central nervous system–produced muscle contraction), trigger point therapy, and increasing blood flow to tissues with decreased circulation.[134-140]

Intensity

An increase in intensity of the electrical stimulus results in a greater penetration of the tissues. High-voltage stimulators are capable of a deeper penetration than low-voltage stimulators.[131]

Duration

By increasing the duration, or length of time that the stimulus is applied, a greater number of nerve fibers are stimulated.

The efficacy of neuromuscular electrical stimulation in increasing muscle strength is recognized, and this is the method used in most clinical applications of electrical stimulation of the muscle. Neuromuscular electrical stimulation (NMES) is either as effective as,[141,142] or more effective,[143] than isometric exercises in increasing muscle strength. These strength gains have been reported in atrophied[144] and normal muscles.[145,146] However, the efficacy of neuromuscular electrical stimulation in combination with an exercise therapy regimen compared with an exercise therapy regimen alone has produced contradictory findings.

Any electrical stimulator, whether it be high voltage, low voltage, alternating current, or TENS, can produce a muscle contraction. The degree of muscle force induced by the stimulator can be controlled using the intensity and frequency parameters. Higher frequencies and intensities produce a stronger contraction and a quicker fatigue of the muscle. To minimize the degree of fatigue, the rest time between contractions should be at least 60 seconds for every 10 seconds of contraction time.[147]

TENS

Despite the fact that low back pain is one of the most common medical problems in western society,[148] current analgesic therapies remain largely unsatisfactory. Conservative intervention with anti-inflammatory drugs and exercise is effective for many patients with acute low back pain.[149] However, when the pain symptoms persist, they can interfere with both physical activity and sleep patterns. Although analgesic medications can provide temporary pain relief, these drugs do not necessarily improve physical function, and are associated with well-known adverse effects. Interest in nonpharmacologic alternatives has led to evaluations of transcutaneous electrical nerve stimulation (TENS),[150] and therapeutic exercise.[151-158]

TENS was first introduced in the early 1950s to determine the suitability of patients with pain as candidates for the implantation of dorsal column electrodes. Despite highly optimistic initial reports and a wide spectrum of indications,[159,160] unsatisfactory results of this procedure in recent years have limited its range of application in pain intervention. The reasons why TENS is only effective in some patients and why numerous patients discontinue TENS therapy are not known. A few aspects of these phenomena have been examined, but a comprehensive and satisfactory explanation has not been provided so far.[160]

The percentage of patients who benefit from short-term TENS pain intervention has been reported to range from 50% to 80%.[161-164] Good long-term results with TENS have been observed in 6% to 44% of patients.[161,165-167]

In one review of TENS, Long[168] concluded the following: TENS has a beneficial effect on patients suffering from pain of diverse origins; in chronic pain syndromes, TENS has a short-term benefit in approximately 50% of patients; and for about 25% of TENS users, TENS is the only therapy needed for years after the intervention begins. In addition, Long concluded that the effect of TENS stimulation is beyond that which can be explained by placebo, but there are few long-term follow-up studies of TENS use.[168]

A more recent literature review by Fishbain and associates[169] indicates that 58% to 72% of patients with chronic pain report an initial positive effect from TENS; at 6 months, 13% to 74% continue to report a positive effect; and at 1 year, 27% to 66% of users still report a reduction in pain. Most of these types of TENS studies rely solely on subjects' pain reports to establish efficacy and rarely on other outcome measures such as activity, socialization, or medication use.[170]

As with the use of other electrical modalities, incorrect use through a lack of understanding may contribute to cases in which a lack of benefit is reported. TENS units typically deliver symmetric or balanced asymmetric biphasic waves of 100- to 500-msec pulse duration, with zero net current to minimize skin irritation,[171] and may be applied for extended periods.

Three modes of action are theorized for the efficacy of this modality: (1) gate control, (2) endogenous opiate control, and (3) central biasing.

Gate Control Theory

This concept of pain control, discussed in Chapter 4, was first introduced by Melzack and Wall in 1965.[114] This theory postulates that electrical stimulation of the large myelinated A-α fibers inhibits transmission of the smaller pain transmitting unmyelinated C fibers, and myelinated A-delta (δ) fibers. As long as the stimulation is applied, the pain fiber transmission will be inhibited unless accommodation to the electrical stimulation occurs.[172,173] The inhibition of the pain fiber transmission takes place primarily in the substantia gelatinosa of the dorsal horn of the spinal column. These large A fibers have a low threshold for stimulation and, therefore, are easily activated by TENS.[171]

Sensory level stimulation, in contrast, employs amplitudes and durations of stimulation that are sufficient to activate cutaneous tactile sensory fibers. Electrotherapy at sensory levels produces a cutaneous paresthesia (pins-and-needles sensation) if the frequency of stimulation is greater than about 10 or 15 pulses per second. If the frequency of sensory level stimulation is below 7 to 10 pulses per second, subjects generally report a tapping sensation. The reported magnitude of the paresthesia or tapping during sensory level stimulation increases as either the stimulus amplitude or pulse duration settings are increased. This increase in the awareness of stimulation is produced as progressively greater numbers of cutaneous sensory axons are recruited. The upper limit of sensory level stimulation lies just below the amplitude that is sufficient to evoke a muscular contraction. Sensory level stimulation for pain control delivered at higher frequencies (50 to 125 pulses/sec) is commonly referred to as *conventional TENS*.

Endogenous Opiate Control

When subjected to certain types of electrical stimulation of the sensory nerves, there may be a release of enkephalin from local sites within the central nervous system, and the release of beta (β)-endorphin from the pituitary gland into the cerebrospinal fluid.[171] To stimulate the release of these opiates, the electrical stimulus must be applied to acupuncture or trigger points both distal and proximal to the painful area.[174,175] If successful, the analgesic effect should last for several hours. Once sufficient current is generated in tissues to activate the axons innervating skeletal muscle, muscle contraction is produced and the stimulation is described as being motor level stimulation. If the frequency of stimulation at motor level is low (less than 5 pulses/sec), twitchlike contractions of muscle are produced. As the frequency of stimulation is increased during motor level stimulation, the contraction first becomes partially fused (tremorlike) and later becomes fused, producing either a smooth isometric or an isotonic tetanic contraction. As the amplitude of stimulation is increased during motor level stimulation, muscle contractions become stronger as greater numbers of motor

axons or muscle fibers are activated. In pain control applications, motor level stimulation is generally applied using low frequencies (2 to 4 pulses/ sec) of stimulation; this is commonly referred to as *strong, low rate (SLR) TENS*.

Central Biasing

Intense electrical stimulation, approaching a noxious level, of the smaller C or pain fibers produces a stimulation of the descending neurons. The central biasing mechanism is discussed in detail in Chapter 4. When stimulation amplitude is increased to a level described by subjects as painful, noxious level stimulation has been reached. This uncomfortable form of stimulation is generally associated with the electrical activation of pain fibers near the site of stimulation. Cutaneous paresthesias and muscular contraction persist as one progresses from motor level to noxious level stimulation. If noxious level stimulation is used at relatively high frequencies (50 to 100 pulses/sec) for pain control; this form of stimulation has been called *brief intense TENS*.

Iontophoresis

Iontophoresis has proved to be valuable in the intervention of musculoskeletal disorders. Delivery of local anesthetics, anti-inflammatory agents, and vasoconstrictive agents to maintain medicament concentration to the joints and associated musculature, as well as ligaments, tendons, and nerve tissue, has been reported to be of therapeutic benefit.[176–178]

The principle of drug iontophoresis is that an electrical potential difference will actively cause ions in solution to migrate according to their electrical charge. Iontophoresis causes an increased penetration of drugs and other compounds into tissues by the use of an applied current through the tissue. Ionized medications or chemicals do not ordinarily penetrate tissues, and if they do, it is not normally at a rate rapid enough to achieve therapeutic levels.[179] This problem can be overcome by administering a direct current energy source that provides penetration and transport.[179,180] Negatively charged ions are repelled from a negative electrode and attracted toward the positive, whereas positive ions are repelled from the positive electrode and attracted toward the negative.[179,180] Iontophoresis has, therefore, been used for the transdermal delivery of drugs.[181] The use of iontophoresis is appealing, because it offers the possibility of the systemic delivery of drugs in a controlled fashion and is potentially effective for any charged molecule.[182] The proposed mechanisms by which iontophoresis increases drug penetration are:

- That the electrical potential gradient induces changes in the arrangement of lipid, protein, and water molecules.[183] The quantity of ions transferred into the tissues is determined by the intensity of the current or current density at the active electrode, the duration of the current flow, and the concentration of ions in solution.[184]

● That the electrical current induces pore formation in the stratum corneum (SC), the outermost layer of the skin.[185,186] Menon and Elias[187] have previously proposed that the lacunae are the penetration pathways for polar and nonpolar molecules across the stratum corneum. The dilated lacunae could act as "pores" for the transit of drugs, which would be the anatomic basis for the pore theory.

● That hair follicles, sweat glands, and sweat ducts act as diffusion shunts with reduced resistance for ion transport.[188,189] Skin and fat are poor conductors of electrical current and offer greater resistance to current flow.

The exact pathway by which ionized drugs transit the stratum corneum has not been elucidated.

Topical drug administration has potential advantages over oral, injection, or intravenous drug delivery. These advantages include convenience, noninvasiveness, and minimal trauma induction. Tightly localized administration is possible, and systemic delivery can be achieved through absorption by the dermal blood supply. The main barrier to cutaneous or transcutaneous drug delivery is the impermeability of the stratum corneum.[190] The cutaneous barrier to both transepidermal water loss and the transcutaneous delivery of drugs resides in the stratum corneum.[191] This permeability barrier is mediated by a series of lipid lamellar membranes in the extracellular spaces of the stratum corneum. If the integrity of the stratum corneum is disrupted, the barrier to molecular transit may be greatly reduced. The primary transdermal iontophoretic route seems to be appendageal or intercellular through preexisting pathways,[189,192] or as a result of low-voltage (less than 5 V)–induced permeabilization of appendageal bilayers.[193]

Iontophoresis can be carried out with a wide variety of chemicals. For a chemical to be successful in iontophoresis, it must solubilize into ionic components. Some of the commonly compounded chemicals for iontophoresis are listed in Table 12–2 on page 252 of this chapter.

Following the basic law of physics that "like poles repel," the positively charged ions are placed under the positive electrode, while the negatively charged ions are placed under the negative electrode. If the ionic source is in an aqueous solution, it is recommended that a low concentration be used (2% to 4%) to aid in the dissociation.[201] Although electrons flow from negative to positive, regardless of electrode size, having a larger negative pad than the positive one will help shape the direction of flow. Current intensity is recommended to be at 5 mA or less for all interventions, and intervention times vary from 10 to 45 minutes. Longer durations produce a decrease in the skin impedance, thus increasing the likelihood of burns.[202] These burns result from an accumulation of ions under the electrodes. An accumulation of negative ions under the positive electrode produce hydrochloric acid, whereas an accumulation of positive ions under the negative electrode produce sodium hydroxide.

Other complications have included prolonged erythema that resolved in 24 hours, and tingling, burning, and pulling sensations that were especially apparent at the start of the current or if the amperage was turned up too rapidly. A metallic taste was noted when iontophoresis was used on the face.[203]

The visible so-called galvanic erythema demonstrates the clear increase of blood flow and the influence of the iontophoresis. This increased blood flow has been proven by different techniques such as plethysmography, thermography, and by means of isotopes.[204–206]

REVIEW QUESTIONS

1. List five general contraindications to spinal manipulation.
2. List three contraindications of manipulation specific to the cervical spine.
3. List three contraindications of manipulation specific to the thoracic spine.
4. List three contraindications of manipulation specific to the lumbar spine.
5. What is the function of grade I and II mobilizations?
6. What is the function of grade III and IV mobilizations?
7. Which of the Maitland grades use a small amplitude?
8. What is the difference between a Maitland grade I and IV mobilization?
9. Where in the range are the larger amplitudes of grades II and III performed?
10. What is another term for a technique that utilizes autogenic inhibition?
11. The technique of contract-relax uses, which type of inhibition?

ANSWERS

1. Spinal cord signs, fourth sacral root impingement (bowel and bladder signs and symptoms), bilateral sciatica unaccompanied by backache, spinal claudication, and anticoagulant medications.
2. Vertebrobasilar insufficiency, craniovertebral transverse ligament instability, bilevel cervical root signs.
3. Possible answers include osteoporosis, costochondritis, visceral symptoms, compression fracture.

4. Cauda equina syndrome, spondylolisthesis, and L1 or L2 root palsy.
5. Pain modulation.
6. Mechanical and neurophysiologic effects.
7. Grades I and IV.
8. Although both involve a small amplitude, the grade I mobilization is performed at the beginning of the range, whereas grade IV is performed at the end of range.
9. Grade II is performed in mid-range, and grade III at the end range.
10. Hold-relax.
11. Reciprocal.

REFERENCES

1. Rothstein J, ed. Guide to physical therapist practice. Phys Ther (Suppl) 1997;77:1163–1650.
2. Van der Muellen JCH. Present state of knowledge of process of healing in collagen structures. Int J Sports Med 1982;3:4–8.
3. van Tulder MW, Koes BW, Bouter LM. A cost-of-illness study of back pain in the Netherlands. Pain 1995;62:233–240.
4. Waddell G. A new clinical model for the treatment of low back pain. Spine 1987;12:632–644.
5. Spitzer WO, LeBlanc FE, Dupuis M, eds. Scientific approach to the assessment and management of activity-related spinal disorders. Spine 1987;(7 Suppl) 1:59.
6. Lamb D. A review of manual therapy for spinal pain. In: Boyling JD, Palastanga N, eds. *Grieve's Modern Manual Therapy: The Vertebral Column*, 2nd ed. Edinburgh, Scotland: Churchill Livingstone; 1994.
7. Evjenth O, Hamberg J. *Muscle Stretching in Manual Therapy; A Clinical manual, Vol 1; The Extremities; Vol 2, The Spinal Column and the TMJ.* Alfta, Sweden: Alfta Rehab Forlag; 1980.
8. Kaltenborn F. *Mobilization of the Spinal Column.* Wellington, New Zealand: New Zealand University Press; 1970.
9. Kaltenborn F. *Manual Therapy for Extremity Joints.* Oslo, Norway: Bokhandel; 1974.
10. Maitland GD. *Vertebral Manipulation*, 5th ed. London, England: Butterworths; 1986.
11. Mennel J. *Joint Pain and Diagnosis Using Manipulative Techniques.* New York, NY: Little, Brown; 1964.
12. Taniqawa M. Comparison of the hold-relax procedure and passive mobilization on increasing muscle length. Phys Ther 1972;52:725–735.
13. Barak T, Rosen E, Sofer R. Mobility: Passive orthopedic manual therapy. In: Gould J, Davies G, eds. *Orthopedic and Sports Physical Therapy.* St Louis, Mo: CV Mosby; 1990.
14. Maitland G. *Vertebral manipulation.* London, England: Butterworths; 1978.
15. Maigne R. *Orthopedic Medicine.* Springfield, Ill: Charles C Thomas; 1972.
16. Kaltenborn FM. *Manual Therapy for the Extremity Joints*, 3rd ed. Oslo, Norway: Bokhandel; 1980.
17. Cyriax J. *Textbook of Orthopedic Medicine*, vol 1, 8th ed. London, England: Balliere Tindall and Cassell; 1982.
18. Mennell J. *Science and Art of Joint Manipulation*, vol 2, London, England: Churchill; 1952.
19. Stoddard A. *Manual of Osteopathic Technique.* London, England: Hutchinson; 1983.
20. Evjenth O, Hamberg J. *Muscle Stretching in Manual Therapy*, vols I and II. Alfta, Sweden: Alfta Rehab; 1984.
21. Meadows JTS. The principles of the Canadian approach to the lumbar dysfunction patient. In: *Management of Lumbar Spine Dysfunction.* APTA Independent Home Study Course, Orthopedic Section, APTA Inc.; 1999.
22. Hertling D, Kessler RM. *Management of Common Musculoskeletal Disorders*, 2nd ed. Philadelphia, Pa: JB Lippincott; 1983.
23. Shiotz EH, Cyriax J. *Manipulation Past and Present.* London, England: Heinemann; 1975.
24. Marlin T. *Manipulative Treatment.* London, England: Edward Arnold; 1934.
25. Mennel JM. *Back Pain.* Boston, Mass: Little, Brown; 1960.
26. Rahlmann JF. Mechanisms of intervertebral joint fixation: A literature review. J Manipulative Physiol Ther 1987;10:177–187.
27. Knott M, Voss D. *Proprioceptive Neuromuscular Facilitation: Patterns and Techniques.* New York, NY: Harper & Row; 1968.
28. Prentice W. A comparison of static stretching and PNF stretching for improving hip joint flexibility. J Ath Train 1983;18:56–59.
29. Mitchell FL. *An Evaluation and Treatment Manual of Osteopathic Muscle Energy Procedures*, 1st ed. Valley Park, Mo: Mitchell, Moran, Pruzzo; 1979.
30. Korr I. Somatic dysfunction, osteopathic manipulative treatment, and the nervous system. J Am Osteopath Assoc 1986;86:109–114.
31. Wyke B. The neurology of joints: A review of general principles. Clini Rheum Dis 1981;7:223–239.
32. Patterson MM. A model mechanism for spinal segmental facilitation. J Am Osteopath Assoc 1976;76:62–72.
33. Sherrington C. The integrative action of the nervous system. New Haven, Conn: Yale University Press; 1961.
34. Lewit K, Simons DG. Myofascial pain: Relief by postisometric relaxation. Arch Phys Med Rehabil 1984; 65:452–456.

35. Goodridge JP. Muscle energy technique: Definition, explanation, methods of procedure. J Am Osteopath Assoc 1981;81:249–254.

36. Kabat H, Licht S, eds. Proprioceptive facilitation in therapeutic exercise. In: *Therapeutic Exercise*, 2nd ed. New Haven, Conn: New Haven Press; 1961.

37. Sullivan PE, Markos PD, Minor MAD. *An Integrated Approach to Therapeutic Exercise; Theory and Clinical Application*. Reston, Va: Reston Pub Co; 1982:138–140.

38. Markos PD. Ipsilateral and contralateral effects of proprioceptive neuromuscular techniques on hip motion and electromyographic activity. Phys Ther 1979;59:1366–1373.

39. Basmajian J. *Therapeutic Exercise*. Baltimore, Md: Williams & Wilkins; 1978.

40. Pettman E. *Level Two and Three Course Notes from North American Institute of Orthopedic Manual Therapy*. Portland, Ore: North American Institute of Orthopedic Manual Therapy; 1990.

41. van Tulder MW. The effectiveness of acupuncture in the management of acute and chronic low back pain: A systematic review within the framework of the Cochrane Collaboration Back Review Group. Spine 1999;24:1113.

41a. Bagnall KM, et al. "The histochemical composition of vertibral muscle." Spine 1984;9:470–473.

42. Lao L. Acupuncture techniques and devices. J Alternative Complementary Med 1996;2:23–25.

43. Melzack R, Wall PD. On the nature of cutaneous sensory mechanisms. Brain 1962;85:331–356.

44. Melzack R. The gate theory revisited. In: LeRoy PL, ed. *Current Concepts in the Management of Chronic Pain*. Miami, Fla: Symposia Specialists; 1977.

45. Chu LSW, Yeh SDJ, Wood DD. *Acupuncture Manual: A Western Approach*. New York, NY: Marcel Dekker; 1979:154–165.

46. Stux G, Pomeranz B. *Basics of Acupuncture*. Berlin, Heidelberg, Germany: Springer-Verlag; 1988:14–18.

47. Rogers J. The controversy of cranial bone motion [literature review]. Orthop Sports Phys Ther 1997;26:95–103.

48. Holenberry S, Dennis M. An introduction to craniosacral therapy. Physiotherapy 1994;80:528–532.

49. Holmes P. Cranial osteopathy. Nursing Times 1991;87:36-38.

50. Upledger J, Vredevoogd JD. *Craniosacral Therapy*. Seattle, Wash: Eastland Press; 1983.

51. Porter RW, Trailescu IF. Diurnal changes in straight leg raising. Spine 1990;15:103.

52. Adams MA, Dolan P, Hutton WC, Porter RW. "Diurnal changes in spinal mechanics and their clinical significance." J Bone Joint Surg [Br] 1990;72(2):266–270.

53. Murphy DR. *Conservative Management of Cervical Spine Disorders*. New York, NY: McGraw-Hill; 2000:545–546.

54. Cameron M. *Physical Agents in Rehabilitation*. Philadelphia, Pa: WB Saunders; 1999.

55. Knight KL. *Cryotherapy in Sports Injury Management*. Champaign, Ill: Human Kinetics; 1995:3–98.

56. Meeusen R, Lievens P. The use of cryotherapy in sports injuries. Sports Med 1986;3:398–414.

57. Merrick MA, Knight KL, Ingersoll CD, Potteiger JA. The effects of ice and compression wraps on intramuscular temperatures at various depths. J Athl Train 1993;28:236–245.

58. Reed B. Wound healing and the use of thermal agents. In: Michlovitz S, ed. *Thermal Agents in Rehabilitation*, 3rd ed. Philadelphia, Pa: FA Davis; 1996.

59. Abramson DI. Physiologic basis for the use of physical agents in peripheral vascular disorders. Arch Phys Med Rehabil 1965;46:216–244.

60. Barcroft H, Edholm OG. The effect of temperature on blood flow and deep temperature in the human forearm. J Physiol 1943;102:5–20.

61. Bennett D. Water at 67° to 69° Fahrenheit to control hemorrhage and swelling encountered in athletic injuries. Athl Train 1961;1:12–14.

62. Clarke R, Hellon R, Lind A. Vascular reactions of the human forearm to cold. Clin Sci 1958;17:165–179.

63. Baker R, Bell G. The effect of therapeutic modalities on blood flow in the human calf. JOSPT 1991;13:23.

64. Basset SW, Lake BM. Use of cold applications in the management of spasticity. Phys Ther Rev 1958;38:333–334.

65. Hartviksen K. Ice therapy in spasticity. Acta Neurol Scand Suppl 1962;3:79–84.

66. Jones DP. Renal metabolism during normoxia, hypoxia, and ischemic injury. Ann Rev Physiol 1986;48:33–50.

67. Jozsa L, Reffy A, Balint BJ, Jarvinen M, Kvist M. Ischemic-hypoxic changes in muscles with tendon injuries. Magy Traumatol Orthop Helyreallito Sebesz 1981;24:218–226.

68. Sapega AA, Heppenstall RB, Sokolow DP, et al. The bioenergetics of preservation of limbs before replantation: The rationale for intermediate hypothermia. J Bone Joint Surg 1988;70-A:1500–1513.

69. Leadbetter WB. An introduction to sports-induced soft-tissue inflammation. In: Leadbetter WB, Buckwalter JA, Gordon SL, eds. *Sports Induced Inflammation*, Chicago, Ill: American Academy of Orthopedic Surgeons; 1990:3–23.

70. Knight KL. Effects of hypothermia on inflammation and swelling. Athl Train 1976;11:7–10.

71. Merrick MA, Rankin JM, Andres FA, Hinman CL. A preliminary examination of cryotherapy and

secondary injury in skeletal muscle. Med Sci Sports Exerc 1999;31:1516–1521.

72. Belitsky RB, Odam SJ, Hubley-Kozey C. Evaluation of the effectiveness of wet ice, dry ice, and cryogen packs in reducing skin temperature. Phys Ther 1987; 67:1080–1084.

73. Oosterveld FGJ, Rasker JJ, Jacobs JWG, Overmars HJA. The effect of local heat and cold therapy on the intraarticular and skin surface temperature of the knee. Arthritis Rheum 1992;35:146–151.

74. Zemke JE, Andersen JC, Guion WK, McMillan J, Joyner AB. Intramuscular temperature responses in the human leg to two forms of cryotherapy: Ice massage and ice bag. J Orthop Sports Phys Ther 1998; 27:301–307.

75. Cwynar DA, McNerney T. A primer on physical therapy [review]. Prim Care Pract 1999;3:451–459.

76. Griffin JG. Physiological effects of ultrasonic energy as it is used clinically. J Am Phys Ther Assoc 1966; 46:18.

77. Lehmann JF, Silverman DR, et al. Temperature distributions in the human thigh produced by infrared, hot pack and microwave applications. Arch Phys Med Rehabil 1966;47:291.

78. Abramson DI, Tuck S, Lee SW, et al. Comparison of wet and dry heat in raising temperature of tissues. Arch Phys Med Rehabil 1967;48:654.

79. Kimura IF, Gulick DT, Shelly J, Ziskin MC. Effects of two ultrasound devices and angles of application on the temperature of tissue phantom. J Orthop Sports Phys Ther 1998;27:27–31.

80. Danzell M. *The Physiotherapists Armamentarium. Current Therapy in Sports Medicine.* Philadelphia, Pa: Decker; 1986.

81. Lehmann J, Delateur B, Stonebridge J, Warren CG. Therapeutic temperature distribution produced by ultrasound as modified by dosage and volume of tissue exposed. Arch Phys Med Rehabil 1967;48:662–666.

82. McDiarmid T, Burns PN. Clinical applications of therapeutic ultrasound. Physiotherapy 1987;73:156–161.

83. Arnheim D. Therapeutic modalities. In: Arnheim D, ed. *Modern Principles of Athletic Training.* St Louis, Mo: Times Mirror/Mosby; 1989:350–367.

84. Lehmann J, Warren CG, Scham S. Therapeutic heat and cold. Clin Orthop 1974;99:207–226.

85. Prentice W. Therapeutic ultrasound. In: Prentice W, ed. *Therapeutic Modalities in Sports Medicine.* St Louis, Mo: Times Mirror/Mosby; 1990:129–140.

86. Weber DC, Brown AW. Physical agent modalities. In: Braddom RL, ed. *Physical Medicine and Rehabilitation.* Philadelphia, Pa: WB Saunders; 1996:454–456.

87. Hartley A. *Ultrasound, a Monograph.* Chattanooga, Tenn: Chattanooga Group; 1991:1–35.

88. Lehman JF. *Therapeutic Heat and Cold.* Baltimore, Md: Williams & Wilkins; 1982:353–403.

89. Webster DF, Pond JB, Dyson M, et al.: The role of cavitation in the "in vitro" stimulation of protein synthesis in human fibroblasts by ultrasound. Ultrasound Med Biol 1978;4:343.

90. Bly N. The use of ultrasound as an enhancer for transcutaneous drug delivery: Phonophoresis. Phys Ther 1995;6:89–103.

91. Dyson M. Non-thermal cellular effects of ultrasound. Br J Cancer 1982;45(suppl V):165–171.

92. Nyborg WL. Ultrasonic microstreaming and related phenomena. Br J Cancer 1982;45(suppl V):156–160.

93. Piersol GM, Schwann HP, Pennell RB, Carstensen EL. Mechanism of absorption of ultrasonic energy in blood. Arch Phys Med Rehabil 1952;33:327–331.

94. Schwann HP. *Absorption of Ultrasound by Tissues and Biological Matter.* Unpublished manuscript; 1959.

95. Cummings GS, Tillman LJ. Remodeling of dense connective tissue in normal adult tissues. In: Currier DP, Nelson RM, eds. *Dynamics of Human Biologic Tissues.* Philadelphia, Pa: FA Davis; 1992:68–69.

96. Arnheim D. Therapeutic modalities. In: Arnheim D, ed. *Modern Principles of Athletic Training.* St Louis, Mo: Times Mirror/Mosby; 1989:350–367.

97. Stewart H. Survey of use and performance of ultrasonic therapy equipment in Pinellas County, Florida. Phys Ther 1974;54:707–714.

98. Wessling KC, DeVane DA, Hylton CR. Effects of static stretch versus static stretch and ultrasound combined on triceps surae muscle extensibility in healthy women. Phys Ther 1987;67:674–679.

99. Reed B, Ashikaga T. The effects of heating with ultrasound on knee joint displacement. J Orthop Sports Phys Ther 1997;26:131–137.

100. Ward AR. *Electricity, Fields and Waves in Therapy.* Marrickville, Australia: Science Press; 1986.

101. Ziskin MC, McDairmid T, Michlovitz SL. Therapeutic ultrasound. In: Michlovitz SL, ed. *Thermal Agents in Rehabilitation,* 2nd ed. Philadelphia, Pa: FA Davis; 1990.

102. Lehmann JF, DeLateur BJ. Therapeutic heat. In: Lehmann JF, ed. *Therapeutic Heat and Cold,* 4th ed. Philadelphia, Pa: FA Davis; 1990.

103. Jackins S, Jamieson A. Use of heat and cold in physical therapy. In: Lehmann JF, ed. *Therapeutic Heat and Cold,* 4th ed. Philadelphia, Pa: FA Davis; 1990.

104. Bradnock B. Long-wave ultrasound in soft-tissue injury. Int J Sports Med Soft Tissue Trauma 1994;6:6–7.

105. Ward AR, Robertson VJ. Comparison of heating of nonliving soft tissue produced by 45 kHz and 1 MHz frequency ultrasound machines. J Orthop Sports Phys Ther 1996;23:258–266.

106. Michlovitz S, Ziskin M, McDiarmid T. Therapeutic ultrasound. In: Michlovitz S, ed. *Thermal Agents in Rehabilitation*. Philadelphia, Pa: FA Davis; 1990:134–164.

107. Castel JC. Therapeutic ultrasound. Rehabil Ther Prod Rev 1993;Jan/Feb:22–32.

108. Draper DO, Ricard MD. Rate of temperature decay in human muscle following 3 MHz ultrasound: The stretching window revealed. J Athl Train 1995;30: 304–307.

109. Gersten J. Effect of ultrasound on tendon extensibility. Am J Phys Med 1955;34:362–369.

110. Lehmann J, Delateur B. *Therapeutic Heat and Cold.* Baltimore, Md: Williams & Wilkins; 1990.

111. Paaske WP, Hovind H, Sejrsen P. Influence of therapeutic ultrasnic irradiation on blood flow in human cutaneous, subcutaneous and muscular tissue. Scand J Clin Invest 1973;31:388.

112. Wyper DJ, McNiven DR, Donelly TJ. Therapeutic ultrasound and muscular blood flow. Physiotherapy 1978;64:321.

113. Falconer J, Hayes KW, Chang RW. Therapeutic ultrasound in the treatment of musculoskeletal conditions. Arthritis Care Res 1990;3:85–91.

114. Melzack R, Wall PD. Pain mechanisms: A new theory. Science 1975;150:971–979.

115. Bonica JJ. *The Management of Pain.* Philadelphia, Pa: Lea & Febiger; 1990:1776–1781.

116. Okeson JP. *Bell's Orofacial Pain*, 5th ed. Chicago, Ill: Quintessence Publishing; 1995:197–201.

117. Lloyd JJ, Evans JA. A calibration survey of physiotherapy ultrasound equipment in North Wales. Physiotherapy 1988;74(2):56–61.

118. Stewart H. Survey of use and performance of ultrasonic therapy equipment in Pinellas County, Florida. Phys Ther 1974;54:707–714.

119. Allen KGR, Battye CK. Performance of ultrasound therapy equipment in Pinellas County. Phys Ther 1978;54:174–179.

120. Fyfe MC, Parnell SM. The importance of measurement of effective transducer radiating area in the testing and calibration of therapeutic ultrasonic instruments. Health Phys 1982;43:377–381.

121. Hekkenberg RT, Oosterbaan WA, van-Beekum WT. Evaluation of ultrasound therapy devices. Physiotherapy 1986;72:390–394.

122. Repacholi MH, Benwell DA. Using surveys of ultrasound therapy devices to draft performance standards. Health Phys 1979;36:679–686.

123. Ross RN, Sourkes AM, Sandeman JM. Survey of ultrasound therapy devices in Manitoba. Health Phys 1984;47:595–601.

124. McDiarmid TM, Ziskin MC, Michlovitz SL. Therapeutic ultrasound. In: Michlovitz SL, ed. *Thermal Agents in Rehabilitation*, 3rd ed. Philadelphia, Pa: FA Davis; 1996:168–212.

125. Lowden A. Application of ultrasound to assess stress fractures. Physiotherapy 1986;72:160–161.

126. Cosgrove K, Alon G. The electrical effect of two commonly used clinical stimulators on traumatic edema on rats. Phys Ther 1992;72:227–233.

127. Benton L, Baker L, Bowman B. *Functional Electrical Stimulation: A Practical Clinical Guide*, Downey, Calif: Rancho Los Amigos Hospital; 1980.

128. Nelson R, Currier D. *Clinical Electrotherapy*. Norwalk, Conn: Appleton & Lange; 1987.

129. Prentice WE. *Therapeutic Modalities for Allied Health Professionals*. New York, NY: McGraw-Hill; 1998.

130. Watkins A. *A Manual of Electrotherapy*, 3rd ed. Philadelphia, Pa: Lea & Febiger; 1968.

131. Alon G, DeDomeico G. High voltage stimulation: An integrated approach to clinical electrotherapy. Chattanooga, Tenn: Chattanooga Corp; 1987.

132. Wolf SL. *Electrotherapy: Clinics in Physical Therapy.* New York, NY: Churchill Livingstone; 1981:1–24,99–121.

133. Murphy GJ. Electrical physical therapy in treating TMJ patients. J Craniomand Pract 1983;2:67–73.

134. Okeson JP. *Management of Temporomandibular Disorders and Occlusion.* St Louis, Mo: Mosby-Year Book; 1993: 345–378.

135. Friedman MH, Weisberg J. *Temporomandibular Joint Disorders: Diagnosis and Treatment.* Chicago, Ill: Quintessence Publishing; 1985:119–140.

136. Bettany JA, Fish DR, Mendel FC. Influence of high voltage pulsed direct current on edema formation following impact injury. Phys Ther 1988;4:219–224.

137. Reed BV. Effect of high voltage pulsed electrical stimulation on microvascular permeability to plasma proteins. Phys Ther 1988;4:491–495.

138. Sohn N, Weinstein MA, Robbins RD. The levator syndrome and its treatment with high-voltage electrogalvanic stimulation. Am J Surg 1982;144:580–582.

139. Barrett NVJ, Martin JW, Jacob RF, King GE. Physical therapy techniques in treating head and neck patients. J Prosthet Dent 1988;3:343–346.

140. Rocabado M, Iglarsh ZA. *Musculoskeletal Approach to Maxillofacial Pain.* Philadelphia, Pa: JB Lippincott; 1991:174–182.

141. Laughman RK, Youdas JW, Garrett TR, Chao EYS. Strength changes in the normal quadriceps femoris muscle as a result of electrical stimulation. Phys Ther 1983;63:494–499.

142. McMiken DF, Todd-Smith M, Thompson C. Strengthening of human quadriceps muscles by cutaneous electrical stimulation. Scand J Rehabil Med 1983;15:25–28.

143. Delitto A, Rose SJ, McKowen JM, et al. Electrical stimulation versus voluntary exercise in strengthening

thigh musculature after anterior cruciate ligament surgery. Phys Ther 1988;68:660–663.

144. Gould N, Donnermeyer BS, Pope M, Ashikaga T. Transcutaneous muscle stimulation as a method to retard disuse atrophy. Clin Orthop 1982;164:215–220.

145. Currier DP, Mann R. Muscular strength development by electrical stimulation in healthy individuals. Phys Ther 1983;63:915–921.

146. Selkowitz DM. Improvement in isometric strength of quadriceps femoris muscle after training with electrical stimulation. Phys Ther 1985;65:186–196.

147. Binder-MacLeod S, Snyder-Mackler L. Muscle fatigue: Clinical implications for fatigue assessment and neuromuscular electrical stimulation. Phys Ther 1993;73:902–910.

148. Hadler NM. Workers with disabling back pain. N Engl J Med 1997;337:341–343.

149. Frymoyer JW. Back pain and sciatica. N Engl J Med. 1988;318:291–300.

150. Melzack R, Vetere P, Finch L. Transcutaneous electrical nerve stimulation for low back pain. Phys Ther 1983;63:489–493.

151. Faas A. Exercises: Which ones are worth trying, for which patients, and when? Spine 1996;21:2874–2878.

152. Manniche C. Assessment and exercise in low back pain with special reference to the management of pain and disability following first time disc surgery [review]. Dan Med Bull 1995;42:301–313.

153. Manniche C, Lundberg E, Christensen I, Hesselsoe G. Intensive dynamic back exercises for chronic low back pain: A clinical trial. Pain 1991;47:53–63.

154. Frost H, Klaber Moffet JA, Moser JS, Fairbank JCT. Randomised controlled trial for evaluation of fitness programme for patients with chronic low back pain. BMJ 1995;310:151–154.

155. Hansen FR, Bendix T, Skov P, et al. Intensive, dynamic back-muscle exercises, conventional physiotherapy, or placebo-control treatment of low-back pain. Spine 1993;18:98–107.

156. Koes BW, Bouter LM, Beckerman H, van der Heijden GJMG, Knipschild PG. Physiotherapy exercises and back pain, a blinded review. BMJ 1991;302:1572–1576.

157. Lindstrom I, Ohlund C, Eek C, Wallin L, Peterson L, Nachemson A. Mobility, strength, and fitness after a graded activity program for patients with subacute low back pain. Spine 1992;17:641–652.

158. Manniche C, Hesselsoe G, Bentzen L, Christensen I, Lundberg E. Clinical trial of intensive muscle training for chronic low back pain. Lancet 1988;2: 1473–1476.

159. Loeser JD, Black RG, Christman A. Relief of pain by transcutaneous stimulation. J Neurosurg 1975;42: 308–314.

160. Woolf JC, Thompson JW. Stimulation-induced analgesia: Transcutaneous electricial nerve stimulation (TENS) and vibration. In: Wall PD, Melzack R, eds. *Textbook of Pain.* London, England: Churchill-Livingstone; 1984:1191–1208.

161. Eriksson MBE, Sjölund BH, Nielzen S. Long-term results of peripheral conditioning stimulation as an analgesic measure in chronic pain. Pain 1979;6:335–347.

162. Long DM. Stimulation of the peripheral nervous system for pain control. Clin Neurosurg 1983;31:323–343.

163. Eriksson MBE, Sjölund BH, Sundbärg G. Pain relief from peripheral conditioning stimulation in patients with chronic facial pain. J Neurosurg 1984;61:149–155.

164. Ishimaru K, Kawakita K, Sakita M. Analgesic effects induced by TENS and electroacupuncture with different types of stimulating electrodes on deep tissues in human subjects. Pain 1995;63:181–187.

165. Fried T, Johnson R, McCracken W. Transcutaneous electrical nerve stimulation: Its role in the control of chronic pain. Arch Phys Med Rehabil 1984;65:228–231.

166. Kreczi T, Klingler D. Transkutane Nervenstimulation bei chronischen Schmerzzuständen nach Verletzung peripherer Nerven. Analyse der Therapieversager. Anaesthesist 1985;34:549.

167. Langohr HD, Gläser N, Mayer K. Ergebnisse einer Behandlung von schmerzhaften Mono- und Polyneuropathien mit psychotropen Medikamenten und transkutaner Nervenstimulation. Schmerz 1983;1:1216.

168. Long DM. Fifteen years of transcutaneous electrical stimulation for pain control. Stereotact Funct Neurosurg 1991;56:2–19.

169. Fishbain DA, Chabal C, Abbott A, et al. Transcutaneous electrical nerve stimulation (TENS) treatment outcome in long term users. Clin J Pain 1996;12: 201–214.

170. Gersh MR, Wolf SL. Applications of transcutaneous electrical nerve stimulation in the management of patients with pain: State-of-the-art update. Phys Ther 1985;65:314–336.

171. Murphy GJ. Utilization of transcutaneous electrical nerve stimulation in managing craniofacial pain. Clin J Pain 1990;6:64–69.

172. Lampe G. Introduction to the use of transcutaneous electrical nerve stimulation devices. Phys Ther 1978;58:1450–1454.

173. Wolf S. Neurophysiological mechanisms in pain modulation: relevance to TENS. In Manheimer J, Lampe G (eds). Clinical Applications of TENS. Philadelphia, FA Davis 1984.

174. Clement-Jones V. Increased β endorphin but not metenkephalin levels in human cerebrospinal fluid after acupuncture for recurrent pain. Lancet 1980;8: 946–948.

175. Salar G. Effect of transcutaneous electrotherapy on CSF β-endorphin content in patients without pain problems. Pain 1981;10:169–172.

176. Gangarosa LP, Haynes M, Qureshi S, Selim MM, Ozawa A, Hayakawa K. Treatment of post herpetic neuralgia by iontophoresis. Pain 1985:263–265.

177. Gangarosa LP. Defining a practical solution for iontophoretic local anesthetic of skin. Methods Find Exp Clin Pharmacol 1981;3:83–94.

178. Costello CT, Jeske AH. Iontophoresis: Applications in transdermal medication delivery. Phys Ther 1995;6: 104–113.

179. Gangarosa LP. Iontophoresis in dental practice. Chicago, Ill: Quintessence Publishing; 1982:13–20.

180. Coy RE. *Anthology of Craniomandibular Orthopedics*, vol 2. Seattle, Wash: International College of Craniomandibular Orthopedics; 1993:41–85.

181. Burnette RR: Iontophoresis. In: Hadgraft J, Guy RH, eds. *Transdermal Drug Delivery: Developmental Issues and Research Initiatives.* New York, NY: Marcel Dekker; 1989:247–291.

182. Green PG, Flanagan M, Shroot B, Guy RH. Iontophoretic drug delivery. In: Walters KA, Hadgraft J, eds. *Pharmaceutical Skin Penetration Enhancement.* New York, NY: Marcel Dekker; 1993:311–333.

183. Chien YW, Siddiqui O, Shi M, Lelawongs P, Liu JC: Direct current iontophoretic transdermal delivery of peptide and protein drugs. J Pharm Sci 1989;78: 376–384.

184. Cummings J. Iontophoresis. In: Nelson RM, Currier DP, eds. *Clinical Electrotherapy.* Norwalk, Conn: Appleton & Lange; 1991.

185. Grimnes S. Pathways of ionic flow through human skin in vivo. Acta Dermatol Venereol (Stockh) 1984; 64:93–98.

186. Burnette RR, Ongpipattanakul B. Characterization of the pore transport properties and tissue alteration of excised human skin during iontophoresis. J Pharm Sci 1988;77:132–137.

187. Menon GK, Elias PM. Penetration pathways through the stratum corneum interstices localize to lacunar domains [abstract]. J Invest Dermatol 1996;106:917.

188. Burnette RR, Marrero D. Comparison between the iontophoretic and passive transport of thyrotropin releasing hormone across excised nude mouse skin. J Pharm Sci 1986;75:738–743.

189. Lee RD, White HS, Scott ER. Visualization of iontophoretic transport paths in cultured and animal skin models. J Pharm Sci 1996;85:1186–1190.

190. Scheuplein RJ, Bronaugh RL. Percutaneous absorption. In: Goldsmith LA, ed. *Biochemistry and Physiology of the Skin.* New York, NY: Oxford University Press; 1983:1255–1295.

191. Su MH, Srinivasan V, Ghanem AH, Higuchi WI. Quantitativein vivo iontophoretic studies. J Pharm Sci 1994;83:12–17.

192. Edwards DA, Langer R. A linear theory of transdermal transport phenomena. J Pharm Sci 1994;83: 1315–1334.

193. Chizmadzhev YA, Indenbom AV, Kuzmin PI, Galichenko SV, Weaver JC, Potts RO. Electrical properties of skin at moderate voltages: Contribution of appendageal macropores. Biophys J 1998;74:843–856.

194. Weider D. Treatment of traumatic myositis ossificans with acetic acid iontophoresis. Phys Ther 1992;72: 133–137.

195. Banta C. A prospective nonrandomized study of iontophoresis, wrist splinting, and anti-inflammatory medication in the treatment of early mild carpal tunnel syndrome. J Orthop Sports Phys Ther 1995;21: 120.

198. Boone D. Hyaluronidase iontophoresis. J Am Phys Ther Assoc 1969;49:139–145.

199. Tannenbaum M. Iodine iotophoresis in reduction of scar tissue. Phys Ther 1980;60:792.

200. Kahn J. Calcium iontophoresis in suspected myopathy. JAPTA 1975;55:276.

201. O'Malley E, Oester Y. Influence of some physical chemical factors on iontophoresis using radioisotopes. Arch Phys Med Rehabil 1955;36:310.

202. Zeltzer L, Regalado M, Nichter LS, Barton D, Jennings S, Pitt L. Iontophoresis versus subcutaneous injection: A comparison of two methods of local anesthesia delivery in children. Pain 1991;44: 73–78.

203. Maloney JM, Bezzant JL, Stephen RL, Petelenz TJ. Iontophoretic administration of lidocaine anesthesia in office practice. An appraisal. J Dermatol Surg Oncol 1992;18:937–940.

204. Schnizer W, Manert W, Kleinschmidt J, et al. Effects of electric current by transcutaneous application to human peripheral blood vessels (Untersuchung zur Frage der transkutanen Wirkung des elektrischen Stromes auf das periphere Gefä[beta]system des Menschen [in German, English summary]). Z Phys Med Baln Med Klim 1980;9:238–244.

205. Danz J, Callies R. Thermographic objectivation of a differentiated direct current therapy (Thermographische Objektivierung einer differenzierten Gleichstromtherapie [in German, English summary]). Z Physiother 1980;32:15–20.

206. Hupka J. Changes of the capillary blood supply of the peroneal muscles after the application of several types of current (Veränderungen der Kapillardurchblutung des Wadenmuskels nach Applikation mancher Stromtypen [in German]). Z Physiother 1981;33:421.

CHAPTER THIRTEEN

THE LUMBAR SPINE

Chapter Objectives

At the completion of this chapter, the reader will be able to:

1. Describe the anatomy of the vertebra, ligaments, muscles, and blood and nerve supply that comprise the lumbar intervertebral segment.
2. Describe the biomechanics of the lumbar spine, including coupled movements, normal and abnormal joint barriers, kinesiology, and the reactions to various stresses.
3. Describe the common pathologies and lesions of this region.
4. Perform a detailed objective examination of the lumbar musculoskeletal system, including palpation of the articular and soft tissue structures, specific passive mobility and passive articular mobility tests for the intervertebral joints, and stability tests.
5. Interpret the results from the examination and establish the definitive biomechanical diagnosis.
6. Design a plan of care based on the Direct Interventions of manual therapy, therapeutic exercise, and electrotherapeutic modalities and thermal agents.
7. Apply mobilization techniques to the lumbar spine, using the correct grade, direction, and duration, and explain the mechanical and physiologic effects.
8. Evaluate intervention effectiveness in order to progress or modify the intervention.
9. Plan an effective home program including spinal care, and instruct the patient in same.

OVERVIEW

At some time in their lives, most people will experience low back pain (LBP).[1,2] One study, published in 1987, estimated that eight million Americans suffered from chronic low back pain.[3] Low back pain is second only to the common cold as a reason for outpatient visits, representing the most common, and the most expensive, source of compensated work-related injury in modern industrialized countries.[4–6] Moreover, both the rate and the degree of disability accruing from LBP are increasing worldwide.[7,8]

Despite the many studies examining low back pain, several key issues concerning occurrence and prognosis remain unanswered. This is due in part to the fact that it is a difficult problem to investigate, because of its variable natural history which is thought to be multifactorial in origin, and the broad range of risk factors involved in its cause and course.[9,10]

For a patient, the first episode of back pain can have differing results: 88% will be asymptomatic in 6 weeks, 98% in 24 weeks, and 99% in 52 weeks; 97% of causes are unknown, 2% attributed to disc problems, and 1% to apophyseal disorders.[11] No more than 29% will require conservative measures, 1% will require surgery, and the remainder will recover spontaneously.[11] These often-quoted percentages have fueled a recommendation of essentially "benign" neglect in the first several months of occurrence when pain is more easily managed.[12] Recent literature supports the concept that although many patients experience improvement, up to 75% have one or more relapses and 72% continue to have pain at 1 year.[13,14]

There appear to be a number of "red flags" that can predict a complicated course, which include:[15]

- Age older than 50 years at first episode of back pain
- History of malignancy
- History of intravenous drug use
- Corticosteroid use
- Fever
- Weight loss
- Adenopathy
- Hematuria
- Signs or symptoms of systemic disease
- Sciatica

● Neurologic deficit on examination
● History of severe acute trauma

Low back pain in general, and disc herniation specifically, are influenced by many factors including age and gender.[16] Without including the work situation as a factor, the incidence of low back pain shows little difference between men and women.[17] But when the work situation is included, one study found that 35% of women and 19.1% of men in physically heavy jobs had low back pain.[18] About 30% of all workers will, at some time, miss work because of a back ailment, and 2% to 4% will actually change jobs at least once because of a back problem, in addition to the ones who become disabled.[19]

In longitudinal studies, lack of social confidence, poor social support, low level of education, poor work content, demands on physical strength, smoking, and a back pain history have been shown to be related to LBP.[20–23] People who are simultaneously subjected to demanding physical and psychosocial conditions have more LBP than people with only demanding physical or only demanding psychosocial conditions.[24,25]

Physical load on the back has commonly been implicated as a risk factor for LBP, and in particular, for work related LBP. Certain occupations and certain work tasks seem to have a higher risk of LBP.[26–29] Repeated lifting of heavy loads is considered a risk factor for low back pain,[30] especially if combined with side-flexion and twisting.[31,32] A study of static work postures found that there was an increased risk of low back pain if the work involved a predominance of sitting.[33]

There are several hypotheses relating to a link between obesity and LBP. Increased mechanical demands resulting from obesity have been suspected of causing LBP through excessive wear and tear,[34–38] and it has been suggested that metabolic factors associated with obesity may be detrimental.[34]

From a clinical perspective, it is worth noting that strength, flexibility, aerobic conditioning, and posture have all been found to have a significant preventative effect on the occurrence and recurrence of back injuries. One study demonstrated that weak trunk musculature and decreased endurance were recognized risk factors in the development of back problems.[39] Nachemson summarized a variety of data indicating that motion, rather than rest, may be beneficial in healing soft tissues and joints.[40] Thus, physical therapy, with its emphasis on the restoration of functional motion, strength, and flexibility, should be the cornerstone of both the treatment and the preventative processes. The treatment approach should be active and should direct the responsibility of the rehabilitative process toward the patient. Extrapolating the information from Chapter 4, each mechanical, manual, or active technique initiates an abundance of afferent inputs into the central nervous system, all of which

have the potential to both modulate pain and alter the state of a muscle contraction.

Given the numerous causes and types of low back pain, a clinician evaluating and treating this region must have a sound understanding and knowledge of the anatomy and biomechanics. Although this knowledge is not the sole determinant of the approach to low back pain, it does provide a solid framework on which to build successful management.

ANATOMY

The lumbar spine, consisting of five lumbar vertebrae, is clinically characterized as the region from T10 down to the sacral base. Although three cardinal planes of motion are available, 6 degrees of freedom are often cited.[41] Flexion and extension are relatively pure motions, with the axis just posterior to the disc nucleus. Another axis occurs at the zygapophysial joints. The impure motions of this region are rotation and side-flexion, and they are coupled motions.

In general, the vertebrae, increase in size from C1 to L5 to accommodate progressively increasing loads. Nutrient foramens, represented by one or more large holes, are found on the posterior surface of the vertebral body, and serve to transmit the nutrient arteries of the vertebral body and the basivertebral veins.

Vertebral Body

The anterior part of each vertebra is called the vertebral body (Figure 13–1). The vertebral body, with its slightly concave anterior and lateral surfaces and flattish top, bottom, and posterior surfaces, is kidney shaped when viewed from above or below. The vertebral body is the weight-bearing unit of the vertebra and it is well designed for this purpose. Although a solid bone structure would provide the vertebral body with sufficient strength, especially for static loads, it would be too heavy, and would not be suitable for dynamic load bearing.[42] Conversely, a strong outer layer and hollow cavity would be equally unsuitable to sustain longitudinally applied loads, unless a source of reinforcement was present. The reinforcement is provided by vertical and horizontal struts called vertical and transverse trabeculae.

During the aging process, a gradual decrease in cortical bone of 3% per decade can be expected for both sexes, whereas an 6% to 8% decrease in trabecular bone per decade can be expected to begin between 20 and 40 years of age for both sexes.[43] Consequently, there is a dramatic effect on the load-bearing capacity of the cortical cancellous bone after the age of 40.[44] Before the age of 40, approximately 55% of the load-bearing capacity exists in the cancellous bone, which decreases to around 35% after the age of 40, with bone strength decreasing more rapidly than bone quantity.[45]

3RD LUMBAR VERTEBRA

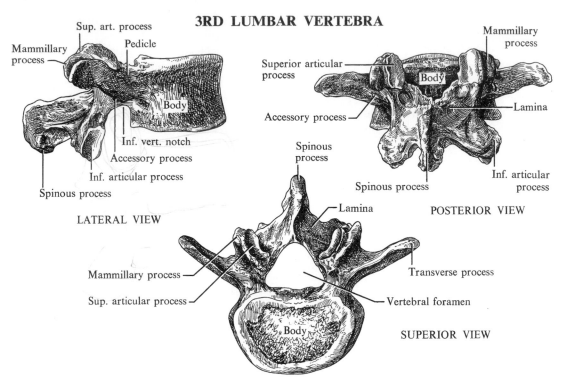

FIGURE 13–1 A typical lumbar vertebra. (*Reproduced, with permission from Pansky B: Review of Gross Anatomy, 6/e. McGraw-Hill, 1996*)

Two robust shafts of bone, each called a pedicle (see Figure 13–1), project from the posterior aspect of the vertebral body. Attached to the back of the vertebral body is an arch of bone aptly called the neural arch. Viewing a vertebra from above, it can be seen that the neural arch and the back of the vertebral body surround a space called the vertebral canal, in which the spinal cord lies.

The pedicles, the only connection between the posterior components and the vertebral bodies, deliver both tensile and bending forces. If the vertebral body slides forward, the inferior articular processes of that vertebra will lock against the superior articular processes of the next lower vertebra and resist the slide.[42] These resistive forces are transmitted to the vertebral body along the pedicles. Noticeably, all the muscles that act on a lumbar vertebra pull downward, transmitting the muscular action to the vertebral body through the pedicles, which act as levers, and are, thus, subjected to a certain amount of bending.[42]

Extending medially from each pedicle is the lamina (see Figure 13–1). The two laminae meet and fuse with one another, forming the so-called roof of the neural arch. The centrally placed lamina function to absorb the various forces that are transmitted from the spinous and articular processes. The part of the lamina located between the superior and inferior articular processes on each side is called the pars interarticularis. The biomechanical significance of the pars interarticularis is that it connects the vertically oriented lamina and the horizontally extending pedicle, which exposes it to appreciable bending forces.[42]

A spinous process extends posteriorly from the junction of the two laminae. Each vertebra has four articular processes. Projecting upward from the junction of the lamina and pedicle on each side is a superior articular process and, from the lower lateral corner of the lamina, the inferior articular process extends (see Figure 13–1). On the medial surface of each superior articular process and on the lateral surface of each inferior articular process is the articular facet.

A transverse process projects laterally from the junction of the pedicle and the lamina on each side of the vertebral body (see Figure 13–1). Both the transverse and spinous processes provide areas for muscle attachments.

Ligaments

Anterior Longitudinal Ligament

This ligament covers the anterior aspects of the vertebral bodies and discs (Figure 13–2).[46] It extends from the sacrum along the anterior aspect of the entire spinal column and

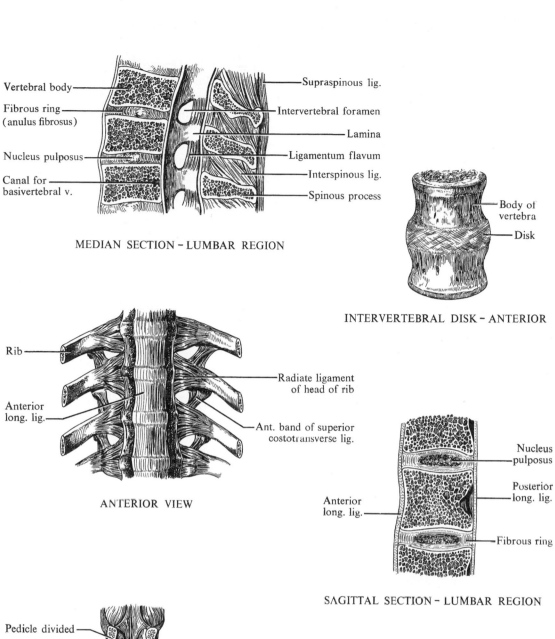

Vertebral body

Fibrous ring
(anulus fibrosus)

Nucleus pulposus

Canal for
basivertebral v.

Supraspinous lig.

Intervertebral foramen

Lamina

Ligamentum flavum

Interspinous lig.

Spinous process

MEDIAN SECTION – LUMBAR REGION

Body of
vertebra

Disk

INTERVERTEBRAL DISK – ANTERIOR

Rib

Anterior
long. lig.

Radiate ligament
of head of rib

Ant. band of superior
costotransverse lig.

ANTERIOR VIEW

Nucleus
pulposus

Posterior
long. lig.

Anterior
long. lig.

Fibrous ring

SAGITTAL SECTION – LUMBAR REGION

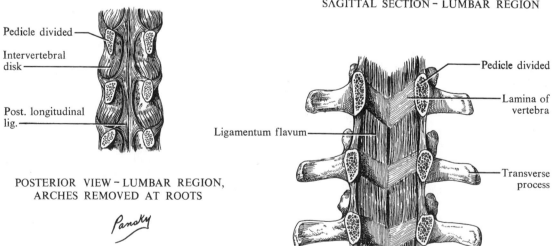

Pedicle divided

Intervertebral
disk

Post. longitudinal
lig.

POSTERIOR VIEW – LUMBAR REGION,
ARCHES REMOVED AT ROOTS

Pansky

Pedicle divided

Lamina of
vertebra

Ligamentum flavum

Transverse
process

FRONT VIEW – BODIES OF VERTEBRAE REMOVED

FIGURE 13–2 The common ligaments of the vertebral column. (*Reproduced,
with permission from Pansky B: Review of Gross Anatomy, 6/e. McGraw-Hill, 1996)*

becomes thinner as it ascends. Some of the ligament fibers insert directly into the bone or periosteum of the centrum.[47] Because of these attachments and the pull on the bone from the ligament, it is proposed that the anterior aspect of the vertebral body becomes the site for osteophytes. The remaining ligament fibers cover two to five segments, attaching to the upper and lower ends of the vertebral body. The ligament is only indirectly connected with the anterior aspect of the disc by loose areolar tissue.[42]

The ligament is innervated by recurrent branches of the grey rami, and functions to prevent over extension of the spinal segments, in addition to functioning as a minor assistant in limiting anterior translation and vertical separation of the vertebral body.

Posterior Longitudinal Ligament
This ligament is found throughout the spinal column and covers the posterior aspect of the centrum and disc (see Figure 13–2). Its deep fibers span two segments, from the superior border of the inferior vertebra, to the inferior margin of the superior. They mesh with, and penetrate, the superficial annular fibers to attach to the posterior margins of the vertebral bodies.[48] The more superficial fibers span up to five segments. In the lumbar spine, the ligament becomes constricted over the vertebral body and widens out over the disc. It does not attach to the concavity of the body but is separated from it by a fat pad, which acts to block the venous drainage through the basivertebral vein during flexion, as the ligament presses it against the opening of the vein. Although the posterior ligament is rather narrow, and is not as massive as the anterior longitudinal ligament, it is important in preventing disc protrusion.[41] Both the anterior longitudinal and the posterior longitudinal ligaments have the same tensile strength per unit area.[49]

Innervated by the sinuvertebral nerve, the ligament tends to tighten in traction and posterior shearing of the vertebral body, and acts to limit flexion over a number of segments.

Ligamentum Flavum
The ligamentum flavum connects two consecutive laminae (see Figure 13–2). This is a bilateral ligament with a medial aspect that attaches superiorly to the lower anterior surface of the lamina and inferior surface of the pedicle, and inferiorly to the back of the lamina and pedicle of the next inferior vertebra.[50] Its lateral portion attaches to the articular process and forms the anterior capsule of the zygapophysial joint.

It is formed primarily from elastin (80%), with the remaining 20% being collagen.[51] It is, therefore, an elastic ligament that is stretched during flexion and it recovers its length with the neutral position or extension.

The function of this ligament is to resist separation of the lamina during flexion, but there is also appreciable strain in the ligament with side-flexion.[42,52] While it seems unlikely that the ligament contributes to an extension recovery from flexion, it does appear to prevent the anterior capsule from becoming nipped between the articular margins as it recoils during extension.[42]

Interspinous Ligament
The interspinous ligament lies deeply between two consecutive spinal processes and is important for the stability of the spine (see Figure 13–2). It represents a major structure for the posterior column of the spine. Unlike the longitudinal ligaments, it is not a continuous fibrous band, but consists of loose tissue that fills the gap between the bodies of the spinous processes.[55,56] It is often disrupted in traumatic cases in which the posterior column becomes unstable. In the 1950s, it was reported that rupture of the interspinous ligament was found frequently in patients undergoing disk surgery, and that disk prolapse was secondary to ligamentous damage.[53,54] An extensive anatomic study on the interspinous ligament showed that degenerative changes start as early as the late second decade. The ruptures occur in more than 20% of the subjects older than 20 years, particularly at L4–5 and L5–S1.[54]

The ligament has three distinct parts: ventral, middle, and dorsal; of which, the middle has the most clinical significance because it is the part where ruptures occur.[52] The dorsal part consists of fibers that run from the posterior upper half of the lower spinous process behind the posterior border of the superior spinous process to form the supraspinous ligament.

Supplied by the medial branch of the dorsal rami, this ligament, thought at one time to resist lumbar flexion movements, more likely functions to resist separation of the spinous processes during flexion.[57]

Palpable tenderness of this structure is often indicative of a segmental hypermobility or instability.[58]

Supraspinous Ligament
This is a single mid-line ligament that bridges the interspinous gaps (see Figure 13–2). The supraspinous ligament is broad, thick and cord-like, but is only well developed in the upper lumbar region.[42] It joins the tips of two adjacent spinous processes and merges with the insertions of the lumbar dorsal muscles. As mentioned, part of the ligament is derived from the posterior part of the interspinous ligament, whereas the rest runs from tip to tip of the spinous processes.[55] Its arrangement allows it to function in a way similar to that of suspension bridge as the spine flexes, the supraspinous ligament is tightened and, in turn, increases the tension on the tethering strands, which pull the vertebra backward and prevent excessive

anterior translation.[42] Because this ligament is the most superficial of the spinal ligaments and farthest from the axis of flexion, it has the greater potential for sprains.[59] As with the interspinous ligament, palpable tenderness of this structure is often indicative of a segmental hypermobility or instability.[58]

Iliolumbar Ligament

The iliolumbar ligament is one of the three vertebropelvic ligaments, the others being the sacrotuberous and the sacrospinous ligaments. While the functional role of the iliolumbar ligament is well known (it restrains flexion, extension, axial rotation, and side-flexion of L5 on S1),[60] its anatomic structure is controversial. The ligament is believed to be a degenerate part of the quadratus lumborum or the iliocostalis. Starting out as a muscle bundle,[61] its initial development begins at about 7 years and is a structure unique to humans. It does not fully develop until the age of 30 years and then begins to deteriorate and have fatty deposits, soon after.[42] An injury to this ligament which often occurs during a bending and lifting maneuver, has a similar history and findings to those of a disk herniation and/or a strain of the thoracolumbar fascia.

Many books and articles describe the iliolumbar ligament differently. According to Testut and Latarjet[62] and Broudeur and colleagues,[63] the ligament always arises from the transverse processes of the L4 and L5 vertebra. These two parts join to form a single large ligament that inserts on the anterior margin of the iliac crest.

Luk and co-workers,[61] Chow and colleagues,[60] and Uhthoff[64] maintain that the ligament only sometimes originates from the L4 transverse process, and always from the L5 transverse process. According to Luk and co-workers and Chow and co-workers, the anterior band inserts on the anterior margin of the iliac crest, and the posterior band inserts on the posterior margin of the iliac crest. According to Uhthoff, the anterior band inserts on the anterior aspect of the iliac wing, and the posterior band inserts from the anterior margin to the apex of the iliac crest.

Hanson and Sonesson[65] describe the ligament to be made up of two bands that originate only from the L5 transverse process, with the anterior band inserting on the upper part of the iliac tuberosity below the medial part of the iliac crest, and the posterior band inserting on the anterior part of the iliac tuberosity above the anterior part of the ligament.

Maigne and Maigne[66] also describe the ligament as originating only from the L5 transverse process, formed by a single band, inserted on the anterior margin of the iliac crest. *Testut's Anatomy*[62] and *Gray's Anatomy*[46] describe some other accessory bands, often called lumbosacral ligaments.

Shellshear and associates have proposed that it consists of five parts[67]:

1. *Anterior.* The anterior part runs posterior-laterally from the anterior-inferior corner of the transverse process to the anterior surface of the iliac crest. This part is thickened superiorly to afford attachment for the lower end of quadratus lumborum. Degenerative disc disease of L5 can lead to an increase tension on these fibers which, when working unilaterally, function to prevent ipsilateral side-flexion,[68] and, when working bilaterally, prevent forward translation of L5 on the sacrum.

2. *Superior.* The superior portion is formed from the membranous anterior fascia surrounding the quadratus lumborum, and it attaches to the anterior-superior border of the transverse process, near its tip. It passes behind the quadratus lumborum to blend with the anterior fibers at the iliac crest. This portion works as a triangular ligament through its attachments to the anterior and posterior parts.

3. *Posterior.* The posterior part of the ligament comes from the tip and posterior aspect of the transverse process to attach to the ilium behind the origin of quadratus lumborum, and give rise to the deep fibers of the longissimus lumborum, forming a triangle with the anterior fibers. The posterior band is thinner and has a narrower insertional site on the iliac crest than the anterior band. It works bilaterally to prevent flexion movements and rotary twisting. Its insertion on the apex of iliac crest permits the local examination, by rubbing it, and to apply deep friction on its insertional site.

4. *Inferior.* The inferior fibers of the ligament arise from the inferior part of the transverse process, pass inferior-laterally in an oblique direction, across the anterior sacroiliac ligament, to attach to the upper part of the iliac fossa. This portion is relatively weak and has a questionable function.

5. *Vertical.* The vertical fibers come from the anterior-inferior border of the transverse process and descend vertically to attach to the iliopectineal line, and have a questionable function.

Considering how difficult it is to study the soft tissue anatomy of the lumbosacral junction, these controversial anatomic observations are not surprising. This area has numerous, complex, varied anatomic structures, but it is important to understand how these structures are arranged to comprehend the clinical and biomechanic repercussions.

The spatial disposition of the iliolumbar ligament is probably important for the stability of the lumbosacral junction, because when it is missing, degenerative instability and isthmic lumbar spondylolisthesis increase.[69,70]

Pseudo-Ligaments

These consist of the intertransverse, transforaminal, and mamillo-accessory ligaments.

Intertransverse Ligaments

These run between transverse processes and appear more membranous than ligamentous.[48] The ligament splits into dorsal and ventral portions between which is a fat-filled recess. The fat in the recess communicates with the intra-articular fat of the apophyseal joints.[42,46] During flexion and extension movements, the fat can be displaced to accommodate the repositioning of the articular zygapophysial joint. The main function of the ligament appears to be to compartmentalize the anterior and posterior musculature.[42]

Transforaminal Ligaments

Occurring in about 47% of subjects, the transforaminal ligaments traverse the lateral end of the intervertebral foramen.[71] They include:

A. Superior corporotransverse. At L5, the fifth lumbar nerve root runs between the ligament and the ala of the sacrum. With marked forward slip and downward descent of L5, or with a loss of disk height, the ligament can have guillotine effect on the fifth nerve root.[72] Symptoms mimic those of an L4–5 disc herniation and can include:
1. Numbness in one dermatome with standing
2. Abatement of symptoms with lying or seated traction

B. Inferior corporotransverse

C. Superior transforaminal

D. Inferior transforaminal

E. Mid transforaminal

Mamillo-Accessory Ligament

This ligament runs from the accessory process to the mammillary process of the same vertebra, bridging the gap between them, and may be a vestige of the semispinalis tendon in the lumbar spine.[73] It forms a tunnel for the medial branch of the dorsal ramus, thereby, preventing it from lifting off the neural arch. In about 10% of cases at L5, it ossifies to form a bony tunnel.[73]

MUSCLES

The lumbar muscles may be divided into intrinsic and extrinsic muscles. Intrinsic muscles attach only to the spinal column, whereas the extrinsic ones are generally limb muscles that originate from the vertebral column. The less familiar terms of hypoaxial and epiaxial refer to muscle position in relation to the vertebral column, rather than the attachment points, with the epiaxial muscle (epimere) lying dorsal to the transverse process, and the hypoaxial musculature (hypomere) anterior to them. The epimere is supplied by the dorsal rami. The hypomere is supplied by the ventral rami.[42]

Hypomere

Psoas Major

This muscle, combined with the iliacus muscle, directly attaches the lumbar spine to the femur,[74] and originates from:

- The anterior-lateral aspects of the vertebral bodies
- The disks of T12 to L5
- The transverse processes of L1 to L5
- The tendinous arch spanning the concavity of the sides of the vertebral bodies

The layered muscle belly runs down the anterior-lateral aspect of the spinal column to form a common tendon with the iliacus that attaches to the lesser trochanter of the femur.

The iliacus is attached superiorly to the iliac fossa and the inner lip of the iliac crest. Joining with the psoas major, the combined tendon passes over the superior lateral aspect of the pubic ramus and attaches to the lesser trochanter of the femur.

Action The psoas major is electromyographically active in many different positions and movements of the lumbar spine. Its activity adds a compressive effect to the intervertebral disc.[75] From a clinical perspective, the iliacus and psoas major are considered together.

The iliopsoas, working bilaterally with the insertion fixed, produces an increase in the lumbar lordosis.[76] With the insertion fixed and the muscle working unilaterally, the iliopsoas side-flexes the spine ipsilaterally.[76] Working from a stable spine above (origin fixed), the iliopsoas muscle flexes the hip joint by flexing the femur on the trunk.[76] It may also assist in external rotation and abduction of the hip joint.[76] Bilateral action of the iliopsoas muscle with the insertion fixed, produces flexion of the trunk on the femur as in the sit-up from supine position or in bending over to touch the toes.[76]

Biomechanically, the iliacus and psoas major serve different functions. With the foot fixed on the ground, contraction of the iliacus produces an anterior torsion of the ilium and extension of the lumbar zygapophysial joints. If there is a decrease in the length of the iliacus due to adaptive shortening or increased efferent neural input to the muscle, the result is an anteriorly rotated pelvis, producing the compressive and anterior shear stresses on the lumbosacral and lumbar zygapophysial joints as they move towards increased extension.[77] With the foot fixed on the ground, contraction of the psoas major produces an anterior shear, which has the potential to increase the lumbar lordosis and increase flexion of the lumbar-pelvic unit on the femur.[77] Porterfield and DeRosa[77] suggest that the "toe-out" gait pattern, adopted by the pregnant female or the patient with a weak and pendulous abdomen, is a compensatory pattern to decrease the muscle tension in the psoas major, thereby reducing the compression and anterior shear to the lumbar spine.

Trunk flexion by the iliopsoas, which involves fixation of the insertion, involves a change in the amount of lumbar lordosis, and is dependent on the lumbar-pelvic rhythm.[78] The first 60 degrees of forward bending, on the average, are due to flexion of the lumbar motion segments, which is followed by an additional movement at the hip joints of about 25 degrees.[79] The psoas major is innervated by the ventral rami of L1 and L2.

Psoas Minor

This is a small inconsistent muscle that arises from the T12 and L1 disc to attach to the iliopubic eminence. It weakly flexes the lumbar spine when working from a fixed pelvis, and helps tilt the pelvis posteriorly when working from a stable spine.

Quadratus Lumborum

The muscle attaches to:

- The inferior anterior surface of the twelfth rib
- The anterior surface of the upper four transverse processes
- The anterior iliolumbar ligament
- The iliac crest lateral to the attachment of the iliolumbar ligament

The quadratus lumborum competes with the iliocostalis muscle as the origin of the iliolumbar ligament.[80] The muscle is large and rectangular with its fibers passing medially upwards. It is supplied by the ventral rami of T12–L2.[46]

Action The muscle is active during inspiration where it fixes the lowest rib to afford a stable base from which the diaphragm can act. Working unilaterally, it side-flexes the lumbar spine. It is essentially a static stabilizer and works very hard when a heavy weight is held in the opposite hand.

Epimere

Not all of the following muscles have a lumbar vertebral attachment, but all have a very definite effect on the lumbar spine.

Interspinales

These are located either side of, and connect to, adjacent spinous process. There are four pairs, and they can act with multifidus to produce the rocking component of extension. They are supplied by the medial branch of the dorsal ramus.

Action Probably angular extension and control of flexion, as a result of their attachment to the spinous process.

Intertransversarii Mediales

Considered by many to be true back muscles, these muscles originate from the accessory and mammillary process and the connecting accessory ligament, and insert into the mammillary process of the vertebra below. They are supplied by the dorsal ramus of the spinal nerve.[81]

Action As they are very small muscles and lie close to the axis of motion, it seems unlikely that they can directly contribute very much to either side-flexion or extension. It is more likely that they have proprioceptive mechanisms, with their muscle spindles monitoring and helping control the movements of larger better placed muscles.[82]

Multifidus

Over the past several decades, there has been much research regarding the multifidus with particular reference to its relationship to low back pain, and its importance in rehabilitation. This is the largest of the intrinsic muscles and lies most medially in the spinal gutter. It is a fascicular muscle with each fascicle layered on another, giving it a laminated appearance.[42] It originates in three groups, arising from the same vertebra.

1. Laminar fibers from the inferior-posterior edge of the lamina
2. Basal fibers from the base of the spinous process
3. Common tendon fibers from a common tendon attached to the inferior tip of the spinous process

It has a complicated insertion:[83,84]

	Laminar	Basal	Common Tendon
L1	m.p. L3	m.p. L4	m.p. L5, S1, and PSIS
L2	m.p. L4	m.p. L5	m.p. S1 and ant-lateral aspect of PSIS
L3	m.p. L5	m.p. S1	inferior to the PSIS and lateral sacrum
L4	m.p. S1	as c.t.	sacrum, lateral to foramina
L5	as c.t.	as c.t.	sacrum, medial to foramina

m.p. = mammillary process.
c.t. = common tendon.
PSIS =posterior superior iliac spine.

The muscle has the distinction of being innervated segmentally by the medial branch of the dorsal ramus of the same level or level below the originating spinous process.[85,86]

Being of segmental origin and innervation, any impairment of the multifidus can produce hypertonus from segmental facilitation of this muscle. As each muscle is only supplied from its own segment, hypertonicity will direct the examiner to this segment.

Action Working bilaterally, it will produce the rocking component of extension, but due to its vertical orientation, it cannot produce the accompanying translation. Additionally, the muscle, by "bow stringing" over a number of segments, can increase the lumbar lordosis, working in a postural role.[87]

Unilaterally, it should be able to produce side-flexion and rotation. However, its horizontal vector is very small and it is unlikely to be an efficient rotator of the spine.[42] It is consistently active during both ipsilateral and contralateral spinal rotation and may act as a stabilizer.[88] That is, both are simultaneously active regardless of which way the spine is turning. It is believed that this is a synergistic function opposing the flexing moment of the abdominals as they rotate the trunk.[89]

The multifidus is active in nearly all antigravity activities and appears to contribute to the stability of the lumbar spine by compressing the vertebra together.[90] Indeed, recruitment of the multifidus during lumbar hyperextension has been found to be markedly different in patients with chronic low back pain compared with normal.[91]

The multifidus also shares a close association with the gluteus maximus, the sacrotuberous ligament that is thought to enhance sacroiliac joint and lumbar spine stability.

Erector Spinae

This is a composite muscle consisting of the iliocostalis lumborum and the thoracic longissimus. Both muscles have a thoracic and lumbar component and are subdivided into the lumbar and thoracic longissimii and iliocostallii.[42] The innervation of the erector spinae muscles is by the medial branch of the dorsal ramus of the thoracic and lumbar spinal nerves.

Longissimus Thoracis Pars Lumborum

This is a fascicular muscle arising from the accessory processes of the lumbar vertebrae to insert into the posterior superior iliac spine and the iliac crest lateral to it. The upper four tendons converge to form the lumbar aponeurosis, which inserts lateral to the L5 fascicle.

Action The muscles have both a vertical and horizontal vector, each with a relative size that varies for each fascicle.

The vertical vector is much the larger of the two, and will produce extension or side-flexion depending on whether it is functioning bilaterally or unilaterally.[92] However, due to its attachment to the transverse rather than the spinous process, it is much less efficient than the multifidus to produce posterior sagittal rotation, due to its reduced leverage.[93] The horizontal vector is much larger and more posterior than the multifidus and so this muscle is eminently capable of producing the posterior translation of extension.[93] It is a poor axial rotator because its line of action is directed in line with the axis of motion. Because it is attached to a single vertebra, its action in increasing the lordosis will be minimal. Mathematic analysis of the lumbosacral portion of the muscle suggests that the net effect would be an anterior, not posterior, shear.[42]

Iliocostalis Lumborum Pars Lumborum

There are four overlying fascicles arising from the tip of the upper four transverse processes and the adjoining middle layer of the thoracolumbar fascia. The fibers insert onto the iliac crest, with the lower fibers being deepest, and attach laterally to the posterior superior iliac spine. The other fibers are lateral to this.[93]

There is no muscular fiber from L5, but it is believed that this is represented by the iliolumbar ligament, which, as previously mentioned, is completely muscular in children, becoming collagenous by 30 years of age.

Action The vectors and actions of this muscle are similar to those of longissimus. However, the more lateral attachment of the lower fibers and their attachment to the transverse processes produce strong axial rotation (probably the only intrinsic muscles to do so) and act with the multifidus as synergists during abdominal muscle action to produce rotation.[93]

Longissimus Thoracis Pars Thoracis

This muscle group consists of 11 to 12 pairs of muscles extending from the transverse processes of T2 and their ribs. It runs inferior-medially to attach to the spinous processes of L3–5 and the sacral spinous processes, as well as the posterior superior iliac spine.

Action The orientation and various attachments of this muscle group allow it to act indirectly on the lumbar spine, which, by a bowstring action, can increase the lordosis. The main action of the muscle appears to be the extension of the thoracic spine on that of the lumbar. An anatomic-mathematical study[94] suggests that 70% to 80% of the force required to extend the upper lumbar spine is produced from the thoracic fibers of the erector spinae, which also generate 50% of the force in the lower levels.

Iliocostalis Lumborum Pars Thoracis

The thoracic iliocostalis serves as the thoracic part of the iliocostalis lumborum and not the iliocostalis thoracic. It is a layered muscle consisting of inferior-medially orientated fascicles and attached to the following points.[93]

- The lateral part of the lower eight rib angles
- Posterior superior iliac spine
- Dorsal surface of the sacrum, distal to the multifidus

Actions This muscle completely spans the lumbar spine. It is in an excellent position to extend and side-flex the spine as well as increase the lordosis. It is a weak rotator because the amount of rib separation on ipsilateral rotation is minor, but on contralateral rotation, it is better. It is, therefore, possible that the muscle is an effective derotator of the spine.[42]

Thoracolumbar Fascia

The fascia extends in the lumbar region, from the spinous process of T12, to the posterior superior iliac spine and iliac crest. It consists of three layers of connective tissue that envelop the lumbar muscles and separates them into anterior, middle, and posterior compartments or layers.[95]

The anterior layer is derived from, and covers, the anterior surface of the quadratus lumborum muscle. It is attached to the anterior transverse processes, and then to the intertransverse ligaments. On the lateral side of the quadratus lumborum, it blends with the other layers of the fascia.

The middle layer is posterior to the quadratus lumborum, with its medial attachment to the tips of the transverse processes and the intertransverse ligaments. Laterally, it gives rise to, or is attached to, the transverse abdominal aponeurosis.

The posterior layer covers the lumbar musculature and arises from the spinous processes, wrapping around the muscles. It blends with the other layers of the fascia along the lateral border of iliocostalis lumborum in a dense thickening of the fascia called the lateral raphe.[95] This layer consists of two laminae, a superficial one with its fibers orientated inferior-medially, and a deep lamina with fibers that are inferior-lateral. The superficial fibers are derived from the latissimus dorsi.

Action
- Provides muscular attachment.
- Stabilizes the spine against anterior shear and flexion moments.
- Resists segmental flexion via tension generated by the transverse abdominis on the spinous process.
- Assists in transmission of extension forces during lifting.

The posterior ligamentous system has been proposed as a model to explain some of the forces required for lifting. It is believed to transmit forces by passive resistance to flexion, from the joint capsule and extracapsular ligaments, and from the more dynamic effects of the thoracolumbar fascia.[96]

The passive elements are strong enough to withstand very high forces, allowing most of the lifting force to be generated by the hip extensors on the pelvis provided that the lumbar spine is preflexed and remains that way. The abdominal muscles maintain this flexion and also, perhaps incidentally, raise the intra-abdominal pressure. The thoracolumbar fascia is a factor in lifting and has been speculated to provide this assistance in three different ways.[97]

1. By attaching to the ilium and sacrum, the fibers running from the spinous processes of L4 and L5 would afford an indirect connection between the hip extensors and the spine
2. The pull of the transverse abdominis on the lateral raphe increases the tension in the posterior layer and, due to the cross-hatch arrangement of the layer's fibers, limits intersegmental flexion and anterior translation.
3. The complete envelopment of the back muscles by the fascia's middle and posterior layers increases the tension generated in these muscle during their contraction, which also reduces the amount of flexion available. It is termed the hydraulic amplifier.[98] Recently, the effect of this amplifier has been shown to be a minor contribution.[99]

Intervertebral Joint

The articulations between two consecutive lumbar vertebrae form three joints, one between the two vertebral bodies, and the other two by the articulation of the superior articular process of one vertebra, with the inferior articular processes of the vertebra above, known as the zygapophysial joints. The only formal name for the joints between the vertebral bodies is the classification to which the joints belong—symphysis or intervertebral amphiarthrosis.[42]

Zygapophysial Joint

As mentioned, these are the posterior joints of the three-joint complex that make up the intervertebral joint. They are formed by the inferior and superior articular processes of adjacent vertebrae and demonstrate the features of a typical synovial joint.

In the intact lumbar vertebral column, the primary function of the zygapophysial joints is to resist the forces of anterior shear and the torque of the vertebral bodies.

Their additional function includes production of coupling movements.

The superior articulating facet of the inferior vertebra is slightly concave and faces medially and posteriorly. In general, there is a change from a relatively sagittal orientation at L1 to L3, to a more coronal orientation at L5 and S1.

From an anterior-posterior perspective, the joints appear straight, but when viewed from above, they are seen to be curved into a "J" or "C" shape. Their orientation varies both with the level and with the individual subject. It is thought that this orientation serves to maximally restrict anterior and rotary movements, and that the C-shaped joints do better in preventing anterior displacement than the J-shaped joints, due to the curvature of the joint surfaces where the superior-medial end of the superior facet limits anterior motion.[42] Both shapes competently prevent rotation.

A fibrous capsule surrounds the joint on all of its aspects except the anterior aspect, which consists of the ligamentum flavum. Posteriorly, the capsule is reinforced by the deep fibers of the multifidus.[100] In lumbar extension, the posterior capsule can become pinched between the apex of the inferior facet and the lamina below. To prevent this, some fibers of the multifidus blend with the posterior capsular fibers and appear to keep the capsule taut.

Superiorly and inferiorly, the capsule is very loose. Superiorly, it bulges toward the base of the next superior transverse process while, inferiorly, it does so over the back of the lamina. In both the superior and inferior poles of the capsule, there is a very small hole that allows the passage of fat from within the capsule to the extra-capsular space.[101] There are three types of intra-articular meniscoids

- A connective tissue rim. Merely a wedge-shaped thickening of the internal capsule that fills the joint space.
- An adipose tissue pad. These are found at the anterior-superior and inferior-posterior parts of the joint, and consist of fat and blood vessels contained in a fold of synovium that project into the joint cavity. These structures tend to increase in size with age.
- A fibroadipose meniscoid. This is the largest of the internal structures, projecting into the superior and inferior aspect of the joint.

It is thought that the function of the intra-articular meniscoid is the following

1. Fill the joint cavity
2. Increase the articular surface area without reducing flexibility

3. Protect the articular surfaces as they become exposed during extreme flexion and extension

Their ability to cause symptoms is thought to occur when they fail to return to their original position on recovery from a flexion or extension movement, blocking the joint toward the neutral position.

Age Changes

The subchondral bone of the zygapophysial joint increases in thickness during the first two thirds of life, reaching a maximum at about 50 years, after which it begins to thin.[102,103] The articular cartilage, on the other hand, continues to thicken throughout life. The area of cartilage most involved in resisting anterior shear forces is the anterior-medial part of the superior zygapophysial joint, and it is this area that is most vulnerable to fibrillation.[42] The tangential splitting and vertical tearing of the cartilage that occurs with age are believed to reflect these forces, and are part of the normal degeneration of the joint.[42]

In addition to the changes to the articular cartilage, the hypertrophy and spreading of its edges appears to represent a response to repeated rotatory stresses that might otherwise damage the articular margins. As a consequence to these stresses, osteophytes can form, fortuitously producing an increase in the load-bearing surface area of the joint.

Nerve Supply of the Lumbar Segment

The nerves of the lumbar spine follow a general pattern (Figure 13–3).

Disc

The outer half of the disc is innervated by the sinuvertebral nerve[104] (Figure 13–4) and the grey rami communicants,[105] with the posterior-lateral aspect being innervated by both the sinuvertebral nerve[106] and the grey rami communicants. The lateral aspect receives only sympathetic innervation. The nerve endings are both simple and complex, encapsulated and nonencapsulated, existing as free nerve endings and in plexi, loops, and meshes.

It has been suggested that apart from a nociceptive function, these nerve endings may also have a proprioceptive one,[107] although a study in cats did not find any evidence for this.[108] Due to the extremely small number of blood vessels in the disc, a vasomotor or vasosensory function is unlikely. For a more detailed description of the intervertebral disc, the reader should refer to Chapter 7.

Ligaments

The posterior longitudinal ligament is innervated by the sinuvertebral nerve, whereas the anterior longitudinal ligament

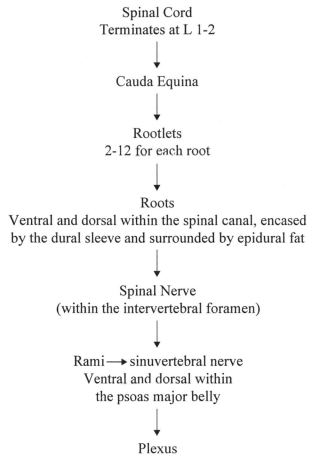

Spinal Cord
Terminates at L 1-2

↓

Cauda Equina

↓

Rootlets
2-12 for each root

↓

Roots
Ventral and dorsal within the spinal canal, encased
by the dural sleeve and surrounded by epidural fat

↓

Spinal Nerve
(within the intervertebral foramen)

↓

Rami ⟶ sinuvertebral nerve
Ventral and dorsal within
the psoas major belly

↓

Plexus

FIGURE 13–3   Nerve supply of the lumbar segment.

reccives its supply from the grey rami communicants. The ligamentous flavum, interspinous and supraspinous ligaments, are innervated by the medial branch of the dorsal ramus.

Dural Sleeve
Only the anterior aspect of the dural sleeve is innervated,[109] and this by the sinuvertebral nerve. Although innervation occurs from both the immediate and the

superior and inferior nerves,[110] the bulk of the supply is from the nerve of the same level.

Zygapophysial Joint
Zygapophysial joints are innervated by the medial branches of the dorsal rami.[81,104,111,112] Therefore, the distributions of referred pain must be considered in relation to the neurologic supply of the dorsal rami.

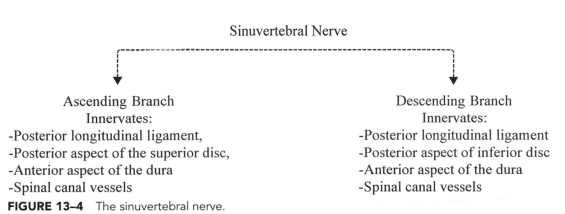

Sinuvertebral Nerve

Ascending Branch
Innervates:
-Posterior longitudinal ligament,
-Posterior aspect of the superior disc,
-Anterior aspect of the dura
-Spinal canal vessels

Descending Branch
Innervates:
-Posterior longitudinal ligament
-Posterior aspect of inferior disc
-Anterior aspect of the dura
-Spinal canal vessels

FIGURE 13–4   The sinuvertebral nerve.

The L1–4 dorsal rami form three branches, medial, lateral, and intermediate, in the intertransverse space.[81] The L1–4 medial branches curve around the root of the superior articular process, passing through a notch bridged by the mamillo-accessory ligament. Thereafter, they supply articular branches to the caudal aspect of the joint above, and to the cranial aspect of the joint below, and ramify in multifidus.[81,104] Each joint receives its nerve supply from the corresponding medial branch above and below the joint.[81,104] For instance, the L4–5 joint receives its nerve supply from the medial branches of L3 and L4.

The lateral branches cross the subjacent transverse process and pursue a sinuous course caudally, laterally, and dorsally, through the iliocostalis lumborum.[81] They innervate that muscle, and eventually the L1–3 lateral branches pierce the dorsal layer of thoracolumbar fascia and become cutaneous. They emerge from the iliocostalis, cross the iliac crest, and supply the skin over the lateral buttock as far as the greater trochanter.[89,104] The L1–2 lateral branches cross the iliac crest in the subcutaneous tissue parallel to the T12 cutaneous branch. The L3 lateral branch is bound to the iliac crest by a bridge of connective tissue just lateral to the origin of the iliocostalis lumborum. The L4 lateral branch remains entirely intramuscular.[81]

The intermediate branches run dorsally and caudally from the intertransverse spaces and are distributed to the longissimus thoracis; the intermediate branches form a series of intersegmental communications within the longissimus thoracis.[81,104]

The L5 dorsal ramus runs dorsally and caudally over the ala of the sacrum, lying in the groove formed by the junction between the ala and the root of the superior articular process of the sacrum.[81,104]

Along this course, it divides into two branches, a medial branch and an intermediate branch. It lacks a lateral branch. The medial branch curves medially around the caudal aspect of the lumbosacral zygapophysial joint, supplies the multifidus muscle, and ends there.[81,104] The intermediate branch innervates the longissimus thoracis and communicates with the S1 dorsal ramus.[81] The iliocostalis does not caudally extend as far as the L5 spinal nerve and so does not receive a supply from it.[104]

Thus, the L1–4 medial branches are distributed to the zygapophysial joints and to the multifidus. Consequently, given that the medial branches supply other structures in addition to the zygapophysial joints, the reproduction of pain after medial branch stimulation does not exclusively point to the zygapophyseal joint as the source of pain in patients. The joint is innervated by a direct articular branch from the dorsal ramus (Figure 13–5) for the anterior aspect.[113] The nerve endings suggest proprioceptive and nociceptive functions.

Lumbar Spine Vascularization

The blood supply for the lumbar spine is provided by the lumbar arteries (Figure 13–6). Its venous drainage occurs via the lumbar veins (Figure 13–7).

BIOMECHANICS

Three cardinal planes exist in this area; sagittal (flexion and extension), coronal (side-flexion), and transverse (rotation). This area has varying degrees of segmental motion. The greatest amount of flexion/extension (20 to 25 degrees) occurs at L4–5, and at L5–S1, and decreases cranially.[41,42]

The human lumbar facets are capable of only two major motions, gliding upward and gliding downward. If these movements occur in the same direction, flexion or extension occurs. If in opposite directions, side-flexion occurs. Most of the side-flexion of the lumbar spine occurs in the mid-lumbar area. Rotation, which occurs with

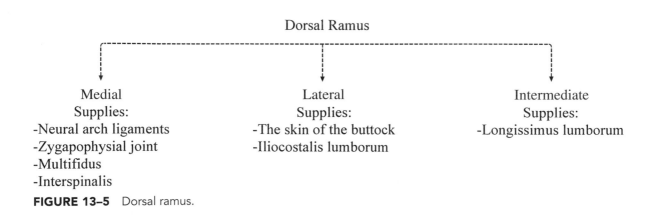

FIGURE 13–5 Dorsal ramus.

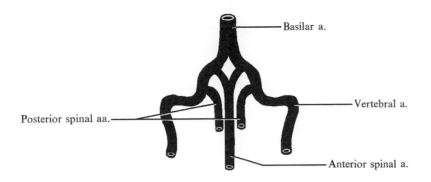

ORIGIN OF SPINAL ARTERIES (SCHEMATIC)

ARTERIES OF SPINAL CORD

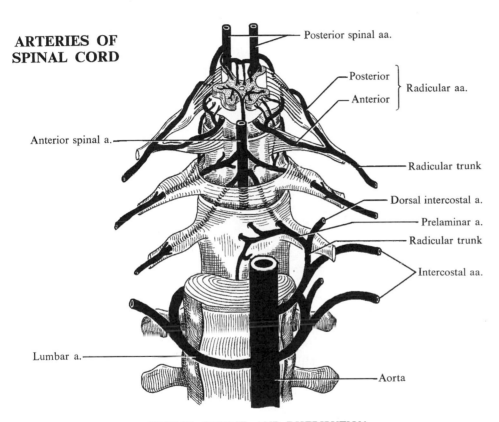

SOURCE, COURSE, AND DISTRIBUTION

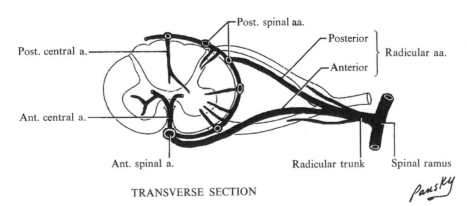

TRANSVERSE SECTION

FIGURE 13–6 Arteries of the spinal cord. *(Reproduced, with permission from Pansky B: Review of Gross Anatomy, 6/e. McGraw-Hill, 1996)*

285

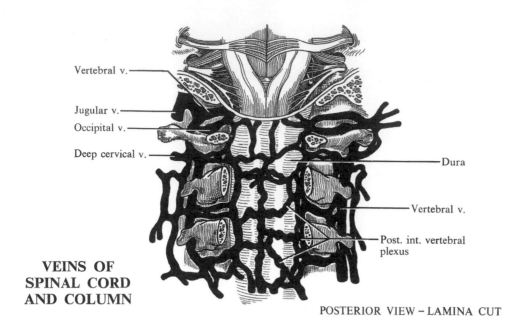

VEINS OF SPINAL CORD AND COLUMN

Vertebral v.

Jugular v.

Occipital v.

Deep cervical v.

Dura

Vertebral v.

Post. int. vertebral plexus

POSTERIOR VIEW – LAMINA CUT

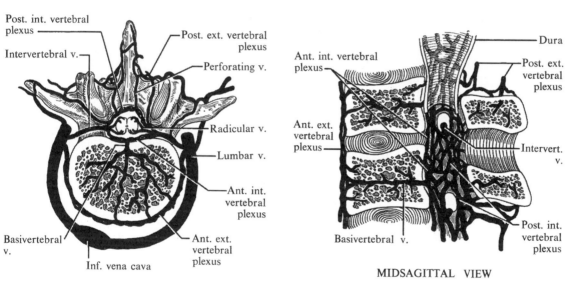

Post. int. vertebral plexus

Intervertebral v.

Post. ext. vertebral plexus

Perforating v.

Radicular v.

Lumbar v.

Ant. int. vertebral plexus

Basivertebral v.

Inf. vena cava

Ant. ext. vertebral plexus

TRANSVERSE VIEW

Ant. int. vertebral plexus

Ant. ext. vertebral plexus

Basivertebral v.

Dura

Post. ext. vertebral plexus

Intervert. v.

Post. int. vertebral plexus

MIDSAGITTAL VIEW

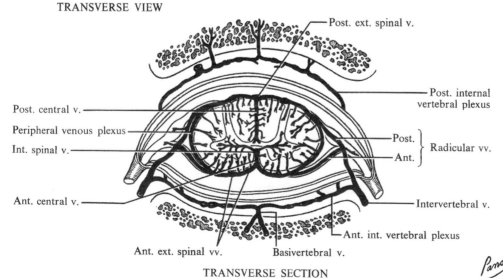

Post. ext. spinal v.

Post. central v.

Peripheral venous plexus

Int. spinal v.

Ant. central v.

Post. internal vertebral plexus

Post.

Ant. } Radicular vv.

Intervertebral v.

Ant. int. vertebral plexus

Ant. ext. spinal vv.

Basivertebral v.

TRANSVERSE SECTION

FIGURE 13–7 Veins of the spinal cord and column. *(Reproduced, with permission from Pansky B: Review of Gross Anatomy, 6/e. McGraw-Hill, 1996)*

side-flexion as a coupled motion, is minimal, and occurs most at the lumbosacral junction. The amount of range available decreases with age as the elastin changes to collagen. There are a number of forces that the spine, as well as the intervertebral disc, must withstand. These are axial compression, axial traction, and anterior, posterior, and lateral shears. A force that produces a translation is called a shear. A force that causes a rotation is called torque.

Kinematics of Flexion

The lumbar spine is well designed for flexion. During flexion, the entire lumbar spine leans forward, producing a combination of an anterior roll and an anterior glide of the vertebral body.[114] During flexion, the lumbar spine tips forward on the sacrum, resulting in a straightening, or minimal reversal of, the lordosis. At L4–5, reversal may occur, but at the L5–S1 level, the joint will straighten, but not reverse,[115] unless there is pathology present. A separation of the laminae and spinous processes also occurs.

During the anterior rocking motion of the segment that occurs with flexion, the inferior facets of the superior vertebra lift upward and backward, opening a small gap between the facets. The superior vertebra slides forward, closing the gap, producing anterior translation. The zygapophysial joints are, therefore, vital in the limitation of this anterior shear, with the anterior-medial portion of the superior zygapophysial joint taking most of the stress.[116] In addition, stability is enhanced by the 5 to 7 millimeters of slide,[88] producing tension of the joint capsule and a capsular end feel. Flexion is also limited by the decreased compression ability of the anterior structures and by the decreased extensibility of the posterior structures (ligaments, disc, and muscles). With hyperflexion, the nucleus material can become lodged in the outer fibers of the anulus and become a space-occupying lesion. These outer layers of the anulus, which are attached to the end plate of the vertebral body, can be avulsed. In addition, hyperflexion can produce a meniscus entrapment and cause the zygapophysial joint to lock.

Kinetics of Flexion

The zygapophysial joints play a major role in the stability of spine during flexion. The simultaneous contribution by the various structures to the resistance of segmental flexion is resisted by the following.[117]

- The joint capsule resists about 39%
- The supraspinous and interspinous ligaments resist about 19%.
- The ligamentum flavum ligament resists about 13%.

- The intervertebral disc resists about 29%.
- The compressibility of the structures anterior to the fulcrum

An anterior sagittal translation, or shear, is generated by:

- Sequential flexion
- Nonsequential extension (lordosing)
- Weight bearing in neutral at the lumbosacral junction
- Extension at the lumbosacral junction
- Gravity

This translation or shear force is resisted by:

- The superior-anterior orientation of the lateral fibers of the anulus.
- The iliolumbar and supraspinous ligaments at the L5–S1 segment, with the longitudinal ligaments helping to a lesser extent.
- The semisagittal and sagittal orientation of the zygapophysial joints, which cause the superior facet to come against the inferior one during an anterior shear, with the highest pressure occurring on the medial end of zygapophysial joint surface.
- The horizontal vector of the erector spinae, and the multifidus, act to pull the vertebrae backward.
- The development of osteophytes, which increase the load-bearing area

While much emphasis has been placed on the strengthening of the rectus abdominus to protect against anterior shearing, recent research has suggested that it is the contraction of the hoop-like transversus abdominis that creates a rigid cylinder, resulting in enhanced stiffness of the lumbar spine.[90,118] The cross-hatch arrangement of the thoracolumbar fascia creates a pressurized visceral cavity anterior to the spine when the transversus abdominis contracts, resulting in the production of a force against the apex of the lumbar lordosis. This force increases the stability of the lumbar spine during a variety of postures and movements.[119]

Kinematics of Extension

Extension movements of the lumbar spine produce a converse of those that occur in flexion. Theoretically, true extension of the lumbar spine is pathologic, and depends on the definition used. Pure extension involves a posterior roll and glide of the vertebra, and a posterior and inferior motion of the zygapophysial joints, but not necessarily a change in the degree of lordosis. The inferior zygapophysial joint of the superior vertebra moves downward, impacting with the lamina below, producing a bony end feel[120] and a buckling of the interspinous ligament between the two spinous processes. This impaction, accentuated when the joint is subjected to the action of the back muscles,[121] serves to block extension. However, if the extending force continues to be applied, especially unilaterally, the superior facets can pivot on their inferior counterparts, producing a strain on the opposite zygapophysial joint and potentially damaging or tearing the capsule. Repetitive contact of these spinous processes can lead to a periostitis called "kissing spine" or Baastrup's disease,[122] with resulting ligamentous laxity and hypermobility of the segment.[123]

An increase in the lumbar lordosis involves the anterior motion of the vertebrae and their associated structures. While seemingly esoterical, this has clinical implications during the examination when the clinician is assessing the ability of the patient to assume the extended position of the lumbar spine. Pure lumbar extension involves the patient leaning back at the waist. Patients with low back pain tend to utilize a protective guarding mechanism against the compression and shearing forces generated by simply hyperextending the hips. By applying a compressive force through the patient's shoulders during the backward bending, the clinician can induce a small increase in the lumbar lordosis. Pure extension is limited by the:

- Ability of structures anterior to the fulcrum to be elongated
- Ability of the intervertebral disc to allow compression

Hyperextension injuries, which are almost always traumatic in origin, produce a shearing force in a posterior direction. The same mechanisms that resist extension assist, with some additional help from:

- Joint capsule tension
- A passive restraint from the psoas major muscle

Axial Rotation
Axial rotation of the lumbar spine involves the following.

- Twisting or torsion of the disc, a gapping of the ipsilateral zygapophysial joint, and a compression of the contralateral joint. For example, with left axial rotation, the right inferior zygapophysial joint will impact on the superior zygapophysial joint of the bone below.
- Stress on those annular fibers inclined toward the direction of rotation

Because collagen can only elongate 4% before damage, maximum segmental rotation at each segmental level is limited to about 3 degrees.[79]

The axis of rotation passes through the aspect of the disc and vertebral body.[124] In normal segments, the zygapophysial joints protect the disc from torsional injuries, becoming impacted before microfailure of the disc can occur. During axial rotation, tension is built in the interspinous and supraspinous ligaments, and the contralateral joint becomes impacted after less than 1 degree of rotation. Further movement is accommodated by compression of the articular cartilage. It has been calculated that about 0.5 mm of compression must occur for each 1 degree of rotation to occur, and that to allow 3 degrees of rotation, the cartilage must be compressed to about 62% of its resting thickness.[125] If this 3-degree range is exceeded, further rotation is impure, forcing the upper vertebra to pivot backward on the impacted joint, around a new axis of rotation. This causes the vertebra to swing laterally and backward, exerting a lateral shear on the anulus. At this extreme, the impacted joint is compressed, the disc is vulnerable to torsional and shear forces, and the other joint capsule is placed under severe tension. Failure can occur in any of these structures. If the force continues, microscopic damage occurs in the form of minute cartilaginous fissuring and microscopic tearing of the anulus fibrosus. Continued torsion can result in macroscopic damage with compression fractures of the contralateral lamina, subchondral fractures, fragmentation of the articular surface and tearing, avulsion of the ipsilateral joint capsule, or a pars interarticularis fracture.[42] Axial torsion of the intact intervertebral disc is resisted by various structures.[126]

- About 65% of the resistance comes from a combination of tension and impaction of the zygapophysial joint and tension of the supraspinous and interspinous ligaments.
- The disc contributes about 35% of the resistance.
- If rotation occurs with flexion, the likelihood of an anulus injury increases in forward flexion[127] due to the minimal contact of the zygapophysial joints, reducing their protective mechanism.

Forced Rotation		
1 degree	Free axial rotation	No damage
2 degrees	Hyaline compression	No damage
4 degrees	Hyaline and anulus	Micro damage
7 degrees	Hyaline, anulus, lamina subchondral, and bone fractures	Macro damage

Side-Flexion
This movement is a coupled movement involving rotation. The means of how this is achieved has been the subject of debate for many years and it is difficult to ascertain how an impaired segment would behave as compared to a healthy one.

The ranges in Table 13–1 are the average for live normal males aged 25 to 36 years[128]

TABLE 13–1 AVAILABLE SEGMENTAL MOTION

SEGMENTAL LEVEL	SIDE FLEX L : R	ROTATION L : R	FLEXION°	EXTENSION°	COMBINED FLEXION AND EXTENSION°
L1–2	5 : 6	1 : 1	8	5	13–5
L2–3	5 : 6	1 : 1	10	3	13–2
L3–4	5 : 6	1 : 2	12	1	13–2
L4–5	3 : 5	1 : 2	13	2	16–4
L5–S1	0 : 2	1 : 0	9	5	14–5

COMMON LESIONS AND PATHOLOGIES OF THE LUMBAR SPINE

Intervertebral Disc Lesions

These lesions are covered in depth in Chapters 7 and 10.

Spondylolisthesis

Forward slipping of one vertebral body (and the remainder of the spinal column above it) in relation to the vertebral segment immediately below it is referred to as spondylolisthesis. This forward slip of the vertebra is resisted by the bony block of the posterior facets, by an intact neural arch and pedicle, and, in the case of the L5 vertebra, the iliolumbar ligament. The disc at the level of the spondylolisthesis is subjected to considerable anteriorly directed shear forces, and is the main structure that opposes these shear forces, functioning to prevent against further slippage and keeping the spinal motion segment in a stable equilibrium.

The most common site for spondylolysis and spondylolisthesis is L5–S1.

Age appears to be an important factor in the natural history of spondylolisthesis. Children under the age of 5 years rarely present with spondylolysis and severe spondylolisthesis is equally rare. The period of most rapid slipping is between the ages of 10 and 15, with no more slipping occurring after the age of 20.[129] Higher grade olisthesis is twice as common in girls as in boys.[130]

Degenerative spondylolisthesis is the only disorder of the adult spine in which a distinct difference between genders has been observed. It is approximately four times more common in women than men. One study found a 4.1% incidence of degenerative spondylolisthesis in adults.[131] The most common site for this type of spondylolisthesis is the fourth lumbar vertebra.

There are two prevailing theories as to the etiology of degenerative spondylolisthesis

1. *Dysfunction of the disc.*[132,133] It is postulated that slip progression after skeletal maturity is almost always related to disc degeneration at the slip level. As the biochemical and biomechanical integrity of the disc is lost, the lumbosacral slip becomes unstable and progresses. Disc degeneration at the slip level and adult slip progression are likely to develop during the fourth and fifth decades of life. This unstable mechanical situation leads to symptoms of low back and sciatic pain.

2. *Horizontalization of the lamina and the facets and/or sacrum morphology.* One study found a more trapezoidal shape of the vertebral body, and/or a dome-shaped contour of the top of the sacrum are found in individuals with slipping.[134] Another study found that patients with degenerative spondylolisthesis had greater anterior flexion of the lumbar spine than normal individuals of comparable age,[135] whereas a further study postulated that a segment of the population is predisposed to degenerative spondylolisthesis by the sagittal orientation of their facet joints.[136] If the lamina and the facets are horizontalized, the vertebra is more likely to slip, but this condition alone does not produce slipping according to a study by Nagaosa and co-workers,[137] who found that almost all of the patients in their study of spondylolisthesis demonstrated disc degeneration and intervertebral instability, but that not every case progressed to spondylolisthesis. In addition, it is unlikely that there is a group of people who develop these anomalies. In fact, one study indicated that the greater angles seen in degenerative spondylolisthesis are not developmental but are acquired as a result of remodeling associated with the arthritic process, and, that the steeper angles are the effect of anterior wear of the facet joints rather than being a cause of the forward subluxation.[138] Other factors, such as the lumbosacral angle, ligamentous laxity, previous pregnancy, and hormonal factors, impose an increased stress on the L4–L5 facet joints and, as most of the stress is placed anteriorly on the inferior facet of L4, the wear pattern is concentrated at this point, creating a more sagittally orientated joint by way of remodeling.[138]

Whatever the cause, if the syndesmosis maintains the bonds between the two halves of the neural arch, there is no mechanical instability and the patient is asymptomatic. If the syndesmosis is loose, separation occurs during flexion. Repetitive flexion strains can give rise to both local and referred pain in a sciatic distribution, due to nerve root irritation or degenerative changes occurring in the underlying disc.

The spectrum of neurologic involvement runs from rare to more common in the higher grade slips, with the majority of neurologic deficits being an L5 radiculopathy with an L5–S1 spondylolisthesis. Cauda equina impairments can occur in grade III or IV slips. Symptoms, if they do occur, usually begin in the second decade but cannot be correlated with the degree of slip and, often, the pain may not originate from the spondylolisthetic segment. This is due to the fact that with a forward slip of the vertebral body, the intervertebral foramen is generally enlarged. It is only when the neural arch rotates on the pivot formed by its articulation with the sacrum, or there are anterior osteophytes, that encroachment occurs resulting in root irritation. Isthmic spondylolisthesis develops as a stress fracture. In more advanced slips, there is a palpable soft tissue depression immediately above the L5 spinous process on passing the fingers down the lumbar spine and a segmental lordosis. If an asymptomatic slip reaches 50%, vigorous contact sports and other activities carrying a high risk of back injury should be avoided.

X-ray findings for these patients can be misleading. In a lateral view, taken while the patient is supine, the forward displacement often appears trivial as it is only when the patient is standing that the true degree of slip is appreciated. Consequently, if spondylolisthesis is suspected, a lateral spot view of the lumbosacral junction must be taken while the patient stands upright, and during flexion and extension of the trunk.[139] However, a patient with low back pain who demonstrates a spondylolisthesis on x-ray may have an asymptomatic spondylolisthesis, and the back pain may be coming from other causes.

The intervention depends on the severity of the slip and the symptoms and ranges from conservative to surgical. The average case is one of a limited slip and sparse clinical findings.

Degenerative Spinal Stenosis

Degenerative spinal stenosis is predominantly a disorder of the elderly that is being diagnosed more frequently because of widespread use of sophisticated noninvasive imaging techniques.[141] This condition was initially described by Verbiest.[142] Initially the depth of the canal that constituted narrowing was an anterior-posterior measurement. More recently, the lateral width of the spinal canal has been studied. Both the subjective complaints and the examination findings are very specific and these patients typically respond very well to the intervention, provided that the condition is not advanced.

The radicular canal is the lateral aspect of the spinal canal and begins at the point where the nerve root sheath emerges from the dural sac and ends at the intervertebral foramen. The following serve as its borders.

- The posterior border is formed by the ligamentum flavum, superior articular process, and lamina.
- The anterior border is formed by the vertebral body and disc.
- The dural sac forms the medial wall and the internal aspect of the pedicle and lateral wall.

The radicular canal can be classified according to its location.[143]

- Entrance zone—medial and anterior to the superior articular process
- Mid zone—under the pars interarticularis of the lamina and below the pedicle
- Exit zone—the area surrounding the intervertebral foramen

The radicular canal may be narrowed by different mechanisms but the usual mechanism is a combination of factors. A compression of the nerve within the canal results in a limitation of the arterial supply or claudication due to the compression of the venous return. The compression of the foraminal contents in the canal occurs from several sources.[144]

- The length of the canal is shorter in lumbar lordosis than kyphosis.
- The canal is also shortened by disc degeneration at several levels resulting in the cauda equina bunching up, producing a constriction.
- The foramen is already narrowed by anterior osteophytes, posterior exostosis of the foramen, a bunching up of the ligamentum flavum, or from a hypertrophic superior facet of the inferior vertebra.
- In extension of the lumbar spine, the foramen is mechanically narrowed.

The claudication, therefore, results in nerve root ischemia and symptomatic claudication. Any impingement on the nerve root is intermittent and is related to dynamic changes in the lateral recess during changes in posture and trunk movement. Most of the compression occurs when the canal is at its narrowest diameter, with relief occurring when the diameter increases. Extension and, to a lesser degree, side-flexion of the lumbar spine toward the involved side produces a narrowing of the canal. A flexion of the lumbar spine reverses the process, returning both the venous capacity and blood flow to the nerve.

Failure to respond to conservative treatment is an indication for nerve root and sinuvertebral nerve infiltration.[145] Permanent relief in lateral recess stenosis has been reported with an injection of local anesthetic around the nerve root.[146]

When nerve root infiltration fails, surgical decompression of the nerve root is indicated. One study, albeit inconclusive, found that, at a 1-year follow-up, patients with severe lumbar spinal stenosis who were treated surgically had greater improvement than patients treated nonsurgically.[147] However, studies have found a dwindling of benefit from surgery after 2 or more years of follow-up, and that the more definite the myelographic stenosis in patients with no prior surgical intervention, comorbidity of diabetes, hip joint arthrosis, preoperative fracture of the lumbar spine, or postoperative complications, the greater the chances of achieving a good outcome after surgical management of lumbar spinal stenosis.[148] The overall success rates for performing a second surgery on patients in whom initial back surgery failed have also been highly variable, ranging from 25% to 80%.[149] Another study found that a patient's perception of improvement had a much stronger correlation with long-term surgical outcome than structural findings seen on postoperation magnetic resonance imaging, and that degenerative findings had a greater effect on a patient's walking capacity than stenotic findings.[150]

Instability

Lumbar instability is considered to be a significant factor in patients with chronic low back pain.[151] However, there is considerable controversy as to what exactly constitutes spinal instability, although Panjabi has attempted to redefine it in terms of a region of laxity around the neutral resting position of a spinal segment called the neutral zone.[152] The neutral zone is the position of the segment in which minimal tension is occurring in the passive and active structures that control it. This neutral zone is shown to be larger with intersegmental injury and intervertebral disc degeneration[153,154] and smaller with simulated muscle forces across a motion segment.[155,156] Thus, the size of the neutral zone is determined by passive and active control systems, which in turn are controlled by the neural system.[152]

- *Passive system:* consists of the vertebrae, intervertebral discs, zygapophysial joints, and ligaments.
- *Active system:* consists of the muscles and tendons surrounding and acting on the spinal column. The particular role of the active components at static equilibrium is to enable a choice of posture, independent of the

distribution and magnitude of the outer load, albeit within physiologic limits.
- *Neural system:* consists of the nerves and central nervous system that direct and control the active system in providing dynamic stability.

Panjabi[152] defined spinal instability as a significant decrease in the capacity of the stabilizing systems of the spine to maintain intervertebral neutral zones within physiologic limits, so there is no major deformity, neurologic deficit, or incapacitating pain.

Panjabi and colleagues[155] studied the effect of intersegmental muscle forces on the neutral zone and range of motion of a lumbar functional spinal unit subjected to pure moments in flexion-extension, lateral bending, and rotation. The simulated muscle forces were applied to the spinous process of the mobile vertebra of a single motion segment using two equal and symmetrical force vectors directed laterally, anteriorly, and inferiorly. The simulated muscle force maintained or decreased the motions of the lumbar segment for intact and injured specimens with the exception of the flexion range of motion, which increased.

Tencer and Ahmed[157] and Wilder and co-workers[158] refer to the concept of a "balance point" and define the balance point for a single lumbar motion segment as the point of application of a compressive load that minimizes coupled flexion-extension rotations caused by the segmental bending moment.

Wilke and colleagues[156] compared the effect on the stability of a single lumbar motion segment of five muscle pairs acting separately or simultaneously. They simulated a constant muscle force value of 80 N per pair. The simulated muscle action generally decreased the range of motion and neutral zone, particularly for flexion and extension.

The recent research of Gardner-Morse and associates[159] and O'Sullivan and co-workers[160] lends support to the hypothesis of a balance point or neutral zone, revealing that a reduction of motion segment stiffness of as little as 10% can compromise the stability of the spine. They concluded that factors such as pathologic reduction in motion segment stiffness, as well as poor neuromuscular control of the spinal musculature and reduction of muscle stiffness, could result in a state of spinal instability. Cholewicke and McGill[161] reported that lumbar stability is maintained in vivo by increasing the activity (stiffness) of the lumbar segmental muscles, and highlighted the importance of motor control to coordinate muscle recruitment between large trunk muscles and small intrinsic muscles during functional activities to ensure that stability is maintained.

From the mechanical point of view, the spinal system is highly complex and statically highly indeterminate. The concept of different trunk muscles playing differing roles in the provision of dynamic stability to the spine was proposed by Bergmark,[162] who proposed that two muscle systems are engaged in the equilibrium of the lumbar spine.

1. *Global muscle system:* consisting of large torque producing muscles that act on the trunk and spine without being directly attached to it. These muscles, with origins on the pelvis and insertions on the thoracic cage, include the rectus abdominis, external oblique, and the thoracic part of lumbar iliocostalis. They provide general trunk stabilization but are not capable of having a direct segmental influence on the spine.

2. *Local muscle system:* consisting of muscles that have insertions and/or origins at the lumbar vertebra and are responsible for providing segmental stability and directly controlling the lumbar segments. These muscles include the lumbar multifidus, transversus abdominis, and the posterior fibers of the internal oblique

The lumbar multifidus, transversus abdominis, and the posterior fibers of the internal oblique are known to be tonically active during upright postures and active motions of the trunk,[163,164] with the transversus abdominis capable of tonic activity irrespective of trunk position, direction of movement, or loading of the spine.[165] Recent research indicates that it may also be the first trunk muscle to become active before movement initiation,[166] or perturbation,[167] and is the primary muscle involved in the initiation and maintenance of intra-abdominal pressure.[165] The lumbar multifidus is considered to have the greatest potential to provide dynamic control to the motion segment, particularly in its neutral zone.[168,169] The co-contraction of the deep abdominal muscles with the lumbar multifidus has the potential to provide a dynamic corset for the lumbar spine, enhancing its segmental stability.

As with any system, the potential for breakdown exists. Research has shown that it is the local system that is particularly vulnerable to breakdown with both lumbar multifidus[170,171] and deep abdominal[172,173] muscle inhibition, resulting in altered patterns of synergistic control or coordination of the trunk muscles.[174,175]

The ligamentous spine is known to be unstable at loads far less than that of body weight.[176] The neuromuscular system must therefore fulfill the role of maintaining postural stability while simultaneously controlling and initiating movement. Instability, whether ligamentous or articular, is perhaps the most difficult of the motion impairments to treat. A stiff or jammed joint is a relatively simple problem of selecting and applying a mobilization or manipulation technique. But, instability is a permanent, or at best, a semipermanent state that can only be managed, and the effectiveness of the management is very dependent on the

patient's motivation, compliance, and body awareness sense.[83] It is also dependent on time constraints placed upon the clinician by a busy caseload, as reeducation can be very labor intensive.

The following clinical findings (anywhere in the spinal or peripheral joints) may indicate the presence of instability, and its pertinence to the presenting complaints of the patient.

History
- Trauma
- Repeated unprovoked episode(s) of feeling unstable or giving way, following a minor provocation
- Inconsistent symptomatology
- Minor aching for a few days after a sensation of giving way
- Compression symptoms (vertebrobasilar, spinal cord) that are not associated with a disc- or stenotic-like history
- Consistent clicking or clunking noises
- Protracted pain (with full range of motion)

Observation
- Creases posteriorly or on abdomen (spondylolisthesis)
- Spinal ledging
- Spinal angulation on full range of motion
- Inability to recover normally from full range of motion, commonly flexion
- Excessive active range of motion

Hypermobility

One of the limitations with the clinical diagnosis of lumbar instability is the unreliability of conventional radiological testing in detecting abnormal or excessive intersegmental motion.[177,178] As with all movement impairments, instabilities or hypermobilities can be symmetrical or asymmetrical but, in contrast to the hypomobilities, the principles of intervention for these are not dependent on the degree of symmetry. Hypermobility is usually the most difficult impairment to diagnose in the spine as it is not a matter of stiffness but a relative degree of looseness. However, once discovered, hypermobility is the most easily treated impairment as the hypermobile joint is, unless irritable when it is treated with modalities, not treated at all. The recovery from the hypermobile state is simply a matter of removing abnormal stresses from the joint and then waiting for adaptive shortening to tighten the attenuated tissue.[83] If the underlying cause of the articular hypermobility is deemed to be a localized hypomobility, then this latter impairment must logically be dealt with first. Having attended to this, or indeed, if the hypermobility is of a primary origin, the main consideration is how to make the segment more stable. The aim of the intervention of a hypermobility is to prevent it becoming unstable. The patient is asked to avoid any activities or postures that would move the joint into its hypermobile range. The clinician treats any associated hypomobilities that might be placing abnormal stress on the joint. If necessary, an external support is used as a temporary measure.

Hypomobility

Hypomobility in the lumbar spine can have a variety of causes including ligament tears,[179] muscle tears or contusions,[180] lumbago,[181] intra-articular meniscoid entrapment,[182] zygapophysial joint capsular tightness, and zygapophysial joint fixation or subluxation.[183] A disc protrusion and prolapse and anular tear[184] can also produce a hypomobility and are discussed in Chapters 7 and 10.

Ligament Tears

As with elsewhere in the body, ligament tears of the lumbar spine are traumatically induced. Ligaments function to limit the motion of one bone on another especially at the extremes of motion. A knowledge of the various restraints to the various motions of the lumbar spine can aid in determining which ligament has the potential to be sprained with a given mechanism. The iliolumbar ligament, an extremely important structure that stabilizes the lumbar spine on the sacrum and functions to anchor the L5 vertebra onto the S1 vertebral body,[61] is commonly injured with a mechanism of forward bending combined with twisting.

Muscle Contusions and Tears

Muscle contusions and tears present with a history of trauma and are capable of producing a significant degree of discomfort. Muscle tears can complicate a contusive injury. Two sites are commonly involved, and can occur with relatively little trauma.[185]

- The point where the erector spinae group of muscles join to their common tendon just above and medial to the posterior superior iliac spines.
- At the gluteal origin on the ala of the ilium, just lateral to the posterior iliac spines.

However, muscle pain can also be produced from excessive muscle activity or the muscle guarding that follows an injury to the spine.

Lumbago

The term *lumbago* is used to describe local back pain of a discogenic origin, but can also be used to describe a sudden onset of persistent low back pain, marked by a restriction of lumbar movements and reports of "locking." The mechanism of mechanical locking is still a contentious issue.[186,187] The severity of each episode varies, from incapacitating to minor discomfort. Although it can occur at any age, lumbago typically affects those in the ages of between 20 and 45 years. The mechanism of injury usually involves a sudden unguarded movement of the lumbar spine involving either flexion or extension combined with rotation and/or side-flexion.

Hypomobilities can be classified as symmetrical or asymmetrical. If both sides of the joint are involved, the lesion is symmetrical, whereas if only one side is involved, the lesion is asymmetrical.

Symmetric Movement Dysfunctions

There are two main types of symmetrical impairments.

- Those caused by acute pain, where both zygapophysial joints are equally inflamed, or those where the segment is so painful due to articular or extra-articular impairments that motion is lost symmetrically.
- Those caused by myofascial and articular tissue shortening from a fixed postural impairment.

A symmetrical impairment will not be apparent in the flexion and extension position tests because, as both are equally impaired, there is no deviation from the path of flexion or extension, but rather the path is shortened or lengthened depending on which type of impairment (hypo- or hypermobility) is present. In addition, there is no apparent loss of side-flexion or rotation, and both sides appear equally hypomobile or hypermobile.

Asymmetric Movement Dysfunction

The asymmetrical movement dysfunctions include unilateral zygapophyseal joint hypomobilities, disc protrusions, and unilateral myofascial shortening.

BIOMECHANICAL EXAMINATION OF THE LUMBAR SPINE

At this stage of the examination, a number of diagnoses should have been ruled out, either by the subjective history and/or by the scan examination. A number of diagnoses still need to be ruled out and these include:

- Zygapophysial joint pathology. Although it is difficult to envision a zygapophysial joint impairment without having a disc impairment, it is possible to have a disc impairment without a zygapophysial joint impairment because the disc is a primary stabilizer.

- Hypomobility, hypermobility or instability of the joint complex
- Bursitis
- Chronic musculotendinous impairment
- Articular impairment
- Capsular impairment
- Ligamentous impairment

A biomechanical diagnosis, such as those just outlined, is the goal for this part of the examination. The components of the biomechanical examination are the same for the spine as they are for other joints. They include:

- An examination of active, and passive range of motion
- Over pressure applied at the end of range to detect the end feel
- An emphasis not only on plane movements but also on movement combinations
- Reproduction of the patient's symptoms

The examination of coupling or combined movements introduces the importance of lumbar spine position, that is, whether the spine is in neutral, flexion, or extension. A great deal of controversy exists with regard to the concept of spinal coupling and which coupling occurs with each of the spinal positions. It is generally agreed that the following occurs.

- *Neutral:* side-flexion and rotation occur to opposite sides.
- *Flexion:* side-flexion and rotation occur to the same side.
- *Extension:* side-flexion and rotation occur to opposite sides initially, but at the extremes of extension, they occur to the same side.
- At L5, because of the influence of the iliolumbar ligament, the coupling varies.

Whereas the segment can flex, extend, side flex, and rotate, the only motion that can occur at the zygapophysial joints is a superior, or inferior glide, with varying degrees of anterior or posterior inclination depending on how flexed or extended the spine is at the time. Thus, rotation or side-flexion of the segment is associated with flexion of one joint and extension of the other.

LOCKING TECHNIQUES FOR THE LUMBAR SPINE BASED ON COUPLING

Two types of locking techniques are used to isolate a specific segment for either examination or treatment, and each is named according to the combination of rotation and side-flexion that are used in the technique.

If the rotation used is to the same side as the side-flexion, then the technique is termed congruent (other names used include physiological and zygapophysial joint locking). For example, a congruent locking technique would be right side-flexion with right rotation, in flexion.

If the rotation used is not to the same side, then the technique is termed incongruent (other names used include nonphysiologic and ligamentous locking). For example, an incongruent locking technique would be right side-flexion with left rotation, in flexion.

Thus, there are *four* possible locking combinations.

1. Congruent extension
2. Incongruent extension
3. Congruent flexion
4. Incongruent flexion

In the techniques described, it is assumed that at the extreme of flexion and extension, the rotation occurs to the same side as the side-flexion. Since there is much disagreement as to the coupling that occurs in neutral, locking in this position is avoided.

The rotational component used in a specific mobilization is always opposite to the side the patient is lying on, as rotation to the same side will render the patient's body mass difficult to control. Therefore, the direction of rotation is a constant when determining whether to use a congruent or incongruent technique. For example, if the patient is in right side-lying, the rotation employed must be to the left, and a congruent technique for flexion or extension would involve left side-flexion.

Locking from Above

Locks from above are achieved through the use of an arm pull. When locking from above, the rotation, side-flexion, and flexion and extension movements are done simultaneously. Since rotation is a constant, the only concerns are:

A. How to produce side-flexion to either the right or left.

B. Which side-flexion to use in conjunction with either flexion or extension.

1. Locking from above—extension: The patient is positioned in side lying, facing the clinician. The patient's hips and knees are slightly flexed. To facilitate the upper lock of extension, the upper arm of the patient should be placed in a position with the elbow flexed and shoulder extended, so that the arm is *posterior to the trunk* (Figure 13–8). To ensure that the upper spine is positioned in extension, the patient's lower arm is drawn *vertically toward the ceiling* (Figure 13–8).

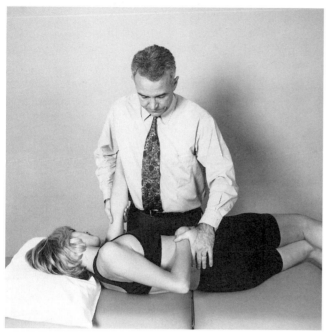

FIGURE 13–8 An upper extension lock with the patient lying on left side.

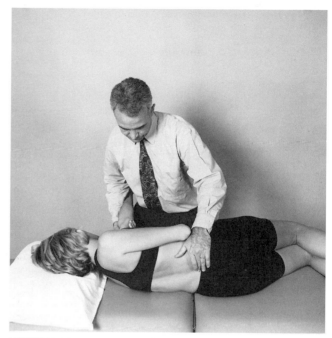

FIGURE 13–9 An upper flexion lock with the patient lying on left side.

2. Locking from above—flexion: the patient is positioned in side-lying, facing the clinician. The patient's hips and knees are slightly flexed. The clinician places the patient's upper arm *anterior to the trunk* in such a way that the palm is flat on the bed and adjacent to the patient's waist. The lower arm and shoulder girdle are then drawn forward, *parallel to the table* (Figure 13–9).

3. Right side-flexion in flexion/extension: the patient is positioned in side lying, facing the clinician. The patient's hips and knees are slightly flexed. If the patient is in right side-lying, then the *right arm is drawn toward the feet* (i.e., caudal; Figure 13–10).

An Upper Lock Utilizing Left Side-Flexion

The patient is positioned in side-lying, facing the clinician. The patient's hips and knees are slightly flexed. If the patient is in right side-lying, then the *right arm is drawn superiorly toward the head,* keeping the arm parallel to the bed.

An Upper Lock Combining Side-flexion with Flexion/Extension

When performing locking techniques from above, the side-flexion positioning is performed with the flexion and extension simultaneously by combining arm movements.

Congruent Left side-flexion and Extension With the patient in right side-lying, the right arm and shoulder girdle are drawn in a direction that is the oblique resultant of a

cranial and vertical pull (Figure 13–11). This technique, with the location of the end feel, can be used to test the joint's ability to achieve the full range of motion, or it can be used to position a patient to mobilize one side of a joint.

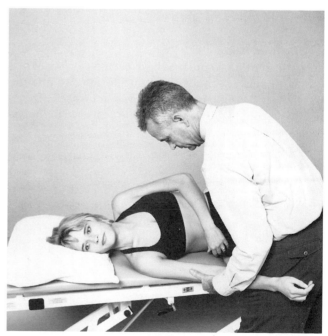

FIGURE 13–10 A right side flexion upper lock with the patient lying on right side.

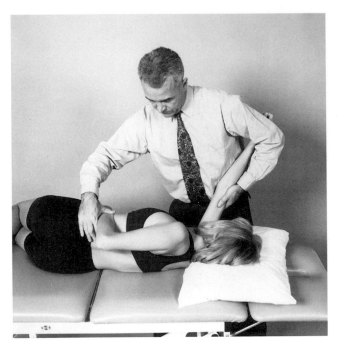

FIGURE 13–11 An extension and left side flexion lock with the patient lying on right side.

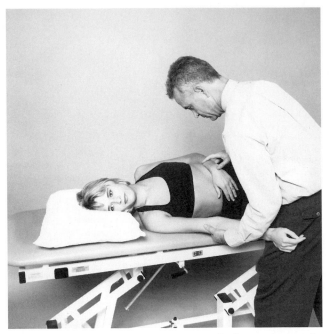

FIGURE 13–12 A flexion and right side flexion lock with the patient lying on right side.

Incongruent Right side-flexion and Flexion With the patient right side-lying, the patient's right arm and shoulder girdle are drawn in a direction that is the oblique resultant of a *caudal and horizontal pull* (Figure 13–12). This technique, with the location of the end feel, can be used to test the joint's ability to achieve the full range of motion, or it can be used to position a patient to mobilize one side of a joint.

Locking from Below

So far, the locking techniques have been *from above*. When locking *from below*, simultaneous side-flexion and rotation with flexion and extension is not easily controlled. Therefore, it is recommended that the spine be locked in the following sequence.

1. Flexion or extension
2. Side-flexion
3. Rotation

Lower Lock: Flexion and Extension

Most easily performed to the correct level, as per the PPIVM technique, with the knees flexed.

Lower Lock: Side-flexion

Assuming the patient is in left side-lying:

- *Left side-flexion:* the patient's upper (right) leg is encouraged, or drawn, inferiorly (Figure 13–13).

- *Right side-flexion:* the patient's lower (left) leg is encouraged, or drawn, inferiorly (Figure 13–14).

Lower Lock: Rotation

Assuming the patient is in right side-lying. As with locking techniques from above, the locking from below involves a

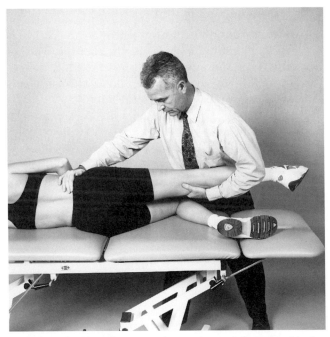

FIGURE 13–13 The upper leg is drawn inferiorly with the patient lying on left side.

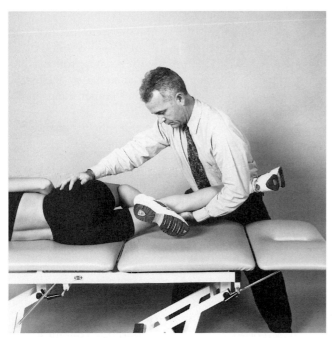

FIGURE 13–14 The lower leg is drawn inferiorly with the patient lying on left side.

constant of rotation. For example, right side-lying must be accompanied by left rotation. When locking from below, the rotation occurs to the side that the patient is lying on (right side-lying is accompanied by right rotation) and is controlled by the motion of the pelvis, either directly, by drawing the pelvis forward into the clinician's body, or indirectly, by allowing the upper (left) leg to drop toward the ground.

It will be seen later that there are the same four possible combinations of locking techniques from below, as there were from above, and this would appear to present the clinician with a daunting sixteen possible combinations! In reality, however, one seldom needs to worry about making the right choices. Many clinicians develop a favored combination that seems to work "most of the time." On the other hand, the patients who have reacted adversely to mobilizations are just the ones who probably require some special consideration when selecting the appropriate locking technique. On these occasions, one is grateful for the variable options available.

Listed below are some of the guidelines for locking.

- An attempt should always be made to keep the segment to be mobilized in neutral until the slack in those segments above and below has been removed by the locking techniques.
- In mobilizations, generally, it is stated that one must fix one bone while mobilizing another. A detailed biomechanical examination of the spine will reveal which "end" will be fixated and which will be used as a lever to mobilize.

- During locking, it must be remembered to incorporate the direction of the mobilization into the locking technique of the lever arm. For example, if L3–4 were hypomobile in left extension, the fixated part of the spine may be locked with any of the combinations just mentioned since the L3–4 will be kept in neutral. However, the lever arm must incorporate into its locking technique the motions of extension and left side-flexion. So, for example, if the patient is in right side-lying, the technique used for the lever arm would be left congruent extension.
- As a general rule, one may fix through a hypermobility, but not lever through it. Ideally, the clinician should place any hypermobilities in a flexion lock, which is less firm than an extension lock. Where possible, though, the clinician should lock with extension as it tends to produce a firmer lock. One should neither fix nor lever through an unstable segment.

A review of the flow diagram in Figure 13–15 will be a helpful guide to the reader. The flow diagram assumes that the clinician has taken the history and performed a scan, if appropriate, but has yet to determine a diagnosis.

The Examination Components

Active Weight-bearing Movement Testing
The amount of range available depends on a number of factors, including age and stage of healing. Even in so-called 'normal' spines there is a great deal of variability.[188] Some individuals are able to touch their toes with only hip and/or thoracic motion. However, the focus of the examination is the quality of the motion, the symptoms the motions provoke, and the end feel. The reader should refer to Chapter 10 for details about what to observe during the planar motions.

At the end of each of the active motions, passive over pressure is applied, and resistance tests are performed with the muscles in the lengthened positions. In cases of low back pain, the results of the isometric tests for the most part are negative, and when positive, are more likely due to the compressive effect that they have on the injured segmental tissues.[189] However, if the active or passive test reproduced pain or other symptoms, do not have the patient perform an isolated contraction at the end of range, since the resulting compression may do more damage to the segmental structures.[189]

The same planar motions that were used in the lumbar scan are used, but if the planar motions fail to reproduce symptoms, combined motions are introduced in both

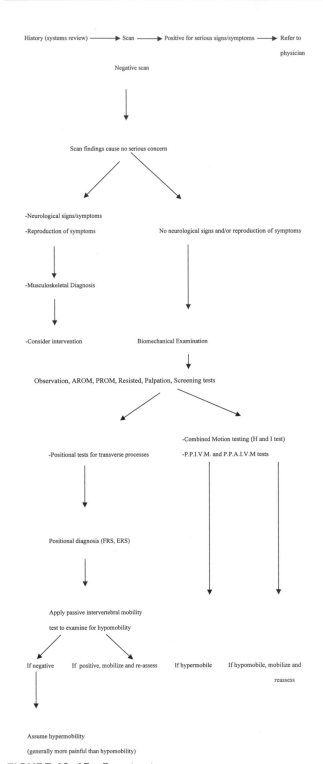

FIGURE 13–15 Examination sequence.

flexion and extension, and a note is made about whether deviations occur before, or subsequent to, the end of range. These combined motion tests are called H and I tests, and the findings from these tests determine the sequence for the rest of the examination.

H and I Tests[83]

These are biomechanical tests for the spine, testing both the range and the function of the joint complex using combined motions. The tests get their name from the pattern produced by the motions that make up each test. They are used to detect biomechanical impairments in the chronic or subacute stages of healing.

These tests are quite useful as a quick test once the limitations of screening tests are understood.

- False negatives
- They are non discriminatory and will highlight irrelevant instabilities.
- They do not differentiate between instabilities.
- They do not tell the clinician which segment is at fault, only the motion that reproduces the pain, or is restricted.

As discussed in Chapter 11, combined motion tests can reproduce the pain in a structure that is either being compressed or stretched, and the findings from these tests are used to formulate a working hypothesis as to the patient's condition. While the patient's pain and its location are of interest at this stage, these tests primarily assess the quality and quantity of motion.

H Test

This test involves starting the patient with side-flexion of the lumbar spine, followed by extreme forward flexion of the lumbar spine (Figure 13–16). From this position, the patient maintains the side-flexion, and moves into extreme extension of the lumbar spine (Figure 13–17). The test is then repeated using side-flexion to the other side, and repeating the flexion and extension motions while maintaining the side-flexion.

The range of motion and end feels are compared. It is important that the clinician observe the curvature of the lumbar spine during these maneuvers, and look for any compensations that the patient might unintentionally use to achieve the ranges.

I Test

This test involves starting the patient with extreme forward flexion of the lumbar spine before moving into side-flexion of the lumbar spine (see Figure 13–16). From this position, the patient side-flexes the trunk to the other side. The test is then repeated using extreme extension and side-flexion to both sides (see Figure 13–17), and the range of motion and end feels are compared. It is important to observe the curvature of the lumbar spine and to look for any protective compensations that the patient might unintentionally use to achieve the range.

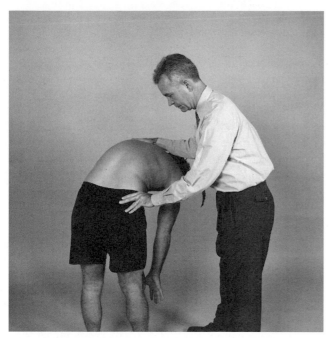

FIGURE 13–16 The H test.

It can be seen from these tests that each of H and I maneuvers test both sides of the anterior and posterior quadrants using two different combined movements.

1. *Anterior quadrants.* These are tested in the I test when the patient is asked to actively flex forward as far as possible and then side-flex in one direction, and in the

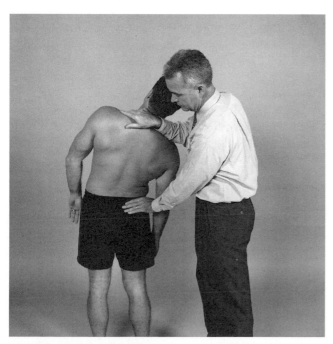

FIGURE 13–17 The I test.

H test, when the patient is asked to side-flex in one direction and then flex fully.

2. *Posterior quadrants.* These are tested in the I test when the patient is asked to actively extend as far as possible and then side flex in one direction, and in the H test, when the patient is asked to side-flex in one direction, and then extend fully.

These tests should provide the clinician with a working hypothesis as to whether the patient's condition results from too little, or too much, motion, and further testing can be used in the biomechanical examination to either confirm or refute the hypotheses.

Example: Hypomobility. If there is a hypomobility into the posterior left quadrant, the patient demonstrates difficulty moving into that quadrant, whether via extension and left side-flexion or left side-flexion followed by extension.

If a particular quadrant is suspected for hypomobility after the H and I test, further testing is performed to determine the segment at fault using position testing (see later discussion). It is the position testing or the passive mobility testing that indicates to the clinician the level of the impairment. For example, if during the H and I test, the patient was unable to extend and right side-flex, and the position tests or PPIVM tests (see later discussion) confirmed the impairment to be an FRSL (flexed, rotated, side-flexed left) at L4, the clinician positions the patient in side-lying so that L4 can be taken to the extreme of extension and right side-flexion to confirm the hypothesis.

Example: Hypermobility. The medical definition of instability is "an abnormal response to applied loads, characterized by movements in the motion segment beyond normal constraints."[190] Using this definition, a hypermobility can be defined as excessive angular motion at a joint where the joint retains its stability and functions normally under physiological loads. Instability, hypermobility, and hypomobility are described in detail in Chapter 11.

An inconsistent *hypomobility* appears to be a common characteristic of directional instabilities.[192] That is, if the joint is moved in one direction, the movement may be hypermobile, but it does not sublux into the instability and become hypomobile. However, when it is moved in the opposite direction, it subluxes into the instability and becomes hypomobile. If a left lateral hypermobility is present at one segment, the first part of the H test (side-flexion) does not demonstrate a hypomobility. However, as the patient tries to flex or extend, a reduction in motion would occur as the resulting subluxation would jam the joint and prevent further motion from occurring. However, if the I test is used, initiating with flexion, and then side-flexion, no loss of motion would be apparent.

In the lumbar spine, a simple test further demonstrates this phenomenon. The patient is asked to forward bend at the waist. If an anterior instability is present, the patient is able to bend forward with little, if any, trouble. However, after reaching the full range of flexion, the patient demonstrates difficulty extending from this position, often using his or her hands to walk up the thighs.

The subjective history should support the hypothesis of instability. If the instability does not cause symptoms either directly or indirectly, then an intervention is almost certainly not required. In the case of the spine, the instability should be associated with a clinically detectable hypermobility.[192] If the instability is not sufficiently gross to produce a discernible hypermobility, then it is unlikely to be a cause of symptoms or impairment and does not require an intervention.

A positive finding in one of the H and I tests but not the other (a loss of motion detected in the I test but no loss detected in the H test) can mean one of three conclusions.

1. Instability
2. Anomaly
3. Hypermobility

Not only can the H and I test be used to pick up instabilities, but it can also help differentiate the direction of the instability.

The I test is used to detect anterior or posterior instabilities, whereas the H test is used to detect lateral instabilities. These findings are then confirmed with a stress test. (see later).

- A loss of motion with flexion in the I test probably indicates posterior disc fiber weakness and, therefore, a possible anterior translation instability. This can be confirmed by performing the anterior stress test.
- A loss of motion with extension in the I test probably indicates a weakness of the anterior disc fibers and, therefore, a posterior translation instability. This can be confirmed with the posterior stress test in sitting. It is worth noting that if both of the posterior quadrants are implicated, then this may indicate a central weakness of the anterior disc fibers.
- A positive finding in the H test, without one in the I test, could indicate a lateral or side-flexion instability. This can be confirmed with the lateral stability test.

At the completion of the H and I test, the clinician will know with a good deal of certainty if the patient's condition involves a hypomobility or hypermobility and instability. If a hypomobility is suspected, passive physiologic intervertebral motion (PPIVM) tests are carried out

to test segmental mobility. If a hypermobility is suspected, stress tests are performed into the suspected range.

Nonweight Bearing (NWB) H and I Test[83]
The nonweight-bearing H and I test applies the same principles as the weight-bearing version just described, although it does offer some distinct advantages for the detection of hypermobilities and hypomobilities. It is also used to confirm the findings of the weight-bearing test. A positive weight-bearing H and I test but a negative nonweight-bearing H and I test probably indicates the presence of instability. The patient is positioned side-lying.

H Test   The patient's lumbar spine is locked from above using either an extension and rotation lock or a flexion and side-flexion lock, depending on which quadrant is being assessed.

I Test   The patient's lumbar spine is locked from below using either a flexion or extension lock and is locked from above using a rotation lock.

For example, if impairment into the right posterior quadrant was found in the weight-bearing H and I test, the patient is positioned in left side-lying. The clinician locks down from above with an extension and right side-flexion lock, by pulling the patient's bottom arm up to the ceiling and toward the head of the bed at the same time. Both of the patient's lower extremities are then moved into gross lumbar extension, extending through the segment to be tested.

The H part of the test is applied into the impaired quadrant (right posterior in this example).

- While maintaining the upper lock of extension and right side-flexion, the clinician moves the patient's lower extremities from full extension to neutral, and back again into extension.
- Normal motion involves a gradual and smooth motion of the segment. A hypermobility will display a very quick movement of the spinous process at the point when the patient's lower extremities are moved out of extension toward the neutral position.

The I part of the test is applied into the impaired quadrant (right posterior in this example).

- Both of the patient's lower extremities are positioned in sufficient extension to extend the lumbar spine through the segment. Maintaining the extension, the clinician then moves the patient's trunk and lumbar spine in and out of the right side-flexion, *not* rotation. Although this motion resembles thoracic rotation, the clinician's force is directed cranially. If a hypomobility exists, the two adjoining spinous processes will appear to move together, instead of independently, as in a normal segment.

POSITION TESTING

Referring to the flow diagram in Figure 13–15, the position tests are performed after the active motion tests, instead of the combined motion tests and the passive physiologic intervertebral motion tests (refer to the Chapter 11).

Procedure
The clinician must be very familiar with "layer palpation," to be sure that the palpating fingers are monitoring the positions of the transverse processes. Tests need to be performed in:

- Hyperextended prone
- Flexion (Figure 13–18), or hyperflexion
- Neutral prone

The transverse processes are layer-palpated, and if there is a rotational element to the flexion or extension, it will be palpated as a much firmer end feel to the palpation on that side. The rotation is a result of the altered axis of rotation produced by the stiffer of the two sides of the segment. The direction of the rotation is toward the more posterior of the two transverse processes and the positional name is an osteokinematic one, having no established relationship with any joint.

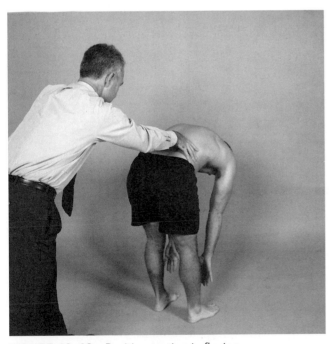

FIGURE 13–18 Position testing in flexion.

A. Positional testing in hyperextension[83]
1. If a marked segmental rotation is evident at the limit of extension, this would indicate that one of the facets is unable to complete its inferior motion (i.e., it is being held in a relatively flexed position). The direction of the resulting rotation (denoted in terms of the anterior part of the vertebral body) would tell the clinician which of the facets is not moving.
2. If the segment is rotated to the LEFT when palpated in extension, then it must be the RIGHT zygapophysial joint that is not moving normally.
3. This impairment can be named in one of two ways.
   a. The right zygapophysial joint cannot extend.
   b. The segment "cannot close" on the right.
      (1) Positional impairment: the right zygapophysial joint is Flex*ed* (F), Rotat*ed* (R), and Side-flex*ed* (S) Left (L) around the axis of the right zygapophysial joint. FRS or extension impairments give more dramatic findings in the positional tests than ERS ones. This is because there is less overall motion available into extension.
      (2) Motion impairment: the right zygapophysial joint demonstrates a restriction of extens*ion*, right side-flex*ion*, and right rotat*ion*.

B. Positional testing in flexion/hyperflexion[83]
1. Similarly, if a marked segmental rotation were evident in full flexion, this would indicate that one of the facets could not complete its superior motion.
2. If the segment is rotated to the left when palpated in flexion, then it must be the left zygapophysial joint that is not moving normally.
3. Terminology
   a. The left zygapophysial joint cannot flex.
   b. The segment "cannot open" on the left.
      (1) Positional impairment: the left zygapophysial joint is extended (E), Rotated (R), and Side-flexed (S) Left (L)
      (2) Motion impairment: the left zygapophysial joint demonstrates a restriction of flexion, right rotation, and right side-flexion.

C. Positional testing in neutral[83]—Performed for three reasons
1. If a rotational impairment of a segment only exists in neutral, and is not evident in either full flexion or full extension, it would indicate that the cause of the impairment is probably not mechanical in origin, but rather neuromuscular. These neuromuscular impairments are usually found where ascending and descending spinal decompensations "meet."
2. If a marked rotation is evident at a segment, and this rotation is consistent throughout flexion, extension and neutral, then the cause is probably an anatomical anomaly, not articular, (e.g., scoliosis).

3. If the cause of the rotational impairment is articular (zygapophysial joint), positional testing in neutral gives the clinician an idea as to the starting position of the corrective technique.

   Note: the terminology used to describe the dysfunctional motion describes the positional and kinetic impairments only. It does not indicate what the pathology might be. However, when these tests are used in conjunction with other aspects of the total examination, a biomechanical diagnosis can be determined.

Evaluation of Positional Findings

A. *Disc lesion* (e.g., a right posterior-lateral protrusion)

1. In FLEXION—ERS left and ERS right found with position testing: theoretically, the presence of pain protectively prevents a compression of the anterior aspect of the disc, as this would push the protrusion out further. As a result, the zygapophysial joints cannot flex into either of the anterior quadrants.

2. In EXTENSION—FRS left found with position testing: theoretically, the right zygapophysial joint is prevented from extending by the mechanical block of the protruding disc. Therefore, it is flexed, rotated, and side bent left.

3. In NEUTRAL: a rotational deviation may be present in neutral, but is generally most marked towards full flexion and extension. The key sign is the loss of motion to the same side in both extremes.

Intervention: Treat the extension impairment (see later)

B. *Zygapophysial joint lesions*, these impairments fall into one of three categories.

1. The hypomobile zygapophysial joint: the specific cause is differentiated with the end feel. The key sign is the loss of motion in one quadrant only, for example, the loss of extension in the right zygapophysial joint, but normal flexion in the right zygapophysial joint.

   a. Osseous fusion (no motion felt at zygapophysial joint) producing a bony end feel
   b. Gross capsular fibrosis (posterior transverse process) producing a capsular end feel
   c. An intra-articular loose body producing a springy end feel
   d. A muscle hypertonus producing a elastic end feel
   e. An articular subluxation producing a hard, jammed end feel

   The key sign is a loss of motion occurring simultaneously in diagonally opposite quadrants. For example an ERSR combined with an FRSL produces a loss of motion in both directions, but only one of the zygapophysial joints is locked.

2. Hypermobile zygapophysial joint, a hypermobility can occur as a result of macrotrauma or microtrauma. Three of the most common causes are:

   a. Post-trauma
   b. Post-partum
   c. Secondary to the presence of a hypomobile segment above or below.

   This is the most difficult impairment to identify because it mimics an FRS or ERS impairment. However, it is usually very reactive, and if testing is done kinetically, with careful observation during active motion tests, the rotational impairment appears markedly at the very end of range. The impairment is usually inculpated by the findings of the PPIVM (see later discussion). A difference in findings between positional testing and passive physiologic mobility may be found as a result of adaptive changes produced by the body in response to the local impairment.

Kinetic Positional Testing

Position testing does not have to be a static procedure and in many respects it is more accurate if it is not. Some clinicians have a better sense of relative depth and they should use the static version of the test. Other clinicians are better at detecting motion and, thus, the kinetic positional tests are more suitable.

The patient is asked to stand with the hands by their sides. While the clinician palpates a segmental level, the patient is asked to look over the left shoulder, and then the right shoulder (Figure 13–19). This head turning induces the correct motion in the lumbar spine. The segment being palpated should rotate to the ipsilateral side during the head turning.

PASSIVE PHYSIOLOGIC INTERVERTEBRAL MOVEMENT TESTING

Passive physiologic intervertebral movement (PPIVM) tests are most effectively carried out if the combined motion tests locate a hypomobility, or if the position tests are negative (see later discussion), rather than as the entry tests for the lumbar spine. This is because the vast majority of patients presenting for an intervention are symptomatic due to asymmetrical impairments. This is not to imply that postural impairments are unimportant, but if present, they are usually masked by the more painful impairment. In any case, the symptomatic problem should be addressed first, or at least concurrently with any postural intervention, as this is the reason the patient came for an intervention.

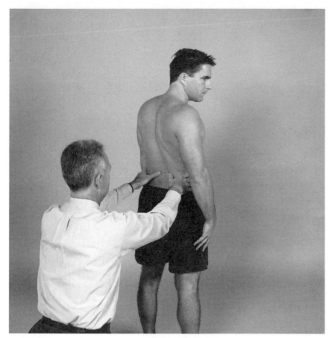

FIGURE 13–19 Kinetic positional testing using head turn.

The passive physiologic movement tests are performed into:

- Flexion
- Extension
- Rotation
- Side-flexion

The adjacent spinous processes of the segment are palpated simultaneously, and movement between them is assessed as the segment is passively taken through its physiologic range. If both spinous processes move simultaneously, there is no movement occurring at the segment and a hypomobility exists. As indicated by the flow diagram in Figure 13–15 the hypomobility is tested by the appropriate PPAIVM test (see later). If too much movement occurs, a hypermobility is likely. If a symmetrical impairment exists, then flexion and/or extension and both rotations, and both side-flexions, will be limited or excessive.

The test is used for acute and subacute patients who have pain in the cardinal motion planes. For the tests, the patient is positioned in side-lying, facing the clinician. The clinician locates the patient's lumbosacral junction using one of the following methods.

- By locating the L5 spinous process, which is short, sharp, and thick compared to the others, and moving inferiorly.
- By locating the PSIS and moving superiorly and medially.
- By locating the spinous process of T12 and counting down to the correct level using the spinous processes.

- By locating the iliac crest, which is level with L4, and counting down one.
- By having the patient perform a pelvic tilt during the palpation, to help locate the lumbosacral junction.

Once located, the neutral position of the spine for flexion and extension is found by palpating the L5 spinous process and alternatively flexing and extending the hips until it is felt to rock around the flexion and extension point.

Flexion

The patient is positioned in side-lying, close to the clinician, with the underneath leg slightly flexed at the hip and knee. A small pillow or roll can be placed under the patient's waist to maintain the lumbar spine in a neutral position with respect to side-flexion. The test can be performed by flexing one or both of the patient's legs, but it is generally easier to use one leg. The clinician, facing the patient, palpates between two adjacent lumbar spinous processes in the interspinous space, with the cranial hand, while the other hand grasps the patient's ankles or the knee of the uppermost leg if one leg is being used. The patient's lower extremities are moved into hip and lumbar flexion, and returned to neutral by the clinician, as the motion between segments is palpated (Figure 13–20A). Using this general technique, the clinician works up and down the lumbar spine getting a sense of the overall motion available. Although there is a high degree of variability in patients, segmental motion should decrease from L5 to L1. A generalized hypermobility demonstrates more motion in all of the segments, whereas an isolated hypermobile segment demonstrates more motion at only that level. Each segment is then checked one at a time, while moving the lumbar spine passively from neutral to full flexion.

For a greater degree of accuracy, once the lumbar spine is flexed up to the desired level, the spinous process of that level is pinched and side-flexion of the lumbar spine is added by grasping the patient's uppermost leg and raising it to the ceiling. The spinous process should be felt to tilt toward the table. For the mid and upper lumbar segments, this technique can be modified for the larger patient by performing it with the patient sitting up.

Extension

While flexion and extension can be tested together, it is more accurate to assess them separately. The patient is positioned as just described, but diagonally on the bed, so that the pelvis is close to the edge while the shoulder is moved further from the edge. A small pillow or roll can be placed under the patient's waist to maintain the lumbar spine in a neutral position with respect to side-flexion.

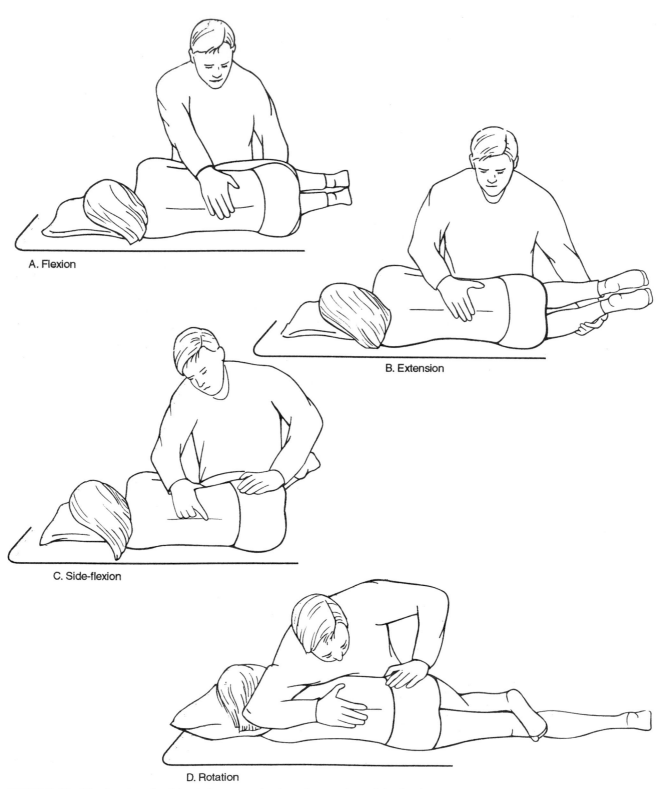

A. Flexion

B. Extension

C. Side-flexion

D. Rotation

FIGURE 13–20 Passive physiologic intervertebral motion testing of the lumbar spine.

The clinician locates two adjacent spinous processes with the cranial hand while the caudal arm flexes the patient's knees as much as possible before extending the patient's hips (see Figure 13–20B). As the patient's knees move off the table, the clinician supports them on his or her thighs. When the patient's legs are on the table, the clinician's caudal arm is used to produce the hip extension. The pelvis motion is felt and the spine is returned to its neutral position each time. At the end of the extension motion, a cranial pressure through the patient's thighs is produced by the clinician. This produces a posterior tilt of the superior zygapophysial joint and is used to produce an end feel, allowing the clinician to discriminate between a pure extension movement and an extension and rotation movement.

Again, for greater accuracy, the whole lumbar spine is placed into extension by moving the bottom leg into both hip and lumbar spine extension. The spinous process of the level to be tested is located and pinched between the thumb and index finger of the cranial hand. The uppermost thigh and leg of the patient is grasped and the lumbar spine is side-flexed by raising the patient's thigh up to the ceiling while maintaining the lumbar spine extension.

This technique can be modified for the larger patient if the clinician is unable to flex the patient's knee. The patient's lower extremity is fixed and the extension force is applied through the pelvis to test extension (Figure 13–21). To

introduce the side-flexion component, the clinician can push the patient's pelvis cranially through pressure at the superior innominate.

Side-Flexion

The patient is positioned as just described with the knees and hips flexed, and the thighs supported on the table, and the lower legs off the table. The lumbar spine should be in a position of neutral in relation to flexion and extension. The clinician, facing the patient, places his or her cranial arm between the patient's arm and body and palpates the interspinous spaces, while the caudal hand grasps the patient's feet and ankles as in Figure 13–20B for extension. As the patient's feet and ankles are lifted toward the ceiling, the superior spinous process should be felt to move toward the table, as the lumbar spine is side-flexed away from the table. The opposite occurs if the patient's feet are lowered off the table as the lumbar spine side-flexes toward the table. The direction of the leg lift represents the direction of the side-flexion. For example, with the patient positioned in right side-lying, right side-flexion (and left rotation) is introduced by lowering the feet and ankles off the table. The procedure is repeated for the other side and the two sides are compared.

If the patient is unable to tolerate having the lower extremity moved toward the ceiling, the clinician places his or her caudal hand around the patient's upper pelvis, under the inferior/posterior aspect of the patient's uppermost greater trochanter, (see Figure 13–20C) and, if possible, under the patient's ischial tuberosity.

The clinician firmly grasps the patient's pelvis and upper thigh with the caudal hand and, using a rhythmical motion of his or her own trunk, applies a force in a superior direction toward the patient's head, thereby inducing a side-flexion movement from below-upward by rocking the pelvis.

If the patient is unable to tolerate having the lower extremity lowered off the table, the clinician can grasp the patient's ASIS (anterior superior iliac spine) (closest to the table). While placing the armpit of the caudal arm over the patient's uppermost ASIS, the clinician can apply an inferior force, thereby inducing side-flexion of the lumbar spine into the table.

Unfortunately, these tests do not completely exclude such intersegmental impairments as minor end range asymmetrical hypomobilities, or hypermobilities, because the application of side-flexion or rotation in neutral does not fully flex or extend the zygapophysial joints. Also it is not possible to fully flex or extend both zygapophysial joints simultaneously. To completely flex a particular joint, the opposite joint has to move out of the fully flexed position by utilizing side-flexion, and allowing the increased

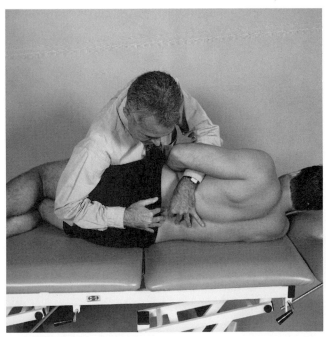

FIGURE 13–21 Symmetrical passive physiologic intervertebral motion testing of extension.

superior glide of the superior zygapophysial joint on the opposite joint.

A further problem with using symmetrical tests in the presence of an asymmetrical impairment is that the vertebra will tend to rotate as the restriction is encountered and, unless the clinician is sensitive to this, the movement of the spinous process that occurs during the rotation may be mistaken for normal, and the test considered negative.

All of these techniques can be modified and used as mobilization techniques, using the appropriate grade of movement based on the findings on the examination.[193] These interventions can also be given in conjunction with the examination rather than waiting until the examination is completed.

Rotation

The patient is positioned in spinal neutral, with both knees just off the table. A small pillow or roll can be placed under the patient's waist to maintain the lumbar spine in a neutral position. The interspinous spaces are palpated with the cranial hand, which is placed along the lower thoracic spine with a reinforced finger resting against adjacent spinous processes from underneath. The caudal hand rests on the patient's greater trochanter (Figure 13–20D). One of two methods can now be used.

1. The patient's thorax is stabilized by the clinician's cranial hand, while the patient's pelvis is rocked backward and forward, so that the pelvis and lumbar spine rotate (see Figure 13–20D). As the patient's pelvis is rocked backward, the spinous process of the lower segment should be felt to rotate toward the table compared to the spinous process of the upper segment.
2. The patient's pelvis is stabilized by the caudal hand, while the patient's thorax is rotated toward and away from the clinician, using the cranial hand. As the patient's thorax is rotated away, the spinous process of the upper segment should be felt to rotate toward the table compared to the spinous process of the lower segment.

The spine is returned to neutral each time and the clinician progresses up the spine. More rotation should be available in the lower lumbar spine. The process is repeated with the patient side-lying on the opposite side.

PPIVM TESTING WITH POSITION TESTING RESULTS[189]

If the PPIVM to be tested is determined from the position test, then rotation can be used instead of side-flexion, since now the clinician is looking to see if the segment can be derotated in the extended or flexed position. If it cannot be derotated, the flexion or extension is probably

limited, whereas if it can be derotated, it is probably not restricted. At first, an assumption is made that the ERS or FRS is the result of a hypomobility. For example, if the left transverse process was found to be posterior in the flexion position test, a hypothesis is generated that the cause of the abnormality is a hypomobility on the left side of the segment (ERSL). This hypothesis is then tested.

The patient is put into a position that would tend to force the hypomobile joint into its reduced range. In this case, the patient would be laid on the left side because this is the side of the posterior transverse process. The hips are flexed so that flexion is felt to occur throughout the entire lumbar spine. Further lumbar flexion and rotation are produced from above by pulling the lower arm of the patient parallel to the bed and perpendicular to the patient's trunk. The patient's upper arm hangs down over the trunk. Further rotation can be obtained by partly extending the lower leg without extending the spine and rotating the pelvis toward the floor using the forearm of the caudal arm (Figure 13–22). The lumbar spine is now fully flexed and rotated to the right. The segment of interest is tested by rotating it to the right through its spinous process (Figure 13–22) and evaluating the end feel. If the end feel is abnormal, the PPAIVM is assessed by gliding the superior bone superiorly and anteriorly on the stabilized lower bone and again assessing the end feel. If the end feel is normal, the hypomobility is caused by an extra-articular dysfunction, whereas if the PPAIVM is abnormal, the restriction lies in the periarticular structures. If the end feel is normal compared to the segments above and below it, there is no hypomobility present and flexion of that

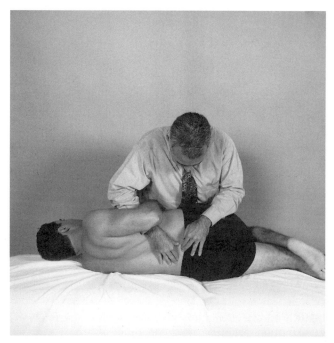

FIGURE 13–22   ERSL testing with patient in left side-lying

side of the segment is normal, so a second hypothesis must be considered—that the right side of the segment is hypermobile into flexion. To test for hypermobility, the examining movements essentially exaggerate the positional asymmetry. The patient lies on the other side (the right in this case), and flexion is again produced by the same means, but this time it is the right side of the segment that is being tested by evaluating its rotation via its end feel. If there is a spasm end feel or a soft capsular end feel, then hypermobility is present. If the end feel is normal, and given the result of the first segmental test, flexion of the segment is normal.

If the position test demonstrated a posterior left transverse process in extension (FRSL), the hypomobility is considered to be on the right side. To test this hypothesis, the patient lies on the left side (the posterior transverse process downward) and the lumbar spine is extended from below by extending the hips, with the top most one being flexed. To extend and right rotate the lumbar spine from above, the upper arm is placed backward behind the patient, while the lower one is pulled upward toward the ceiling in a plane that is neither caudal nor cranial. To increase rotation, the pelvis is rotated downward toward the floor. The lumbar spine is now fully extended and right rotated. The PPIVM is tested by specifically right rotating the segment through its spinous process and assessing the end feel. If the end feel is normal compared to the segments above and below it, there is no extension hypomobility present. If abnormal, then the right side of the segment is hypomobile and the PPAIVM will determine if the hypomobility is caused by articular or extraarticular restrictions. If no hypomobility is found, hypermobility is tested by positioning the patient in the extended and rotated position but with the patient lying on the other side.

Interpretation of Findings

TABLE 13–2 CAUSES AND FINDINGS OF AN ERSL

CAUSES OF AN ERSL	ASSOCIATED FINDINGS
Isolated left joint flexion hypomobility (ERSL)	PPIVM and PPAIVM tests in the right flexion quadrant are reduced
Tight left extensor muscles (ERSL)	PPIVM test in the right flexion quadrant is decreased, the PPAIVM is normal
Arthrosis/itis left joint/ capsular pattern (ERSL < FRSL)	PPIVM and PPAIVM tests are equally reduced in the right flexion and left flexion quadrants
Fibrosis left joint (ERSL = FRSL)	PPIVM and PPAIVM tests equally reduced in the right and left flexion quadrants
Right posterior-lateral disc protrusion (ERSL < FRSL)	PPIVM tests in the right extension quadrant reduced with a springy end feel; both flexion quadrants appear normal

An ERSR would have the same causes and findings, but on the opposite side.

TABLE 13–3 CAUSES AND FINDINGS FOR AN FRSR

CAUSES OF AN FRSR	ASSOCIATED FINDINGS
Isolated left joint extension hypomobility (FRSR)	PPIVM and PPAIVM tests in the left extension quadrant are reduced
Tight left flexor muscles (FRSR)	PPIVM test in the left extension quadrant is decreased; PPAIVM test is normal
Arthrosis/itis left joint/capsular pattern (ERSL < FRSR)	PPIVM and PPAIVM tests in the right flexion quadrant are more reduced than in the left extension quadrant
Fibrosis left joint (ERSL = FRSR)	PPIVM and PPAIVM tests equally reduced in the right flexion and left extension quadrants
Left Posterior-lateral disc protrusion (ERSR < FRSR)	PPIVM tests in the left extension quadrant are reduced with a springy end feel; both flexion quadrants are normal

PASSIVE PHYSIOLOGIC ARTICULAR INTERVERTEBRAL MOVEMENT TEST

Passive physiologic articular intervertebral movement (PPAIVM) tests investigate the degree of linear or accessory glide that a joint possesses, and are used on segmental levels where there is a possible hypomobility to help determine if the motion restriction is articular, periarticular, or myofascial in origin. In other words, they assess the amount of joint motion as well as the quality of the end feel.

The motion is assessed, in relation to the patient's body type and age and the normal range for that segment, and the end feel is assessed for:

- Pain
- Spasm/hypertonicity
- Resistance

A number of techniques have been proposed over the years to assess segmental mobility of the T10–L5 segments, including posterior-anterior pressure techniques. The posterior-anterior pressure techniques, advocated by Maitland,[194] involve the application of pressure applied against the spinous, mammillary, and transverse processes of this region. Although these maneuvers are capable of eliciting pain, restricted movement, and/or muscle spasm, they are fairly nonspecific in determining the exact level involved or the exact cause of the symptoms. Consider the following example with the patient positioned in prone.

- A posterior-anterior pressure is applied simultaneously to both transverse processes of the L3 segment. Biomechanically, this produces a relative extension movement of L2 on L3, while producing a flexion movement of L3 on L4.

- If the spinous process of L3 is pushed to the right, inducing a left rotation of L3, this produces a relative right rotation of L2 on L3, but a left rotation of L3 on L4.

If either of these procedures elicits symptoms, it becomes very difficult to determine which of the segments, or motions, are at fault.

The techniques outlined as follows are more specific and will yield a more definitive diagnosis to the clinician. A pillow or towel roll should be placed under the lumbar spine of the patient if side-flexion of the lumbar spine appears to be occurring when the patient is placed in the side-lying position.

Flexion

The patient is positioned in side-lying, close to the edge of the bed, the spine supported in the neutral position, thighs on the table, and the head resting on a pillow. The clinician faces the patient. Using the patient's leg(s) as in the PPIVM test to produce motion of flexion from below, the suspected level is located. The clinician flexes down to that segment by pulling the patient's lower arm out horizontally from the table. The patient's trunk is stabilized with the cranial arm, while the cranial hand palpates the superior vertebra of the joint complex to be assessed. The interspinous space is palpated with the index finger of the caudal hand, while the caudal forearm supports the lower lumbar spine and pelvic girdle. The clinician's lower thorax supports the patient's abdomen and iliac crest.

Stabilizing the spinous process of the superior segment with the cranial hand, the clinician straddles the transverse processes of the inferior segment with the index and middle fingers of the caudal hand, and pulls the segment inferiorly using the caudal hand and forearm, thereby indirectly assessing the full superior linear glide of the superior segment (Figure 13–23). At the end of flexion, the articular surfaces roll and anteriorly glide, and the superior zygapophysial joint tilts posteriorly.

Extension

The patient and clinician are positioned as with the flexion test, but with the patient positioned diagonally on the bed, the hips forward, knees well flexed, and the head resting on a pillow. Having located the suspected level, the clinician extends the patient's spine down to that level by pulling the lower arm of the patient out from the table and toward the ceiling. The superior spinous process of the segment is pinched and the joint complex is passively taken into full extension by straddling the transverse processes, as for the flexion technique, and pushing the caudal vertebra anteriorly. At the end of the available range, the transverse processes of the inferior segment are glided in a cranial direction to test the full linear glide

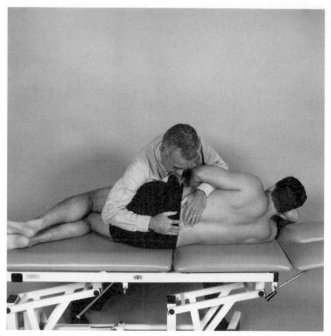

FIGURE 13–23 Symmetrical passive physiological intervertebral accessory motion testing-flexion.

(Figure 13–24). The caudal forearm, and clinician's lower thorax, guide the anterior roll/translation of the caudal vertebra, and stress the posterior shear component, while the spinous process of the superior segment is felt to move inferiorly and posteriorly.

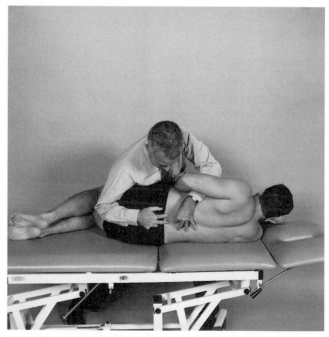

FIGURE 13–24 Symmetrical passive physiological intervertebral accessory motion testing-extension.

Side-Flexion/Rotation

Patient is positioned in side-lying close to the edge of the bed, the spine supported in the neutral position, thighs on the table, and the head resting on a pillow. The clinician faces the patient. Using the patient's leg(s) as in the PPIVM test, the suspected level is located. The clinician rotates the patient's lumbar spine down to the segment by pulling the lower arm out at a 45-degree angle to the table. With the thumb of the cranial hand, the lateral aspect of the spinous process of the cranial vertebra is palpated. The cranial forearm supports the patient's arm. The clinician, using the cranial forearm and thumb, passively side-flexes and rotates the segment around the appropriate axis, while the caudal hand pinches the spinous process of the inferior segment, preventing motion occurring at the inferior segment. This test may be performed in varying degrees of flexion and extension. The procedure is repeated on the other side.

PALPATION

Before palpating this region, it is well worth noting any alterations in the alignment of the spinous processes that could suggest the presence of a spondylolisthesis. Evidence of tenderness during palpation can highlight an underlying impairment.

- Specific pain elicited from one segment can be indicative of an instability.[195]
- Acute unilateral tenderness of the posterior inferior iliac spine is a useful confirmatory sign if it is well localized.[196]
- A well-localized and painful point at the gluteal level of the iliac crest may indicate the presence of Maigne's syndrome.[197] The point is located 8 to 10 cm from the midline. According to Maigne, referred pain may be mediated by the cluneal nerves, the posterior rami of the T12, or L1 spinal nerves.[198]
- Hardness of the gluteals accompanied by tenderness with pressure may implicate the gluteals as a source of low back pain.[199]
- Normally, the skin can be rolled over the spine and gluteal region with ease. Tightness or pain produced with the skin rolling indicates some underlying pathology.

INTERVERTEBRAL STRESS TESTING

If the passive physiologic intervertebral motion (PPIVM) tests demonstrate a hypermobility, the presence of an underlying instability should be suspected, and its possibility investigated. If a symmetrical instability (that is anterior or posterior) exists, flexion and/or extension, both rotations

TABLE 13–4 COMMON FINDINGS FOR INSTABILITY AND HYPERMOBILITY[192]

MOVEMENT	STRESS	INSTABILITY
L1–S1 flexion	anterior	symmetrical
L5–L1 flexion	posterior	symmetrical
S1–L5 flexion	posterior	symmetrical
L1–L5 extension	posterior	symmetrical
L5–S1 extension	anterior	symmetrical
RIGHT rotation	RIGHT torsion	Asymmetrical
LEFT rotation	LEFT torsion	Asymmetrical
RIGHT side-flexion	RIGHT lateral	Asymmetrical
LEFT side-flexion	LEFT lateral	Asymmetrical

and both side-flexions will be hypermobile. If the instability is asymmetrical (rotational or lateral), one rotation and/or side-flexion will be hypermobile, and this hypermobility will preclude normal flexion and/or extension. It should, therefore, be possible to select a stress test from the results of the PPIVM tests that is specific to a particular instability. However, it is wise to carry out all of the stress tests for that segment in case the PPIVM test, or the clinician, has missed a hypermobility.

For a segment to be unstable, all of the important segmental structures that control the effect of the stress must be inadequate. For example, there may be degradation or degeneration of the disc, but if the zygapophysial joints are stable, they will prevent abnormal anterior migration of the vertebra.

Although translations and axial rotations occur as part of the normal segmental motion they only occur in very small amounts. If the stability is within normal limits, the degree of movement during the stress test is imperceptible if proper pretest positioning is carried out.

The determination of the relevance of an instability is based on the judgment of the clinician, who must appraise the importance of the instability in light of the entire musculoskeletal examination (using both the selective tissue tension tests and the biomechanical examination).

The Tests

The key to these tests is to take up the slack of the angular motion first, before attempting to gain a further linear glide, or (in the case of rotation and side-flexion) a torsional motion for the test. A positive test produces excessive motion, shifting, and/or pain.

With all of the stability tests, the clinician should feel a firm end feel if the segment is stable. A loose end feel, especially if accompanied by crepitation, is considered a sign of instability. It must be realized, however, that this interpretation of instability does not correspond to the grosser, visually obvious instabilities diagnosed through x-rays, which only begin their grading with a 25% slippage. There is a certain irony in the clinical observation that the most painful instabilities are those that possess more intact inert tissue to resist the stresses of everyday life. As the peak incidence for disabling symptoms in the low back occurs between ages 35 and 55 years,[197] one might conclude that the last stage of degeneration, the stabilization phase of Kirkaldy-Willis, has a protective effect to the functional spine unit.[200]

Anterior Stability

Taking up the slack in flexion is a little difficult in the lower three lumbar segments because of the antishearing mechanism of the supraspinous ligament. So, the test is performed initially in a position just short of tightening the supraspinous ligament, and then again with the ligament taut in full lumbar flexion (full posterior pelvic tilt). Using this approach, the clinician can tell if the supraspinous antishearing mechanism is working well enough to be utilized as part of the intervention through the posterior pelvic tilt.

- *Patient position:* side-lying, knees and hips drawn up into flexion, the clinician resting his or her thighs against the patient's knees.
- *Fixation:* The upper spinous process is fixed, using the index finger and middle finger of the cranial hand, and is stabilized by placing the other hand over it (Figure 13–25). The inferior interspinous space is palpated with the ring finger of the caudal hand.

- *Stress:* to test L4 and L5, the clinician pushes with his or her thighs, through the patient's knees, along the line of the femur. At L3, the patient's hips are flexed up to 90 degrees prior to testing so that the line of force is parallel to the vertebral body joint line. The angle of the vertebral bodies is about 45 degrees for T12–L3, 30 degrees for L4, and 40 degrees for L5. The process is repeated for L2 and L1. If instability is found, the patient's hips are flexed up to 90 degrees, they are asked to perform and maintain a pelvic tilt, and all of the levels are retested (especially L4 and L5).

Posterior Stability

- *Patient position:* sitting on the edge of the bed in a position of lumbar lordosis. The patient's forearms are flexed and pronated and placed on the shoulders of the clinician (Figure 13–26). Starting at the mid-low thoracic spine, the clinician moves caudally applying an anterior force to the lower segment as the lumbar spine is extended. The lordosis position takes up the available linear glide, and the hyperextension, applied by the clinician, locks the joint.
- *Fixation:* the spinous process of the inferior vertebra is fixed, while the interspinous space above is palpated
- *Stress:* while maintaining the lordosis, the patient is instructed to try to gently push the clinician away using their forearms.

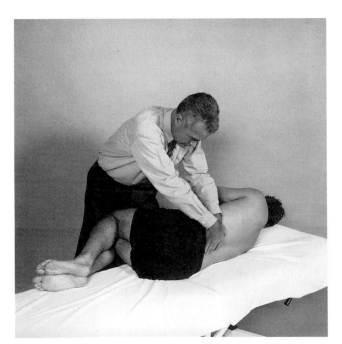

FIGURE 13–25 Anterior stability test position.

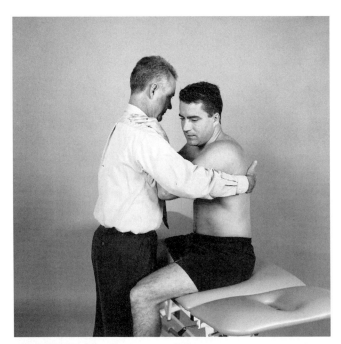

FIGURE 13–26 Posterior stability test position.

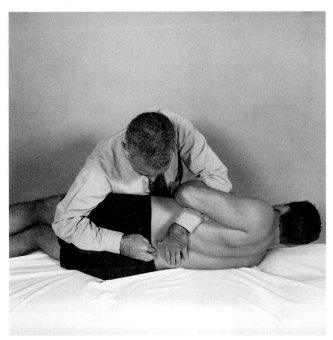

FIGURE 13–27 Rotation stability test position.

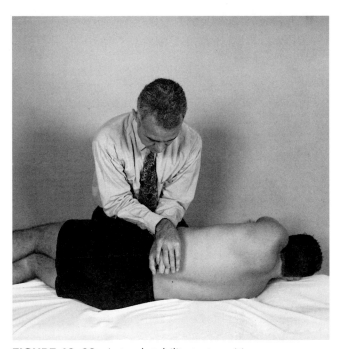

FIGURE 13–28 Lateral stability test position.

Rotational Stability
- *Patient position:* side-lying with their hips flexed to about 45 degrees; the lumbar spine in neutral throughout. The clinician pulls the patient's lower arm out at a 45-degree angle to horizontal and locks through the lumbar spine.
- *Fixation:* the inferior vertebra of the segment is fixed by blocking the side of the spinous process closest to the bed with the caudal hand.
- *Stress:* the clinician pushes the superior spinous process down toward the bed with the thumb of the cranial hand. (Figure 13–27). Very little, if any, motion should be felt.

Lateral Stability
This test does not rely on the objectivity of a specific end feel. Instead, an indirect shearing test is used as it appears to give a consistent result. Lateral instability is a fairly common finding in postpartum females.

- *Patient position:* side-lying, facing the clinician, the lumbar spine positioned in neutral, and the hips and knees flexed to about 45 degrees.
- *Stress:* the clinician, using the fleshy part of forearm, applies a downward pressure to the lateral aspect of the patient's trunk at the level of the L3 transverse process (Figure 13–28). This produces a lateral translation of the entire lumbar spine in the direction of the bed. The pressure is applied until an "end feel" is detected. The test is repeated with the

patient side-lying on the opposite side. The reproduction of pain is a positive finding.

Vertical Stability (Compression)
The same test as described in Chapter 10 is used to assess vertical stability. The patient is positioned in supine with the hips and knees flexed. The clinician stands at the patient's side. Using the cranial arm, the clinician cradles the patient's knees and controls the amount of hip and knee flexion. The clinician rests the caudal forearm on the soles of the patient's feet.

Test
- Maintaining the lumbar spine in the neutral position, the clinician applies a compressive force with the caudal forearm in a cranial direction, with the direction of the force parallel to the floor. The clinician notes any reproduction of any symptoms.
- The test is repeated with the lumbar spine in full flexion. The clinician notes the reproduction of any symptoms.
- The test is repeated with the lumbar spine in full extension. A roll may be used under the lumbar spine to maintain the full extension. The clinician notes the reproduction of any symptoms.

Vertical Stability (Traction)
The patient is positioned in supine with the hips and knees flexed, and the feet placed close to the end of the table.

The clinician stands at the end of the table, facing the patient. With the fingers interlaced, the clinician places his or her hands on the patient's calves. A towel wrapped around the patient's calves may also be used.

Test A traction force is applied in a caudal direction through the patient's calves. The angle of pull may be altered in accordance with the level being tested and the patient's response. The clinician notes the reproduction of any symptoms.

Coronal Plane Stability: Left Iliolumbar Ligament (Posterior Fibers)

The patient is positioned in prone with the clinician standing at the patient's right side. Stabilization is provided by placing the thumb against the right side of the L5 spinous process to prevent the left rotation of L5 from occurring. With the caudal hand, the clinician palpates the left aspect of the left ASIS and iliac crest and the lateral aspect of the left thigh, distal to the hip.

Test Fixing the L5 vertebra with the thumb of the cranial hand, the clinician pulls the left ilium posteriorly and caudally with the caudal hand, thereby applying a side-flexion force in the coronal plane to the pelvic girdle (Figure 13–29). This is performed until the motion barrier of right side-flexion at L5–S1 has been reached, and the force is sustained until the end feel is perceived. The

quantity of motion at the end feel, as well as the reproduction of symptoms, are noted.

Examination Conclusions

Following the biomechanical examination, a working hypothesis is established based on a summary of all of the findings. As mentioned, the focus of the biomechanical exam is to elicit a movement diagnosis and to determine:

- Which joint is impaired
- The presence and type of movement impairment
- The resultant functional impairment

At the completion of the biomechanical examination, the clinician should have information concerning the motion state of the joint, and should be able to determine whether the joint is myofascially and pericapsularly hypomobile, subluxed, hypermobile, or ligamentously and articularly unstable.

The following tables summarize the typical findings in a patient with a movement diagnosis, highlighting both the similarities and the differences between each.

TABLE 13–5 REDUCED MOVEMENT[83]

MYOFASCIAL	JOINT/PERICAPSULAR

Cause
  Muscle shortening
  (scars,contracture,
  adaptive)
	Cause
	  Capsular or ligamentous
	  shortening due to
	  Scars
	  Adaptation to a chroni-
	  cally shortened position
	  Joint surface adhesions

Findings
  Reduced movement or
  hypomobility may have an
  insidious or sudden onset;
  the presence or absence
  of pain depends on the
  level of chemical and/or
  mechanical irritation of the
  local nociceptors, which in
  turn, is a function of the
  stage of healing
  Pain is usually aggravated
  with movement and
  alleviated with rest
  Negative scan
PPIVM and PAIVM Findings
  Reduced gross PPIVM but
  PPAIVM normal
Intervention:
  Muscle relaxation
  techniques
  Transverse frictions
  Stretches
	Findings
	  Reduced movement or
	  hypomobility may have an
	  insidious or sudden onset;
	  the presence or absence
	  of pain depends on the
	  level of chemical and/or
	  mechanical irritation of the
	  local nociceptors, which in
	  turn, is a function of the
	  stage of healing
	  Pain is usually aggravated
	  with movement and
	  alleviated with rest
	  Negative scan
	PPIVM and PAIVM Findings
	  Reduced gross PPIVM *and*
	  PPAIVM
	Intervention
	  Joint mobilizations at
	  specific level

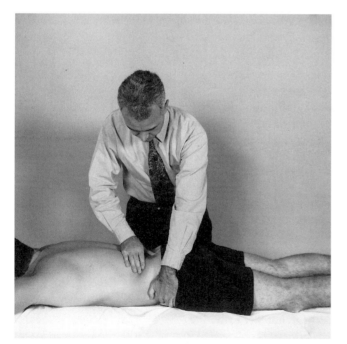

FIGURE 13–29 Left iliolumbar ligament test position.

TABLE 13–6 REDUCED MOVEMENT[83]

PERICAPSULAR/ARTHRITIS	DISC PROTRUSION
Cause	Cause
Degenerative or degradative changes	Cumulative stress
	Low level but prolonged overuse
	Sudden macrotrauma
Findings	Findings
Negative scan	Positive scan
Reduces gross PPIVM in all directions except flexion	Key muscle fatigable weakness
Active motion restricted in a capsular pattern	Hyporeflexive DTRs
(decreased extension and equal limitation of	Sensory changes in dermatomal distribution
rotation and side-flexion)	Subjective complaints of radicular pain
PPIVM and PAIVM Findings	PPIVM and PAIVM Findings
Reduced gross PPIVM but PPAIVM normal	Reduced gross PPIVM *and* PPAIVM
Intervention:	Intervention
Capsular and muscle stretching	Traction
Active exercises and PREs	Active exercises in to spinal extension
Anti-inflammatory modalities if necessary	Positioning
Joint protection techniques	

INTERVENTIONS

Manual Techniques

Numerous manual therapy techniques are available to the clinician for this region and the reader is encouraged to explore as many as possible. In fact, all of the examination techniques that are used to assess joint mobility can also be employed as treatment techniques. However, the intent of the technique changes from one of assessing the end feel to one where the application of graded mobilizations or muscle

TABLE 13–7 EXCESSIVE MOVEMENT[83]

HYPERMOBILITY	INSTABILITY
Causes	Causes
Cumulative stress due to neighboring hypomobility	Sudden macrotrauma (ligamentous)
Low level but prolonged overuse	Hypermobility allowed to progress (ligamentous)
Sudden macrotrauma that is not enough to produce instability	Degeneration of interposing hyaline or fibrocartilage (articular)
Findings	Findings
Subjective complaints of catching	Subjective complaints of catching
Good days and bad days	Good days and bad days
Symptoms aggravated with sustained positions	Symptoms aggravated with sustained positions
Negative scan	Negative scan
PPIVM Findings	PPIVM Findings
Increase in gross PPIVM with pain at end range	Increase in gross PPIVM with pain at end range
	Presence of nonphysiologic movement (positive stress test)
	Recurrent subluxations
Intervention	Intervention: falls into three areas
Educate the patient to avoid excessive range	1. Global stabilization
Take stress off joint (mobilize hypomobility)	Educate patient to stay out of activities likely to take him or her
Anti-inflammatory modalities if necessary	into the instability
Stabilize if absolutely necessary	Total body neuromuscular movement pattern reeducation
	Work or sports conditioning and rehabilitation
	2. Local stabilization
	Muscular splinting of the region (lifting techniques, twisting on
	feet, chin tucking when lifting)
	Bracing with supports (collars, corsets, splints, and braces)
	Regional neuromuscular movement pattern reeducation
	3. Segmental stabilization
	PNF and active exercises to the segment

energy techniques are applied at the appropriate joint range. Manual techniques can be used with hypomobilities, hypermobilities, instabilities, and soft tissue injuries.

Myofascial Hypomobility

These types of hypomobility respond well to muscle energy techniques and stretching.

Joint Hypomobility

The purpose of these techniques is to be able to isolate a mobilization to a specific level, and in so doing:

- Reduce stresses through both the fixation and leverage components of the spine.
- Reduce stresses through hypermobile segments.
- Reduce the overall force needed by the clinician, thus giving greater control.

Choice of Manual Technique

The selection of a manual technique is dependent on a number of factors including: (1) the acuteness of the condition; (2) the goal of treatment, and (3) whether the restriction is symmetric or asymmetric.

Acuteness of the Condition If the structure is acutely painful (pain is felt before resistance or pain is felt with resistance), pain relief, rather than a mechanical effect, is the major goal. The manual techniques that can provide pain relief include:

- Joint oscillations (grade I and II) that do not reach the end of range. The segment or joint is left in its neutral position and the mobilization is carried out from that point. There is no need for, and in fact every reason to avoid, muscle relaxation techniques to help reach the end of range.
- Gentle passive range of motion

These techniques can be supplemented with the use of modalities. Heat can be applied to the specific area prior to the manual technique.

- A moist heat pack causes an increase in the local tissue temperature, reaching its highest point about 8 minutes after the application.[201] Wet heat produces a greater rise in local tissue temperature compared to dry heat at a similar temperature.[202]
- Ultrasound is the most common clinical deep-heating modality used to promote tissue healing.[203–205]

Another modality is electrical stimulation. For the manual therapist, electrical stimulation can be used:

- To create a muscle contraction through nerve or muscle stimulation

- To decrease pain through the stimulation of sensory nerves (TENS)
- To maintain or increase range of motion
- To stimulate tissue healing by creating an electrical field in biological tissue
- Muscle re-education or facilitation by both motor and sensory stimulation
- To drive ions into or through the skin (iontophoresis)

Goal of the Treatment[189] If stretching of the mechanical barrier rather than pain relief is the immediate objective of the treatment, a mobilization technique is carried out at the end of the available range. To achieve this, the antagonist muscle must be relaxed and this is most easily accomplished by the hold and relax technique. After this has been gained (and sometimes before and after), there is some minor pain to be dealt with using grade IV oscillations, after which, the joint capsule can be stretched using either grade IV++ or prolonged stretch techniques. The prolonged stretch or the strong oscillations are continued for as long as the clinician can maintain good control. At the point where control is about to be lost, several isometric contractions to the agonists and the antagonists are demanded of the patient's muscles in the new range to give the central nervous system information about the newly acquired range. To complete the reeducation, concentric and eccentric retraining is carried out through the whole range of the joint. Active exercises are continued at home and at work on a regular and frequent basis to reinforce the reeducation.

Symmetric versus Asymmetric Restriction Whether the restriction is symmetric, involving both sides of the segment or asymmetric, involving only one side of the segment, influences the manual technique used. It is unwise to use a symmetrical mobilization for an asymmetrical impairment. If the right joint cannot extend and a symmetrical extension mobilization technique is applied, there is a risk of mobilizing the normal joint, leading to hypermobility. In addition to this risk, is the technique's inadequacy, as full range extension or flexion can only be achieved unilaterally.

Symmetric Restrictions Symmetrical restrictions are usually the result of a postural dysfunction. A number of manual techniques can be used to increase motion at a lumbar spine segment.

A. Symmetrical Restriction of Flexion. Symmetrical impairments can effectively be treated with symmetrical mobilizations, at least for all but the extreme parts of the zygapophysial joint ranges. Nonacute symmetrical impairments can be better treated using bilateral symmetrical techniques. The L3–4 segment is used in the following example.

1. *Mobilization technique:* the patient is positioned in side-lying, with the lumbar spine supported in a neutral position, and the head resting on a pillow. The clinician faces the patient. Using the palpating finger of the cranial hand, the clinician palpates the interlaminar spaces of the L3–L4 segment. Using the caudal hand, the clinician flexes the patient's hips, knees, and the lower lumbar spine until L4 is felt to move. With the palpating finger of the caudal hand, the clinician palpates the interlaminar spaces of the L3–L4 segment. The clinician locks the upper lumbar spine by pulling through the patient's lower most arm until L3 is felt to move. The direction of the arm pull determines whether the lock occurs in flexion, extension, or neutral, and whether a congruent or incongruent lock is used. The L3–L4 segment remains in its neutral position. The clinician fixes L3 and flexes the L3–L4 segment to the motion barrier using the caudal hand and forearm (Fig. 13–23). A grade I–IV force is applied to produce a superior-anterior glide of the zygapophysial joints at L3–L4.

2. *High velocity thrust technique:* this classic lumbar technique involves the patient side-lying and the clinician standing in front of the patient. A ligamentous lower lock of flexion is used with an upper lock of rotation, leaving the segment to be treated in a neutral position.

To accomplish the lower lock using flexion and rotation up to, but not including, the segment to be treated, the ankle of the top leg is held by the clinician, using the hand closest to the patient's feet, and the patient's thigh is flexed up to L4. This is achieved by flexing the upper most leg of the patient through the segment in question, allowing the thigh to adduct, before unflexing the lock back to the L4 segment. The ankle of the upper leg is then placed behind the knee of the lower leg.

The upper lock of flexion and rotation down to L3 is completed by pulling the bottom arm of the patient either horizontally (for flexion) or vertically (for extension), while the top arm is resting on top of the trunk (for extension) or in the front of (for flexion). The clinician then threads their cranial arm under the patient's upper most arm. The patient is then log-rolled toward the clinician so that the trunk is more vertical to the bed, while making sure that the lock is not lost. Fine-tuning of the lock is completed by slightly rotating the patient's pelvis toward the clinician. A four-point contact of the clinician on the patient occurs.

1. The thumb and index finger of the clinician's cranial hand fix the L3 spinous process.
2. The index and middle finger of the clinician's caudal hand are placed over the transverse processes of L4.
3. The clinician's body leans against the anterior aspect of the patient's trunk.
4. The forearm of the clinician's caudal arm is placed between the patient's greater trochanter and under the patient's iliac crest of the upper most leg and parallel/in line with, the patient's spine.

The high velocity, low amplitude thrust is then delivered by the caudal hand and arm posteriorly and inferiorly in an oblique direction that matches the plane of the L3–L4 joint.

If the patient's condition is hyperacute and a flexion or extension mobilization is too painful to perform, a technique called specific traction can be employed (see later discussion).

B. Symmetrical restriction of extension. The L3–L4 segment is used in these examples. As mentioned previously, the end feel and the stage of healing are used as guides to determine the intensity of the treatment.

1. *Mobilization technique:* the patient is positioned in side-lying, with the lumbar spine supported in a neutral position and the head resting on a pillow. The clinician faces the patient. Using the palpating finger of the cranial hand, the clinician palpates the interlaminar spaces of the L3–L4 segment. Using the caudal hand, the clinician extends the patient's hip until L4 is felt to move. The patient's upper most hip and knee are flexed while the lower most leg is extended. With the palpating finger of the caudal hand, the clinician palpates the interlaminar spaces of the L3–L4 segment. Using the cranial hand and forearm, the clinician locks the lumbar spine by pulling through the patient's lower most arm until L3 is felt to move. The direction of the arm pull determines whether the lock occurs in flexion, extension, or neutral, and whether a congruent or incongruent lock is used. The L3–L4 segment remains in its neutral position. The spinous process of L3 is fixed using a pinch grip of the cranial hand. The clinician mobilizes L4 by applying a posterior-anterior force to the articular pillars of the L3 vertebra using the index and long finger of the caudal hand (Figure 13–30). A grade I–IV force is applied to produce a posterior-inferior glide of the zygapophysial joints at L3–L4, using the cranial hand and forearm.

2. *High velocity thrust technique:* this classic technique involves the patient side-lying and the clinician standing in front of the patient. A ligamentous lower lock of flexion is used with an upper lock of rotation, leaving the segment to be treated in a neutral position.

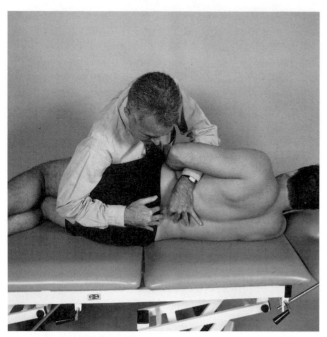

FIGURE 13–30 Patient and clinician position for symmetrical mobilization into extension.

To accomplish the lower lock using flexion and rotation up to, but not including, the segment to be treated, the ankle of the top leg is held by the clinician, using the hand closest to the patient's feet, and the patient's thigh is flexed up to L4. This is achieved by flexing the upper most leg of the patient through the segment in question, allowing the thigh to adduct before unflexing the lock back to the L4 segment. The patient's ankle of the upper leg is then placed behind the knee of the lower leg.

The upper lock of flexion and rotation down to L3 is completed by pulling the bottom arm of the patient either horizontally (for flexion) or vertically (for extension), while the top arm is resting on top of the trunk (for extension) or in front (for flexion). The clinician then threads the cranial arm under the patient's upper most arm. The patient is then log-rolled toward the clinician so that the trunk is more vertical to the bed, while making sure that the lock is not lost. Fine-tuning of the lock is completed by slightly rotating the patient's pelvis toward the clinician. A four-point contact of the clinician on the patient occurs.

   i. The thumb and index finger of the clinician's cranial hand fix the L3 spinous process.
   ii. The index and middle finger of the clinician's caudal hand rest over the transverse processes of L4.
   iii. The clinician's body leans against the anterior aspect of the patient's trunk.

   iv. The forearm of the clinician's caudal arm is placed between the patient's greater trochanter and under the patient's iliac crest of the upper most leg and parallel/in line with the patient's spine.

     The palm of the caudal arm is placed on the spine, with the hypothenar eminence placed over L4. The thrust is then delivered to L4 anteriorly and superiorly in an oblique direction, matching the plane of the joint.

3. *Asymmetrical (quadrant) techniques:* in the case of asymmetrical hypomobility, the approach can be either to mobilize the stiff combined movement or to ascertain which joint and which glide is restricted and mobilize that directly, while, at the same time, safeguarding the other segments from the effect of the mobilization. For example, if right rotation and side-flexion and flexion is restricted, the segment can be mobilized using a flexion and right rotation mobilization technique. Alternatively, the same result would be achieved if the segment was positioned in flexion and right side-flexion and a side-flexion mobilization applied to increase the superior glide of the superior zygapophysial joint of the left zygapophysial joint.

   Asymmetrical techniques can be used for any condition that allows the barrier to movement to be encroached upon. These conditions include unilateral zygapophysial joint hypomobilities, disc protrusions, bilateral zygapophysial joint impairments (such as a fixed postural hypomobility), noninflamed systemic arthritis, and unilateral and bilateral myofascial shortening. If an appropriate bilateral hypomobility is to be treated, the clinician can utilize a bilateral asymmetrical technique rather than the often-awkward symmetrical technique. The only conditions that cannot be treated with asymmetrical techniques are the acutely painful ones where sub-barrier grades of mobilization must be used.

4. *Restriction of extension and side-flexion (posterior quadrant restrictions):* These impairments occur when the zygapophysial joint cannot extend and side-flex. The patient typically presents with one-sided pain that is aggravated with extension and side-flexion toward the painful side. This impairment is also known as a closing restriction.

   i. Technique using a hi-low table. The patient is positioned in side lying on their pain-free side. The table is adjusted so that the head and foot parts are raised, which produces a side-flexion of the patient's lumbar spine towards the painful side. The patient's lumbar spine is extended, rotated, and side-flexed from below by placing their lowermost leg in hip extension, while their upper leg is flexed until motion is felt at the inferior aspect of the segment. The patient's lumbar spine is extended, rotated, and side-flexed from above by pulling the patient's lowermost arm out and up towards the ceiling until the spinous process of the superior segment is felt to move. The clinician places his or her arms against the patient's shoulder and pelvis, and rotates the patient's shoulder back while counter rotating the pelvis and monitoring the segment to be treated.

The cranial hand of the clinician monitors the spinous process of the superior segment while the caudal hand monitors the spinous process of the inferior segment. Once the segment has been located, the clinician pushes down on the spinous process of the superior segment using the thumb of the cranial hand while pulling up on spinous process of the lower segment with the fingers of the caudal hand. (Fig. 13-22) The motion barrier is felt and a hold and relax technique is used to move to the new motion barrier. The process is repeated until a further increase in range is noted.

ii. Seated technique. A seated technique can be used if the patient-to-clinician size ratio is too great. In this example, the patient has a restriction into the right posterior quadrant. The patient is positioned in sitting with a cushion under the left buttock. This positions the lower lumbar spine in right side-flexion. The clinician stands on the right side of the patient. The patient is asked to sit up and straighten the back while the clinician palpates at the level of the impairment and encounters the motion barrier by fixing the spinous process of the inferior segment. With the clinician supporting the patient's shoulder girdle, the patient is asked to side-flex and rotate toward the clinician until the spinous process of the upper segment is felt to move. At that point a hold and relax technique is easily delivered by giving the patient the command, "Don't let me lift your shoulder." Upon relaxation, the new motion barrier is reached and the procedure is repeated as necessary.

iii. Standard mat table. For this example, the right zygapophysial joint at L3–4 has a restriction of extension, right side bending and rotation, or to use the osteopathic description, an FRSL, or the right zygapophysial joint at L3–4 cannot "close." The patient is positioned in left side-lying with the side of the impairment upper most, the lumbar spine in neutral, and the head resting on a pillow. The clinician, who is standing facing the patient, palpates the interlaminar spaces of the L3–L4 segment with the cranial hand. With the caudal hand, the clinician extends the lower lumbar spine by extending

the lower most leg at the hip until L3 is felt to begin moving. The patient's upper most hip and knee remain flexed while the lower most leg is extended. With the palpating finger of the caudal hand, the clinician palpates the interlaminar spaces of the L3–L4 segment. Using the cranial hand and forearm, the clinician locks the upper lumbar spine using lateral flexion and rotation by pulling through the patient's lower most arm until L3 is felt to move. The direction of the arm pull determines whether the lock occurs in flexion, extension, or neutral, and whether a congruent or incongruent lock is used. The L3–L4 segment remains in its neutral position. The clinician fixes L4 by applying a posterior-anterior force to the articular pillars using the index and middle finger of the caudal hand. The clinician extends, right side-flexes, and rotates the L3–L4 segment to the motion barrier, using the thumb of the cranial hand, which exerts a force on the inferior articular process of L3, while the cranial forearm is applied to the lower lateral thorax. A grade I–V force is applied to produce a posterior-inferior glide of the right zygapophysial joint at L3–L4.

5. *Restriction of flexion and side-flexion (anterior quadrant restrictions):* these impairments occur when the zygapophysial joint cannot flex and side-flex away from the side of the pain. The patient typically presents with one-sided pain and complaints of pain with flexion and side-flexion away from the painful side. This impairment is also known as an "opening" restriction. The technique is identical to the posterior quadrant impairment, except that the patient is positioned in flexion.

i. Technique using a hi-low table. The patient is positioned in side-lying on their pain-free side. The table is positioned so that head and feet sections are lowered, producing a side-flexion of the lumbar spine toward the nonpainful side. Monitoring the inferior segment with the cranial hand, the clinician flexes the patient's knees and hips until the motion barrier is felt. The lower most leg remains in this position, while the upper most leg is placed in a figure-4 position, tucking its foot behind the knee of the lower most leg. To position the patients lumbar spine in flexion from above, the patient's upper most elbow is placed forward of the patient's trunk, the underneath arm being drawn horizontally toward the clinician. The clinician places the arms against the patient's shoulder and pelvis and places the fingers against the inferior side of superior and inferior segment. Using both elbows, the clinician pushes down toward the table while lifting the spinous processes with the finger tips.

ii. Seated technique. The seated techniques can be used if the patient-to-clinician size ratio is too great. In this example, the patient has a restriction into the left anterior quadrant. A pillow is placed under the patient's right buttock, thereby, producing a left side-flexion of their lower lumbar spine. Standing to the left of the patient, the clinician stabilizes the lateral aspect of the L3 spinous process with one hand. The patient is asked to side-flex toward the clinician until L2 is felt to move. The patient is then passively flexed and rotated toward the clinician until L2 is felt to move on L3. Using a contract and relax (CR) or a hold and relax (HR) technique, the right side at the L2–L3 level is maximally opened.

iii. *Standard mat table.*

Mobilization—the right zygapophysial joint at L3–4 has a restriction of flexion, left side bending and rotation, or to use the osteopathic description, an ERSR, or the right zygapophysial joint at L3–4 cannot open. The patient is positioned in left side-lying, with the side of the impairment upper most, the lumbar spine in neutral, and the head resting on a pillow. The clinician, who is standing facing the patient, palpates the interlaminar spaces of the L3–L4 segment with the cranial hand. With the caudal hand, the clinician flexes hips, knees, and the lower lumbar spine until L4 is felt to begin moving. The patient's upper most hip and knee remain flexed while their lower most leg is extended. With the palpating finger of the caudal hand, the clinician palpates the interlaminar spaces of the L3–L4 segment. Using the cranial hand and forearm, the clinician locks the upper lumbar spine using side-flexion by pulling through the patient's lower most arm until L3 is felt to move. The direction of the arm pull determines whether the lock occurs in either flexion, extension, or neutral, and whether a congruent or incongruent lock is used. The L3–L4 segment remains in its neutral position. The clinician fixes L4 with the caudal hand. The clinician flexes, left side-flexes, and rotates the L3–L4 segment to the motion barrier. A grade I–V force is applied to produce a superior-anterior glide of the right zygapophysial joint at L3–L4.

Muscle energy—the left zygapophysial joint at L2–3 cannot open. The patient is positioned in side-lying with the impairment side up. If the left zygapophysial joint at L2–3 cannot open, the patient is positioned in right side-lying. A pillow placed under the pelvis can be used to accentuate the side-flexion. The clinician locks down to L2 using rotation to the left by pulling the bottom arm out at an angle of 45 degrees. The clinician then locks from the bottom by flexing the patient's hips up until L3 is felt to move. The patient's heels are lowered off the bed, which introduces right side-flexion into the lumbar spine, until L3 is felt to move on L2. Gravity is now used to open the segment while the clinician controls the descent of the legs, or, the patient can attempt to raise the feet toward the ceiling against the resistance of gravity or the clinician.

6. *Restriction of extension and side-flexion* and *flexion and side-flexion at the same segment:* It is assumed that following a fibrotic distortion of the capsule, motion is restricted equally in both flexion and extension, to the same side. It is also assumed that this fibrosis is stretched maximally by a separation of the articular surfaces of the affected joint. To achieve this, the patient's spine must be positioned in neutral. When palpating motion at the interspinous level, there is a point in the lumbar spine where the inferior spinous process no longer moves superiorly but begins to move posteriorly, an indication that extension at the zygapophysial joint has begun. It is at this point that the segment can be considered to be in neutral. To treat a left zygapophysial joint, the patient is positioned in right-side lying, and, having gained a neutral position for the segment in question, the upper spine is rotated and side-flexed to the left. Osteokinematically, the lower spine is rotated and side-flexed to the right. This will bring the segment in question to a position that will maximally stretch the left zygapophysial joint capsule. A hold/relax/stretch technique should, theoretically, stretch the affected capsule and, subsequently, regain motion at that segment.

Soft Tissue Injuries

These injuries usually respond well to a combination of electrotherapeutic modalities, thermal agents, soft tissue techniques, and relaxation.

Electrotherapeutic Modalities and Thermal Agents The anticipated benefits to the soft tissues from the use of electrotherapeutic modalities and physical agents are used primarily in the acute and subacute phases of injury to the soft tissues to help control swelling and interrupt the pain cycle so the individual can begin to exercise. In the chronic stages of rehabilitation, modalities generally play a more secondary role to therapeutic exercise procedures. The application of modalities alone is not recommended because it fosters dependence on the clinician for relief of symptoms, rather than self-management and independence.

Soft Tissue Techniques   These techniques have the specific purpose of improving the vascularity and extensibility of the tissues and include massage, myofascial release, and strain and counterstrain.

Pelvic Shift Correction

As mentioned in Chapter 10, patients commonly present with a pelvic shift or list. The shift is thought to be a protective mechanism due to:

- An irritation of a zygapophysial joint
- An irritation of a spinal nerve and/or its dural sleeve, due to a disc herniation[206] and the resulting muscle spasm.[207]

The correction can be done a number of ways depending on the type of shift. There are three types of shifts, and each is dealt with differently.

Lateral Shift

1. While the patient is standing, have him or her shift further into the shift rhythmically and repeatedly.
2. As the patient is standing, manually correct the shift by pushing the pelvis into its correct position (McKenzie shift correction[208]).
3. Apply strain and counterstrain techniques to the quadratus lumborum and iliacus muscles by placing the muscles in a shortened position.

Quadratus Lumborum   Patient is positioned in prone with the clinician standing on the opposite side to the involved side. The quadratus lumborum muscle fibers on the side opposite to the direction of the shift are palpated from the 12th rib to the lateral aspect of the iliac crest. At varying parts along the muscle's length, the clinician pushes the fibers toward the table and pulls them up toward the ceiling, attempting to find the most comfortable direction. Once found, the clinician holds the stretch in that direction for about 90 seconds. For a reciprocal inhibition, the patient abducts the contralateral leg against the clinician's resistance.

Iliacus   To relax the iliacus, the patient is positioned in prone and each iliacus in turn is palpated at its origin just inferior to the ASIS. The pelvis is lifted by the clinician on the tested side, toward the ceiling, and each side is assessed for tightness. On the tighter side, the clinician uses a hold-relax technique by asking the patient to push the ASIS into the bed against the clinician's resistance for 3 to 5 times. Once the quadratus lumborum and iliacus are relaxed, the patient is positioned in side-lying with the convexity of the curve uppermost. Using the soft part of the forearm, the clinician pushes down gently on the convexity

and gradually reducing the shift. A towel roll placed under the lumbar spine will prevent over-correction for those patients with an additional anterior or posterior instability. Once the shift is corrected, erector spinae strengthening is initiated with the patient remaining in prone.

Posterior Shift

With this patient type, the structures that resist a posterior translation of the segment are compromised. If the dysfunction is unilateral, the patient presents with pain during extension and side-flexion to one side.

The intervention for the quadratus lumborum and iliacus is the same as just described except that the correction utilizes the anterior shear test position (Figure 13–25). The patient is positioned in side-lying and a force is applied longitudinally through the length of the femur to move the shift in the opposite direction to that of the instability.

Anterior Shift

With this patient type, the structures that resist anterior translation of the segment are compromised. If the dysfunction is unilateral, the patient presents with pain during flexion and side-flexion to one side. To relax the kyphosis, the quadratus lumborum and iliacus are treated as just discussed and then the shift is corrected using the position to test for posterior instabilities (Figure 13–26), that is, with the patient seated, elbows flexed, and forearms pronated, with the clinician standing in front of the patient. The patient rests the forearms on the clinician's chest and the clinician reaches behind the patient with both hands and stabilizes the inferior segment while the patient pushes against him or her with the forearms.

Specific Traction

The technique of specific traction is used for patient's whose condition is acute. It is an excellent technique to aid in the relief of pain when applied correctly.

The patient is positioned in side-lying, close to the front edge of the bed and the clinician close to the patient. The segment to be treated is identified by flexing the patient's hips and knees while palpating. The clinician places his or her cranial hand/arm between the patient's arm and body. While palpating the segmental level with the cranial hand, the patient is asked to lift both lower extremities off the table with the clinician helping as needed. Alternatively, the patient can push the foot of the lowermost leg to the bottom end of the table. Both of these maneuvers induce a side-flexion of the lumbar spine away from the bed. Passive pulling on the lowermost hip or leg by the clinician can also induce the slight side-flexion away from the table. While the patient's pelvis is tilted toward the table, the clinician stabilizes it there by placing the armpit of their caudal arm under the patient's uppermost ASIS.

The clinician flexes the patient's uppermost leg to 90 degrees of hip flexion while palpating at the segmental level. The patient's lower most arm is pulled out at an angle of 45 degree with the cranial hand, while the caudal hand palpates for rotation at the segment. The segment is locked down to, but not in to. The patient's lower most arm is tucked behind the patient's head. The upper most leg is flexed up to, but not into the segment. Once the patient is in this position, fine tuning is applied by rotating from either above and/or below. With cranial hand, the clinician applies a pincer grip on the spinous process of the superior segment while stabilizing the lower segment with the index and middle finger of the caudal hand. As the specific traction is applied, the clinician pivots over the patient's lower trochanter by pushing down with the armpit on the patient's pelvis, thereby returning the lumbar spine to neutral in terms of the sideflexion. The traction is applied by moving the pelvis toward the patient's feet with an appropriate grade for the problem.

Therapeutic Exercises

The exercises outlined in this section are designed to address imbalances of flexibility or strength. The exercises that are prescribed to increase the strength of the surrounding musculature are referred to as "stabilization" exercises.

Stabilization Exercises

Stabilization exercises can be categorized as segmental or regional.

Segmental Exercises A recent focus in the rehabilitation of patients with chronic low back pain has been the specific training of those muscles surrounding the lumbar spine with a primary role that is considered to be the provision of dynamic stability and segmental control to the spine.[209] These are the deep abdominal muscles (internal oblique and transversus abdominis) and the lumbar multifidus. The importance of the lumbar multifidus regarding its potential to provide dynamic control to the motion segment in its neutral zone is now well acknowledged,[168] and its co-activation with the oblique and transverse abdominals provide an important stiffening effect on the lumbar spine, enhancing its dynamic stability.[210] The internal oblique and the transversus abdominis are known to be primarily active in providing rotational and lateral control to the spine while maintaining adequate levels of intra-abdominal pressure and imparting tension to the thoracolumbar fascia.[165] Recent studies indicate that the deep

abdominal muscles undergo changes in their functional performance in populations with low back pain.[172, 173] In addition, studies have described subtle changes or shifts in the pattern of abdominal muscle activation in subjects with chronic low back pain where there is an overriding activation of the rectus abdominis during attempts to preferentially recruit the deep abdominal muscles,[209, 211] such as the transversus abdominis.

Thus, particular emphasis should be placed on strengthening exercises for the quadratus lumborum, transversus abdominis, internal oblique and lumbar multifidus.

A. Internal oblique and transversus abdominis
   1. Research investigating different abdominal exercises has confirmed that some exercises are more specific for activating the deep abdominal muscles than others.[164] The abdominal drawing-in, or hollowing maneuver, is one exercise known to result in preferential activation of the internal oblique and transversus abdominis, with little contribution by the rectus abdominis in the pain-free population.[164] Researchers have pointed out that an inability to perform the abdominal drawing-in maneuver differentiated chronic low back pain from pain-free subjects.[212]
   2. The exercise is performed in the following manner:
      a. The patient is positioned in supine crook-lying with the hips flexed to 45 degrees.
      b. The patient is instructed to contract the deep abdominal muscles by drawing the navel up in a cranial direction and in toward the spine, so as to draw in the lower abdomen.
      c. The patient's head and upper trunk must remain stable. He or she is not permitted to flex forward, push through the feet, or tilt the pelvis.

B. Quadratus lumborum
   1. The patient is prone and the quadratus lumborum is palpated.
   2. The patient resists while the clinician attempts to side-flex the patient away from the tested side by pushing on the shoulder.
   3. The muscle can also be tested in standing by having the patient resist as the clinician attempts to pull his or her arm/hand to the floor.

C. Multifidus. The multifidus can be strengthened using resisted spinal extension/hyperextension exercises. These exercises include:[200]
   1. Back extension and hyperextension over a high bench
   2. Modified "dead lift" (knees flexed to about 20 degrees)

3. Seated rows
4. Squats
5. Dumbbell overhead cleans
6. Back extension machines (with the pelvis fixated)

Manual Approach to Segmental Stabilization This is the most difficult part of the stabilization therapy and requires thousands of repetitions by the patient. Manual segmental stabilization is for circumstances when the strengthening exercises have failed to prevent the joint from moving into its unstable range. It is essential at this juncture that the rate and degree of movement into the instability are controlled and minimized as much as possible. To do this, modified PNF (proprioceptive neuromuscular facilitation) techniques to reeducate the muscles controlling segmental movement are initiated. The muscles that govern the impaired segment are required to produce smooth, well-controlled, isometric concentric and eccentric contractions into and out of the instability in response to eventually arbitrary demands from the clinician.

Example: In this example the patient has been diagnosed with a left zygapophysial joint hypermobility into extension. The patient is positioned in right side-lying, facing the clinician. The patient's lumbar spine is initially placed into the hypermobile extreme (extension and left side-flexion). The segment is then moved out of the hypermobile range into the normal range. The first command is for the patient to "hold" against a force, which would tend to bring the segment back into its hypermobile extreme. The magnitude of the clinician's force is dictated by the reaction of the segmental paraspinal muscles on the opposite side. Eccentric exercises are performed throughout the "normal" range and the patient is asked to hold at the new end range each time. The next command is for the patient to slowly allow the movement into the hypermobile range. Monitoring the segmental range of motion, the clinician avoids the hypermobile extreme but increases the force to a maximum at what is judged to be the "normal limit" of motion. The clinician performs passive range of motion throughout the range giving hold commands at various parts in the range.

All exercises should be tailored to the patient's diagnosis. In general, pain aggravated by sustained or repeated flexion should benefit from extension exercises and press-ups,[213] whereas pain aggravated with repeated or sustained extension should benefit from flexion exercises.

Regional Exercises The patient must be encouraged and educated to avoid the activities or postures that promote movement of the segment into the unstable range. For example, any patient with an anterior instability at L5–S1 should be counseled to avoid all lifting, not to stand for prolonged periods, not to run long distances, and to avoid activities that increase the lordosis of the lumbar spine. If the activity or posture cannot be avoided, as is usually the case, then the patient must learn how to protect the region of the spine if it is inadvertently or unavoidably stressed into the instability. If for example, the patient with the anterior instability at L5–S1 must lift, then he or she should be taught to lift with a posterior pelvic tilt to produce a posterior shear at the lumbar segments. If prolonged standing is unavoidable, then putting one foot up on a box and alternating periodically is suggested. If the patient insists on continuing to run, then the difficult chore of teaching running in a posterior pelvic tilt falls to the clinician.

The following protocols for regional strengthening have proven useful over the years in treating lumbar instabilities, and the reader is encouraged to investigate these further while individually tailoring their intervention depending on clinical findings.

Edelman, B. Conservative treatment considered best course for spondylolisthesis. Orthopedics Today 9(1): 6–8, 1989.

Morgan, D. Concepts in functional training and postural stabilization for the lowback-injured. Top Acute Care Trauma Rehabil 2(4):8–17. Aspen publishers, 1988.

Saal, J.A. Rehabilitation of sports related lumbar spine injuries. In Saal J.A. (ed). Physical Medicine and Rehabilitation: State of the Art Reviews 1(4):613–638 Hanley and Belfus, Inc. Philadelphia, 1987.

White, A.H. Conservative care of low back pain. In Genant, H. (ed). Spine Update 1987:283–285. University of California, San Francisco Press, 1987.

White, A.H. Principles for physical management of work injuries. In Isenhagen S. (ed). Work Injury. Aspen publishers, 1988.

Level 1
Protection of the lumbar spine needs to be provided during these exercises to prevent an excessive amount of lordosis from occuring. For example, the exercises in the prone position should be performed with a pillow underneath the patient's abdominals.

Abdominal Strengthening
● *Curl-up:* the patient is positioned in supine with their legs bent at the knees and the feet flat on the floor. The arms are folded across the chest. Concentrating on curling the upper trunk as much as possible, the patient

is asked to perform a posterior pelvic tilt and then to raise the head and shoulders off the bed by about 30 to 45 degrees (Figure 13–31). After holding this position for 2 to 3 seconds, the patient returns to the initial position. The muscles strengthened with this exercise include the upper rectus abdominis and the internal and external obliques.

- *Partial sit-up:* the patient is asked to cross the arms on their chest and to lift the chin toward the chest. The patient is then asked to attempt to lift the shoulders straight up from the table until the lower back starts to move toward the table before slowly lowering the shoulder to the table.
- *Rotational partial sit-up:* the patient is asked to cross the arms on the chest and to lift the chin toward the chest. The patient is then asked to attempt to lift the right shoulder up from the table while twisting the trunk to the left before slowly lowering the shoulder to the table.
- *Reverse sit-up:* the patient is positioned in supine with the legs bent at the knees and the feet flat on the floor. The arms are by the sides. The patient is asked to raise the feet off the bed until the thighs are vertical. This is the start position. From this position, the patient is asked to raise the pelvis up and toward the shoulders, keeping the knees bent tightly, until the knees are as close to the chest as possible (Figure 13–32). The patient is allowed to push down on the bed with the hands. After holding

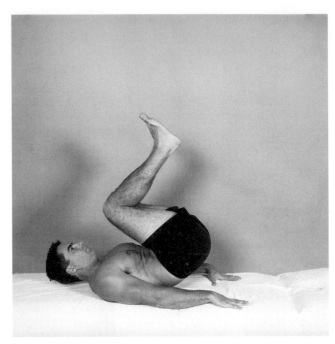

FIGURE 13–32 Reverse sit up.

this position for 2 to 3 seconds, the patient returns to the start position.

Hip and Spinal Extensors
A. Gluteus maximus
  1. *Isometric:* Patient positioned in prone with a pillow under their stomach. The patient is asked to tighten the buttock muscles and to hold the contraction for 6 seconds, then relax.
  2. *Alternating hip extension:* Patient positioned in prone with a pillow under the stomach. The patient is asked to tighten the buttock and abdominal muscles and to lift one leg 1 inch off the table. They then lower the leg and perform a lift with the other leg. The knees should be kept straight, or bent, depending on the degree of difficulty. From the prone position, the patient is asked to flex the knee to around 90 degrees, and then to raise the thigh off the bed as high as is comfortable and without introducing rotation at the lumbar spine (Figure 13–33). The end position is held for 2 to 3 seconds and then the thigh is returned to the bed. The exercise can be made more difficult by extending the knee and raising the straight leg from the bed.
B. Erector spinae. The patient is positioned in prone. From this position, the patient is asked to raise the arms alternately. The patient is then asked to raise the legs alternately. Finally, the patient is asked to raise an alternate arm and leg together (Figure 13–34).

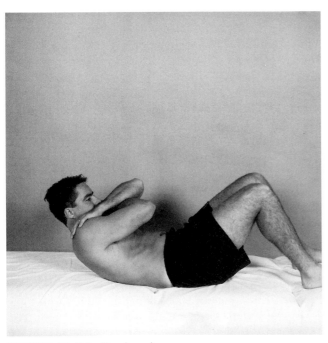

FIGURE 13–31 Trunk curl up.

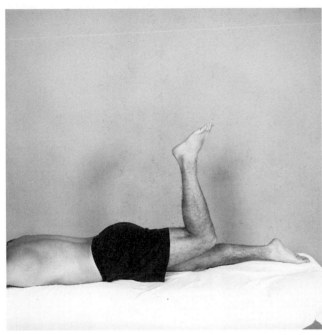

FIGURE 13–33 Exercise to strengthen the hip extensors, particularly the gluteus maximus.

General Stabilization—Patient Supine Unless Otherwise Indicated

A. *Cervical flexion:* The patient is asked to lift the head from the table attempting to touch the chin to the chest.

B. *Bilateral shoulder flexion:* The patient is asked to start with the arms toward the ceiling. Keeping the elbows

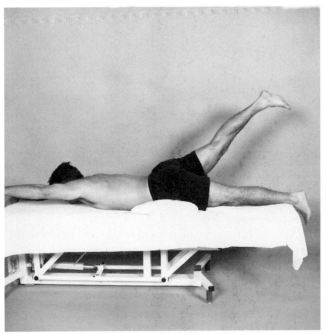

FIGURE 13–34 Alternate arm and leg raise.

straight, the patient is asked to slowly lower the arms overhead until they feel the lower back lifting away from the table. The patient is asked to slowly return the arms to the starting position.

C. *Alternating shoulder flexion:* The patient is asked to start with the arms toward the ceiling. Keeping the elbows straight, the patient is asked to slowly lower one arm overhead until they feel the lower back lifting away from the table. The patient is asked to slowly return the arm to the starting position.

D. *Bilateral knees to chest:* With their arms at the sides, the patient is asked to slide both of the feet along the table toward their buttocks. The patient is then asked to lift both of the knees toward the chest until the lower back starts to move toward the table. The patient is asked to return to the starting position.

E. *Alternate knees to chest:* With the arms at the sides, the patient is asked to slide one leg along the table toward the buttock. The patient is then asked to lift the knee toward the chest until the lower back starts to move toward the table.

F. *Alternating shoulder flexion:* The patient is positioned in prone with a pillow under the stomach. The patient is asked to position the arms overhead with the elbows straight and then to tighten the abdominal muscles and lift one arm toward the ceiling before lowering the arm to the table.

G. *Bridging:* The patient is positioned in supine with arms by the sides. The patient is asked to keep the knees bent and feet flat and to lift the buttocks from the floor. Maintaining this position, the patient is asked to perform:
   a. *Isometric gluteus maximus:* the patient is asked to tighten buttocks and hold for 5 seconds, and then to lower the hips to table.
   b. *Alternating one-legged stance:* the patient is asked to keep the pelvis level by placing a cane across the front of the hips.
   c. *Hip abduction/adduction:* the patient is asked to keep the pelvis level by placing a cane across the front of the hips while allowing the knees to spread apart, then bring them together.

H. *Quadriped:* The patient is positioned in the quadriped position (on their hands and knees) and is asked to maintain the neutral zone during the following activities:
   a. *Unilateral shoulder flexion:* the patient is asked to reach one arm out in front of, and to prevent the hips/pelvis from rotating.

b. *Unilateral hip extension:* the patient is asked to reach one leg out behind without allowing the hips and pelvis to rotate.

c. *Weight shifting:* the patient is asked to move the body forward and backward as far as possible while maintaining the neutral zone.

I. *High kneeling:* The patient is positioned in high kneeling with the hips and trunk straight. The patient is asked to maintain the neutral zone during the following activities:

a. *Bilateral shoulder flexion:* with the elbows straight, the patient is asked to raise the arms overhead as far as possible while tightening the abdominal muscles. The patient is then asked to slowly lower the arms while maintaining the neutral zone throughout the exercise.

b. *Alternating shoulder flexion:* with their elbows straight, the patient is asked to raise one arm overhead as far as possible while tightening the abdominals. The patient is then asked to slowly lower the arms while maintaining the neutral zone throughout the exercise.

c. *Forward bending:* the patient is asked to lower the buttocks to touch the heels of the feet and to place the palms of the hands on the floor in front of them. The patient is then asked to return to the starting position by reversing the motions while maintaining the neutral zone.

J. The patient is standing.

a. *Bilateral shoulder flexion:* with the elbows straight, the patient is then asked to raise the arms overhead as far as possible while tightening their abdominal muscles before slowly lowering their arms, while maintaining the neutral zone throughout the exercise.

b. *Alternating shoulder flexion:* with the elbows straight, the patient is asked to raise one arm overhead as far as possible while tightening their abdominal muscles. The patient is then asked to slowly lower the arm while maintaining the neutral zone throughout the exercise.

c. *Wall slides:* with the back against a wall, the patient is asked to perform a squat until the knees are bent to 60 degrees, (Figure 13–35) then return to standing while maintaining the neutral zone throughout the exercise.

d. *Lateral weight shifting:* while maintaining the neutral zone throughout the exercise, the patient is asked to shift the hips from side to side while bending at the knees.

e. *Forward lunge:* while maintaining the neutral zone throughout the exercise, the patient is asked to step forward with one leg and lower the opposite knee to the ground.

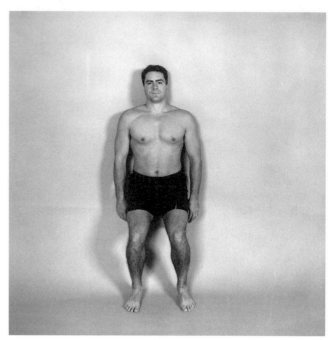

FIGURE 13–35   Wall slide.

f. *Backward lunge:* while maintaining the neutral zone throughout the exercise, the patient is asked to step backward with one leg and lower the same knee to the ground before returning to the starting position.

Level II

A. The patient is positioned in supine with the knees straight and legs flat on the table.

1. The patient is asked to start with arms and legs straight with arms overhead. Keeping the right elbow straight, the patient brings the arm to waist level while bringing the left knee toward their chest. The patient is then asked to touch the left knee with the right hand before returning to the starting position.

2. The patient is asked to start in the same starting position as the previous example. Keeping the elbows straight, the patient brings both knees and arms to the waist. The patient touches the knees with the hands before returning to the starting position.

B. The patient is positioned in prone.

1. *Bilateral arm swim:* the patient is asked to perform the arm motions for the swimmer's breast stroke.

2. *Bilateral arm swim with hip extension:* the patient is asked to perform same technique as in the previous exercise while raising one leg slightly up from the table and keeping the knee straight.

3. *Superman:* with the arms overhead and knees straight, the patient is asked to raise both arms and legs

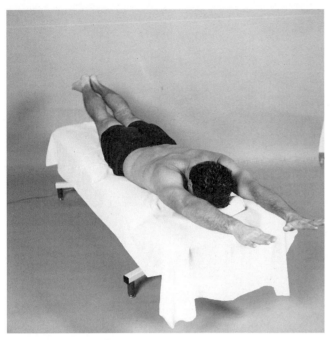

FIGURE 13–36 Superman position.

toward the ceiling while keeping their head resting on the table (Figure 13–36).

C. The patient performs a bridge—with the arms by the sides, knees bent, and feet flat, they lift the buttocks from the table. While maintaining this position he or she performs:

1. *Alternating unilateral stance:* the patient is asked to keep the pelvis level by placing a cane across the front of their hip, and to raise one foot off the table before returning to the starting position. The clinician can add weight onto the stomach to increase the resistance.

D. The patient is positioned in the 'quadriped' position. While maintaining this position they perform:

1. *Unilateral shoulder flexion and hip extension:* the patient is asked to attempt to reach one arm forward and the opposite leg backward at the same time. The patient is asked to return to the starting position before performing the same motion with the other arm and leg.

2. *Weight shifting and reaching:* the patient is asked to move the body forward and backward as far as possible while maintaining the neutral zone. The patient is asked to attempt to reach one arm out in different directions while the body is moving.

E. The patient is asked to sit with the knees bent and arms on the table behind the body. While maintaining this position he or she performs:

1. *Alternating hand and leg lift:* the patient is asked to raise one hand and the opposite leg off the ground before returning to the starting position.

2. *Bilateral hand and leg lift:* the patient is asked to raise both hands and legs off the ground and to hold the position for 6 to 8 seconds.

F. The patient is standing. While maintaining this position:

1. The patient is asked to hold a stick in both hands and to place the arms overhead before lowering them to the waist level. The patient is asked to kneel on one knee, then both knees. The patient is asked to lower the stick to the floor and reach it out in front. The movement is reversed until the patient is standing with the stick overhead.

2. Mimic sporting swing (i.e., golf, tennis).

Aerobic Exercise Programs

It has been shown that activity in large muscle groups yields an increased amount of endorphins in both the blood stream and the cerebrospinal fluid.[214] This in turn lessens the pain sensitivity.[215] Additional benefits of aerobic exercise include relieving depression,[216] increased mental alertness,[217] sleep,[218] and stamina.[219] The following aerobic exercises are recomended:

- Walking and jogging on soft, even ground
- Indoor cross-country skiing machines
- Water aerobics
- Swiss ball exercises

Dynamic Abdominal Bracing

Beryl Kennedy[220] proposed the technique of dynamic abdominal bracing (DAB), which makes use of intra-abdominal pressure to give stability and protection to the lumbar spine during both weight-bearing postures and movements. Pelvic tilting, using the abdominal muscles combined with breathing exercises, incorporate the principles of DAB. The progression of exercises include bridging, cross-arm knee pushing, knee raising, double knee raising, sit ups, oblique sit ups, and alternate straight leg raising and lowering with the opposite knee bent and the foot resting on the floor.

Back School

Several back schools and back rehabilitation programs have been developed to teach people proper lifting technique and body mechanics according to currently accepted ergonomic principles.[221] These programs are aimed at groups of patients and include the provision of general information on the spine, recommended postures and activities, preventative measures,[222,223] and exercises for the back. The efficacy of back schools, however, remains controversial.[224,225] Cohen[226] concluded that there is insufficient evidence to recommend group education for people with low back pain. Revel[227] claimed that back school interventions have no effect.

Flexibility Exercises

Occasionally, stretching both the anterior and posterior thigh muscles is beneficial. However, most of the time, only one should be stretched and the decision is based on the biomechanical diagnosis.

A. The patient with spinal stenosis, spondylolisthesis, or a painful extension hypomobility who responds well to lumbar flexion exercises should be taught how to stretch the hip flexors and rectus femoris while protecting the lumbar spine from lordosis.

B. The patient with a painful flexion hypomobility or disc herniation who responds well to lumbar extension exercises should be taught how to stretch the hamstrings while protecting the lumbar spine from flexing.

   1. *Stretch for the hip flexors and rectus femoris:* although a number of exercises have been advocated to stretch these muscle groups, because of their potential to either increase the anterior shear of the lumbar vertebrae directly or indirectly, the standing/kneeling position is preferred. A pillow is placed on the floor and the patient kneels down on the pillow with the other leg placed out in front in the typical lunge position. The patient is asked to perform a posterior pelvic tilt and to maintain an erect position with respect to the trunk. From this start position, the patient glides the trunk anteriorly, maintaining the trunk in the near vertical position (Figure 13–37). A stretch on the upper aspect of the anterior thigh of the kneeling leg

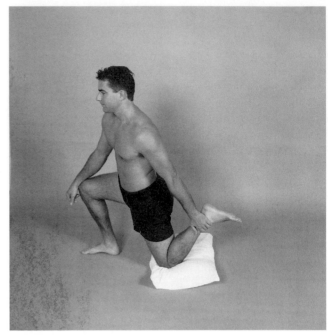

FIGURE 13–38   Standing rectus femoris and hip flexors stretch.

will be felt. The rectus femoris can be stretched further from this position by grasping the ankle of the kneeling leg and raising the foot toward the buttock (Figure 13–38).

   2. *Stretching of the hamstrings:* a number of techniques have evolved over the years to stretch the hamstrings. The problem with most of these techniques is that they do not afford the lumbar spine much protection while performing the stretch. The patient should be taught to perform the stretch in the supine position with a small towel roll placed under the lumbar spine to maintain a slight lordosis. The uninvolved leg is kept straight while the patient is asked to flex the hip of the side to be tested to about 90 degrees. From this position, the patient extends the knee on the tested leg until a stretch is felt on the posterior aspect of the thigh. This position is maintained for about 30 seconds before allowing the knee to flex slightly. As the patient progresses to doing the stretch in the standing position, he or she must be reminded to maintain an anterior pelvic tilt during the stretch.

Case Study: Central Low Back Pain with Occasional Right Radiation

Subjective

A 58-year-old female presented with a gradual onset of low back and sacroiliac joint pain and whose chief complaint was

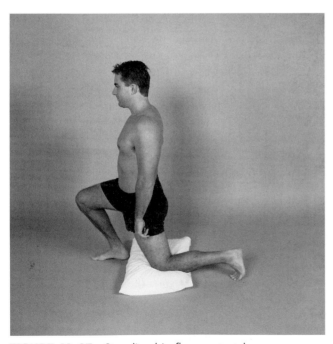

FIGURE 13–37   Standing hip flexors stretch.

a "stiff" back, especially in the morning. The patient had experienced mild discomfort over a number of years but had noticed a recent increase in its intensity over the last few months. The pain was reported as being worse with prolonged standing, lifting, bending, and walking, and was relieved by sitting and lying down. The pain was occasionally felt in the right buttock, hip, and thigh. A recent x-ray revealed the presence of "arthritic changes" in the lumbar spine.

Questions

1. What structure(s) could be at fault with complaints of low back and sacroiliac joint pain?
2. What does the history of morning stiffness tell the clinician?
3. Why do you think the patient's symptoms are worsened with prolonged standing, lifting, bending, and walking, and improved with sitting or lying?
4. What questions would you ask to help rule out a cauda equina impairment?
5. What questions would you ask to help rule out a spinal cord impairment?
6. What is your working hypothesis at this stage? List the various diagnoses that could present with low back and sacroiliac joint pain, and the tests you would use to rule out each one.
7. Does this presentation and history warrant a scan? Why or why not?

Examination

Because of the insidious nature of the low back pain, a lumbar scan was performed with the following positive finding.

- Upon observation, it was noted that the patient stood with her knees slightly flexed, had a pronounced lumbar lordosis, and slightly flattened buttocks.
- Active range-of-motion testing revealed a restriction of forward bending and pain reproduced with excessive lordosis positioning.
- There was limited extensibility of the hamstrings[228] with the straight leg raise but no neurologic findings.
- On palpation, the L5 spinous process was prominent and tender and pressure against the lateral aspect of the spinous process of L5 toward the right side produced radiating pain in the L5 nerve root distribution. The pain subsided when the spinous process was pressed in the opposite direction.[229]

Questions

1. Given the findings from the scanning examination, can you determine the diagnosis, or is further testing warranted in the form of special tests? What information would be gained with further testing?

2. What is the significance of the findings from the spinous process motion tests?
3. Why is there a decrease in the extensibility of the hamstrings?

Evaluation

A provisional diagnosis could be made on the strength of the subjective history—an older patient with low back pain, or radicular paresthesia, or pain, that is reproduced by increasing the lordosis and disappears on reducing the lordosis. The findings from the scanning examination confirmed the diagnosis and indicate the presence of a degenerative spondylolisthesis of L5.

Questions

1. Having confirmed the diagnosis, what will be your intervention?
2. How would you describe this condition to the patient?
3. How will you determine the intensity of the exercises for the intervention?
4. What would you tell the patient about your intervention?
5. Which manual techniques are appropriate for this condition? Why?
6. Estimate this patient's prognosis.
7. What modalities could you use in the intervention of this patient? Why?
8. What exercises would you prescribe? Why?

Intervention

A call was placed to the above patient's physician to ask if a series of flexion-extension x-rays could be taken based on the examination findings, and the patient was advised to stand in the x-ray waiting room before the x-ray to ensure that the slippage would not reduce during sitting. The x-rays revealed a grade II slippage. The patient returned to physical therapy for a trial period of conservative intervention.

- Electrotherapeutic modalities and thermal agents. With the exception of symptomatic pain relief, the thermal agents were not felt to be of benefit for this patient. A TENS unit was issued to help the patient perform activities of daily living.
- Manual therapy. Often, the only manual intervention with this patient type is the correction of any muscle imbalances. Stretching of the hip flexors and rectus femoris while protecting the lumbar spine were performed on this patient. The hamstrings were not stretched. Why?
- Therapeutic exercises. A lumbar stabilization progression was initiated with this patient. Aerobic exercises using a stationary bike and upper body ergometer (UBE) were also prescribed. Why?

- Patient-related instruction. Explanation was given as to the cause of the patient's symptoms. The patient was advised against the extremes of motion, especially lumbar hyperextension. Prolonged standing was to be accompanied with the patient raising one foot onto a stool. Instructions to sleep on the side with a pillow between the knees were given. The patient was educated on the positions and activities to avoid. The patient was advised to continue the exercises at home 3 to 5 times each day and to expect some post-exercise soreness. The patient also received instruction on the use of heat and ice at home.
- Goals and outcomes. Both the patient's goals from the treatment and the expected therapeutic goals from the clinician were discussed with the patient. It was concluded that the clinical sessions would occur 3 times per week for 1 month, at which time, a decision would be made as to the effectiveness of the lumbar stabilization exercise progression. With a strict adherence to the instructions and exercise program, it was felt that the patient would improve their functional status and the control of their pain.

Case Study: Low Back Pain

Subjective

A 40-year old male presented with a 3-month history of gradual onset of low back pain with no specific mechanism of injury. He reported no pain in the morning upon arising but the low back pain began soon after reporting to work as a cashier in a grocery store. The pain worsened with activities that involved prolonged standing, walking, or prone lying. The pain was felt across the low back, but was eased by sitting in a slumped position. The patient had radiographs taken recently, which showed nothing remarkable.

Examination

Upon observation, it was noted that the patient stood with a flattened lumbar lordosis. Because of the insidious nature of the low back pain, a lumbar scan was performed with the following positive findings.

- Full and pain-free range of all movements
- No dural or nerve root signs present but prone knee bending test reproduced the low back pain

The biomechanical examination revealed the following.

- Overpressure in to full extension was painful and, with the addition of side-flexion to either side, during the H and I tests, the pain worsened on each side

- The application of passive bilateral knee flexion with the patient in prone (Pheasant test) increased the symptoms. This test introduces an anterior pelvic tilt and increase in lordosis in a nonweight-bearing position through the pull of the rectus femoris. The clinician needs to ensure that sufficient knee flexion is used to produce the pelvic tilting. If full knee flexion is achieved before the tilting occurs, the patient is positioned in the prone on elbows position and the test is repeated. Patients who test positive for this maneuver tend to have the following subjective complaints: pain with supine lying with the legs straight, unless the rectus and hip flexors are especially flexible; pain with prone lying; pain with sitting erect; and pain with prolonged standing.
- PPIVM testing indicated good mobility at all levels.
- PPAIVM testing indicated good mobility, with the exception of the extension glides of L3 on L4 bilaterally, which were reduced.
- Weakness of the abdominals.
- Tightness of the hip flexors, hamstrings, and rectus femoris.

Evaluation

It would appear from the examination that an otherwise healthy mobile spine began to hurt when the tissues restraining extension were stressed producing a painful symmetrical impairment. The patient actually slumps into lumbar extension while standing by "hanging" on the anterior ligaments. The goal of the intervention should be the removable of the aggravating stresses and the resumption of the extension motion.

Intervention

- Electrotherapeutic modalities and thermal agents. A moist heat pack was applied to the lumbar spine when the patient arrived for each treatment session. Electrical stimulation with a medium frequency of 50 to 120 pulses per second was applied with the moist heat to aid in pain relief. Ultrasound at 1 MHz was administered following the moist heat. An ice pack was applied to the area at the end of the treatment session
- Manual therapy. Following the ultrasound, soft tissue techniques were applied to the area followed by a specific mobilization of the L3–L4 segment into symmetrical extension.
- Therapeutic exercises to strengthen the abdominals, the gluteals, the multifidus, and the erector spinae were prescribed. Aerobic exercises using a stationary bike and upper body ergometer (UBE) were also prescribed. The patient was instructed on how to stretch the hip flexors and rectus femoris. The hamstrings were not stretched. Why not?

- Patient-related instruction. Explanation was given as to the cause of the patient's symptoms. The patient was advised against sitting or standing upright. Prolonged standing was to be accompanied with the patient raising one foot onto a stool. Instructions to sleep on the side were given. The patient received instructions regarding the use of posterior pelvic tilting during activities of daily living and correct lifting techniques. The patient was advised to continue the exercises at home, 3 to 5 times each day and to expect some post-exercise soreness. The patient also received instruction on the use of heat and ice at home.

- Goals and outcomes. Both the patient's goals from the treatment and the expected therapeutic goals from the clinician were discussed with the patient. It was concluded that the clinical sessions would occur 3 times per week for 1 month, after which time, the patient would be discharged to a home exercise program. With adherence to the instructions and exercise program, it was felt that the patient would make a full return to function.

Case Study: Unilateral Low Back Pain[230]

Subjective

A 20-year-old male complained of a sudden onset of unilateral low back pain that prevented him from standing upright. He had bent forward quickly to catch a ball near his left foot and he was unable to straighten because of sharp back pain. He had no past history of back pain and no spinal radiographs had been taken.

Examination

There was no pain when his back was held in slight flexion but on standing upright, pain was experienced to the right of the L5 spinous process. He was prevented by pain from extending, side-flexing, or rotating his low lumbar spine to the right. The other movements were full and painless. PPIVM and PPAIVM testing revealed an inability to produce the painful movements at the L4–5 segment with marked spasm on attempting to do so. Unilateral posterior-anterior pressures over the right L4–5 zygapophysial joint produced marked pain and spasm.

Evaluation

With this patient, the quick movement into flexion and left side-flexion gapped the right lumbar zygapophysial joints, following which, there was a mechanical blocking of the movements that normally appose the articular surfaces (extension, side-flexion, and rotation of the trunk to the right).

Intervention

- Electrotherapeutic modalities and thermal agents. A moist heat pack was applied to the lumbar spine when the patient arrived for each treatment session. Electrical stimulation with a medium frequency of 50 to 120 pulses per second was applied with the moist heat to aid in pain relief. Ultrasound at 1 MHz was administered following the moist heat. An ice pack was applied to the area at the end of the treatment session.

- Manual therapy. Following the ultrasound, soft tissue techniques were applied to the area followed by an asymmetrical mobilization (grade III–IV) to gap the right L4–5 zygapophysial joint. Immediately after, the patient could fully extend, side-flex, and rotate to the right with some soreness experienced at the extreme of these motions. This soreness was lessened by gentle, large amplitude posterior-anterior pressures performed unilaterally over the right L4–5 zygapophysial joint.

- Therapeutic exercises to promote spinal extension were prescribed. These consisted of a progression from prone lying, to prone on elbow, to prone push-ups. Aerobic exercises using a stationary bike and upper body ergometer (UBE) were also prescribed.

- Patient-related instruction. Explanation was given as to the cause of the patient's symptoms. The patient was advised against sudden bending and twisting movements. Instructions to sleep on the side were given. The patient received instructions regarding correct lifting techniques. The patient was advised to continue the exercises at home, 3 to 5 times each day and to expect some post-exercise soreness. The patient also received instruction on the use of heat and ice at home.

- Goals and outcomes. Both the patient's goals from the treatment and the expected therapeutic goals from the clinician were discussed with the patient. It was concluded that the clinical sessions would occur 3 times per week for two weeks, after which time, the patient would be discharged to a home exercise program. With adherence to the instructions and exercise program, it was felt that the patient would make a full return to function.

Case Study: Central Low Back Pain

Subjective

A 45-year-old woman was referred for low back pain. She complained of pain across the center of her back at the waistline. The pain, which had started gradually many years ago, had not spread from this small area but it had increased in intensity. The increase in intensity resulted from a bending and lifting injury a few years previously and, since that incident, the patient reported having difficulty straightening up from the bent over position. Twisting maneuvers, whether in standing, sitting, or lying, also produced the pain, but otherwise she was able to sit, stand, or walk for long periods without pain.

Examination

Although this patient presented with an insidious onset of pain, the onset had been many years ago and the area of pain had not changed over those years. Although the intensity had increased, there was no evidence of radiation and the pain appeared to be related to movement, and thus only a modified scan was performed with the following result.

- Flexion was full range and pain free, although the return from flexion was painful, especially the initiation. All other motions were full and pain-free.
- Compression, distraction, and posterior-anterior pressures were all pain-free.
- Positive Pheasant test
- No evidence of neurologic compromise was found.

The biomechanical examination revealed the following.

- Characteristic H and I pattern for hypermobility and instability, with a positive finding in the anterior aspect of the I test, but no findings in the H test.
- Nonweight-bearing Hand I test was negative.
- PPIVM tests revealed good mobility at all levels of the lumbar spine.
- PPAIVM, testing into extension of the L5–S1 segment produced a spasm end feel.
- Segmental stability testing was positive for an extension hypermobility with an anterior instability.
- Decreased flexibility of the hip flexors, rectus femoris, and hamstrings.

Evaluation

The history of this patient suggested instability. The possibilities of a disc herniation, degenerative changes, and zygapophysial joint impairment needed to be eliminated. In this case, the absence of neurologic symptoms and the pattern of motion restriction helped. More serious impairments could also be ruled out by the number of years that the patient had the problem. The subjective history suggested instability and the objective tests confirmed it.

Intervention

- Electrotherapeutic modalities and thermal agents. With the exception of symptomatic pain relief, the thermal agents were not felt to be of benefit for this patient. A TENS unit was issued to help the patient perform activities of daily living.

- Manual therapy. Often, the only manual intervention with this patient type is the correction of any pelvic shift that is present and the correction of any muscle imbalances. Stretching of the hip flexors and rectus femoris while protecting the lumbar spine were performed on this patient. The hamstrings were not stretched. Why?
- Therapeutic exercises. A lumbar stabilization progression was initiated with this patient. Aerobic exercises using a stationary bike and upper body ergometer (UBE) were also prescribed.
- Patient-related instruction. Explanation was given as to the cause of the patient's symptoms. The patient was advised against the extremes of motion, especially lumbar hyperextension. Prolonged standing was to be accompanied with the patient raising one foot onto a stool. Instructions to sleep on the side with a pillow between the knees were given. The patient was educated on the positions and activities to avoid. The patient was advised to continue the exercises at home, 3 to 5 times each day and to expect some post-exercise soreness. The patient also received instruction on the use of heat and ice at home.
- Goals and outcomes. Both the patient's goals from the treatment and the expected therapeutic goals from the clinician were discussed with the patient. It was concluded that the clinical sessions would occur three times per week for a month, at which time a decision would be made as to the effectiveness of the lumbar stabilization exercise progression. With a strict adherence to the instructions and exercise program, it was felt that the patient would improve their functional status and the control of their pain.

Case Study: Leg Pain with Walking

Subjective

A 65-year-old male presented with an insidious onset of right leg symptoms that followed a period, or distance, of walking, or after a period of standing, and that disappeared when he sat down. The patient also complained of pain at night, especially when he slept on his stomach. Further questioning revealed that the patient had a history of back pain related to an occupation involving heavy lifting but was otherwise in good health and had no reports of bowel or bladder impairment.

Questions

1. Given the age of the patient and the subjective history, what is your working hypothesis?
2. Why do you think the patient has pain with prone lying?

3. Is the pain at night a cause for concern in this patient? Why?
4. Does this presentation and history warrant a scan? Why or why not?

Examination

The diagnosis for this patient is made on the strength of the subjective history—an elderly patient with root pain or paresthesia that is reproduced in the erect position and immediately disappears on sitting or bending forward. This is a classic syndrome of the elderly. The physical examination revealed the following.

The patient was of a medium build. His standing posture revealed a flattened lumbar spine and slight flexion at the hips and knees, but was otherwise unremarkable. Despite the fact that the patient appears to fit the pattern of a syndrome, it is well worth taking the time to perform a scan, particularly in view of the insidious onset of symptoms and the presence of leg symptoms. A lumbar scan revealed the following result.

● Active range-of-motion tests demonstrated a capsular pattern of restriction for the spine, that is, normal trunk flexion, a decrease in lumbar extension with rotation, and side-flexion equally limited bilaterally. During the spinal extension, no symptoms were reported but closer observation revealed very little motion occurring at the lumbar spine during this maneuver.
● When the patient was asked to perform an anterior pelvic tilt to increase the lumbar lordosis, the paresthesias into the leg were reproduced, and reversing the lordosis relieved the symptoms.
● The distribution of the paresthesia included the lateral and medial aspect of the leg and dorsum of the foot and great toe.
● The straight leg raise test was normal.
● Hip range of motion revealed a decrease in hip extension range of motion bilaterally.
● Abdominal muscle strength testing revealed weakness.
● The bicycle test of van Gelderen[231] was used to help confirm the diagnosis and to help rule out arterial claudication.

Evaluation

The findings for this patient indicate the presence of a lateral recess spinal stenosis at the L4–L5 level on the right side.

Questions

1. Having confirmed the diagnosis, what will be your intervention?
2. How would you describe this condition to the patient?
3. In order of priority, and based on the stages of healing, list the various goals of your intervention?

4. What would you tell the patient about your intervention?
5. Is an asymmetrical or symmetrical technique more appropriate for this condition? Why?
6. Estimate this patient's prognosis.
7. What modalities could you use in the intervention of this patient?
8. What exercises would you prescribe?

Intervention

● Electrotherapeutic modalities and thermal agents. A moist heat pack was applied to the lumbar spine when the patient arrived for each treatment session. Electrical stimulation with a medium frequency of 50 to 120 pulses per second was applied with the moist heat to aid in pain relief. Ultrasound at 1 MHz was administered following the moist heat. An ice pack was applied to the area at the end of the treatment session.
● Manual therapy. Asymmetrical manual traction (see below) was performed initially. As the patient appeared to obtain good results from this, mechanical traction was introduced (see below).
● Therapeutic exercises incorporating lumbar flexion were prescribed. These included posterior pelvic tilts, single and bilateral knees to chest, and seated flexion. Aerobic exercises using a stationary bike and upper body ergometer (UBE) were also prescribed.
● Patient-related instruction. Explanation was given as to the cause of the patient's symptoms. The patient was advised against sitting or standing upright. Prolonged standing was to be accompanied with the patient raising one foot onto a stool. Instructions to sleep on the right side were given. Why? The patient received instructions regarding the use of posterior pelvic tilting during activities of daily living and correct lifting techniques. The patient was advised to continue the exercises at home, 3 to 5 times each day and to expect some post-exercise soreness. The patient also received instruction on the use of heat and ice at home.
● Goals and outcomes. Both the patient's goals from the treatment and the expected therapeutic goals from the clinician were discussed with the patient. It was concluded that the clinical sessions would occur 3 times per week for 1 month, at which time, the patient would be discharged to a home exercise program. With adherence to the instructions and exercise program, it was felt that the patient would make a full return to function.

Manual Traction   The patient is placed in a left side-lying position with the spine in a neutral position in relation to flexion and extension. A small pillow is placed under the patient's waist to prevent any unwanted side-flexion from occurring. The clinician, while palpating the spinous process of L4 with the caudal hand, pulls the patient's lower arm out at a 45-degree angle to the bed with the other hand. The patient's trunk is thereby rotated from top to bottom down to the L4 level. The clinician now palpates the spinous process of L5 with the cranial hand and, using the patient's uppermost leg, flexes the lumbar spine up to the L5 level. The L4–5 segment is in neutral as the lock went down to L4 and up to L5, but not into the L4–5 space. The clinician places the cranial hand on the underside of the L4 spinous process and places the caudal hand on the underside of the L5 spinous process. The clinician applies an upward force away from the table on both spinous processes simultaneously while placing the armpit of the caudal arm over the patient's ASIS and applying an inferior force using their body to reinforce the side-flexion to the left and into the table.

Mechanical Traction   The patient is positioned in supine and 90/90. Sustained or intermittent traction is used. The goal is to decrease inflammation and edema, not change the size of the foramen.

Case Study: Right Buttock Pain

Subjective

A 21-year-old female presented with low back pain that had occurred while playing tennis, and she had felt a sharp pain in the right buttock area. She was able to carry on playing and the sharp pain subsided until the following morning when she awoke and attempted to weight bear through the right leg. The pain again subsided after a hot shower and her walk to work. That evening, she went jogging and was forced to stop after about a mile secondary to the return of the sharp pain in the buttock. A hot soak eased the pain but was replaced by a dull ache, which lasted several days, at which time, she sought medical advice and was referred to physical therapy. When asked to indicate where her pain was, she pointed to a small area, medial to the right trochanter, over the piriformis muscle. Further questioning revealed that the patient had no previous history of back pain and was otherwise in good health with no reports of bowel or bladder impairment.

Questions

1. What structure(s) could be at fault with complaints of buttock pain?
2. What does the history of the pain tell the clinician?
3. What is your working hypothesis at this stage? List the various diagnoses that could present with buttock pain, and the tests you would use to rule out each one.

4. Does this presentation and history warrant a scan? Why or why not?

Examination

The pain was of a traumatic origin and its intensity and behavior suggests a biomechanical cause, so a lumbar scan is not warranted. Observation revealed nothing remarkable. The biomechanical examination demonstrated the following.

- Straight plane active range of motion revealed a restriction of right side-flexion of 75% and a slight restriction of extension.
- The H and I test revealed a restriction of the right posterior quadrant—the combined motion of right side-flexion and extension at 50%, compared to extension and left side-flexion, with a reproduction of the patient's pain.
- A posterior-anterior pressure applied over L5 produced local tenderness.
- The PPIVM tests were positive for hypomobility at the L4–5 and L5–S1 levels.
- The PPAIVM test was positive for hypomobility for extension and right side-flexion at the L5–S1 level.

Questions

1. What information is gained from a positive H and I test?
2. Did the biomechanical examination confirm your working hypothesis? How?
3. If the biomechanical examination had not confirmed your working hypothesis, what would be your course of action?
4. Given the findings from the biomechanical examination, what is the diagnosis, or is further testing warranted in the form of special tests? What information would be gained with further testing?
5. How can you determine whether the loss of motion is due to an articular restriction or a myofascial restriction?

Evaluation

The patient was diagnosed as having an articular hypomobility of extension and right side-flexion at the L5–S1 level. The clinician determined the diagnosis from the H and I tests, which indicated a hypomobility into the posterior right quadrant. This was confirmed with the PPIVM. The question remained as to whether the hypomobility was the result of a myofascial or articular restriction. The answer to this was provided by the positive PPAIVM indicating that the joint glide was restricted, which would highlight that the loss of motion was articular in origin and not myofascial.

Questions

1. Having confirmed the diagnosis, what will be your intervention?
2. How would you describe this condition to the patient?
3. In order of priority, and based on the stages of healing, list the various goals of your intervention?
4. How will you determine the amplitude and joint position for the intervention?
5. What would you tell the patient about your intervention
6. Is an asymmetrical or symmetrical technique more appropriate for this condition? Why?
7. What modalities could you use in the intervention of this patient?
8. What exercises would you prescribe?

Intervention

- Electrotherapeutic modalities and thermal agents. A moist heat pack was applied to the lumbar spine when the patient arrived for each treatment session. Electrical stimulation with a medium frequency of 50 to 120 pulses per second was applied with the moist heat to aid in pain relief. Ultrasound at 1 MHz was administered following the moist heat. An ice pack was applied to the area at the end of the treatment session
- Manual therapy. Following the ultrasound, soft tissue techniques were applied to the area. Given the fact that the joint glide was restricted in an asymmetrical pattern, an asymmetrical mobilization technique was performed to increase extension and right side-flexion at the L5–S1 level. Initially, grades I–II were used. Later grades III–IV were introduced.
- Therapeutic exercises. The following exercises were prescribed: (1) prone hip extension on the right, (2) supine pelvic rotations in the hook-lying position, (3) standing side-flexion and rotation to the right, and (4) aerobic exercises using a stationary bike and upper body ergometer (UBE).
- Patient-related instruction. Explanation was given as to the cause of the patient's symptoms. Instructions to sleep on the side were given. The patient received instructions regarding correct lifting techniques. The patient was advised to continue the exercises at home, 3 to 5 times each day and to expect some post-exercise soreness. The patient also received instruction on the use of heat and ice at home.
- Goals and outcomes. Both the patient's goals from the treatment and the expected therapeutic goals from the clinician were discussed with the patient. It was concluded that the clinical sessions would occur 3 times per week for 1 month, at which time, the patient would be discharged to a home exercise program. With adherence to the instructions and exercise

program, it was felt that the patient would make a full return to function.

Case Study: Symmetric Low Back Pain

Subjective

A 30-year-old female presented with a 3-month history of gradual onset of pain with no specific mechanism of injury. She reported no pain in the morning upon arising, but by mid afternoon her low back began to ache. The pain worsened with activities that involved sustained flexion and when lifting. Sitting and lying eased the pain. The patient had radiographs taken recently that were normal.

Examination

Upon observation, it was noted that the patient stood with a normal lumbar lordosis. Because of the insidious nature of the low back pain, a lumbar scan was performed with the following findings.

- Full and pain-free range of all movements.
- No dural or nerve root signs present.

The biomechanical examination revealed the following.

- Overpressure in to full flexion was painful and with the addition of side-flexion to either side, the pain worsened on each side.
- PPIVM testing indicated good mobility at all levels.
- PPAIVM testing indicated good mobility, with the exception of the flexion glides of L3 on L4 bilaterally, which were reduced.
- Weakness and slackness of the gluteals, erector spinae, and abdominals.
- Moderate tightness of the hamstrings with a straight leg raise of 75 degrees bilaterally.

Evaluation

It would appear from the examination that an otherwise healthy and mobile spine began to hurt when the tissues restraining flexion were stressed producing a painful symmetrical impairment. These structures include the posterior ligamentous and zygapophysial joint structures that were receiving poor dynamic support from the abdominals and gluteals.

Intervention

This patient's condition was non-acute and the intervention was relatively straight-forward.

- Explanation as to the cause of the patient's symptoms was given as well as exercises to strengthen the lower abdominals, the gluteals, and the erector spinae and exercises to stretch the hamstrings. This was complemented with instructions on anterior pelvic tilting and correct lifting techniques.

- The L3–4 segment was mobilized into symmetrical flexion.
- As the patient experienced difficulties performing the exercises correctly, a biofeedback unit was used to help teach the patient when the correct muscle is being activated, and neuromuscular (functional) electrical stimulation (NMS) was used to activate the appropriate muscles.
- The patient received patient education on the maintenance of ideal body mechanics (line of gravity, use of hip, load close to body, etc.) during lifting considering pathology, signs, patient ability, lifting required, and potential for change.
- The patient was taught the "position of power" by using a dynamic pelvic tilt in the following sequence: (1) the patient is positioned in supine, in the hook-lying position and is asked to perform a pelvic tilt and to find the neutral zone—the point in the range of the pelvic tilt where the pain is minimized. This exercise teaches the patient about an awareness of neutral with respect to flexion or extension. While holding the tilt, the patient is asked to straighten one leg and abduct it. (2) The patient is positioned in sitting. The patient is asked to find the neutral zone using a pelvic tilt. Once the patient has achieved this, he or she is asked to stand against a wall and to find the neutral zone using a pelvic tilt. Once this is mastered, the patient is asked to maintain the neutral zone and to walk away from the wall.

REVIEW QUESTIONS

1. Which of the two longitudinal ligaments gives the best support to the anulus?
2. Which lumbar ligament, consisting of five bands, prevents anterior shearing of L5 on S1?
3. At what vertebral level does the spinal cord turn into the cauda equina?
4. Name the six common spinal ligaments, from superficial to deep.
5. The most limited motion in the *lumbar* spine is
   a. Flexion
   b. Side-flexion
   c. Rotation
   d. Extension
   e. The lumbar spine is not limited in any direction of movement.

6. Which muscles make up the erector spinae?
   a. Spinalis thoracis
   b. Longissimus thoracis
   c. Iliocostalis lumborum
   d. a and c
   e. All of the above are included.
7. Patient is a 58-year-old male whose chief complaint is back pain. Radiology examination reveals a gradual slipping of one vertebra on another in the lumbar spine. The term that generally applies to this disorder as seen on a radiologic examination is?
   a. Scoliosis
   b. Spondylolisthesis
   c. Lumbar spine stenosis
   d. Kyphosis
8. Which motions does the multifidus muscle produce?
9. Which lumbar level is the most susceptible to anterior shearing?
10. Describe the kinematics of the vertebra that occur during lumbar flexion.
11. How many degrees of rotation are available at the lumbar segment?
12. Which component of the vertebral complex is more susceptible to a compression overload?
13. Approximately what is the normal amount of lumbar range of motion with flexion and extension?
14. Describe the four boundaries of the intervertebral foramina.
15. What are the contents of the intervertebral foramina?

ANSWERS

1. Anterior.
2. Iliolumbar.
3. L1–2
4. Supraspinous; interspinous, ligamentum flavum; posterior longitudinal; annulus, anterior longitudinal.
5. c.
6. e.
7. b.
8. Lumbar extension; ipsilateral side-flexion and contralateral rotation of the lumbar spine.
9. L4–5.
10. An anterior sagittal rotation and anterior sagittal translation.
11. 3.
12. The end plate.
13. 60 degrees of flexion, 25 degrees of extension.
14. The vertebral notch represents both the inferior and superior boundary. The zygapophyseal joint capsule represents the posterior boundary. The vertebral body represents the anterior boundary.

15.
1. Mixed spinal nerve and sheath.
2. Two to four sinuvertebral nerves.
3. Variable spinal arteries.

REFERENCES

1. Deyo RA, Cherkin D, Conrad D, et al. Cost, controversy, crisis: low back pain and the health of the public. *Annu Rev Public* Health 1991;12:141–156.

2. Royal College of General Practitioners. Morbidity statistics from general practice; fourth national survey 1991/2. London: HMSO, 1994.

3. Steiner C, Staubs C, Ganon, M. et al. Piriformis syndrome: pathogenesis, diagnosis and treatment. *J Am Osteopath Assoc* 1987;87:318–323.

4. Dagi FT, Beary JF. Low back pain. In: Beary JF, ed. *Rheumatology and Outpatient Orthopedic Disorders: Diagnosis and Therapy.* 2nd ed. Boston: Little, Brown, & Co; 1987;97–103.

5. Frank JW, Kerr MS, Brooker A-S, et al. Disability resulting from occupational low back pain. Part I: what do we know about primary prevention? A review of the scientific evidence on prevention before disability begins. *Spine* 1996;21:2908–2917.

6. Accident Rehabilitation and Compensation Insurance Corporation. Injury statistics 1998. Wellington: New Zealand; 1998.

7. Frymoyer JW, Cats-Baril WL. An overview of the incidences and costs of low back pain. *Orthop Clin North Am* 1991;22:263–271.

8. Waddell G. Low back pain disability: a syndrome of western civilization. *Neurosurg Clin North Am* 1991; 2:719–738.

9. Michel A, Kohlmann T, Raspe H. The association between clinical findings on physical examination and self-reported severity in back pain. Results of a population-based study. *Spine* 1997;22:296–304.

10. Waddell G, Somerville D, Henderson I, Newton M. Objective clinical evaluation of physical impairment in chronic low back pain. *Spine* 1992;17:617–628.

11. Lageard P, Robinson M. Back pain: current concepts and recent advances. *Physiotherapy* 1986;72:105.

12. Frymoyer JW, Durett CL. The economics of spinal disorders. In: Frymoyer JW, Ducker TB, Hadler NM, Kostuik JP, Weinstein JN, Whitecloud TS III, eds. *The Adult Spine: Principles and Practice.* vol 1. 2nd ed. Philadelphia: Lippincott; 1997;143–150.

13. van der Hoogen HJ, Koes BW, van Eijk JT, Bouter LM, Deville W. On the course of low back pain in general practice: a one year follow up study. *Ann Rheum Dis* 1998;57:13–19.

14. Wahlgren DR, Atkinson JH, Epping-Jordan JE, et al. One-year follow-up of first onset low back pain. *Pain* 1997;73:213–221.

15. Wipf JE, Deyo RA. Low back pain. *Med Clin North Am* 1995;79:231–246.

16. Biering-Sorenson F. Low back trouble in a general population of 30-, 40-, 50- and 60 year old men and women: study design, representiveness and basic results. *Dan Med Bull* 1982;29:289–299.

17. Horal J.: The clinical appearance of low back pain disorders in the city of Goteborg, Sweden: comparison of incapacitated probands and matched controls. *Acta Orthop Scand* 1969;(suppl 118):1–109.

18. Magora A. Investigation of the relation between low back pain and occupation: 2. work history. *Ind Med Surg* 1970;39:504–510.

19. Valkenberg HA, Haanen HCM. The epidemiology of low back pain. In: White, A.A., Gordon, S.L. eds. *American Academy of Orthopedic Surgeons Symposium on Idiopathic Low Back Pain.* St Louis: C.V. Mosby; 1982:9–22.

20. Bigos SJ, Battié M, Spengler DM, et al. A prospective study of work perceptions and psychosocial factors affecting the report of back injury. *Spine* 1991;16:1–6.

21. Dehlin O, Berg S. Back symptoms and psychological perception of work. *Scand J Rehab Med* 1977;9:61–65.

22. Leino PI, Hänninen V. Psychosocial factors in relation to back and limb disorders. *Scand J Work Environ Health* 1995;21:134–142.

23. Viikari-Juntura E, Jouri J, Silverstein BA, Kalimo R, Kuosma E, Videman T. A lifelong prospective study on the role of psychosocial factors in neck-shoulder and low back pain. *Spine* 1991;16:1056–1061.

24. Linton S. Risk factors for neck and back pain in a working population in Sweden. Work and stress. 1990;4:41–49.

25. Bildt Thorbjörnsson CO, Alfredsson L, Fredriksson K, et al. Psychosocial and physical risk factors associated with low back pain: a 24-year follow-up among women and men in a broad range of occupations. *Occup Environ Med* 1998;55:84–90.

26. Riihimaki H. Epidemiology and pathogenesis of nonspecific low back pain: what does the epidemiology tell us? *Bull Hosp Jt Dis* 1996;55:197–198.

27. Smedley J, Egger P, Cooper C, et al. Prospective cohort study of predictors of incident low back pain in nurses. *BMJ* 1997;314:1225–1228.

28. Kraus JF, Gardner L, Collins J, et al. Design factors in epidemiologic cohort studies of work-related low back injury or pain. *Am J Ind Med* 1997;32:153–163.

29. Macfarlane GJ, Thomas E, Papageorgiou AC, et al. Employment and physical work activities as predictors of future low back pain. *Spine* 1997;22: 1143–1149.

30. Kelsey JL, An epidemiological study of the relationship between occupations and acute herniated lumbar intervertebral discs. *Int J Epidemiol* 1975;4: 197–205.

31. Tichauer ER. *The Biomedical Basis of Ergonomics: Anatomy Applied to the Design of the Work Situation.* New York, Wiley Inter-Sciences; 1978.

32. Magora A. Investigation of the relation between low back pain and occupation: 4. physical requirements: bending, rotation, reaching and sudden maximal effort. *Scand J Rehabil Med* 1973;5:186–190.

33. Magora A. Investigation of the relation between low back pain and occupation: 3. physical requirements: sitting, standing and weight lifting. *Ind Med Surg* 1972;41:5–9.

34. Aro S, Leino P. Overweight and musculoskeletal morbidity: a ten-year follow-up. *Int J Obesity* 1985;9: 267–275.

35. Böstman OM. Body mass index and height in patients requiring surgery for lumbar intervertebral disc herniation. *Spine* 1993;18:851–854.

36. Deyo RA, Bass JE. Lifestyle and low-back pain. The influence of smoking and obesity. *Spine* 1989;14: 501–506.

37. Heliövaara M. Body height, obesity, and risk of herniated lumbar intervertebral disc. *Spine* 1987;12: 469–472.

38. Kelsey JL. An epidemiological study of acute herniated lumbar intervertebral discs. *Rheumatol Rehabil* 1975;14:144–159.

39. Kahanovitz N, Nordin M, Verderame R, et al. Normal trunk muscle strength and endurance in women and the effect of exercises and electrical stimulation: Part 2. comparative analysis of electrical stimulation and exercise to increase trunk muscle strength and endurance. *Spine* 1987;12:112–118.

40. Nachemson AL. Work for all: for those with low back pain as well. *Clin Orthop* 1983;179:77–85.

41. White AA, Panjabi MM. *Clinical Biomechanics of the Spine,* 2nd ed. Philadelphia: Lippincott-Raven; 1990.

42. Bogduk N, Twomey LT. *Clinical Anatomy of the Lumbar Spine and Sacrum.* 3d ed. Edinburgh: Churchill Livingstone; 1997;2–53;81–152;171–176.

43. Mazess, RB. On aging bone loss. *Clin Orthop* 1983;165:237–252.

44. Rockoff SD, Sweet E, Bluestein, J. The relative contribution of trabecular and cortical bone to the strength of the human vertebrae. *Calcif Tissue Res* 1969;3:163–175.

45. Bell GR, Dunbar O, Beck SJ, et al. Variation in strength of vertebrae with age and their relation to osteoporosis. *Calcif Tissue Res* 1967;1:75–86.

46. Williams PL, Warwick R. eds. *Gray's Anatomy.* 38th ed. Edinburgh: Churchill Livingstone; 1995.

47. Francois RJ. Ligament insertions into the human lumbar vertebral body. *Acta Anat* 1975;91:467–480.

48. Vallois HV. Arthrologie. In: Nicolas A, ed. *Pourier and Charpy's Traite d'Anatomie Humaine,* vol 1. Paris: Masson; 1926.

49. Tkaczuk H. Tensile properties of human lumbar longitudinal ligament. *Acta Orthop Scand* 1968; (suppl) 115:9–69.

50. Yong-Hing K, Reilly J, Kirkaldy-Willis WH. The ligamentum flavum. *Spine* 1976;1:226–234.

51. Yahia LH, Garzon, S, Strykowski, H, Rivard, C-H. Ultrastructure of the human interspinous ligament and ligamentum flavum: a preliminary study. *Spine* 1990;15:262–268.

52. Panjabi MM, Goel, VK, Takata, K. Physiologic strains in the lumbar ligaments: an in vitro biomechanical study. *Spine* 1983;7:192–203.

53. Köhler R. Contrast examination of the lumbar interspinous ligaments. *Acta Radiol* 1959;52:21–27.

54. Newman PH. Sprung back. *J Bone Joint Surg* [Br] 1952;34:30–37.

55. Rissanen PM. The surgical anatomy and pathology of the supraspinous and interspinous ligaments of the lumbar spine with special reference to ligament ruptures. *Acta Orthop Scand* 1960;46(Suppl):1–100.

56. Heylings DJA. Supraspinous and interspinous ligaments of the human spine. *J Anat* 1978;125:127–131.

57. Hukins DWL, Kirby MC, Sikoryn TA, Aspden RM, Cox AJ. Comparison of structure, mechanical properties, and function of lumbar spinal ligaments. *Spine* 1990;15:787–795.

58. Lamb DW. Personal communication, 1992.

59. Kapandji IA. *The Physiology of the Joints, Vol 3: The Trunk and Vertebral Column.* New York: Churchill Livingstone; 1974.

60. Chow DHK, Luk KDK, Leong JCY, Woo CW. Torsional stability of the lumbosacral junction: significance of the iliolumbar ligament. *Spine* 1989;14: 611–615.

61. Luk KDK., Ho HC, Leong, JCY. The iliolumbar ligament. A study of its anatomy, development and clinical significance. *J Bone Joint Surg* 1986;68B: 197–200.

62. Testut L, Latarjet A. *Trattato di Anatomia Umana.* ed 5. Torino: UTET; 1972.

63. Broudeur P, Larroque CH, Passeron R, Pellegrino I. Le syndrome ilio-lombaire. Une syndesmo-périostite de la créte iliaque. Arguments cliniques, radiologiques, thérapeutiques. Diagnostic avec la lombo-sciatique. 440 observation. *Rev Rhum* 1982;49: 693–698.

64. Uhthoff H. Prenatal development of the iliolumbar ligament. *J Bone Joint Surg Br* 1993;75:93–95.

65. Hanson P, Sonesson B. The anatomy of the iliolumbar ligament. *Arch Phys Med Rehabil* 1994;75: 1245–1246.

66. Maigne JY, Maigne R. Trigger point of the posterior iliac crest: painful iliolumbar ligament insertion or cutaneous dorsal ramus pain? An anatomic study. *Arch Phys Med Rehabil* 1991;72:734–737.

67. Shellshear JL, Macintosh, NWG. The transverse process of the fifth lumbar vertebra. In: Shellshear JL, Macintosh NWG, eds. Surveys of Anatomical Fields. Sydney: Grahame; 1949:21–32.

68. Leong JCY, Luk KDK, Chow DHK, Woo CW. The biomechanical functions of the iliolumbar ligament in maintaining stability of the lumbosacral junction. *Spine* 1987;12:669–674.

69. Kirkaldy-Willis WH, Farfan HF. Instability of the lumbar spine. *Clin Orthop* 1982;165:110–123.

70. Seitsalo S, Osterman K, Hyvarinen H, Tallroth K, Schlenzka D, Poussa M. Progression of the spondylolisthesis in children and adolescents. *Spine* 1991;16:417–421.

71. Golub BS, Silverman, B. Transforaminal ligaments of the lumbar spine. *J Bone Joint Surg* 1969;51A: 947–956.

72. McNab I. *Backache.* Baltimore: Williams and Wilkins; 1978;98–100.

73. Bogduk N. The lumbar mamillo-accessory ligament. Its anatomical and neurosurgical significance. *Spine* 1981;6:162–167.

74. Bogduk N, Pearcy M, Hadfield G. Anatomy and biomechanics of psoas major. *Clin Biomech* 1992;7:109–119.

75. Nachemson A. Electromyographic studies of the vertebral portion of the psoas muscle. *Acta Orthop Scand* 1966;37:177.

76. Kendall FP, Kendall KM, Provance PG. *Muscles. Testing and Function.* 4th ed. Baltimore: Williams & Wilkins; 1993.

77. Porterfield JA, DeRosa C. *Mechanical Low Back Pain,* 2nd ed. Philadelphia: Saunders; 1998

78. Cailliet R. *Soft Tissue Pain and Disability.* Philadelphia: Davis; 1977.

79. White AA, Panjabi MM. *Clinical Biomechanics of the Spine.* 2nd ed. Philadelphia: Lippincott-Raven; 1990;106–108.

80. Poirier P. Myologie. In: Nicolas A, ed. *Pourier and Charpy's Traite d'Anatomie Humaine,* 3rd ed, vol 2, fasc 1. Paris: Masson; 1912;139–140.

81. Bogduk N, Wilson A.S, Tynan W. The human lumbar dorsal rami. *J Anat* 1982;134:383–397.

82. Bastide G, Zadeh J, Lefebvre D. Are the "little muscles" what we think they are? *Surg Radiol Anat* 1989;11:255–256.

83. Meadows J, Pettman, E. *Manual Therapy: NAIOMT Level II & III Course Notes* Denver, 1995.

84. Bogduk N. In: Twomey LT, Taylor J, eds. Innervation, pain patterns, and mechanisms of pain production. *Physical Therapy of the Low Back.* 2d ed. Melbourne: Churchill Livingstone; 1994:116–120.

85. McIntosh JE, Valencia F, Bogduk N, Munro, R.R. The morphology of the lumbar multifidus muscles. *Clin Biomech* 1986;1:196–204.

86. Shindo H. Anatomical study of the lumbar multifidus muscle and its innervation in human adults and fetuses. *J Nippon Med School* 1995;62:439–446.

87. Kalimo H, Rantenan J, Vilgarnen T, Einola S. Lumbar muscles: structure and function. *Ann Med* 1989; 21: 353–359.

88. Lewin T, Moffet B, Viidik A. The morphology of the lumbar synovial intervertebral joints. *Acta Morph* 1962;4:299–319.

89. Kalimo H, Rantenan J, Vilgarnen T, Einola S. Lumbar muscles: structure and function. *Ann Med* 1989; 21:353–359.

90. Farfan HF.: *Mechanical Disorders of the Low Back.* Philadelphia: Lea & Febiger; 1973.

91. Flicker PL, Fleckenstein J, Ferry K, et al. Lumbar muscle usage in chronic low back pain. *Spine* 1993; 18:582.

92. Bogduk N. A reappraisal of the anatomy of the human lumbar erector spinae. *J Anat* 1980;131: 525–540.

93. McIntosh JE, Bogduk N. The morphology of the lumbar erector spinae. *Spine* 1986;12:658–668.

94. Bogduk N, Macintosh JE, Pearcy, MJ. A universal model of the lumbar back muscles in the upright position. *Spine* 1992;17:897–913.

95. Bogduk N, Macintosh J. The applied anatomy of the thoracolumbar fascia. *Spine* 1984;9:164–170.

96. Gracovetsky S, Farfan HF, Lamy C, The mechanism of the lumbar spine. *Spine* 1981;6:249–262.

97. Gracovetsky S, Farfan HF, Helleur C. The abdominal mechanism. *Spine* 1985;10:317–324.

98. Gracovetsky S, Farfan HF, Lamy C. A mathematical model of the lumbar spine using an optimal system to control muscles and ligaments. *Orthop Clin North Am* 1977;8:135–153.

99. Ross E, Parnianpour M, Martin D. The effects of resistance level on muscle coordination patterns and movement profile during trunk extension. *Spine* 1995;20:2645–2651.

100. Lewin T. Osteoarthritis in lumbar synovial joints. *Acta Orthop Scand Supp* 1964;73:1–112.

101. Lewin T, Moffet B, Viidik A. The morphology of the lumbar synovial intervertebral joints. *Acta Morphol Neerlando-Scand* 1962;4:299–319.

102. Taylor JR, Twomey LT. Age changes in the subchondral bone of human lumbar apophyseal joints. *J Anat* 1985;143:233.

103. Taylor JR, Twomey LT. Age changes in lumbar zygapophyseal joints. *Spine* 1986;11:739–745.

104. Bogduk N. The innervation of the lumbar spine. *Spine* 1983;8:286–293.

105. Hovelacque A. *Anatomie des Nerf Craniens et Rachdiens et du Systeme Grande Sympathetique* Paris: Doin; 1927.

106. Bogduk N, Tynan W, Wilson AS. The nerve supply to the human intervertebral discs. *J Anat* 1981;132: 39–56.

107. Malinsky J. The ontogenetic development of nerve terminations in the intervertebral discs of man. *Acta Anat* 1959;38:96–113.

108. Kumar S, Davis PR. Lumbar vertebral innervation and intra-abdominal pressure. *J Anat* 1973;114: 47–53.

109. Groen G, Baljet B, Drukker J. The innervation of the spinal dura mater: anatomy and clinical implications. *Acta Neurochir* 1988;92:39–46.

110. Edgar MA, Nundy S. Innervation of the spinal dura mater. *J Neurol Neurosurg Psychiatry* 1964;29:530–534.

111. Mooney V, Robertson J. The facet syndrome. *Clin Orthop* 1976;115:149–156.

112. Bradley KC. The anatomy of backache. *Aust N Z J Surg* 1974;44:227–232.

113. Lazorthes G, Zadeh J, Galey E, Roux P. [Cutaneous territory of the posterior branches of spinal nerves. A review of Dejerine's scheme] [French] Neuro-Chirurgie 1987; 33(S):386–390.

114. Twomey LT, Taylor J. Sagittal movements of the human vertebral column: a quantitative study of the role of the posterior vertebral elements. *Arch Phys Med Rehab* 1983;64:322–325.

115. Pearcy M, Portek I, Shepherd J. The effect of low back pain on lumbar spinal movements measured by three-dimensional x-ray analysis. *Spine* 1985;10:150–153.

116. Dunlop RB, Adams, MA, Hutton WC. Disc space narrowing and the lumbar facet joints. *J Bone Joint Surg* 1984;66B:706–710.

117. Adams MA, Hutton, W.C. The resistance to flexion of the lumbar intervertebral joint. *Spine* 1980;5:245–253.

118. McGill SM, Norman RW. Low back biomechanics in industry: the prevention of injury through safer lifting. In: Grabiner MD, ed. *Current Issues in Biomechanics.* Champaign II: Human Kinetics Publishers; 1993: 69–120.

119. Aspden RM. The spine as an arch: a new mathematical model. *Spine* 1989; 14:266–274.

120. Adams MA, Dolan P, Hutton WC. The lumbar spine in backward bending. *Spine* 1988;13:1019–1026.

121. El-Bohy AA, Yang KH, King AI. Experimental verification of load transmission by direct measurement of facet lamina contact pressure. *J Biomech* 1989;22: 931–941.

122. Grieve GP. Clinical features. In: Grieve GP, ed. *Common Vertebral Joint Problems.* 2nd ed. New York: Churchill Livingstone; 1988:159–209.

123. Jungham H. Spondylolisthesen ohne Spalt im Zwischengelenkstuck (pseudospondylolisthesen). *Arch Orthop Unfall Chir* 1930;29:118–123.

124. Cossette JW, Farfan HF, Robertson GH, Wells RV. The instantaneous center of rotation of the third intervertebral joint. *J Biomech* 1971;4:149–153.

125. Ham AW, Cormack DH. *Histology.* 8th ed. Philadelphia: Lippincott; 1987; 373.

126. Farfan HF, Cossette JW, Robertson GH, Wells RV, Kraus H. The effects of torsion on the lumbar intervertebral joints: the role of torsion in the production of disc degeneration. *J Bone Joint Surg* 1970;52A:468–497.

127. Pearcy MJ. Twisting mobility of the human back in flexed postures. *Spine* 1993;18:114–119.

128. Pearcy M, Portek I, Shepherd J. Three-dimensional analysis of normal movement in the lumbar spine. *Spine* 1984;9:294–297.

129. Friberg S. Studies on spondylolisthesis. *Acta Chir Orthop* 1939:60–65(suppl):1.

130. Dandy DJ, Shannon, MJ. Lumbosacral subluxation. *J Bone Joint Surg* 1971; 53B:578–582.

131. Farfan HF. The pathological anatomy of degenerative spondylolisthesis: a cadaver study. *Spine* 1980; 5:412–418.

132. Guntz E. Erkrankungen der Zwischenwirbelgelenke. *Arch Orthop Unfall-Chir* 1934;34:333–341.

133. Rosenberg NJ. Degenerative spondylolisthesis. *J Bone Joint Surg* [Am] 1975;57:467–474.

134. Vallois HV., Lozarthes G. Indices lombares et indice lombaire totale. *Bull Soc Anthropol* 1942;3:117–120.

135. Matsunaga S, Sakou T, Morizonon Y, Masuda, A, Demirtas AM. Natural history of degenerative spondylolisthesis: pathogenesis and natural course of slippage. *Spine* 1990;15:1204–1210.

136. Grobler LJ, Robertson PA, Novotny JE, Pope MH. Etiology of spondylolisthesis: assessment of the role played by lumbar facet joint morphology. *Spine* 1993; 18:80–91.

137. Nagaosa Y, Kikuchi S, Hasue M, Sato S. Pathoanatomic mechanisms of degenerative spondylolisthesis: a radiographic study. *Spine* 1998; 23:1447–1451.

138. Love TW, Fagan AB, Fraser RD Degenerative spondylolisthesis: developmental or acquired? *J Bone Joint Surg* 1999;8/B(4):670–674.

139. Meschan I. Spondylolisthesis: a commentary on etiology and on improved method of roentgenographic mensuration and detection of instability. *AJR* 1945;55:230.

140. Boxall D, et al. Management of severe spondylolisthesis in children and adolescents. *J Bone Joint Surg* 1979;61A:479.

141. Kent DL, Haynor DR, Larson EB, Deyo RA. Diagnosis of lumbar spinal stenosis in adults: a meta-analysis

of the accuracy of CT, MR, and myelography. *AJR Am J Roentgenol* 1992;158:1135–1144.

142. Verbiest H. A radicular syndrome from developmental narrowing of the lumbar vertebral canal. *J Bone Joint Surg* 1954;26B:230–235.

143. Lee CK, Rauschning W, Glenn W. Lateral lumbar spinal canal stenosis: classification, pathologic anatomy and surgical decompression. *Spine* 1988;13:313–320.

144. Cailliet R. *Low Back Pain Syndrome.* 4th ed. Philadelphia: Davis; 1991:263–268.

145. Dooley JF, McBroom RJ, Taguchi T, Macnab I. Nerve root infiltration in the diagnosis of radicular pain. *Spine* 1988;13:79–83.

146. Tajima T, Furakawa K, Kuramochi E. Selective lumbosacral radiculography and block. *Spine* 1980;5:68–77.

147. Atlas SJ, Deyo RA, Keller RB, et al. The Maine Lumbar Study, Part III: 1-year outcomes of surgical and nonsurgical management of lumbar spinal stenosis. *Spine* 1996;21(15):1787–1794.

148. Airaksinen O, Herno A, Turunen V, Saari T, Suomlainen O. Surgical outcome of 438 patients treated surgically for lumbar spinal stenosis. *Spine* 1997;22:2278–2282.

149. Kim SS, Michelson CB. Revision surgery for failed back surgery syndrome. *Spine* 1992;17:957–960.

150. Herno A, Partanen K, Talaslahti T, et al. Long-term clinical and magnetic resonance imaging follow-up assessment of patients with lumbar spinal stenosis after laminectomy. *Spine* 1999;24:1533.

151. Friberg O. Lumbar instability: a dynamic approach by traction-compression radiography. *Spine* 1987;12:119–129.

152. Panjabi MM. The stabilizing system of the spine. Part 1. function, dysfunction adaption and enhancement. *J Spinal Disord* 1992;5:383–389.

153. Kaigle A, Holm S, Hansson, T. Experimental instability in the lumbar spine. *Spine* 1995;20:421–430.

154. Mimura M, Panjabi M, Oxland T, Crisco J, Yamamoto I, Vasavada A. Disc degeneration affects the multidirectional flexibility of the lumbar spine. *Spine* 1994;19:1371–1380.

155. Panjabi M, Abumi K, Duranceau J, Oxland T. Spinal stability and intersegmental muscle forces. A biomechanical model. *Spine* 1989;14:194–199.

156. Wilke H, Wolf S, Claes L, Arand M, Wiesend A. Stability increase of the lumbar spine with different muscle groups. *Spine* 1995;20:192–198.

157. Tencer AF, Ahmed AM. The role of secondary variables in the measurement of the mechanical properties of the lumbar intervertebral joint. *J Biomech Eng* 1981;103:129–137.

158. Wilder DG, Pope MH, Seroussi RE, Dimnet J, Krag MH. The balance point of the intervertebral motion segment: an experimental study. *Bull Hosp Joint Dis* 1989;49:155–169.

159. Gardner-Morse M, Stokes I, Laible J. Role of muscles in lumbar spine stability in maximum extension efforts. *J Orthop Res* 1995;13:802–808.

160. O'Sullivan, P, Twomey L, Allison G. Evaluation of specific stabilizing exercise in the treatment of chronic low back pain with radiologic diagnosis of spondylolysis or spondylolisthesis. *Spine* 1997;22:2959–2967.

161. Cholewicke J, McGill S. Mechanical stability of the in vivo lumbar spine: implications for injury and chronic low back pain. *Clin Biomech* 1996;11:1–15.

162. Bergmark A. Stability of the lumbar spine. A study in mechanical engineering. *Acta Orthop Scand* 1989;230(suppl 60):20–24.

163. Oddsson L, Thorstensson A. Task specificity in the control of intrinsic trunk muscles in man. *Acta Physiol Scand* 1990;139:123–131.

164. Strohl K, Mead J, Banzett R, Loring S, Kosch P. Regional differences in abdominal muscle activity during various manoeuvres in humans. *J Appl Physiol* 1981;51:1471–1476.

165. Cresswell A, Grundstrom H, Thorstensson A. Observations on intra-abdominal pressure and patterns of abdominal intra-muscular activity in man. *Acta Physiol Scand* 1992;144:409–418.

166. Hodges P, Richardson C. Contraction of transversus abdominis invariably precedes upper limb movement. *Exp Brain Res* 1997;114:362–370.

167. Cresswell A, Oddsson L, Thorstensson A. The influence of sudden perturbations on trunk muscle activity and intra-abdominal pressure while standing. *Exp Brain Res* 1994;98:336–341.

168. Goel V, Kong W, Han J, Weinstein J, Gilbertson L. A combined finite element and optimization investigation of lumbar spine mechanics with and without muscles. *Spine* 1993;18:1531–1541.

169. McGill S. Kinetic potential of the trunk musculature about three orthogonal orthopaedic axes in extreme postures. *Spine* 1991;16:809–815.

170. Bierdermann HJ, Shanks GL, Forrest WJ, Inglis J. Power spectrum analysis of electromyographic activity. *Spine* 1991;16:1179–1184.

171. Lindgren K, Sihvonen T, Leino E, Pitkanen M. Exercise therapy effects on functional radiographic findings and segmental electromyographic activity in lumbar spine stability. *Arch Phys Med Rehabil* 1993;74:933–939.

172. Hodges P, Richardson C. Inefficient muscular stabilisation of the lumbar spine associated with low back pain: a motor control evaluation of transversus abdominis. *Spine* 1996;21:2540–2650.

173. Hodges P, Richardson C, Jull G. Evaluation of the relationship between laboratory and clinical tests of transversus abdominis function. *Physiother Res Int* 1996;1:30–40.

174. Edgerton V, Wolf S, Levendowski D, Roy R. Theoretical basis for patterning EMG amplitudes to assess muscle dysfunction. *Med Sci Sports Exerc* 1996; 28:744–751.

175. O'Sullivan P, Twomey L, Allison G. Altered patterns of abdominal muscle activation in chronic back pain patients. *Aust J Physiother* 1997;43:91–98.

176. Nachemson A. The load on lumbar discs in different positions of the body. *Clin Orthop* 1966;45:107–122.

177. Dvorak J, Panjabi M, Novotny J, Chang D, Grob D. Clinical validation of functional flexion-extension roentgenograms of the lumbar spine. *Spine* 1991; 16:943–950.

178. Pope M, Frymoyer J, Krag M. Diagnosing instability. *Clin Orthop* 1992;296:60–67.

179. Burnell A. Injection techniques in low back pain. In: Twomey LT, ed. *Symposium: Low Back Pain.* Perth: Western Australian Institute of Technology; 1974:111–116.

180. Strange FG. Debunking the disc. *Proc R Soc Med* 1966; 9:952–956.

181. Cyriax J. *Textbook of Orthopedic Medicine.* Vol 1, 8th ed. London: Balliere Tindall and Cassell; 1982.

182. Kraft GL, Levinthal DH. Facet synovial impingement. *Surg Gynecol Obstet* 1951;93:439–443.

183. Seimons LP. *Low Back Pain: Clinical Diagnosis and Management.* Norwalk, CT: Appleton-Century-Crofts; 1983.

184. Ciric I, Milhael MA, Tarkington JA, et al. The lateral recess syndrome: a variant of spinal stenosis. *J Neurosurg* 1980;53:433–443.

185. Mennell JM. *Back Pain.* Boston: Little Brown; 1960.

186. Bogduk N, Jull G. The theoretical pathology of acute locked back: a basis for manipulative therapy. *Man Med* 1985;1:78.

187. Twomey LT, Taylor JR. Age changes in the lumbar articular triad. *Aust J Physio* 1985;31:106–112.

188. Allbrook D. Movements of the lumbar spinal column. *J Bone Joint Surg Br* 1957;39:339–345.

189. Meadows JTS. The principles of the Canadian approach to the lumbar dysfunction patient. In: *Management of Lumbar Spine Dysfunction.* APTA Independent Home Study Course, 1999:1–26.

190. American Academy of Orthopaedic Surgeons. A *Glossary on Spinal Terminology.* Chicago: American Academy of Orthopaedic Surgeons; 1985:34.

191. Muhlemann D. Hypermobility as a common cause for chronic back pain. *Ann Swiss Chiro Assoc* (accepted).

192. Meadows JTS. *Manual Therapy: Biomechanical Assessment and Treatment Advanced Technique.* Lecture and video supplemental manual. Swodeam Consulting, Alberta, Canada; 1995.

193. Paris SV. Mobilization of the spine. *Phys Ther* 1979; 59:988–995.

194. Maitland GD. *Vertebral Manipulation.* 5th ed. London: Butterworths; 1986.

195. Nachemson A, Bigos SJ. The low back. In: Cruess RL, Rennie WRJ, eds. *Adult Orthopedics.* Vol 2. New York: Churchill Livingstone; 1984:843–938.

196. Grieve GP. *Mobilization of the Spine: Notes on Examination, Assessment and Clinical Methods.* 4th ed. New York: Churchill Livingstone; 1986.

197. Kirkaldy-Willis WH, ed. *Managing Low Back Pain.* 2nd ed. New York: Churchill Livingstone; 1988.

198. Maigne R. Manipulation of the spine. In: Rogoff JB, ed. *Manipulations, Traction and Massage.* 2nd ed. Baltimore: Williams & Wilkins; 1980: 59–120.

199. Maign R. *Orthopaedic Medicine.* Springfield IL: Charles C. Thomas; 1976.

200. Porterfield JA, DeRosa C. *Mechanical Low Back Pain.* 2nd ed. Philadelphia: WB Saunders; 1998.

201. Lehmann JF, Silverman DR, Baum BA, Kirk NL, Johnston VC. Temperature distributions in the human thigh produced by infrared, hot pack and microwave applications. *Arch Phys Med Rehabil* 1966; 47:291.

202. Abramson DI, Tuck S, Lee SW, et al. Comparison of wet and dry heat in raising temperature of tissues. *Arch Phys Med Rehabil* 1967;48:654.

203. Arnheim D. Therapeutic modalities. In: Arnheim D, ed. *Modern Principles of Athletic Training.* St. Louis: Times Mirror/Mosby College Publishing; 1989: 350–367.

204. Lehmann J, Warren CG, Scham S. Therapeutic heat and cold. *Clin Orthop* 1974;99:207–226.

205. Prentice W. Therapeutic ultrasound. In: Prentice W, ed. *Therapeutic Modalities in Sports Medicine.* St. Louis: Times Mirror/Mosby College Publishing; 1990: 129–140.

206. Bianco AJ. Low back pain and sciatica. Diagnosis and indications for treatment. *J Bone Joint Surg Am* 1968;50:170.

207. Maigne R. *Diagnosis and Treatment of pain of Vertebral Origin.* Baltimore: Williams & Wilkins; 1996.

208. McKenzie RA. *The Lumbar Spine: Mechanical Diagnosis and Therapy.* Waikanae, New Zealand: Spinal Publications Limited; 1989.

209. Richardson C, Jull G. Muscle control-pain control. What exercises would you prescribe? *Manual Ther* 1995;1:2–10.

210. Aspden R. Review of the functional anatomy of the spinal ligaments and the lumbar erector spinae muscles. *Clin Anat* 1992;5:372–387.

211. Robison R. The new back school prescription: stabilization training. Part 1. *Occup Med* 1982;7:17–31.

212. Richardson C, Jull G, Richardson B. A dysfunction of the deep abdominal muscles exists in low back pain patients. In: *Proceedings of the 12th International Congress of the World Confederation for Physical Therapy.* Washington, June 25–30, 1995. Washington, DC: American Physical Therapy Association; 1995:932.

213. Kendall PH, Jenkins JM. Exercises for back ache: a double blind controlled study. *Physiotherapy* 1968; 54:154–157.

214. Almay BG, Johansson F, Von Knorring L, et al Endorphins in chronic pain: I. differences in CSF endorphin levels between organic and psychogenic pain syndromes. *Pain* 1978;5:153–162.

215. Mayer DJ, Price DD. Central nervous system mechanisms of analgesia. *Pain* 1976;2:379–404.

216. Folkins CH, Sime WE. Physical fitness training and mental health. *Am Psychol* 1981;36:373–389.

217. Young RJ. The effect of regular exercise on cognitive functioning and personality. *Br J Sports Med* 1979; 3:110–117.

218. Smith AE. Physical activity: a tool in promoting mental health. *J Psychiatr Nurs* 1979;11:24–25.

219. Kavanagh T. Exercise: the modern panacea. *Ir Med J* 1979;72:24–27.

220. Kennedy B. An Australian programme for management of back problems. *Physiother* 1980;66:108.

221. Schenk RJ, Doran RL, Stachura JJ. Learning effects of a back education program. *Spine* 1996;21:2183–2189.

222. Aberg J. Evaluation of an advanced back pain rehabilitation program. *Spine* 1982;7:317–318.

223. Fisk, J, Dimonte, P., Courington, S.: Back schools. *Clin Orthop* 1983;179:18–23.

224. Daltroy LH, Iversen MD, Larson MG, et al. A controlled trial of an educational program to prevent low back injuries. *N Engl J Med* 1997;337:322–328.

225. Hall H. Point of view. *Spine* 1994;21:2189.

226. Cohen JE, Goel V, Frank JW, Bombardier C, Peloso P, Guillemin F. Group education interventions for people with low back pain: an overview of the literature. *Spine* 1994;19:1214–1222.

227. Revel M. Rehabilitation of low back pain patients: a review. *Revue Du Rhumatisme* (English Edition) 1995; 62(1):35–44.

228. Barash HL, Galante JO, Lambert CN, Ray RD. Spondylolisthesis and tight hamstrings. *J Bone Joint Surg* 1970;52:1319.

229. Spring WE. Spondylolisthesis—a new clinical test. Proceedings of the Australian Orthopedics Association. *J Bone Joint Surg* 1973;55B:229–233.

230. Trott PH, Grant R, Maitland GD. Manipulative therapy for the low lumbar spine: technique selection and application to some syndromes. In: Twomey LT, Taylor JR, eds. *Clinics in Physical Therapy; Vol 13: Physical Therapy of the Low Back.* Churchill Livingstone; 1987:216–217.

231. Dyck P, Doyle JB. "Bicycle test" of van Gelderen in diagnosis of intermittent cauda equina compression syndrome. *J Neurosurg* 1077;46:667–670.

CHAPTER FOURTEEN

THE CERVICAL SPINE

Chapter Objectives

At the completion of this chapter, the reader will be able to:

1. Describe the anatomy of the vertebra, ligaments, muscles, and blood and nerve supply that comprise the cervical intervertebral segment.
2. Describe the biomechanics of the cervical spine, including coupled movements, normal and abnormal joint barriers, kinesiology, and reactions to various stresses.
3. Perform a detailed objective examination of the cervical musculoskeletal system, including palpation of the articular and soft tissue structures, specific passive mobility and passive articular mobility tests for the intervertebral joints, and stability tests.
4. Perform and interpret the results from combined motion testing.
5. Analyze the total examination data to establish the definitive biomechanical diagnosis.
6. Apply active and passive mobilization techniques, and combined movements to the cervical spine in any position, using the correct grade, direction, and duration, and explain the mechanical and physiologic effects.
7. Assess the dynamic postures of the cervical spine, and implement the appropriate correction.
8. Evaluate intervention effectiveness to progress or modify the intervention.
9. Plan an effective home program including spinal care, and instruct the patient in same.
10. Describe the intervention strategies based on clinical findings and established goals.

OVERVIEW

Neck and upper extremity pain are common in the general population, with surveys finding the 1-year prevalence rate for neck and shoulder pain to be 16% to 18%.[1,2] Almost 85% of all neck pain results from acute or repetitive neck injuries or chronic stresses and strain.[3]

Cervical impairments have the same causes as any other areas of the spine, that is, microtraumatic and macratraumatic impairments of the structures that compose the joint complex. The cervical spine appears particularly vulnerable as its anatomy indicates that stability has been sacrificed for mobility. Progressive degenerative changes are expected to appear over time on radiographs as part of the natural history of the aging spine. Radiographic evidence of cervical degeneration is observed in some 30-year-olds and is present in more than 90% of people more than 60 years of age.[4,5] Although aging of the cervical spine is ubiquitous, controversy remains about whether the process of spondylosis may be accelerated in patients with a history of soft-tissue injuries to the neck and persistent pain. However, in the absence of pain, the finding of degenerative changes on radiographs should not be misconstrued as pathologic. Thus, the intervention of patients with musculoskeletal neck and upper extremity pain must include education regarding the natural history of neck pain and radiographic findings in the cervical spine as it ages.

Given that the cause of the various cervical disorders is not fully understood,[6] intervention for chronic neck disorders has varied from the traditional methods of pain management and manipulative therapy, to group gymnastics, neck-specific strengthening exercises, and ergonomic changes at work.

Although strengthening exercises have been advocated for the intervention of neck pain,[7,8] only a few controlled intervention studies have been conducted to examine their benefit for neck problems. In addition, the efficacy of group gymnastics, active exercises, and passive physical therapy has been partly disappointing.[9–11] However, in a recent randomized study, investigators found that a multi-modal intervention of postural, manual, psychological, relaxation, and visual training techniques was superior to traditional approaches of modalities.[12] The patients returned to work earlier, and they had better results in pain intensity, emotional response, and postural disturbances.[12]

One of the problems of extrapolating conclusions from studies is that very little description is devoted to explaining how the various diagnoses were arrived at. It goes without saying that correct intervention to an incorrect diagnosis bears little fruit, and that a more precise biomechanical examination of the cervical spine may provide additional insight into the nature of various injuries and degenerative disorders, as well as aid in determining the effects of different forms of intervention aimed at altering the mechanical function of the neck.

Anatomically and biomechanically, the cervical spine can be divided into two areas, the upper or craniovertebral region and the mid-lower cervical region. For the sake of ease, these two regions are described separately. The mid-lower cervical spine is described in this chapter, whereas the craniovertebral area is described in the chapter of the same name.

ANATOMY

The majority of the anatomy of this region can be explained in reference to the functions that the head and neck perform on a daily basis. To perform these various tasks, the head has to be provided with the ability to perform extensive, detailed and, at times, very quick motions. These motions allow for precise positioning of the eyes and the ability to respond to a host of postural changes that result from a stimulation of the vestibular system.[13] In addition to providing this amount of mobility, the cervical spine has to afford some protection to some very vital structures, including the spinal cord.

Vertebra

The vertebrae included in the cervical spine proper are the inferior aspect of C2 down to the inferior aspects of the C7 vertebra. Compared with the rest of the spine, the vertebral bodies of the cervical spine are small, and consist predominantly of trabecular (cancellous) bone.[13]

The third to sixth cervical vertebrae can be considered typical, whereas the seventh is atypical. The third, fourth, and fifth vertebrae are almost identical. The sixth has enough minor differences to distinguish it from the others.

The typical cervical vertebra has a larger transverse than anterior-posterior dimension (Figure 14–1). The superior aspect of the centrum is concave transversely and convex anterior-posteriorly, forming a sellar surface that reciprocates with the inferior surface of the centrum, superior to it. The superior surface of the vertebral body is characterized by superiorly projecting processes on the superior-lateral aspects. Each of these hook-shaped processes is called an uncinate process. The uncinate process, described later, is the raised lip of the superior-lateral aspect of the body that articulates with a reciprocally curved surface at the synovial uncovertebral joint that develops by the end of the first decade of life, and which is beveled so the bones are separated, at least in the neutral position.[13] The inferior surface of the disc is concave, and the inferior-anterior surface of the centrum projects downward to partly cover the anterior disc.[13]

The vertebral body has a convex anterior surface, the margin of its disc giving attachment to the anterior longitudinal ligament. This surface can be palpated by the clinician by gently coming around the neck, and is often

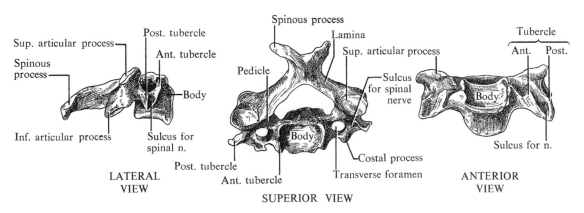

CERVICAL VERTEBRA

FIGURE 14–1 Typical cervical vertebra. *(Reproduced, with permission from Pansky B: Review of Gross Anatomy, 6/e. McGraw-Hill, 1996)*

tender in the presence of instability. The posterior surface is flat or slightly concave, and its discal margins are attached to the posterior longitudinal ligament.

Variations in the lower cervical vertebrae are most commonly found in the spinous and transverse processes. The transverse processes are short and project anterior-laterally and slightly inferiorly, and are typified by a foramen in each. The transverse process consists of two parts.

1. The anterior part, or costal process, ends laterally as the anterior tubercle. The longus capitis, scalenus anterior, and longus colli are attached to this tubercle, and the tubercle, particularly in the most inferior vertebra C7, may be enlarged, forming a cervical rib. The cervical rib may be formed from either bone or fibrous tissue and, thus, may or may not be visible radiologically. The carotid tubercle, the anterior tubercle of the C6 vertebra, is particularly large, and is so-called because the carotid pulse is taken at this point. The anterior border of the transverse process also serves as the attachment site for the scalenus minimus.

2. The posterior part, considered the true transverse process, ends laterally as the posterior tubercle and has the muscles of the splenius longissimus cervicis, iliocostalis cervicis, levator scapulae, and scalenus medius and posterior attached to it.

With the exception of vertebra C2, the superior aspect of the transverse process has a deep groove that mimics the orientation of the transverse process and transmits the spinal nerve, both of which are parallel with the intervertebral foramen. The inferior-lateral orientation of the transverse process, and the fact that the spinal nerves are firmly anchored in the gutters, makes the nerves vulnerable to a stretch injury around the distal end of the transverse process with distraction of the cervical vertebra.[13]

The transverse processes of vertebrae C2 through C6 are posterior and lateral to the transverse foramina through which the vertebral artery accessory vertebral vein, the vertebral venous plexus, and the vertebral nerve all pass.

The articular pillar is formed by the superior and inferior articular processes of the zygapophysial joint, which bulge laterally at the pedicle-lamina junction. The articular facets on the superior articular process are concave, and face superior-laterally to articulate with the reciprocally curved and orientated facet on the inferior articular process of the vertebra above. The articular pillars bear a significant proportion of axial loading.[14]

The pedicles project backwards and laterally, while the long narrow laminas run posteriorly and medial, to terminate in a short bifid spinous process.[14] Although the usual

spinous process is bifid and the two projections are of equal length, they often are unequal in size. As in the rest of the spine, the pedicles and laminae form the neural arch that encloses the vertebral foramen.

The spinous processes project slightly inferiorly. According to Hoppenfeld,[15] all of the spinous processes below C2 are usually palpable. The interval between the external occipital protuberance and the spine of C2 contains the posterior arch of vertebra C1, which is very deeply located and usually not palpable. The C2 spinous process can be palpated in the midline below the external occipital protuberance, the prominent midline elevation on the posterior-inferior aspect of the occipital bone. Occasionally, because of a bifid spine that is not symmetrical, the spine may appear to be lateral to the midline, or two bony prominences may be felt at a single level between C3 and C6. C7 is usually the longest spinous process, being referred to as the vertebra prominens, although, the spinous process of either C6 or T1 might be quite long as well. The spinous process of C7 is located by either counting down to the correct level or by using a motion test. The motion test involves the clinician feeling for the largest spinous process located at the base of the neck and then asking the patient to extend their neck. The C6 spinous process will be felt to move anteriorly with neck extension, whereas the spinous process of C7 will not. In addition to possessing a much longer and monoid spinous process, the seventh cervical vertebra varies from the typical cervical vertebra, and has wider transverse processes, no inferior uncinate facet, and no transverse foramen.[13] The spinous process ends in a prominent tubercle to which the ligamentum nuchae attaches (Figure 14–2).

As in the rest of the vertebral column, the cervical vertebrae form a portion of the vertebral canal that both

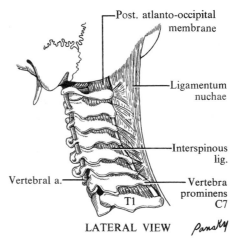

FIGURE 14–2 Lateral view of the cervical spine. *(Reproduced, with permission from Pansky B: Review of Gross Anatomy, 6/e. McGraw-Hill, 1996)*

houses and protect the spinal cord, and they provide dependable landmarks for the surface locations of a variety of soft tissue structures.[13,15]

The articular pillars and zygapophysial (facet) joints of vertebrae C2–7 are located approximately an inch lateral to the spinous processes. The mass of muscle on the posterior aspect of the neck is very thick and consists of the trapezius most superficially, and the underlying levator scapulae.

Articulations

The structure of the cervical vertebrae combined with the orientation of the zygapophysial facets provides very little bony stability, and the lax soft tissue restraints permit large excursions of motion.[13] Given the narrow space between the spinal cord and the vertebral canal walls in this region, in addition to the very small amount of extra space in the intervertebral foramina, a relatively small change to either the vertebral canal or the intervertebral foramen dimensions can result in significant compression of the spinal cord or spinal nerve.[38]

Each pair of vertebrae in this region of the cervical spine is connected by three articulations. Posteriorly, there is a pair of zygapophysial joints, and anteriorly there is the intervertebral disc. The orientation of the zygapophysial joints permit the motions of flexion and extension, and encourage the coupling motions of rotation and side-flexion to the same side (see later).

Forward flexion occurs with rotation below the C5–6 level. Extension occurs with rotation above the C4–5 level. The net result is that whenever cervical spine rotation occurs, the greatest degree of weight bearing is on the anterior edge of the vertebral bodies below the C5–6 segments and on the posterior edge above C4–5 (this factor has been implicated in the cause of spondylosis in these areas). The amount of available motion varies at each segment and is a consequence of the height of the intervertebral discs and tightness of the soft tissue constraints that interconnect the vertebrae.

Motion within the mid-lower cervical segments involves an average of about 15 degrees of sagittal range per segment, compared to an average of about 10 degrees per segment in the lumbar spine,[16] but this can vary significantly depending on the instructions given to subjects.[17] The greatest amount of motion occurs at the C5–6 segment, with the C4–5 and C6–7 segments a close second.[18] A coupled translation of between 2 and 3.5 mm occurs with flexion and extension. Side-flexion averages about 10 degrees to each side in the mid-cervical segments, decreasing in the caudal segments. There is significant flexion centering around C5–6, and extension around C6–7.

Zygapophysial Joints

There are 14 zygapophysial joints from the occiput to the first thoracic vertebra. These joints are typical synovial joints because the articular surfaces (the facets) are covered with hyaline cartilage and a closed joint space is formed by a joint capsule. The anterior capsule is strong but lax in neutral and extension,[19] allowing for translation between facets, whereas the posterior capsule is thin and weak. The major constraints and supports of these joints are the ligaments of the vertebral column and the intervertebral disc. Even though the most lateral part of the ligamentum flavum does blend with the joint capsule, it is not considered a ligament of the joint per se, and does not appear to have any nociceptive nerves.[13,20]

Vascular, fat-filled synovial intra-articular inclusions[21] have been observed in these joints, and have been described as fibro-adipose meniscoids, synovial folds, and capsular rims. These inclusions act as space fillers in the triangular spaces around the joint margins. They are theorized to play some role in protecting the articular surfaces as they are sucked in or expelled during movements and are also prone to entrapment, playing a potential role in intra-articular fibrosis and cervical spine pain.[22]

The orientations of the zygapophysial joint planes are oblique between the frontal and transverse planes.[23] The articular facets are teardrop-shaped with the superior facet facing up and posteriorly, whereas the inferior one faces down and anteriorly. The orientation changes depending on the level. It is 45 degrees at C2–3, reducing to 10 degrees at C7–T1. Clinically, the orientation can be thought of passing through the patient's nose. This orientation permits considerable flexibility, allowing a combined sagittal range of 30 to 60 degrees.[18] The articular facets are coronally positioned and should allow large quantities of rotation. This movement, however, is constrained and modified by the sagittal orientated uncinate processes. These butt against each other during rotation, limiting axial rotation and causing side-flexion to occur, producing an ipsilateral coupled motion (i.e., side-flexion and rotation occurring to the same side). In addition, the uncinate processes are responsible for a contralateral translation that occurs during side-flexion, which serves to prevent excessive amounts of spinal stretching and kinking, thereby relieving the stress on the disc, ligaments, joint capsule, and arteries.

At the zygapophysial joint level, the restriction of rotation by the uncinate processes means that the only significant arthrokinematic available to them is an inferior, medial glide of the inferior articular process of the superior facet during extension, and a superior, lateral glide during flexion. Segmental side-flexion is, therefore, extension of the ipsilateral joint and flexion of the contralateral joint. Rotation, coupled with ipsilateral side-flexion, involves extension of the ipsilateral joint and flexion of the contralateral.

The capsular pattern of the zygapophysial joint is a limitation of extension and equal loss of rotation and side-flexion, with flexion unaffected.

Joints of Luschka

From C3–T1 there is a total of ten saddle-shaped, di-arthrodial articulations between the uncinate process and the adjacent body known as uncovertebral joints, or joints of Luschka.[24] These joints are formed from the clefts between each uncinate process and the beveled inferior-lateral aspect of the vertebral body above.[25] The uncinate processes, together with the superior aspect of the body, form a sagitally oriented furrow in which the body of the vertebra above can translate anteriorly and posteriorly, as it does during flexion and extension. This furrow also tends to ensure that translation between bodies is limited to the sagittal plane.[26,29] There is some doubt as to whether their development occurs within true disc tissue or as a cleft in the looser connective tissue immediately lateral to the anulus.[25] Some authorities do not classify this joint as a synovial joint because although there is a joint capsule, there is no synovial sheath. However, although the joint is considered by most anatomists as a pseudo-joint, motion does occur between the two bony surfaces. Panjabi et al[27] reported that the mean area of the superior articulating surface of the uncovertebral joint is 44 mm,[28] approximately twice that of the inferior articulating surface.

The joint's medial aspect is bounded by the disc and laterally by the joint's capsule. Two of these joints of Luschka are found between each pair of adjacent vertebrae in the cervical spine proper, and their presence emphasizes the fact that the cervical intervertebral discs do not occupy the complete interval between vertebral bodies.

The lateral portion of the uncinate process is composed of the medial wall of the transverse foramina. The cervical nerve roots are closely related to the posterior aspect of the uncovertebral joints as they course through the intervertebral foramina to emerge anterior-laterally.

The uncovertebral joint is located in front of the axilla of the nerve root and lateral portion of the cord. The angle of inclination of the uncovertebral joint increases from C5 to C7 in the frontal plane.[27]

Cervical rotation, which is an impure motion at this joint, produces a posterior rotation at the ipsilateral joint and an anterior rotation at the contralateral joint. With the onset of degenerative changes, gliding motion at the uncovertebral joints is substituted by hinge motion, with the pivot point on the contralateral side.[13] Thus, the lever arm may lengthen and lead to a considerable increase in the reaction force.

The space between the uncinate process and the vertebral body above is less than the height of the intervertebral disc. With a loss of disc height, the potential for repeated contact between the bony surfaces of the Luschka's joint increases, producing the hypertrophic changes in the form of osteophytes.[13] A combination of the higher uncinate process, the smaller anterior-posterior diameter of the intervertebral foramina, the longer course of nerve roots in close proximity to the uncovertebral joints at C4 to C6 levels, and the greatest mobility occurring at C5 and C6, the nerve roots at these levels are more predisposed to compression by these osteophytes.

The vertebral artery also may be compromised in the degenerative cervical spondylotic process, which has been shown to occur more commonly at the mid-cervical spine level rather than at the lower cervical level,[30] but the reasons for involvement of the vertebral artery at a higher level than the nerve roots are not clear.

Cervical Curve

The cervical spine forms a lordotic curve that develops secondary to the response of an upright posture. The center of gravity for the skull lies anterior to the foramen magnum. The zygapophysial joint and disc planes largely determine the degree of lordosis. With a reduced curve, more weight has to be borne on the vertebral bodies and discs. An increased lordosis increases the compressive load on the zygapophysial joints and posterior elements. The C5 vertebra C4–5 interspace is considered to be the midpoint of the curve.

Intervertebral Foramina

The intervertebral foramina serve as the principal routes of entry and exit to and from the vertebral canal and to the rest of the body. Intervertebral foramina are found between all vertebrae of the spine, except in the upper cervical spine.

The anterior boundaries of the foramen are the intervertebral disc and portions of both bodies.

Posteriorly, the articular process and/or the zygapophysial joint serve as the boundaries. The medial to lateral depth of the posterior wall is formed by the lateral aspect of the ligamentum flavum.

The pedicles form the boundaries superiorly and inferiorly.

The cervical intervertebral foramina are 4 to 5 mm long and 8 to 9 mm high, and extend obliquely anteriorly and inferiorly from the spinal canal at an angle of

45 degrees in the coronal plane and 10 degrees caudally in the axial plane.[36] Within each foramen are a segmental mixed spinal nerve, from two to four recurrent meningeal nerves or sinuvertebral nerves, variable spinal arteries, and plexiform venous connections.

The lower cervical spinal nerves are quite large in diameter and nearly fill the foramina. As the dimensions of the intervertebral foramen decrease with full extension of the cervical spine, the nerve roots occupy a more cranial part of the foramen,[37,38] and uncovertebral osteophytes may compress the nerve root and cervical cord posteriorly.

Posteriorly, the spinal nerves are in close proximity to both the ligamentum flavum and zygapophysial joint. Inflammation secondary to arthritis or an hypertrophic ligamentum flavum can cause posterior impingement.

Vertebral Canal

In the cervical region, the vertebral canal contains the entire cervical part of the spinal cord as well as the upper part of the first thoracic spinal cord segment. There are eight cervical spinal cord segments and, thus, eight cervical spinal nerves on each side, but only seven cervical vertebrae.[13]

Ligaments

Both the function and location of the ligaments in this region are similar to that of the rest of the spine. For the purposes of these descriptions, the short ligaments that interconnect adjacent vertebrae are classified as segmental, whereas those that attach to the peripheral aspects of all of the vertebrae are classified as continuous.

Continuous Ligaments

Anterior Longitudinal The anterior longitudinal ligament is a strong band, extending along the anterior surfaces of the vertebral bodies and intervertebral discs from the front of the sacrum to the anterior aspect of C2. The ligament is narrower in the upper cervical spine and wider in the lower cervical spine. The ligament is firmly attached to the superior and inferior end plates of the cervical vertebrae, but not to the cervical discs. In the waist of the centrum, the ligament thickens to fill in the concavity of the body. The anterior longitudinal ligament functions to restrict spinal extension and is thus vulnerable to hyperextension traumas.

Posterior Longitudinal Lying on the anterior aspect of the vertebral canal, the posterior longitudinal ligament, (PLL) extends from the sacrum to the body of the axis

(C2) where it is continuous with the tectorial membrane. It travels over the posterior aspect of the centrum, attaching to the superior and inferior margins of the body, but is separated from the waist of the body by a fat pad and the basivertebral veins. In addition, this ligament attaches firmly to the posterior aspect of the intervertebral discs, laminae of hyaline cartilage, and adjacent margins of vertebral bodies. The ligament, which is broader and thicker in the cervical region than it is in the thoracic and lumbar regions, functions to prevent disc protrusions, as well as flexion of the vertebral column. The dura mater is strongly adhered to the PLL at C3 and above, but this attachment diminishes at lower levels.

Ligamentum Nuchae This bilaminar fibroelastic intermuscular septum spans the entire cervical spine, extending from the external occipital protuberance to the spinous process of the seventh cervical vertebra, but its connections between the occipital base and foramen magnum to the atlas and axis are considered to be the most significant (Figure 14–2).[32] From this layer, laminae are given off that attach to the posterior tubercle of the atlas and the spines of the remaining cervical vertebrae, and its importance as a posterior restraint is well accepted.[34] When the atlanto-occipital joint is flexed, the superficial fibers tighten and pull on the deep laminae, which in turn, pull the vertebrae posteriorly, limiting the anterior translation of flexion and, therefore, flexion itself.

Segmental Ligaments

The interspinous ligaments are thin and, almost membranous, interconnecting the spinous processes. The ligament is poorly developed in the upper cervical spine but well developed in the lower (see Figure 14–2).[31]

The ligamentum flavum runs perpendicularly to the spine, from C1–2 to L5–S1 connecting the laminae of successive vertebrae, from the zygapophysial joint, to the root of the spinous process. It is formed by collagen and yellow elastic tissue and, therefore, differs from all other ligaments of the cervical spine. The ligamenta flava of the cervical spine are fairly long, allowing an appreciable amount of flexion to occur, while being able to maintain tension when the head and neck are in neutral. Scarring, or fatty infiltration to the ligament in this region can compromise the degree of elasticity, making the ligament lax, particularly with cervical extension. This laxity increases the potential for the contents of the vertebral canal to be compressed by the ligament as it buckles.[35] Enlargement of the ligament increases the likelihood of a spinal nerve and/or its posterior root becoming impinged.[13] The ligament appears to function as a passive extensor force of the neck.

Muscles

The majority of the muscles in the neck function to support and move the head. A muscle's function is the role that it plays in a specific activity.

All muscles of the neck have the action of ipsilateral side-flexion. Intrinsic muscles of the neck act on the axial skeleton only, whereas other muscles act on the shoulder girdle. For the purposes of the following section, the muscles of the cervical spine are separated into the superficial muscles, the lateral muscles, and the deep muscles of the back.

Superficial Muscles

The trapezius muscle (Figure 14–3) is the most superficial back muscle. It is a flat triangular muscle that extends over the back of the neck and well beyond the cervical region, arising from most of the thoracic spinous processes. Its origin, which runs from the superior nuchal line and external occipital protuberance of the occipital bone, to the spinous process of T_{12} is the longest muscle attachment in the body. Its insertion can be traced from the entire superior aspect of the spine of the scapula, the medial aspect of the acromion, and the posterior aspect of the lateral third of the clavicle.

This muscle is traditionally divided into upper middle, and lower parts according to anatomy and function.

- The middle part originates from C7 and forms the cervicothoracic part of the muscle.
- The lower part, attaching to the apex of the scapular spine, is relatively thin.
- The upper part is very thin and yet it has the most mechanical and clinical importance to the cervical spine.[40] The trapezius is innervated both by the cranial (accessory) nerve XI and fibers from spinal cord segments C2 through C4, with the former speculated to provide the motor innervation, and the latter the sensory innervation.[41] The greater occipital nerve occasionally travels through the trapezius near its superior border to reach the scalp.[23]

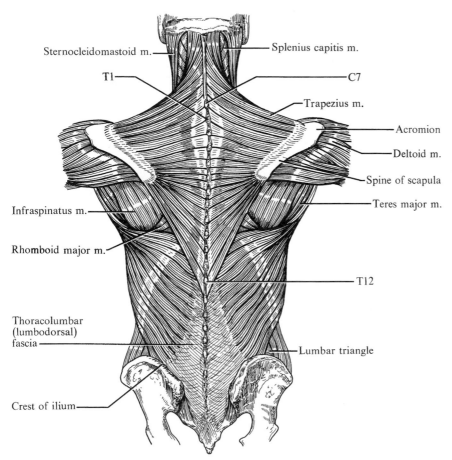

FIGURE 14–3 The superficial muscles of the back. *(Reproduced, with permission from Pansky B: Review of Gross Anatomy, 6/e. McGraw-Hill, 1996)*

The different parts of this muscle provide a variety of actions on the shoulder girdle including elevation, and retraction of the scapula. Also, when the shoulder girdle is fixed, it produces ipsilateral side-flexion and contralateral rotation of the head and neck, whereas bilateral activity causes symmetrical extension of the neck and head.[42] Its major actions are scapular adduction (all three parts) and upward rotation of the scapula (primarily the superior and inferior parts).

The sternocleidomastoid (SCM) (Figure 14–4), a fusiform muscle, descends obliquely across the side of the neck forming a distinct landmark for palpatory purposes. It is the largest muscle in the anterior neck, and it is the muscle involved in torticollis, a postural deformity of the neck. It is attached inferiorly by two heads, arising from the posterior aspect of the medial third of the clavicle and the manubrium of the sternum. From here, it passes superiorly and posteriorly to attach on the mastoid process of the temporal bone. The motor supply for the muscle is from the accessory nerve (CN XI), while the sensory innervation is supplied from ventral rami of C2 and C3.[11] This muscle can provide the clinician with information regarding the severity of symptoms and postural impairments because of its tendency to become prominent when hypertonic.

In broad terms, the actions of this muscle are flexion, side-flexion and contralateral rotation of the head and neck.[42] Acting together, the two muscles, draw the head forward, and can also raise the head when the body is supine. This action is a combination of upper cervical extension and lower cervical flexion. The muscle is active on resisted neck flexion. With the head fixed, it is also an accessory muscle of forced inspiration.

The levator scapulae (Figure 14–5) is a slender muscle attached by tendinous slips to the posterior tubercles of the transverse processes of the upper cervical vertebrae (C1–4). The levator, located deep to both the upper and middle parts of the trapezius, can be palpated just deep to the superior border of the trapezius. It descends posteriorly, inferiorly, and laterally to the superior angle and medial border of the scapula between the superior angle and the base of the spine. The levator is the major stabilizer and elevator of the superior angle of the scapula, and its contraction is readily palpable over its superior portion. With the scapula stabilized, the levator produces rotation and side-flexion of the neck to the same side; while acting bilaterally, weak cervical extension is produced.[42] With a forward head posture, the potential for this extension moment increases.[13] If the levator is shorter on one side, it can provoke contralateral suboccipital muscle spasms and subsequent headaches.[13] A quick test to determine the extensibility of the levator involves positioning the patient in erect sitting.[44] The patient is asked to place one hand on top of the head. For example if the length of the left levator is to be tested, the patient is asked to place the right hand on the head. The patient's neck and head is positioned in neutral and the patient is asked to abduct the left arm as far as possible. Normal extensibility of the

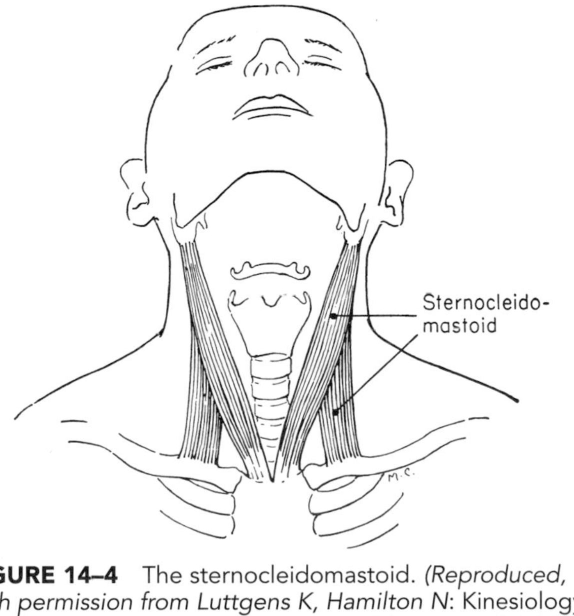

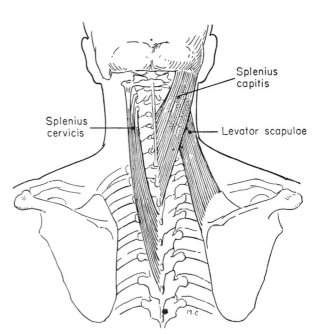

FIGURE 14–4 The sternocleidomastoid. *(Reproduced, with permission from Luttgens K, Hamilton N: Kinesiology: Scientific Basis on Human Motion, 9e McGraw-Hill, 1997)*

FIGURE 14–5 The levator scapulae and splenius cervicis. *(Reproduced, with permission from Luttgens K, Hamilton N: Kinesiology: Scientific Basis on Human Motion, 9e McGraw-Hill, 1997)*

levator and the absence of shoulder girdle pathology should allow the patient to abduct the arm so that it touches the ipsilateral ear. An inability to achieve full range would indicate an adaptive shortening or hypertonus of the levator.[44] The test is repeated on the other side for comparison. It might be argued that the rhomboids are also tested with this maneuver and from an anatomic viewpoint this is true, however, from a clinical viewpoint, it is unusual to find a decrease in flexibility of the rhomboids, especially given the propensity for the typically adopted round-shouldered posture. However, the clinician should be aware that the extensibility of the rhomboids might be a factor.

The levator is supplied by direct branches of C3 and C4 cervical spinal nerves, and from C5 through the dorsal scapular nerve. It is heavily innervated with muscle spindles.

The rhomboideus major is a quadrilateral sheet of muscle, and the rhomboideus minor muscle is small and cylindrical (Figure 14–6). Together, they form a thin sheet of muscle that fills much of the interval between the medial border of the scapula and the midline. Although the rhomboid minor, with its attachment to the spinous

processes of C7 and T1, has a slight association with the cervical spine, the rhomboid major, arising from the spinous processes of T1–5, is inactive during isolated head and neck movements. The two muscles descend from their points of origin, passing laterally to the posterior aspect of the vertebral border of the scapula, from the base of the spine to the inferior angle. Both of these muscles are covered by the trapezius. Innervation for these muscles is supplied by the dorsal scapular nerve. The major action of these muscles is to work with the levator scapulae to control the position and movement of the scapula, and they are involved with concentric contractions during rowing exercises, or other activities involving scapular retraction.

Lateral Muscles

Scalenes The scalenes extend obliquely like ladders (*scala* means ladder in Latin) and share a critical relationship with the subclavian artery (Figure 14–7). Tightness of these muscles will affect the mobility of the upper cervical spine and, due to their distal attachments to the first and

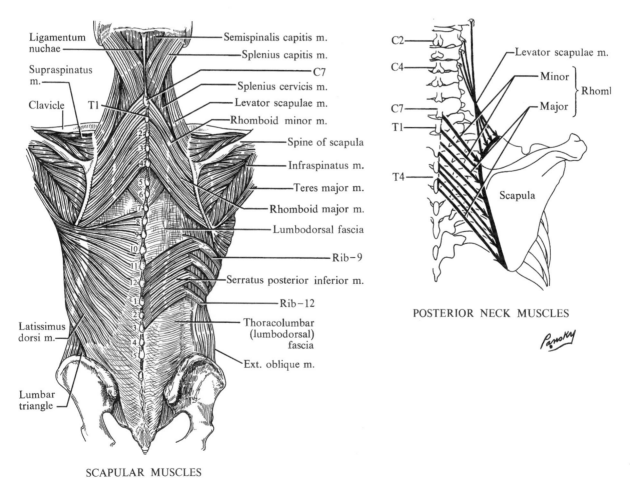

SCAPULAR MUSCLES

FIGURE 14–6 The scapular muscles and the rhomboid muscles. *(Reproduced, with permission from Pansky B: Review of Gross Anatomy, 6/e. McGraw-Hill, 1996)*

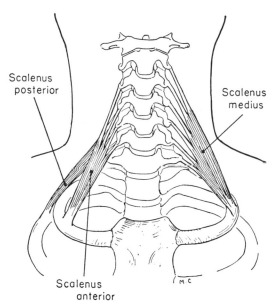

FIGURE 14–7 The scalenes. *(Reproduced, with permission from Luttgens K, Hamilton N: Kinesiology: Scientific Basis on Human Motion, 9e McGraw-Hill, 1997)*

second ribs, if in spasm, they can, elevate the ribs and be implicated in the thoracic outlet syndrome.

- *Scalenus anterior.* The scalenus anterior runs vertically, behind the sternocleidomastoid on the lateral aspect of the neck. Arising from the anterior tubercles of the C3, C4, C5, and C6 transverse processes, it travels to the scalene tubercle on the inner border of the first rib. The osteal portion of the vertebral artery and stellate ganglion run laterally to it. Acting from above, the scalenus anterior, like the rest of the scalenes, is an inspiratory muscle, even with quiet breathing, [45] when it fixes the first rib so that the diaphragm can exert its action on the lung. Working bilaterally from below, it flexes the spine. Unilaterally, it ipsilaterally side-flexes and contralaterally rotates the spine.[42] It is supplied by the ventral rami of C4, C5, and C6.
- *Scalenus medius.* The scalenus medius is the largest and longest of the group, attaching to the transverse processes of all of the cervical vertebra except the atlas (although it often attaches to this), and runs to attach to the upper border of the first rib. It is separated from the anterior scalene by the carotid artery and cervical nerve, and is pierced by the nerve to the rhomboids and the upper two roots of the nerve to the serratus anterior (long thoracic nerve). Working unilaterally on the cervical spine, it is an ipsilateral side flexor, whereas bilaterally, it is a flexor. Working from a fixed spine, it elevates or fixes the first rib during inspiration.

- *Scalenus posterior.* The scalenus posterior is the smallest and deepest of the group, running from the posterior tubercles of C4–6 transverse processes, to attach to the outer aspect of the second rib. It functions to elevate or fix the second rib and ipsilaterally side-flex the neck. It is supplied by the ventral rami of C5, C6, and C7.
- *Scalenus minimus (pleuralis).* The scalenus minimus is a small muscle slip running from the transverse process of C7 to the inner aspect of the first rib and the dome of the pleura. It is the supra pleural membrane that is often considered to be the expansion of the tendon of this muscle. It functions to elevate the dome of the pleura during inspiration and is innervated by the ventral ramus of C7.

The broad sheet of the platysma muscle is the most superficial muscle in the cervical region, where it covers most of the anterior-lateral aspect of the neck, the upper parts of the pectoralis major and deltoid. It extends superiorly to the inferior margin of the body of the mandible. As a muscle of facial expression, it does not affect bony motion, except perhaps as a passive restraint to head extension. It is supplied by the cervical branch of the cranial (facial) nerve VII.

Deep Muscles of the Back
The deep, or intrinsic, muscles of the back are the primary movers of the vertebral column and head, and are located deep to the thoracolumbar fascia. The muscles in all of these groups are segmentally innervated by the lateral branches of the dorsal rami of the spinal nerves.[23]

The splenius capitis (Figure 14–5) extends upward and laterally from the dorsal edge of the nuchal ligament and the spines and spinous processes of the lower cervical and upper thoracic vertebrae (T4–C7), to the mastoid process of the occipital bone just inferior to the superior nuchal line, and deep to the SCM muscle.

The splenius cervicis (Figure 14–5) is just inferior and appears continuous with the capitis, extending from the spines of the third to the sixth thoracic vertebrae, to the posterior tubercles of the transverse processes of the upper cervical vertebrae. The splenius capitis and splenius cervicis muscles are two important head and neck rotators. By their attachments, it is clear that both are capable of ipsilateral rotation, side-flexion, and extension at the spinal joints they cross.

Erector Spinae
The erector spinae complex spans multiple segments, forming a large musculotendinous mass consisting of the iliocostalis, longissimus, and spinalis muscles.

The iliocostalis cervicis appears to function as a stabilizer of the cervicothoracic junction and lower cervical spine. The semispinalis has thoracis, cervicis, and capitis divisions. The obliquus capitis superior and inferior and the

TABLE 14–1 PRIME MOVERS OF THE CERVICAL SPINE—ROTATORS AND SIDE-FLEXORS

ROTATOR AND SIDE-FLEXOR MUSCLES

Ipsilateral side flexion	*Ipsilateral rotation*
Longissimus capitis	Splenius capitis
Intertransversarii posteriores cervices	Splenius cervices
	Rotatores breves cervices
Multifidus	Rotatores longi cervices
Rectus capitis lateralis	Rectus capitis posterior major
Intertransversarii anteriores cervices	Obliquus capitis inferior
	Ipsilateral side flexion and
Scaleni	*contralateral rotation*
Contralateral rotation	Sternocleidomastoid
Obliquus capitis superior	
Ipsilateral side flexion and	
ipsilateral rotation	
Iliocostalis cervices	
Longus coli	

rectus capitis posterior major and minor lie underneath the semispinalis capitis and splenius capitis muscles.[46] The semispinalis cervicis is a stout muscle that extends superiorly to the spinous process of vertebra C2, functioning as a strong extensor of the lower cervical spine.[13]

The interspinales and intertransversarii, which interconnect the processes for which they are named, produce only minimal motion as they can influence only one motion segment, and are more likely to function as sensory organs for reflexes and proprioception.[177] (Tables 14–1 and 14–2).

TABLE 14–2 PRIME MOVERS OF THE CERVICAL SPINE—EXTENSORS AND FLEXORS

EXTENSOR MUSCLES		FLEXOR MUSCLES
PRIME MOVERS	ACCESSORY MUSCLES	PRIME MOVERS
Trapezius	Multifidus	Sternocleidomastoid-anterior fibers
Sternocleidomastoid-posterior	Suboccipitals Rectus capitis posterior	Accessory muscles
Iliocostalis cervices	Obliquus capitis superior	Prevertebral muscles Longus coli
Longissimus cervices	Obliquus capitis inferior	Longus capitis
Splenius cervices		Rectus capitis anterior
Splenius capitis		Scalene group
Interspinales cervices		Scalenus anterior
Spinalis cervices		Scalenus medius
Spinalis capitis		Scalenus posterior
Semispinalis cervices		Infrahyoid group
Semispinalis capitis		Sternohyoid
Levator scapulae		Omohyoid
		Sternothyroid
		Thyrohyoid

Segmental Biomechanics

Although it may be clinically useful to describe the motions that occur at the cervical spine as separate motions, these motions correspond to the motion of the head alone, and do not describe what is occurring at the various segmental levels. It should be obvious that the range of head movement bears no relation to the range of neck movement, and that the total range is the sum of both the head and the neck motions.[47]

Flexion is described as an anterior osteokinematic rock/tilt of the superior vertebra in the sagittal plane, a superior-anterior glide of both superior facets of the zygapophysial joints, and an anterior translation/slide of the superior vertebra on the intervertebral disc. The produces a ventral compression and a dorsal distraction of the cervical disc. The uncovertebral joint lies on, or very near to, the axis of rotation for flexion and extension. Consequently, the main arthrokinematic motion that seems likely to be occurring here is an anterior spin (or very near spin).[48] This appears especially probable because impairments of the uncovertebral joint seem to be unaffected by flexion or extension. It can be assumed then that the uncovertebral joint is only involved with side-flexion, and that uncovertebral restrictions will be detected in all cervical positions, although flexion partly disengages the joint due its posterior position on the vertebra.[48]

Although all of the following anatomic movement restrictors act to some degree on most of the components of flexion, the following act particularly on the associated movement component.

- The anterior osteokinematic—restrained by the extensor muscles and the posterior ligaments (posterior longitudinal, interspinous, ligamentum flavum).
- The superior-anterior arthrokinematic is restrained by the joint capsule, whereas the translation is restrained by the disc and the nuchal ligament.

Extension is described as a posterior osteokinematic sagittal rock, an inferior-posterior glide, and approximation of the superior facets of the zygapophysial joints, and a posterior translation of the vertebra on the disc. The uncovertebral joint undergoes a posterior arthrokinematic spin. The restrictors of the extension movement are the anterior prevertebral muscles and the anterior longitudinal ligament, which limit the osteokinematic; and the zygapophysial joint capsule, which restrains the arthrokinematic.[48] The disc limits the posterior translation.

Side-flexion is an ipsilateral osteokinematic rock, a superior-anterior glide of the contralateral superior facet, a posterior-inferior glide of the ipsilateral facet, a contralateral translation of the vertebra on the disc, an inferior-medial

FIGURE 14–8 Schematic representation of the motion that occurs at the uncovertebral joint.

glide of the ipsilateral uncovertebral joint, and a superior-lateral glide of the contralateral uncovertebral joint. A composite curved translation results. It is formed by the superior-inferior linear glides of the zygapophysial joints, the oblique inferior-medial and superior-medial glides of the uncovertebral joints, and the linear translation across the disc (Figure 14–8).[48]

The osteokinematic rock can be limited by the contralateral scalenes and intertransverse ligaments. The uncovertebral and zygapophysial arthrokinematics can be limited by the joint capsule and the translation by the disc. If the side-flexion is limited, but the translation is okay, it is unlikely that the joint complex (the zygapophysial joint, disc, or uncovertebral joint) is impaired, and would tend to implicate muscle tightness.[48] However, if the translation is also limited, there exists a problem with the joint complex.

Rotation is chiefly an osteokinematic rotation of the vertebra about a vertical axis that is coupled with ipsilateral side-flexion. Presumably, the translation follows the side-flexion, which is contralateral, resulting in the same uncovertebral and zygapophysial arthrokinematics that side-flexion does.[48] With right rotation, the vertebral bodies (not the zygapophysial joints) of C2–4 flex and the vertebral bodies of C5–7 extend.

The clinician should be able to differentiate between a disc or zygapophysial joint impairment by using the end feel. A disc protrusion will result in a springy end feel, whereas a zygapophysial joint restriction will have an abrupt end feel.[48]

COMMON PATHOLOGIES AND LESIONS

There are a variety of causes for head, neck, shoulder, and arm pain. An appropriate history and physical examination must be performed to exclude fracture, instability, inflammatory disorders, postoperative pain, and tumors.[49] After excluding the extrinsic causes, the clinician must determine the intrinsic causes of the symptoms.

The most likely pain candidates are assessed first. They include the bone, muscles, ligaments, zygapophysial joints, and intervertebral discs. Neural structures, including the dorsal root ganglia and nerve roots, may also mediate pain.

In acute sprains and strains, patients typically relate an activity that precipitated the onset of their symptoms. This may be lifting or pulling a heavy object, an awkward sleeping position, or prolonged static postures. In whiplashassociated disorders, patients generally describe an accident in which they were unexpectedly struck from the rear, front or side by a vehicle traveling at low to moderate speed. Rotational injuries can occur in all types of impact, with a delayed onset of pain a common occurrence (refer to Chap. 19).[49]

A common physician diagnosis for acute neck pain, in the absence of fracture or radicular symptoms, is a sprain and strain of the cervical tissues. This is far too generalized for the clinician, who must ascertain the specific cause of the patients impairment.

Zygapophyseal Joint

The cervical zygapophysial (facet) joints can be responsible for a significant portion of chronic neck pain. Established referral zones for the cervical zygapophysial joint[50,51] overlap both myofascial and dermatomal pain patterns. Cervical zygapophysial joint pain is typically unilateral, and described as a dull ache. Occasionally, the pain can be referred into the craniovertebral or interscapular regions. Palpation just lateral to the midline often indicates regional soft tissue changes in response to the underlying zygapophysial joint injury, and motion testing shows a pattern corresponding to the injured zygapophysial joint.[52] Traditional images (plain radiographs, computed tomography, magnetic resonance imaging) are typically unremarkable, and clinical suspicions of zygapophysial joint injuries are best confirmed by diagnostic intra-articular zygapophysial joint injections or block of the zygapophysial joint's nerve supply.[53]

Posture

Cervical pain not associated with traumatic injuries may arise from poor posture, which in turn, results in abnormal forces and strain on the structures that balance and control the head.[54] Persistent pain may be caused by an inadequately addressed compensatory posture, such as the forward head. Over time, the body attempts to keep the eyes horizontal using greater capital extension.[55–57] Normal motion undertaken in this poor postural environment produces abnormal strain, particularly of the joint capsule, ligaments, intervertebral discs, and the levator scapulae, upper trapezius, sternocleidomastoid, scalene, and suboccipital muscles.[48] Other adaptations associated with this posture include rounded shoulders and protracted scapulae with tight anterior muscles and stretched posterior muscles.[58,59] The traumatized muscles may cause pain, which in turn, causes the patient to restrict motion. Patients with these postural abnormalities may experience secondary myofascial pain that can cause referral zone pain.[40] (Refer to Chapter 11)

Muscle Tear

A cervical strain is produced by an overload injury to the muscle-tendon unit because of excessive forces on the cervical spine, which result in the elongation and tearing of muscles or ligaments, secondary edema, hemorrhage, and inflammation. Many cervical muscles do not terminate in tendons but instead, attach directly to bone by myofascial tissue that blends into the periosteum.[60] Muscles respond to injury in a variety of ways, including reflex contraction, which increases the resistance to stretch and serves as a protection to the injured muscle.

Cervical Disc

Cervical radiculitis, most commonly associated with disc herniations, can usually be treated successfully without surgery.[61] The intervention of cervical discogenic pain includes oral medications, cervical traction, soft cervical collar, and therapeutic exercise. Surgical intervention is reserved for those patients with persistent radicular pain, who do not respond to conservative measures.[62] (Refer to Chapter 7)

Myofascial Pain

The basic pathologic impairment in myofascial pain has yet to be substantiated,[63] although it is thought to involve pain and autonomic responses referred from hyperirritable areas, or a secondary tissue response to disc or zygapophysial joint injuries.[64] These hyperirritable areas, which are painful to compression and can give rise to referred pain, tenderness and autonomic responses, are defined as myofascial trigger points.[40] Trigger points are classified as either active or latent. Active trigger points are believed to spontaneously cause pain, whereas latent trigger points are said to restrict range of motion and produce weakness of the affected muscle, with the patient unaware of the tender area until it becomes activated. Latent trigger points may persist for years after a patient recovers from an injury, and may become active and create acute pain in response to minor overstretching, overuse, or chilling of the muscle.[40,57]

Fibromyalgia

Primary fibromyalgia is a common but poorly understood complex of generalized body aches that may cause pain or paresthesias, or both, in a non-radicular pattern.[65] For a diagnosis of fibromyalgia, pain should be present in at least 11 of 18 tender sites for at least 3 months.[65]

Fibromyalgia symptoms are often reported to be worse in the morning, and during humid weather. Sleep is usually poor, and sleep studies show that stage IV sleep is the most interrupted.[66] The trigger points and pain associated with fibromyalgia typically respond to spray and stretch, microstimulation, and massage.[65]

Torticollis

Torticollis is classified into congenital and acquired types.[67–69] Congenital muscular torticollis (CMT) is the most common type of congenital torticollis.[70] Several causes are implicated, including fetal positioning, difficult labor and delivery, cervical muscle abnormalities, Sprengel's deformity, and Klippel-Feil syndrome.[71] Abnormal fetal head and neck positioning and passage through the birth canal is thought to selectively injure the sternocleidomastoid (SCM) by kinking the muscle, leading to a compartment syndrome. The resultant edema and muscle injury cause progressive fibrosis and contracture of the muscle. In one study where the laterality of birth head position was noted, the laterality of the torticollis was the same.[72] This proposal is in contrast to other birth trauma theories that purport that difficult labor and delivery cause tearing and bleeding of the SCM, resulting in reparative fibrosis and contracture,[73] even though histologic studies have not demonstrated evidence of acute or chronic bleeding or hematomata in or near the SCM.

Acquired torticollis, which include spasmodic torticollis, is clinically similar but has different etiologies. Acquired torticollis in children may be related to trauma or infections, as in Grisel's syndrome, which occurs after head and neck infections.[74] In this syndrome, the soft-tissue inflammation associated with pharyngitis, mastoiditis, or tonsillitis results in accumulation of fluid in the nearby cervical joints. This edema may then lead to subluxation of the atlantoaxial joint (refer to Chap. 18). Children with ocular abnormalities often develop torticollis in an attempt to compensate for diplopia or diminished visual acuity.

Spasmodic torticollis is the involuntary hyperkinesis of neck musculature causing turning of the head on the trunk, sometimes with additional forward flexion (anterocollis), backward extension (retrocollis), or lateral flexion (laterocollis). It is also marked by abnormal head postures. Idiopathic spasmodic torticollis usually has an insidious onset that begins in the fourth or fifth decade of life with no strong gender predominance.[75,76]

Pure retrocollis (6% of cases) and pure anterocollis (3%) represent symmetrical involvement of muscles:[77] most cases are asymmetrical and the involved hypertrophied muscles can readily be palpated and compared with the contralateral normal musculature. The sternocleidomastoid muscle is involved in 75% of cases and the trapezius in 50%. Other muscles that might become involved include the rectus capitis, obliquus inferior, and splenius capitis.[77] In some cases, the spasm generalizes to the muscles of the shoulder, girdle, trunk, or limbs.[78]

Neck movements can vary from jerky to smooth[75,78] and are aggravated by standing, walking, or stressful situations, but usually do not occur with sleep. Pain in the neck and shoulders can accompany spasmodic torticollis, but it is unusual as a presenting symptom.[77] Pain can develop later, however, as the result of degenerative joint disease of the cervical spine or as a result of muscle spasm. Patients will often observe that they can reduce or eliminate the spasms by a physical stimulus, such as placing their hands or pillow on the back of the neck or chin.[77,78]

Spontaneous remissions (partial or complete) have been reported in up to 60% of patients in some series;[75] others note full remission in 16%, with sustained remission for 12 months of 6 to 12%.[76,79]

Although the cause of torticollis remains unknown and no consistent structural, biochemical, or molecular abnormality has so far been identified, recent psychophysical studies have revealed abnormalities in the way patients with torticollis judge the position of their bodies in space.[80,81]

Most intriguingly, patients do not always recognize "straight ahead" in the way normal individuals do,[82] or, they can have subtle difficulties in recognizing when they are in a vertical state (the "postural vertical")[83] and in recognizing when a line is vertical (the "visual vertical").[80,81] These abnormalities do not seem to be due to the patients' abnormal head position because their performance still differs from that of normal controls who assume similar head positions. The overall conclusion from these studies is that patients with torticollis rely less on the position of their heads than do normal individuals, and that they process the afferent signals from the vestibular apparatus and from proprioceptors in the neck and body in an abnormal way.[80,81]

Torticollis appears to have a genetic component, with 5 to 15% of patients with a positive family history of a movement disorder.[84,85] A small percentage of patients have a history of serious head and neck trauma[77] or a long history of neuroleptic drug use,[76] but in most cases, the spasmodic torticollis is idiopathic.

Rondot and associates[76] found that 61% of patients suggested a discrete event associated with the onset of spasmodic torticollis. In order of frequency, these events included emotional stress, medical problems, vocational upsets, head trauma, a neuroleptic prescription, or a febrile infection.

The location of the human gene for idiopathic torsion dystonia[86] might help to clarify questions about etiology.

Various treatments for torticollis have been described. Spencer and co-workers[87] described a single-subject study using behavioral therapies that consisted of progressive relaxation, positive practice, and visual feedback. The patient had significant improvements in all areas, which were maintained at a 2-year follow-up examination.

Agras and Marshall[88] used massed negative practice (i.e., repeating the spasmodic positioning) of 200 to 400 repetitions of the movement daily, which achieved full resolution of symptoms in 1 of 2 patients. Results persisted for 22 months.

Another single-case study used positive practice (exercising against the spasming muscle groups) in a bedridden woman who had 8 years of spasmodic torticollis symptoms. After 3 months of positive practice, she was able to ambulate unassisted; her therapeutic gains were maintained at a 1-year follow-up examination.[87]

Biofeedback has been used by several researchers: Leplow[89] reviewed 184 biofeedback sessions in 10 patients. Considerable improvements occurred during this study; however, they occurred during the instructional phase or very early in the biofeedback training. This finding suggests that cognitive processes and visual feedback (i.e., mirrors) might play an important role in the treatment of spasmodic torticollis, and that the biofeedback might only be of secondary importance.

Headaches

More than 90% of people in the United States experience a headache[90,91] during a given 1-year period.[92] Most treat themselves with over-the-counter medications.[93,94] An estimated 1.7 to 2.5% of patient visits to the emergency department are for complaints of headache.[95]

Headaches can be grouped into two main divisions, benign and nonbenign. Of the benign headaches, approximately 20% are of vascular origin,[96] with the remainder being variously attributed to tension, psychogenic overlay, fatigue, depression, and cervical spine impairment.[90]

Chronic daily headaches following trauma to the head or neck are a common occurrence.[97–99] The duration of these headaches is unrelated to the severity or type of trauma.[100,101]

Neurologic conditions, including headache (migraine, cluster, tension, chronic daily, occipital, rebound, posttraumatic, postlumbar puncture), atypical facial pain, trigeminal and glossopharyngeal neuralgia, and reflex sympathetic dystrophy, have also been shown to be the cause of head and neck pain.[90] The systemic conditions of osteoarthritis, rheumatoid arthritis and related rheumatoid arthritis variants, dermatomyositis, temporal arteritis, Lyme's disease, and fibromyalgia have been indicated as additional sources of head and neck pain.[90]

Neck pain and headache are the cardinal features of whiplash,[102] but these symptoms are musculoskeletal and not neurologic in origin. According to the international classification, headache after whiplash is best classified as cervicogenic (group 11.2.1) and, thus, related to injured structures around the cervical spine.[103] (Refer to Chap. 19)

Neck pain can arise from injuries of the cervical muscles, ligaments, discs, and joints. From lower cervical segments, the pain may be referred to the shoulder and upper limb. From upper segments, neck pain may be referred to the head and present as headache. The incidence of headache after whiplash injury is said to decrease during the first 6 months after trauma.[104] Particularly relevant is the relation between a history of headache and the development of a trauma-related headache after whiplash injury. In addition, psychological variables, which may be important in idiopathic headache,[105,106] should be evaluated in relation to the development and recovery from headache after whiplash.

Although the cervical spine can play a frequent role in headaches, especially the upper region, considerable controversy still exists about whether cervical disease plays any part in headache syndromes.[107–109] Headaches that are cervical in origin tend to be unilateral accompanied by tenderness of the C2–3 articular pillars on the affected side.[110] Other causes include:

- Trigeminal nerve irritation
- Epidural bleed (post trauma); the clinical presentation for this is diffuse pain, drowsiness, and a decrease in intellectual function
- Fracture of cribriform plate
- Alar ligament sprain
- Migraine (see discussion below)
- Cluster headaches (see discussion below)
- Sinus pressure
- Retro-orbital; if isolated (only complaint), then likely to be problem with eye and vision

Types

Migraine headaches are found equally distributed among genders in childhood, but two out of every three adults with migraine headaches are women.[90] The International Headache Society has described migraine headaches as a headache disorder which consists of episodes lasting 4 to 72 hours.[111] The symptoms of a migraine headache are typically unilateral and have a pulsating quality of moderate or severe intensity. Migraines are aggravated by routine physical activity, and are associated with nausea, photophobia, and phonophobia.[112]

Cluster headaches are described as a severe unilateral retro-orbital headache, often accompanied by nasal congestion, discharge, and ptosis (drooping eyelid) on the symptomatic side.[112,113] Unlike migraine sufferers, who feel obliged to lie down during a severe headache, these individuals

feel better during a headache by remaining in an erect posture and moving about.[90] As their name suggests, cluster headaches occur in groups or clusters, and at predictable times of day. The daily bouts of headache usually subside and then disappear, only to reoccur after several months.[113]

Tension-type headache is the term designated by the International Headache Society to describe what was previously called tension headache, muscle contraction headache, psychomyogenic headache, stress headache, ordinary headache, and psychogenic headache. The International Headache Society defines tension-type headache more precisely, distinguishing between the episodic and the chronic varieties, and divides them into two groups, those associated with a disorder of the pericranial muscles and those not associated with this type of disorder.

Tension headaches constitute up to 70% of headaches, occurring more often in women than in men.[114,115] They are characterized by a bilateral steady ache in the frontal or temporal areas.

Occipital headache is felt by many clinicians to be referred pain from a cervical disorder,[117–119] especially when cervical traction, temporarily decreases the pain.[120] The underlying musculoskeletal mechanism for the pain is often structural, including cervical hypomobility or hypermobility, joint subluxation, degenerative bony changes, or postural, with or without forward head position. Postures, movements, or activities that put strain on the neck have been associated with headaches.[126] In one study, 51% of patients associated their headaches with particular sustained neck flexion during reading, studying, or typing and driving a car. Sixty-five percent of headache patients reported a chronic course running between 2 to 20 years, and only 7% reported pain of less than 1 week duration.[127] The general misunderstanding, that there is no cervical sensory reference to the head area as the C1 dorsal ramus has no sensory component, has led to the belief that only the trigeminal nerve has sensory input to the vertex and frontal regions. In fact, there is considerable sensory input into the C1 root, but not from a cutaneous source.[121] Experiments have confirmed a close trigeminocervical relationship.[122,123] Because the head and neck are one functional unit, cervical musculoskeletal disorders can refer as headache, temporomandibular, or facial pain with or without neck pain.[124] Occipital hyperextension of the cranium on the cervical spine has been related to head and neck pain. A postural/pain relationship has recently been described by Willford and co-workers[125] in people wearing multifocal corrective lenses.

Chronic daily headache is a syndrome consisting of a group of disorders and can be subclassified into primary and secondary types.[128] The primary chronic daily headache disorders, including transformed migraine, chronic tension-type headache, new daily persistent headache, and hemicrania continua, are defined as a constant tension headache with migrainous exacerbations.[129,130] Chronic daily headache usually evolves over time from episodic migraine, but the cause is still controversial.

Secondary causes of chronic daily headache include, cervical spine disorders, headache associated with vascular disorders, and nonvascular intracranial disorders.

Individuals suffering from chronic daily headache frequently suffer from rebound headache as well. Rebound headache is the worsening of head pain in chronic headache sufferers. It is caused by the frequent and excessive use of non-narcotic analgesics.[131] In a recent review of chronic daily headaches, Mathew[132] stressed that 73% of 630 patients with chronic daily headache suffered from drug-induced or rebound headache. Omitted from these totals were patients with post-traumatic headache.

Trauma was reported in 44% of 6000 headache patients in one study[135] and in 40% of 96 in another,[127] with 16% of the 96 having been involved in a motor vehicle accident. One study,[136] categorizing patients who had been involved in rear-end vehicle collisions in a similar fashion to the Quebec Task Force grades 1, 2, and 3, found that headaches persisted in a 20 month follow-up in 70% of the group 3 patients and 37% of group 1 and 2. The role of trauma may be understated as, frequently, the trauma may occur some considerable time before the onset of the headache and so may be forgotten. Tension headaches may well initiate a headache in a patient predisposed by some previous and forgotten traumatic incident.

In addition to the immediate pain following a head injury, *post-traumatic headache*, a more prolonged and enduring headache, may develop.[134] This condition, resembling either migraine or tension-type headache, may last for weeks, months, or years. It may also be associated with post-traumatic syndrome, which includes a variety of symptoms such as irritability, insomnia, anxiety, depression, and reduced ability to concentrate.[134] A diagnosis of chronic post-traumatic headache should never be made unless analgesic rebound has been excluded.[133]

Atypical facial pain is considered by many neurologists as a neuralgia characterized by typically unilateral and relatively constant facial pain that is unrelated to jaw function.[137] This condition, recently reclassified as facial pain by the International Headache Society, is not well understood and often defies all modes of intervention.[112] Many authorities believe that facial pain is psychogenic.[138,139] However, it has recently been reported that intraoral edema and trigeminal V2 nerve distribution area tenderness were consistently found in individuals with atypical facial pain.[137] Furthermore, these individuals experienced relief of their symptoms in response to low-level helium-neon laser therapy.[140]

BIOMECHANICAL EXAMINATION

The cervical spine proper, composed of muscles, zygapophysial joints, discs, and uncovertebral joints, is more complicated than the craniovertebral region. Consequently, its examination is somewhat more detailed and complex. A review of the flow diagram in Figure 14–9 will be a helpful guide to the reader. The flow diagram assumes that the clinician has taken the history and performed a scan, if appropriate, but has yet to determine a diagnosis.

For the purposes of the assessment, it is important to establish a baseline of symptoms so that the clinician is able to determine whether a particular movement has aggravated or lessened the patient's symptoms. A movement restriction is a loss of movement in a specific direction. A movement toward or away from the restriction may alter the degree and location of those symptoms.

Observation

Static observation of general posture, as well as the relationship of the neck on the trunk and the head on the neck, is observed while the patient is standing and

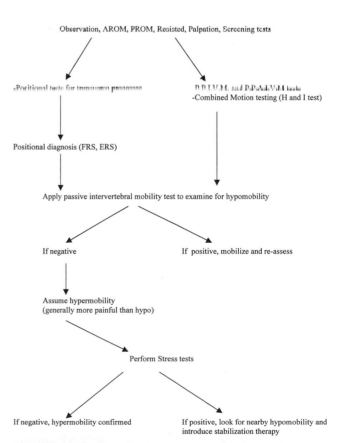

FIGURE 14–9 Examination sequence for the cervical spine.

sitting, both in the waiting area, and in the examination room.

Side View

● The forehead should be vertical.

● The tip of the chin should be perpendicular with the manubrium. If the chin is anterior to the manubrium, a forward head is present. A forward head places the head ahead of the center of gravity (COG) and is often the result of a thoracic hypomobility.[48] For each inch that the head is forward in relation to the COG, the weight of the head is added to the load needed to be borne by the cervical structures.[141] For example, the average head weighs 10 pounds. If the chin is 2 inches anterior to the manubrium, 20 pounds is added to the load. These additional forces can be transmitted to the lumbar spine, increasing the amount disc compression, especially at L5–S1.[142,143] The forward-head posture has been linked with a number of syndromes including temporomandibular arthralgia,[144-148] probably as the result of an alteration in bite biomechanics.[146] (Refer to Chap. 11)

The clinician should:

● Measure the difference in inches. A computer-assisted slide digitizing system, postural analysis digitizing system (PADS), can be used to determine characteristic values for head and shoulder girdle posture and characteristic range of motion for head protraction-retraction and shoulder protraction-retraction.[149] PADS is a modification of a two-dimensional slide digitizing system developed for measuring trunk range of motion. The patient is photographed in a neutral position, the maximally protracted position, and the maximally retracted position of the head and scapula. The slide photographs are then analyzed using a computer-assisted digitizing system. Other posture measuring devices have been cited.[150]

● Check if the forward head is reducible by applying a passive chin tuck. The chin tuck is performed by passively retracting the patient's head while keeping the chin level, thereby flattening the cervical lordosis. Although the chin tuck is a good assessment tool, its use as a cervical exercise is under review. As with any exercise, the potential for harm exists if the exercise is performed overzealously, and although as yet unproven, there are strong suspicions that the chin tuck can induce instability to the cervical spine.

● Check thoracic mobility.

Back View

1. The clinician should assess muscular asymmetry, especially in the upper trapezius and sternocleidomastoid.

2. The spinous process of the axis should be in mid-line.

3. As the patient rotates the head to each side, the tips of the transverse processes of the atlas should be felt to rotate anteriorly and then posteriorly. Both sides are compared. The procedure is repeated for side-flexion. The transverse process should become less prominent and should approximate the mastoid process on the side of the side-flexion.

Front View

A. The clinician should assess whether the patient's head is shifted to one side. A cervical disc protrusion (C3–4 or C4–5) can produce a horizontal side shift of the head.[48] This side shift allows the patient to maintain eye level.

B. A slight tilt of the head is normal.
1. Split the mass of the head into two vertical halves. Cerebral asymmetries in form and volume, associated with cranial asymmetries, are a common feature of the human race and are often associated with facial asymmetries.[151-153] In many cases, this asymmetry is, related to asymmetric cerebral growth, which is mostly accomplished in utero.[154,156] Although they may also have a local origin, for instance, in the case of mandibular asymmetry.
2. Look for tilts but do not straighten them—tilt your head to match.
   a. Does the patient's head appear to be moving in the opposite direction to the chin?
   b. Is the face "moving toward one ear"—indicative of a trigeminal nerve impairment?[48]
3. The head and jaw should move in opposite directions.
4. The head and eyes should move in opposite directions.

C. Check eye levels, depths, and sizes.

D. Check the symmetry of the nasal bone—is it positioned evenly between the eyes?

E. Check for nostril defects.

F. Check the mouth:
1. For tilts and upturns
2. For dry and cracked lips—indicating a *mouth breather*[48]

G. Palpate the midline symphysis (not always where the dimple is).

H. Check if the teeth are visible.
1. An overbite pushes the head of mandible up and back.

2. If the tongue is visible, this is further confirmation of a mouth breather.[48]

I. Check the chin muscles—they should look relaxed.

Active Range of Motion

An assessment of gross range of motion of cervical flexion, and extension is performed (Figure 14–10), and the clinician makes note of any motion that reproduces or enhances the symptoms and the location of the symptoms. The weight of the head should provide sufficient overpressure for all motions except rotation. Considerable emphasis should be placed on the amount of flexion available and the symptoms it provokes, as flexion is the only motion tolerated well by the normal spine. In addition, the clinician should note the quality of movement. When interpreting the motion findings, the position of the joint at the

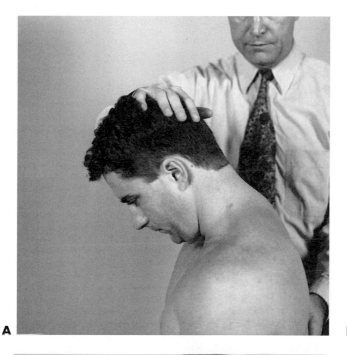

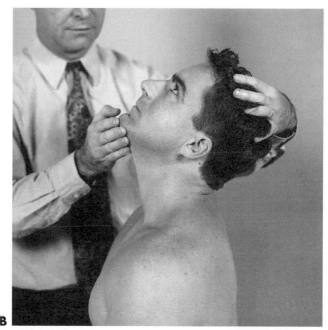

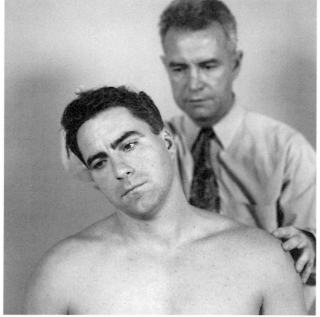

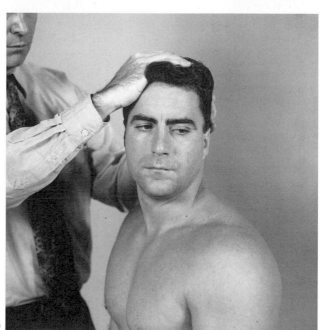

FIGURE 14–10   Active range of motion of the cervical spine.

beginning of the test should be correlated with the subsequent mobility noted since alterations in joint mobility may merely be a reflection of an altered starting position.

According to Cyriax,[157] the capsular pattern of the cervical spine is full flexion in the presence of limited extension and symmetrical limitation of rotation and side-flexion. The presence of a capsular pattern indicates arthritis. If end-range flexion is immediately painful, meningitis or acute radicular pain should be ruled out. If the pain is felt after a 15- to 20-second delay, ligament pain should be suspected. The most common restricter of cervical flexion is upper thoracic/cervicothoracic, or occipitoatlantal joint impairment, but flexion can also be limited by acute/severe trauma (muscle spasms straighten the lordosis), fracture/dislocations, or disc impairments.

Three screening tests can be used to highlight the level of a rotation restriction. All of the tests utilize rotation of the neck with the neck in various amounts of flexion.

1. Rotation with the neck in full flexion tests the C1–2 level.
2. Rotation with the neck in a chin tuck tests the C2–3 level.[158]
3. Rotation with the neck in full extension tests the levels below C3. The more extension, the lower the level of involvement.

Normal extension motion allows the face to be parallel with the ceiling. With rotation, the chin should be in line with the acromioclavicular joint at the end of rotation (see Figure 14–10). If a patient is able to maintain eye level during rotation, this rules out any atlantoaxial involvement. If, during active rotation the patient side-flexes to achieve full motion (Figure 14–10D), there is likely a problem with the atlantoaxial joint or thorax. However, if during rotation, they are unable to side-flex to achieve the full motion, the problem is in the mid to low cervical spine.

Side-flexion is performed to the left and right while the ipsilateral shoulder is stabilized by the clinician (see Figure 14–10C; stabilizing the contralateral shoulder merely tests the length of the upper trapezius).

Active elevation of each upper extremity is then assessed to rule out symptom reproduction from the shoulder movements.

Clinicians need to look for a painless restricted motion, or normal motion that is painful, indicating a hypermobility. Pain that is produced by the motion that is restricted indicates an acute/subacute injury, whereas pain that is produced by the motion that is not restricted, or excessive, indicates a hypermobility.

The next stage in the examination process depends on the clinician's background. For those clinicians heavily influenced by the muscle energy techniques of the osteopaths,[159]

position testing is used to determine which segment to focus on. Other clinicians omit the position tests and proceed to the combined motion and passive physiologic tests.

Position Testing

The position tests are screening tests that like all screening tests, are valuable in focusing the attention of the examiner to one segment, but are not appropriate for making a definitive statement concerning the movement status of the segment. However, when combined with the results of the passive movement testing, they help to form the working hypothesis.

The patient is positioned in sitting and the clinician stands behind the patient. Using the thumbs, the clinician palpates the articular pillars of the cranial vertebra of the segment to be tested. The patient is asked to flex the neck, and the clinician assesses the position of the cranial vertebra relative to its caudal neighbor and notes which articular pillar of the cranial vertebra is the most dorsal (Figure 14–11). A dorsal left articular pillar of the cranial vertebra relative to the caudal vertebra is indicative of a left rotated position of the segment in flexion.[159]

The patient is asked to extend the joint complex while the clinician assesses the position of the C4 vertebra relative to C5 by noting which articular pillar is the most dorsal. A dorsal left articular pillar of C4 relative to C5 is indicative of a left rotated position of the C4–5 joint complex in extension.[159]

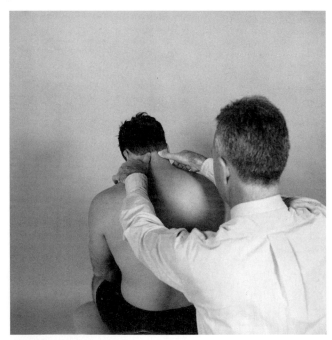

FIGURE 14–11 Patient and clinician position for testing at C3–4 for flexion.

This test may also be performed with the patient supine, but in sitting, the clinician can better observe the effect of the weight of the head on the joint mechanics.

Combined Motions and Passive Physiologic Tests

These tests are screening tests which, as with any other screening test, quickly demonstrate the need for more exhaustive testing and to focus the examiner's attention on a specific level(s) and specific movement(s). There are a number of screening tests that can be employed, each with its own strengths and weakness.

● H and I tests or Figure-of-8 test—combined motion test
● Translational glides—passive physiologic motion test

H and I Tests

The H and I tests, described in Chapter 13, can also be used in the cervical spine with the same interpretations made about the findings. Closing restrictions produce a restriction of cervical extension, side-flexion, and rotation to the same side in the tests.

Opening restrictions are slightly more difficult to identify in the cervical spine because, frequently, there is no actual restriction of cervical flexion, but rather, a restriction of rotation and side-flexion along with reproduction of pain on the contralateral side.

Referred symptoms, which are cervical in origin, can occur in the upper extremities, the thoracic spine, the scapula, and occasionally, the upper chest. The most common pattern producing the distal symptoms is the closing restriction, but a limitation in cervical flexion accompanied by the production of distal symptoms can also occur. This finding has to be differentiated from restricted flexion, which produces central symptoms in the upper thoracic area. Side-flexion to the opposite side of the pain can also reproduce upper extremity symptoms.

In some instances, there may be findings in the movement examination that indicate the need for mobility testing using translational glides.

Figure-of-8 Test

The figure-of-8 test is a useful tool, once the occipito-atlantal (O-A), atlanto-axial (A-A), and the first three thoracic levels have been cleared, in helping to elicit the presence of any hypomobilities and/or arthrotic instabilities in the cervical spine. It is similar to the H and I tests in that it can only be used on the nonacute patient. However, unlike the H and I tests, which do not examine each level segmentally, the figure-of-8 test can be used at a specific level once the general test has proved to be positive. The figure-of-8 test can be performed with the patient seated or supine, with the clinician standing behind the patient. The clinician's hand rests on top of the patient's head while the other hand palpates the base of the patient's neck. The neck is moved through a figure-of-8 pattern, first with flexion and then with extension, and crepitus is felt for. The following sequence is normally used.

Flexion The clinician passively flexes the patient's neck. While maintaining the flexion, left side-flexion is introduced (Figure 14–12). Maintaining the side-flexion, the clinician, moves the patient's head and neck into extension before returning the head and neck to the neutral, or start, position. From this position, the neck is flexed and side-flexed to the right, followed by the cervical extension motion while maintaining the side-flexion. The head is then returned to neutral. The whole series of movements is performed in a flowing manner and in the pattern of a figure 8.

Extension The clinician passively extends the patient's neck and then introduces left side-flexion, then cervical flexion, before returning the head and neck to the neutral, or start, position. From the neutral position, the head and neck are again extended, but then side-flexed to the right, followed by cervical flexion while maintaining the side-flexion. The head is then returned to neutral.

Positive findings for this test include:

● *Crepitus*: if crepitus in the neck is felt during the test, the test is repeated at each level with the clinician

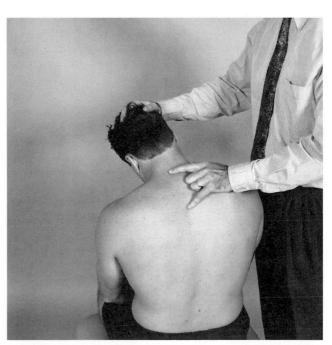

FIGURE 14–12 Patient and clinician position for cervical flexion and left side flexion during Figure of 8 test.

palpating the posterior tubercles of each level, to localize the source of the crepitus. Once the level is localized, the test is repeated with the inferior segment stabilized, making sure to allow enough room for the zygapophysial joints of the superior segment to glide posteriorly.

- *Motion block*: a block in one motion or direction but no block when the quadrant is approached from a different direction.
- *Pain at the extreme ranges*: this could indicate a hypermobility.
- *Unusual shunts and shifts felt by the clinician*: these may indicate the presence of instability.

Translational Glides

The correct axis of motion for this test can be visualized by using imaginary rods pointing vertically from each vertebral body.

To test the passive mobility of the mid-cervical region, the patient's neck is placed in the neutral position of the head on the neck, and the neck on the trunk, after which lateral glides are performed, beginning at C2 and progressing inferiorly (Figure 14–13). The glides are typically tested in one direction before repeating the process on the other side. Lateral glides result in a relative side-flexion of the cervical spine in the opposite direction to the glide. Light pressure from the clinician's body can be applied against the top of the patient's skull to hold the head in position. This reinforces the stabilization caused

by the weight of the patient's thorax against the plinth. Each spinal level is glided laterally to the left and right while the examiner palpates for muscle guarding, range of motion, end feel, and the provocation of symptoms. Lateral glides are performed as far inferiorly as is possible. Following this procedure, the areas of involvement are targeted and repetition of the lateral glides is performed from the extended and then flexed positions, rather than from neutral. Because the cervical spine usually tolerates flexion, gross cervical flexion may be used. Since extension is poorly tolerated by the injured cervical spine, segmental extension rather than gross extension is utilized. With the patient supine, and their occiput cupped, the segment is extended by lifting the superior vertebra forward (obviating the need to extend the entire spinal region) and allowing the patient's head and neck to bend over the fulcrum created by the examiner's fingers. While maintaining the extended position (by pushing the transverse processes of the segment anteriorly), the segment is side-flexed left and then right around its axis of motion and translated contralaterally (Figure 14–14). During the translation, very slight head motion should occur and a slight tilting around each segmental axis occurs, using gentle pressure via the finger tips or the fleshy part of the second metacarpophalangeal (MCP) joint. The slight side-flexion before the translation is to fix the axis at that segmental level. During left side-flexion, the left side of the segment is maximally extended while the right side is moved toward its neutral position. If, for example, left

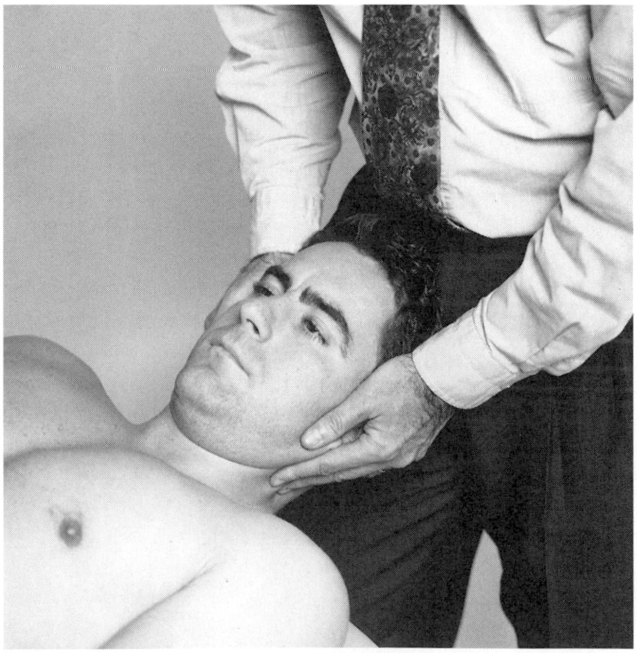

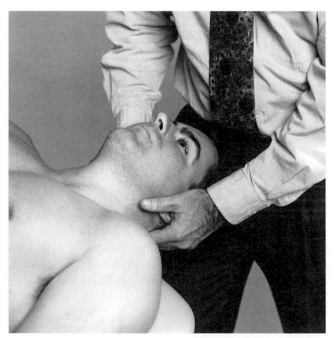

FIGURE 14–13 Patient and clinician position for cervical side glides performed in neutral.

FIGURE 14–14 Patient and clinician position for cervical side glides performed in extension.

side-flexion is restricted, restriction of the flexor muscles or one of the joints on the left is the problem. If the end feel of the translation is normal but the side-flexion is restricted, the hypomobility is extra-articular (myofascial). The range of motion of the side-flexion and the end feel of the translation is evaluated for normal, excessive, or reduced motion states. As the procedure is repeated, the examiner once again assesses the same parameters previously described, except that the greatest difference of movement in the lateral glide from one side to the other is determined. This is compared to the same movement from a different starting position (i.e., neutral versus flexion versus extension). Due to the unreliability of mobility testing in extension, the information gleaned from the motion testing is more likely to be more reliable in determining the side of the closing restriction.[44]

The same considerations are pertinent for flexion hypomobilities. To test in flexion, the patient's head and neck are flexed without allowing a chin tuck, which would tighten the nuchal ligament. If left side-flexion is restricted in flexion, the right side of the segment is not flexing sufficiently. As previously mentioned, cervical spine motion is a combination of zygapophysial and uncovertebral joint glides. Clinically, it would appear that the zygapophysial joints are more involved with the rotational aspect of the coupling, functioning to prevent excessive rotation, whereas the uncovertebral joints appear to be more involved with pure side-flexion motions. While this concept may not hold up to scientific scrutiny, it tends to work well in the clinic. Thus, a glide restriction found in flexion, extension, and neutral would tend to implicate a problem with the uncovertebral joint. Occasionally, the side-flexion appears normal but the translation is restricted in all three positions. The likeliest cause of this is an uncovertebral joint impairment.

Having tested the whole complex with the translations, it is now necessary to individually test each of the segments that produced positive results with the translations. Because of the influence of the uncovertebral joints in the upper segments (C2–4), these need to be tested by first isolating the segment, and then testing its ability to side-flex and rotate, as well as its ability to perform a pure side-flexion. If, for example, a reduced right translation was found at C3–4, the joint is tested at that level with left rotation and then left side-flexion. If the side-flexion is more restricted than the rotation, the uncovertebral joint could be at fault, whereas if the rotation appears to be more restricted than the side-flexion, the zygapophysial joint is more likely to be at fault. However, before this can be ascertained, the zygapophysial joint has to be treated. Once the zygapophysial joint motion has been restored, the translation to the right, in extension, is reassessed. If the translation is still restricted, the uncovertebral joint glides are assessed and treated.

TABLE 14–3 MOVEMENT RESTRICTION AND POSSIBLE CAUSES[48]

MOVEMENT RESTRICTED	POSSIBLE REASON
Extension and right side-flexion	Right extension hypomobility
	Right flexor muscle tightness
	Right anterior capsular adhesions
	Right subluxation
	Right small disc protrusion
Flexion and right side-flexion	Left flexion hypomobility
	Left extensor muscle tightness
	Left posterior capsular adhesions
	Left subluxation
Extension and right side-flexion > Extension and left side-flexion	Left capsular pattern—arthritis/osis
Flexion and right side-flexion = Extension and left side flexion	Left arthro-fibrosis (very hard) Capsular end feel
Side-Flexion in neutral, flexion, and extension	Uncovertebral hypomobility or anomaly

Although it is not necessary to make a biomechanical diagnosis from these tests because there are direct arthrokinematic tests available for all of the articular components of the segments, some useful deductions can be made and these will direct the ensuing arthrokinematic tests to the appropriate joint (Table 14–3).

Passive Physiologic Articular Intervertebral Motion Testing

If the motion is determined as being reduced (hypomobile), passive physiologic articular intervertebral mobility (PPAIVM) testing is performed to determine whether the reduced motion is a result of an articular or extra-articular restriction. With few exceptions, muscles cannot restrict the glides of a joint, especially if the glides are tested in the loose pack position of a peripheral joint and, at the end of available range, in the spinal joints. Thus, if the joint glide is restricted, the cause is an articular restriction, such as the joint surface or capsule. If the glide is normal, then the restriction must be from an extra-articular source, such as a periarticular structure or muscle.

Zygapophysial Joints
The patient is laid supine and if extension is to be tested, the superior vertebra of the segment is lifted to gain extension and the clinician's fingers are put over the inferior articular processes of the superior vertebra. The two zygapophysial joint surfaces of the hypomobile side are compressed against each other as the superior facet is pushed inferiorly and the end feel assessed by comparing it with the other side and/or the joints above and below.

For flexion, the segment is flexed and the suspected hypo-mobile joints superior facet is pulled superiorly again to assess the end feel.

Example: A Suspected Extension and Right Side-Flexion Restriction Extension and right side-flexion is performed to the barrier. The superior zygapophysial joint on the right is pushed caudally with the pads of the index finger while the inferior zygapophysial joint on the opposite side is pulled up cranially (Figure 14–15).

For a flexion restriction, the head is flexed and side-flexed away from the side of the suspected impairment. The superior zygapophysial joint is pulled cranially while the zygapophysial joint, on the opposite side, is pushed caudally.

Uncovertebral Joints

The orientation of the uncovertebral joint is inferior-medial and superior-lateral in a mainly sagittal plane and its axis of motion travels through the vertebral body. With the patient supine, the superior articular surface is glided inferior-medially in the direction of the restricted transla-tion. The end feel is assessed by comparisons with the other side and/or the joints above and below.

The uncovertebral arthrokinematic can be restricted by a small disc protrusion. This can be determined by combining the results from the other findings. The find-ings for a disc protrusion will be positive ipsilaterally in

extension but not in flexion or neutral. There will be a springy end feel and an associated loss of the side-flexion.

Example: A Patient with a Decreased Left Translation in Flexion, Extension, and Neutral at C3–4 The patient is positioned in supine and the occiput is cupped in the clin-ician's hands.

1. The clinician stabilizes the left side of C4 while an in-ferior medial glide of C3 on C4 is performed using the index MCP joint in a direction toward the patient's opposite hip to test the inferior glide of C3 on the right side.[160]
2. The clinician stabilizes the right side of C3 while an in-ferior medial glide of C4 toward the opposite hip is performed to test the superior-lateral glide of C4 on C3 on the left side.

Cervical Stress Tests

Depending on the irritability of the segment, a variety of tests can be used to assess for instability. It is worth-while to start gently with segmental palpation and gentle posterior-anterior pressures before progressing to the other techniques.

Segmental Palpation

The patient lies supine and the clinician stands at the patient's head. The patient's head is rested against the clin-ician's thigh. Using the index fingers, the clinician slides the fingers under the sternocleidomastoid and begins to palpate the anterior aspect of the cervical vertebral bodies (from C7 to C3) for tenderness. The posterior aspects can be palpated with the other hand. If palpation reveals some tenderness, the clinician can further stress the segment by gently applying a posterior-anterior pressure.[160] This is ac-complished using the hand under the neck and applying an anterior shear at each segmental level. This should result in a slight increase in the cervical lordosis. If it results in an anterior glide at the segment, the test can be considered positive and a stability test of that segment should be performed.

The patient is laid supine and the following tests carried out for stability.

Transverse Shear

The transverse shear test should not be confused with the lateral glide tests previously mentioned. The lateral glide tests are used to assess joint motion, whereas the transverse shear test assesses the stability of the segment. While mo-tion is expected to occur in the lateral glide test, no motion should be felt to occur with the transverse shear test.

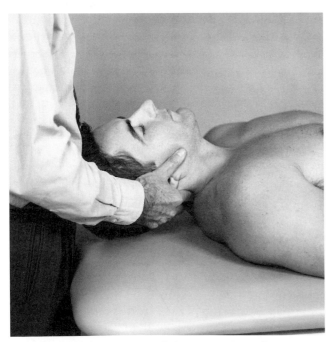

FIGURE 14–15 Patient and clinician position for passive physiologic intervertebral accessory motion testing into extension and right side flexion.

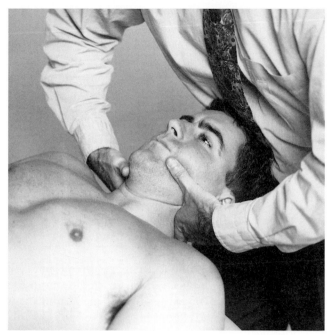

FIGURE 14–16 Patient and clinician position for transverse shear at C4–5.

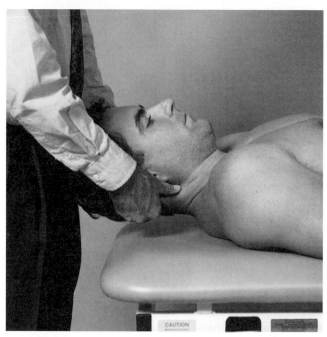

FIGURE 14–17 Patient and clinician position for anterior-posterior shear test.

Example: C1–5 The soft aspect of one second metacarpal head is placed on the opposite transverse processes and laminae of C4 and C5, with the palms facing each other. C4 is stabilized and the clinician attempts to translate C5 transversely using the soft part of the MCP joint of the index finger[160] (Figure 14–16). No movement should be felt, and the end feel should be a combination of capsular and slightly springy. The other side of C4 is then stabilized and C5 is translated in the other direction. The test is repeated at each segmental level.

Anterior-Posterior Shear

For anterior stability testing, the clinician places the thumbs over the anterior aspects of the transverse processes of the inferior vertebra of the segment being tested. The index finger tips are then applied to the posterior neural arch of the superior segment (Figure 14–17). The superior vertebra is then pushed anteriorly on the stabilized inferior vertebra, and the clinician feels for movement, especially for any slippage.[160]

For posterior stability testing, the position of the fingers and thumbs are simply reversed so that the thumbs are on the anterior aspect of the superior vertebra and the index fingers are on the posterior aspect (neural arch) of the inferior.[160] The inferior vertebra is then pushed anteriorly on the superior one, producing a relative posterior shear of the superior segment.

To keep this test comfortable, the thumbs must be under (posterior) the sternocleidomastoid and merely function to stabilize, exerting no pushing force.

Vertical Shear

The vertical shear test examines the five-joint complex—the intervertebral disc, the two zygapophysial joints, and both uncovertebral joints.

The patient is supine and the clinician stands at the patient's head. The clinician cups the patient's occiput in one hand and rests the anterior aspect of the ipsilateral shoulder on the patient's forehead. The other hand stabilizes at a level close to the base of the neck[160] (Figure 14–18). A traction-compression-traction force is initially applied as the clinician palpates for a consistent clicking. If this occurs, each segment is then individually tested in the same manner to localize the instability by stabilizing the lower segment and applying the traction and compression above the segment. Once the instability is localized, the patient is asked to perform and hold a chin tuck to test the ability of the nuchal ligament to stabilize the segment while the level is retested.

The test is performed in:

1. Flexion
2. Extension
3. Neutral

Special Tests

Foraminal compression and distraction or "quadrant" tests with axial compression can be applied at the end of all four quadrants. Quadrant tests fully open or close zygapohysial joints and formina, in addition to stressing the

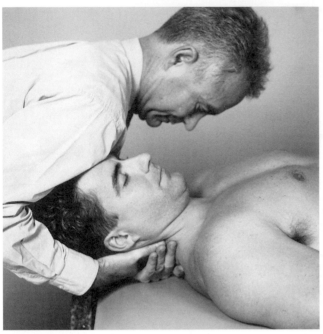

FIGURE 14–18 Patient and clinician position for general traction.

disc. These tests are only used when the cardinal movements are pain free and there are no complaints of radicular pain.

Flexion combined with side-flexion away tests the integrity of the disc, whereas extension combined with side-flexion toward the tested side tests for foraminal encroachment. Overpressure and resistance can also be applied.

Compression of the spine gives an indication of vertical irritability. A reproduction of pain with this test suggests the presence of:

- A disc herniation
- An end plate fracture
- A vertebral body fracture
- Acute arthritis or joint inflammation of a zygapophysial joint
- Nerve root irritation, if radicular pain is produced

A reproduction of pain with cervical distraction suggests the presence of:

- A spinal ligament tear
- A tear or inflammation of the anulus fibrosus
- Dural irritability (if nonradicular arm, or leg pain is produced)

Examination Conclusions

Following the biomechanical examination, a working hypothesis is established based on a summary of all of the

findings. As mentioned, the focus of the biomechanical examination is to elicit a movement diagnosis and to:

- Determine which joint is impaired
- Determine the presence and type of movement impairment

At the completion of the biomechanical examination, the clinician should have information concerning the motion state of the joint and can determine whether the joint is myofascially/pericapsularly hypomobile, subluxed, hypermobile, or ligamentously/articularly unstable.

INTERVENTION

Based on a working hypothesis, an intervention is initiated and typically includes education, activity modification, and therapeutic exercise. Topical agents, oral medications, psychological support and counseling, or the multidisciplinary approach used in treating chronic pain may also be prescribed by the physician.

General Considerations

Patients with neck and extremity pain must be evaluated and treated comprehensively. The goals of treating neck pain are to decrease pain, to restore motion if biomechanically possible, and to improve strength and function.

The intervention of cervical strains and sprains is nonsurgical. Many patients improve within 8 weeks, although complete resolution is less common.[49] If pain persists for more than 3 months, more severe ligamentous, disc, or associated zygapophysial joint injuries should be suspected. If significant neck pain persists past 6 to 8 weeks, flexion and extension radiographs may be useful to exclude or confirm instability.

Cervical Collars
Soft cervical collars do not rigidly immobilize the cervical spine and have not been shown to be of benefit in the intervention of acute neck pain.[161,162] They can, however, provide much needed support to the head and, if used for a brief period, can help in the reduction of symptoms.

Bed Rest
Bed rest has not been shown to improve recovery and, when compared with mobilization or patient education, rest tends to prolong symptoms.[163,164]

Therapeutic Exercise
Active or passive ranges of motion are typically more effective for the mechanical component of pain.[49] Aerobic

exercise increases the general sense of well-being and should be a part of all exercise programs. The intervention for chronic cervical strain must include postural reeducation, strengthening, and stretching.

Strengthening often begins with isometric contractions in the cardinal planes against manual resistance applied by the clinician and then by the patient.

Exercise programs for patients with disc herniations are individualized;[165] however, most patients obtain analgesia using the controlled use of cervical retraction or posterior gliding of the lower cervical spine in combination with extension of the lower cervical spine and flexion of the upper cervical spine (chin-tuck).[49] As mentioned previously, this exercise has the potential to cause harm and should only be used as long as the patient is achieving benefit.

Ischemic compression is advocated for myofascial trigger-points and is achieved by sustaining direct pressure over a trigger point for 60 to 180 seconds, using the thumb to apply pressure.[49] To facilitate self-treatment for inaccessible regions, such as the rhomboid muscles, lying on a tennis ball or using the handle of a cane can be substituted for direct manual compression.[49]

Ergonomics

Work station ergonomics should be addressed. A chair that provides adequate support and encourages the patient to maintain a lumbar lordosis provides a stable platform for the cervical spine.[54] The feet should easily touch the floor and the thighs should be horizontal to the ground. Computer monitors should be positioned to allow a slight 20 degree downward slope of the eyes.

Electrotherapeutic Modalities and Thermal Agents

Physical therapy has been shown to be beneficial in reducing neck pain and improving mobility.[167–169] Modalities such as heat, electrical stimulation, and ultrasound may be used to relax the muscles in the acute period (less than 4 weeks) after cervical soft tissue injury, but for the most part, the efficacy of their use has not been subjected to scientific clinical trials.[162] Cervical traction has been advocated for neck sprains, but no clinical or statistically significant change in pain or overall range of motion has been identified.[166] The pain of radiculopathy may be treated with cervical traction.[165,170,171] The efficacy of traction has not been scientifically proved in a randomized controlled trial, but it is commonly used and thought to be of benefit in reducing radicular pain.[49] Return to activities should be encouraged and begin within 2 to 4 days after the injury. However, the use of mobilization in the first 4 weeks after injury remains controversial.[49]

Manual Therapy

Numerous manual therapy techniques are available to the clinician, each with its own uses. These techniques can be used with hypomobilities, hypermobilities, instabilities, and soft tissue injuries.

Myofascial Hypomobility

These types of hypomobility respond well to muscle energy techniques and stretching.

Joint Hypomobility

The purpose of these techniques is to be able to isolate a mobilization to a specific level, and in so doing:

● Reduce stresses through both the fixation and leverage components of the spine.
● Reduce stresses through hypermobile segments.
● Reduce the overall force needed by the clinician, thus giving greater control.

The selection of a manual technique is dependent on a number of factors including:

A. The acuteness of the condition and the restriction to the movement that is encountered. If the structure is acutely painful (pain is felt before resistance or pain is felt with resistance), pain relief rather than a mechanical effect is the major goal. Manual techniques that can provide pain relief include:
  1. Joint oscillations (grade I and II) that do not reach the end of range. The segment or joint is left in its neutral position and the mobilization is carried out from that point.
  2. Gentle passive range of motion
  3. Modalities

B. The goal of the treatment.

C. Whether the restriction is symmetrical, involving both sides of the segment, or asymmetrical, involving only one side of the segment.

A number of specific manual techniques can be employed. Some clinicians use the recognized coupling for locking whereas others rely on translations. The vast majority of cases involving biomechanical dysfunction of the neck present with a posterior quadrant dysfunction, that is, a loss of extension and a loss of side-flexion and rotation to one side or both. A loss of cervical flexion should always lead the clinician to suspect a cervical disc, a cervicothoracic dysfunction, or a craniovertebral dysfunction. However, for completeness, the techniques described here address a loss in both the anterior and posterior quadrants. The C4–5 level will be used in the following examples.

Techniques to Restore Motion in the Posterior Quadrant

Translation Technique to Restore Extension and Left Side-flexion/Rotation By treating with translation, the whole joint complex (zygapophysial joint, uncovertebral, etc.) is addressed. The patient is seated and the clinician stands on the left side. The segments above are locked incongruently by right side-flexing and flexing. The clinician, using a full lumbrical grip of the left hand, grasps and stabilizes C5. The right hand reaches around the head, securing it to the clinician's chest, and its fifth finger is applied to the left transverse process and neural arch of C4. The C4–5 segment is then left side-flexed, extended, and right translated to barrier the left joint. The mobilization is carried out by the clinician applying pressure against the left transverse process and neural arch of C4 with the metacarpophalangeal joint of the little finger, producing a right translation.

Seated Mobilization Technique to Restore Extension and Left Side-flexion/Rotation If the clinician has large hands, mobilizing into extension can be a problem as the stabilizing hand prevents the full glide into extension from occurring. To alleviate this problem, the stabilizing inferior hand is performed by pushing the thumb up against the side of the spinous process, thereby preventing the rotation induced by the mobilization of the superior segment. For example, if the left side of C4–5 is being mobilized into extension, left side-flexion, and left rotation by the upper hand, the thumb of the inferior hand is pushed against the right side of the C5 spinous process, preventing rotation of C5 to the right (Figure 14–19).

Supine Mobilization Technique to Restore Extension and Right Side-flexion/Rotation[160] The patient is positioned in supine with the head supported on a pillow. The clinician stands at the patient's head, facing the shoulders. With the radial aspect of the right index finger, the clinician palpates the spinous process and the right inferior articular process of the C4 vertebra. With the other hand, the clinician supports the head and neck superior to the level being treated. An incongruent lock of the superior segment is accomplished by right side-flexing and left rotating the C3–4 joint complex, leaving the craniovertebral joints in a neutral position. The motion barrier for extension/right side-flexion/right rotation of C4–5 is then localized by pushing the right inferior articular process of C4 posterior-inferior-medially on C5.

- *Passive.* The clinician applies a grade I to V force to the C4 vertebra to produce a posterior-inferior-medial glide of the right zygapophysial joint at C4–5.
- *Active.* From the motion barrier, the patient is asked to turn the eyes in a direction that facilitates further

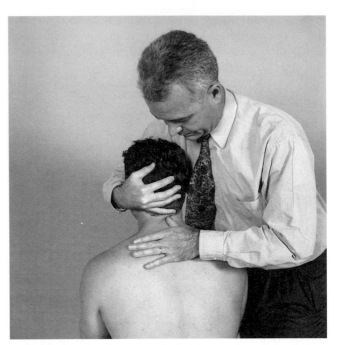

FIGURE 14–19 Patient and clinician position for seated mobilization technique into extension and left side-flexion at C4–5.

extension/right side-flexion/right rotation. The isometric contraction is held for up to 5 seconds and followed by a period of complete relaxation. The joint is then passively taken to the new motion barrier. The technique is repeated three times and followed by a reexamination.

Supine Thrust Technique to Increase Right Rotation at C4–5 The patient is positioned in supine, with the clinician at the head of the table. The clinician supports the patient's head with both hands. The posterior arches of C4 are located with both index fingers, and each thumb rests on the patient's jaw line. The index fingers maintain contact with C4, while the C4–5 segment is lifted toward the ceiling and placed into an extended position using both hands. The lock from above is applied using a combined motion of side-flexion to the left and rotation to the right, until motion is felt at C4 by the right index finger (Figure 14–20). The slack is taken up by the clinician, and the thrust is applied by moving the neck and C4 posteriorly and inferiorly (in the direction of the left hip) into right rotation (extension at the right joint of C4–5), thereby moving the right facet along the plane of its joint. This is an arthrokinematic mobilization. The technique can be graded from I to V. Care must be taken not to be over aggressive with this technique as the joint is in its close-packed position and the bones could be excessively impacted.

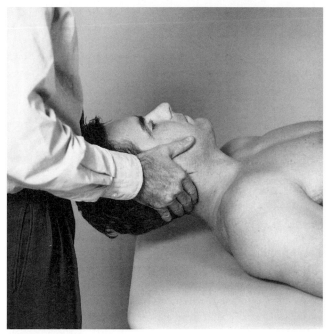

FIGURE 14–20 Patient and clinician position for supine thrust technique at C4–5.

Uncovertebral Mobilization As these joints do not flex or extend to any significant degree, but take part in side-flexion by gliding inferior medially on the ipsilateral side and superior-laterally on the contralateral side, it really does not matter whether the segment is flexed or extended. However, these impairments may actually be a disc protrusion that has been incorrectly diagnosed. To still do the right thing for the wrong reasons, the technique is better applied in extension.[48]

This is an axial technique utilizing the arthrokinematics of the affected side-flexion. The segment is extended, ipsilateral side-flexed, and contralaterally translated. The clinician stabilizes the segments below with one hand and applies a graded inferior-medial pressure to the ipsilateral transverse process while maintaining the translation force.

Techniques to Restore Motion in the Anterior Quadrant

Mobilization Technique to Restore Flexion, Left Side-flexion/Rotation in Supine The patient is positioned in supine with the head supported, and the clinician stands at the head of the table facing the patient. The C4–5 segment is flexed, left side-flexed, and right translated to bring the right joint to its flexion barrier. The clinician hooks a finger tip under the right articular process and lays a finger tip pad over the articular process on the left. The mobilization is achieved by pulling the right process cranially as

steady, light pressure is applied to the back of the left process to maintain a normal axis of motion.

Mobilization Technique to Restore Flexion, Left Side-flexion/Rotation in Supine[160] The patient is positioned in supine with the head supported, and the clinician stands at the head of the table facing the patient. With the radial aspect of the right index finger, the clinician palpates the inferior articular process and lamina of the C4 vertebra on the right. With the other hand, the clinician supports the head and neck cranial to the level being treated. An incongruent lock of the cranial segment is accomplished by applying right side-flexing and left rotating the C3–4 joint complex, leaving the craniovertebral joints in a neutral position. The motion barrier for flexion, left rotation, and left side-flexion of C4–5 is localized by passively gliding the right inferior articular process of the C4 vertebra superior-anterior-medially on the superior articular process of C5.

- *Passive.* A grade I to V mobilization force is applied to the C4 vertebra to produce a superior-anterior-medial glide of the right zygapophyseal joint at C4–5.
- *Active.* At the motion barrier, the patient is asked to turn the eyes in a direction that facilitates further flexion/left side-flexion/rotation at C4–5. The isometric contraction is held for up to 5 seconds and followed by a period of complete relaxation. The joint is then passively taken to the new motion barrier. This technique is repeated three times and followed by a reexamination function.

Mobilization Technique to Restore Flexion, Left Side-flexion/Rotation in Sitting The patient is positioned in sitting and the clinician stands on the right side. With one hand, the clinician stabilizes the C5 segment using a lumbrical grip. The other hand reaches around the head of the patient, securing it to the clinician's chest, and the fifth finger is applied to the left transverse process and neural arch of C4. The C4–5 segment is then left side-flexed, flexed, and right translated to the barrier of the right joint. The mobilization is carried out by the clinician applying pressure against left transverse process and neural arch of C4, producing right translation.

Mobilization Technique to Restore Flexion, Left Side-flexion/Rotation in Sitting[160] The patient is positioned in sitting and the clinician stands on the right side. With one hand, the clinician stabilizes the C5 segment using a lumbrical grip. The other hand reaches around the head of the patient, securing it to the clinician's chest, and the ulnar border of the fifth finger is applied to the laminae and inferior articular processes of the C4 vertebra. The rest of the hand supports the cranium and the upper cervical spine. While fixing C5, the neck is flexed into the C4–5 segment motion barrier.

● *Passive.* A grade I to IV mobilization force is applied to the C4 vertebra to produce a superior-anterior glide at the zygapophyseal joints, thus flexing the C4–5 joint complex and feeling the spinous processes separate.

● *Active.* At the motion barrier, the patient is instructed to turn the eyes in a direction that facilitates further flexion at C4–5. The isometric contraction is held for up to 5 seconds and followed by a period of complete relaxation. The joint is then passively taken to the new motion barrier. The technique is repeated three times and followed by a reexamination of function.

Distraction Thrust Technique to Restore Anterior Glide on the Right The patient is positioned in supine, with the clinician at the head of the table. The clinician supports the patient's head in the hands and contact is made, using a wide lumbrical pinch grip of the right hand, with the upper bone of the segment to be mobilized (C4). The clinician places the right hand on the patient's right cheek. The patient's neck is then fully flexed up from below, beyond the cranial bone (C4) before being unflexed (extended), so that the segment to be mobilized (C4–5) is in neutral (feels slack), thereby utilizing a ligamentous lock of the neck below the caudal bone of the segment in question. Locking from above then takes place. While the clinician maintains contact with the right hand grip on C4, he or she moves to the right-hand side of the patient. The clinician then supports the patient's head with the left arm and forearm, wrapping around the left side of the patient's face and grasping the chin. Noncongruent locking from above is achieved with right side-flexion and then slight left rotation down to the point where motion is felt to occur at the upper segment (C4). Three possibilities now exist for the clinician.

1. A distraction thrust, applied with the thrusting arm parallel to the sternum and the other hand and arm moving in concert.

2. A "glide thrust," applied in line with the plane of the C4–5 zygapophyseal joint, toward the opposite eye of the patient.

3. A thrust applied across the segment, at right angles to the joint, thereby gapping the joint on the opposite side to the direction of the side-flexion (in this case, the left joint) into further side-flexion. This technique is only used if the side-flexion cannot be obtained to the side of the thrust.

Thrust Technique to Restore Right Rotation at C3–4 The patient is positioned in supine, with the clinician at the head of the table. The clinician supports the patient's head in both hands. Contact of the posterior arches of C3 is made with both index fingers, each thumb resting on the patient's jaw line. C3 is then lifted toward the ceiling into extension, thereby increasing the lordosis. The joints below C3 are now flexed. The barrier on the left is engaged from above through side-flexion to the left and rotating to the right down to C3. Once the slack has been taken up, the thrust is then applied by "flicking" the neck into right rotation in the direction of the right eye, thereby moving the left facet along the plane of its joint.

Specific Traction

The specific traction technique is used for acutely painful joints, for a trial traction treatment, or if mechanical traction is not feasible for one reason or another and the condition of the other segments in the neck demands that they be protected. The technique can be applied either in sitting or supine, with the force easier to control in sitting, but more force available in lying. Specific technique produces a distraction between the centra and a superior glide at the zygapophysial joint. A symmetrical lock of flexion or extension is used and will depend on the tolerance of the patient. The C4–5 level is used in the following example.

The patient is seated and the clinician stands to the side of the patient. Using one hand, the clinician stabilizes C5 with full lumbrical grip. Using the other hand, the clinician wraps around the front of the patient's face and places the little finger around as much of the C4 segment as possible. The patient's head is gently squeezed against the chest of the clinician and is gently flexed until the C4 segment is felt to move. To perform a grade I distraction, the clinician takes a deep breath. The technique is continued for a few minutes and the patient's response is monitored.

Soft Tissue Techniques

A variety of soft tissue techniques are at the disposal of the clinician.[177] The choice of technique depends on the goals of the treatment and the dysfunction being treated.

Reflex Spasm This is an involuntary muscle contraction and serves as a protective mechanism in the presence of intense nociception. The muscle is typically tender to palpation. Deep tissue massage is one of the most effective tools to reduce spasm[178] and promote pain reduction.[179] It is recommended that the patient's symptomatic response to the treatment be closely monitored, as there is a risk of further traumatizing the tissues in a patient with an acute soft tissue injury.

Myofascial Trigger Points A myofascial trigger point is a localized contracture of a fascicle of muscle fibers that causes congestion to develop in a focal area, leading to ischemia and metabolite accumulation. Arguably the best method for treating a myofascial trigger point is the application of direct pressure to the trigger point to produce an ischemic compression. It is important that the pressure applied is not so great as to cause significant pain for the patient. The pressure is held for 5 to 7 seconds and then quickly withdrawn. The procedure is repeated on each trigger point. After each trigger point has been treated, the clinician returns to the first trigger point. The procedure is repeated three times on each trigger point.

Muscle Tightness   A tight muscle is a muscle that is hypertonic in addition to being shortened. The recommended treatment for muscle tightness is the postfacilitation stretch (PFS) technique developed by Janda.

- The patient and the muscle being treated must be completely at rest.
- The clinician is positioned so that he or she can provide resistance to a strong muscle contraction by the patient.
- The muscle to be treated is placed in its mid-range.
- The patient is asked to perform a maximal contraction of the muscle. If the clinician is unable to resist a maximal contraction, a submaximal one is used. The contraction is held for 10 seconds. After the contraction, the patient is instructed to completely let go of the muscle.
- When the clinician is sure that the muscle is completely relaxed, a fast stretch is applied to it and the stretch is held for 10 to 15 seconds.
- The muscle is returned to its mid-range.
- The procedure is repeated 3 to 5 times.

Case Study: Neck Pulsing

Subjective
A 37-year-old woman presented to the office complaining that her head "wanted to go back." Her symptoms began approximately 6 months earlier with painless "pulsing" on the left side of her neck that became worse with stressful situations and physical activity, but were relieved by relaxation and sleep. She could briefly stop the pulsing by placing her hand on the right posterior aspect of the neck. Her symptoms had progressed to an extension of the neck with spasm, which caused her to lean forward to maintain eye contact with others. She also noted an occasional "eye tic," which seemed to come and go spontaneously. She denied any paresthesias, weakness, dysphasia, visual changes or hearing loss, or bowel or bladder changes. Although she had no family history of specific neurologic problems, the patient

reported a maternal aunt who had "facial tics." The patient had a medical history notable for anxiety and several phobias for which she had received psychological counseling.

Objective
On physical examination, her neck was extended, side-flexed slightly to the left, and rotated to the right, and there was a palpable spasm and hypertrophy of the left cervical paravertebral musculature. She had full range of motion of the neck in all planes with infact motor strength, and there were no other motor or sensory deficits. Cranial nerve tests and reflexes were normal bilaterally, and no other tremor, tic, or dystonia was observed.

Evaluation
A diagnosis of spasmodic torticollis was made. Given the fact that this patient had no sensory, motor, or range-of-motion deficits, the case was discussed with her physician. The physician agreed to a trial period of physical therapy using the principles of positive practice.[87]

Intervention

- Electrotherapeutic modalities and thermal agents. A moist heat pack was applied to the left side of the cervical spine when the patient arrived for each treatment session. Ultrasound at 3 MHz was administered to the cervical musculature on the left side of the neck for 10 minutes following the moist heat.
- Manual therapy. Following the ultrasound, soft tissue techniques of massage and gentle stretching were performed. The neck was gently stretched into flexion, right side-flexion, and left rotation.
- Therapeutic exercises. The patient performed repetitive active range-of-motion exercises into the combined motion of flexion, right side-flexion, and left rotation against the spasming muscle group.
- Patient-related instruction. Explanation was given as to the potential causes of the patient's symptoms. The patient was advised to perform the active range-of-motion exercises as many times as possible when in the upright position. Her husband was instructed on the stretching and massage techniques. The patient also received instruction on the use of heat at home. Instructions to sleep on the left side using a medium sized pillow were given.
- Goals and outcomes. Both the patient's goals from the treatment and the expected therapeutic goals from the clinician were discussed with the patient. It was concluded that the clinical sessions would occur until the patient, and her husband, felt comfortable being able to perform the treatment protocol independently, at which time, the patient would be discharged

to a home exercise program. The patient attended therapy sessions for six visits. At a 2-month follow-up, the patient reported a marked improvement in her symptoms, but noticed that they returned in a few days if the exercise regime was not continued.

Case Study: Right-sided Neck Pain

Subjective

A 45-year old woman awoke with right-sided neck pain 3 days earlier. The pain was felt over the right neck on an intermittent basis. She related that the pain was worse with head turning to the right, and further aggravated with activities involving cervical extension. She described no neurologic pain or paresthesia. The pain sites and intensity were unchanged since the onset.

Further questioning revealed that the patient was otherwise in good health and had no reports of bowel or bladder impairment, night pain, dizziness, or radicular symptoms.

Questions

1. What structure(s) could be at fault with complaints of right-sided neck pain?
2. What should the motion pattern of the pain tell you?
3. What is your working hypothesis at this stage? List the various diagnoses that could present with right-sided neck pain and the tests you would use to rule out each one.
4. What do the questions with regard to night pain and dizziness pertain to?
5. Does this presentation and history warrant a scan? Why or why not?

Examination

There was nothing suggestive in the history that would indicate the need for a scan at this time. A biomechanical examination was initiated and revealed the following.

- Active range of motion into flexion and left rotation and left side-flexion were normal.
- Extension was limited to about 50% of normal and reproduced the right-sided neck pain.
- Right rotation and right side-flexion were limited to about 50% of normal and reproduced the pain in the right neck and supraspinatus fossa.
- Passive physiologic intervertebral mobility tests revealed a hypomobility at the right zygapophysial joints of C3–4.
- The pain in the right side of the neck and supraspinatus fossa was reproduced with passive articular intervertebral mobility test with posterior glides of the right zygapophysial joints of C3–4.

Questions

1. Did the biomechanical examination confirm your working hypothesis? How?
2. Given the findings from the biomechanical examination, what is the diagnosis, or is further testing warranted in the form of special tests?

Evaluation

The findings from the biomechanical examination indicate an extension and right side-flexion hypomobility at C3–4.

Questions

1. Having confirmed the diagnosis, what will be your intervention?
2. How would you describe this condition to the patient?
3. In order of priority, and based on the stages of healing, list the various goals of your intervention?
4. How will you determine the amplitude and joint position for the intervention?
5. What would you tell the patient about your intervention
6. Is an asymmetrical or symmetrical technique more appropriate for this condition? Why?
7. Estimate this patient's prognosis.
8. What modalities could you use in the intervention of this patient?
9. What exercises would you prescribe?

Intervention

- Electrotherapeutic modalities and thermal agents. A moist heat pack was applied to the cervical spine when the patient arrived for each treatment session. Ultrasound at 3 MHz was administered for 5 minutes over the right side of the C3–4 segment following the moist heat. An ice pack was applied to the area at the end of the treatment session.
- Manual therapy. Following the ultrasound, soft tissue techniques were applied to the area followed by a specific asymmetrical mobilization of the C3–4 segment into extension and right side-flexion.
- Therapeutic exercises of active range of motion of the cervical spine were prescribed. These were progressed to isometric resistive throughout the range. Exercises for the major muscle groups of the neck and shoulder were also prescribed. In addition, aerobic exercises using a stationary bike and upper body ergometer (UBE) were prescribed.
- Patient-related instruction. Explanation was given as to the cause of the patient's symptoms. The patient was advised against sudden turning of the head to the

right. The patient was advised to continue the exercise at home, 3 to 5 times each day and to expect some post-exercise soreness. The patient also received instruction on the use of heat and ice at home.

- Goals and outcomes. Both the patient's goals from the treatment and the expected therapeutic goals from the clinician were discussed with the patient. It was concluded that the clinical sessions would occur three times per week for 1 month, at which time, the patient would be discharged to a home exercise program. With adherence to the instructions and exercise program, it was felt that the patient would make a full return to function.

REVIEW QUESTIONS

1. Contraction of one sternocleidomastoid muscle results in:
   a. Rotation of the face to the same side
   b. Lateral flexion of the head and neck to the same side
   c. Flexion of the head and neck
   d. Rotation of the face to the opposite side
2. The scalene muscles act to produce lateral neck flexion or rotation to the opposite side. Which structure(s) pass(es) between the scalenus anticus and scalenus medius muscles?
   a. Thoracic duct
   b. Subclavian artery
   c. Carotid artery
   d. Brachial plexus
3. Functions of the subclavius muscle include:
   a. Depression of the clavicle
   b. Helping to retain the sternal end of the clavicle in place
   c. Affording protection to the subclavian artery in fractures of the clavicle
   d. Assisting in flexion of the shoulder when the shoulder is internally rotated
4. The following group of muscles perform cervical rotation to the opposite side?
   a. Longus capitis, rectus capitis anterior and posterior
   b. Splenius cervicis, splenius capitis
   c. Sternocleidomastoid, scalenus anterior, rectus capitis
   d. Sternocleidomastoid, scalenus anterior, rectus capitis anterior
5. Muscle that is thin and sheet-like with fibers that extend from the chest upward over the neck is:
   a. Levator scapula
   b. Buccinator
   c. Orbicularis oris
   d. Platysma
6. T___F___ The nerve supply for the platysma is the accessory nerve.
7. What are the nerve roots for the phrenic nerve?
8. T___ F___ The trapezius rotates the glenoid cavity of the scapula downward.
9. What is the action of the SCM?
10. In the mid-lower cervical spine, an ERS L would produce which motion restrictions?
11. Which process is thought to help prevent cervical disc protrusions?

ANSWERS

1. c.
2. c.
3. a.
4. c.
5. d.
6. False.
7. C3–5.
8. False.
9. Ipsilateral side-flexion, contralateral rotation.
10. Flexion, right rotation, and right side-flexion.
11. Uncinate.

REFERENCES

1. Takala J, Sievers K, Klaukka T. Rheumatic symptoms in the middle-aged population in southwestern Finland. *Scand J Rheumatol* 1982;47(suppl):15–29.
2. Westerling D, Jonsson BG. Pain from the neck-shoulder region and sick leave. *Scand J Soc Med* 1980;8:131–136.
3. Jackson R. Cervical trauma: Not just another pain in the neck. *Geriatrics* 1982;37:123–126.
4. Heine J. Uber die arthritis deformans. *Virchows Arch Pathol Anat* 1926;260:521–663.
5. Schmorl G, Junghann H. Clinique et radiologic de la colonne vertébrale normale et pathologique Paris, Doin ed. 1956.
6. Takala EP. Assessment of neck-shoulder disorders in occupational health care practice. Helsinki: University of Helsinki; 1991:69.
7. Berg HE, Berggren G, Tesch PA. Dynamic neck strength training effect on pain and function. *Arch Phys Med Rehabil* 1994;75:661–665.
8. Dyrssen T, Svedenkrans M, Paasikivi J. Muskelträning vid besvär I nacke och skuldror effektiv behandling för att minska smärtan. Läkartidningen 1989;86:2116–2120.
9. Aker PD, Gross AR, Goldsmith CH, Peloso P. Conservative management of mechanical neck pain: systematic overview and meta-analysis. *BMJ* 1996;313:1291–1296.

10. Gross AR, Aker PD, Goldsmith CH, Peloso P. Conservative management of mechanical neck disorders. A systematic overview and meta-analysis. *Online J Curr Clin Trials* 1996;doc no. 200–201.

11. Levoska S, Keinänen-Kiukaanniemi S. Active or passive physiotherapy for occupational cervicobrachial disorders? A comparison of two treatment methods with a 1-year follow-up. *Arch Phys Med Rehabil* 1993; 74:425–430.

12. Provinciali L, Baroni M, Illuminati L, Ceravolo G. Multimodal treatment of whiplash injury. *Scand J Rehabil Med* 1996;28:105–111.

13. Pratt N. *Anatomy of the Cervical Spine*. APTA Orthopedic Section, Physical Therapy Home Study Course LaCrosse, Wisconsin 96-1;1996:1–26.

14. Pal GP, Sherk HH. The vertical stability of the cervical spine. *Spine* 1988;13:447.

15. Hoppenfeld S. *Physical Examination of the Spine and Extremities*. New York, Appleton-Century-Crofts; 1976.

16. Taylor JR, Twomey L. Sagittal and horizontal plane movement of the lumbar vertebral column in cadavers and in the living. *Rheum Rehab* 1980;19:223.

17. Van Mameren H, Drukker J, Sanches H, Beurgsgens J. Cervical spine motions in the sagittal plane. I: ranges of motion of actually performed movements, an x-ray cine study. *Eur J Morphol* 1990;28:47–68.

18. Penning L: *Functional Pathology of the Cervical Spine*. Excerpta Medica Foundation. Baltimore: Williams & Wilkins; 1968.

19. Lysell E. Motion in the cervical spine: an experimental study on autopsy specimens. *Acta Orthop Scand* 1969;123:1.

20. Ashton IK, Ashton BA, Gibson SJ, et al. Morphological basis for back pain: the demonstration of nerve fibres and neuropeptides in the lumbar facet joint but not in ligamentum flavum. *J Orthop Res* 1992;10:72–78.

21. Mercer S, Bogduk N. Intra-articular inclusions of the cervical synovial joints. *Br J Rheumat* 1993;32: 705–710.

22. Giles LG, Taylor JR. Innervation of human lumbar zygapophysial joint synovial folds. *Acta Orthop Scand* 1987;58:43–46.

23. William PL, Warwick R, Dyson M, Bannister LH. *Gray's Anatomy*. 37th ed. Edinburgh: Churchill Livingstone; 1989.

24. Orofino C, Sherman MS, Schechter D. Luschka's joint—a degenerative phenomenon. *J Bone Joint Surg* 1960;5A:853–858.

25. Hayashi K, Yabuki T. Origin of the uncus and of Luschka's joint in the cervical spine. *J Bone Joint Surg* 1985;67A:788–791.

26. Porterfield JA, DeRosa C. *Mechanical Neck Pain*. Philadelphia: Saunders; 1995.

27. Panjabi MM, Duranceau J, Goel V, et al. Cervical human vertebrae. Quantitative three-dimensional anatomy of the middle and lower regions. *Spine* 1991;16:861–869.

28. Bayley JC, Yoo JU, Kruger DM, et al. The role of distraction in improving the space available for the cord in cervical spondylosis. *Spine* 1995;20:771–775.

29. Milne N. The role of zygapophysial joint orientation and uncinate processes in controlling motion in the cervical spine. *J Anat* 1991;178:189–201.

30. Argenson C, Francke JP, Sylla S, et al. The vertebral arteries (segment VI and V2). *Anat Clin* 1980;2:29–41.

31. Johnson RM, Crelin ES, White AA, et al. Some new observations on the functional anatomy of the lower cervical spine. *Clin Orth Rel Res* 1975;111:192–200.

32. Buckworth J. Anatomy of the suboccipital region. Vernon H, ed. In *Upper Cervical Syndrome*. Baltimore: Williams & Wilkins; 1998.

33. Hollinshead WH. *Anatomy for Surgeons: Vol 3, The Back and Limbs*. Philadelphia: Lippincott; 1982.

34. Fielding JW, Burstein AA, Frankel VH. The nuchal ligament. *Spine* 1976;1:3–11.

35. Penning L. Normal movements of the cervical spine. *J Roentgenol* 1978;130:317–326.

36. Hadley LA. Intervertebral joint subluxation, bony impingement and foramen encroachment with nerve root changes. *Am J Roentgenol* 1951;65:377–402.

37. Ferguson RJ, Caplan LR. Cervical spondylitic myelopathy: history and physical findings. Neurologic clinics 1985;3(2):373–382.

38. Yoo, JU, Zou, D, Edwards T, et al. Effect of cervical motion on the neuroforaminal dimensions of the human cervical spine. *Spine* 1992;17:1131–1136.

39. Le Gros Clark WE. Central nervous system. Hamilton WJ, ed. In *Textbook of Human Anatomy* 2nd ed. Saint Louis; CV Mosby, 1976

40. Travell JG, Simons DG. *Myofascial Pain and Dysfunction—The Trigger Point Manual*. Baltimore: Williams & Wilkins; 1983.

41. Fitzgerald MJT, Comerford PT, Tuffery AR. Sources of innervation of the neuromuscular spindles in sternomastoid and trapezius. *J Anat* 1982;134:471–490.

42. Kendall FP, Kendall KM, Provance PG. *Muscles: Testing and Function*. 4th ed. Baltimore: Williams & Wilkins; 1993.

43. Porterfield JA, DeRosa. *Mechanical Neck Pain*. Philadelphia: Saunders; 1995.

44. Ehrhardt R, Bowling R. Treatment of the cervical spine. APTA Orthopedic Section, Physical Therapy Home Study Course LaCrosse, Wisconsin 96-1, 1996: 1–28.

45. Raper AJ, Thompson WT, shapiro W, et al. Scalene and sternomastoid muscle function. *J Appl Physiol* 1966;21:497–502.

46. Hiatt JL, Gartner LP. *Textbook of Head and Neck Anatomy.* Baltimore: Williams & Wilkins; 1987.

47. Adams CBT, Logue V. Studies in spondylotic myelopathy 2. The movement and contour of the spine in relation to the neural complications of cervical spondylosis. *Brain* 1971;94:569–586.

48. Meadows J, Pettman E, Fowler C. *Manual Therapy: NAIOMT Level II & III Course Notes.* Denver 1995.

49. Dreyer SJ, Boden SD. Nonoperative treatment of neck and arm pain. *Spine* 1998:23:2746–2754.

50. Aprill C, Dwyer A, Bogduk N. Cervical zygapophyseal joint pain patterns II: a clinical evaluation. *Spine* 1990;15:458–561.

51. Dwyer A, Aprill C, Bogduk N. Cervical zygapophseal joint pain patterns I: a study in normal volunteers. *Spine* 1990;15:453–457.

52. Jull G, Bogduk N, Marsland A. The accuracy of manual diagnosis for cervical zygapophyseal joint pain syndromes . *Med J Aust* 1988;148:233–236.

53. Barnsley L, Bogduk N. Medial branch blocks are specific for the diagnosis of cervical zygapophyseal joint pain. *Reg Anesth* 1993;18:343–350.

54. Black KM, McClure P, Polansky M. The influence of different sitting positions on cervical and lumbar posture. *Spine* 1996;21:65–70.

55. Grieve G. Common patterns of clinical presentation. In: Grieve GP, ed. *Common Vertebral Joint Problems.* 2nd ed. London: Churchill Livingstone; 1988:283–302.

56. Kendall FP, Kendall-McCreary E. *Muscles: Testing and Function.* 3rd ed. Baltimore: William & Wilkins; 1983.

57. Stratton SA, Bryan JM. Dysfunction, evaluation, and treatment of the cervical spine and thoracic inlet. In: Donatelli B, Wooden M, eds. *Orthopaedic Physical Therapy.* 2nd ed. New York: Churchill Livingstone; 1993:77–122.

58. Janda V. *Muscle Function Testing.* London: Butterworths; 1983.

59. Saunders H. *Evaluation, Treatment and Prevention of Musculoskeletal Disorders.* 2nd ed. Minneapolis: Viking Press; 1985.

60. Press JM, Herring SA, Kibler WB. *Rehabilitation of Musculoskeletal Disordres. The Textbook of Military Medicine.* Washington, DC: Borden Institute. Office of the Surgeon General; 1996.

61. Bush K, Hillier S. Outcome of cervical radiculopathy treated with periradicular/epidural corticosteroid injections: a prospective study with independent clinical review. *Eur Spine J* 1996;5:319–325.

62. Dillin W, Booth R, Cuckeler J, Balderston R, Simeon F, Roth R. Cervical radiculopathy: a review. *Spine* 1986;11:988–991.

63. Bogduk N, Lord SM, Barnsley L. Authors response letter re: chronic zygapophyseal joint pain after whiplash: a placebo-controlled prevalence study. *Spine* 1997;22:1420–1421.

64. Hubbard DR, Berkhoff GM Myofascial trigger points show spontaneous needle EMG activity. *Spine* 1993; 18:1803–1807.

65. Freundlich B, Leventhal L. The fibromyalgia syndrome. In: Schumacher HR, Klippel JH, Koopman WJ, eds. *Primer on the Rheumatic Diseases.* 10th ed. Atlanta: Arthritis Foundation; 1993:227–230.

66. Farney RJ, Walker JM. Office management of common sleep/wake disorders. *Med Clin North Am.* 1995; 79:391–414.

67. Smith DL, DeMario MC. Spasmodic torticollis: a case report and review of therapies. *J Am Board Fam Pract* 1996;9:435–441.

68. Britton TC. Torticollis—what is straight ahead? *Lancet* 1998;351:1223–1224.

69. Ackerman J, Chau V, Gilbert-Barness E. Pathological case of the month. Congenital muscular torticollis. *Arch Pediatr Adolesc Med.* 1996;150:1101–1102.

70. Kiesewetter WB, Nelson PK, Pallandino VS, Koop CE. Neonatal torticollis. *JAMA* 1955;157:1281–1285.

71. Gorlin RJ, Cohen MM, Levin LS. *Syndromes of the Head and Neck.* 3rd ed. New York: Oxford University Press; 1990.

72. Davids JR, Wegner DR, Mubarak SJ. Congenital muscular torticollis: sequela of intrauterine or perinatal compartment syndrome. *J Pediatr Orthop* 1993;13: 141–147.

73. Morrison DL, MacEwen GD. Congenital muscular torticollis: observations regarding clinical findings, associated conditions, and results of treatment. *J Pediatr Orthop* 1982;2:500–505.

74. Wilson BC, Jarvis BL, Haydon RC. Nontraumatic subluxation of the atlantoaxial joint: Grisel's syndrome. *Larynoscope* 1987;96:705–708.

75. Lowenstein DH, Aminoff MJ. The clinical course of spasmodic torticollis. *Neurology* 1988;38:530–532.

76. Rondot P, Marchand MP, Dellatolas G. Spasmodic torticollis—review of 220 patients. *Can J Neurol Sci* 1991;18:143–151.

77. Colbassani HJ Jr, Wood JH. Management of spastic torticollis. *Surg Neurol* 1986;25:153–158.

78. Adams RD, Victor M. *Principles of Neurology.* 5th ed. New York: McGraw-Hill; 1993:93–94.

79. Jahanshahi M, Marion MH, Marsden CD. Natural history of adult-onset idiopathic torticollis. *Arch Neurol* 1990;47:548–552.

80. Leplow B, Stubinger C. Visuospatial functions in patients with spasmodic torticollis. *Percept Motor Skill* 1994;78:1363–1375.

81. Anastasopoulos D, Bhatia K, Bronstein AM, Marsden CD, Gresty MA. Perception of spatial orientation in spasmodic torticollis. Part 2: the visual vertical. *Mov Disord* 1997;12:709–714.

82. Anastasopoulos D, Nasios G, Psilas K, Mergner Th, Maurer C, Lucking CH. What is straight ahead to a patient with torticollis? *Brain* 1998;121:91–101.

83. Anastopoulos D, Bhatia K, Bisdorff A, Bronstein AM, Marsden CD, Gresty MA. Perception of spatial orientation in spasmodic torticollis. Part 1: the postural vertical. *Move Disord* 1997;12:561–569.

84. Anderson TJ, Rivest J, Stell R, et al. Botulinum toxin treatment of spasmodic torticollis. *J R Soc Med* 1992;85:524–529.

85. Boghen D, Flanders M. Effectiveness of botulinum toxin in the treatment of spasmodic torticollis. *Eur Neurol* 1993;33:199–203.

86. Ozelius L, Kramer PL, Moskowitz CB, et al. Human gene for torsion dystonia located on chromosome 9q32-q34. *Neuron* 1989;2:1427–1434.

87. Spencer J, Goetsch VL, Brugnoli RJ, Herman S. Behavior therapy for spasmodic torticollis: a case study suggesting a causal role for anxiety. *J Behav Ther Exp Psychiatry* 1991;22:305–311.

88. Agras S, Marshall C. The application of negative practice to spasmodic torticollis. *Am J Psychiatry* 1965;121:579–582.

89. Leplow B. Heterogeneity of biofeedback training effects in spasmodic torticollis: a single-case approach. *Behav Res Ther* 1990;28:359–365.

90. Friedman MH, Nelson AJ Jr. Head and neck pain review: traditional and new perspectives. *J Orthop Sport Phys Ther.* 1996;24:268–278.

91. Meadows J: *Manual Therapy: Biomechanical Assessment and Treatment—a Rationale and Complete Approach to the Acute and Sub-acute Post-MVA Cervical Patient.* Supplement to Swodeam Consulting Video Series, Alberta, Canada 1995.

92. Barton CW. Evaluation and treatment of headache patients in the emergency department: a survey. *Headache* 1994;34:91–94.

93. Robinson. R. Pain relief for headaches: is self-medication a problem? *Can Fam Physician* 1993;39:867–872.

94. Oates LN, Scholz MJ, Hoffert MJ. Polypharmacy in a headache centre population. *Headache* 1993;33:436–438.

95. Thomas SH, Stone CK. Emergency department treatment of migraine, tension and mixed-type headache. *J Emerg Med* 1994;12:657–664.

96. Appenzeller O. Getting a sore head from banging it on the wall. Editorial. *Headache* 1973;13:77–78.

97. Raskin NH. *Headache.* 2nd ed. New York: Churchill Livingstone, 1988:269–281.

98. Lance JW. *Mechanism and Management of Headache.* 5th ed. Oxford: Butterworth-Heinemann, 1993;206–214.

99. Appenzeller O. Post-traumatic headaches. In: Dalessio DJ, ed. *Wolff's Headache and Other Head Pain.* 5th ed. New York: Oxford University Press, 1987: 289–303.

100. Yamaguchi M. Incidence of headache and severity of head injury. *Headache* 1992;32:427–431.

101. Packard RC. Posttraumatic headache: permanency and relationship to legal settlement. *Headache* 1992;32:496–500.

102. Barnsley L, Lord S, Bogduk N. The pathophysiology of whiplash. In: Malanga GA, ed. *Cervical Flexion-Extension/Whiplash Injuries. Spine: State of the Art Reviews.* Vol 12. Philadelphia: Hanley & Belfus; 1998: 209–242.

103. Headache Classification Committee of the International Headache Society. Classification and diagnostic criteria for headache disorders, cranial neuralgias and facial pain. 1st ed. *Cephalalgia* 1988;7:1–551.

104. Maimaris C, Barnes MR, Allen MJ. "Whiplash injuries" of the neck: a retrospective study. *Injury* 1988;19:393–396.

105. Martin PR, Nathan PR, Milech D, van Keppel M. The relationship between headaches and mood. *Behav Res Ther* 1988;26:353–356.

106. Arena JG, Blanchard EB, Andrasik F. The role of affect in the etiology of chronic headache. *J Psychosom Res* 1984;28:79–86.

107. Edmeads J. The cervical spine and headache. *Neurology* 1988;38:1874–1878.

108. Bellavance A, Belzilc G, Bergeron Y, Huot J, Meloche J, Morand M. Cervical spine and headaches. *Neurology* 1989;39:1269–1270.

109. Boquet J, Boismare F, Payenneville G, Leclerc D, Monnier J-C, Moore N. Lateralization of headache: possible role of an upper cervical trigger point. *Cephalalgia* 1989;9:15–24.

110. Maigne R. La céphalée sus-orbitaire. Sa fréquente origine cervicale. Son traitement. *Ann Med Phys* 1968;39:241–246.

111. International Headache Society. Headache classification and diagnostic criteria for headache disorders, cranial neuralgias, and facial pain. *Cephalalgia* 1988;8 (suppl):19–22, 71, 72.

112. Mumenthaler M. *Neurology.* Stuttgart: Thieme Medical Publishers; 1990.

113. Ekbom K. Some observations on pain in cluster headache. *Headache* 1975;13:219–225.

114. Cohen MJ, McArthur DL. Classification of migraine and tension headache from a survey of 10,000 headache diaries. *Headache* 1981;21:25–29.

115. Friedman AP. Characteristics of tension headache: a profile of 1420 cases. *Psychosomatics* 1979;20:451–461.

116. Cohen MJ, McArthur DL. Classification of migraine and tension headache from a survey of 10,000 headache diaries. *Headache* 1981;21:25–29.

117. Fredriksen TA, Hovdal H, Sjaastad O. Cervicogenic headache: clinical manifestation. *Cephalalgia* 1987; 7:147–160.

118. Hunter CR, Mayfield FH. Role of the upper cervical roots in the production of pain in the head. *Am J Surg* 1949;48:743–751.

119. Wilson PR. Chronic neck pain and cervicogenic headache. *Clin J Pain* 1991;7:5–11.

120. Friedman MH, Weisberg J. Screening procedures for temporomandibular joint dysfunction. *Am Fam Physician* 1982;25:157–160.

121. Kimmel DL. The cervical sympathetic rami and the vertebral plexus in the human foetus. *J Comp Neurol* 1959;112:141–161.

122. Kerr FWL, Olafsson RA. Trigeminal cervical volleys: convergency on single units in the spinal gray at C1 and C2. *Arch Neurol* 1961;5:171–178.

123. Abrahams VC, Richmond FJR, Rose PK. Absence of monosynaptic reflex in dorsal neck muscles of the cat. *Brain Res* 1975;92:130–131.

124. Friedman MH, Weisberg J. *Temporomandibular Joint Disorders.* Chicago: Quintessence Publishing; 1985: 35,86–91,101–106.

125. Willford CH, Kisner C, Glenn TM, Sachs L. The interaction of wearing multifocal lenses with head posture and pain. *J Orthop Sports Phys Ther* 1996;23: 194–199.

126. Lewit K. Vertebral artery insufficiency and the cervical spine. *Br J Geriatr Prac* 1969;6:37–42.

127. Jull GA. Headaches associated with cervical spine: a clinical review. In Boyling JD, Palastanga N, eds. *Grieve's Modern Manual Therapy.* 2 ed. Edinburgh: Churchill Livingstone; 1994:333–347.

128. Silberstein SD. Tension-type headaches. Headache. 34(8):S2–7,1994

129. Mathew NT, Subits E, Nigam M. Transformation of migraine into daily chronic headache. Analysis of factors. *Headache* 1982;22:66–68.

130. Sheftell FD. Chronic daily headache. *Neurol* 1992;42 (suppl 2):32–36.

131. Kudrow L. Paradoxical effects of frequent analgesic use. *Adv Neurol* 1982;33:335–341.

132. Mathew NT. Chronic refractory headache. *Neurology* 1993;43(suppl 3);S26–S33.

133. Warner JS, Fenichel GM. Chronic post-traumatic headache often a myth? *Neurology* 1996;46:915–916.

134. Saper JR, Magee KR. *Freedom from Headaches.* New York: Simon & Schuster; 1981.

135. Braaf MM, Rosner S. Trauma of the cervical spine as a cause of chronic headache. *J Trauma* 1975;15:441–446.

136. Norris SH, Watt I. The prognosis of neck injuries resulting from rear-end vehicle collisions. *J Bone Joint Surg* 1983;65:608–611.

137. Friedman MH. Atypical facial pain: the consistency of ipsilateral maxillary area tenderness and elevated temperature. *J Am Dental Assoc* 1955;126:855–860.

138. Feinman C, Harris M, Cawley R. Psychogenic facial pain: presentation and treatment. *Br Med J* 1984;288: 436–438.

139. Solomon S, Lipton RB. Atypical facial pain: a review. *Semin Neurol* 1988;8:332–338.

140. Friedman MH, Weintraub MI, Forman S. Atypical facial pain: a localized maxillary nerve disorder? *Am J Pain Man* 1995;4:149–152.

141. Cailliet R. *Neck and Arm Pain.* 3rd ed. Philadelphia: Davis; 1990.

142. Christie HJ, Kumar S, Warren SA. Postural aberrations in low back pain. *Arch Phys Med Rehabil.* 1995; 76:218–224.

143. Nachemson A. In vivo discometry in lumbar discs with irregular nucleograms. Some differences in stress distribution between normal and moderately degenerated discs. Acta Orthop Scand 1965;36(4):418–34.

144. Kirk WS Jr, Calabrese DK. Clinical evaluation of physical therapy in the management of internal derangement of the temporomandibular joint. *J Oral Maxillofac Surg.* 1989;47:113–119.

145. Visscher CM, Huddleston Slater JI, Lobbezoo F, Naeije M. Kinematics of the human mandible for different head postures. *J Oral Rehabil.* 2000;27:299–305.

146. Higbie EJ, Seidel-Cobb D, Taylor LE, Cummings GS. Effect of head position on vertical mandibular opening. *J Orthop Sport Phys Ther.* 1999;29:127–130.

147. Gonzalez HE, Manns A. Forward head posture: its structural and functional influence on the stomatognathic system, a conceptual study. Cranio 1996; 14:71–80.

148. Lee WY, Okeson JP, Lindroth J. The relationship between forward head posture and temporomandibular disorders. *J Orofac Pain* 1995;9:161–167.

149. Braun BL, Amundson LR. Quantitative assessment of head and shoulder posture. *Arch Phys Med Rehabil.* 1989;70:322–329.

150. Willford CH, Kisner C, Glenn TM, Sachs L. The interaction of wearing multifocal lenses with head posture and pain. *J Orthop Sport Phys Ther* 1996;23: 194–199.

151. Geschwing N, Levitsky W. Human brain: left-right asymmeties in temporal speech region. *Science* 1968; 161:186–187.

152. Galaburda AM, Le May M. Right left asymmetries in the brain. *Science* 1978;199(4331):852–856.

153. Le May M. Morphological cerebral asymmetries of modern man, fossil man and nonhuman promate. In: Bledschmidt M, ed. *Ann N Y Acad Sci* 1976;280: 349–366.

154. Bledschmidt M. Principles of biodynamic differentiation in human. In: *Development of the Basicranium*. vol. 4. Bethesda, MD: Nat. Inst. Health; 1976:54–80.

155. Enlow DH. The prenatal and postnatal growth of the basicranium. In: *Development of the Basicranium*. vol. 12. Bethesda, MD: Nat. Inst. Health; 1976:192–204.

156. Delaire J. Malformations faciales et asymétries de la base du crâne. *Rev Stomatol* 1965;66:379–396.

157. Cyriax J. *Textbook of Orthopedic Medicine*. Vol 1, 8th ed. London: Balliere Tindall and Cassell; 1982.

158. Jirout J. The rotational component in the dynamics of the C2–3 spinal segment. *Neuroradiology* 1979; 17:177–181.

159. Mitchell F, Moran PS, Pruzzo NA. *An Evaluation and Treatment Manual of Osteopathic Muscle Energy Procedures*. ICEOP Missouri 1979.

160. Lee DG, Walsh MC. *A Workbook of Manual Therapy Techniques for the Vertebral Column and Pelvic Girdle*. 2nd ed. Vancouver: Nascent; 1996.

161. Gennis P, Miller L, Gallagher EJ, Giglio J, Carter W, Nathanson N. The effect of soft cervical collars on persistent neck pain in patients with whiplash injury. *Acad Emerg Med* 1998;3:568–573.

162. Quebec Task Force on Spinal Disorders. Scientific approach to the assessment and management of activity-related spinal disorders: a monograph for clinicians. Report of the Quebec Task Force on Spinal Disorders. *Spine* 1987;12(suppl):S1–S59.

163. McKinney LA. Early mobilisation and outcome in acute sprains of the neck. *BMJ* 1989;299:1006–1008.

164. McKinney LA, Dornan JO, Ryan M. The role of physiotherapy in the management of acute neck sprains following road-traffic events. *Arch Emerg Med* 1989; 6:27–33.

165. Saal JS, Saal JA, Yurth EF. Nonoperative management of herniated cervical intervertebral disc with radiculopathy. *Spine* 1996;21:1877–1883.

166. Zylbergold RS, Piper MC. Cervical spine disorders. A comparison of three types of traction. *Spine* 1985;10: 867–871.

167. Foley-Nolan D, Moore K, Codd M, Barry C, O'Connor P, Coughlan RJ. Low energy high frequency pulsed electromagnetic therapy for acute whiplash disorders. A double blind randomized controlled study. *Scand J Rehabil Med* 1992;24:51–59.

168. Giebel GD, Edelmann M, Huser R. Sprain of the cervical spine: early functional vs. immobilization treatment (in German). *Zentralbl Chir* 1997;122:512–521.

169. Koes BW, Bouter LM, van Mameren H, et al. The effectiveness of manual therapy, physiotherapy and treatment by the general practitioner for nonspecific back and neck complaints: a randomized clinical trial. *Spine* 1992;17:28–35.

170. Colachis SC, Strohm BR. Cervical traction: relationship of traction time to varied tractive force with constant angle of pull. *Arch Phys Med Rehabil* 1965;46: 815–819.

171. Ellenberg MR, Honet JC, Treanor WJ. Cervical radiculopathy. *Arch Phys Med Rehabil* 1994;75:342–352.

172. Lehmann JF, Silverman DR, et al. Temperature distributions in the human thigh produced by infrared, hot pack and microwave applications. *Arch Phys Med Rehabil* 1966;47:291.

173. Abramson DI, Tuck S, Lee SW, et al. Comparison of wet and dry heat in raising temperature of tissues. *Arch Phys Med Rehabil* 1967;48:654.

174. Arnheim D. Therapeutic modalities. In: Arnheim D, ed. *Modern Principles of Athletic Training*. St. Louis: Times Mirror/Mosby College Publishing; 1989: 350–367.

175. Lehmann J, Warren CG, Scham S. Therapeutic heat and cold. *Clin Orthop* 1974;99:207–226.

176. Prentice W. Therapeutic ultrasound. In: Prentice W, ed. *Therapeutic Modalities in Sports Medicine*. St. Louis: Times Mirror/Mosby College Publishing; 1990: 129–140.

177. Murphy DR. *Conservative Management of Cervical Spine Syndromes*. New York: McGraw-Hill; 2000.

178. Sullivan SJ, Williams LRT, Seaborne DE, Morelli M. Effects of massage on alpha motorneuron excitability. *Phys Ther* 1991;71:555–560.

179. Roy S, Irvin R. *Sports Medicine. Prevention, Evaluation, Management and Rehabilitation*. Englewood Cliffs, NJ: Prentice-Hall; 1983.

180. Cohen JH, Schneider MJ. Receptor-tonus technique. An overview. *Chiro Tech* 1990;2:13–16.

CHAPTER FIFTEEN

The Cervicothoracic Junction

Chapter Objectives

At the completion of this chapter, the reader will be able to:

1. Perform a detailed objective examination of the cervicothoracic musculoskeletal system, including palpation of the articular and soft tissue structures, specific passive mobility and passive articular mobility tests for the intervertebral joints, and stability tests.
2. Perform and interpret the results from combined motion testing.
3. Describe the biomechanics of the cervicothoracic junction, including coupled movements, normal and abnormal joint barriers, kinesiology, and reactions to various stresses.
4. Describe the anatomy of the vertebra, ligaments, and blood and nerve supply that comprise the cervicothoracic junction intervertebral segments.
5. Analyze the total examination data to establish the definitive biomechanical diagnosis.
6. Apply active and passive mobilization techniques and combined movements to the cervicothoracic junction in any position using the correct grade, direction, and duration, and explain the mechanical and physiologic effects.
7. Assess the dynamic postures of the cervicothoracic junction and implement the appropriate correction.
8. Evaluate intervention effectiveness to progress or modify intervention.
9. Plan an effective home program including spinal care, and instruct the patient in same.
10. Record examination data, problems, plans, and procedures in a standardized format.
11. Develop self-reliant examination and intervention strategies.
12. Describe intervention strategies based on clinical findings and established goals.

OVERVIEW

The spine contains four junctions. Each junction is different in posterior element orientation, spinal curvature, and coupling. These junctions, described by Schmorl and Junghanns[1] as ontogenically restless, are often rich in anomalies.[2]

- *Craniovertebral junction:* located between the cervical spine and the atlas, axis, and head. An entire chapter is devoted to this region. (Chapter 18)
- *Cervicothoracic junction:* located between the cervical spine, with its great mobility and the limited motion of the superior thoracic spine. It is the area where the powerful muscles of the upper extremities and shoulder girdle insert. The cervicothoracic junction is detailed in this chapter.
- *Thoracolumbar junction:* located between the thoracic spine and its large capacity for rotation and the lumbar spine with its limited rotation. This region is described in Chapter 16.
- *Lumbosacral junction:* located between the lumbar spine, with its ability to flex and extend and the relative stiffness of the sacrum. The components of this region are described in Chapters 13 and 17.

ANATOMY

As the anatomy of both the cervical and thoracic spines are detailed in other chapters, only the differences specific to these areas are mentioned here.

The cervicothoracic junction, consisting of the C7–T2 levels, forms the thoracic outlet. It is structurally and functionally related to both the cervical and thoracic regions. It is also the area through which the neurovascular structures of the upper extremities pass.

This area is considered by Lewitt[3] to be the third major area of the body for musculoskeletal problems, with the cranioverterbal area and the lumbosacral junction being first and second, respectively.

Notable structural changes in this region include spinous processes that are more elongated, point inferiorly, and lose the characteristic bifid appearance of the cervical spine. In addition, there is typically no transverse foramen and, in the more caudal regions, the uncinate processes diminish in size, before disappearing completely. The costotransverse and costovertebral articulations are found in this region as well as an increasing inclination of the articular facets of the zygapophysial joints. This creates a 60-degree angle toward the coronal plane and a 20-degree turn toward the sagittal plane. The presence of the ribs reduce the amount of available motion while providing additional stability, and movements in all directions between C6 and T3 decrease. The coupling in this area mimics that of the cervical spine.

Manubrium

The manubrium is broad and thick superiorly, and narrower and thinner inferiorly, where it articulates with the body. On either side of the suprasternal notch are articulating facets for the clavicles and below these, are facets for the first rib. On the immediate inferior-lateral aspects of the manubrium are two more small facets for the cartilage of the second rib. The articulation between the manubrium and the superior aspect of the sternum is usually a symphysis, with the ends of the bones being lined with hyaline cartilage, although in about 30% of the population, the joint is synovial.

T1 Vertebra

The first thoracic vertebra (T1) resembles that of C7 and has a whole circular superior costal facet (as opposed to the usual demifacet) for articulation with the whole of the first rib, and a small facet on its inferior aspect for articulation with the second rib. The centrum demonstrates a larger transverse than anterior-posterior dimension of the cervical body, being almost twice as wide as it is long. The spinous process is usually as least as long as that of C7. There are about 32 structures that attach to the first rib and body of T1.[4] Because of the ring-like structure of the thoracic cage, movements of the thoracic vertebrae produce movement anywhere along the ring. This fact is exploited where the palpation of the manubrium can be used as an evaluation tool (see later).

Ribs

The first rib is small but massively built. Being the most curved and the most inferiorly orientated, it slopes sharply downward from its vertebral articulation to the manubrium. The head is small and rounded and articulates only with the T1 vertebra. The second rib, longer than the first, is atypical, with a lack of a twist through its shaft and a small facet on the tubercle. It is attached to the joint by an intra-articular disc and ligament. In about 30% of the population, the disc is reabsorbed and the junction resembles a synovial joint.

The first costal cartilage is the shortest and this, together with the fibrous sternochondral (S-C) joint, contributes to the overall stability of the first ring. The first rib attaches to the manubrium just under the S-C joint and the second rib articulates with the sternum at the sternum-manubrial junction.

Ligaments

The common spinal ligaments are present in the cervicothoracic spine and they perform much the same function as they do elsewhere in the spine.

Muscles

The muscles of the cervicothoracic spine and scapula are described in Chapter 14.

Nerves

The main branches of the spinal nerve are the ventral and dorsal rami. The ventral rami from T2 through T11 become intercostal nerves and supply the body wall of the thorax and part of the abdomen. The ventral rami above T2 and below T11 form the somatic plexuses that innervate the extremities [the anterior primary ramus innervates the skin (dermatome), muscles (myotome), and bone (sclerotome) of the extremities, anterior-lateral trunk, and neck via its lateral and anterior branches]. The distribution of all dorsal rami is similar. The branches of these rami supply the skin of the medial two thirds of the back and neck, the deep muscles of the back and neck (lateral branches), the zygapophysial joints (medial branches),[5] and the ligamentum flavum. As elsewhere, the dermatomes of this region are considered to represent the cutaneous region innervated by one spinal nerve through both of its rami.[6]

BIOMECHANICS

The cervicothoracic junction shares some biomechanical and anatomic features with the cervical and thoracic spines.

The presence of the manubrium makes this junction unique. Movements of the manubrium in young athletes have been measured to average a total range of 2 degrees from full inspiration to full expiration. In the normal population, because the second rib is longer than the first, during inspiration, the superior aspect of the manubrium is forced to tilt posteriorly as its inferior edge is moved anteriorly. As the top of the manubrium tilts back, the clavicle rolls anteriorly. It is this motion that is often lost in the early stages of ankylosing spondylitis.

Traumatic disruption of the manubrium-sternal joint most often occurs via one of two mechanisms. The first, and most common, results from direct compression injury to the anterior chest. The direction of applied force displaces the fragment posteriorly and downward. The second type follows hyperflexion with compression injury to the upper thorax. The force is transmitted to the sternum through the clavicles, the chin, or the upper two ribs. There are two main types of manubrium-sternal dislocations. In type I, the body of the sternum is displaced posteriorly. In type II, which is more common, the body of the sternum is anterior in relation to the manubrium.[39,40]

The superior aspect of the spinous process is in line with the T1–T2 zygapophysial joints. The superior aspect of the vertebral body has two uncinate processes that articulate with the inferior aspect of the body of C7 to form an uncovertebral joint. It is the presence of these uncinate processes that has many manipulators of this area utilizing side-flexion, rather than rotation techniques, to decrease the risk of injury.

The zygapophysial facets of the superior articular process (SAP) lie in the coronal body plane, whereas those of the inferior articular process (IAP) present a gentle curve in both the transverse and sagittal planes. Both the zygapophysial and costotransverse joints are synovial.

In the mobile thorax, flexion in this region consists of[7]:

● Anterior rotation of the head of the rib
● A superior-anterior glide of the zygapophysial joints

In the mobile thorax, extension and arm elevation in this region consists of[7]:

● A posterior sagittal rotation and posterior translation of the superior vertebra. This action pushes the superior aspect of the head of the rib posteriorly at the costovertebral joint, producing a posterior rotation of the rib (the anterior aspect travels superiorly, whereas the posterior aspect travels inferiorly), except at those levels where the superior costovertebral joint does not exist (T1, T11, and T12).
● An inferior-posterior glide of the superior thoracic vertebra.

● A posterior translation and coupled posterior sagittal rotation of the inferior zygapophysial joint

In the mobile thorax, side-flexion at this region consists of[7]:

● The same pattern as the mid-cervical region, which is side-flexion coupled with ipsilateral rotation. The head of the first rib does not articulate with C7 so the superior-inferior glide of the ribs and the conjunct rotation cannot influence the direction of coupling between C7 and T1, and T1–2.
● An inferior glide of the transverse process, relative to the rib on the right, during right side-flexion of the head and neck, and superiorly relative to the rib on the left.

In the mobile thorax, rotation at this region consists of the same pattern as the mid-cervical region.[7]

During unilateral elevation of the arm, the zygapophysial joints side-flex and slightly extend to the same side as the elevated arm, producing a rotation of the T1 and T2 vertebrae to the same side.

The biomechanics of these regions have thus far been described for a normal thorax. Pathologic or aging processes however can stiffen the thorax and produce the following biomechanical changes.

Stiff Thorax[7]

Flexion. The anterior aspect of the rib travels inferiorly, whereas the posterior aspect travels superiorly.

Costotransverse joints of T1–T2. The concave facets of the transverse process of T1–2 glide superiorly relative to the tubercle of the ribs, resulting in a relative inferior glide of the tubercle of the rib.

Extension. Initially, the anterior aspect of the rib travels superiorly and the posterior aspect travels inferiorly. In addition, a posterior rotation of the ribs occurs, whereas an inferior-posterior glide of zygapophysial joints also occurs, but with less posterior translation of the zygapophysial joints.

A superior glide of the tubercle occurs at the costotransverse joints of T1–2.

COMMON PATHOLOGIES AND LESIONS

The cervicothoracic junction is an area subject to many forces, usually rotational, and is also vulnerable to postural impairments. While the coupled motions of rotation and side-flexion are ipsilateral (occur to the same side) in the cervical spine, the coupled motions of the thoracic spine vary according to which motion initiates. Thus, the cervicothoracic region becomes a transition area for these conflicting coupled motions. Incongruent rotations that occur in the spine produce dysfunction in the tissues.[7] Examples of this transfer between congruent and incongruent rotations can be seen in sports.

- A left-handed batter at the termination of the swing demonstrates rotation of the head to the left and rotation of the thoracic and lumbar spine to the right—the area for a potential breakdown is the cervicothoracic junction.
- A right handed quarterback in football, with the throwing arm cocked, demonstrates rotation of the head to the left, rotation of the upper to mid thoracic spine to the right—the area of potential breakdown is the cervicothoracic junction.
- A baseball pitcher with the throwing arm cocked, produces changes in rotation occurring at both the cervicothoracic and thoracolumbar-lumbar junctions.
- A golfer at the termination of the back swing produces a potential breakdown of the cervicothoracic junction.

The dysfunction in the tissues results when one or more of the segments within the junction becomes hypomobile. However, because the cervical spine is very mobile, this loss of motion can be compensated for, allowing the necessary motions to take place. Theoretically, this compensation usually results in a nearby hypermobility. For example, if the T1 segment became hypomobile from a habitual forward head posture and was held in a symmetrical flexed position, the C7 segment would compensate during cervical extension. Not only does the C7 segment have to provide extension at its own segment, but it now has to provide it for the T1 segment and, over time, becomes hypermobile and painful. The novice clinician locating the pain to the C7 segment would begin to mobilize this segment. Unfortunately, this would result in further pain as the C7 segment became more hypermobile. The experienced clinician, recognizing this syndrome and locating the offending hypomobile segment, would mobilize the correct segment and alleviate the patient's symptoms. In addition to mobilizing the segment, a therapeutic exercise program is initiated to strengthen the larger muscles of this area, including the levator scapula, trapezius, and rhomboids (see later discussion).

Forward Head

The stoop-shouldered individual with the forward head demonstrates certain characteristics.

- The cervical curve is decreased and the thoracic curve increased by the flexion.
- The shoulders are drawn forward and the chest is flattened.

An underlying cycle of abnormal relaxation in some muscles, with shortening, stretching, and a loss of tone in others, occurs during this process, with resultant joint strain and dysfunction. This cycle of events is further perpetuated by the natural cycle of aging of the spine, which involves degeneration of the disc, vertebral wedging, ligamentous calcification, and a reduction in the cervical and lumbar lordoses, producing a position of spinal flexion, or stooping.

Habitual movement patterns or positions also contribute to the development of these changes, producing muscular hyperactivity, ligamentous stress, and alteration of the anatomic relationship of the joints, thus, frequently becoming a source of pain.

As the head is brought forward by flexing the cervical segments, the scalene muscles are permitted to adaptively shorten, thus, lessening the support of the upper ribs, and the chest wall flattens anteriorly. The cervical flexion is followed by an increase of the thoracic curvature and the tension of the spinal musculature increases.[8,9] The scapulae become abducted and the weight of the shoulder girdle and upper extremity reinforce the spinal deformity. These altered relations increase the distance between the origin and insertion of the trapezius, the rhomboid major and minor, and the levator scapulae, which result in strain. The abduction of the scapulae causes a lowering of the coracoid process, which brings the origin and insertion of the pectoralis minor closer together, adaptively shortening it and further depriving the anterior chest wall of support. The tips of the shoulders have now assumed a position that is downward and forward, bringing the origin and insertion of the serratus anterior and of the pectoralis major closer together.[10] After a period of relaxation, their chronic adaptive shortening takes place.

Further down the spine an exaggeration of the lumbar curve is accompanied by a shift of the weight to the posterior part of the vertebral bodies and to the articular processes. The weight is delivered to the pelvis through the lumbosacral junction, producing maximum joint strain of this transitional area and a forward inclination of the pelvis. Whether the excessive anterior shearing force of L5 on the sacrum could eventually lead to a spondylolisthesis has yet to be demonstrated.

The increased forward inclination of the pelvis produces a shortening of the erector spinae group and flexors of the hip, accompanied by a lengthening of the abdominal and hamstring muscles—muscular imbalances that serve to maintain the deformity.[11]

Some of the more serious consequences of a poor posture are segmental hypermobility and instability. With a forward head posture, this commonly occurs at the C4–5 level, with C4 sliding anterior in relation to C5. This anterior translation probably occurs because of a slackening of the nuchal ligament, which normally undergoes increased tension in craniovertebral flexion and cervicothoracic extension.[12]

Other segments will become affected, often due to soft tissue tightness. The so-called "weekend warrior," with poor posture from inactivity, is often vulnerable to injury. Forced extension of the hip during an activity such as stride walking can pull on a shortened, and therefore tight, iliopsoas muscle. The iliopsoas has the potential to transmit this force to the lumbar spine, creating an anterior shear force. Theoretically, this anterior shear force can pull the lumbar spine into a position of increased lordosis, rendering it more susceptible to spondylolisthesis. Any further activity that increases the lumbar lordosis perpetuates the breakdown, eventually producing pain and forcing the individual to seek help.

Thoracic Outlet Syndrome

No discussion of this area can occur without a mention of thoracic outlet syndrome (T.O.S.). Thoracic outlet syndrome has many names, most of which describe the numerous potential sources for its compression, and include cervical rib syndrome, scalenus anticus syndrome, hyperabduction syndrome, costoclavicular syndrome, pectoralis minor syndrome, and first thoracic rib syndrome.[13]

It was Hunald in 1743, who associated the cervical rib with the development of thoracic outlet syndrome. In 1927, Adson[16] stressed the role of the scalene muscles in neurovascular compromise and in 1945 Wright[15] showed that shoulder hyperabduction could produce thoracic outlet obstruction. However, it was Peet et al[17] who coined the term "thoracic outlet syndrome" in 1956. Then, in the early 1960s Roos[18] emphasized the importance of the first rib and its muscular and ligamentous attachments in causing thoracic outlet obstruction.[13]

Thoracic outlet syndrome is defined as a clinical syndrome characterized by symptoms attributable to compression of the neural or vascular anatomic structures that pass through the thoracic outlet.

The thoracic outlet is bordered by the first thoracic rib, the clavicle, and the superior border of the scapula, through which the great vessels of the upper extremity, and the nerves of the brachial plexus pass. The nerve trunks of the brachial plexus pass through an interscalene triangle, which is formed anteriorly by the anterior scalene muscle, posteriorly by the middle scalene muscle, and inferiorly by the first rib. These trunks divide behind the clavicle before re-uniting to form cords that surround the axillary artery as it passes deep to the pectoralis minor tendon. The motor and sensory branches of the brachial plexus typically divide distal to the pectoralis minor

tendon. The lowest trunk of the plexus, consisting of the C8 and T1 nerve roots, lies above the first rib and behind the subclavian artery and is the most commonly compressed neural structure in thoracic outlet syndrome.[13]

From the interscalene triangle, the brachial plexus and subclavian artery pass behind the clavicle into the costoclavicular space. From there, they pass over the first rib between the anterior and middle scalene muscle insertions.

Thus, the course of the neurovascular bundle can be subdivided into three different sections, based on the areas of entrapment.

1. As the brachial plexus and subclavian artery pass through the interscalene triangle. The subclavian vein is not involved at this entrapment site, as it usually passes anterior to the anterior scalene muscle. Interscalene triangle compression can result from injury of the scalene or scapular suspensory muscles. In some cases, fibromuscular bands can develop between the anterior and middle scalenes, or connect from the elongated transverse processes of the lower cervical vertebrae, and these may produce entrapment.[19]

   Entrapment at this site can also result from cervical ribs, which are present in 0.2% of the population and occur bilaterally in 80% of those affected.[18] However, the presence of a cervical rib does not always precipitate signs and symptoms, with fewer than 10% of individuals with cervical ribs ever experiencing problems.[18]

2. As it passes the first rib, the clavicle and the subclavius— the costoclavicular interval. Entrapment in this space that lies between the rib cage and the posterior aspect of the clavicle, can occur with clavicle depression, ribelevation (due to scalene hypertonicity) or a first rib clavicular deformity. A post-fracture callus formation of the first rib or clavicle can increase the potential for entrapment.

3. As it passes the coracoid process, pectoralis minor, and the clavipectoral fascia, to enter the axillary fossa. At the point where the neurovascular bundle enters the axillary fossa, the subclavian artery and vein become the axillary artery and vein. At this third site, the neurovascular bundle can be compromised with arm abduction or elevation, especially if external rotation is superimposed on the motion.

   Pectoralis minor tendon compression is associated with shoulder hyperabduction. During hyperabduction, the tendon insertion and the coracoid act as a fulcrum about which the neurovascular structures are forced to change direction. Hypertrophy of the pectoralis minor tendon has also been noted as a cause of outlet compression.[15]

   There may be multiple points of compression of the peripheral nerves between the cervical spine and hand, in addition to the thoracic outlet. When there are multiple compression sites, less pressure is required at each site to produce symptoms. Thus, a patient may have concomitant thoracic outlet syndrome, ulnar nerve compression at the elbow, and carpal tunnel syndrome. This phenomenon has been called the multiple crush syndrome.[20]

Symptoms vary from mild to limb threatening, and might be ignored by many physicians as they mimic common, but difficult to treat conditions, such as tension headache or fatigue syndromes.[14] The chief complaint is usually one of diffuse arm and shoulder pain, especially when the arm is elevated beyond 90 degrees. Potential symptoms include pain localized in the neck, face, head, upper extremity, chest, shoulder, or axilla; and upper extremity paresthesias, numbness, weakness, heaviness, fatiguability, swelling, discoloration, ulceration, or Raynaud phenomenon.[14] Neural compression symptoms occur more commonly than vascular symptoms.[21]

Karas[22] described four symptom patterns of thoracic outlet syndrome characterized by the primary structures compressed. The lower trunk pattern reflects lower plexus compression and manifests with pain in the supraclavicular and infraclavicular fossae, back of the neck, the rhomboid area, the axilla and the medial arm, and may radiate into the hand, and fourth and fifth fingers. Subjective complaints include feelings of coldness, or electric shock sensations in the C8-T1 nerve root, or ulnar nerve distributions. The upper trunk pattern results from upper plexus compression and is distinguished by pain in the anterolateral neck, shoulder, mandible and ear, and paresthesias that radiate into the upper chest and lateral arm in the C5–7 dermatomes.[18,22,23]

With venous involvement, the signs and symptoms can include swelling of the entire limb, non-pitting edema, bluish discoloration, and venous collateralization across the superior chest and shoulder. Arterial involvement produces coolness, ischemic episodes, and exertional fatigue.[22] Finally, the mixed pattern consists of a combination of vascular and neurologic symptoms.[22]

Twenty-one to 75 percent of thoracic outlet syndrome patients have an association with trauma,[23] whether that be macrotrauma, as in the case of a motor vehicle accident, or microtrauma, as in the case of a muscle strain of the scapular stabilizers due to repetitive overhead activities.[26,27,28,29,30]

During the normal growth of children and adolescents, the scapulae gradually descend on the posterior thorax, with the descent being slightly greater in women than in men. A strain injury to the scapular suspensory muscles, which lengthen in conjunction with scapular descent during normal development, is known to be associated with thoracic outlet syndrome, and helps to explain the rarity of symptomatic thoracic outlet syndrome until after puberty and the increased prevalence in women.[13,31]

Occipitofrontal tension headache, previously thought to have no clear anatomic explanation, has been shown to be related to spasm in the upper cervical muscles; fibers of rectus capitis posterior minor insert into the occipital dura and can cause headache.[32]

Neurophysiologic tests are useful to exclude coexistent pathologies, such as peripheral nerve entrapment or cervical radiculopathy; an abnormal reflex F wave conduction and decreased sensory action potentials in the medial antebrachial cutaneous nerve may be diagnostic.[33]

Lower plexus thoracic outlet syndrome is surgically treated by first rib and (if present) cervical rib excision.[34]

Although it has been suggested that the insured patient is more likely to have an operation, results are independent of any associated litigation.[35]

Thoracic outlet syndrome is a clinical diagnosis made almost entirely on the basis of the history and physical examination. To rule out other conditions that can mimic thoracic outlet syndrome, the physical examination should include the following.

- A careful inspection of the spine, thorax, shoulder girdles, and upper extremities for postural abnormalities, shoulder asymmetry, muscle atrophy, excessively large breasts, obesity, and drooping of the shoulder girdle.
- The supraclavicular fossa should be palpated for fibromuscular bands, percussed for brachial plexus irritability, and auscultated for vascular bruits that appear by placing the upper extremity in the position of vascular compression.
- The neck and shoulder girdle should be assessed for active and passive ranges of motion, areas of tenderness, or other signs of intrinsic disease.
- A thorough neurologic examination of the upper extremity should include a search for sensory and motor deficits and abnormalities of deep tendon reflexes.

Assessment of:

- Respiration to ensure that the patient is using correct abdominodiaphragmatic breathing.
- Suspensory muscles—middle and upper trapezius, levator scapulae, and sternocleidomastoid—thoracic outlet "openers." These muscles need to be strengthened as part of the intervention approach.
- Scapulothoracic muscles—anterior and middle scalenes, subclavius, pectoralis minor and major—thoracic outlet "closers." These muscles are stretched as part of the intervention approach.
- First rib position or the presence of a cervical rib.

- Clavicle position and history of prior fracture, producing abnormal callous formation or malalignment.
- Scapula position, acromioclavicular joint mobility, and sternoclavicular joint mobility.

Diagnostic Maneuvers. Unfortunately, the majority of tests for thoracic outlet obstruction carry high false-positive rates.[31] The aim of these tests should be to reproduce the patient's symptoms rather than to obliterate the radial pulse, as more than 50% of normal, asymptomatic people will exhibit obliteration of the radial pulse during classic provocative testing.[23]

1. *Adson's vascular test:*[16] The patient extends their neck, turns their head toward the side being examined, and takes a deep breath (Figure 15–1).[16] This test, if positive, tends to implicate the scalenes because this test increases the tone of the anterior and middle scalenes.
2. *Allen's pectoralis minor test:* The Allen test increases the tone of the pectoralis minor muscle. The seated patient is positioned in 90 degrees of glenohumeral abduction, 90 degrees of glenohumeral external rotation, and 90 degree of elbow flexion on the tested side. While the radial pulse is monitored, the patient is asked to turn the head away from the tested side. This test, if positive, tends to implicate pectoralis tightness as the cause for the symptoms.
3. *Costoclavicular:* During this test, the shoulders are drawn back and downward in an exaggerated military

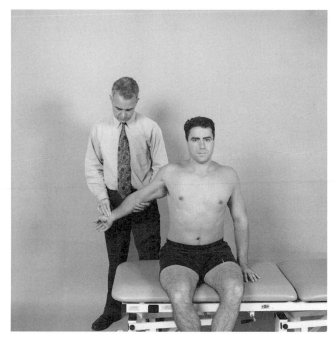

FIGURE 15–2 Costoclavicular test.

position so as to reduce the volume of the costoclavicular space (Figure 15–2).
4. *Cyriax maneuver:* Patient seated on the edge of a table and the clinician grasps the arm on the symptomatic side, passively depresses the shoulder girdle, and then pulls the arm down toward the floor while palpating the radial pulse (Figure 15–3). This test, if positive, implicates heavy lifting as the cause.

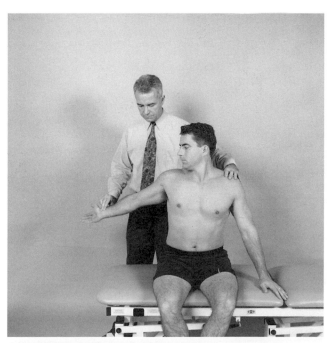

FIGURE 15–1 Adson's test.

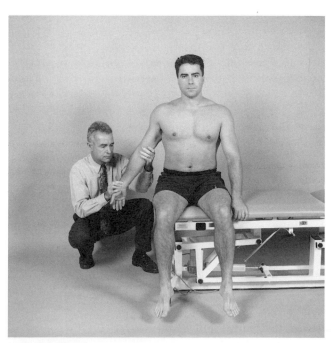

FIGURE 15–3 Cyriax test.

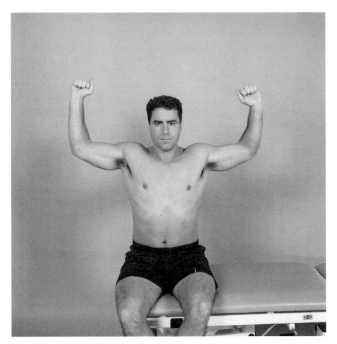

FIGURE 15–4 Roos test.

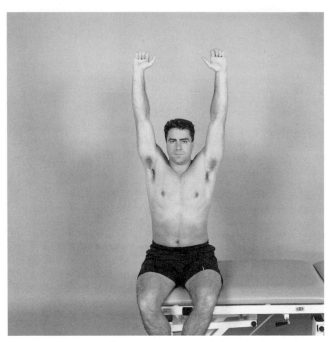

FIGURE 15–5 Full arm elevation with hands clasped.

5. *Roos/EAST/"hands-up" test:* Abduction, elbow flexion, and external rotation of the upper limb in the coronal plane, with slow finger clenching for 3 minutes reproduces the symptoms, which occur when the patient works with the arm elevated (Figure 15–4). The radial pulse may be reduced or obliterated during this maneuver and an infraclavicular bruit may be heard. However, patients with severe neurologic symptoms can be overlooked if the examiner focuses too closely on positional pulse changes.

6. *Overhead test:* The overhead exercise test is useful to detect thoracic outlet arterial compression. During this test, the patient elevates both arms overhead and then rapidly flexes and extends the fingers (Figure 15–5). A positive test is achieved if the patient experiences heaviness, fatigue, numbness, tingling, blanching, or discoloration of a limb within 20 seconds.[13]

7. *Hyperabduction:* The Wright test, or the hyperabduction maneuver, tests several points along the thoracic outlet for compression and is considered by many to be the best provocative test for thoracic outlet compression caused by the pectoralis minor. The test is performed by asking the patient to turn the head away from the side being examined and take a deep breath while the examiner passively abducts and externally rotates the patient's arm (Figure 15–6).

8. *Brachial plexus examination:* Percussion of supraclavicular area, infraclavicular area, and the ipsilateral side of the neck.

- Firm thumb pressure (30 seconds) over the brachial plexus in the supraclavicular area.
- Manual muscle testing, especially the C7 and C8–T1 muscles.

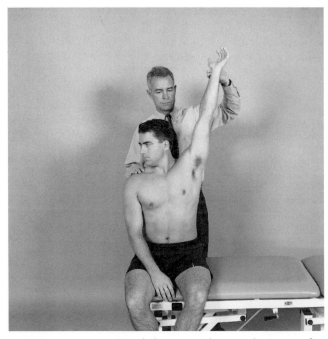

FIGURE 15–6 Passive abduction and external rotation of the arm. The patient turns the head away from the tested side.

● Touch and pin prick sensation in inner forearm, ulnar side of hand, and fingers (occasionally on the dorsum of first web space, radial aspect).

9. A simple, but effective, test to help rule out thoracic outlet syndrome is to have the patient shrug up the shoulder. This slackens the plexus on that side but closes the cervical foramen. Changes in symptoms are noted. The patient is then asked side-flex the head and neck to the opposite side with the shoulder relaxed. This maneuver stretches the plexus but opens the foramen. Changes in symptoms are noted.

Intervention

Conservative intervention should be attempted before surgery and should be directed toward muscle relaxation, relief of inflammation, and attention to posture. This may require a change of occupation as thoracic outlet syndrome is more common in those who stoop at work. Aggressive physical therapy, particularly traction, may make matters worse, and a trial of conservative management is essential.[36]

The focus of nonsurgical intervention is the correction of postural abnormalities of the neck and shoulder girdle, strengthening of the scapular suspensory muscles, stretching of the scapulothoracic muscles, and mobilization of the whole shoulder complex and first and second ribs.

If symptoms progress or fail to respond within 4 months, surgical intervention should be considered.[21]

Kenny and co-workers[38] prospectively evaluated a group of eight patients comprised largely of middle-aged women whose thoracic outlet syndrome was treated with a supervised physical therapy program of graduated resisted shoulder elevation exercises. All patients showed major symptomatic improvement.

EXAMINATION

After a scan, the biomechanical examination of this area should include the following.

Posture Examination

This is an area highly prone to postural dysfunctions, and the postural examination alone can often give the clinician a working hypothesis.

Screening Tests

Two screening tests are commonly used.

1. The assessment of manubrial motion
2. Arm elevation

Manubrium

It is worth remembering that in the elderly populations, the manubrium will often be fused to the sternum[41] invalidating this test. In the younger population, assessing the position and motion of the manubrium during certain movements enables the clinician to screen for an impairment in the following areas.

● Thoracic spine impairments, especially T1–3.
● First, second, and third ring of the thoracic spine and rib complex.
● Clavicle (acromioclavicular joint and sternoclavicular joint joints).
● Scapulothoracic "joint."

Apley's Scratch Test. The patient is asked to try to put the palm of one hand on the back of the neck while placing the dorsum of the other hand in the small of the back. The patient is then asked to try to touch one hand with the other (Figure 15–7). The arms are then switched, the procedure is repeated, and comparisons are made. An inability to touch hands indicates a problem with one of the above areas and is considered a positive test. If the test is positive, the manubrium is palpated (under the clavicle and on the costal cartilage of the 1st rib) (Figure 15–8) during the following sequence of motions.

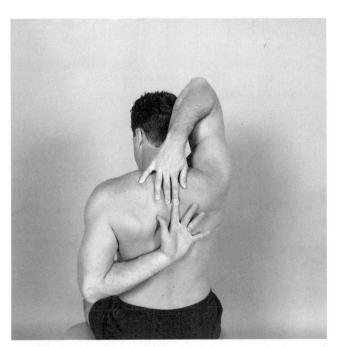

FIGURE 15–7   The manubrium screen test (Apley's scratch test).

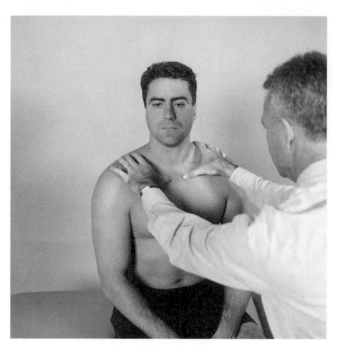

FIGURE 15–8   Palpation of the manubrium.

1. *Cervicothoracic spine flexion, extension, and side flexion:* Cervicothoracic flexion and extension tests the mobility of the first ring. During active flexion and extension of cervicothoracic spine, the manubrium mimics the movements of the spine. During extension, T1 and the manubrium move posteriorly, whereas during flexion they both move anteriorly. A hypomobility at T1 results in a change of motion at the manubrium. With extension, the ring complex should posteriorly rotate, and anteriorly rotate with flexion. With cervicothoracic side-flexion, the manubrium should side flex in the same direction as the cervicothoracic spine, and thus a positional fault in the manubrium should be matched by the same impairment in the cervicothoracic spine. The manubrial impairment can be described using the ERS and FRS terminology. For example, a closing restriction on the left at T1 [flexed rotated side-flexed right (FRSR)] will produce the following findings when the patient extends the neck.

• The ring will rotate to the right making the left side of the manubrium appear to move anteriorly. However, with flexion, there will be no significant changes.

• Extended, rotated, side-flexed (ERS) (opening) restriction—the manubrium rotates toward the side of the impairment. For example, an ERSL impairment

causes the right side of the manubrium to move anteriorly as the ring rotates to the left during head and neck flexion. However, with extension, there will be no significant changes. The second and third "rings" can be assessed in the same manner.

2. *Respiration:* The manubrium should elevate with inspiration and depress with expiration. In addition, during inspiration, the superior aspect of the manubrium tilts posteriorly, whereas the inferior aspect moves anteriorly. The process reverses during expiration. If a problem exists here, the first rib is assessed for an impairment and treated. If the rib motion is restricted, the manubrium/ring will side-flex and rotate away from the side of the fixed rib during respiration. For example, if the right rib is unable to glide inferiorly at the manubrium-costal junction during inspiration, the manubrium/ring will rotate and side-flex to the left during inspiration.

3. The glides of the acromioclavicular and sternoclavicular joints. If a problem exists here, the specific joint glide is restored.

Arm Elevation

Elevation of the arm produces extension, side-flexion, and rotation of T1–2 to the ipsilateral side.[7] In addition to assessing the affect of arm elevation on the vertebrae and/or manubrium, the clinician should examine the position of the scapular at rest and during forward elevation. The medial border of the scapula should be more or less parallel with the T2–7 spinous processes and about 2 ½ to 3 inches away from those processes. The resting position of the scapula, and its ability to function correctly, is determined by the length-strength relationship of a number of muscles. The levator scapulae and the rhomboids are usually prone to tightness. The serratus anterior and the upper and lower trapezii, are usually found to be weak.

During forward elevation, or abduction of the arm, the clinician should note any winging and/or tilting that occurs, which would indicate a weakness of the serratus anterior.

The next stage in the examination process depends on the clinician's background. For those clinicians heavily influenced by the muscle energy techniques of the osteopaths,[42] position testing is used to determine which segment to focus on. Other clinicians omit the position tests and proceed to the active mobility and passive physiologic tests (Figure 15–9).

Position Testing

A. Zygapophysial joints. The patient is positioned in sitting with the clinician standing behind the

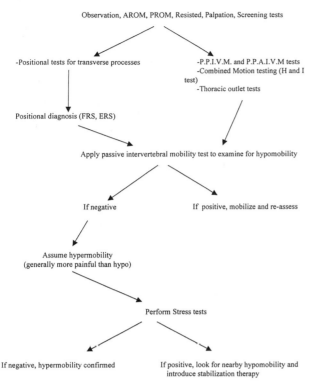

Observation, AROM, PROM, Resisted, Palpation, Screening tests

-Positional tests for transverse processes

-P.P.I.V.M. and P.P.A.I.V.M tests
-Combined Motion testing (H and I test)
-Thoracic outlet tests

Positional diagnosis (FRS, ERS)

Apply passive intervertebral mobility test to examine for hypomobility

If negative

If positive, mobilize and re-assess

Assume hypermobility
(generally more painful than hypo)

Perform Stress tests

If negative, hypermobility confirmed

If positive, look for nearby hypomobility and introduce stabilization therapy

FIGURE 15–9 Examination sequence for the cervicothoracic junction.

patient. With the thumbs, the clinician palpates the transverse processes of the T1 vertebra.

1. The clinician passively flexes the joint complex and then assesses the position of the T1 vertebra relative to T2 by noting which transverse process is the most posterior. A more posterior left transverse process of T1 relative to T2 is indicative of a left rotated position of the T1–2 complex in flexion.

2. The clinician passively extends the joint complex and assesses the position of the T1 vertebra in relation to T2 by noting which transverse process is the most posterior. A posterior left transverse process of T1 relative to T2 is indicative of a left rotated position of the T1–2 joint complex in extension.

   The clinician needs to remember that this region is prone to symmetrical impairments that will not be detected with position testing.

B. Ribs

1. Posterior aspect. The patient is positioned in sitting with the clinician standing behind patient. With the thumbs, the clinician palpates the ribs just lateral to the tubercle and medial to the angle. The superior-inferior, anterior-posterior relationship of the two ribs, left and right is noted.

2. Anterior aspect. The patient is positioned in sitting with the clinician standing in front of the patient.
   a. First rib. With the index fingers or thumbs, the clinician palpates the anterior aspect of the first ribs at the manubrium-costal junction
   b. Second rib. With the index fingers or thumbs, the clinician palpates the anterior aspect and then the cranial aspect of the second ribs at the manubrium-costal junction

The superior-inferior, anterior-posterior relationship of the two ribs, left and right is noted.

Active Mobility Testing

A. Zygapophysial joints
1. Flexion. The following test is used to determine the mobility of two adjacent thoracic or cervical vertebrae during flexing of the head and trunk.
   a. The transverse processes of two adjacent vertebrae are palpated with the index finger and thumb of both hands.
   b. The patient is asked to flex the head and trunk and the quantity of motion, as well as the symmetry of motion, is noted during flexion of the segment (Figure 15–10). Both index fingers should travel superiorly an equal distance.

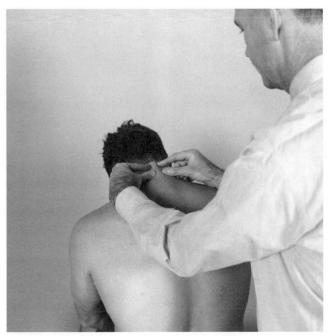

FIGURE 15–10 Patient and clinician position for active mobility testing of cervical flexion.

c. When interpreting the mobility findings, the position of the joint at the beginning of the test should be correlated with the subsequent mobility noted because alterations in joint mobility may merely be a reflection of an altered starting position.[7]

d. To determine the position of the superior vertebra, the posterior-anterior relationship of the transverse processes to the coronal body plane is noted and compared with the level above and below. If the left transverse process of the superior vertebra is more posterior than the left transverse process of the inferior vertebra, then the segment is left rotated.[42] If the left transverse process of the superior vertebra is less posterior than the left transverse process of the inferior vertebra, but more posterior than the right transverse process of the superior vertebra, then the superior vertebra is relatively right rotated compared to the level below, but left rotated when compared to the coronal body plane.[42] This is a typical compensatory pattern seen when a superior segment is derotating or unwinding a primary rotation at a lower level.[7]

e. The same palpation points are used for testing extension, side-flexion, and rotation.

2. Although active mobility testing helps to determine asymmetrical impairments, it is of limited value in the detection of symmetrical impairments unless the clinician has the ability to compare the amount of motion that occurred with the segment above and below with the segment being tested. Remember, this is an area prone to symmetrical impairments, particularly into extension.

B. Ribs

1. The following test is used to determine the mobility of a rib relative to the vertebra of the same number during flexion of the head/trunk.

a. The clinician palpates the transverse process with the thumb of one hand.

b. With the thumb of the other hand, the rib is palpated just lateral to the tubercle and medial to the angle. The index finger of this hand rests along the shaft of the rib.

c. The patient is instructed to flex the head and trunk and the relative motion between the transverse process and the rib is noted (Figure 15–11).

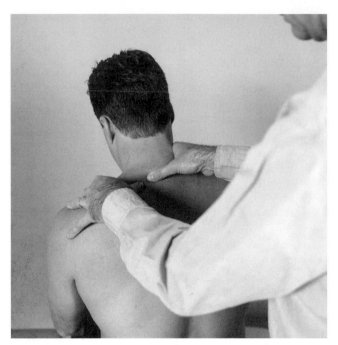

FIGURE 15–11 Patient and clinician position for active mobility testing of the rib.

d. The same palpation points are used for testing cervicothoracic extension, side-flexion, and rotation.

2. Respiration. Active movements of the first rib are tested during respiration by palpating the angle of the rib with the thumbs, and asking the patient to inspire and expire. A normal finding is a slight inferior-anterior motion (depression) occurring at the angle during inspiration, the reverse (elevation) occurring with expiration. Abnormal findings include:

a. Superior glide felt with inspiration—probable subluxation or scalenus shortening

b. Either motion reduced—pericapsular or myofascial

c. Both motions reduced—pericapsular

Note: Scalenus shortening will also demonstrate an obvious lack of rib tubercle elevation with expiration.

3. The first rib can sublux anteriorly, posteriorly or, more commonly, superiorly. If the motion is perceived as abnormal, passive movement testing should be performed.

a. The arthrokinematic is tested with the patient seated and the clinician standing behind.

b. Using the medial aspect of the MCP joint of the index finger, the clinician applies an anterior-inferior-medial glide of the rib to assess the inspiration glide, whereas a posterior-superior-lateral glide is applied to assess the expiration glide.

   c. The end feel is assessed. If it is abrupt and hard (pathomechanical) in both glide directions, then the problem is a subluxation. If it is stiff (hard capsular) in both directions, then a pericapsular restriction is present. If both glides are normal, then the problem is likely to be myofascial.

Passive Physiologic Intervertebral Mobility (PPIVM)

A variety of methods can be employed to assess the passive physiological mobility of this region.

Seated Techniques

1. The patient is seated with the clinician standing to the side. With the index finger of the posterior hand (behind the patient), the clinician palpates the interspinous space of the segment being tested. The ulnar border of the fifth finger of the other hand palpates the lamina and inferior articular pillar of the cranial vertebra. The rest of the hand is cupped, and supports the cervical spine while the arm cradles the cranium (Figure 15–12). The clinician passively flexes, extends, side-flexes, and rotates the segment, noting the quantity and quality of the motion compared to the other levels. With the flexion component, an anterior glide is applied at the end of range. At the end of the extension component, the clinician blocks the inferior spinous process and applies a posterior glide to the superior segment using their chest. At the end of the side bend, a lateral glide is applied. Distraction of the joints can also be tested in this position.

2. The patient is seated. In this example, left side-flexion is tested. The patient is seated with their right hand placed behind the neck. The clinician is seated on the right side of the patient. The clinician places the point of the patient's right elbow against the clinician's chest. The clinician then reaches around the front of the patient and places his or her anterior hand over the patient's hand, which is behind the patient's neck (Figure 15–13). Monitoring the segment with the other hand, the clinician side-flexes the segment away from him or her, using pressure at the right elbow of the patient. Extension and rotation (Figure 15–13) can also be tested in this position.

Side-Lying Technique

The patient is positioned in left side-lying, facing the clinician. The lower arm of the patient hangs off the end of the bed. Placing a cupped hand in the cervical lordosis, the clinician cradles the patient's head in the crook of the right arm. The segment to be tested is monitored with

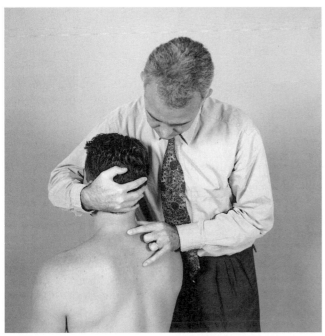

FIGURE 15–12 Patient and clinician position for passive physiologic intervertebral motion testing of the cervical spine.

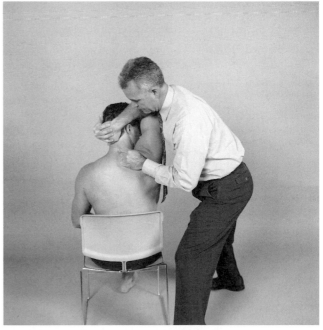

FIGURE 15–13 Seated passive physiologic intervertebral motion testing of the cervical spine.

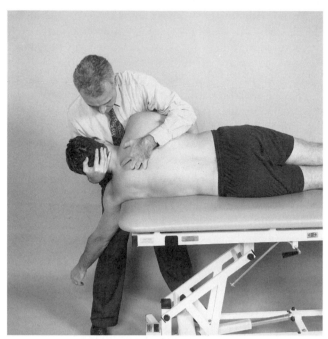

FIGURE 15–14   Side lying technique for passive physiologic intervertebral motion testing.

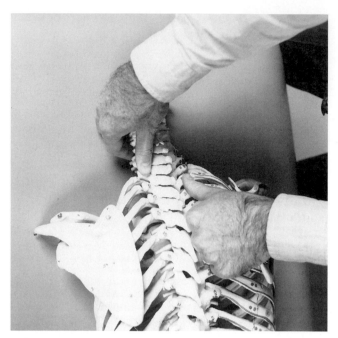

FIGURE 15–15   Hand position for testing the inferior joint glide on the right side of T1–2.

the index finger or thumb of the left hand (Figure 15–14). The patient's head is then side-flexed up to the ceiling, making sure that the motion is occurring only at the segment, and not through the rest of the cervical spine. Rotation, flexion, and extension of the segment can also be tested in this position. The other side is then tested.

Passive Physiologic Articular Intervertebral Motion (PPIAVM)

Zygapophysial Joints

Superior Glide.   The superior glide of the right zygapophysial joint at T1–2 is tested to determine the ability of the right inferior articular process of T1 to glide superiorly relative to the superior articular process of T2.

The patient is positioned in prone-lying with the thoracic spine in neutral. With the left thumb, the clinician palpates the inferior aspect of the left transverse process of T2. The right thumb palpates the inferior aspect of the right transverse process of T1. Using the left thumb, the clinician fixes T2, and a superior-anterior glide is applied to T1 with the right thumb. The quantity and end feel of motion is noted and compared to the levels above and below. The superior glides of this area are usually normal.

Inferior Glide.   The inferior glide of the right zygapophysial joint at T1–2 is tested to determine the ability of the right

inferior articular process of T1 to glide inferiorly relative to the superior articular process of T2.

The patient is positioned in prone-lying with the thoracic spine in neutral. With the left thumb, the clinician palpates the inferior aspect of the left transverse process of T2. The right thumb palpates the inferior aspect of the right transverse process of T1. Using the left thumb, the clinician fixes T2, and an inferior glide is applied to T1 with the right thumb (Figure 15–15). The quantity and end feel of motion is noted and compared to the levels above and below, and at the same level on the opposite side. This technique can be used for all thoracic segments. Special care should be taken with the inferior glides because these are usually reduced symmetrically.

Costotransverse Joints (Passive Articular Mobility)

Inferior Glide.   The inferior glide of the right first rib at the costotransverse joint is tested to determine the ability of the right first rib to glide inferiorly relative to the transverse process of T1.

The patient is positioned in prone with the forehead comfortably resting on a pillow, while the clinician stands at the head of the bed. Using the thumb of the right hand, the clinician palpates the superior aspect of the left transverse process of T1. With the thumb of the right hand, the clinician palpates the superior aspect of the left first rib just lateral to the costotransverse joint. The thumb of the right hand fixes T1, and an inferior-anterior glide (allowing for

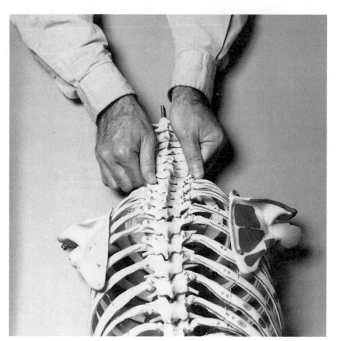

FIGURE 15–16 Hand position for testing the inferior joint glide of the costotransverse joint of the 1st rib.

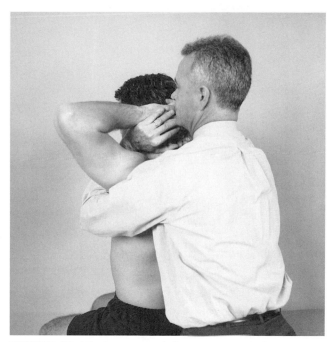

FIGURE 15–17 Patient and clinician position for testing distraction stability of the cervicothoracic junction.

the conjunct posterior rotation to occur) is applied to the first rib using the thumb of the left hand (Figure 15–16). The quantity and end feel of motion is noted and compared to the opposite side.

The superior glide of the right first rib at the costotransverse joint is tested to determine the ability of the right first rib to glide superiorly relative to the transverse process of T1.

The patient is positioned in prone-lying with the head and neck comfortably supported on a pillow. Using the right thumb, the clinician palpates the superior aspect of the right transverse process of T1. The index and middle fingers of the right hand palpate and fix the inferior aspect of the right first rib. A posterior-inferior glide (allowing the conjunct anterior rotation of the rib to occur) is applied to the transverse process of T1, thus producing a relative superior glide of the first rib at the costotransverse joint. The quantity and end feel of motion is noted and compared to the opposite side.

Passive Stability Testing[7]

Distraction

This test stresses the structures that resist vertical force. A positive response is the reproduction of the patient's pain. The patient is sitting with the hands behind the head with fingers interwoven. The cervicothoracic spine is in neutral. The clinician stands behind the patient and winds both arms under the patient's axilla, placing both hands over the patient's

hands. While gripping the thorax under the axilla with the inner arms, the clinician applies a vertical traction force to the lower cervical and upper thorax (Figure 15–17). This technique is also used to mobilize the segments in this area.

Compression

A compression force is applied to the lower cervical spine and upper thorax by applying a vertical force through the top of the patient's head.

Anterior Translation—Spinal

This test stresses the structures that resist anterior translation of a segmental spinal unit. A positive response is the reproduction of the patient's symptoms together with an increase in the quantity of motion and a decrease in the resistance at the end of the range of motion.

With the patient positioned in prone-lying, the transverse processes of the superior vertebra are palpated. With the other hand, the transverse processes of the inferior vertebra are fixed (Figure 15–18). A posterior-anterior force is applied through the superior vertebra while fixing the inferior vertebra (see Figure 15–18). The quantity of motion, the reproduction of any symptoms, and the end feel of motion is noted and compared to the levels above and below. The findings from this test should be correlated with those of the posterior translation test to determine the level of the instability because excessive anterior translation of the T4 vertebra could be due to either an anterior instability of T4–5 or a posterior instability of T3–4.

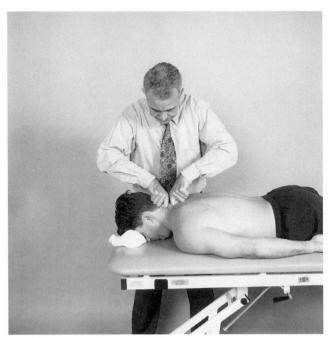

FIGURE 15–18 Patient and clinician position for anterior stability test.

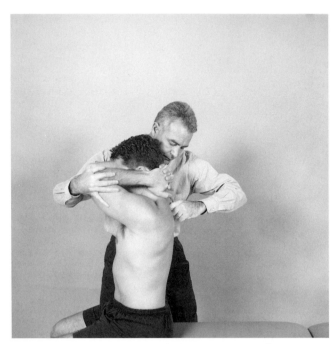

FIGURE 15–19 Patient and clinician position for posterior stability test.

Posterior Translation—Spinal

This test stresses the structures that resist posterior translation of a segmental spinal unit. A positive response is the reproduction of the patient's symptoms, together with an increase in the quantity of motion and a decrease in the resistance at the end of the range of motion.

The patient is seated with the hands clasped behind the neck, with the clinician standing to the side. The clinician fixes the transverse processes of the inferior vertebra with the index finger and thumb of the left hand, and wraps the right arm around the patient's head. Static stability is tested by applying an anterior-posterior force to the superior vertebra while fixing the inferior vertebra (Figure 15–19). The quantity of motion, the reproduction of any symptoms, and the end feel of motion is noted and compared to the levels above and below. The findings from this test should be correlated with those of the anterior translation test to determine the level of the instability.

Dynamic stability of the spinal unit can be tested by resisting the patient during elevation of the crossed arms. If the segmental musculature is able to control the excessive posterior translation during this maneuver, no posterior translation will be felt and the instability is dynamically stable.[7]

Transverse Rotation—Spinal

This test stresses the structures that resist rotation of a segmental spinal unit. A positive response is the reproduction of the patient's symptoms together with an increase in the quantity of motion and a decrease in the resistance at the end of the range of motion.

The patient is positioned in prone-lying, and the clinician palpates the transverse process of the superior vertebra. With the other hand, the contralateral transverse process of the inferior vertebra is fixed (Figure 15–20). A transverse plane rotation force is applied through the superior vertebra

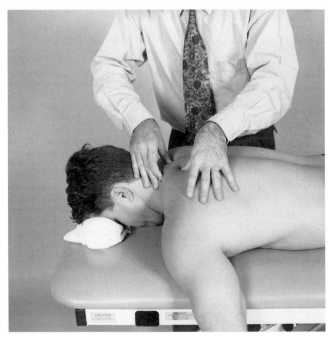

FIGURE 15–20 Patient and clinician position for transverse rotation stability test.

by applying a unilateral posterior-anterior pressure while fixing the inferior vertebra. The quantity of motion, the reproduction of any symptoms, and the end feel of motion is noted and compared to the levels above and below.

Anterior Translation—Posterior Costals
This test stresses the structures that resist anterior translation of the posterior aspect of the rib relative to the thoracic vertebrae to which it attaches. A positive response is the reproduction of the patient's symptoms together with an increase in the quantity of motion and a decrease in the resistance at the end of the range of motion.

The patient is positioned in prone-lying, and the clinician palpates the contralateral transverse processes of the thoracic vertebrae to which the rib is attached. For example, when testing the first rib on the left, the right transverse process of T1 is palpated and fixed. With the thumb of the other hand, the rib is palpated just lateral to the tubercle. A posterior-anterior force is applied to the rib while fixing the thoracic vertebrae (Figure 15–21). The quantity of motion, the reproduction of any symptoms, and the end feel of motion is noted and compared to the levels above and below.

Inferior Translation—Posterior Costals
This test stresses the structures that resist inferior translation of the rib relative to the thoracic vertebrae to which it attaches. A positive response is the reproduction of the patient's symptoms together with an increase in the quantity of motion and a decrease in the resistance at the end of the range of motion.

With the patient positioned in prone-lying, the clinician palpates the contralateral transverse process of the

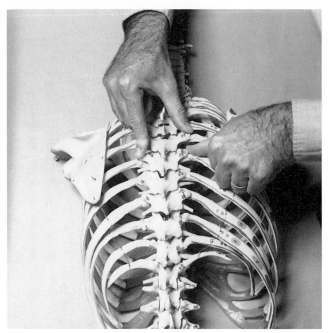

FIGURE 15–22 Clinician hand position for inferior translation of the posterior costals.

thoracic vertebra at the same level as the rib. With the other hand, the superior aspect of the rib, just lateral to the tubercle, is palpated (Figure 15–22). An inferior force is applied through the rib while fixing the thoracic vertebrae. The quantity of motion, the reproduction of any symptoms, and the end feel of motion is noted and compared to the levels above and below.

Superior Inferior Translation–Anterior Costal
This test stresses the structures that resist superior-inferior translation of the costal cartilage relative to the sternum and the rib relative to the costal cartilage. When the sternocostal and/or costochondral joints have been separated, a gap and a step can be palpated at the joint line. The positional findings are noted prior to stressing the joint. A positive response is the reproduction of the patient's symptoms together with an increase in the quantity of motion and a decrease in the resistance at the end of the range of motion.

With one thumb, the clinician palpates the anterior aspect of the sternum and costal cartilage. A superior-inferior force is applied to the costal cartilage and rib with the other thumb (Figure 15–23). The quantity of motion, the reproduction of any symptoms, and the end feel of motion is noted and compared to the levels above and below.

Anterior-Posterior Translation—Sternochondral and Costochondral
The patient is position in supine-lying with the clinician standing at the patient's side. With one thumb, the clinician palpates the anterior aspect of the sternum and costal cartilage. The anterior aspect of the costal cartilage and rib is

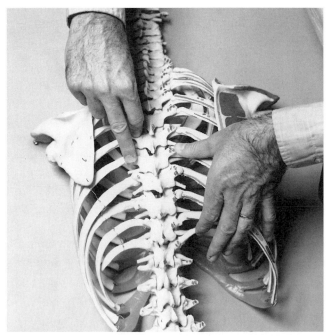

FIGURE 15–21 Clinician hand position for anterior translation of the posterior costals (seventh rib).

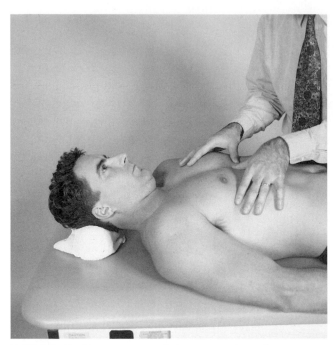

FIGURE 15–23 Patient and clinician position for superior-inferior translation of the anterior costals.

palpated with the other thumb (Figure 15–24). An anterior-posterior force is applied to the:

1. Manubrium (manubrial-costal junction)
2. Sternal end of the costal cartilage (manubrial costal junction)

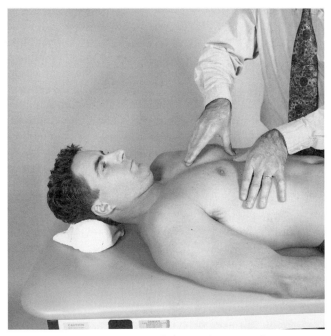

FIGURE 15–24 Patient and clinician position for anterior-posterior translation of the anterior costals.

3. Costal end of the costal cartilage (costochondral junction)
4. Cartilaginous end of the rib (costochondral junction)

The force is sustained until the end feel is perceived and the quantity and quality of motion is noted.

INTERVENTION

Manual Therapy

The selection of an intervention technique for hypomobility is dependent on two main factors.

- The acuteness of the condition
- The barrier to the movement encountered

Mobilization is used in the neck (as elsewhere) for two main purposes, to decrease pain using grade I and II techniques and to increase range of motion using all the various grades of mobilization. There are two main types of mobilization, axial and specific. The specific technique involves stabilization of the joints above and below, either by locking or by the clinician's hands, so that the only segment that moves is the one being treated. Axial techniques rely on the clinician confining the movement to the segment, and does not involve locking, or any form of stabilization, apart from maintaining the axis of motion.

If the joint is acutely painful and pain relief rather than a mechanical effect is the major consideration when selecting a mobilization technique, then oscillations that do not reach the end of range are adopted. The segment or joint is left in its neutral position and the mobilization is carried out from that point. There is no need for, and in fact every reason to avoid, muscle relaxation techniques to help reach the end of range.

If stretching of the mechanical barrier rather than pain relief is the immediate objective of the mobilization, the technique is performed at the end of the available range to be mobilized.

General Techniques

Prone. The patient is positioned in prone, with the clinician standing to the side of the patient. The following areas are massaged.

- *Paraspinal gutter*: the clinician uses a thumb to apply a deep massage to the entire length of the paraspinal gutter.

- *Upper trapezius*: the clinician uses the heel of the palm and massages the upper trapezius. The clinician can also use the fingers to knead the upper trapezius muscle along the directions of its fibers.

Side-lying. With the patient positioned in side-lying, the clinician stands and faces the patient. Reaching over the back of the patient, the clinician grasps the scapula by sliding his or her fingers underneath, and manually distracts the patient's scapula away from their back (Figure 15–25).

Supine. The patient is positioned in supine with the shoulder slightly over the edge, with the clinician standing to the side of the patient. The clinician takes the patient's arm and tucks it between his or her arm and trunk. Reaching over the patient, the clinician grasps the whole shoulder girdle and rotates it in a full circle. This is done repeatedly, producing a rhythmic motion.

The patient is positioned in supine, with the clinician at the head of the bed. The clinician wraps both hands around the back of the patient's neck, attempting to get as low on the cervical spine as possible. The clinician then leans forward so that the front of his or her shoulder rests on the patient's forehead. By compressing the patient's head and gently grasping the back of the neck, a longitudinal distraction is applied.

Seated. The patient is seated with the arms crossed and forearms grasped and resting the head on the hands. The

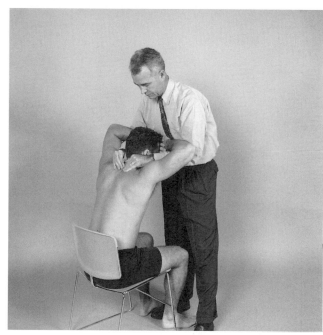

FIGURE 15–26   Seated mobilization technique for the cervicothoracic junction.

clinician stands in front of the patient and threads his or her arms through the patient's arms, before resting both of the hands on the top and back of each of the patient's shoulders (Figure 15–26). By gently leaning the patient forward, the cervical spine is extended until the stiff segment is located at the cervicothoracic junction. Gradually, the clinician increases the amount of cervicothoracic extension by gently kneading the area. Distraction, side-flexion, or rotation motions can also be introduced. Care should be taken to avoid increasing the lordosis of the lumbar spine during this technique by pulling the patient too far forward.

Another seated technique can be used to increase motion at the cervicothoracic junction. In this example, flexion and right rotation is produced. The patient is seated with both hands behind the neck. The clinician stands to the right side of the patient. The clinician places the point of the index finger on the segment to be monitored. The clinician then reaches around the front of the patient and places his or her right hand over the patient's left elbow. Monitoring the segment with the other hand, the clinician now passively flexes and right rotates the segment to the point where motion is felt to occur. A contract-relax technique can be used to gain further motion (Figure 15–27).

Semi-Specific and Specific Techniques
These techniques are employed when the clinician wants to restore motion to one side of the joint at the T1–4 levels.

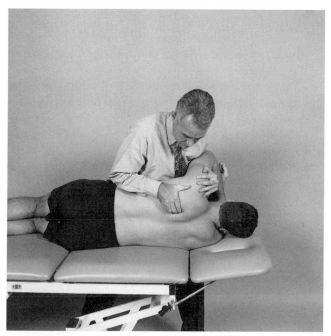

FIGURE 15–25   Patient and clinician position for manual distraction of the scapula.

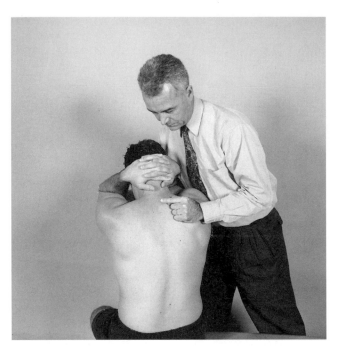

FIGURE 15–27 Seated mobilization technique for the cervicothoracic junction.

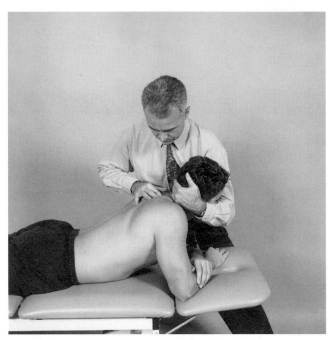

FIGURE 15–28 Mobilization of the cervicothoracic junction with the patient in prone position.

In these examples, the left side of the joint is treated, unless otherwise specified.

The patient is positioned in prone with the clinician standing on the opposite side to the side being treated—the right side in this case.

1. To increase flexion. The clinician reaches over the patient and places his or her caudal hand between the patient and the table, grasping the coracoid process of the patient's shoulder. The patient's shoulder is lifted slightly, thus stabilizing the shoulder girdle and preventing it from moving down onto the table. The clinician uses the cranial hand to mobilize the cervicothoracic junction into flexion and right rotation by pushing the zygapophysial joints, along their joint planes, in the direction of the table.

   A slight modification to this technique can make the technique more specific. In this example the right side of the joint is treated. The patient is positioned in prone, on the elbows, with the clinician standing to the side of the patient, in this example, to the patient's left. This patient position stabilizes the ribs and shoulder girdle. The clinician reaches around the front of the patient's face with the left hand, and wraps the hand around the patient's neck, placing the little finger along the posterior arch of the superior bone of the segment to be treated. The clinician, stabilizes the inferior segment (Figure 15–28) using a pinch grip of

the right hand, or the index finger of the right hand can be placed against the superior aspect of the transverse process of the inferior segment. The anterior aspect of clinician's left shoulder rests against the patient's head. The clinician, using the left hand, pulls the patient's superior segment into flexion and left rotation.

2. To increase extension. The patient is positioned in prone, with the clinician standing on the opposite side to the side being treated. The clinician reaches over the patient and places his or her caudal hand on top of the opposite shoulder girdle, preventing it from raising off the table during the procedure. With the cranial hand, the clinician applies an extension and left rotation mobilization to the zygapophysial joints cervicothoracic junction by gliding them, along their joint planes, away from the table and toward the clinician.

A slight modification to this technique can make the technique more specific. The patient is positioned in prone, on the elbows, with the clinician standing to the side of the patient, in this example, to the patient's left. This patient position stabilizes the ribs and shoulder girdle. The left side of the patient's neck can be encouraged into extension and left rotation using the same patient and clinician position (see Figure 15–28), except that the clinician's right hand stabilizes the left side of the inferior segment's spinous process. Using the left hand and the body, the clinician mobilizes the left joint into extension and left rotation.

Seated Distraction Technique (C6–T2 Levels)

The patient is positioned in sitting or standing with both of the hands behind the neck, fingers interlaced, and the index fingers at the level of the superior segment to be treated. The clinician, standing behind the patient, winds both of his or her arms beneath the patient's axillae through the triangular space created by the flexed elbows. The fingers are interlaced and placed over the patient's hands. The thorax is gently gripped by adducting the arms. The patient is instructed to look forward and the clinician ensures that the ligamentum nuchae is not in full stretch (Figure 15–29). From this position, a grade III to V longitudinal traction technique is applied by rocking the patient backward and forward until a pendular-type motion is produced. Gravity provides the distractive force that will distract the discs and glide the facets. A high velocity, low amplitude thrust technique is applied, in a superior direction, at the apex of the descent when the patient's body weight is dropping.

Rotational Technique to Increase Rotation

The advantage of rotational techniques is that they tend to produce a pure separation of the zygapophysial joints on the side to which the rotation occurs. Rotation to the left at C7–T1 will be used for the example.

Side-Lying Thrust Technique (Upper Thoracic Segments)

For this technique to be successful, mobility must be able to occur throughout the patient's thoracic spine, so the patient is positioned in-side lying (right in this case) with the axilla of the bottom arm off the top end of the bed and the bottom arm hanging down. The clinician supports the patient's head and chin with his or her left arm and hand, respectively. The patient's head is either flexed or extended down to, but not into, the segment to be treated. It is then side-flexed and rotated down to, but not into, the segment. The clinician supports the patient's head on his or her left thigh to prevent overthrusting the patient's head into excessive rotation (particularly important if the neck is positioned in extension). Using a wide lumbrical pinch grip, the right hand is placed, palm down, on the patient's neck, engaging the upper aspect of the caudal spinous process and neural arch (Figure 15–30). After the slack has been taken up, a mobilizing force is applied to the left side of the T1 spinous process, by the right hand of the clinician, in a direction toward the floor, producing a rotation to the right at T1, but a relative left rotation of the cranial bone (C7) and a gapping of the zygapophysial joint on the left side. This is an arthrokinematic mobilization. The technique can be graded from I to V.

Home Exercise Program

In addition to the strengthening and flexibility exercises performed in the clinic, specific exercises are given as part of the home exercise program. It is very important that the following exercises are performed correctly to ensure that

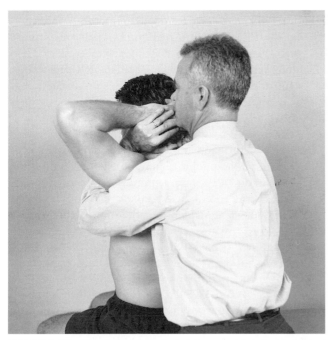

FIGURE 15–29 Patient and clinician position for a seated distraction thrust of the cervicothoracic junction. (MISSING ART)

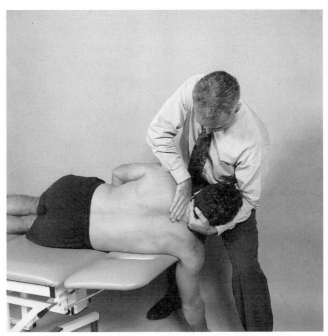

FIGURE 15–30 Thrust of the cervicothoracic junction with the patient positioned on his side.

the hypomobile segment is being mobilized, and not the hypermobile segment.

1. To increase the posterior glides of cervicothoracic extension. A high-backed chair is used to stabilize the thoracic spine, and the patient is seated in the correct posture. The patient places the hands around the mid-cervical spine with the fingers clasped together and the forearms parallel to the floor. The patient is asked to perform chin retraction by pushing his or her neck in a backward direction while maintaining the arms parallel to the floor.

2. To strengthen the cervicothoracic stabilizers. The patient is positioned in prone with the head off the end of the bed and supported in a protracted position of the neck. The patient is asked to retract the chin from this position, raising the head toward the ceiling, maintaining the face parallel to the floor.

3. To increase the side glide of the cervical spine. The patient is positioned in the raised side-lying position, resting on the elbow, so that the body is raised at a 45-degree angle with the bed. From this position, the patient performs a side glide of the neck toward the bed, without allowing any side flexion to occur. This exercise can be progressed to the upright position, where the patient elevates both arms and clasps the palm of the hands together. The side glide motion is performed to both sides. To add resistance to this exercise, the patient is positioned in complete side-lying and the side glide is performed away from the bed. In each of these exercises, it is important that the patient incorporate a minimum amount of side-flexion of the neck.

4. To increase cervicothoracic extension. A high-backed chair is used to stabilize the thoracic spine, with the top of the high back positioned level with the segment just inferior to the hypomobile segment. The patient places the hands around the mid-cervical spine with the fingers clasped together and the forearms parallel to the floor. The index fingers of the patient's clasped hands are placed over the hypermobile segment, and the exercise is performed by asking the patient to raise the chin and forearms together while simultaneously maintaining the thoracic spine against the chair back as the hypomobile segment is extended over the fulcrum produced by the back of the chair. A slight anterior force can be applied by the index fingers to prevent the hypermobile segment from extending too far. A towel can also be used in place of the index fingers.

Electrotherapeutic Modalities and Physical Agents

The same considerations for the use of electrotherapeutic modalities and physical agents are used here as in the cervical spine.

Therapeutic Exercise

Strengthening of Muscles

- *Rhomboids*: the function of the rhomboid is to adduct and elevate the scapula, and rotate it so that the glenoid cavity faces caudally.[43]
- *Middle trapezius*: the function of the middle trapezius is to adduct and stabilize the scapula.[43]
- *Lower trapezius*: the function of the lower trapezius is to depress the scapula and to rotate the scapula so that the glenoid cavity faces cranially.[43]
- *Upper trapezius*: the function of the upper trapezius is to elevate the scapula and to rotate the scapula so that the glenoid cavity faces cranially.[43] It also functions to extend, side-flex, and rotate the vertebra so that the face turns toward the opposite side.[43]
- *Serratus anterior*: the function of the serratus anterior is to abduct the scapula, rotate the inferior angle laterally, and the glenoid cavity cranially.[43] It also functions to hold the medial border of the scapula against the rib cage.[43]

While it is possible to isolate and strengthen these muscles individually, because they work together in functional activities, it is more prudent to strengthen them together.

- Shoulder shrugs. These are initiated without resistance. Once they can be performed without pain, weights are added to the hands. The shrug strengthens the upper trapezius, levator scapulae, and rhomboids.
- Shoulder circles. These are initiated without resistance. Once they can be performed without pain, weights are added to the hands. The shoulder circles strengthen the upper trapezius, levator scapulae, and rhomboids.
- Scapular retraction in internal and external rotation of the glenohumeral joint. This exercise can be performed in prone or standing and is initiated without resistance. Once it can be performed without pain, resistance is added. Scapular retraction in internal rotation of the glenohumeral joint (Figure 15–31) strengthens the infraspinatus, teres minor, middle and posterior deltoids, and the rhomboids. Scapular retraction in external rotation of the glenohumeral joint (Figure 15–32) strengthens the infraspinatus, teres minor, middle and posterior deltoids, and the middle trapezius.
- Serratus punch—end-range shoulder protraction. This is performed initially with the patient supine, the shoulder flexed to 90 degrees and the elbow extended. From this position, the patient raises the hand and protracts the shoulder girdle toward the ceiling. This exercise can be progressed by adding a weight to the hand, to being performed against a wall or a chair, before progressing to a push-up on the floor.

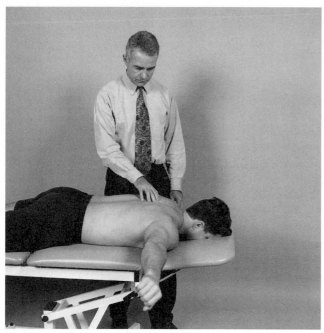

FIGURE 15–31   Strength test for scapular retraction in internal rotation.

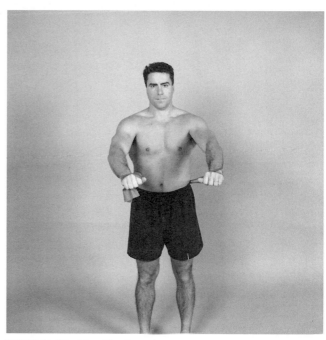

FIGURE 15–33   The 'tree-hug'.

- Tree hug. The patient is asked to wrap a length of elastic tubing around their back and to hold the two ends with the thumbs pointing forward, and the arms in about 60 degrees of abduction (Figure 15–33). From this position, the patient is asked to imagine hugging

a tree and to reproduce that motion. This is a very good exercise for the serratus anterior.

- Upright rows (Figure 15–34). The muscles involved with this exercise include the deltoids, supraspinatus, clavicular portion of the pectoralis major, long head of the biceps, the upper and lower portions of the trapezius, the levator scapulae, and the serratus anterior.

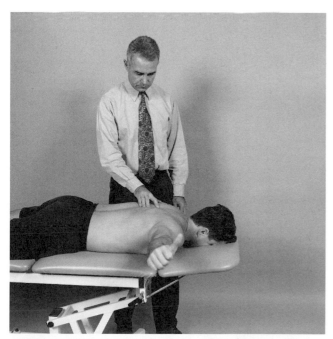

FIGURE 15–32   Strength test for scapular retraction in external rotation.

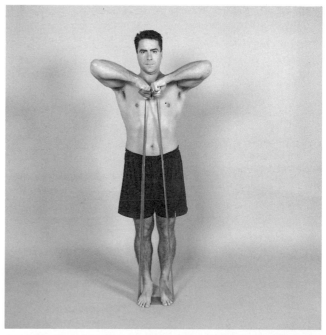

FIGURE 15–34   The upright row.

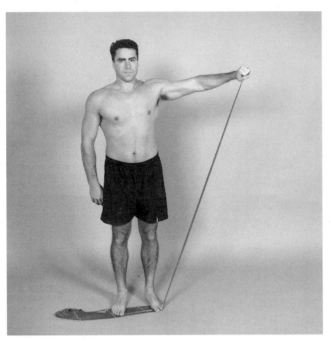

FIGURE 15–35 Lateral arm raise.

- Lateral arm raises (Figure 15–35). These are initiated without resistance. Once they can be performed without pain, resistance in the form of tubing, or hand weights, is added. Lateral arm raises involve the deltoid, supraspinatus, the serratus anterior, and the upper and lower trapezius.

- Front arm raises (Figure 15–36). These are initiated without resistance. Once they can be performed without

pain, resistance in the form of tubing, or hand weights, is added. Front arm raises involve the anterior deltoid, pectoralis major (upper portion), coacobrachialis, serratus anterior, and the upper and lower trapezius.

Soft Tissue Techniques

Muscle Stretching

- *Sternocleidomastoid:* The patient is seated or supine. The patient is asked to perform a chin tuck. From this position, the clinician induces side-flexion of the neck to the contralateral side, and extension of the neck. The clinician stabilizes the scapula and rotates the patient's head and neck toward ipsilateral side (Figure 15–37).

- *Anterior and middle scalene:* the patient is supine. Stabilizing the first two ribs with the heel of one hand, the clinician performs passive cervical extension, contralateral side-flexion, and ipsilateral rotation (Figure 15–38).

- *Levator scapulae:* the stretch can be passively applied by the clinician. The patient is positioned in supine, with the head at the edge of the table. The elbow and hand of the side to be treated are placed above the head. The clinician stands at the head of the table and presses his or her thigh against the point of the patient's elbow, fixing it caudally. Using both hands, the clinician then flexes the neck and side-flexes the patient's head to the opposite side, until resistance is felt (Figure 15–39). The patient is then asked to look

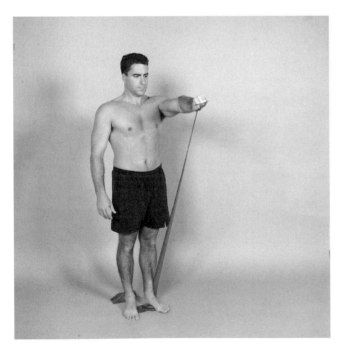

FIGURE 15–36 Front arm raise.

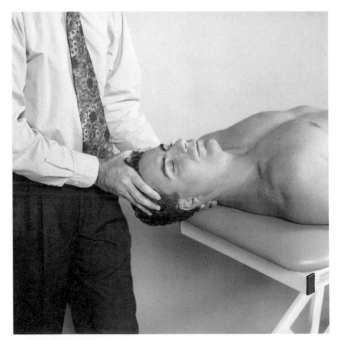

FIGURE 15–37 Patient and clinician position for the stretch of the sternocleidomastoid.

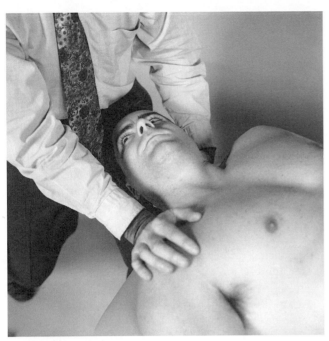

FIGURE 15–38 Patient and clinician position for the stretch of the scalenes.

toward the treated side, a motion that is resisted by the clinician. When the patient relaxes, the clinician moves the head into further side-flexion and flexion.

● *Home exercise:* the patient is positioned in supine with their head on a pillow, placing the cervical spine in flexion. The patient's head is positioned in side-flexion

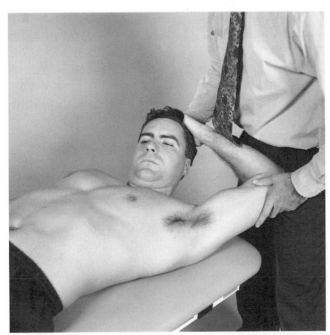

FIGURE 15–39 Patient and clinician position for the stretch of the levator scapulae.

and rotation in the opposite direction of the muscle to be stretched. A stretching cord with a loop at each end is given to the patient. The patient grasps one of the loops on the side of the muscle to be stretched, and places the foot on the same side of the muscle to be stretched in the loop at the opposite end of the cord. The cord is adjusted so that it is taut with the knee flexed. The patient is asked to elevate the scapula on the same side of the muscle to be stretched and holds that position for 5 to 8 seconds before relaxing. The patient is then asked to extend the knee to exert a downward force on the scapula, via the cord, moving it into depression. The stretch is repeated 3 to 5 times.

● *Upper trapezius:* The procedure for this is similar to that of the levator scapulae except that the starting position of the neck is modified by reducing the amount of cervical flexion. The patient is positioned in supine, with the head at the edge of the table. The elbow and hand of the side to be treated are placed above the head. The clinician stands at the head of the table and presses his or her thigh against the point of the patient's elbow, fixing it caudally. Using both hands, the clinician then flexes the neck and side-flexes the patient's head to the opposite side. Rotation to the ipsilateral side is then added until resistance is felt. The patient is then asked to look toward the treated side, a motion that is resisted by the clinician. When the patient relaxes, the clinician moves the head into further flexion, side-flexion, and rotation.

● *Pectoralis minor:* These can be effectively stretched using a corner and placing the forearms on the walls. The patient needs to avoid adopting a forward head posture during the stretch. The patient attempts to move the shoulders, against the wall, into horizontal adduction and internal rotation (Figure 15–40). The clinician is cautioned against using this exercise with any patient with shoulder pathology, especially an anterior instability.

● *Pectoralis major:* The pectoralis major can be specifically stretched if the orientation of its fibers are considered (clavicular and costosternal) by having the patient lie supine and extending the arm off the table in either approximately 140 degrees of shoulder abduction (costosternal fibers) or 45 to 50 degrees of abduction (clavicular fibers).

Case Study: Neck Pain and Arm Paresthesias

Subjective

A 21-year-old female presented to the clinic with complaints of right neck and shoulder pain and paresthesias

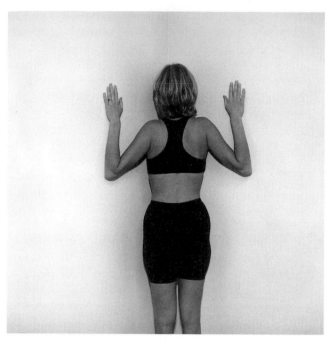

FIGURE 15–40   The wall corner stretch position.

that often radiated into the medial arm, forearm, and fourth and fifth fingers. The patient also reported that her right arm often felt tired and heavy, and that her right hand would occasionally appear to have a weak grip. The patient reported that her symptoms began shortly after she was involved in a motor vehicle accident about 2 months ago. The patient denied any history since the accident of dizziness, blurred vision, or headaches.

Examination
- Pain elicited with manual muscle testing of the trapezius, levator scapulae, sternocleidomastoid, and rhomboids on the right, which were also weak.
- Decreased flexibility of the anterior and middle scalenes and pectoralis minor and major.
- Tenderness to palpation over the brachial plexus.
- Rounded and depressed shoulders
- No evidence upon palpation of a cervical rib
- Negative Tinel sign at right wrist
- Diminished grip strength of the right hand that worsened when the right arm was raised overhead.
- Weakness of C7–T1 muscles
- Positive Allen's test
- Positive Adson's test
- Positive hyperabduction test
- Decreased mobility of the first and second ribs, but glides were normal compared to the other side.

Evaluation
It would appear from the findings that the patient has thoracic outlet syndrome.

Intervention
- *Electrotherapeutic modalities and thermal agents.* A moist heat pack was applied to the right side of the neck when the patient arrived for each treatment session.
- *Manual therapy.* Following the application of heat, the clinician mobilized the whole shoulder girdle complex and first and second ribs. The first rib was tested to see if it was elevated in relation to the other side. This was determined by palpating the first rib while passively rotating the patient's head away from the test side (rib may elevate slightly) and then extending and side-flexing it ipsilaterally (rib should descend). The head is then side-flexed contralaterally (rib should elevate). If the rib remains elevated with the ipsilateral side-flexion of the head, a mechanical impairment is suspected rather than a soft tissue one. The anterior and middle scalenes and pectoralis minor and major muscles were manually stretched, taking care not to stress the glenohumeral joint.
- *Therapeutic exercises* to strengthen the trapezius, levator scapulae, sternocleidomastoid, and rhomboids on the right were prescribed.
- *Patient-related instruction.* Explanation was given as to the cause of the patient's symptoms. The patient received instructions regarding correct posture during activities of daily living and exercises to stretch and strengthen those muscles treated in the clinic. The patient was advised to continue the exercises at home 3 to 5 times each day and to expect some post-exercise soreness. The patient also received instruction on the use of heat and ice at home.
- *Goals and outcomes.* Both the patient's goals from the treatment and the expected therapeutic goals from the clinician were discussed with the patient. It was concluded that the clinical sessions would occur 3 times per week for 1 month, at which time, the patient would be discharged to a home exercise program. With adherence to the instructions and exercise program, it was felt that the patient would make a full return to function.

Case Study: Low Neck Pain

Subjective
A 33-year old female presented with a diagnosis of low neck and upper back pain, which over the last few weeks, had become constant. Initially, the pain had been minimal but had progressively worsened. The pain was localized to the mid-line at the base of the neck, and there was no report of arm pain or symptoms. The patient worked as a computer operator for a local bank. Sleeping had become difficult, and all motions of the neck were reported to

reproduce the symptoms. The patient denied any dizziness or nausea, or history of neck trauma.

Questions

1. What structure(s) could be at fault with complaints of mid-line neck pain?
2. What should the gradual onset of the pain tell the clinician?
3. What is your working hypothesis at this stage? List the various diagnoses that could present with mid line neck pain, and the tests you would use to rule out each one.
4. Should the reports of night pain concern the clinician?
5. Does this presentation and history warrant a scan? Why or why not?

Examination

Although the onset for these symptoms had been gradual and there was reported night pain, there were no reports of pain radiation or radiculopathy. Given the localization of the pain and the patient's occupation, an irritated postural dysfunction is suspected. With this working hypothesis, an examination is performed with the following findings.

- Active range of motion of the cervical spine was limited in a noncapsular pattern of decreased flexion, both rotations, both side-flexions, and extension. Flexion was limited by 50%, both rotations and side-flexions by 30%, and extension by 70%. All of the motions reproduced the mid-line neck pain.
- The position tests were negative.
- The passive physiologic intervertebral mobility tests were positive for hypomobility at the C7–T1 segment during extension.
- The passive physiologic mobility (PPM) and passive articular mobility tests of the first two ribs were negative.
- The pain was reproduced with passive physiologic articular intervertebral mobility testing with posterior glides of both zygapophysial joints of C7 with a pathomechanical end feel.
- The passive physiologic articular intervertebral mobility testing of the upper cervical joints (refer to Chapter 18) revealed a bilateral loss of the posterior glide at both of the OA joints with a pathomechanical end feel.
- The Adson maneuver was positive bilaterally for a diminished pulse.
- Postural examination revealed a forward head posture.
- Point tenderness was elicited over the C7 segment, the origins of both levator scapulae, and the muscle bellies of both upper trapezii.

- Flexibility testing revealed bilateral tightness of the sternocleidomastoid, scalenes, and pectoralis minor and major.
- Muscle testing revealed a weakness of the rhomboids, middle and lower trapezius, and serratus anterior at 4/5.

Questions

1. Did the biomechanical examination confirm your working hypothesis? How?
2. Given the findings from the biomechanical examination, what is the diagnosis, or is further testing warranted in the form of special tests?

Evaluation

The findings from the biomechanical examination indicate an extension hypomobility at C7–T1 and muscle imbalances of the neck and shoulder complex.

Questions

1. Having confirmed the diagnosis, what will be your intervention?
2. How would you describe this condition to the patient?
3. In order of priority, and based on the stages of healing, list the various goals of your intervention?
4. How will you determine the amplitude and joint position for the intervention?
5. Is an asymmetrical or symmetrical technique more appropriate for this condition? Why?
6. Estimate this patient's prognosis.
7. What modalities could you use in the intervention of this patient?
8. What exercises would you prescribe?

Intervention

A fairly global intervention is required for this syndrome.

A. The flexibility and strength deficits of the muscles are addressed.

B. The hypomobile joints at C7–T1 and the OA segments are mobilized.

C. The patient is educated on the importance of good postural habits.
   1. Forward head. Special attention should be applied to manually increasing extension at the cervicothoracic junction and increasing the flexion of the upper cervical joints. The soft tissues that commonly need to be addressed include the following.
      a. Increasing the flexibility of:
         1. The suboccipital extensors
         2. The cervicothoracic flexors
         3. The pectoralis minor
         4. The sternocleidomastoid

   b. Correction of:
   1. The impaired levator scapulae and medial scapula muscles
   2. Any muscle imbalance
   3. Any facilitated hypertonicity

These patients need to be thoroughly assessed and treated. One of the best and most natural ways of improving posture, with little manual or other intervention by the clinician, is for the patient to initiate a walking program. Improvement should occur within a week or two unless there is an underlying biomechanical impairment. For more active intervention and reeducational purposes, the hypomobile joints need to be mobilized and the hypermobile ones protected. It is probably better to start the reeducational correction in the lumbar spine and thorax, addressing the cervical spine later.

A home exercise program is issued to reinforce the treatment.

REVIEW QUESTIONS

1. Approximately how many structures attach to the first rib and vertebral body of T1?
2. In the mobile thorax, arm elevation produces which translation of the superior vertebra of T1–2?
3. Which nerve trunk of the brachial plexus is the most commonly compressed neural structure in TOS?
4. Which tendon compresses the neurovascular bundle with shoulder hyperabduction?
5. List the "suspensory" muscles which are strengthened as part of the intervention for TOS?
6. Which diagnostic maneuver for TOS tests the flexibility of the scalenes?
7. In what position are the head and neck placed in order to stretch the sternocleidomastoid?
8. Weakness of the hand intrinsics, and accompanying TOS signs and symptoms would tend to implicate which nerve trunk of the brachial plexus?

ANSWERS

1. 32
2. Posterior
3. Lowest (C8–T1)
4. Pectoralis minor
5. Middle and upper trapezius, levator scapulae and sternocleidomastoid
6. Adson's
7. Occipito-atlantal flexion, contralateral side-flexion and extension of the neck, and ipsilateral rotation of the head and neck.
8. Lower

REFERENCES

1. Schmor G, Junghanns H. The Human Spine in Health and Disease. 2nd. New York: Grune & Stratton; 1971: 55–60.
2. Wigh R. The thoracolumbar and lumbosacral transitional junctions. *Spine* 1980;5:215–222.
3. Lewitt K. Manipulative Therapy in Rehabilitation of the Locomotor System. 2nd ed, Oxford: Butterworth-Heinemann; 1996.
4. Williams PL, Warwick R, Dyson M, Bannister LH: Gray's Anatomy. 37th Ed. Churchill Livingstone, Edinburgh.
5. Bogduk N, Marsland A. The cervical zygapophysial joint as a source of neck pain. *Spine* 1988;13:610.
6. Haymaker W, Woodhall B. Peripheral Nerve Injuries, 2nd ed. Philadelphia: Saunders; 1953.
7. Lee D. Manual Therapy for the Thorax—A Biomechanical Approach. Delta Publishers, B. C., Canada: 1994.
8. Goldberg ME, Eggers HM, Gouras P. The ocular motor system. In: Kandel ER, Schwartz JH, Jessell TM, eds. *Principles of Neural Science.* 3rd ed. Norwalk, C: Appleton & Lange; 1991:660–677.
9. Scariati P. Neurophysiology relevant to osteopathic manipulation. In: DiGiovanna E, ed. *Osteopathic Approach to Diagnosis and Treatment.* Philadelphia: Lippincott; 1991.
10. Mannheimer JS. Prevention and restoration of abnormal upper quarter posture. In: Gelb H, Gelb M, eds. Postural Considerations in the Diagnosis and Treatment of Cranio-Cervical-Mandibular and Related Chronic Pain Disorders. St. Louis, Mo: Ishiyaku EuroAmerica; 1991:93–161.
11. Troyanovich SJ, Harrison DE, Harrison DD. Structural rehabilitation of the spinc and posture: rationale for treatment beyond the resolution of symptoms. *J Manip Phys Ther* 1998;21:37–50.
12. Visscher CM, deBoer W, Naeije M. The relationship between posture and curvature of the cervical spine. *J Manip Phys Ther* 1998;21:388–391.
13. Nichols AW. The thoracic outlet syndrome in athletes. *J Am Board Fam Prac* 1996;9:346–355.
14. Thompson JF, Jannsen F. Thoracic outlet syndromes. *Br J Surg* 1996;8:435–436.
15. Strukel RJ, Garrick JG. Thoracic outlet compression in athletes: a report of four cases. *Am J Sports Med* 1978;6:35–39.
16. Anonymous. The Classic surgical treatment for symptoms produced by cervical ribs and the scalenus anticus muscle. By Alfred Washington Adson. 1947. *Clin Orthop* 1986;207:3–12.
17. Peet RM, Hendriksen JD, Anderson TP, Martin GM. Thoracic outlet syndrome: evaluation of the therapeutic exercise program. *Proc Mayo Clin* 1956;31:281–287.

18. Roos DB. The place for scalenectomy and first-rib resection in thoracic outlet syndrome. *Surgery* 1982;92:1077–1085.

19. Wood VE, Twito R, Verska JM. Thoracic outlet syndrome. The results of first rib resection in 100 patients. *Orthop Clin North Am* 1988;19:131–146.

20. Mackinnon SE, Dellon AL. *Surgery of the Peripheral Nerve.* New York: Thieme, 1988.

21. Roos, DB. Thoracic outlet nerve compression in Rutherford, RB (ed). Vascular surgery. 3rd ed. Philadelphia WB Saunders, 1989;858–875.

22. Karas SE. Thoracic outlet syndrome. *Clin Sports Med* 1990;9:297–310.

23. Selke FW, Kelly TR. Thoracic outlet syndrome. *Am J Surg* 1988;156:54–57.

24. Riddell DH, Smith BM. Thoracic and vascular aspects of thoracic outlet syndrome. *Clin Orthop* 1986;207:31–36.

25. Sanders RJ, Jackson CG, Banchero N, Pearce WH. Scalene muscle abnormalities in traumatic thoracic outlet syndrome. *Am J Surg* 1990;159:231–236.

26. McCarthy WJ, Yao JST, Schafer MF, et al. Upper extremity arterial injury in athletes. *J Vasc Surg* 1989;9:317–327.

27. Vogel CM, Jensen JE. "Effort" thrombosis of the subclavian vein in a competitive swimmer. *Am J Sports Med* 1985;13:269–272.

28. Cikrit DF, Haefner R, Nichols WK, Silver D. Transaxillary or supraclavicular decompression for the thoracic outlet syndrome. A comparison of the risks and benefits. *Am Surg* 1989;55:347–352.

29. Lindgren KA, Oksala I. Long-term outcome of surgery for thoracic outlet syndrome. *Am J Surg* 1995;169:358–360.

30. Lindgren KA. Thoracic outlet syndrome with special reference to the first rib. *Ann Chir Gynaecol* 1993;82:218–230.

31. Leffert RD. Thoracic outlet syndrome and the shoulder. *Clin Sports Med* 1983;2:439–452.

32. Thompson VP. Anatomical research lives. *Nat Med* 1995;1:297–298.

33. Nishida T, Price SJ, Minieka MM. Medial antebrachial cutaneous nerve conduction in true neurogenic thoracic outlet syndrome. *Electromyogr Clin Neurophysiol* 1993;33:285–288.

34. Crawford FA. Thoracic outlet syndrome. *Surg Clin North Am* 1980;60:947–956.

35. Sanders RJ, Johnson RF. Medico-legal matters. In: Sanders RJ, Haug CE, eds. *Thoracic Outlet Syndrome: A Common Sequela of Neck Injuries.* Philadelphia: Lippincott; 1991:271–277.

36. Cuetter AC, David MB. The thoracic outlet syndrome: controversies, over diagnosis, over treatment, and recommendations for management. *Muscle Nerve* 1989;12:410–419.

37. Stanton PE Jr, Vo NM, Haley T, Shannon J, Evans J. Thoracic outlet syndrome: a comprehensive evaluation. *Am Surg* 1988;54:129–133.

38. Kenny RA, Traynor GB, Withington D, Keegan DJ. Thoracic outlet syndrome: a useful exercise treatment option. *Am J Surg* 1993;165:282–284.

39. Thirupathi R, Husted C. Traumatic disruption of the manubriosternal joint. *Bull Hosp Jt Dis* 1982;42:242–247.

40. Cameron HU. Traumatic disruption of the manubriosternal joint in the absence of rib fractures. *J Trauma* 1980;20:892.

41. Fowler C. Manual therapy: NAIOMT level II & III course notes. Denver: 1995.

42. Mitchell F, Moran PS, Pruzzo NA. An Evaluation and Treatment Manual of Osteopathic Muscle Energy Procedures. ICEOP, Missouri. 1979.

43. Kendall FP, Kendall KM, Provance PG. Muscles: Testing and Function. 4th ed. Baltimore: Williams & Wilkins; 1993.

CHAPTER SIXTEEN

THE THORACIC SPINE

Chapter Objectives

At the completion of this chapter, the reader will be able to:

1. Describe the anatomy of the vertebra, ligaments, muscles, and blood and nerve supply that comprise the thoracic intervertebral segment.
2. Describe the biomechanics of the thoracic spine, including coupled movements, normal and abnormal joint barriers, kinesiology, and reactions to various stresses.
3. Perform a detailed objective examination of the thoracic musculoskeletal system, including palpation of the articular and soft tissue structures, combined motion testing, specific passive mobility and passive articular mobility tests for the intervertebral joints, and stability tests.
4. Analyze the total examination data to establish the definitive biomechanical diagnosis.
5. Apply active and passive mobilization techniques and combined movements to the thoracic spine, in any position, using the correct grade, direction, and duration, and explain the mechanical and physiologic effects.
6. Describe intervention strategies based on clinical findings and established goals.
7. Evaluate intervention effectiveness to progress or modify intervention.
8. Plan an effective home program including spinal care, and instruct the patient in same.
9. Develop self-reliant examination and intervention strategies.

OVERVIEW

In the thoracic spine, protection and function of the thoracic viscera take precedence over intersegmental spinal mobility. Without the ribs, the joints of the thoracic segments would be unmodified ovoids, capable of a vast amount of motion. However, because of the presence of the ribs, the thoracic spine is the least mobile part of the spinal column. It is also an area that is very prone to postural impairments.

ANATOMY

The thoracic region differs from the cervical and lumbar spines in the following ways.

- The presence of a demi facet on the centrum and a costal articular facet on the transverse process that articulate with the ribs. The head of the rib develops an upward projection similar to the uncinate process of the cervical spine.
- The transverse processes possess articular facets for the rib at the costotransverse joint.
- The presence of a small spinal canal for the size of its contents.
- A somewhat deficient blood supply to the spinal cord.
- Coronally orientated articulating facets that facilitate rotation at the segment.

The thoracic spine forms a kyphotic curve of less than 55 degrees,[1] with an accepted range of 20 to 50 degrees,[2] and an average of 45 degrees.[3] It is a structural curve, that is present from birth and considered as a persisting curve of the embryonic axis.[4] Unlike the lumbar and cervical regions, which derive their curves from the corresponding differences in intervertebral disc heights, the thoracic curve is maintained by the wedge-shaped vertebral bodies that are about 2 mm higher posteriorly. The thoracic curve begins at T1–2 and extends down to T12, with the T6–7 disc space as the apex.[5] The kyphotic curve is more prone to be unstable in flexion, and is also vulnerable to alterations from postural habits or disease. Juvenile kyphosis (Scheuermann's disease) and osteoporosis both result in an increase in thoracic kyphosis. Changes in the thoracic curve have an impact on the other spinal curves. For example, an increase in the thoracic kyphosis produces an increased lumbar lordosis and an anterior shifting in the cervical curve.

In addition to the kyphosis, a slight lateral curve in the coronal plane may be present. It is thought that this curve may result from right-hand dominance or the presence of the aorta.[6]

Vertebra

The vertebrae of this region are classified as typical or atypical, with reference to their morphology. The typical thoracic vertebrae are found at T2–9, although T9 may be atypical in that its inferior costal facet is frequently absent. The atypical thoracic vertebrae are the first, tenth, eleventh, and twelfth (and often the ninth)— the upper and lower vertebrae tend to show signs of transition, from a cervical form to a lumbar form, respectively. All of the vertebrae consist of the usual elements (Figure 16–1).

- *Centrum or body*: the typical vertebral body is heart-shaped in cross section and, on each of its lateral aspects, has a superior and inferior costal facet for articulation with the ribs (costovertebral joint). The body is roughly as wide as it is long so that its anterior-posterior and medial-lateral dimensions are of equal length.[7] The body is also very high and strongly constricted about its anterior and lateral aspects. The anterior surface of the body is convex from side to side whereas the posterior surface is deeply concave.[7]

- *Neural arch*: the neural arch is constructed out of two short pedicles and two short, thick laminae, the latter joining to form the spinous process.

- *Transverse and articular processes*: The transverse processes are posteriorly oriented (point backward) and are located directly between the inferior articulating process and superior articulating process of the zygapophysial joints of each level, which make them useful as palpation points when mobility testing in the mid thorax. The costotransverse joint is formed by an oval facet on the lateral aspects of all of the transverse processes, to which the rib attaches, except for T11 and T12, to which no ribs are attached.

The thoracic vertebrae increase in size caudally, their angle of inclination changing depending on their level.

- The upper segments are inclined at 45 to 60 degrees horizontally.
- The middle segments are inclined at 90 degrees horizontally.
- The lower segments are inclined as in the lumbar spine.

The third vertebra is typical but it is the smallest of all of the thoracic vertebra. The T9 vertebra may have no demi facets below, or it may have two demi facets on either side (in which case, the T10 vertebra will have demi facets only at the superior aspect). The T10 vertebra has one full rib facet located partly on the body of the vertebra and partly on the tubercle. It does not articulate with the eleventh rib and so does not possess inferior demi facets and, occasionally, there is no facet for the rib at the costotransverse joint. The tenth rib is very variable. The T11 vertebra has complete costal facets but no facets on the transverse processes

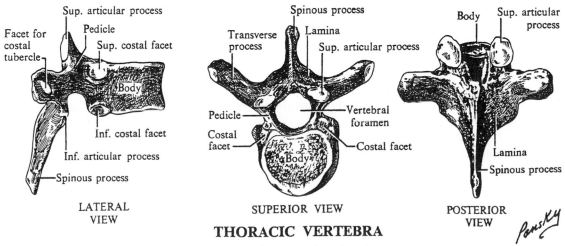

FIGURE 16–1 A typical thoracic vertebral body. (Reproduced, with permission from Pansky B: Review of Gross Anatomy, 6/e. McGraw-Hill, 1996)

for the rib tubercle. This vertebra also begins to take on the characteristics of a lumbar vertebra (the spinous process is short and almost completely horizontal). The T12 vertebra only articulates with its own ribs, and does not possess inferior demi facets. The facets on the inferior articular processes of T12 are lumbar in orientation and concavity. The orientation of the zygapophysial facets changes in orientation by 90 degrees at either T11 or T12, allowing for pure axial rotation to occur. Pure axial rotation (twisting) can only occur at two points in the spine, the thoracolumbar (T–L) and cervicothoracic (C–T) junctions.

The spinous processes of the thoracic region are long, slender, and triangular shaped in cross section. They point obliquely downward, overlapping each other in the mid-thoracic region. This degree of obliquity varies. The first three spinous processes, and the last three are almost horizontal, while those of the mid-thorax are long and steeply inclined.

The common spinal ligaments are present in the thoracic spine and they perform much the same function as they do elsewhere in the spine. However, the anterior longitudinal ligament in this region is narrower but thicker compared to the rest of the spine,[7] whereas the posterior longitudinal ligament, strongly developed at the thoracic level, is wider here at the disc level, but narrower at the vertebral body than in the lumbar region.[8]

The intervertebral disc is narrower and thinner than those in the cervical and lumbar levels, and gradually increases in size from superior to inferior.

The costospinal joints have ligaments unique to this area (Figure 16–2).

- *Costotransverse joint*: the costotransverse ligament, superior costotransverse ligament, and lateral costotransverse ligament
- *Costovertebral joint*: the radiate ligament and intra-articular ligament

Nerve Roots

In the thoracic spine, the segmental nerve roots are situated mainly behind the inferior-posterior aspect of the upper vertebral body rather than behind the disc, which reduces the possibility of root compression in impairments of the thoracic disc.[6] As at the cervical and lumbar level, the thoracic spinal nerves emerge from the cord as a large ventral, and a smaller dorsal, ramus, which join together to form a short spinal nerve root. There are no plexuses in this area and the spinal nerves form the intercostal nerves.[7] The intraspinal course of the upper thoracic nerve root is almost horizontal (as in the cervical spine). Therefore, the nerve can only be compressed by its corresponding disc. However, moving

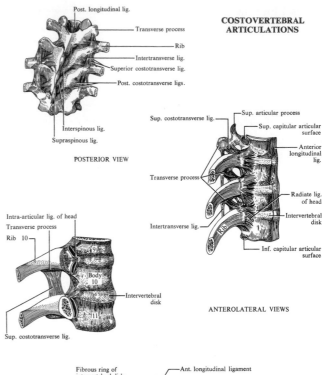

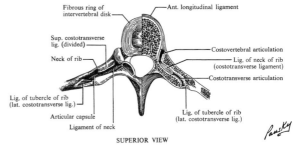

FIGURE 16–2 The thoracic joints and their ligaments. (Reproduced, with permission from Pansky B: Review of Gross Anatomy, 6/e. McGraw-Hill, 1996)

more inferiorly in the spine, the course of the nerve root becomes more oblique, and the lowest thoracic nerve roots can be compressed by disc impairments of two consecutive levels (T12 root by eleventh or twelfth disc). Central disc protrusions are more common in the thoracic region than in other regions of the spine and because the nucleus is small in the thorax, protrusions are invariably of the anular type and nuclear protrusions are rare. Because the intervertebral foramina are quite large at these levels, osseous contact with the nerve roots is seldom encountered in the thoracic spine. As the dermatomes in this region have a fair amount of overlap, they cannot be relied upon to determine the specific nerve root involved.

As at the lumbar and cervical levels, innervation of the spinal canal is by the sinuvertebral nerve which arises from the nerve root and reenters the epidural space. It is formed by a spinal and a sympathetic root. Typically, the spinal root arises from the lateral end of the spinal nerve but, in 25% of cases, the spinal root is made up of two parts that arise from the superior border of the spinal nerve.[9]

Ribs

Twelve pairs of ribs, together with the sternum, the clavicle, and the thoracic spine, form the bony thoracic cage. Each rib consists of a head, neck, and body. The head of the rib consists of the slightly enlarged posterior end, normally carrying two demi facets for the synovial costovertebral joints. All ribs are different sizes, widths, and curvatures. The first rib is the shortest. The rib length increases further inferiorly until the seventh rib, after which they become progressively shorter. The ribs are classified as typical or atypical based on morphology and attachment sites.

Typical
The typical rib[7] has a posterior end containing the head, neck, and tubercle. Its convex shaft is connected to the neck at the rib angle. The upper border of the shaft is round and blunt, whereas the inferior aspect is thin and sharp. The head is divided by a horizontal ridge that affords attachment for the intra-articular ligament. The head of the rib projects upward in a very similar manner to that of the uncinate process in the cervical spine and, in fact, develops in much the same way during childhood, appearing to play a similar mechanical role. The tubercle of the rib lies on the outer surface, where the neck joins the shaft, and is more prominent in the upper parts than in the lower. The articular portion of the tubercle presents an oval facet for articulation at the costotransverse joint. The anterior end of the shaft has a small depression at the tip for articulation at the costochondral joint.

Atypical
The first, second, tenth, eleventh, and twelfth ribs are atypical[7] in that they only articulate with their own vertebra via one full facet, and the lower two do not articulate with the costochondrium anteriorly. The tenth rib has only a single facet on its head due to its lack of articulation with the vertebra above. The eleventh and twelfth ribs do not present tubercles and have only a single articular facet on their heads. The tip of the shortened shafts do not articulate with the costochondrium and so are pointed and covered with cartilage.

The attachment of the ribs to the sternum is variable. The upper five, six, or seven ribs have their own cartilaginous connection.[7] The cartilage of the eighth rib ends by blending with the seventh. The same situation pertains for the ninth and tenth ribs, so giving rise to a common band of cartilage and connective tissue. As mentioned, the eleventh and twelfth ribs remain unattached anteriorly, but end with a small piece of cartilage.

The strong ligamentous attendance, and the presence of the two joints (costovertebral and costotransverse) at each level, severely limits the amount of movement permitted here to slight gliding and spinning motions, morphology determining the function of each rib.[7] The orientation of the ribs increases from being horizontal at the upper levels to being more downwardly oblique in the more inferior levels of the thoracic spine (worth remembering when palpating). The ribs of the midthorax have two demi facets.[7] The shapes of the articular facets of the upper six ribs would suggest that the upward and downward gliding movements that occur would produce spinning of the neck of the rib. In fact, the main movement in the upper six ribs is one of rotation of the neck of the rib, with only small amounts of superior and inferior motion. In the seventh through tenth ribs, the principal movement is superior, posterior, and medial motion during inspiration, with the reverse occurring during expiration.[11]

Zygapophysial Joints

The superior and inferior facets of the zygapophysial joints arise from the upper and lower part of the pedicle of the thoracic vertebra. The superior facet lies superiorly with the articular surface on the posterior aspect, whereas the inferior facet lies inferiorly with the articular surface on the anterior aspect. The facet joint of the thoracic spine is quite different from that of the cervical and lumbar spines because it is oriented in a more coronal direction (see Figure 16–1). It forms an angle of about 60 degrees to the coronal plane and only 20 degrees to the sagittal plane, following the surface of a sphere. Studies have shown that the thoracic facets play an important role in stabilization of the thoracic spine during flexion loading.[12,13]

The degree of superior-inferior and medial-lateral orientation is slight (see Figure 16–1). The superior facet arises from near the lamina-pedicle junction and faces posteriorly, superiorly, and laterally, with the degree of superior-lateral orientation being slight. It is slightly convex posteriorly.

The inferior facet arises from the laminae to face inferiorly, medially, and anteriorly, lying posterior to the superior facet of the vertebra below. The facet surfaces are concave anteriorly and convex posteriorly, bringing the axis of rotation through the centrum rather than through the spinous process, as in the lumbar vertebrae. This concavity means that the biomechanical center of rotation coincides with the actual center formed by body weight.[10] This arrangement (unmodified ovoid) would allow for large amounts of almost pure axial rotation were it not for the effect of the ribs, which restrict and modify the rotation, resulting in coupling.

Costovertebral Joint

This is a hyalinated, synovial joint that forms a relationship between the head of the rib and the lateral side of the vertebral body (see Figure 16–2). Although the joint cannot be palpated, it only has one motion—spinning.[10] The first, tenth, eleventh, and twelfth ribs articulate with their own vertebrae, whereas the remainder articulate with both their own and the vertebra above. Running between the head of the rib and the disc, is the intra-articular ligament and disc. The effect of these structures is to divide the joint into superior and inferior compartments and make this joint both a compound and a complex one. Before the age of about 13 years, there is no superior costovertebral joint, as ossification of the head of the rib has not occurred (hence the vast amount of thoracic rotation and side-flexion that a 8 to 12 year-old gymnast demonstrates).

The radiate ligament (see Figure 16–2) connects the anterior aspect of the rib head to the bodies of two vertebrae and their intervening disc. Each of the three bands of the fan-shaped radiate ligament have different attachments. The superior part runs from the head of the rib to the body of the superior vertebral. The inferior part runs to the body of the inferior vertebra. The intermediate part runs to the intervening disc.

The functional spinal unit (FSU),[14] consisting of two vertebrae and the interconnecting soft tissue, is considered to be the smallest working unit in the cervical and lumbar spine. However, the biomechanical aspects of the thoracic spine are different from those of the cervical and lumbar spine. The thoracic spine is connected to the rib cage by the costovertebral joints, which consist of the costotransverse joints and joints of the head of the ribs (see Figure 16–2). The thoracic vertebrae are connected to their adjacent vertebrae by the bilateral costovertebral joints (see Figure 16–2). Thus, from an anatomic point of view, the FSU should not be regarded as the smallest working unit in the thoracic spine. The costovertebral joints and their surrounding ligaments, such as the costotransverse, superior costotransverse, radiate, and intra-articular ligaments (Figure 16–2), connect adjacent vertebrae and ribs. The "rib cage" consists of these ligaments, the thoracic vertebrae, ribs, and sternum. Various studies have demonstrated that additional structural stability may be provided to the thoracic spine by the costovertebral joints and rib cage.[13,15,16] From a mechanical point of view, destruction of the costovertebral joint would represent damage to the connections between the thoracic spine and the rib cage. Panjabi and colleagues[12] also reported that the costovertebral joints play a pivotal role in stabilizing the functional spinal units of the thoracic spine, and that if there is evidence of costovertebral joint destruction in clinical situations, the ability of the spine to carry normal physiologic loads should be questioned.

Costotransverse Joint

This is a synovial joint between an articular facet on the posterior aspect of the rib tubercle and an articular facet on the anterior aspect of the transverse process (see Figure 16–2). It is supported by a thin fibrous capsule. In the lower two vertebral segments, this articulation does not exist. The fibrous capsule attaches to the edges of the articular surfaces and is a thin membrane. The neck of the rib lies along the length of the posterior aspect of the transverse process. The short, deep costotransverse ligament runs from the posterior aspect of the neck of the rib posteriorly, to the anterior aspect of its transverse process, and fills the costotransverse foramen between the rib neck and its adjacent transverse process (see Figure 16–2).

The superior costotransverse ligament (also called the interosseous, or ligament of the neck of the rib) is formed in two layers (see Figure 16–2). The anterior layer, which is continuous with the internal intercostal membrane laterally, runs from the neck of the rib, up and laterally, to the inferior aspect of the transverse process above. The posterior layer runs up and medially from the posterior aspect of the rib neck to the transverse process above. Jiang et al[17] reported that the superior costotransverse ligaments are very important in maintaining the lateral stability of the spine.

The lateral costotransverse ligament (see Figure 16–2) runs from the tip of the transverse process laterally to the tubercle of its own rib. It is short, thick, and strong but is often damaged with direct blows to the chest (punch, kick, etc.), responding well to ultrasound and transverse friction massage.

Sternum

This is formed in three parts.

- The manubrium (refer to the Chapter 15)
- The body (mesosternum)
- The xiphisternum (xiphoid process)

The body of the sternum is made up of the fused elements of four sternal bodies and the vestiges of these are marked by three horizontal ridges. The upper end of the body articulates with the manubrium at the sternal angle. A facet at the superior end of the body laterally provides a joint surface common with the manubrium for the second costal cartilage. On each lateral border are four other notches that articulate with the third through sixth cartilages. A synchondrosis joins the manubrium and sternal body. It protrudes slightly anteriorly and is known as the sternal angle of Louis. This is an important landmark because the second rib is attached to the sternum at this level. T7 articulates both with the sternum and the xiphoid. The third rib has the deepest fossa on the sternum, indicating that it may serve as the axis for rotation and side-flexion during arm elevation.

The xiphisternum is the smallest part of the sternum. It begins life in a cartilaginous state but, in adulthood, the upper part ossifies. The symphysis usually becomes synostotic after 40 years, but may remain separate even in extreme old age.

Andriacchi[15] and co-workers performed a computer simulation analysis to determine the effect of the rib cage on the stiffness properties of the normal spine during flexion, extension, side-flexion, and axial rotation, and found them to be greatly enhanced by the presence of the rib cage for all four motions, especially extension. The effect of removal of the entire sternum from the intact thorax was also studied, and the result was an almost complete loss of the stiffening effect of the thorax.[16]

Sternocostal Joint

This joint is classified as a synarthrosis. In all of these joints, the periosteum of the sternum and the perichondrium of the costal cartilage is continuous. Synovial joints exist between the costal cartilages and the sternum (except for the first joint, which is a synchondrosis). A thin fibrous capsule is present in the upper seven joints, and attaches to the circumference of the articular surfaces, blending with the sternocostal ligaments. The surface of the joints are covered with fibrocartilage and are supported by capsular, radiate sternocostal or xiphicostal and intra-articular ligaments. The joint is capable of slight motion during full inspiration and full expiration allowing for excursion of the sternum in these activities.

Respiratory Muscles

Connections to the respiratory mechanism have been found to exert a strong influence on areas such as the shoulder and pelvic girdles, as well as the head and neck. Restoration of the respiratory mechanism is an essential element of thoracic intervention.

Respiratory muscles are skeletal muscles that are morphologically and functionally similar to locomotor muscles. Their primary task is to displace the chest wall and, therefore, move gas in and out of the lungs to maintain arterial blood gas and pH homeostasis. The importance of normal respiratory muscle function can be appreciated by considering that respiratory muscle failure due to fatigue, injury, or disease could result in an inability to maintain blood gas and pH levels within an acceptable range and could have lethal consequences.

The function of the ventilatory muscles is an active area of research, but the key finding is that the ventilatory pump is a multimuscle pump. The actions of various ventilatory muscles, which are broadly classified as inspiratory or expiratory based on their mechanical actions, are highly redundant and provide several means by which air can be effectively displaced under a host of physiologic and pathophysiologic conditions.[18,19] For example, even at rest, movement of air into and out of the lungs is the result of the recruitment of several muscles.[20,21] In resting humans, the tidal volume is the result of the coordinated recruitment of the diaphragm, the parasternal intercostal, and the scalene muscles.[22,23] Even the expiratory phase of breathing at rest can be associated with active muscle participation.[24] Despite the fact that quiet breathing involves several muscles, under normal circumstances, breathing demands only a small effort.[25]

Although some have argued that respiratory muscle performance does not limit exercise tolerance in normal healthy adults,[26,27] heavy or prolonged exercise has been shown to impair respiratory muscle performance in humans.[28,29] Furthermore, patients with chronic obstructive lung disease often exhibit respiratory muscle weakness and/or reduced respiratory endurance. This is clinically significant because individuals with reduced respiratory muscle endurance are predisposed to respiratory failure or to a pulmonary limitation to exercise.[30,31]

Because of the potential for respiratory muscle fatigue in both health and disease, interest in the adaptability of respiratory muscles to endurance-type exercise has grown significantly during the last decade.

The diaphragm is the primary muscle of respiration, and may be the only muscle actively elevating the ribs during quiet respiration.[32] It is important to be able to accurately assess the diaphragm for weakness. Patients with bilateral diaphragm paralysis or severe weakness present a striking clinical picture, with orthopnea as the major symptom. Lesser degrees of diaphragm weakness, however, are hard to detect and need specific testing. Vital capacity may be reduced, but this is a nonspecific and relatively insensitive measure, and diaphragm weakness has to be moderately severe before there is a substantial reduction.[34,35]

Beside sharing all common mechanical characteristics with the skeletal muscles of the limbs, the ventilatory muscles are prone to fatigue and are also endowed with the capacity to adapt to altered conditions, including physical exercise.[35,36] Whether or not fatigue or weakness occurs in the respiratory muscles as a result of heavy whole-body exercise has been debated for many decades.[37,38] Although several other respiratory muscles are recruited with whole-body exercise (i.e., external intercostals, scalenes, and sternocleidomastoid muscles), the diaphragm is the most effective pressure generator for increasing alveolar ventilation and, thus, provides the best index of respiratory system muscle function.[39,40]

Despite some similarities, the ventilatory muscles are distinct from the skeletal muscles of the limbs in several aspects.[41,42] First, whereas skeletal muscles of the limbs overcome inertial loads, the ventilatory muscles overcome primarily elastic and resistive loads. Second, the ventilatory muscles are under both voluntary and involuntary control. The third distinguishing feature is that the ventilatory muscles, which represent only 3% of body weight,[43] are like the heart muscles, in that they have to contract rhythmically and generate the required forces for ventilation throughout the entire life of the individual. The ventilatory muscles, however, do not contain pacemaker cells and are under the control of mechanical and chemical stimuli, requiring neural input from higher centers to initiate and coordinate contraction.

The last distinguishing feature of the respiratory muscles is related to their anatomic resting position. Fenn[41] points out that the resting length of the respiratory muscles is a relationship between the inward recoil forces of the lung and the outward recoil forces of the chest wall. Changes between the balance of recoil forces will result in changes in the resting length of the respiratory muscles. Thus, simple and every-day life occurrences, such as changes in posture, will alter the operational length and the contractile strength of the ventilatory muscles. If uncompensated, these length changes would lead to decreases in the output of the muscles and a reduction in the ability to generate volume changes. The skeletal muscles of the limbs, on the other hand, are not constrained to operate at a particular resting length.

Diaphragm

The diaphragm has a phrenic C3–C4 motor innervation and a sensory supply by the lower six intercostal nerves. Functionally and metabolically, the diaphragm can be classified as two muscles[44,45]: the crural (posterior) portion that inserts into the lumbar vertebrae and the costal portion that inserts into the xiphoid process of the sternum and into the margins of the lower ribs. Anatomically, the muscle may be divided into sternal, costal, and lumbar parts.

- The sternal fibers originate from two slips at the back of the xiphoid process.
- The costal fibers originate from the lower six ribs and their costal cartilages.
- The lumbar fibers originate from the crura of the lumbar vertebra and the medial and lateral arcuate ligaments.

Thus, the muscle is attached around the thoracoabdominal junction circumferentially. From these attachments, the fibers arch toward each other centrally to form a large tendon.

Contraction of the diaphragm pulls the large, central tendon inferiorly, producing diaphragmatic inspiration (see later). The other primary muscles of respiration are the sternocostal, and the intercostals, the secondary ones being the anterior and medial scalenes, serratus posterior, pectoralis major and minor, and, with the head fixed, the sternocleidomastoid.

Intercostals

Between the ribs are the intercostal spaces, which are both deeper in front and between the upper ribs. The intercostal muscles connect the ribs to each other and are primary respiratory muscles.[6] The intercostal muscles, together with the sternalis (or sternocostalis or transversalis thoracis), phylogenically form from the hypomeric muscles, and correspond to their abdominal counterparts with the sternalis being homologous to the rectus abdominous, and the intercostals homologous to the external oblique.

- *External intercostals*: the external intercostal muscles, of which there are eleven, are laid in a direction that is superior-posterior to inferior-anterior (run inferiorly and medially in the front of the thorax and inferiorly and laterally in the back). They attach to the lower border of one rib and the upper border of the rib below, extending from the tubercle to the costal cartilage. Posteriorly, the muscle is continuous with the posterior fibers of the superior costotransverse ligament. Due to the oblique course of the fibers, and the fact that leverage is greatest on the lower of the two ribs, the muscle pulls the lower rib towards the upper rib, which results in inspiration. The action of the external intercostals is believed to be entirely inspiratory, although it also counteracts the force of the diaphragm, preventing the collapse of the ribs. Innervation of this muscle is supplied by the adjacent intercostal nerve.
- *Internal intercostals*: the internal intercostals, which also number eleven, have their fibers in a inferior-posterior

to a superior-anterior direction. They are found deep to the external intercostals and also run obliquely, but perpendicular, to the externals. They extend from the posterior rib angles to the sternum, where they end posteriorly. They are continuous with the internal membrane, which then becomes continuous with the anterior part of the superior costotransverse ligament. The action of the internal intercostals is believed to be entirely expiratory. They pull the upper rib down, but only during enforced expiration. Innervation of this muscle is supplied by the adjacent intercostal nerve.

- *Transverse intercostals (intima)*: the deepest of the intercostals, it is attached to the internal aspects of two contiguous ribs. They become progressively more significant and developed further down the thorax. This muscle is used during forced expiration.

Levator Costae

These consist of twelve strong, short muscles that turn obliquely (inferior-laterally), parallel with the external intercostal, from the tip of the transverse process to the angle of the rib. They extend from the C7 to T11 transverse processes. These muscles, innervated by the lateral branch of the dorsal ramus of the thoracic nerve, function to raise the rib, but their importance in respiration is argued. They may also be segmentally involved in rotation and side-flexion of the thoracic vertebra.

Serratus Posterior Superior

The serratus posterior superior runs from the lower part of the ligamentum nuchae, the spinous processes of C7, T1–3, and their supraspinous ligaments, to the inferior border of the second through fifth ribs, lateral to the rib angle. It receives its nerve supply from the second through fifth intercostal nerves. Its function is unclear but it is thought to elevate the rib.

Serratus Posterior Inferior

This muscle arises from the spines and supraspinous ligaments of the two lower thoracic and the two or three upper lumbar vertebrae. It attaches to the inferior border of the lower four ribs, lateral to the rib angle. It receives its nerve supply from the ventral rami of the ninth through twelfth thoracic nerves. Its function is unclear but it is thought to pull the ribs downward and backward.

THORACIC BIOMECHANICS

The biomechanics of the thoracic spine can be expected to be considerably different from those of the lumbar and cervical regions due to the modifying influence of the ribs.[15]

Flexion

There are about 2 to 4 degrees of flexion available at each thoracic segment[46] (25 to 45 degrees total). Flexion is initiated by the abdominal muscles and, in the absence of resistance, and in the erect position, continued by gravity with the spinal erector muscles eccentrically controlling the descent. Flexion may also occur during bilateral scapular protraction. Clinically, three movement patterns can occur and are dependent upon the relative flexibility between the vertebrae and the rib cage. In the mobile thorax, during flexion, the superior facets (i.e., the inferior articular processes of the superior vertebra of the segment) glide superiorly and anteriorly.[47]

This motion at the zygapophysial joint is accompanied by an anterior translation of the superior vertebra, and slight distraction of the centra at the disc. It seems likely that the anterior vertebral rotation and the anterior translation produces a similar rotation in the ribs and a superior glide at the costotransverse joint.[47] During flexion, the anterior aspects of the ribs approximate each other, whereas the posterior aspects separate. One study found that by transecting the various posterior structures sequentially, flexion failure occurred only when the costovertebral joint was affected.[12] Flexion is resisted by the posterior half of disc and anulus, and by the impaction of the zygapophysial joints.

Extension

A total of 15 to 20 degrees of extension is available at 1 to 2 degrees per segment. Extension is produced principally by the lumbar extensors, and results in an inferior glide of the superior facet of the zygapophysial joint. However, bilateral shoulder elevation and scapular retraction are capable of producing extension. During this zygapophysial motion, there occurs a posterior translation of the vertebra and a slight compression of the centrum. The ribs are rotated posteriorly, and an inferior glide at the costotransverse joint results.[47] The posterior aspects of the ribs approximate, and the anterior separate. One study found that sequential transection of the anterior structures, including the anterior half of the disc and the costotransverse joints, had little affect on the stability, until the *posterior* longitudinal ligament was cut.[12] Extension in the thoracic spine is limited by the anterior ligaments, including the anterior longitudinal ligament, the posterior longitudinal ligament, the anterior aspect of the disc, impaction of the inferior facet onto the lamina below, and by further impaction of the spinous processes. The posterior translation that occurs with extension is controlled by the posteriorly directed lamellae of the anulus, and by the capsule of the zygapophysial joint.

Side-Flexion

A total of 25 to 45 degrees of side-flexion is available in the thoracic spine, at an average of about 6 degrees to each side per segment, with the lower segments averaging slightly more at 7 to 9 degrees each.[48] Side-flexion is initiated by the ipsilateral abdominals and erector muscles, and continued by gravity. At the zygapophysial joints, it is mainly the ipsilateral superior facet gliding inferiorly, and the contralateral gliding superiorly. In effect, the ipsilateral zygapophysial joint extends while the contralateral flexes. Side-flexion occurs in the upper thoracic spine and is associated with ipsilateral rotation and ipsilateral translation.[49] This coupling also appears to occur in the rest of the thoracic spine but only if the side-flexion is slight.[50] The coupling that occurs with larger motions in the mid-low thoracic spine depends on which of the two coupling motions initiates the movement.[47] If side-flexion initiates the movement, it is called latexion, and the biomechanics follow the coupling pattern of the lumbar region, which consists of side-flexion, contralateral rotation, and ipsilateral translation.[51] The mechanism of this coupling, or actually tripling, is not known for certain and the clinician must guard against strong conclusions. The postulated mechanism is as follows.[47] With side-flexion, a contralateral convex curve is produced. This causes the ribs on the convex side of the curve to separate and those on the concave side to approximate. Trunk side-flexion is essentially halted either by soft tissue tension or approximation, or both, and the ribs become fixed. Further side-flexion is modified by the fixed ribs. The ipsilateral articular facet of the transverse process, glides inferiorly on its rib, resulting in a relative anterior rotation of the neck of the rib, whereas the contralateral transverse process glides superiorly, producing a posterior rotation of the rib neck.[47] The effect of these bilateral rib rotations is to force the superior vertebra into rotation away from the direction of side-flexion.

Rotation

Axial rotation of 35 to 40 degrees[52] is available in the thoracic spine, with segmental axial rotation averaging 8 to 9 degrees in the upper thoracic area, decreasing slightly in the middle thoracic spine, before significantly increasing to 12 degrees in the last two or three segments.[53] Axial rotation is produced either by the abdominal muscles and other trunk rotators, or by unilateral elevation of the arm. This latter maneuver results in ipsilateral rotation, and produces a curve that is convex ipsilaterally, suggesting that segmental side flexion is occurring ipsilaterally. According to an anatomic study,[10] thoracic segmental rotation is coupled with contralateral side-flexion and contralateral translation.

However, this deviates from what is generally observed clinically. There are, of course, two reasons why clinical observation may differ from anatomic studies. If the clinical view is correct, then the study does not possess external validity and this may be a result of the procedures used. In the quoted study, the anterior aspect of the ribs were resected and this must alter the biomechanics.[47] On the other hand, the clinical observation may be incorrect, a not entirely unheard of situation.

Respiration

The ribs form levers with fulcrums that are placed at the rib angle and effort arm that is the neck. The load arm is the shaft. Because of the relatively small size of the rib neck, a small movement at the rib neck will produce a large degree of movement in the shaft. When the ribs elevate, they rise upward while the rib neck drops down. In the upper ribs, this results in anterior elevation (pump handle) and in the middle and lower ribs (excluding the free ribs), lateral elevation (bucket handle). The former movement will increase the anterior-posterior diameter of the thoracic cavity, and the latter increases the transverse. It is the diaphragm that produces these two kinds of thoracic motion. The first and second rib move only slightly during quiet respiration and it is thought that their function is principally to maintain the stability of the top of the thoracic cavity, preventing it from collapsing as air pressure is reduced during inspiration. The third through sixth ribs increase the anterior-posterior and transverse diameters of the chest. The seventh through tenth ribs act to increase the abdominal cavity free space to afford space for the descending diaphragm. As the ends of these ribs are elevated, they push up on each other, lifting each successive rib upward and, finally, lifting the sternum. The two lower ribs are depressed by the quadratus lumborum to provide a stable base of action for the diaphragm.

Inspiration

The diaphragm descends and pulls the central tendon inferiorly through the fixed twelfth ribs and L1–L3. When the extensibility (distension) of the abdominal walls is reached, the central tendon becomes stationary, and further contraction of the diaphragm produces an elevation and posterior rotation of the lower six ribs, with torsion of the anterior costal cartilage, and an anterior-superior thrust of the sternum (and eventually the inferior aspect of the manubrium). Because of the longer lower ribs, the inferior sternum moves further anteriorly than the superior section during inspiration. The sternum-manubrium junction acts as the hinge for this motion. If this joint stiffens or ossifies, respiratory function will suffer. In addition, if the central tendon stiffens, inspiration will have to be accomplished with the ribs moving laterally. Forced inspiration produces an increase in the activity level of the diaphragm, intercostals, scaleni, and quadratus lumborum. In addition, activity occurs in the sternomastoid, trapezius, both pectorals, and the serratus anterior. During inspiration, the ribs (T1–7) move with the sternum in an upward and forward direction, increasing the anterior-posterior diameter of the chest while their respective rib tubercles and costotransverse joints glide inferiorly. The ribs of T8–10 move upward, backward, and medially (or downward, forward, and laterally), increasing the lateral dimension while their respective rib tubercles and costotransverse joints glide inferiorly, laterally, and anteriorly. T11–12 remain stationary, except for slight caliper motion increasing the lateral dimension. Quiet respiration involves very little zygapophysial joint motion.

Expiration

Quiet expiration occurs passively. During forced expiration, there is activity in the abdominals and latissimus dorsi. During expiration, the ribs anteriorly rotate and the tubercles and costotransverse joints of:[47]

- T1 through T7 glide superiorly.
- T8 through T10 glide in a posterior-medial-superior direction.
- T11 and T12 remain stationary.

During a patient's respiration, it is possible to detect a subluxation of the costotransverse joints by palpating the ipsilateral transverse process, and rib, during inspiration and thoracic side-flexion. For example, a superior subluxation of the right rib will produce:

- A decreased inferior glide—a motion that is required for inspiration.
- A decrease in thoracic motion in the directions of left side-flexion and right rotation.

Biomechanical Regions

The thorax can be divided into four regions according to their respective anatomic and biomechanical differences.[47] (Table 16–1)

Vertebromanubrial (Pectoral Ring)

This area includes the first two thoracic vertebra, the first and second ribs, and the manubrium, and is described in Chapter 15.

Vertebrosternal

The vertebrosternal region consists of T3–T7 and the sternum. This region has the potential for multidirectional movement if it were not for the presence of the ribs. A feature of this region includes long, thin overlapping spinous processes, which are up to three-finger widths inferior to the transverse process, making the transverse processes in this region better situated for intervertebral motion palpation.

In the mobile thorax, flexion at this region consists of the following.[47]

- The costotransverse joints of T3–T7 are convex-concave, respectively (the facet on the transverse processes is concave). The pattern of motion that occurs in this region appears to vary between individuals, and can either be a combination of an anterior rotation and superior glide or, more commonly, a combination of a superior glide of the rib neck and tubercle (T3–T7) and a conjunct anterior rotation.
- Anterior translation and anterior sagittal rotation of the vertebral body.
- Superior-anterior glide at the zygapophysial joints.

In the mobile thorax, extension and arm elevation at this region consists of:[47]

- A variety of motion patterns between individuals, which can be a combination of either a posterior rotation and superior glide or, more commonly, a combination of a posterior rotation of the rib neck and an inferior glide of the tubercle at the costotransverse joint.
- An inferior glide of the tubercle results in a posterior rotation of the neck of the rib due to the concave-convex orientation of the costotransverse joints of T3–7 in both the sagittal and transverse plane. Posterior translation is coupled with backward sagittal rotation.

In the mobile thorax, side-flexion to the right at this region consists of the following.[47]

- A left convex curve.
- A right side-flexion of the thoracic vertebrae, while the right transverse process moves inferiorly.
- An approximation of the rib tubercles on the right.
- The ribs on the right move superiorly and conjunctly rotate anteriorly, a motion that can be palpated at the costotransverse joint, while the rib tubercles on the left separate at their lateral margins, inferiorly glide, and rotate posteriorly.

In the mobile thorax, rotation to the right at this region consists of right rotation and left translation of the superior vertebra.[47] The right rotation of the superior vertebra produces a "pulling" of the superior aspect of the left rib head forward (anterior-medially) at the costovertebral joint. This, in turn, produces an anterior rotation of the left rib neck (and a superior glide at the left costotransverse joint). It also "pushes" the superior aspect of the right rib head backward (posterior-laterally) at the costovertebral joint, producing a posterior rotation of the right rib neck (and an inferior glide at the right costotransverse joint). At the limit of this horizontal translation, both the costovertebral and the costotransverse joints are tensed. As just described, if the region is stable, further rotation of the superior vertebra to the right occurs when the superior vertebral body tilts to the right (a superior glide at the left superior costovertebral joint and an inferior glide at the right superior costovertebral joint), producing a right side-flexion of the superior vertebra during right rotation.

Vertebrochondral

This region consists of the T8–T10 levels and features shorter spinous processes.

In the mobile thorax, flexion at this region consists of:[47]

- A superior-medial-posterior (SMP) glide of the rib tubercle (due to the planar costotransverse joints, which are oriented in a anterior-lateral and superior direction) but does not induce an anterior rotation of the neck of the rib to the same degree as the middle and upper ribs.

In the mobile thorax, extension and arm elevation at this region consists of:[47]

- An inferior-lateral-anterior glide (ILA) of the rib tubercle. The tubercle does not induce a posterior rotation of the neck of the rib to the same degree as the middle and upper ribs.

In the mobile thorax, side-flexion to the right at this region is dependent on the position of the apex of the curve produced with the side-flexion.[47]

- If the apex of the side-flexion curve is in line with the ipsilateral greater trochanter, all of the thoracic vertebra side-flex to the same side as the direction of the side-flexion, while the right ribs approximate, and the left ribs separate. Thus, side-flexion of the vertebra to the right results in a superior glide of the tubercle of the left rib, coupled with a SMP glide on the right and an ILA glide on the left side of the rib. The vertebrae are free at this level to follow the rotation, which is congruent with the levels above and below.

- If the apex of the side-flexion curve is located within the thorax, the thoracic vertebra below the apex of the curve (T9–12) side-flex to the opposite side of the side-flexion, producing an ILA glide on the right and a SMP glide on the left.
- The vertebrae behave as above—follow the rotation that is congruent with the levels above and below.

In the mobile thorax, rotation to the right at this region consists of the following.[47]

- A superior-lateral glide of the zygapophysial joints of the superior vertebra on the left and an inferior-medial glide on the right
- A SMP glide on the left costotransverse joint and an ILA glide on the right costotransverse joint

Thoracolumbar Junction

This region consists of the T11 and T12 levels and features short, stout spinous processes that are contained entirely within the lamina of their own vertebra, and which are more reliable than the spinous processes for palpation during intervertebral motion. The transverse processes of this region have small tubercles, and the mammillary processes are larger and more superficial. The zygapophysial facets of T11 resemble those of both the vertebrosternal and vertebrochondral regions. The facets on the inferior articular processes of T12 resemble the lumbar region but have both a coronal and sagittal orientation, with a 90-degree change occurring. The joints in this region are designed to rotate with minimal restriction of ribs. Rotation can be ipsilateral or contralateral to the side-flexion.[47]

The biomechanics of this region has thus far been described for a normal thorax. As elsewhere, pathologic or aging processes can stiffen the thorax and produce the following biomechanical changes.

Stiff Thorax[47]

Flexion

- The ribs are less mobile than the vertebral column when the stiffer thorax is flexed. The anterior aspect of the rib travels inferiorly, whereas the posterior aspect travels superiorly.
- The zygapophysial arthrokinematics remain the same as in the mobile thorax.
- Costotransverse joints of T3–T7: the concave facets of the transverse process of T3–7 glide superiorly relative to the tubercle of the ribs, resulting in a relative inferior glide of the tubercle of the rib.
- At the vertebrochondral and costotransverse joints of T8–T10, an ILA glide occurs with flexion.

Extension. Initially, the anterior aspect of the rib travels superiorly, whereas the posterior aspect travels inferiorly. In addition, a posterior rotation of the ribs occurs, whereas an inferior-posterior glide of zygapophysial joints also occurs, but with less posterior translation of the zygapophysial joints.

● A superior glide of the tubercle at the costotransverse joints of T3–7.
● At the vertebrochondral region (T8–10), the facets of the costotransverse joints are planar and the relative glide of the rib is thus SMP.

Rigid Thorax[47]

Flexion. The glides of the zygapophysial joints match those of the mobile thorax, but very little, if any, posterior-anterior translation occurs. No palpable movement appears to occur between the thoracic vertebra and ribs.

Extension. Some inferior gliding of the zygapophysial joints occurs, but very little anterior-posterior translation. No palpable movement is found between the thoracic vertebra and ribs.

Right Side-Flexion. In both the mobile and the stiffer thorax, the ribs appear to stop moving before the vertebra, as a result of tissue tension on the left and bone approximation on the right. As the thoracic vertebrae continue to side-flex to the right, the zygapophysial joints produce a superior-medial glide of the left inferior articular process of the superior thoracic vertebra, and an inferior-lateral glide on the right to facilitate right side flexion. As the rib on the right is connected to the inferior aspect of the body of the superior vertebra, its resultant anterior rotation takes the superior vertebral body with it, producing a left rotation of the superior vertebra in the presence of right side-flexion. No anterior-medial or posterior-lateral glide of the ribs, relative to the transverse processes to which they attach, appears to occur during side-flexion of the trunk (Table 16–1).

TABLE 16–1 BIOMECHANICS OF THE THORAX

MOTIONS	Z JOINT	RIB MOTION	COSTOTRANSVERSE JOINT
		VERTEBROMANUBRIAL (T1–2)	
Flexion	Superior-anterior	Anterior Rotation	—
Extension	Inferior-posterior	Posterior Rotation	—
Latexion	Ipsilateral Coupling	—	—
Rotexion	Ipsilateral Coupling	—	—
Inspiration	—	Elevation	—
Expiration	—	Depression	—
		VERTEBROSTERNAL (T3–7)	
Flexion	Superior-anterior	Varies (very mobile) anterior-posterior rotation	Superior-inferior glide (varies)
Extension	Posterior-inferior	Varies (very mobile) anterior-posterior rotation	Superior-inferior glide (varies)
Latexion	Ipsilateral side-flexion	Ipsilateral-anterior rotation	Ipsilateral-superior
	Contralateral rotation	Contra–posterior rotation	Contra-inferior
Rotexion	Ipsilateral side-flexion	Ipsilateral-posterior rotation	Ipsilateral-inferior
	Ipsilateral rotation	Contra-anterior rotation	Contra-superior
Inspiration	—	Posterior rotation	Inferior glide
Expiration	—	Anterior rotation	Superior glide
		VERTEBROCHONRAL (T8–10)	
Flexion	Superior-anterior	Anterior rotation	S.M.P.
Extension	Inferior-posterior	Posterior rotation	I.L.A.
Latexion	Varies		Apex in line with trochanter
			Ipsilateral-S.M.P.
			Contra-I.L.A.
			If not = reverse
Rotexion	Ipsilateral		Ipsilateral-I.L.A. then anterior-medial
			Contra-P.M.S. then posterior-lateral
Inspiration			I.L.A.
Expiration			S.M.P.

BIOMECHANICAL EXAMINATION OF THE RIBS AND THORAX

Although there is some disagreement as to whether the ribs or the intervertebral joints are the major source of impairment in the thoracic region, the approach to be taken should be to clear the larger articulations, thereby giving a better idea on the state of the costal joints. It seems more likely that apparent movement disorders are caused by the larger bones, as these will exert the greater influence. This approach has been supported by clinical experience in that if the rib examination is delayed until the intervertebral joints have been treated, the number of rib impairments decreases dramatically. The reverse has not been experienced by the majority of clinicians. Of course, it may be that the intervention inadvertently cleared the rib impairment, but as this seems to happen so consistently, it really does not matter too much (Figure 16–3).

Subjective/History

As mentioned in Chapter 10, the cause of chest pain can be difficult to determine, especially as there are a number of visceral structures that are capable of referring pain to this region. To help differentiate between visceral pain and musculoskeletal pain in the thoracic region, the clinician should focus on the relationship of specific movements to the pain, and the quality of the pain, rather than attempting to relate the pain to function or activity. Information regarding the onset as well as aggravating factors are also important. The reader is encouraged to review Chapters 8 and 10.

Observation

In addition to those features outlined in Chapter 10, the clinician should assess the presence and impact of any spinal curvatures in the thoracic spine.

Palpation

The spinous processes of the thoracic vertebrae have varying degrees of obliquity and if they are used as landmarks, this obliquity must be understood and exploited. The transverse processes are roughly level with their own bodies. On average, the degree of obliquity is different for different areas of the spine and divides it into four regions in the so-called Rule of Three (Figure 16–4).

● First group of three spinous processes (T1–3). These spinous processes are level with vertebral body of the same level.

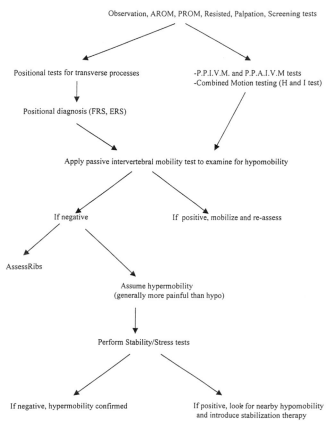

FIGURE 16–3   Examination of the Thoracic Spine.

Observation, AROM, PROM, Resisted, Palpation, Screening tests

Positional tests for transverse processes

-P.P.I.V.M. and P.P.A.I.V.M tests
-Combined Motion testing (H and I test)

Positional diagnosis (FRS, ERS)

Apply passive intervertebral mobility test to examine for hypomobility

If negative

If positive, mobilize and re-assess

AssessRibs

Assume hypermobility
(generally more painful than hypo)

Perform Stability/Stress tests

If negative, hypermobility confirmed

If positive, look for nearby hypomobility and introduce stabilization therapy

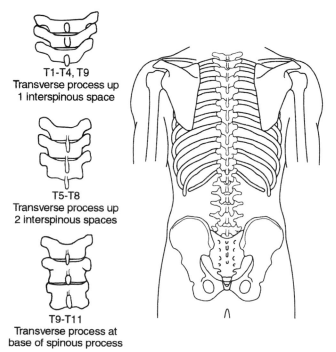

T1-T4, T9
Transverse process up
1 interspinous space

T5-T8
Transverse process up
2 interspinous spaces

T9-T11
Transverse process at
base of spinous process

FIGURE 16–4   The Rule of 3

TABLE 16–2 ANTERIOR AND POSTERIOR PALPATION POINTS

ANTERIOR ASPECT	POSTERIOR ASPECT
Suprasternal notch	Spinous and their associated transverse processes
Sternomanubrial angle	T2 level with base of spine of scapula
Xiphoid process	Spinal gutter (rotatores)
Infrasternal angle	Erector spinae
Sternochondral junctions	Rib angles
Costal cartilage	Rib shafts
	Rib shafts and rib joint line of costotransverse joint
	C6 locate the largest spinous process at the base of the neck, have patient extend the neck; the first spinous process to move anteriorly under the clinician's finger is C6

- Second group of three spinous processes (T4–6). These spinous processes are level with the disc of the inferior level. This can be estimated at about three finger breadths.
- Third group of three spinous processes (T7–9). These spinous processes are level with the vertebral body of the level below.
- The fourth group of three spinous processes reverse the obliquity. T10 is level with the vertebral body of the vertebra below (same as T7–9). T11 is level with the disc of the inferior vertebra (same as T6). T12 is level with its own vertebral body (same as T3).

Landmarks should be palpated as shown in (Table 16–2).

Screening Tests

A few simple screening tests can help differentiate between a rib impairment and a thoracic vertebra impairment. In the examples presented, the mid scapular pain is on the patient's right side and reproduced by thoracic extension and scapular retraction.

1. The patient lies prone and the clinician stands on the left side of the patient. Reaching over the patient, the clinician spreads the length of the thumb over the right rib in question and applies a posterior-anterior force. This is the equivalent of a left rotation of the thoracic spine. The clinician then repeats the posterior-anterior force on the rib using the heel of the palm, except this time, he or she blocks the rotation of the thoracic spine by placing the ulnar border of his or her other hand over a group of left transverse processes (Figure 16–5). Pain produced with this maneuver would implicate the rib, but if the pain is not provoked, then the thoracic spine should be assessed.

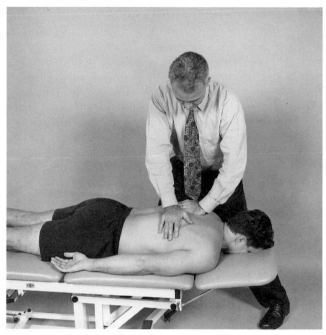

FIGURE 16–5 The rib screen - posterior-anterior pressure on the right side, with the left transverse processes stabilized.

2. The patient is prone and the clinician stands on the left side of the patient. The clinician grasps the patient's right shoulder and raises it off the bed. If this reproduces the pain the test is repeated, except that the thoracic spine is stabilized to prevent it from rotating using the same technique as in the previous example. Reproduction of the pain in the second part of the test would indicate a rib impairment.

3. The patient is seated with the thoracic spine positioned in extreme flexion. The patient is then asked to take a deep breath in. Pain with breathing in would indicate a restricted inferior glide of the rib.

Active Motion

These tests can be performed with the patient seated or standing. The overpressure applied at the end of the available range of motion takes the joint from its physiologic barrier to its anatomic barrier, and an increase in resistance to motion should be felt. Because of the length of the spine in this region, it is important to ensure that all parts of the thoracic spine are involved in the range of movement testing. Active range of motion is initially performed globally, looking for abnormalities. A specific examination is then performed on any region that appeared to have an impairment. Various techniques are used to correctly assess each area of the thoracic spine.

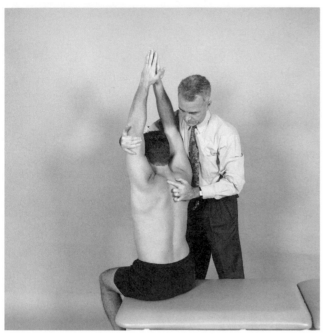

FIGURE 16–6   Patient and clinician position for passive mobility testing.

Upper Thorax

The patient is asked to raise both arms over the head while keeping the palms together. The clinician grasps the patient's arm(s) and, while monitoring the spinous process or transverse processes at a specific level, asks the patient to move into flexion, side-flexion, extension, and rotation at the thoracic segments (Figure 16–6). During these motions the clinician observes for any onset of pain, patterns of restriction, and asymmetries. As in the lumbar and cervical spine, there are a number of classic patterns of restriction.

The right side will be deemed impaired in the following examples.

- Opening [extended, rotated, side-flexed (ERS)] restriction of the zygapophysial joint—demonstrated by a decrease in flexion, left side-flexion, and left rotation.
- Closing [flexed, rotated, side-flexed (FRS)] restriction of the zygapophysial joint—demonstrated by a decrease in extension, right side-flexion, and right rotation.
- A right costotransverse joint (T3–9) restriction—demonstrated by a decreased superior glide of the right costotransverse joint, a decrease in flexion or extension (variable), right side-flexion, and left rotation.
- A right costotransverse joint (T3–9) restriction—demonstrated by a decreased inferior glide of the right costotransverse joint, a decrease in flexion or extension (variable), left side-flexion, and right rotation.

Mid-Low Thorax

- Flexion. The patient is asked to slump forward as though trying to place the forehead on the knees. The clinician observes for any paravertebral fullness, which might indicate hypertonus.
- Extension. The clinician places one hand and arm across the upper chest region of the patient, while the other hand is placed over the spinous processes of the lower thoracic spine. The patient is guided into a backward slump. Overpressure is applied by the arm across the front of the patient while avoiding any anterior translation occurring at the lumbar spine.
- Rotation. The patient is asked to turn to each side at the waist. Overpressure is applied through both shoulders (Figure 16–7). This motion tests the ability of the ribs and the superior vertebra to translate in the direction opposite to the rotation—a motion essential for complete rotation and side-flexion to occur.
- Side-flexion. Using a hand placed against the patient's side, the patient is asked to side-flex over the clinician's hand. Overpressure is applied through the contralateral shoulder while stabilizing the patient's knees (Figure 16–8).
- Inspiration and expiration. The motions of the manubrium are assessed during breathing

Resistance applied at the point of overpressure can give the clinician an indication as to the integrity of the

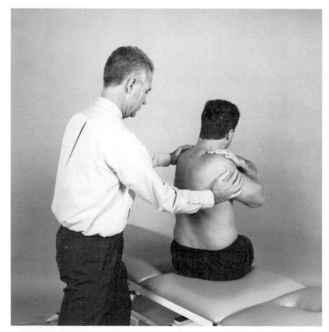

FIGURE 16–7   Patient and clinician position for active range of motion of thoracic rotation. Note the clinician's guiding hand.

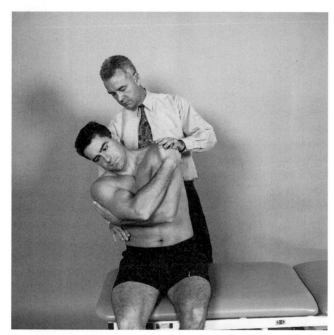

FIGURE 16–8 Patient and clinician position for active range of motion of thoracic side flexion. Note the clinician's guiding hand.

musculotendinous units of this area. Resistance is applied at the end range of flexion, extension, rotation, and side-flexion while the clinician looks for pain, weakness, and/or painful weakness.

The next stage in the examination process depends on the clinician's background. For those clinicians heavily influenced by the muscle energy techniques of the osteopaths,[54] position testing is used to determine which segment to focus on. Other clinicians omit the position tests and proceed to the combined motion and passive physiologic tests.

Position Testing—Spinal

The vertebrae are tested for symmetry. To determine the position of the superior vertebra, the posterior-anterior relationship of the transverse processes to the coronal body plane is noted and compared with the level above and below. If the left transverse process of the superior vertebra is more posterior than the left transverse process of the inferior vertebra, then the segment is left rotated. If the left transverse process of the superior vertebra is less posterior than the left transverse process of the inferior vertebra, but more posterior than the right transverse process of the superior vertebra, then the superior vertebra is relatively right rotated compared to the level below, but left rotated when compared to the coronal body plane.[54] This is a

typical compensatory pattern seen when a superior segment is derotating or unwinding a primary rotation at a lower level.[47]

Symmetrical impairments are more common in the thoracic region than in the lumbar, particularly in the upper and cervicothoracic spine, due to fixed postural impairments. These, of course, will not be apparent on position testing and must be sought after when the position tests are negative. If no asymmetry was found on position testing, then the segment of interest would be separately passively flexed, extended, and rotated in all directions.

Example T7–8. The patient is positioned in sitting with the clinician standing behind the patient. Using the thumbs, the clinician palpates the transverse processes of the T7 vertebra. Each joint is tested in the following manner.

- The joint complex is flexed and an evaluation is made as to the position of the T7 vertebra relative to T8 by noting which transverse process is the most posterior (Figure 16–9). A posterior left transverse process of T7 relative to T8 is indicative of a left rotated position of the T7–8 complex in flexion.
- The joint complex is extended and an evaluation is made as to the position of the T7 vertebra in relation to T8 by noting which transverse process is the most posterior. A posterior left transverse process of T7

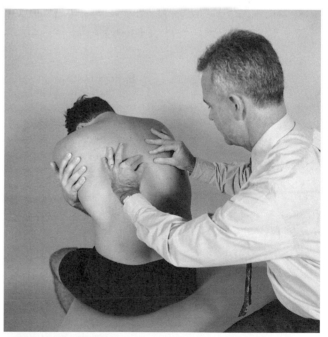

FIGURE 16–9 Patient and clinician position for position testing.

relative to T8 is indicative of a left rotated position of the T7–8 joint complex in extension.

Physiological Mobility and Combined Motions—Spinal

Active mobility tests are used to determine the osteokinematic function of two adjacent thoracic vertebrae during active motions.

Flexion is tested with the patient seated with the arms folded, one hand on top of the shoulder and the other hand under the opposite axilla. The clinician palpates the transverse processes of two adjacent vertebrae with the index finger and thumb of both hands (Figure 16–10). The patient is asked to flex the head/trunk, and the quantity of motion, as well as the symmetry of motion, is noted. Both index fingers should travel an equal distance superiorly. When interpreting the mobility findings, the position of the joint at the beginning of the test should be correlated with the subsequent mobility noted, since alterations in joint mobility may merely be a reflection of an altered starting position. The same palpation points are used for testing extension, side-flexion, rotation, and respiration.

Combined motions are introduced if the planar motions do not reproduce the symptoms, the scan is negative, but posterior-anterior pressures reproduce the pain. Combined motions should be performed remembering that the coupling is determined in this region by the initiating movement. Rotexion, that is, a motion initiated with

rotation, produces the coupling of ipsilateral side-flexion and rotation, whereas latexion, a motion initiated with side-flexion, produces contralateral side-flexion and rotation.[47]

Passive physiologic intervertebral mobility tests are performed primarily to confirm findings in the scanning examination or in the event that there are no symptoms to reproduce. Localization of the correct level is achieved primarily by palpation for any rotatores hypertonus. This is then confirmed by the response (pain and/or muscle guarding) to posterior-anterior pressures of the vertebrae and/or ribs. Localization of the joint, however, is achieved by more accurate use of localized pressures—directing the posterior-anterior pressures on adjacent spinous processes in a superior or inferior direction to ascertain if the intervertebral impairment is in flexion or extension.

Anterior-Posterior Oscillations

The patient is seated with the arms folded and the elbows pointing forward. The clinician stands in front of the patient, and reaching around the back of the patient with one hand, the clinician palpates the interspinous spaces. With the other hand, the clinician grasps the patient and applies a gentle anterior-posterior force, producing a slight posterior glide of the thoracic segments (Figure 16–11).

Posterior-Anterior Oscillations

The patient is seated with the hands behind the neck and the elbows pointing forward. The clinician stands

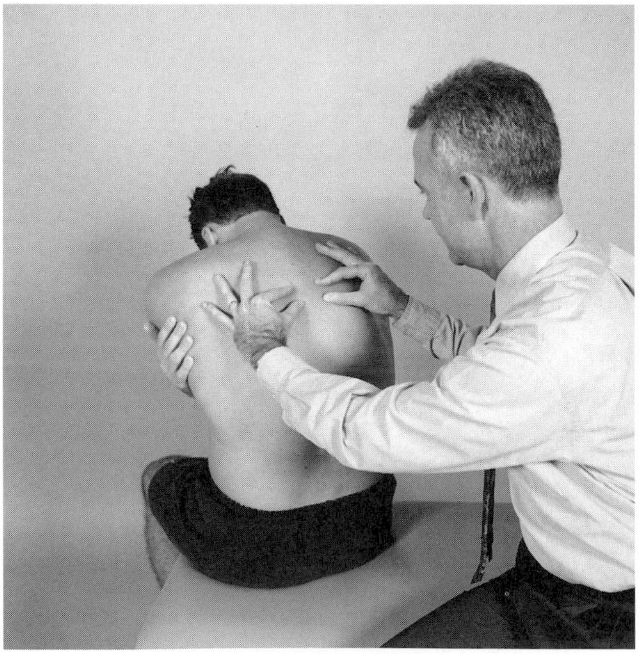

FIGURE 16–10 Active mobility testing.

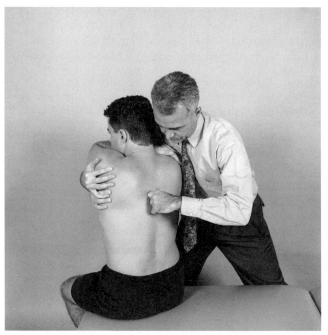

FIGURE 16–11 Anterior-posterior oscillations.

behind the patient and, by using the thumb of one hand, applies a posterior-anterior pressure to one transverse process while stabilizing the thoracic spine by holding the top of the contralateral shoulder with a lumbrical grip. In this position, oscillatory motions can be introduced by pulling the shoulder posteriorly, while palpating each segment with the other hand and thumb, feeling for any hypertonicity. This technique can be modified by having the clinician stand at the patient's side and introducing the thoracic motion via the patient's elbows.

Posterior-anterior pressures can also be performed with the patient prone, using the heel of the clinician's hand. Care should be taken to apply the force gently, by taking up the slack, and then applying the overpressure along the plane of the joint, perpendicular to the thoracic curve.

More specific segmental motion tests, incorporating symmetrical or asymmetrical motions, can be added in the form of passive physiologic intervertebral articular mobility (PPAIVM) tests.

Passive Physiologic Intervertebral Articular Mobility

If the gross physiologic range was found to be restricted, the arthrokinematics need to be assessed to determine if the hypomobility is articular or extra-articular (myofascial).

If an asymmetrical impairment is suspected, the appropriate segmental quadrant is investigated. In the case of an extended, rotated, side flexed right (ERSR), the right joint of the segment is taken into flexion, left side-flexion, and left rotation, and its range and end feel assessed for hypomobility. If this was found to be normal, then the left joint would be taken into flexion right rotation and right side-flexion and would, thus, be evaluated for hypermobility.

Levels T1–4—Unilateral Flexion of Zygapophysial Joints

Seated Technique. The patient is seated with their hands clasped behind their neck. The clinician stands to the side of the patient. While palpating the interspinous spaces or the transverse processes of each level with one hand, the clinician wraps the other arm around the front of the patient. Crouching slightly, the clinician then places his or her anterior shoulder region against the lateral aspect of the patient's shoulder. Side-flexion of the patient's thoracic spine is then performed. The palpating hand palpates the concave side of the curve.

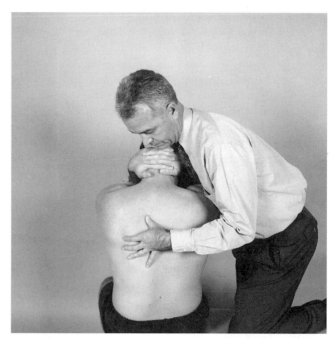

FIGURE 16–12   Seated techniques to correct a T4–5 flexion hypomobility.

For example, with a left flexion hypomobility at T4–5, the clinician flexes, right side-flexes, and right rotates the patient to the motion barrier of the restricted quadrant. Using a thumb, the clinician pushes the left transverse process of T4 superiorly and anteriorly into further flexion (Figure 16–12). The end feel is assessed. The same technique is employed for the intervention, except graded mobilizations, or muscle energy techniques are incorporated at the end range of range.

Prone Technique.   An alternative technique can be used to test the superior glide of the right zygapophysial joint at T4–5 and to determine the ability of the right inferior articular process of T4 to glide superiorly, relative to the superior articular process of T5.[47]

The patient is positioned in prone-lying and the thoracic spine is placed in neutral. The clinician, standing to the left side of the patient, palpates the inferior aspect of the left transverse process of T5 with the left thumb. The right thumb palpates the inferior aspect of the right transverse process of T4. The left thumb is used to fix T5, and a superior-anterior glide is applied to T4 with the right thumb. The quantity and end feel of motion is noted and compared to the levels above and below. This technique can be used for all thoracic segments. The same technique is employed for the intervention, except graded mobilizations, or muscle energy techniques are incorporated at the end range of range.

Levels T1–6—Unilateral Extension of Zygapophysial Joints

Seated Technique. For example, a right extension hypomobility at T5–6. The patient is seated with both hands clasped behind their neck. The clinician stands to the side of the patient. While palpating the interpinous spaces or the transverse processes of each level with one hand, the clinician wraps the other arm around the front of the patient. Crouching slightly, the clinician then places the anterior shoulder region against the lateral aspect of the patient's shoulder.

The patient is moved to the extension barrier using extension right side-flexion and right rotation. At this point, the clinician, using a thumb, tests the superior glide of the left transverse process of T5 (Figure 16–13), or the superior glide of the right transverse process of T6, to test the inferior glide of the right zygapophysial joint of T5 into extension. The same technique is employed for the intervention, except graded mobilizations, or muscle energy techniques are incorporated at the end range of range.

Prone Technique.[47] The patient is positioned in prone and the thoracic spine is placed in neutral to test the inferior glide of the right zygapophysial joint at T4–5 and to determine the ability of the right inferior articular process of T4 to glide inferiorly relative to the superior articular process of T5. The clinician, standing to the left side of

the patient, palpates the inferior aspect of the T5 transverse process with the right thumb. The left thumb palpates the superior aspect of the right transverse process of T4. The right thumb fixes T5 and an inferior glide is applied to T4 with the left thumb. The quantity and end feel of motion is noted and compared to the levels above and below. This technique can be used for all thoracic segments.

Passive Stability—Spinal

Nonspecific stability testing of this area traditionally involved the use of rib springing. The following techniques are more specific.

Vertical (Traction and Compression)

This test stresses the anatomic structures that resist vertical forces. A positive response is the reproduction of the patient's symptoms together with an increase in the quantity of motion, and a decrease in the resistance at the end of the range of motion.

Traction. For the upper half of the spine, traction is applied through the shoulder girdle (see below) and via the lumbar traction test for the lower half. If the test reproduces the patient's symptoms, injury of the longitudinal ligaments may be present or, again, in the acutely painful patient, an inflammation of the zygapophysial joint.

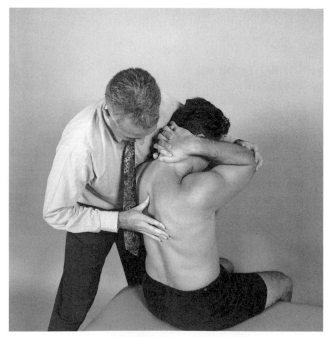

FIGURE 16–13 Seated techniques to correct a T3–4 extension hypomobility.

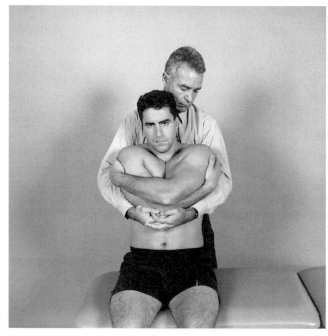

FIGURE 16–14 Vertical distraction stability test.

For the upper-thorax (T1–6), the patient is sitting with the arms crossed such that the arm closest to the chest grasps the scapula. The other arm rests on top of the contralateral shoulder. The thoracic spine is in neutral. The clinician can use a towel over the transverse process of the lower segment and his or her sternum. The clinician stands behind the patient and wraps both of the arms around the patient, grasping the patient's inferior elbow. The patient is asked to lean the head back onto the clinician's upper chest area. The clinician pulls up on the patient's elbow as though attempting to drag the patient up and off the bed (see Figure 16–14). This position is maintained for about 20 seconds.

Compression.   Compression is the more important of the two vertical stress tests. Stress is applied to the upper half of the thoracic spine as the clinician leans on the patient's shoulders (Figure 16–15). The middle and lower thorax is tested using the lumbar compression test described as part of the lumbar scan. Reproduction of the symptoms is considered a positive test and may be indicative of vertical instability. Conditions that would produce a positive test include an end plate fracture, a disc impairment, or a centrum fracture. In the acutely painful patient, a positive test may result from a zygapophysial joint inflammation.

Anterior Translation—Spinal

This test stresses the anatomic structures that resist anterior translation of a segmental spinal unit. Often, the patient presents with a noticeable "step off" in the thoracic

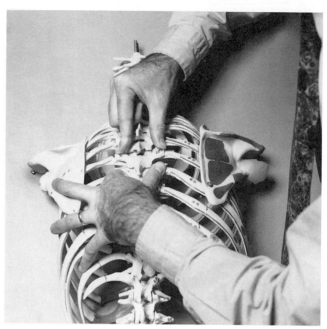

FIGURE 16–16   Clinician hand position for anterior stability test.

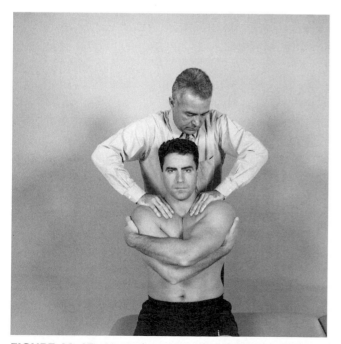

FIGURE 16–15   Vertical compression stability test.

spine during observation. A positive response is the reproduction of the patient's symptoms together with an increase in the quantity of motion and a decrease in the resistance at the end of the range of motion.

Pressure is applied by the clinician over the transverse process of the superior bone of the segment of interest. The pressure will produce an anterior shear force between the bone and its inferior partner, and a posterior shear of its superior (Figure 16–16). Any perceived anterior motion is indicative of instability. An excessive anterior translation of the T4 vertebra could be due to either an anterior instability of T4–5 or a posterior instability of T3–4. It is, therefore, important that the posterior translation is tested, and cleared, before assessing the results of this test.

With the patient prone-lying, the transverse processes of the superior vertebra are palpated and the "nose pinch grip" is used (see Figure 16–16). With the other hand, the transverse processes of the inferior vertebra are fixed by placing the thumb and index finger over the right and left transverse processes. A posterior-anterior force is applied through the superior vertebra, while fixing the inferior vertebra with the fingers (see Figure 16–16). The quantity of motion, the reproduction of any symptoms, and the end feel of motion is noted and compared to the levels above and below.

Posterior Translation—Spinal

This test stresses the anatomic structures that resist posterior translation of a segmental spinal unit. A positive response is the reproduction of the patient's symptoms together with

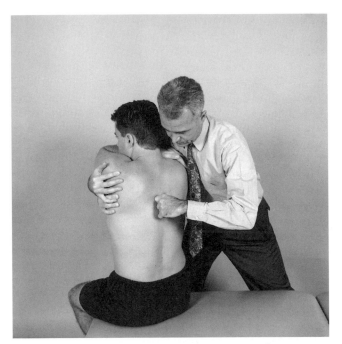

FIGURE 16–17 Patient and clinician position for posterior stability test.

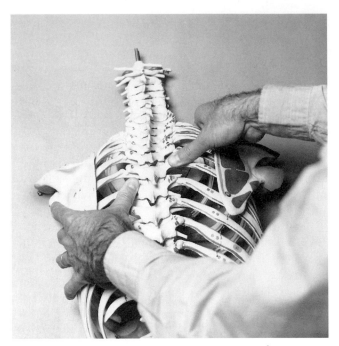

FIGURE 16–18 Patient and clinician position for rotation stability test.

an increase in the quantity of motion and a decrease in the resistance at the end of the range of motion.

The patient is sitting with the arms crossed, hands on opposite shoulders. The clinician, standing to the side of the patient, stabilizes the thorax with the ventral hand and arm under or over (depending on the level) the patient's crossed arms, while the contralateral scapula is grasped. The transverse processes of the inferior vertebra are fixed by the clinician with the dorsal hand. Static stability is tested by applying an anterior-posterior force to the superior vertebra through the thorax (Figure 16–17). The clinician palpates for posterior motion at the segment above the one being stabilized, which would indicate instability. The quantity of motion, the reproduction of any symptoms, and the end feel of motion is noted and compared to the levels above and below. The findings from this test should be correlated with those of the anterior translation test to determine the level and direction of the instability. Dynamic stability can be tested by resisting elevation of the crossed arms. If the segmental musculature is able to control the excessive posterior translation, no posterior translation will be felt and the instability can be deemed dynamically stable.

Rotation—Spinal

This test stresses the anatomic structures that resist rotation of a segmental spinal unit. A positive response is the reproduction of the patient's symptoms together with an

increase in the quantity of motion and a decrease in the resistance at the end of the range of motion.

With the patient positioned in prone-lying, a transverse process of the superior vertebra is palpated. With the other hand, the contralateral transverse process of the inferior vertebra is fixed using the thumb. A transverse-plane rotation force is applied through the superior vertebra by applying a unilateral posterior-anterior pressure, while fixing the inferior vertebra (Figure 16–18). The quantity of motion, the reproduction of any symptoms, and the end feel of motion is noted and compared to the levels above and below.

COSTAL EXAMINATION

As mentioned, it is well worth postponing the costal, or rib, examination until after the thoracic spinal joints have been examined and treated, or the testing of which prove negative.

All of the ribs move with complex combinations of what is often described as "pump-handle," "bucket-handle," and/or caliper motion. Pump-handle (anterior) motion is analogous to flexion and extension, bucket-handle (lateral rib) motion is analogous to adduction and abduction, and caliper motion is analogous to internal and external rotation.

The first rib has an equal proportion of pump- and bucket-handle motion, while the sternal ribs have a greater proportion of pump-handle motion. Ribs 8 through 10 have a greater proportion of bucket handle motion.

Palpation

Surface landmarks can be used to locate the ribs. The first rib is located 45 degrees medially to the junction of the posterior scalene and trapezius. Palpation of the first rib during respiration can detect the presence of asymmetry. The difference in height between each side will help determine the cause of the asymmetry.

- If the difference is 3/8 in. higher, a superior subluxation may be present.
- If the difference is 3/4 in. higher, a cervical rib may be present.
- If one side is higher but the difference is less than 3/8 in., a thoracic rotoscoliosis may be present.

The costal cartilages of the second rib articulate with the junction between sternum and manubrium, or sternal angle. The fifth rib passes directly under, or slightly inferior to, the male mammary nipples.

To palpate the rib angles of the inter-scapular ribs, the shoulders are positioned in horizontal adduction. The rib angles of 3 through 10 can then be felt about 1 to 2 inches lateral to the spinous processes.

When palpating anteriorly, on the sternum, an impairment will be highlighted by the presence of asymmetry, and should be compared with the posterior findings. A prominent rib angle on the back and a depression of that rib at the sternum would indicate a posterior subluxation, the reverse occurring in an anterior subluxation. A rib that is prominent both anteriorly and posteriorly indicates a single-rib torsion.

Position Testing—Costal

Positional testing of the ribs is performed to assess for asymmetry.

Costal (Ventral)

The patient is positioned in supine and the clinician stands to the side of the patient. Using the index fingers or thumbs, the clinician palpates the ventral aspect of the ribs at the sternochondral junction (Figure 16–19). The superior-inferior, anterior-posterior relationship of the two ribs, left and right, is noted.

Active Mobility Examination of Ribs 2 through 10

General

Active movements of these ribs can be assessed by:

1. Observing the motion of the palpating finger over the rib angle. This can be done with the patient in sitting or supine.

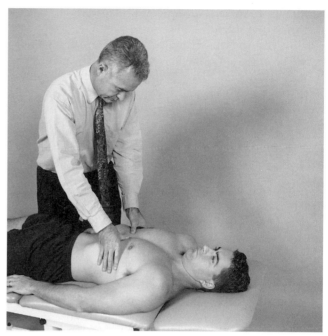

FIGURE 16–19   Patient and clinician position for position testing - costal.

2. Having the patient actively elevate the arm while the clinician palpates the intercostal spaces on the patient's lateral trunk, feeling for the ribs to separate with arm elevation and approximate as the arm descends.

Passive overpressure is applied at the end of ranges.

1. For rib elevation, the overpressure is applied by grasping the patient's arm above the elbow and rocking the arm into hyperabduction for the lower ribs (bucket) and hyper flexion for the upper seven ribs (pump).
2. For the lowering and adducting action, the overpressure is applied via a longitudinal force through the humerus in the abducted or flexed position in the direction of the ribs.

Specific[47]

The following tests are used to determine the osteokinematic function of a rib relative to the vertebra of the same number during active motion.

The transverse process is palpated with the thumb of one hand and the rib is palpated just lateral to the posterior tubercle, but medial to the angle, with the thumb of the other hand. The patient is instructed to forward bend the head and/trunk and the relative motion between the transverse process and the rib is noted. The same palpation points are used for testing extension, side-flexion, rotation.

During respiration, the posterior tubercle of the rib should move inferiorly with inspiration and superiorly with expiration. A detected asymmetry with respiration will not determine the side of the lesion. However, it is proposed that the costovertebral and costotransverse joints move like a typical bicondylar joint, with a distinctive glide along the axis of joint rotation. Although a differentiation between a costotransverse joint impairment and a costovertebral impairment cannot be made, both are treated as a unit.

Passive Articular Motion—Costal

The patient is positioned in prone with the head in the hole of the bed and arms by the side. The clinician spreads the length of his or her thumb along the length of a rib and places the heel of the other hand over the thumb (Figure 16–20). The rib is now pushed anteriorly and then anterior-laterally to test the glides of the costovertebral and costotransverse joints respectively. The top ribs are palpated medial to the medial border of the scapular. Care must be taken with prone techniques to avoid imparting too much force.

Combinations of active motion and passive physiologic motion can be performed, testing the ability of the ribs to perform congruent and incongruent motions. This is achieved with the patient seated and the clinician standing to one side. Using one hand, the clinician flexes the patient's thorax and then side-flexes the patient toward them. If the clinician is standing on the patient's left side, this maneuver produces a congruent left rotation of the thoracic spine. The clinician applies overpressure into further left rotation. Using the MCP of the index finger of the other hand, the clinician palpates the right costotransverse joints. Each level is assessed by pushing the rib anteriorly with the medial aspect of the index finger. While maintaining the left side-flexion, the patient is then rotated incongruently to the right. At the end of the available right rotation, overpressure is applied and the rib is again pushed anteriorly, using the medial aspect of the index finger. The procedure is repeated, initiating with rotation before introducing the side-flexion.

Costotransverse Joints—Inferior Glide

Levels T1–6: Example. To test the inferior glide of the right sixth rib at the costotransverse joint, and to determine the ability of the right sixth rib to glide inferiorly relative to the transverse process of T6.[55]

The patient is positioned in prone, with both arms off the edge of the table and the thoracic spine in neutral. Using the left thumb, the clinician palpates the inferior aspect of the right transverse process of T6. The right thumb is used to palpate the superior aspect of the right sixth rib, just lateral to the tubercle (Figure 16–21). The left thumb fixes T6 and an inferior glide, allowing the conjunct posterior roll to occur, is applied to the sixth rib with the right thumb. The quantity and end feel of motion is noted and compared

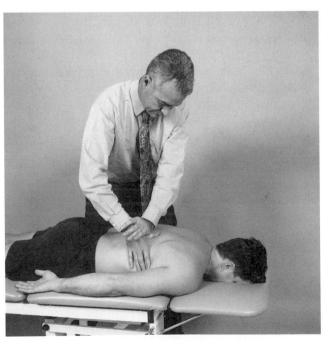

FIGURE 16–20 Patient and clinician position for posterior-anterior pressure. Note the clinician's thumb spread along the shaft of the rib.

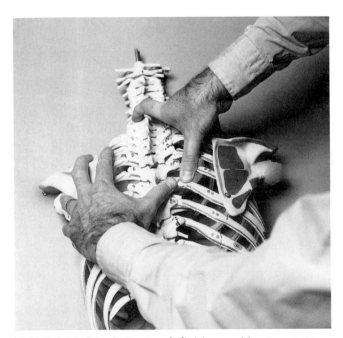

FIGURE 16–21 Patient and clinician position to assess the inferior glide of the costotransverse joint.

to the levels above and below. A loss of the inferior glide would indicate that the rib is held superiorly (inspiratory impairment). The superior rib is treated first.

Levels T7 and T10:   At these levels, the orientation of the costotransverse joint changes, such that the direction of the glide is anterior-lateral-inferior, in more of a sagittal axis. The position of the clinician's right hand is modified to facilitate this change in joint direction so that the thumb of the right hand lies along the shaft of the rib and assists in gliding the rib in an anterior-lateral-interior direction while the left thumb stabilizes the thoracic segment.

Costotransverse Joints—Superior Glide

Levels T1–6:   Example. To test the superior glide of the right sixth rib at the costotransverse joint, and to determine the ability of the right sixth rib to glide superiorly relative to the transverse process of T6.[55]

The patient is positioned in prone-lying as above. Using the right thumb, the clinician palpates the superior aspect of the right transverse process of T6. Using the left thumb, the clinician palpates the inferior aspect of the right sixth rib, just lateral to the tubercle (Figure 16–22). The right thumb fixes T6 and a superior glide, allowing the conjunct anterior roll to occur, is applied to the sixth rib with the left thumb. The quantity and end feel of motion is noted and compared to the levels above and below. A loss of the superior glide would indicate that the rib is held inferiorly (expiration impairment).

Levels T7 and T10:   At these levels, the orientation of the costotransverse joint changes such that the direction of the glide is posterior-medial-superior. The position of the right hand is modified to facilitate this change in joint direction so that the thumb of the right hand lies along the shaft of the rib and fixes the rib. The thumb of the left hand glides the transverse process anterior-lateral-inferiorly, thus producing a relative posterior-medial-superior glide of the rib at the costotransverse joint.

Costal Stability Testing

Anterior Translation—Posterior Costal[55]
This test stresses the anatomic structures that resist anterior translation of the posterior aspect of the rib relative to the thoracic vertebrae to which it attaches (the vertebra of its own number and the vertebra above). A positive response is the reproduction of the patient's symptoms together with an increase in the quantity of motion and a decrease in the resistance at the end of the range of motion.

With the patient prone-lying, the contralateral transverse processes of the thoracic vertebrae to which the rib is attached are palpated and fixed, preventing any posterior motion. For example, to test the seventh rib on the right, the left transverse processes of T6 and T7 are palpated and fixed. With the other hand, the rib is palpated just lateral to the tubercle using the thumb (Figure 16–23). A posterior-anterior force is applied to the rib while fixing the thoracic vertebrae at the transverse processes. The

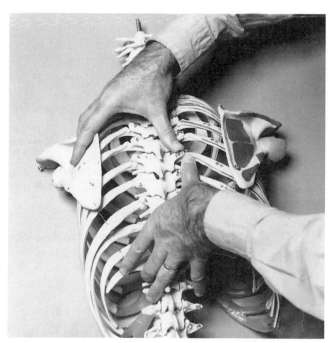

FIGURE 16–22 Clinician hand position to assess the superior glide of the costotransverse joint.

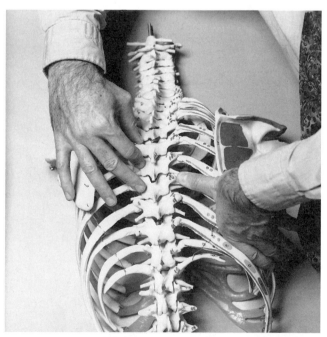

FIGURE 16–23 Patient and clinician position to assess the anterior translation of the 7th rib - posterior costal.

quantity of motion, the reproduction of any symptoms, and the end feel of motion is noted and compared to the levels above and below. A posterior translation can be applied by stabilizing the rib with a lateral distraction force and applying a posterior-anterior force to the ipsilateral transverse process of the same level and number.

Inferior Translation—Posterior Costal: Example—Right Seventh Rib[55]

This test stresses the anatomic structures that resist inferior translation of the rib relative to the thoracic vertebrae to which it attaches, including the superior costotransverse ligament. A positive response is the reproduction of the patient's symptoms together with an increase in the quantity of motion and a decrease in the resistance at the end of the range of motion. With the patient positioned in prone-lying and the clinician standing on the side to be tested, the contralateral transverse process of the thoracic vertebra, at the same level as the rib to be tested (T7 on the right), is palpated and fixed with the index finger pad of one hand to prevent it moving superiorly. With the thumb of the same hand, the ipsilateral transverse process of the thoracic vertebra at the level above the rib to be tested (T6 on the right), is palpated and fixed to prevent it moving. With the other hand, the superior aspect of the rib, just lateral to its tubercle, is palpated using the thumb (Figure 16–24). An inferior force is applied through the rib while fixing the thoracic vertebrae. The quantity of motion, the reproduction of any symptoms, and the end feel

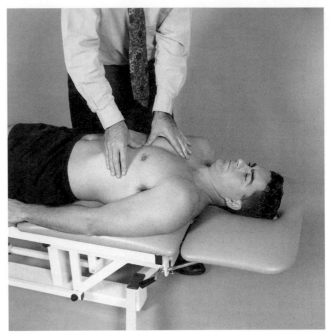

FIGURE 16–25 Patient and clinician position for anterior-posterior pressure of the anterior costals.

of motion is noted and compared to the levels above and below.

Superior-Inferior Translation and Anterior-Posterior Translation—Anterior Costal

This test stresses the anatomic structures that resist a superior-inferior translation of the costocartilage relative to the sternum and the rib relative to the costocartilage. When the sternocostal and/or costochondral joints have been separated, a gap and/or a step can be palpated at the joint line. The positional findings are noted prior to stressing the joint. A positive response is the reproduction of the patient's symptoms together with an increase in the quantity of motion and a decrease in the resistance at the end of the range of motion. With one thumb, the anterior aspect of the sternum and costocartilage is palpated (Figure 16–25). A superior-inferior force is applied to the costocartilage and rib. The quantity of motion, the reproduction of any symptoms, and the end feel of motion is noted and compared to the levels above and below. The technique is modified, except that an anterior-posterior and posterior-anterior force is applied to the costocartilage/rib to access the anterior-posterior translation.

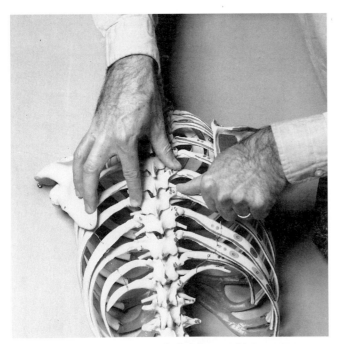

FIGURE 16–24 Patient and clinician position to assess the inferior translation of the 7th rib - posterior costal.

EXAMINATION CONCLUSIONS

Following the biomechanical examination, a working hypothesis should have been established based on a summary of all of the findings. The focus of the biomechanical examination is to elicit a movement diagnosis and to:

1. Determine which costal and/or spinal joint is impaired.
2. Determine the presence and type of movement impairment.

At the completion of the biomechanical examination, the clinician should have information concerning the motion state of the joint and can determine whether the joint is myofascially and pericapsularly hypomobile, subluxed, hypermobile, or ligamentously and articularly unstable.

INTERVENTIONS

Manual Techniques

Numerous manual therapy techniques are available to the clinician for this region and the reader is encouraged to explore as many as possible. In fact, all of the examination techniques that are used to assess joint mobility can be employed as treatment techniques. However, the intent of the technique changes from one of assessing the end feel to one where the application of graded mobilizations or muscle energy techniques is applied at the end of joint range. Manual techniques can be used with hypomobilities, hypermobilities, instabilities, and soft tissue injuries.

Myofascial Hypomobility
These types of hypomobilities respond well to muscle energy techniques and stretching.

General Stretching Techniques for the Thoracic Spine and Ribs
This is an area that is prone to stiffness. There are a number of general techniques that can be used to increase the overall mobility of this area. A few of them are described here.

1. The patient is positioned in supine and the clinician stands at the head of the bed. The clinician rests the heels of his or her palms on both sides of the patient's upper rib cage over the inferior angle of the scapula. The patient is instructed to take a deep breath and to fully exhale. At the end of the exhalation, the clinician applies a gentle anterior-posterior pressure to the rib cage.
2. The patient is positioned in supine and the clinician stands at the head of the bed. The patient elevates both arms over the head and he or she reaches around the back of the clinician's thighs. By having the patient hold onto the two ends of a towel in this position, the

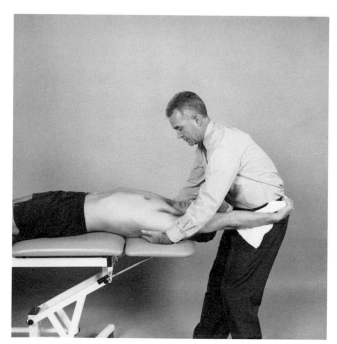

FIGURE 16–26 Patient and clinician position for the general rib cage stretch.

clinician places both of his or her hands under the patient's rib cage and then pulls up on the rib cage in an anterior and cranial direction, into thoracic extension (Figure 16–26).
3. For bucket-handle motion, the patient is positioned in side-lying. The clinician fully abducts the patient's uppermost arm, grasping it above the elbow. The arm is taken into hyper abduction, thereby fully expanding the rib cage on the uppermost side. Muscle energy techniques can also be incorporated. By adjusting the point of stabilization, this technique can be used to treat inspiration and expiration restricted impairments. For example, at ribs 4 and 5:

● Inspiration restriction—pump handle. The clinician stabilizes the fifth rib with the heel of one hand while moving the uppermost arm into sufficient flexion with the other arm.
● Expiration restriction—pump handle. While holding the arm in sufficient flexion with one hand, the clinician uses the heel of the other hand to mobilize the fourth rib inferiorly and distally.

Joint Hypomobility
The purpose of these techniques is to be able to isolate a mobilization to a specific level, and in so doing:

1. Reduce stresses through both the fixation and leverage components of the spine.

2. Reduce stresses through hypermobile segments.
3. Reduce the overall force needed by the clinician, thus giving greater control.

The selection of a manual technique is dependent on a number of factors including the acuteness of the condition and the restriction to the movement that is encountered. If the structure is acutely painful (pain is felt before resistance or pain is felt with resistance), pain relief, rather than a mechanical effect, is the major goal. The manual techniques that can provide pain relief include:

- Joint oscillations (grade I and II) that do not reach the end of range. The segment or joint is left in its neutral position and the mobilization is carried out from that point. There is no need for, and in fact every reason to avoid, muscle relaxation techniques to help reach the end of range.
- Gentle passive range of motion.

Another consideration is whether the restriction is symmetrical, involving both sides of the segment or asymmetrical, involving only one side of the segment. It is unwise to use a symmetrical mobilization for an asymmetrical impairment. If the right joint cannot extend and a symmetrical extension mobilization technique is applied, there is a risk of mobilizing the normal joint, leading to hypermobility. In addition to this risk, is the technique's inadequacy, as full range extension or flexion can only be achieved unilaterally.

The selection of a manual technique or approach also depends on the goal of the treatment. If stretching of the mechanical barrier rather than pain relief is the immediate objective of the treatment, a mobilization technique is carried out at the end of the available range. After this has been gained (and sometimes before and after), there is some minor pain to be dealt with using grade IV oscillations, after which, the joint capsule can be stretched using either grade IV++ or prolonged stretch techniques. Active exercises are continued at home and at work on a regular and frequent basis to reinforce the reeducation.

Symmetrical Techniques to Increase Flexion at T5–6
One of five techniques can be employed to increase flexion at T5–6 based on the stage of healing and other findings.

1. The patient is positioned on the mat table, the buttocks on the edge of the back of the table, and the hands wrapped around themselves. The clinician stands behind the patient and places a small towel roll at the T6 level. The towel roll is held in place by

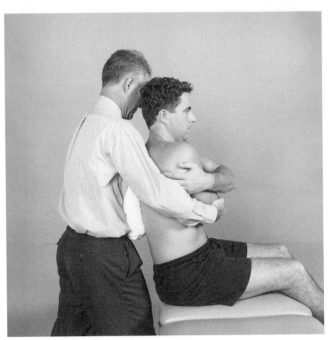

FIGURE 16–27 Patient and clinician position for thrust technique at T5–6.

the clinician's chest. (It is easier if the clinician turns slightly so that the side of the chest is used.) The clinician threads his or her arms around the front of the patient. A stride-stance (one foot in front of the other) is adopted by the clinician (Figure 16–27) and, while keeping their elbows close together, the clinician gently rocks the patient backward and forward. After two or three rocks, the traction force is applied as the clinician shifts their body weight from the forward leg to the back, while lifting the patient and squeezing the forearms toward each other.

2. The patient is positioned as in the previous example. The clinician stands behind the patient and places a small towel roll at the T5 level. The towel roll is held in place by the clinician's chest. (It is easier if the clinician turns slightly so that the side of the chest is used.) The patient is asked to cross the arms over the chest. The clinician reaches around the patient and grasps the patient's lower elbow in both hands and wedges the forearm under the infraglenoid tubercle area of the patient's scapula (Figure 16–28). The segment is flexed as much as is comfortable and the upper body is lifted by a graded squeezing of the arms together underneath the scapula. The patient's buttocks should not be lifted off the bed.

3. Longitudinal traction produces a superior glide of the zygapophysial joint bilaterally. This technique may be done with the patient either supine-lying or sitting. With the patient supine, grade 1 and 2 techniques are

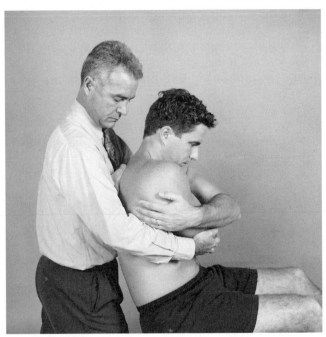

FIGURE 16–28 Patient and clinician position for thrust technique at T5–6.

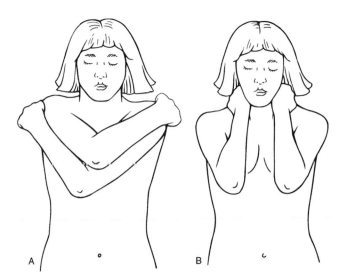

FIGURE 16–29 Arm positions for patient.

better controlled and can be applied for pain relief. The stronger mobilizations can be done with the patient either supine or sitting.

The supine technique is performed as follows:

The patient is side-lying, and the arms crossed to the opposite shoulders. The method of arm crossing depends on the size and flexibility of the patient. The larger, heavier, and less flexible patient, crosses the arms as in Figure 16–29A. The smaller, lighter, and more flexible patient, crosses the arms as in Figure 16–29B. The clinician stands on the side of the patient so that the patient's arm resting on the chest is nearest to the clinician. With the tubercle of the scaphoid bone placed against the lateral aspect of the spinous process, and the flexed PIP joint of the middle finger placed on the other side of the spinous process, the transverse processes of the inferior vertebra are palpated and fixed, blocking the inferior ring complex (Figure 16–30). The other hand and arm lies across and on top of the patient's crossed arms to control the thorax. Segmental localization is achieved by flexing the joint to the motion barrier using the hand and arm controlling the thorax. This localization is maintained by having the clinician's body lean on the patient's elbows as he or she reaches around the neck and back of the patient and supports the thorax as the patient is rolled supine or semisupine (only until contact is made between the table and the dorsal hand; Figure 16–31). The thoracic curve above the treated

segment is maintained either by the clinician or by raising the table end. A minimum amount of the patient's body weight should be resting on the clinician's right hand to prevent a painful compression against the contact hand. From this position, longitudinal traction is applied through the thorax, along the plane of the joint, to produce a superior glide of the zygapophysial joint bilaterally. No posterior-anterior compression should occur. This is an arthrokinematic mobilization. The technique can be graded from 1 to 5.

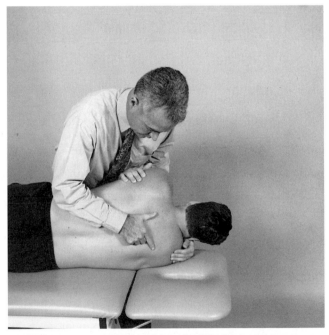

FIGURE 16–30 Hand position for T5–6.

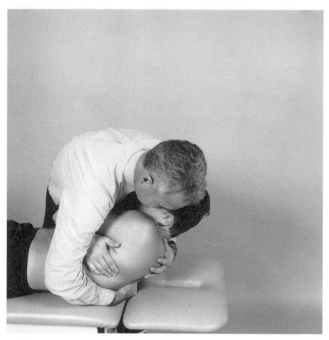

FIGURE 16–31 Patient and clinician pre-thrust position.

An active mobilization assist (muscle energy technique) may be used to effect a change in the muscle tone segmentally. When the motion barrier has been localized, the patient is instructed to gently elevate the crossed arms. The motion is resisted by the clinician and the isometric contraction is held for up to 5 seconds, followed by a period of complete relaxation. The joint is then passively taken to the new motion barrier. The technique is repeated three times and is followed by a reexamination of function.

4. In the supine distraction and gapping technique, the patient is positioned in supine with clinician standing to one side as in technique 3. The patient crosses the arms and places the hands on opposite shoulders (hug themselves), so that the arm closest to them is closest to the clinician. Rolling the patient toward the clinician, he or she places the palm side of the right hand in the classical tripod, or pistol, position (thumb and index finger extended, with the remaining fingers fully flexed), against the patient's thoracic spine, so that the transverse processes of the caudal bone engage the middle finger and thenar eminence. Thus, the spinous process of T5 nestles in the space created by the extended index finger (see Figure 16–30). The clinician's right hand is held firmly against the patient's spine as the patient is rolled back over into a supine position, the body weight being supported by the left arm of the clinician, which is around the back of the patient's neck. As such, the patient, and the clinician's right hand, are lifted back onto the bed,

and the thoracic kyphosis of the patient is maintained (see Figure 16–31). A minimum amount of the patient's body weight should be resting on the clinician's right hand to prevent a painful compression against the contact hand. Two choices now exist. A mobilizing force in a superior direction, up the bed, produces a distraction of the segment, whereas a mobilizing force in a posterior direction, down into the bed, will produce a gapping of the segment. This is an arthrokinematic mobilization. The technique can be graded from 1 to 5.

Techniques to Restore the Extension Glide (on the Left) at the T5–6 Level

Thrust Technique. The patient is positioned in right side-lying, the head supported on a pillow and the arms crossed to the opposite shoulders. With the tubercle of the right scaphoid bone and the flexed PIP joint of the right middle finger, the clinician palpates the left transverse process of T6 and the right transverse process of T5 (Figure 16–32). The other hand and arm lies across the patient's crossed arms to control the thorax. Segmental localization is achieved by extending the joint to the motion barrier with the hand and arm controlling the thorax. The localization is maintained as the patient is rolled supine only until contact is made between the table and the dorsal hand.

The thoracic curve above the treated segment is maintained either by the clinician or by raising the table

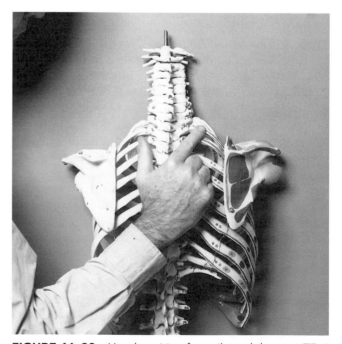

FIGURE 16–32 Hand position for unilateral thrust at T5–6.

end. From this position, a left side-flexion force (coupled with a slight posterior glide) is applied through the thorax to produce an inferior glide of the left zygapophysial joint. By restoring the joint, or linear glide, the angular motion will be restored. The technique can be graded from 1 to 5.

An active mobilization assist (muscle energy technique) may be used to effect a change in the muscle tone. When the motion barrier has been localized, the patient is instructed to gently elevate the crossed arms. The motion is resisted by the clinician and the isometric contraction is held for up to 5 seconds, followed by a period of complete relaxation. The joint is then passively taken to the new motion barrier. The technique is repeated three times and is followed by a reexamination of function.

Side-lying Technique Using Rotation. The patient is positioned in right side-lying, the head supported on a pillow and the arms crossed and hands behind the neck. The clinician grasps the patient's lower arm with one hand and supports the patient's elbows on the lateral pelvis (cranial side). With the other hand, the clinician palpates the segment to be treated. The thoracic spine is now moved into extension as the clinician rotates his or her pelvis toward the patient's head, thereby imparting a posterior force through the patient's elbows. Oscillations at the correct level can be used.

To increase the specificity of this technique for the higher thoracic levels, the clinician rotates the patient's shoulder away and extends the thoracic spine to the correct level. Rotation below the desired level is prevented from occurring by fixing the spinous process of the inferior segment. The upper segment is extended and rotated to the point of restriction and is either mobilized directly, or indirectly by using muscle energy.

To increase the specificity of this technique for the lower segments, the clinician positions the patient's top arm into shoulder flexion, to remove it out of the way, and rotates the patient's rib cage away. The clinician's contact with the patient's rib cage is via the cranial forearm and palm of hand. As before, the caudal hand is used to stabilize the inferior spinous process.

Muscle Energy Technique. When the myofascial structures are thought to be the main cause of the osteokinematic restriction, the following technique can be useful. The patient is sitting with the arms crossed to the opposite shoulders. With the dorsal hand, the intertransverse space is palpated. The ventral hand is placed on the contralateral shoulder. The motion barrier is localized by extending and left side-flexing the thorax (Figure 16–33). From this position, the patient is instructed to hold still while the clinician applies resistance to the trunk. The

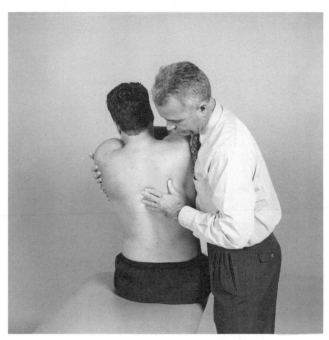

FIGURE 16–33 Patient and clinician position for seated unilateral muscle energy technique into extension and left side flexion.

direction of the applied resistance is determined by the neurophysiologic effect desired from the technique. A hold and relax technique applies the principles of autogenic inhibition and is used primarily for a shortened muscle. The necessary muscle is recruited strongly and then maximally stretched in the immediate post-contraction relaxation phase. A contract and relax technique applies the principles of reciprocal inhibition and is used primarily for a hypertonic muscle. The antagonist muscle is recruited gently, and the contraction results in a reciprocal inhibition of the antagonistic hypertonic muscle. The isometric contraction is held for up to 5 seconds, following which the patient is instructed to completely relax. The new extension and side-flexion barrier is localized and the mobilization repeated three times.

The reader should be able to extrapolate the necessary information from above to treat an FRSL impairment.

Mobilization and Manipulation of the Fifth Rib

Any one of the following techniques could be used.

Mobilization Technique. The patient is sitting with the arms crossed to the opposite shoulders. With the dorsal hand, the fifth rib is palpated. The ventral hand is placed on the patient's ipsilateral shoulder. The motion barrier is localized by right side-flexing and left rotating the thorax

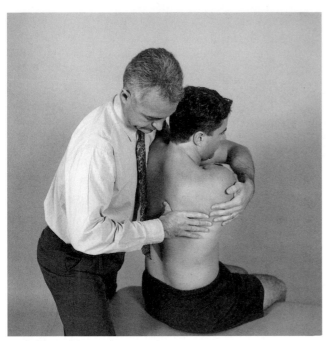

FIGURE 16–34   Patient and clinician position for mobilization of the fifth rib on the right.

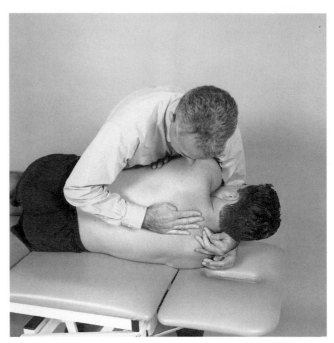

FIGURE 16–35   Patient and clinician position for the rib thrust technique.

(Figure 16–34). From this position, the patient is instructed to hold still while the clinician applies resistance to the trunk. The direction of the applied resistance is determined by the neurophysiologic effect desired from the technique. A hold and relax technique is used primarily for a contractured muscle. The involved muscle is recruited strongly and then maximally stretched in the immediate post-contraction relaxation phase. A contract and relax technique is used primarily for a hypertonic muscle. The antagonist muscle is recruited gently. The contraction results in a reciprocal inhibition of the antagonistic hypertonic muscle. The isometric contraction is held for up to 5 seconds, following which the patient is instructed to completely relax. The new motion barrier is localized and the mobilization repeated three times.

Thrust Technique.   The patient is positioned in side-lying, arms crossed to opposite shoulders (the patient's arm that is closest to the clinician is closest to the patient's chest) while the clinician stands at the patient's side. The clinician tucks the thumb of the stabilizing hand onto the palm of the hand. Maintaining this position, the clinician palpates just lateral to the rib tubercle, on the rib angle, but not as medial as the transverse process, with the tip of the thumb. The fingers of the stabilizing hand are pointed perpendicular to (Figure 16–35), or along the line of the ribs. The first two or three ribs are difficult to access due to the presence of the scapula and the fingers of the stabilizing hand

have to placed perpendicular to the line of the ribs. Lower down the thoracic spine, the scapula is less intrusive and either hand placement can be used, although additional support is provided if the fingers are placed along the line of the ribs. The other hand and arm supports the patient's thorax. This contact is maintained as the patient is rolled into the supine position, only until sufficient contact has been made between the dorsal hand and the table. The thoracic curve above the treated segment is maintained. Specific localization can be used to lock the thoracic spine, so as to prevent the spine from rotating in the same direction. The thorax is axially rotated against the fixed rib. This is a grade 5 technique and minimal force is required to reduce the subluxation.

Muscle Energy Technique to Restore the Posterior Rotation of the Fifth Rib.   When the myofascia is thought to be the main cause of the osteokinematic restriction, the following technique can be useful. The patient is sitting with the arms crossed to opposite shoulders. With the dorsal hand, the fifth rib is palpated. The ventral hand is placed on the patient's contralateral shoulder. The motion barrier is localized by left side-flexing and right rotating the thorax. From this position, the patient is instructed to hold still while the clinician applies resistance to the trunk. The direction of the applied resistance is determined by the neurophysiologic effect desired from the technique. The isometric contraction is held for up to 5 seconds, following which the patient is instructed to completely relax. The new motion barrier is localized and the mobilization repeated three times.

Home Exercise. To maintain the mobility gained, the patient is instructed to perform specific mid thoracic left side flexion and right rotation frequently (up to ten times, ten times per day). The amplitude of the exercise should be in the pain-free range and should not aggravate any symptoms.

Electrotherapeutic Modalities and Physical Agents

The manual techniques can be supplemented with the use of modalities. Heat can be applied to the specific area prior to the manual technique.

● A moist heat pack causes an increase in the local tissue temperature, reaching its highest point about 8 minutes after the application.[56] Wet heat produces a greater rise in local tissue temperature compared with dry heat at a similar temperature.[57]

● Ultrasound is the most common clinically used deep heating modality to promote tissue healing.[58–60]

Other modalities include electrical stimulation. For the manual therapist, electrical stimulation can be used:

● To create a muscle contraction through nerve or muscle stimulation.

● To decrease pain through the stimulation of sensory nerves (TENS).

● To maintain or increase range of motion.

● To stimulate tissue healing by creating an electrical field in biologic tissue.

● Muscle reeducation or facilitation by both motor and sensory stimulation.

● To drive ions into or through the skin (iontophoresis).

Case Study: Right Anterior Chest Pain[61]

Subjective

A 25-year-old male presented at the clinic complaining of pain in his right anterior chest. About 1 month previously, the patient had experienced a sudden and sharp pain in his right posterior chest at the mid-scapular level during a tug of war game at his company's picnic. The posterior chest pain subsided very quickly and did not bother him for the rest of the game. However, the next morning, pain was felt in the anterior aspect of the chest. This anterior chest pain eased off over the next few days with rest, but recurred as soon as the patient returned to weight lifting.

Questions

1. Given the mechanism of injury, what structure(s) could be at fault?

2. Should the report of anterior chest pain concern the clinician in this case?

3. What is your working hypothesis at this stage? List the various diagnoses that could present with anterior chest pain, and the tests you would use to rule out each one.

4. Why did the pain shift from posterior thoracic to anterior thoracic?

5. Does this presentation and history warrant a scan? Why or why not?

Examination

On observation, the patient was a healthy looking male with no obvious postural deficits. The patient had presented with pain following a specific mechanism of injury but as the pain had shifted, a scan was considered to be necessary. A modification of a thoracic and cervical scan revealed the following.

● The patient demonstrated full range of cervical motion.

● The patient demonstrated full range of thoracic motion, although overpressure with rotation to the right produced the anterior chest pain.

● The slump, neck flexion, and scapular retraction tests were all negative.

● The neurologic tests were negative.

● The compression, traction, and posterior-anterior pressures were all pain free.

● Anterior-posterior pressure over the right fifth costochondral joint reproduced the patient's pain.

Questions

1. Did the scanning examinations confirm the working hypothesis? How?

2. Given the findings from the scanning examination, what is the diagnosis, or is further testing warranted in the form of special tests? What information would be gained with further testing?

3. Why did the pain shift from posterior thoracic pain to anterior thoracic?

The results of the scan seemed to indicate a costochondritis of the fifth rib. However, the original mechanism had produced posterior thoracic pain. A biomechanical examination was necessary and it revealed the following.

● The H and I tests for the thoracic spine were inconclusive.

● The position tests for the thoracic spine were negative.

- The screening test was positive for a rib impairment (positioning the thoracic spine in extreme flexion and having the patient take a deep breath in, reproduced the pain, as did positioning the thoracic spine in extreme extension, and having the patient take a deep breath out.)
- The PPIVM tests for the thoracic spine were negative.
- Once the thoracic spine has been cleared, a rib examination must be performed to confirm a musculoskeletal cause for the patient's symptoms.
- The rib examination revealed that the posterior rib joint glides were all full and pain free, except for the fifth rib, which appeared to have lost all of its glides.

Evaluation

The patient was diagnosed with a fifth costotransverse and/or costovertebral joint subluxation, with a loss of anterior rotation of the rib. The costochondritis probably resulted from abnormal stresses being imparted to this area as a result of the subluxation and provides a good example of the silent hypomobile joint producing pain in a nearby joint.

Questions
1. Having confirmed the diagnosis, what will be your intervention?
2. How would you describe your findings to the patient?
3. In order of priority, and based on the stages of healing, list the various goals of your intervention?
4. How will you determine the amplitude and joint position for the intervention?
5. Estimate this patient's prognosis.
6. What modalities could you use in the intervention of this patient?

Intervention

- *Electrotherapeutic modalities and thermal agents.* A moist heat pack was applied to the thoracic spine when the patient arrived for each treatment session. Electrical stimulation with a medium frequency of 50 to 120 pulses per second was applied with the moist heat to aid in pain relief. Ultrasound at 1 MHz was administered to the articulation in question following the moist heat. An ice pack was applied to the area at the end of the treatment session.
- *Manual therapy.* Following the ultrasound, general stretch techniques were applied to the area followed by a mobilization/manipulation of the fifth rib.
- *Therapeutic exercises.* To maintain the mobility gained, the patient is instructed to perform specific mid thoracic right side flexion and left rotation. The amplitude of the exercise should be in the pain-free range and should not aggravate any symptoms. Aerobic exercises using a stationary bike and the treadmill were also prescribed.

- *Patient-related instruction.* Explanation was given as to the cause of the patient's symptoms. The patient was advised to continue the exercises at home, up to ten times, ten times per day and to expect some post-exercise soreness. The patient also received instruction on the use of heat and ice at home.
- *Goals and outcomes.* Both the patient's goals from the treatment and the expected therapeutic goals from the clinician were discussed with the patient. It was concluded that the clinical sessions would occur 3 times per week for 1 month, at which time, the patient would be discharged to a home exercise program. With adherence to the instructions and exercise program, it was felt that the patient would make a full return to function.

Case Study: Bilateral and Central Upper Thoracic Pain

Subjective

A 30-year-old housewife presents at the clinic with a 3-day history of constant central and bilateral upper thoracic pain that is deep, dull and can be felt in the front of the chest when the pain is aggravated. The pain is reported to be worse with flexion motions but is improved with lying on a hard surface. Further questioning revealed that the patient had a history of minor back pain but was otherwise in good health and had no report of bowel or bladder impairment.

Questions
1. What structure(s) could be at fault with central and bilateral upper thoracic pain as the major complaint?
2. Should the report of anterior chest pain concern the clinician in this case?
3. Why was the statement about "no reports of bowel or bladder impairment" pertinent?
4. What is your working hypothesis at this stage? List the various diagnoses that could present with central and bilateral upper thoracic pain and the tests you would use to rule out each one.
5. Does this presentation and history warrant a scan? Why or why not?

Examination

The pain appears to be activity related, is of short duration, and is nonradicular in nature. Therefore, a thoracic scan is not warranted at this time. Active motion testing of the thoracic spine revealed the following.

- Flexion limited and painful, with a minimal loss of rotation and side-flexion bilaterally. Extension appeared normal.

- The thoracic H and I tests revealed an increase in pain with flexion and side-flexion to both sides, and side-flexion to both sides and flexion.
- Position testing was normal.
- Symmetrical PPIVM tests revealed decreased flexion at T5–6.
- Confirmatory posterior-anterior pressures revealed pain over T5 and T6.

Questions
1. Did the active motion confirm the working hypothesis? How?
2. What information was gathered from the H and I tests?
3. Using the results of the H and I tests, is it possible to determine the specific segment at fault?
4. Given the findings from the biomechanical examination, what is the diagnosis, or is further testing warranted in the form of special tests? What information would be gained with further testing?

Evaluation
The patient is presenting with the classic signs of a symmetrical flexion hypomobility at T5–6. A hypomobility may present as a bilateral or unilateral capsular, or noncapsular hypomobility, or as a unilateral or bilateral hypermobility. If a bilateral arthritis is present, then extension and both side-flexions and rotations will be decreased, with flexion being less affected. If it is unilateral, then there will be more loss of extension than flexion and one rotation and side-flexion will be decreased more than the other. A unilateral capsular pattern of the right apophyseal joint will demonstrate, on position testing, as a large FRSL and a smaller ERSR.

Questions
1. Having confirmed the diagnosis, what will be your intervention?
2. In order of priority, and based on the stages of healing, list the various goals of your intervention?
3. How will you determine the amplitude and joint position for the intervention?
4. Is an asymmetrical or symmetrical technique more appropriate for this condition? Why?
5. Estimate this patient's prognosis.
6. What modalities could you use in the intervention of this patient?

Intervention
- *Electrotherapeutic modalities and thermal agents.* A moist heat pack was applied to the thoracic spine when the patient arrived for each treatment session. Electrical stimulation with a medium frequency of 50 to 120 pulses per second was applied with the moist heat

to aid in pain relief. Ultrasound at 1 MHz was administered to the articulation in question following the moist heat. An ice pack was applied to the area at the end of the treatment session.
- *Manual therapy.* Following the ultrasound, general stretch techniques were applied to the area followed by a specific mobilization to increase flexion at T5–6.
- *Therapeutic exercises.* To maintain the mobility gained, the patient is instructed to perform specific mid-thoracic flexion. The amplitude of the exercise should be in the pain-free range, and should not aggravate any symptoms. Aerobic exercises using a stationary bike and the treadmill were also prescribed.
- *Patient-related instruction.* Explanation was given as to the cause of the patient's symptoms. The patient was advised to continue the exercises at home, up to ten times, ten times per day and to expect some post-exercise soreness. The patient also received instruction on the use of heat and ice at home.
- *Goals and outcomes.* Both the patient's goals from the treatment and the expected therapeutic goals from the clinician were discussed with the patient. It was concluded that the clinical sessions would occur 3 times per week for 1 month, at which time, the patient would be discharged to a home exercise program. With adherence to the instructions and exercise program, it was felt that the patient would make a full return to function.

Case Study: Interscapular Pain

Subjective
A 21-year-old female presented with a 1-week history of left-sided inter-scapular pain that started at work. The patient worked as a computer operator. The pain was reported to be aggravated by lying prone, deep breathing in, and standing or sitting erect. Further questioning revealed that the patient had a history of this pain over the last few months but that it had not been as painful. The patient was otherwise in good health and had no reports of bowel or bladder impairment.

Questions
1. List the structures that can produce inter-scapular pain.
2. Given the fact that this patient works at a computer, what could be the cause of her pain?
3. What is your working hypothesis at this stage? List the various diagnoses that could present with inter-scapular pain, and the tests you would use to rule out each one.
4. Does this presentation and history warrant a scan? Why or why not?

Examination

Given the postural history at work and the localization of the pain, a thoracic scan was not performed. Instead a biomechanical examination was initiated with the following results.

- With plane motions, the pain was reproduced with extension, and with left side flexion
- Using the H and I tests, the combined movement of extension, left rotation, and left side-flexion reproduced the pain
- The PPIVM test revealed decreased motion at the T5–6 level into extension and decreased motion into left side-flexion
- Posterior-anterior pressure over T6 revealed extreme tenderness
- With the PPAIVM test, the inferior joint glide at the T5–6 zygapophysial joint was reduced on the left side

Questions
1. Did the active motion confirm the working hypothesis? How?
2. What was the purpose of the H and I tests, if two aggravating motions had already been found?
3. Given the findings from the biomechanical examination, what is the diagnosis, or is further testing warranted in the form of special tests? What information would be gained with further testing?

Evaluation

The results of the examination revealed that the patient had a unilateral restriction of extension at the T5–6 level or an FRSR of T5.

Questions
1. Having confirmed the diagnosis, what will be your intervention?
2. In order of priority, and based on the stages of healing, list the various goals of your intervention?
3. How will you determine the amplitude and joint position for the intervention?
4. Is an asymmetrical or symmetrical technique more appropriate for this condition? Why?
5. Estimate this patient's prognosis.
6. What modalities could you use in the intervention of this patient?

Intervention
- *Electrotherapeutic modalities and thermal agents.* A moist heat pack was applied to the thoracic spine when the patient arrived for each treatment session. Electrical stimulation with a medium frequency of 50 to 120 pulses per second was applied with the moist heat to aid in pain relief. Ultrasound at 1 MHz was administered to

the articulation in question following the moist heat. An ice pack was applied to the area at the end of the treatment session.
- *Manual therapy.* Following the ultrasound, general stretch techniques were applied to the area followed by a specific mobilization to restore the extension glide on the left at the T5–6 level.
- *Therapeutic exercises.* To maintain the mobility gained, the patient is instructed to perform specific mid thoracic left side-flexion in slight extension frequently (up to ten times, several times per day). The amplitude of the exercise should be in the pain-free range and should not aggravate any symptoms. Aerobic exercises using a stationary bike and the treadmill were also prescribed.
- *Patient-related instruction.* Explanation was given as to the cause of the patient's symptoms. The patient was advised to continue the exercises at home, up to ten times, ten times per day and to expect some post-exercise soreness. The patient also received instruction on the use of heat and ice at home.
- *Goals and outcomes.* Both the patient's goals from the treatment and the expected therapeutic goals from the clinician were discussed with the patient. It was concluded that the clinical sessions would occur 3 times per week for 1 month, at which time, the patient would be discharged to a home exercise program. With adherence to the instructions and exercise program, it was felt that the patient would make a full return to function.

REVIEW QUESTIONS

1. T__ F__ The external intercostal muscles run downward and posteriorly.
2. T__ F__ The external intercostals are muscles of exhalation.
3. In the thoracic region, in which plane are the facet joints oriented?
4. Which are the atypical ribs and why?
5. At a typical thoracic segment, what does the rib articulate with?
6. What is the joint where the rib and the vertebra meet called?
7. Which levels contain the typical thoracic vertebra?
8. At the costovertebral joint, where are the demi facets located?
9. Which structures modify and restrict rotation in the thoracic region?
10. Which of the thoracic vertebra is the smallest?
11. The typical vertebrae articulate with which two vertebrae?
12. Which ribs demonstrate bucket handle movement and which display pump handle?

13. Which ribs articulate with the sternum directly?
14. How do the ribs 8 to 10 articulate with the sternum?
15. In the "rule of 3s," the second set of spinous processes (T4–6) are level with what?
16. Which levels are known as the vertebrosternal region?
17. What are the coupling motions for latexion at the T3–T10 levels?
18. Down to which level in the thorax can be treated as a cervical impairment?
19. What are the four areas for concern with patient history in the thoracic spine?
20. With thoracic forward flexion, which motions occur at the head of the rib in the vertebrosternal region?

ANSWERS

1. False, downward and laterally.
2. False.
3. Coronally (to facilitate rotation).
4. 1, 10, 11, 12 (only articulate with their own vertebra and do not possess inferior demi facets).
5. Two adjacent vertebra and the intervening disc.
6. Costovertebral.
7. T2–9.
8. On the centrum.
9. Ribs.
10. T3.
11. Own level and the one above.
12. T1–6, pump handle; T7–12, bucket handle.
13. T1–7.
14. Via the one above them (eleventh and twelfth are free at their lateral ends).
15. The disc below.
16. T3–7.
17. Side-flexion and rotation occur to opposite sides.
18. T3.
19. Elderly patient with no causal factor (tumor), gall-bladder disease, cardiac disease, osteoporosis.
20. Anterior rotation (conjunct).

REFERENCES

1. Macrae JE. *Roentgenometrics in chiropractic.* Toronto: Canadian Memorial Chiropractor College; 1974.
2. Bernhardt M, Bridwell KH. Segmental analysis of the sagittal plane alignment of the normal thoracic and lumbar spines and the thoracolumbar junction. *Spine* 1989;14:717–721.
3. Harrison DE, Harrison DD, Troyanovich SJ, Harmon, S. A normal spinal position: It's time to accept the evidence. Journal of Manipulative and Physiological Therapeutics 2000;23(9):623–644.
4. Frazer JE. Frazer's Anatomy of the Human Skeleton. London: Churchill Livingstone; 1965.
5. Bradford S. Juvenile kyphosis. In: Bradford DS, Lonstein JE, Moe JH, Ogilvie JW, Winter RB, eds. *Moe's Textbook of Scoliosis and Other Spinal Deformities.* Philadelphia: Saunders; 1987:347.
6. Ombregt L, Bisschop P, ter Veer HJ, Van de Velde T. A System of Orthopaedic Medicine. London, WB Saunders, 1995.
7. Williams PL, Warwick R, Dyson M, Bannister LH. Gray's Anatomy. 37th ed. Edinburgh: Churchill Livingstone; 1989.
8. Rouviere H. Anatomie Humaine. Descriptive et Topographique. Paris: Masson; 1927.
9. Hovelacque A. Anatoime des Neufs Craniens et Radichiens et du Sisteme Grand Sympathetique chez L'homme. 1st ed. Paris: Gaston Doin et Cie; 1927.
10. MacConail MA, Basmajian JV. Muscles and Movements: A Basis for Human Kinesiology. Baltimore: Williams & Wilkins; 1969.
11. Lee D. Manual Therapy for the Thorax—A Biomechanical Approach Delta Publishers, BC, Canada; 1994.
12. Panjabi MM, Hausfield JN, White AA. A biomechanical study of the ligamentous stability of the thoracic spine in man. *Acta Orthop Scand* 1981;52:315–326.
13. White AA, Hirsch C. The significance of the vertebral posterior elements in the mechanics of the thoracic spine. *Clin Orthop* 1971;81:2–14.
14. Schmorl G, Junghanns H. The Human Spine in Health and Disease. 2nd American edn. New York: Grune & Stratton; 1971.
15. Andriacchi T, Schultz A, Belytschko T, Galante J. A model for studies of mechanical interactions between the human spine and rib cage. *J Biomech* 1974;7:497–507.
16. Panjabi MM, Brand RA, White AA. Mechanical properties of the human thoracic spine. *J Bone Joint Surg* [Am] 1976;5:642–651.
17. Jiang H, Raso JV, Moreau MJ, Russell G, Hill DL, Bagnall KM. Quantitative morphology of the lateral ligaments of the spine. Assessment of their importance in maintaining lateral stability. *Spine* 1994;19:2676–2682.
18. De Troyer A. Actions and load sharing between respiratory muscles. In: Jones NL, Killian KJ, eds. *Breathlessness: The Campbell Symposium.* Hamilton, Ontario: Boehringer Ingelheim; 1992:13–19.
19. Whitelaw WA. Recruitment patterns of respiratory muscles. In: Jones NL, Killian KJ, eds. *Breathlessness: The Campbell Symposium.* Hamilton, Ontario: Boehringer Ingelheim; 1992:20–26.
20. De Troyer A, Sampson MG. Activation of the parasternal intercostals during breathing efforts in human subjects. *J Appl Physiol* 1982;52:524–529.

21. Estenne M, Ninane V, De Troyer A. Triangularis sterni muscle use during eupnea in humans: effect of posture. *Resp Physiol* 1988;74:151–162.

22. Taylor A. The contribution of the intercostal muscles to the effort of respiration in man. *J Physiol* 1960;151:390–402.

23. Whitelaw WA, Feroah T. Patterns of intercostal muscle activity in humans. *J Appl Physiol* 1989;67:2087–2094.

24. De Troyer A, Ninane V, Gilmartin JJ, Lemerre C, Estenne M. Triangularis sterni muscle use in supine humans. *J Appl Physiol* 1987;62:919–925.

25. Grassino AE. Limits of maximal inspiratory muscle function. In: Jones NL, Killian KJ, eds. *Breathlessness: The Campbell Symposium.* Hamilton, Ontario: Boehringer Ingelheim; 1992:27–33.

26. Brooks G, Fahey T. *Fundamentals of Human Performance.* New York: Macmillan; 1987.

27. Nava S, Zanotti E, Rampulla C, Rossi A. Respiratory muscle fatigue does not limit exercise performance during moderate endurance run. *J Sports Med Phys Fitness* 1992;32:39–44.

28. Mador M, Magalang U, Rodis A, Kufel T. Diaphragmatic fatigue after exercise in healthy subjects. *Am Rev Resp Dis* 1993;148:1571–1575.

29. Johnson B, Babcock M, Dempsey J. Exercise-induced diaphragmatic fatigue in healthy humans. *J Physiol (Lond)* 1993;460:385–405.

30. Rochester D, Arora N. Respiratory muscle failure. *Med Clin North Am* 1983;67:573–597.

31. Roussos C, Macklem P. The respiratory muscles. *N Eng. J Med.* 1982;307:786–797.

32. Agostoni E, Sant' Ambrogio G. The diaphragm. In: Campbell EJM, Agostoni E, Newsom-Davis J, eds. *The Respiratory Muscles: Mechanics and Neurological Control.* 2nd ed. London: Lloyd-Luke; 1970;145–160.

33. Allen SM, Hunt B, Green M. Fall in vital capacity with posture. *Br J Dis Chest* 1985;79:267–271.

34. Mier-Jedrzejowicz A, Brophy C, Moxham J, Green M. Assessment of diaphragm weakness. *Am Rev Respir Dis* 1988;137:877–883.

35. Aubier M, Farkas G, De Troyer A, Mozes R, Roussos C. Detection of diaphragmatic fatigue in man by phrenic stimulation. *J Appl Physiol* 1981;50:538–544.

36. Bellemare F, Grassino A. Effect of pressure and timing of contraction on human diaphragm fatigue. *J Appl Physiol* 1982;53:1190–1195.

37. Bye PTP, Farkas GA, Roussos C. Respiratory factors limiting exercise. *Ann Rev Physiol* 1983;45:439–451.

38. Dempsey JA. Is the lung built for exercise? *Med Sci Sports Exerc* 1986;18:143–155.

39. Babcock MA, Johnson BD, Pegelow DF, Suman OE, Griffin D, Dempsey A. Hypoxic effects on exercise-induced diaphragmatic fatigue in normal healthy humans. *J Appl Physiol* 1995;78:82–92.

40. Babcock MA, Pegelow DF, McClaran SA, Suman OE, Dempsey A. Contribution of diaphragmatic work to exercise-induced diaphragm fatigue. *J Appl Physiol* 1995;78:1710–1717.

41. Fenn, WO. A comparison of respiratory and skeletal muscles. In: *Perspectives in Biology. Houssay Memorial Papers.* Cori CF, Foglia VG, Leloir LF, Ochoa S, eds. Amsterdam: Elsevier; 1963;293–300.

42. Sharp JT. Respiratory muscles: a review of old and new concepts. *Lung* 1980;157:185–199.

43. Rochester D. Respiratory muscles: structure, size, and adaptive capacity. In: Jones NL, Killian KJ, eds. *Breathlessness: The Campbell Symposium.* Hamilton, Ontario: Boehringer Ingelheim; 1992:2–12.

44. Detroyer A, Sampson M, Sigrist S, Macklem P. Action of the costal and crural parts of the diaphragm during breathing. *J Appl Physiol* 1982;53:30–39.

45. Detroyer A, Sampson M, Sigrist S, Macklem P. The diaphragm: two muscles. *Science* 1981;213:237–238.

46. Raou RJP. Recherches sur la Mobilité Vertebrale en Fonction des Types Rachidiens. Paris: Thèse; 1952.

47. Lee D. Manual Therapy for the Thorax—A Biomechanical Approach. Delta Publishers, BC, Canada; 1994.

48. Gonon JP, Dimnet J, Carret JP, Mauroy JO, Fischer LP, Morgues G. Utilité de l'analyse cinématique de radiographies dynamiques dans le diagnostic de certaines affections de la colonne lombaire. In: Simon L, Rabourdin JP. Lombalgies et Médecine de Rééducation. Paris: Masson; 1983;27–49.

49. Panjabi MM, Brand RA, White AA. Three-dimensional flexibility and stiffness properties of the human thoracic spine. *J Biomech* 1976;9:185.

50. Lovett RW. *Lateral Curvature of the Spine and Round Shoulders.* Philadelphia–Bilkeston Beard and Co; 1907.

51. Miles M, Sullivan WE. Lateral bending at the lumbar and lumbosacral joints. *Anat Rec* 1961;139:387–392.

52. Raou RJP. Recherches sur la Mobilité Vertebrale en Fonction des Types Rachidiens. Paris: Thèse; 1952.

53. White AA, Panjab MM. *Clinical Biomechanics of the Spine.* 2nd ed. Philadelphia: Lippincott; 1990.

54. Mitchell F, Moran PS, Pruzzo N. An Evaluation and Treatment Manual of Osteopathic Muscle Energy Procedures. ICEOP, Missouri; 1979.

55. Lee DG, Walsh MC. *A Workbook of Manual Therapy Techniques for the Vertebral Column and Pelvic Girdle.* 2nd ed. Vancouver: Nascent; 1996.

56. Lehmann JF, Silverman DR, Baum BA, Kirk NL, Johnston VC et al. Temperature distributions in the human thigh produced by infrared, hot pack and

microwave applications. *Arch Phys Med Rehabil* 1966; 47:291.

57. Abramson DI, Tuck S, Lee SW, et al. Comparison of wet and dry heat in raising temperature of tissues. *Arch Phys Med Rehabil* 1967;48:654–661.

58. Arnheim D. Therapeutic modalities. In: Arnheim D, ed. *Modern Principles of Athletic Training.* St. Louis: Times Mirror/Mosby College Publishing; 1989:350–367.

59. Lehmann J, Warren CG, Scham S. Therapeutic heat and cold. *Clin Orthop* 1974;99:207–226.

60. Prentice W. Therapeutic ultrasound. In: Prentice W, ed. *Therapeutic Modalities in Sports Medicine.* St. Louis: Times Mirror/Mosby College Publishing; 1990:129–140.

61. Meadows JTS. Orthopedic Differential Diagnosis in Physical Therapy. New York: McGraw-Hill; 1999.

CHAPTER SEVENTEEN

THE SACROILIAC JOINT

Chapter Objectives

At the completion of this chapter, the reader will be able to:

1. Describe the anatomy of the vertebra, ligaments, muscles, and blood and nerve supply that comprise the sacroiliac region.
2. Describe the biomechanics of the sacroiliac joint, including coupled movements, normal and abnormal joint barriers, kinesiology, and reactions to various stresses.
3. Perform a detailed objective examination of the sacroiliac musculoskeletal system, including palpation of the articular and soft tissue structures, specific passive mobility tests, passive articular mobility tests, and stability tests.
4. Analyze the total examination data to establish the definitive biomechanical diagnosis.
5. Describe intervention strategies based on clinical findings and established goals.
6. Apply active and passive mobilization techniques, and combined movements to the sacroiliac joint, in any position, using the correct grade, direction, and duration, and explain the mechanical and physiologic effects.
7. Evaluate intervention effectiveness in order to progress or modify intervention.
8. Plan an effective home program including spinal care, and instruct the patient in same.
9. Develop self-reliant examination and intervention strategies.

HISTORICAL PERSPECTIVE

The pelvic mechanism is the least understood and, therefore, the most controversial area of the spine. The air of mystery surrounding this region dates back to the Middle Ages, a time when the burning of witches was commonplace. After these burnings, it was noticed that three bones were not destroyed, a large triangular bone, and two very small bones. It can only be assumed that some degree of significance was given to the large triangular bone as it was deemed a sacred bone, and was thus called the sacrum. The two smaller bones, were the sesamoid bones of the great toe, but it is unclear what significance was given to these bones.

In the 17th century, it was theorized by the medical community that the high infant mortality rate at that time was due to a narrow birth canal, and crude attempts were made to widen the canal.[1] Not surprisingly, there was no change in the mortality rate but there was a sharp increase in complaints of severe pelvic pain!

Until the mid-20th century, it was widely believed that no motion occurred at the sacroiliac joint, and very little was written about it. This paucity of sacroiliac joint literature can probably be attributed to an article by Mixter and Barr,[2] which attributed the cause of low back pain to the intervertebral disc.

Although mechanical impairments within the pelvic girdle, and their contributions to low back pain, have long been recognized,[3] it was not until about 50 years ago that significant attention was applied to the study of its anatomy and function. The pelvic mechanism began to be explored, and a series of evaluation and intervention techniques were introduced.

Grieve[4] postulated that this articulation, together with the craniovertebral region and the other spinal junctions, is of prime importance in understanding the conservative intervention of vertebral joint problems. Because of its location, the joint has a major biomechanical effect on the lower quadrant, serving as the point of intersection between spinal and peripheral joints, both of which use predominantly different planes of motion, with the former essentially using only one plane of motion, that of flexion and extension, and the latter (the hip) utilizing three, including rotation. Thus, the pelvic area must function to absorb the majority of the lower extremity motion before it reaches the lumbar spine. Although its absorbing capabilities cannot be understated, the pelvic mechanism must also allow for motion,[7] particularly during bipedal gait.[5]

Isolated pelvic impairments are rare, however, findings for them appear to be common. This may be due to the fact that in addition to producing pain on its own, the pelvic mechanism can often refer pain, particularly from its surrounding ligaments.[6] Despite its unusual shape and the fact that there are no muscles that specifically move the joint, the sacroiliac joint is capable of motion.[7]

ANATOMY

The ilium, ischium, and pubic bone fuse at the acetabulum to form each innominate. The two innominates articulate with the sacrum, forming the sacroiliac joint, and with each other at the symphysis pubis.[8] The sacrum, a strong bone located between the two hip joints, provides stability to this area, and transmits the weight of the trunk from the mobile vertebral column to the stable pelvic region. In addition to these more commonly considered bones and joints, are those of the coccygeal spine.

Phylogenically and biomechanically, the innominates are peripheral bones, whereas the sacrum, often referred to as L6, is a spinal bone, so that the joint cannot easily be classified as an axial or appendicular articulation.

Morphologically, the configuration of the sacroiliac joints is extremely variable from person to person.[9] Structurally, the sacroiliac joint is different from other joints in a number of ways, and does not appear to be designed to allow for motion to occur because of the following.

1. It consists of two very incongruent surfaces.
2. It is an area with dense ligamentous support.
3. The presence of an interosseus ligament, normally found with a syndesmosis.

The iliac joint surfaces are formed from fibrocartilage, whereas the sacral surfaces are formed from hyaline cartilage,[10] which is 3 to 5 times thicker than the fibrocartilage.[11] The response of these two surfaces to the aging process appears to differ, with early degenerative changes occurring on the iliac surface rather than on both surfaces of the joint simultaneously.[12] Other changes also occur with aging as the joint begins to develop intra-articular fibrous connections,[13] resembling a joint of the synchondrosis type. However, even with severe degenerative changes, the joint rarely fuses, except in ankylosing spondylitis.[14] Between the sacral and iliac auricular surfaces, the sacroiliac joint is deemed a synovial articulation or diarthrosis.[14]

The sacrum is a triangular bone, with its base above and anterior, and its apex below and posterior (Figure 17–1).

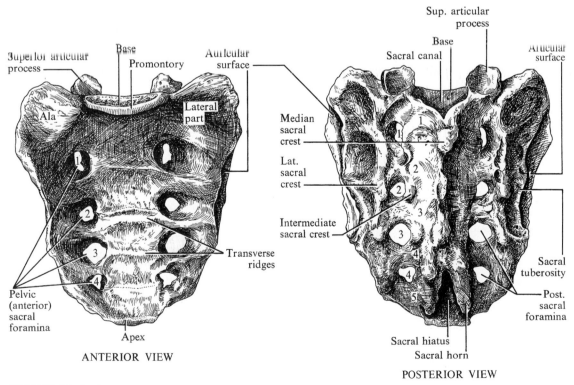

FIGURE 17–1 Sacrum.

Five centra fuse to form the central part of the sacrum, which contains remnants of the intervertebral discs enclosed by bone. The transverse processes of the first sacral vertebrae fuse with the costal elements to form the alae and lateral masses. Anatomic studies of this joint reveal differences between the gender in terms of morphology and mobility.[15,16] These differences are not pathologic, but normal adaptation related to childbearing.[17]

The inverted, L-shaped, auricular, articular surface of the sacrum is contained entirely by the costal elements of the first three sacral segments. The short (superior) arm of this L-shape, lies in a craniocaudal plane within the first sacral segment, and corresponds to the depth of the sacrum (Figure 17–2). It is widest superiorly and anteriorly. The long (inferior) arm of the L-shape lies in an anterior-posterior plane, within the second and third sacral segments, and represents the length of the sacrum from top to bottom. It is widest inferiorly and posteriorly. On the articular surfaces, there are large irregularities on each surface[18] that are roughly, though not exactly, reciprocal, with the sacral contours being generally deeper.[19,20]

In addition to the larger irregularities, there are smaller horizontal crests and hollows running anterior-posterior. These incongruencies do not form until the age of 11 to 15 years and are not fully formed until the late teens or early adult.

The joint is formed in a "V," with the apex pointing anteriorly. The degree of opening of the V is inconsistent between individuals, and even from side to side in the same subject. So common are the variants that they have been classified as type A, being less vertical than type B, and type C as an asymmetrical mixture of types A and B.[21]

Each of these variants can alter the function of the pelvis and its influence on the lumbar lordosis.[22]

The sacral promontory is formed by the ventral projection from the base of the sacrum (see Figure 17–1). The superior articular processes, which are concave and oriented posterior-medial, extend upward from the base, to articulate with the inferior articular processes of the fifth lumbar vertebra. The ala of the sacrum forms the superior-lateral portions of the base.

On the dorsal surface of the sacrum is a midline ridge of bone called the median sacral crest (see Figure 17–1), which represents the fusion of the sacral spinous processes of S1 to S4. Projecting posteriorly from this crest are four spinous tubercles. The fused laminae of S1 to S5, which are located lateral to the median sacral crest, form the intermediate sacral crest. The sacral hiatus (see Figure 17–1) exhibits bilateral downward projections that are called the sacral cornua. These projections represent the inferior articular processes of the fifth sacral vertebra, and are connected to the coccyx via the intercornual ligaments. On the inferior-lateral borders of the sacrum, about $\frac{3}{4}$ in. to either side of the sacral hiatus, are the inferior lateral angles.

The sacral canal (Fig 17–1), which houses the cauda equina, is triangular in shape. There are four intervertebral foramen on each lateral wall of the sacral canal (Fig 17–1) which communicate with the sacral foramina. The sacrum has four pairs of pelvic sacral foramina for transmission of the ventral primary rami of the sacral nerves, and four pairs of dorsal sacral foramina for transmission of the dorsal primary rami.

The joint capsule, consisting of two layers, is extensive and very strong. It attaches to both articular margins of the joint, and is thickened inferiorly.

Ligaments

Like other synovial joints, the sacroiliac joint is reinforced by ligaments, but the ligaments of the sacroiliac joint are some of the strongest and toughest ligaments of the body (Figure 17–3).

- *Anterior sacroiliac (articular).* This ligament is an anterior-inferior thickening of the fibrous capsule, which is relatively weak compared to the rest of the sacroiliac ligaments. It extends between the anterior and inferior borders of the iliac auricular surface and the anterior border of the sacral auricular surface.[14] It is a thin ligament but is better developed near the arcuate line and the posterior inferior iliac spine (PSIS), where it connects the third sacral segment to the lateral side of the preauricular sulcus. Due to its thinness, this ligament is often injured

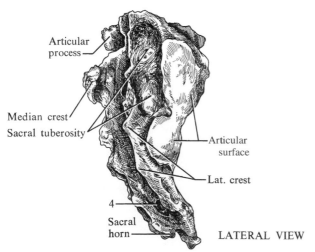

FIGURE 17–2 Lateral view of the sacrum.

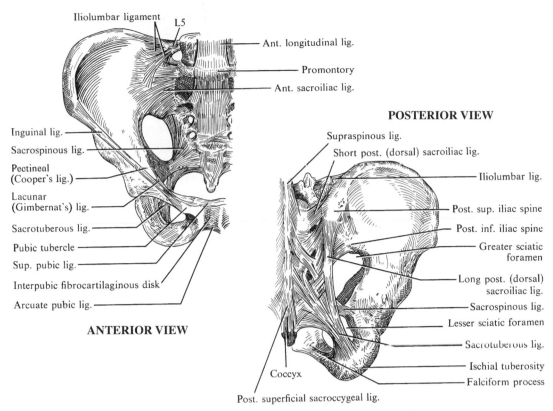

FIGURE 17–3 The ligaments of the sacroiliac joint.

and can be a source of pain. It can be palpated at Baer's SI point[1][23] and can be stressed using the transverse anterior distraction/posterior compression pain provocation test (see discussion later).

● *Interosseus sacroiliac (articular).* This is a strong, short ligament located deep to the dorsal sacroiliac ligament. It forms the major connection between the sacrum and the innominate. Although not officially recognized, it is the largest syndesmosis in the body, and functions as the major bond between the bones filling the irregular space posterior-superior to the joint between the lateral sacral crest and the iliac tuberosity. The deep portion sends fibers cranially and caudally from behind the auricular depressions. The superficial portion is a fibrous sheet connecting the cranial and dorsal margins of the sacrum to the ilium, forming a layer that limits direct palpation of the sacroiliac joint. The interosseus ligament functions to resist anterior and inferior movement of the sacrum.

● *Long dorsal sacroiliac (articular).* The long dorsal sacroiliac ligament (long ligament) (see Figure 17–3), which

is easily palpable in the area directly caudal to the posterior superior iliac spine (PSIS), connects the PSIS (and a small part of the iliac crest) with the lateral crest of the third and fourth segment of the sacrum.[24] This is a very tough and strong ligament. The fibers from this ligament are multidirectional and blend laterally with the sacrotuberous ligament. It also has attachments medially to the erector spinae,[25] multifidus muscle,[26] and the thoracodorsal fascia. Contractions of the various muscles that attach to it can result in a tightening of the ligament. The skin overlying the ligament is a frequent source of pain.[27]

Directly caudal to the PSIS, the ligament is so solid and stout that one can easily think a bony structure is being palpated. The question is raised whether the tension of the long ligament can be increased by displacement in the SI joint and/or by muscle activity. Nutation of the SI joint appears to induce relaxation of the long ligament, whereas counternutation increases tension. This is in contrast to the effect on the sacrotuberous ligament, where nutation leads to an increase of tension, counternutation to relaxation.[28,29]

At the cranial side, the long ligament is attached to the PSIS and the adjacent part of the ilium, at the caudal side to the lateral crest of the third and fourth

---

[1]Baer's SI point has been described as being on a line from the umbilicus to the anterior superior iliac spine 5 cm from the umbilicus.

sacral segments. In some specimens, fibers pass also to the fifth sacral segment.[25] The lateral expansion of the long ligament in the region directly caudal to the PSIS varies between 15 to 30 mm. The length, measured between the PSIS and the third and fourth sacral segments, varies between 42 to 75 mm. The lateral part of the long ligament is continuous with fibers passing between ischial tuberosity and iliac bone.

Since counternutation increases tension in the long ligament, this ligament can assist in controlling counternutation.

- *Sacrotuberous (extra-articular).* This ligament (Fig 17–3) is comprised of three large fibrous bands, broadly attached by its base to the posterior inferior iliac spine and the lateral sacrum, and partly blended with the dorsal sacroiliac ligament. Its oblique, lateral fibers descend and attach to the medial margin of the ischial tuberosity, spanning the piriformis muscle, from which it receives some fibers. The medial fibers, running anterior-inferior-lateral, have an attachment to the transverse tubercles of S3, S4, and S5, and the lateral margin of the coccyx. To the sacrotuberous ligament's posterior surface are attached the lowest fibers of the gluteus maximus, the contraction of which produces increased tension in the ligament.[30] Superficial fibers of its inferior aspect can continue into the tendon of the biceps femoris.[31] This ligament appears to play a significant role in stabilizing against nutation (forward rotation) of the sacrum, and counteracting against the dorsal and cranial migration of the sacral apex during weight bearing.
- *Sacrospinous (extra-articular).* Thinner than the sacrotuberous ligament, this triangular ligament extends from the ischial spine to the lateral margins of the sacrum and coccyx, and laterally to the spine of the ischium (Fig 17–3). The ligament runs anterior (deep) to the sacrotuberous ligament to which it blends, and attaches to the capsule of the sacroiliac joint.[26] Its anterior surface is muscular (coccygeus). Both the sacrotuberous and sacrospinous ligaments oppose forward tilting of the sacrum on the hip bone during weight bearing of the trunk and vertebral column. They convert the greater and lesser sciatic notches into the greater and lesser foramen respectively.

- *Iliolumbar (indirect).* For a detailed description of the anatomy of the iliolumbar ligament, please refer to Chapter 13.

The sacroiliac ligaments work collectively as a force transfer for the hip and trunk muscles, producing innominate and/or sacral movements, in response to induced forces from the femur and/or vertebrae. They also help to prevent the following.

- Craniocaudal dislocation
- Anterior gapping (lateral innominate rotation)
- Posterior gapping (medial innominate rotation)
- Hyperflexion (posterior innominate rotation, or nutation)
- Hyperextension (anterior innominate rotation, or counternutation)

Pubic Symphysis

The pubic symphysis is classified as a symphysis as it has no synovial tissue or fluid and contains a fibrocartilaginous disc (Figure 17–4). The bone surfaces of the joint are covered with hyaline cartilage, but are kept apart by the presence of the disc.

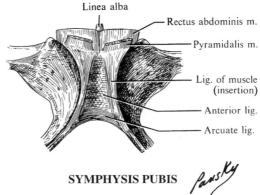

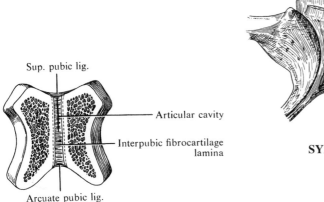

SYMPHYSIS PUBIS

Labels (Figure right): Linea alba, Rectus abdominis m., Pyramidalis m., Lig. of muscle (insertion), Anterior lig., Arcuate lig.

Labels (Figure left): Sup. pubic lig., Articular cavity, Interpubic fibrocartilage lamina, Arcuate pubic lig.

FIGURE 17–4 Pubic symphysis.

The supporting ligaments of this joint are[32]:

- The superior pubic ligament, a thick fibrous band.
- The inferior arcuate ligament, which attaches to the inferior pubic rami bilaterally, and blends with the disc.
- The posterior pubic ligament, a membranous structure that blends with the adjacent periosteum.
- The anterior pubic ligament, a very thick band that contains both transverse and oblique fibers.

Muscles

The impression often given is that muscular control of this joint is either nonexistent, or of no significance. However, Lee[33] lists 35 muscles that attach directly to the sacrum and/or innominate (Table 17–1).

A muscle attaching to a bone has the potential for moving that bone, although the degree of potential varies. The muscles around the pelvis can probably be involved directly or indirectly in providing stability to the sacroiliac joint. Six of the previously listed muscles attach to both the sacrum and the innominate and, therefore, have potential to produce movement at the sacroiliac joint.

Piriformis

The piriformis arises from the anterior aspect of the S2, S3, and S4 segments of the sacrum, as well as the capsule of the sacroiliac joint, and the anterior aspect of the posterior inferior iliac spine of the ilium. It exits from the pelvis via the greater sciatic foramen, before attaching to the greater trochanter of the femur. The muscle is as close to a prime mover of the sacrum as any. It mainly functions to produces external rotation and abduction of the femur, but is also thought to function as an internal rotator of the hip if the hip joint is flexed beyond 90 degrees. It also helps to stabilize the sacroiliac joint, although too much tension from it can restrict motion. The increased tension usually results from SI joint dysfunction.[34,35] The piriformis has been implicated as the source for a number of conditions in this area.

- Entrapment neuropathies of the sciatic nerve
- Trigger points[36]
- Piriformis syndrome[37]

Multifidus

The anatomy of the multifidus muscle is discussed in Chapter 13. Some of the deepest fibers of the multifidus attach to the capsules of the zygapophyseal joints,[38] and are located close to the centers of rotation for spinal motion. They connect the adjacent vertebra at appropriate angles and their geometry remains fairly constant through a range of postures, thereby enhancing spinal stability.[39]

Erector Spinae

For a detailed description of the anatomy of the erector spinae, please refer to Chapter 13. Through its extending effect on the spine and its substantial sacral attachments, it might be thought to promote sacral nutation, although this has not been proven.

Gluteus Maximus

This is one of the strongest muscles in the body. It arises from the posterior gluteal line of the innominate; the dorsum of the lower lateral sacrum and coccyx; the aponeurosis of erector spinae muscle, the sacrotuberous ligament, the superficial laminae of the posterior thoracodorsal fascia, and the fascia covering the gluteus medius muscle; before attaching to the gluteal tuberosity. In the pelvis, it blends with the ipsilateral multifidus, through the raphe of the thoracodorsal fascia,[26] and the contralateral latissimus dorsi, through the superficial laminae of the thoracodorsal fascia.[40] Some of its fibers attach to the sacrotuberous ligament. When these fibers contract, tension in the sacrotuberous ligament is increased.[41]

Iliacus

Arises from the iliac fossa, the ventral sacroiliac ligament, and the inferior fibers of the iliolumbar ligament,[42] in addition to the lateral aspect of the sacrum. As it travels distally, its fibers merge with the lateral aspect of the psoas tendon, and onto the lesser trochanter of the femur, sending some fibers to the hip joint capsule as it passes.

Coccygeus

The coccygeus arises from the pelvic surface of the ischial spine and sacrospinous ligament and inserts on the coccyx margin and side of the lowest segment of the sacrum. Supplied by the muscular branches of the pudendal plexus, it functions to pull forward and support the coccyx.

TABLE 17–1 MUSCLES THAT ATTACH TO THE SACRUM, ILIUM, OR BOTH

Latissimus dorsi	External oblique	Adductor magnus
Erector spinae	Internal oblique	Rectus femoris
Semimembranosus	Transversus abdominis	Quadratus lumborum
Semitendinosus		Pectineus
Biceps femoris	Rectus abdominis	Psoas minor
Sartorius	Pyramidalis	Adductor brevis
Inferior gamellus	Gluteus minimus	Adductor longus
Multifidus	Gluteus medius	Levator ani
Obturator internus	Gluteus maximus	Sphincter urethrae
Obturator externus	Quadratus femoris	Superficial transverse perineal
Piriformis	Superior gemellus	Ischiocavernous
Tensor fascia lata	Gracilis	Coccygeus
	Iliacus	

The latissimus dorsi muscle is linked to this area through its attachment to the thoracolumbar fascia, where it attaches to the contralateral gluteus maximus. The latissimus dorsi and the gluteus maximus appear to function in concert during trunk rotation.[41]

The biceps femoris muscle, as has been mentioned, functions as a tensor of the sacrotuberous ligament. Its importance in relation to gait is discussed later.

Neurology

It remains unclear precisely how the anterior and posterior aspects of the sacroiliac joint are innervated,[43] although the anterior portion of the joint likely receives innervation from the posterior rami of the L2–S2 roots. Contribution from these root levels is highly variable and may differ among the joints of given individuals.[44] Additional innervation to the anterior joint may arise directly from the obturator nerve, superior gluteal nerve, and/or lumbosacral trunk.[45,46] The posterior portion of the joint is innervated by the posterior rami of L4–S3,[47,48] with a particular contribution from S1 and S2.[48] An additional autonomic component of the joint's innervation further increases the complexity of its neural supply, and likely adds to the variability of pain referral patterns.[45] It is the joint's highly variable and complex innervation that produces a very diffuse pattern of pain referral from this area.[49]

BIOMECHANICS

There is very little agreement, either among disciplines, or even within disciplines, about the biomechanics of the pelvic complex. There have been periods where the joint is considered the cause of almost all low back and leg pain, and other times where it is only a problem in pregnancy.

The results from the numerous studies on mobility of the sacroiliac joint have led to a variety of different hypotheses and models of pelvic mechanics over the years.[50] Although sacroiliac joint mobility is, under normal circumstances, very limited, movement has been demonstrated.[51,52] In a more recent study of cadavers, Smidt and colleagues reported that extreme hip positions are necessary to appreciate full sacroiliac joint motion, which can be as high as 15 degrees in the sagittal plane.[53]

Other studies have demonstrated that small movements, especially nutation and counternutation, do occur at the sacroiliac joint (Figure 17–5 and 17–6).[54,55]

It is likely that the movement of the pelvis is in the nature of "squishing," with the pelvic ring deforming in response to body weight and ground-reaction forces, with the motion occurring being similar to that which occurs at a syndesmosis. This motion is facilitated by a number of features.

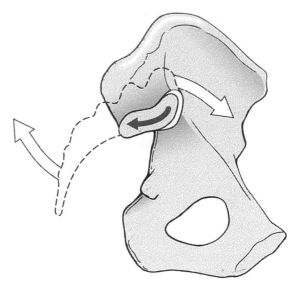

FIGURE 17–5 Sacral nutation.

- The fibrocartilaginous surface of the innominate facets, which are deformable, especially during weight bearing, when the surfaces are forced together.
- The pubic symphysis. If the innominates are moving at the sacroiliac joint, then they must also be moving at their anterior junction, which would allow for an immediate, and almost perfect, reciprocal motion.

A model of pelvic mechanics developed by Illi[56] is still regarded by many as the most complete. He proposed that the sacroiliac joint is most active during locomotion, with movement occurring mainly in the oblique sagittal plane. In this proposal, each sacroiliac joint goes through two full

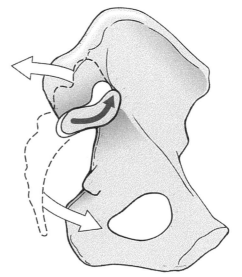

FIGURE 17–6 Sacral counternutation.

cycles of alternating flexion and extension during gait, with the motion at one joint mirrored by the motion at the opposing joint. He suggests that as one innominate flexes, the ipsilateral sacral base moves anterior and inferior, and as the other innominate extends, the sacral base on that side moves posterior and superior. If the described actions of the sacrum are visualized as one continuous motion, it can be viewed as an oblique and horizontal figure of eight. He further postulates that alternating movements of flexion act through the iliolumbar ligament to dampen motion at L5, and hence the whole spine.[57] As the ilium moves posteriorly, L5 is pulled posteriorly and inferiorly through tension in the iliolumbar ligament, and the rest of the lumbar spine undergoes coupled motion in slight rotation and lateral flexion (type I motion).

The following section, mainly from the work of Vleeming[25] and Lee,[33] describes the current status concerning both the known and the proposed biomechanics of the pelvic girdle and incorporates the findings of research and clinical impressions.

It appears that when the sacrum nutates, or flexes, relative to the innominate, a linear glide occurs between the two surfaces. The articular surface of the sacroiliac joint is L-shaped with the two lengths perpendicular to each other (see Figure 17–2). The shorter of the two lengths, level with S1, lies in a vertical plane, whereas the longer length, spanning S2–4, lies in an anterior-posterior plane.

During sacral nutation (see Figure 17–5), the sacrum glides inferiorly down the short length and posteriorly along the long length. This motion is resisted by a number of factors that include:

- The wedge shape of the sacrum
- The ridges and depressions of the articular surfaces
- The friction coefficient of the joint surface
- The integrity of the interosseous and sacrotuberous ligaments, supported by the muscles that insert into the ligaments

When the sacrum counternutates, or extends (see Figure 17–6), the sacrum glides anteriorly along the longer length and superiorly up the shorter length. This motion is resisted by the long dorsal sacroiliac ligament,[25] which is supported by the contraction of the multifidus.

Innominate motion is induced by hip motion, as in extension of the lower extremity, or during trunk motion when bending forward at the waist. When the innominate rotates anteriorly (Figure 17–7), it glides inferiorly down the short length of the "L," and posteriorly along the longer length of the "L" of the sacroiliac joint, in exactly the same way as it occurs during counternutation of the sacrum (see Figure 17–2). When the innominate rotates posteriorly (Figure 17–8), it glides anteriorly along the

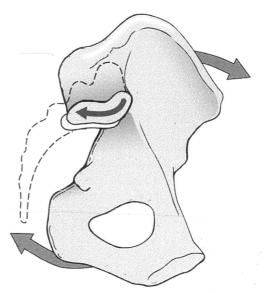

FIGURE 17–7 Anterior rotation of the innominate.

longer length of the "L," and superiorly up the short length of the "L" of the sacroiliac joint, in exactly the same way as it occurs during nutation of the sacrum.

Form Closure and Force Closure

Snijders[60] and Vleeming[15,17] coined the terms form closure and force closure to describe the passive and active forces that help to stabilize the pelvis and the sacroiliac joint. Form closure refers to a state of stability within the pelvic mechanism, with the degree of stability dependent upon its anatomy, with no need for extra forces to maintain the stable state of the system.[59] The following anatomic structures assist with the form closure.

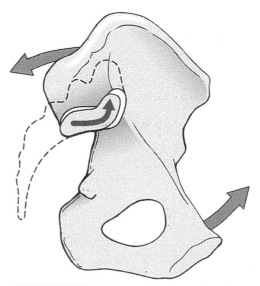

FIGURE 17–8 Posterior rotation of the innominate.

age-shaped sacrum and the friction coefficient e articular cartilage. The incongruent surfaces ovide resistance against horizontal and vertical translation. In infants, the joint surfaces are very planar. Between the ages of 11 and 15 years, the characteristic ridges and humps that make up the mature sacrum are beginning to form on the joint surfaces. By the third decade, the superficial layers of the fibrocartilage are fibrillated, and crevice formation and erosion has begun. By the fourth and fifth decade, the articular surfaces increase irregularity and coarseness, and the wedging is incomplete.[14] Both the coarseness of the cartilage and the complementary grooves and ridges increase the friction coefficient and, thus, contribute to form closure.[20]

- The integrity of the ligaments
- The shape of the closely fitting joint surfaces

The integrity of form closure is clinically evaluated with the long-arm and short-arm shear tests (see later discussion).

Force closure, the need for extra forces to keep an object in place, requires friction to be present.[59] The degree of friction depends on the compressive forces acting through the joint. This dynamic force relies on intrinsic and extrinsic supports involving the osseous, articular, neurologic, and myofascial systems, and gravity. As mentioned, the long dorsal sacroiliac ligament[25] tightens with sacral counternutation, or anterior rotation of the innominate, whereas the sacrotuberous and interosseous ligaments tighten during sacral nutation, or posterior rotation of the innominate. Vleeming and co-workers found that when the sacrum moves towards nutation, the increase in ligament tension facilitates the force closure mechanism.[59]

Kinetic analysis of the pelvic girdle highlights two muscle groups that resist translational forces and help to provide stability, the inner unit and the outer unit.

The inner unit consists of the following.

- The muscles of the pelvic floor
- Transverse abdominis
- Multifidus
- The diaphragm

The outer unit consists of four systems.

- *Posterior oblique.* The gluteus maximus, which blends with the thoracodorsal fascia, and the contralateral latissimus dorsi contribute to force closure of the sacroiliac joint posteriorly by approximating the posterior aspects of the innominates. This oblique system crosses the midline and is a significant contributor to load transference through the pelvic girdle during the rotational activities of gait.

- *Deep longitudinal.* Includes the thoracodorsal fascia the erector spinae muscles, the biceps femoris, and the sacrotuberous ligament. This system counteracts any anterior shear (sacral nutation), as well as facilitating the compression through the sacroiliac joints. As previously mentioned, the biceps femoris muscle controls the degree of nutation via its connections to the sacrotuberous ligaments.[28]

- *Anterior oblique.* Includes the oblique abdominal muscles, the contralateral adductor muscles of the thigh, and the intervening abdominal fascia. The oblique abdominals, acting as phasic muscles, initiate movement[61] and are involved in all movements of the trunk and upper and lower extremities, except when the legs are crossed.[62]

- *Lateral.* Includes the gluteus medius and minimus and the contralateral adductors of the thigh, which function to stabilize the pelvic girdle on the femoral head during gait through a coordinated action. These muscles are reflexively inhibited with an instability of the sacroiliac joint.

It is, therefore, important that the length and strength of each of these structures are assessed, as weakness or insufficient recruitment of these systems can reduce the force closure mechanism and can lead to compensatory movement strategies,[63] resulting in a decompensation in the lumbar spine, hip, and/or knee.

Biomechanics of Functional Movements

The biomechanics of this region, involve an integration of lumbar-pelvic-hip motions.

Forward Bending A combination of anterior and outward rotation of both innominates results in both posterior superior iliac spines (PSIS) approximating, and moving in a superior direction, while the sacrum nutates. Sacral flexion, or nutation, involves an anterior rotation in the sagittal plane, so that the anterior aspect of the sacrum inclines downwards. If this flexion occurs as part of lumbar flexion, and occurs sequentially after L5 is flexed, it results in flexion of the lumbosacral junction. However, if the sacrum flexes under L5, as part of an anterior pelvic tilt, then this nonsequential flexion produces extension of the lumbosacral junction.

After about 60 degrees of forward bending, the innominates continue to anteriorly rotate, but the sacrum no longer nutates, producing a relative counternutation of the sacrum. If the sacrum remains nutated throughout forward bending, the sacroiliac joint remains compressed and stable. If the sacrum counternutates early, as in individuals with tight hamstrings, less compression occurs and the sacroiliac joint has to rely on an increase in motor control, making it more vulnerable for injury.

If the innominate rotates anteriorly, the anterior superior iliac spine (ASIS) faces in a downward position and, if rotated posteriorly, a more upward position. Iliosacral flexion is movement of the innominate on a relatively fixed sacrum, initiated from the lower limbs, as occurs in climbing or walking. If the femur is flexed, the ipsilateral innominate posteriorly rotates while the sacrum rotates to the same side as the flexed femur. If the femur is extended, the ipsilateral innominate anteriorly rotates, and the sacrum rotates to the contralateral side to the extended femur. However, if the anterior rotation of the innominates is generated by an anterior pelvic tilt on a relatively fixed femur, the femur is flexed. The converse holds true for posterior rotation. That is, if the innominate is posteriorly rotated or flexed by the femur, the hip is flexed, but if a posterior pelvic tilt produced the motion, the hip is extended. Thus, the direction of the innominate rotation depends on the initiating movement.

Backward Bending A combination of an anterior displacement of the pelvic girdle and both posterior superior iliac spines moving inferiorly. No innominate rotation occurs and the sacrum remains nutated.

Side-Flexion During right side-flexion, the right innominate rotates anteriorly, while the sacrum right side-flexes and left rotates. A ground-reaction force is probably producing the motion of the innominate. As side-flexion to the right occurs, the right leg takes more weight and is compressed. This downward body-weight force, together with the upward ground-reaction force results in anterior rotation (extension) of the innominate, causing flexion of the hip. This hip flexion, together with the flattening of the foot and hyperextension of the knee, effectively allows the leg to shorten in response to these compressive forces. It is interesting that in nonweight bearing, anterior innominate rotation results in a leg length increase, whereas in weight bearing, an anterior rotation produces a leg length decrease. In fact, it is the same mechanism in both cases.[64] In nonweight bearing, such as in the long sit test, the anterior rotation of the innominate pushes the femur downward. As there is no resistance under the foot, and no force to flex the hip, the leg can lengthen, In weight bearing, ground-reaction forces push the innominate superiorly due to the inability of the leg to lengthen during the side-flexion.

Trunk Rotation During left axial rotation of the trunk, the right innominate anteriorly rotates, whereas the left posteriorly rotates. The sacrum counternutates at the right sacroiliac joint, and nutates at the left. The motion of the innominates during trunk rotation allows the sacrum to osteokinematically rotate while maintaining a more or less vertical orientation. Both hips and the entire pelvis move during these twisting motions. As this motion must also be occurring at the pubis, the axis cannot run through one or both sacroiliac joints but through an area within the pelvic cavity.

Sacral Torsions and Innominate Rotations

Most of the earlier osteopathic models of sacroiliac joint motion considered only sacral flexing (nutation) and extension (counternutation), which occurred around four axes:

- A posterior extra-articular axis
- An anterior extra-articular axis
- An intra-articular axis at the convergence of the limbs
- An axis with a slide along the inferior limb

In addition, three other axes at S1, S2, and S3 were proposed to explain respiratory, sacroiliac, and iliosacral, motions respectively.

Later theories also included two oblique axes about which the sacrum rotated in an oblique fashion. These axes were named after the upper corner of the sacrum from which they emerge. So that the axis running from the superior right corner to the inferior left was termed the right oblique axis and that running from the superior and left corner, to the inferior right, the left oblique axis.

It was proposed that the innominates rotated anteriorly and posteriorly, depending on the motion occurring. A clear distinction was made between a sacroiliac impairment and an iliosacral impairment. Despite the obvious fact that the two lesions were describing an impairment at the same joint, the distinction has survived. Part of this confusion was due to the assumption that the ilium and the sacrum operated around different axes. What has become clearer over time is that these two structures share the same axis and that their impairments do not occur in an isolated fashion but occur together.

By using a simple palpation experiment, it is clear that a problem exists with the originally proposed axes for sacral motion, because if the sacrum is palpated during movement, the axes do not seem to exist.[64] For example, the sacrum is palpated with the patient seated, so that the movement of the upper left corner and the lower right corner can be monitored during trunk rotation. The patient is asked to twist to the left. Under normal circumstances, the upper left corner can be felt to move backward while the lower right corner moves forward. This would appear to be backward rotation to the left, or a Left on Right, using osteopathic terminology. However, if left rotation is carried out again, but this time while palpating the upper left and lower right corners, it will be felt that the right upper corner moves forward, while the lower left moves backward. This would appear to be forward rotation to the left, or a Left on

Left. The sacrum, or any other joint, cannot move using two distinct axes simultaneously. The basis for this misunderstanding relates to the fact that the sacrum articulates with both the sacroiliac and lumbosacral joint simultaneously. Although lumbosacral extension does involve anterior inferior motion of the sacral base, the same movement of the sacrum occurs during sacroiliac flexion, not extension. While it is true that minute motion can occur in either a forward or backward direction due to the shape of the articular surface, this motion does not occur around a pure axis, oblique or otherwise. As mentioned previously, forward motion of the sacrum involves an inferior movement of the sacrum along the short length of each L-shaped articular surface, together with a posterior movement along the longer length of each articular surface. The backward motion of the sacrum is the reverse; an anterior movement of the sacrum along the longer length of each L-shaped articular surface, together with a superior movement along the shorter length of each articular surface. For both sides of the sacrum to move anteriorly and inferiorly simultaneously, the trunk has to be involved with flexion and extension. Trunk motions that involve rotation or side-flexion will produce a torsional motion at the sacroiliac and lumbosacral joints. These latter trunk motions are involved during the normal gait cycle.

Gait Biomechanics An efficient gait requires, among other things, a fully functioning lumbar-pelvic-hip complex.[35,63] The following describes the gait sequence. With the right leg in the swing phase from its position of toe-off:

- The pelvic girdle rotates counterclockwise in the transverse plane, translates anteriorly, and adducts on the femoral head.
- Posterior rotation occurs at the right innominate with anterior rotation occurring at the left innominate. Posterior rotation of the right innominate increases the tension of the sacrotuberous and interosseous ligament. The posterior rotation of the right innominate, produced by tension in the hamstrings, helps to augment the capacity for hip flexion and shock absorption at heel strike. The anterior rotation of the innominate, on the side opposite the leading leg, is produced by tension in the hip flexors of that side.
- The sacrum nutates at the right sacroiliac joint and counternutates at the left sacroiliac joint.[35] Using osteopathic terminology, this would be termed a Right on Left rotation occurring at the sacrum.
- During this phase of the gait cycle, the lower lumbar vertebrae flex and side-flex contralaterally, adopting the same rotation as the sacrum,[65] with the iliolumbar

ligament modifying the motion at the L5–S1 segment.[66] The lumbar rotation and side-flexion appear to occur in an isolated manner, and are out of phase with each other—when the spine is side-flexed maximally, it is rotated the least, and vice versa. This unusual coupling is thought to allow:

1. The facet column on the nonweight-bearing leg to function as a mobile adaptor, so that the spine is in a loose-pack position at heel strike.
2. The opposite facet column to function as a rigid lever, so that the spine is in a close pack position during weight-bearing.
- The rotation of the pelvis during mid-stance reverses the function of the facet columns in preparation for propulsion on the weight-bearing limb and the impact of heel strike on the opposite limb.

Just before the right heel strike and left toe off, the interosseous ligament and the right sacrotuberous ligament tighten. In addition, the biceps femoris[67] is also tightened, and this pulls on the sacrotuberous ligament. This increase in tension contributes to the force closure mechanism while augmenting the form closure mechanism. The tension in the biceps femoris also increases the tension in the peroneus longus, causing it to fire, and the fibula head is pulled inferiorly and internally rotated, while the foot is pulled into, and maintained in, dorsiflexion. A combination of activity, from the biceps femoris, peroneus longus, and anterior tibialis, produces an elastic longitudinal force. At heel strike, this elastic force is transferred downward and helps to propel the leg and foot forward. Just after heel strike, and toward mid-stance, the fibula moves superiorly and externally rotates.

At right heel strike, the right sacral base has rotated anteriorly on the left diagonal axis from a relative position of Right on Left at toe off, into a Left on Left. The lower pole of the left diagonal axis is held by the contraction of the right piriformis, which pulls the right inferior arm of the sacrum into contact with the corresponding articular surface of the innominate. This Left on Left sacral torsion is a compensation for the left rotation and right side-flexion that occurs in the lumbar spine.

From heel strike to mid-stance, the ipsilateral gluteus medius and contralateral adductors are active to stabilize the pelvic girdle on the femoral head. During this period of double support, the lumbar spine is initially in a position of neutral with reference to side-flexion. However, as the left foot comes off the ground, the pelvis lists to the left. This list is controlled by the right hip abductors and left lumbar side-flexors. To compensate for the list, the lumbar spine side-flexes to the right. The pelvis remains in a position of counterclockwise rotation.

During the right single leg stance phase:

- The pelvic girdle rotates clockwise in the transverse plane, translates anteriorly, and adducts on the right femoral head.
- The right innominate begins to anteriorly rotate relative to the sacrum, and the left innominate posteriorly rotates.
- The right sacroiliac joint counternutates, while the left sacroiliac joint nutates. The counternutation occurring at the right joint is resisted by the right dorsal sacroiliac ligament.
- The biceps femoris relaxes and the gluteus maximus becomes more active.[67] Simultaneously, the trunk counter rotates and the contralateral latissimus dorsi fires.[68] The hamstring muscles relax and the gluteus maximus becomes more active. This occurs in conjunction with a counter rotation of the trunk and firing of the contralateral latissimus dorsi. Together, these two muscles tense the thoracodorsal fascia, facilitating the force closure mechanism.

In the early stance phase on the right, with the shoulders in opposite position to the pelvis, the lumbar spine is positioned in right side-flexion and left rotation, rotating in the same direction as the sacrum. The pelvis now begins to rotate in a clockwise direction. At mid-stance on the right, the pelvis has reached a position of neutral rotation in the transverse plane. This motion is controlled by the hip external rotators on the right.

During the late stance on the right leg, the pelvis continues to rotate in a clockwise direction and the lumbar spine is now in a position of full left rotation and slight side-flexion to the right.

The displacement of the center of gravity is exaggerated when the sacroiliac joint is unstable, and compensation results through a transfer of weight laterally over the involved limb (compensated Trendelenburg), thus reducing the vertical shear forces through the joint.[63] In a noncompensated gait pattern, the patient often demonstrates a true Trendelenburg to reduce the vertical shear force.

COMMON PATHOLOGIES AND LESIONS

Sacroiliac joint impairments fall into the same groups as any other joint, that is, the joint can demonstrate reduced motion due to a hypomobility or excessive motion due to a hypermobility and/or instability. The findings for these movement impairments, as with any other joint, will depend on the stage of healing.

These impairments can be further subdivided into two groups: those demonstrable from the primary stress test (major lesions), and those that can only be diagnosed from the biomechanical examination (biomechanical lesions).

Major Lesions

There is an abundance of structures that can produce low back, pelvic, and/or groin pain of a serious nature. Listed as follows are some of the more common ones that should be ruled out before launching into a thorough lumbar-pelvic-hip examination. As with the other joints, the clinician must attempt to link the subjective reports to a biomechanical cause, and a scanning examination should be performed on any patient who presents with an insidious onset of pelvic pain.

Psoriatic Arthritis
Psoriatic arthritis[69] is an inflammatory arthritis associated with psoriasis.[70] It affects men and women with equal frequency. Its peak onset is in the fourth decade of life, although it may occur in children and in older adults. It can present in one of a number of patterns, including distal joint disease (affecting the distal interphalangeal joints of the hands and feet), asymmetric oligoarthritis, polyarthritis (which tends to be asymmetric in half the cases), and arthritis mutilans, which is a severe destructive form of arthritis, and the spondyloarthropathy, which occurs in 40% of the patients, but most commonly in the presence of one of the peripheral patterns.[69] Patients with psoriatic arthritis are less tender over both affected joints and tender points than patients with rheumatoid arthritis.[71]

The spondyloarthropathy of psoriatic arthritis can be distinguished from ankylosing spondylitis (AS) by the pattern of the sacroiliitis. Whereas sacroiliitis in AS tends to be symmetrical, affecting both sacroiliac joints to the same degree, it tends to be asymmetric in psoriatic arthritis,[69] and patients with psoriatic arthritis do not have as severe a spondyloarthropathy as patients with AS.[72]

Another articular feature of psoriatic arthritis is the presence of dactylitis in 35% of the patients. Patients also develop tenosynovitis, often digital, in flexor and extensor tendons, and in the Achilles tendon. Enthesitis is also a feature of psoriatic arthritis.[70] The presence of erosive disease in the distal interphalangeal joints is typical for psoriatic arthritis.[70]

The most common extra-articular feature in psoriatic arthritis is the skin lesion. The majority of patients have psoriasis vulgaris. Nail lesions occur in more than 80% of the patients with psoriatic arthritis, and have been found to be the only clinical feature distinguishing patients with psoriatic arthritis from patients with uncomplicated psoriasis.[73] Iritis occurs in psoriatic arthritis much less frequently than in AS. Urethritis and gastrointestinal complaints can occur. Other extra-articular features include iritis, urethritis, and cardiac impairments similar to those seen in AS, although less frequently.[70]

Psoriatic arthritis may result in significant joint damage and disability.[74]

Reiter's Syndrome and Reactive Arthritis

This form of arthritis usually follows an infection of the genitourinary or gastrointestinal tract, and manifests at least one other extra-articular feature.[69] The association of Reiter's syndrome and reactive arthritis (RS/ReA) with HLA-B27, occurring in 70 to 90% of patients, has been recognized for nearly as long as the association of HLA-B27 with AS.[75]

"Reiter's syndrome" refers to the clinical triad of nongonococcal urethritis, conjunctivitis, and arthritis first described by Reiter in 1916.[76] The onset is most common between the ages of 20 and 40 years, with males predominantly affected.[69]

The arthritis of Reiter's syndrome and reactive arthritis, as in psoriatic arthritis, tends to be asymmetric and there is involvement of the large weight-bearing joints. The joints of the mid-foot, and the metatarsophalangeal and interphalangeal joints of the toes, are the most commonly affected. Dactylitis is also a feature of Reiter's syndrome. Reiter's disease is more commonly associated with conjunctivitis, urethritis, and iritis than is psoriatic arthritis.[69] A high percentage of patients with Reiter's syndrome show radiographic evidence of sacroiliitis,[77] but only a small percentage develop a spondylitis. The clinical evidence of sacroiliac joint involvement may occur as early as 3 months from the onset of the illness.[78]

Reactive arthritis usually runs a self-limited course of 3 to 12 months, although some patients can continue to have a chronic indolent arthritis.[69,79]

Clinical Presentation of Sacroiliac Arthritis

1. Pain: in the posterior aspect of the sacrum, or groin pain alone (uncommon); radiating to the posterior thigh; with walking, either at heel strike or at mid- stance; which frequently wakes the patient when turning in bed.
2. Motion: extension is the most painful; Ipsilateral sideflexion and rotation less so; flexion least of all
3. One leg weight bearing and hopping: the patient stands on one leg and transfers the weight from one foot to another. If no pain is produced, the patient is asked to hop on each leg. If hopping on one leg reproduces the pain on the affected side, but is reduced if an SI belt is worn, the test is positive.
4. Positive primary stress test (see discussion later and Chapter 10)

Groin Pain

Chronic pain in the groin region is a difficult clinical problem to evaluate, and in many cases the cause of the pain is poorly understood. The differential diagnosis of groin pain includes adductor muscle strain, prostatitis, orchitis, inguinal hernia, urolithiasis, ankylosing spondylitis, Reiter's syndrome, hyperparathyroidism, metastasis, osteitis pubis (see later discussion), stress fracture, rheumatoid arthritis tendinitis, degenerative joint disease of the hip bursitis, osteitis, hernias, conjoint tendon strains, inguinal ligament enthesopathy, and entrapment of the lateral cutaneous nerve of the thigh.[80–82]

In addition, compression of the anterior division of the obturator nerve in the thigh has been described recently as one possible cause for adductor region pain.[86]

Other nerve entrapment syndromes have been described previously. The groin area is innervated by the genitofemoral or ilioinguinal nerves, which are terminal branches of the L1 or L2 spinal nerves. Kopell and colleagues[84] described an entrapment neuropathy of the ilioinguinal nerve that causes groin pain; entrapment of this nerve together with the genitofemoral nerve, which also causes groin pain, has been treated successfully by nerve section.[85]

Groin pain is a complaint often present in patients with lumbar disc herniation. On questioning, these patients often describe this pain as a dull ache lying deep beneath the skin, which they usually find difficult to localize with any degree of accuracy. Although the patient often reports pain and numbness on physical examination, the clinician is often unable to discern any objective findings, such as tenderness, muscle weakness, or hypesthesia, except perhaps occasionally a slight hyperalgesia. One study[86] showed that taking subjective complaints and MRI findings into account, elderly patients with protruded herniation of the anulus fibrosus were considered to be more likely to experience groin pain, with the rate of L4–5 disc involvement being higher than that of L5–S1 involvement. These results support conclusions drawn from a study by Murphey,[87] which found that groin and testicular pain are rare with L5–S1 disc disease, but are fairly common with L4–5 disc disease.

The posterior anulus fibrosus, the posterior longitudinal ligament, and the dura are innervated by the sinuvertebral nerve, which is considered to arise from the ventral ramus and the sympathetic trunk.[88] Groen and associates[89] reported that the sinuvertebral nerve originates exclusively from the sympathetic trunk and its ramifications. If the sinuvertebral nerve does indeed originate exclusively from sympathetic nerves, the lumbar disc would be innervated from above the L2 segment.

Osteoarthritis of the hip is one of many causes of groin pain in older patients, and it is important to identify patients with symptomatic OA correctly and to exclude conditions that may be mistaken for or coexist with OA.[90,91] Periarticular pain that is not reproduced by passive motion and direct joint palpation suggests an alternate etiology such as bursitis, tendonitis, or periostitis. The distribution of painful joints is also helpful to distinguish OA from other types of arthritis because MCP, wrist, elbow, ankle, and shoulder arthritis are unlikely locations for OA, except after trauma. Symptoms including prolonged morning stiffness (greater than 1 hour) should raise suspicion for an inflammatory arthritis, such as rheumatoid arthritis. Intense inflammation on examination suggests an infectious or microcrystalline processes such as gout or pseudogout. Weight loss, fatigue, fever, and loss of appetite should be sought out because these are clues to a systemic illness, such as polymyalgia rheumatica, rheumatoid arthritis, lupus, or sepsis.

Typically, osteoarthritis of the hip begins in the fovea capitis area of the hip joint, with proteoglycan damage, and occurs in three stages.

1. Imperceptible cartilage damage or fibrillation.
2. Thinning of the articular cartilage, followed by instability secondary to a buckling of the ligaments, which produces an increase in joint shearing and an early capsular pattern. This instability is usually the first physical sign. Initially, the muscles limit the motion into the joints muscular capsular pattern, which is flexion and adduction; extension and internal rotation. Later on, the fibrosis maintains the capsular pattern.
3. A decrease in the length of femoral head and neck produces a mechanical disadvantage of the muscles resulting in a leg length discrepancy and a Trendelenburg gait pattern. Radiographic changes occur during this stage indicating the presence of osteophytosis and sometimes ankylosis, and traction spurs are formed.

Older people are at high risk for developing disability, gait impairment, and recurrent falls.[92,93] Difficulties with mobility, gait, upper extremity function, household management, and self-care activities have been associated with arthritis and joint pain in several studies of community-residing older persons.[93–95,96–99,100–102]

Osteitis Pubis

Historically and as early as 1827, this process has largely been related to pelvic surgery or obstetrical intervention.[103] In 1924, Beer,[104] a urologist, first detailed osteitis pubis in patients after suprapubic surgery. Many theories have been put forward concerning the etiology and progression of the disease, but the cause of osteitis pubis remains unclear.

Osteitis pubis is seen in athletes who participate in activities that create continual shearing forces at the pubic symphysis, as with unilateral leg support, or acceleration-deceleration forces required during multidirectional activities. These include such activities as running, race walking, gymnastics, soccer, basketball, rugby, and tennis. Pain with walking can be in one or several of many distributions:

perineal, testicular, suprapubic, inguinal, and postejaculatory pain in the scrotum and perineum.[105] Overuse is the most likely etiology of the inflammation and the process is usually self-limiting.[105]

Osteitis pubis has been likened to gracilis syndrome, an avulsion fatigue fracture involving the bony origin of the gracilis muscle at the pubic symphysis, and occurring in relation to the directional pull of the gracilis.[106] However, osteitis pubis does not necessarily involve a fracture. The process could be the result of stress reaction which might be associated with several biomechanical abnormalities.

Osteitis pubis usually appears during the third and fourth decade of life and occurs more commonly in men.[107] The pain or discomfort can be located in the pubic area, one or both groins, and in the lower rectus abdominis muscle. Symptoms of osteitis pubis have been described as "groin burning," with discomfort while climbing stairs, coughing, or sneezing.

During the physical examination, pain can be elicited by having the patient squeeze a fist between the knees with resisted long and flexed adductor contraction. Range of motion in one or both hips may be decreased. An adductor muscle spasm might occur with limited abduction and a positive lateral compression test and positive cross-leg test.[108,109] A soft tissue mass with calcification, and an audible or palpable click over the symphysis might be detected during daily activities.[105]

Correct examination of this region involves examining the position of the pelvic girdle. The normal position for the pelvic bowl is 45 degrees in the sagittal plane and 45 degrees in the coronal plane. Pubic motion is assessed by locating the pubic crest and then gently testing the mobility of each available direction.

Dysfunction of this articulation may be primary or secondary and, when present, is always treated first, as a loss of function, or integrity, of this joint disrupts the mechanics of the entire pelvic complex. The impairment pattern is determined by palpating the position of the pubic tubercles and correlating the findings with the side of the positive kinetic test (see later), with the restricted side indicating the side of the impairment.

An altered positional relationship within the pelvic girdle is significant only if a mobility restriction of the sacroiliac joint and/or pubic symphysis is found. The inguinal ligament is usually very tender to palpation on the side of the impairment. It is common to find the pubic symphysis held in one of the four following positions.

1. Anterior-inferior
2. Posterior-superior
3. Anterior-superior
4. Posterior-inferior

Coccydynia

Coccygeal pain is a fairly common occurrence. The coccyx can move anteriorly or posteriorly. There are a number of ligaments around this area that can become injured and these are the following.

Ventral

● Lateral sacrococcygeal
● Ventral ligament of the coccyx (caudal extension of the anterior longitudinal ligament)

Dorsal

● Superficial dorsal sacrococcygeal (caudal extension of the ligamentum flavum)
● Deep dorsal sacrococcygeal (caudal extension of the posterior longitudinal ligament)
● Intercornual ligament

The dominant muscle in this area is the levator ani, which has connections with:

● Iliococcygeal ligament
● Pubococcygeal ligament

Coccydynia tends to occur when the coccyx becomes stuck into flexion with an accompanying deviation. The causes can be muscle scarring or trauma.

Biomechanical Lesions

Some conditions predispose these joints to isolated impairments, due to either gross trauma or a lack of integrity of the joint surfaces and ligamentous support.

1. Until about the age of 11 years, the sacroiliac joint is quite planar, with very few ridges to provide support to the joint.
2. Due to the release of relaxin during pregnancy, there is a decrease in the tensile strength of all of the ligaments in the body. This ligamentous laxity continues to occur for up to 3 months after the pregnancy.[110] As the pelvic area relies heavily on its ligaments for stability, the area becomes vulnerable to injury, even with minor trauma.
3. Significant high-velocity trauma to the pelvic complex, such as that which occurs during a motor vehicle accident, can produce a subluxation of the sacroiliac joint.

In normal, healthy adults, the pelvic complex is a structure that is not prone to injury. Lesions that do occur in the normal population typically occur as combinations of innominate rotations and sacral torsions, due to the ligamentous relationship that the various joints share. It would appear from the anatomy and biomechanics of this region that the pelvic complex is anatomically and functionally a contiguous circle, or ring, and that isolated impairments to this region probably only occur when a high degree of trauma is involved. With less severe trauma, impairments seem to occur in combinations, with an injury to one part of the ring having repercussions at other parts within the ring. Based on the biomechanics of this complex, the sacroiliac, lumbosacral, and pubic symphysis joints can adopt one of four pathologic positions.

● One side of the sacrum is nutated while the ipsilateral ilium is posteriorly rotated. The pubic tubercle is superior on the side of the posteriorly rotated ilium.
● One side of the sacrum is counternutated while the ipsilateral ilium is anteriorly rotated. The pubic tubercle is inferior on the side of the anteriorly rotated ilium.
● One side of the sacrum is nutated while the ipsilateral ilium is anteriorly rotated. The pubic tubercle is inferior on the side of the anteriorly rotated ilium.
● One side of the sacrum is counternutated while the ipsilateral ilium is posteriorly rotated. The pubic tubercle is superior on the side of the posteriorly rotated ilium.

The biomechanical examination should determine which of the four scenarios is occurring. Two syndromes are recognized, the type I sacral torsion syndrome and the type II sacral torsion syndrome.[111]

Type I Sacral Torsion

The left sacral torsion syndrome exists when the anterior sacrum is held in a left-rotated position and the lumbar vertebrae adapt by following the first law of physiologic spinal motion and side-flex to the right and rotate to the left.[111] A left torsion of the sacrum is defined as an unphysiologic occurrence. Arthrokinematically, the sacrum glides anterior-inferior along the short length on the right joint and posterior-inferior along the long-arm on the left joint.[112] A review of Fryette's laws of physiologic spinal motion[21] help explain the effect on the lumbar spine when the sacrum is held in this unphysiologic position.

Law I Whenever the spine moves from neutral, side-flexion occurs before rotation, except during pure flexion or extension. The side-flexion produces a bending movement about which the rotation occurs. This combined motion is referred to as latexion, and the side-flexion and rotation occur to opposite sides; the vertebral body rotates into the convexity of the curve. Spinal impairments presenting as latexion are referred to as type I impairments.[111] Anterior sacral torsions are classified as type I impairments.[111]

Law II   From a position of full flexion or full extension, rotation precedes side-flexion when movement occurs other than a return to neutral. This combined motion is referred to as rotexion, and the rotation and side-flexion occur to the same side; the vertebral body rotates into the concavity of the curve. Spinal impairments presenting as rotexion are referred to as type II impairments.[111] Posterior sacral torsions are classified as type II impairments.[111]

With the left sacral torsion, the sacrum will have moved inferiorly and posteriorly on the left articular surface, and inferiorly and anteriorly on the right. Relative to the sacrum, the left innominate will have moved superiorly and anteriorly, and the right innominate will have moved posteriorly.[111] If the lumbosacral angle is increased, and the iliolumbar ligaments have, therefore, become taut, the right iliolumbar ligament pulls on the posterior aspect of the right transverse processes of the fifth and, sometimes, the fourth lumbar vertebrae and they will move with the innominates—superiorly and anteriorly on the left and posteriorly on the right.[111] Applying the second law of Fryette, the vertebrae are now in a right rotated and right side-flexed position. The lumbar vertebrae above L5 and L4 gradually counterrotate, producing the appearance of a left convexity.[111]

If the lumbosacral angle is in neutral, with no tension on the iliolumbar ligaments, the fifth lumbar vertebra will be free to follow Fryette's first law of physiologic spinal motion and side-flex to the right and rotate to the left.[111] The remainder of the lumbar spine will follow L5, side-flexing to the right and producing a convexity to the left.

Type II Sacral Torsions

The type II sacral torsion syndrome exists when the anterior surface of the sacrum is held in a left rotated position and the lower lumbar vertebrae follow the second law of physiologic motion; L5 and L4 rotate and side-flex to the right.[111] The clinical appearance of the type II sacral torsion is very similar to the acute lumbar disc prolapse, and the subjective examination is often helpful in differentiating the two (i.e., type II sacral torsion are not aggravated by sitting, whereas the patient with an acute lumbar disc prolapse finds this position intolerable). This impairment occurs more frequently on the right side.

The intervention for these scenarios can then be approached in one of two ways.

1. Addressing all of the deficits simultaneously.
2. Addressing all of the deficits individually.

Thus far, the success of interventions at this joint has been mixed, due in part to the poor reliability of many of the examinations used. It follows that if the examination gives a mixed diagnosis, the intervention will have a mixed result.

OSTEOPATHIC APPROACH TO THE SACROILIAC JOINT

As mentioned, many of the osteopathic tests have been found to have poor reliability and have been poor predictors of diagnosis. It is worth spending some time analyzing these tests and highlighting their shortcomings.

Positional Testing

Positional testing includes palpating the sacral sulcus and contralateral inferior lateral angle (ILA) with the patient positioned in prone-lying, then prone on elbows, and finally, in lumbar flexion. In flexion, if the sacrum position is palpated, and the right sacral sulcus is deeper than the left, and the left posterior corner of the sacrum, or the inferior lateral angle (ILA) is more posterior than the right, this supposedly indicates that instead of flexing normally, the sacrum has rotated to the left, and is in either a Left on Left, or a Left on Right position.[113]

With the prone push-up, or Sphinx test, an extension hypomobility will be apparent at the end of range, or earlier. For example, a patient with a right sacroiliac extension (counternutation) hypomobility, demonstrates a deeper right sulcus and a posterior ILA, as compared to the other side. As the spine is extended sequentially, the axis producing the rotation is through the hypomobile joint (the right) and must be oblique, as the other joint is unaffected. This is the right oblique axis. The palpation of the two sacral corners is maintained, as the patient flexes. An increase in symmetry that occurs with flexion indicates an anterior torsion, whereas a decrease in symmetry indicates a posterior torsion.

The problems with positional testing are:

● Determining whether the asymmetry is normal or abnormal.
● Determining which side is asymmetrical.
● Determining whether the asymmetry is too asymmetrical or not asymmetrical enough.

Standing Flexion Test

The standing flexion test has been used frequently to analyze SI joint mobility,[114] and has been used by most health professions to determine the side of the impairment. However, reliability studies so far lack sufficient diagnostic power.[115,116]

Each posterior superior iliac spine (PSIS) is palpated with a thumb placed on it caudally. Providing that there is no impairment in the sacroiliac joint or the lower lumbar spine, the following is expected to occur.

- As the patient bends forward, both thumbs under each of the PSIS move cranially.

What appears to be happening during the maneuver is that during the initial component of trunk flexion, the sacrum is nutating, or flexing, as the spine takes it in the same direction. Between 45 and 60 degrees of spinal flexion, both innominates rotate anteriorly producing a relative counternutation of the sacrum, or sacroiliac extension. A positive finding for this test is:

- An increase in the cranial migration of the thumb on one side compared to the other
- Iniation of the cranial migration occurring on one side before the other

However, it is apparent that the generally held view that the hypomobile sacroiliac joint is on the side of the posterior superior iliac spine with the greatest cranial movement, cannot be correct, as even a fused joint would result in the innominate and the sacrum moving together, and the innominate being held down by the sacrum, or at best, side-flexing the sacrum upward on that side. The other limitation to this test is that most patients have an equality of hamstring length between sides, allowing for an earlier cranial movement of the PSIS on the more flexible side.

The seated flexion test (Piedallu's sign) is the same test but with the patient sitting, with his or her legs over the end of the table, feet supported.[113] In this position, the innominate motion is severely abbreviated as the sitting position places the innominates near the end of their extension range. This is perhaps the more reliable of the two tests, but it is questionable how much information it gives the clinician, especially as there are more reliable tests that can give the same information.

The Long Sit Test

This test has been used to confirm the side of the impairment using the principle of rotation.[113] Following a positive standing flexion test to determine the side of the impairment, the long sit test is used to indicate the direction of the rotation that the implicated innominate has adopted. If, after noting a leg length discrepancy in supine on the side of the impairment obtained from the standing flexion test, the clinician observes whether the medial malleolus on that side moves distally or proximally during the long sit test. Rotation about a coronal axis, whose resultant movement leads to an increase in the length of a limb, is defined as extension. If it shortens the length of the limb, it is defined as flexion. Thus, if the apparent shorter leg becomes longer during the test, the innominate on that side is held in a posteriorly rotated malposition; if the apparent longer leg becomes shorter during the test, the innominate on that side is held in a anteriorly rotated malposition.

The problems with this test involve the maneuver itself. To ask patients who are in some degree of discomfort to raise themselves off the bed from a supine position into a long sit position without any twisting or use of the arms, is unnecessarily painful. In addition, the patient needs 90 degrees of hip flexion and hamstring length for the test. As with the standing flexion test, there is no allowance made for the length of the hamstrings and their effect on the results. The long sit test also relies heavily on the findings from the standing flexion test, an unreliable test itself.

Leg Length Tests

These are usually performed as part of the bony landmark examination. Anatomic discrepancies in leg length can predispose patients to a pelvic and/or lumbar impairment. Although not an exact measurement of leg length, these tests can highlight any asymmetries. The chiropractor assesses leg length with the patient prone, by observing the comparative length of the heels or medial malleoli. If a discrepancy is noted, the legs are flexed to 90 degrees while maintaining a neutral of hip rotation to screen for a shortened tibia. The leg lengths are then assessed with the patient supine, and then again in the long sit position.

All of the tests just described utilize an indirect process to examine the sacroiliac joint. Given that the sacroiliac joint appears to behave like other joints in that its motions are a combination of linear glides and angular motions, it should be assessed like other joints. Combining the findings from static and dynamic tests should always be incorporated. Dynamic tests that test the ability of a joint to perform its normal motion are more pertinent than static tests, which look at landmarks, especially landmarks that are either very distal to the joint or prone to the effects of muscle imbalances. The tests in the following sequence are designed to examine the various components of a normally functioning lumbar-pelvic-hip complex. These components include a gait and postural analysis, the glides that occur along the short and long lengths of the sacroiliac joint surfaces, the elements of the force and form closure mechanisms, and the normal functional movements that this complex performs on a regular basis. Although most of these tests have yet to be subjected to rigorous scrutiny and scientific research, they have worked well in the clinic and are based on a logical biomechanical model.

BIOMECHANICAL EXAMINATION OF THE SACROILIAC JOINT

The biomechanical examination of the sacroiliac joint is performed if a diagnosis cannot be made from the scanning examination (Figure 17–9). The scanning examination, which includes the primary stress tests (anterior and posterior gapping), can be used to detect ligament tears, sacroiliitis resulting from microtraumatic arthritis, microtraumatic arthritis, or systemic arthritis (ankylosing spondylitis, Reiter's, syndrome etc.), or the more serious pathologies grouped under the sign of the buttock. A positive test would suggest a high degree of inflammation and irritability. The following findings would likely be present.

- A history of sharp pain awakening the patient from sleep upon turning in bed.
- Pain with walking.
- A positive straight leg raise at, or near the end, of range (occasionally early in the range when hyperacute), pain, and, sometimes, limitation on extension and ipsilateral side-flexion of the trunk.

A positive test is one that reproduces unilateral or bilateral sacroiliac pain, either anteriorly or posteriorly.[33] A positive test indicates the presence of inflammation, but does not give any information as to the cause of the arthritis. If either test is positive in the older patient who has recently fallen, there is a possibility that a fracture of the pelvis exists. The clinician should also clear the hip joint before proceeding with an in depth examination of the sacroiliac joint, as the hip joint is a common source of groin and pelvic pain.

Anterior

The anterior stress test, also called the gapping test, is performed with the patient supine with the legs extended. The test is identical to the one performed as part of the lumbar and sacroiliac scan (Fig 17–10).

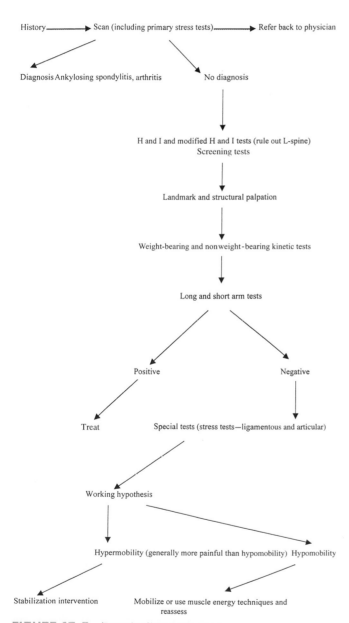

FIGURE 17–9   Examination sequence.

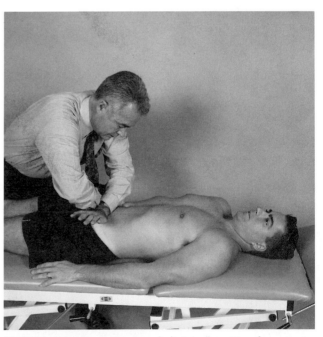

FIGURE 17–10   Patient and clinician position for anterior gapping of the sacroiliac joint.

Posterior

The patient is laid in side-lying and the clinician applies pressure to the lateral side of the ilium, thereby compressing the anterior aspect of the joint and gapping its posterior aspect (Figure 17–11). The posterior and interosseus ligaments are among the strongest in the body and are not usually torn by trauma, but may be attenuated by prolonged or repeated stress. This test is less sensitive for arthritis due to the reduced leverage available to the clinician and, when positive, indicates fairly severe arthritis. This also indirectly tests the ability of the sacrum to counternutate.

Examination Sequence

In most cases, a biomechanical examination of the pelvic joints is of little use if the lumbar spine has not been previously cleared by examination or intervention. When impaired, the lumbar spine, profoundly affects the positions and active movements of the sacroiliac joint. However, if the existing lumbar problem is not improving with adequate intervention, the sacroiliac pathology may be the factor preventing its improvement. In these cases, a sacroiliac joint examination prior to clearing the spine is appropriate.

A patient history and a lumbar scan are performed. The lumbar spine is cleared using the H and I tests, making sure that sacral motion is prevented during the test. However, monitoring the sacrum does not preclude the presence of an impairment at the lumbosacral junction. Because of this relationship, a number of quick screening tests using active range of motion of the lumbar spine can be used.

The patient is asked to stand with the feet shoulder width apart. Crouching behind the patient, the clinician locates the sacral sulcus and the contralateral inferior lateral angle (ILA) and places a thumb over each (e. g., the right sacral sulcus and the left ILA). The patient is asked to forward bend and then to rotate to the left while forward bent.

● Forward bending combined with left rotation produces a Left on Right motion at the sacrum.

The patient is asked to backward bend and then to rotate to the left while backward bent.

● Backward bending and left rotation produces a Left on Left motion at the sacrum.

The test is then repeated using forward bending and right rotation, and backward bending and right rotation. This is a good screening test for the overall function of the lumbar spine and pelvic complex, and if negative, would indicate that these regions are not the source of pain.

Landmark Palpation

The palpation of landmarks is an integral part of the examination, particularly for seeking out tenderness, but the results from these tests should be combined with other examination findings to formulate a working hypothesis, and should not be solely relied upon. Various landmarks of the pelvis are palpated with the patient positioned in standing, sitting, and prone-lying. Pelvic asymmetry is probably the norm and so it should not be surprising that the palpation of landmarks should find so many positive findings. An altered positional relationship within the pelvic girdle should only be significant if a mobility restriction of the sacroiliac joint and/or pubic symphysis is found. There are, therefore, inherent problems with the reliance on static landmarks as the basis for making a diagnosis.[118]

● Determining whether the asymmetry is normal or abnormal. It is generally accepted that, except in small children, a symmetrical pelvis is a rare thing.
● Determining which side is asymmetrical. Is the innominate anteriorly rotated on the right or posteriorly rotated on the left?
● Determining whether the asymmetry is too asymmetrical or not asymmetrical enough. If the innominate is anteriorly rotated compared to the left, is it rotated too much, too little, or just the right amount, when compared to its starting position? As the starting position is not known, then the degree of rotation cannot be assessed.

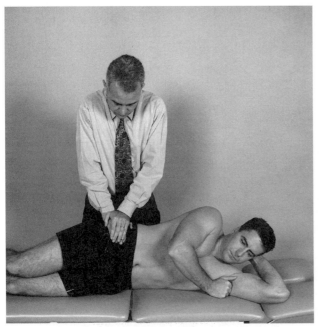

FIGURE 17–11   Patient and clinician position for posterior gapping of the sacroiliac joint.

The following landmarks and structures need to be palpated.

- *Iliac crest:* Typically level with the L4–L5 disc space. The crest heights should be level (Figure 17–12).
- *Anterior superior iliac spine (ASIS)* (Figure 17–13). An inferior ASIS relative to the other side may indicate an anteriorly rotated innominate, whereas a superior ASIS, relative to the other side, may indicate a posteriorly rotated innominate.[113] In supine, if the innominate is anteriorly rotated, the leg will be longer on that side, but shorter if it is posteriorly rotated.[113]
- *Posterior superior iliac spine (PSIS).* Typically located 1 inch beneath the dimples of the lumbar spine (Figure 17–14). The clinician should hook the thumbs under the posterior superior iliac spine (PSIS). A superior PSIS relative to the other side may indicate an anteriorly rotated innominate on that side, whereas an inferior PSIS may indicate a posteriorly rotated innominate on that side.[113]
- *Pubic symphysis and pubic tubercles (lateral to the pubic symphysis)*
- *Thoracodorsal fascial attachments*
- *Long dorsal ligament*
- *Greater trochanter*
- *Ischial tuberosities and sacrotuberous ligament (medial to the tuberosities).* The sacrotuberous ligament is firm on the side of an anteriorly rotated innominate, and taut on the side of a posteriorly rotated innominate.[113] The

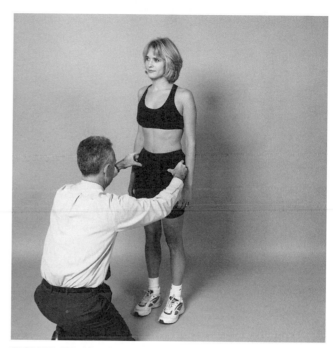

FIGURE 17–13 Anterior-superior iliac spine heights.

patient is positioned in prone and the clinician stands at the patient's side. With the heel of the hands, the clinician locates the ischial tuberosities through the soft tissue at the gluteal folds. Then, with the thumbs, the clinician palpates the inferior-medial aspect of the

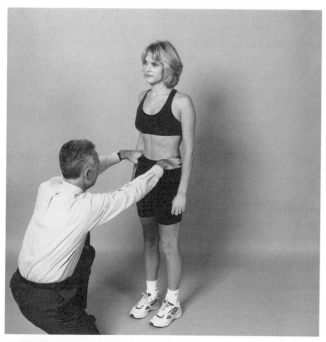

FIGURE 17–12 Iliac crest heights.

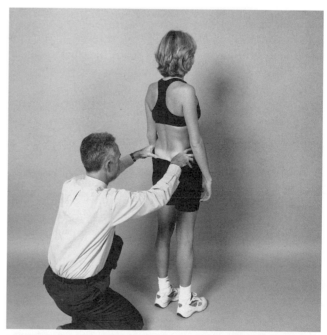

FIGURE 17–14 Posterior-superior iliac spine heights.

ischial tuberosities. From this point, the clinician slides the thumbs superior-lateral and palpates the sacrotuberous ligament. The clinician then compares the relative tension between the left and right side.

- *Sacral sulcus and sacral base.* From the posterior inferior iliac spine, the clinician moves in a thumb's width, and then up a thumb's width.
- *Inferior lateral angle (ILA).* Level with the prominent part of the tail bone.
- *The L5 segment.* The clinician palpates medially along the iliac crest. L5 is level with the point at which the palpating finger begins to descend on the crest.
- *L5–S1 facets.* These are located half way between the L5 spinous process and the ipsilateral posterior inferior iliac spine (PSIS).
- *Lumbosacral angle.* An increased lumbosacral angle on one side may indicate an anteriorly rotated innominate, while a decreased lumbosacral angle on one side may indicate an posteriorly rotated innominate.
- S2 should be level horizontally with the posterior inferior iliac spine (PSIS).

Passive Range of Motion

Passive range of motion of the hip, including internal and external rotation, is performed to help rule out pain referred from the hip joint.

Weight-Bearing Kinetic Tests

These tests were designed to observe the osteokinematics occurring at the sacroiliac joint during patient generated movements. They assess the mobility of the ilium, the ability of the sacrum to nutate (ipsilateral test), and to side-flex (contralateral test). The kinetic tests, as a group, include both weight-bearing and nonweight-bearing tests. As these movements are difficult to observe, bony landmarks are palpated during the movements. The tests for the right side are described.

Ipsilateral Flexion Kinetic Test (Stork Test) The ipsilateral flexion kinetic test[119] assesses the mobility of the short-arm of the auricular surface, and the ability of the ipsilateral ilium to posteriorly rotate. With the patient standing, the inferior aspect of the right posterior superior iliac spine (PSIS) is palpated with one thumb, while the left thumb palpates the median sacral crest (S2) directly parallel. The clinician then asks the patient to flex the right hip to 90 degrees (Figure 17–15). During this movement, the innominate on the ipsilateral side to the hip flexion rotates backward on the fixed sacrum, and the clinician notes the movement of the PSIS relative to the sacrum. To perform this test, the patient has to be able to maintain balance. During this maneuver, the lumbar spine side-flexes contralaterally, to the side of the hip flexion, and rotates ipsilaterally. Substitutions to look for during this test include ipsilateral hip

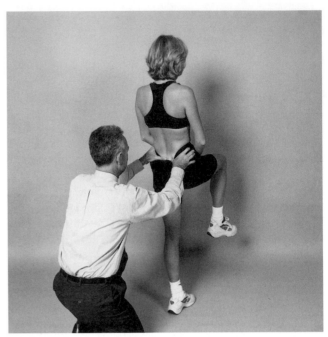

FIGURE 17–15 Patient and clinician position for the ipsilateral weight-bearing kinetic test.

hiking or a leaning away from the tested side. A positive ipsilateral kinetic test is observed when the thumb on the inferior aspect of the posterior superior iliac spine moves cranially instead of caudally, and the patient hikes the right side of the pelvis. When this occurs, an impairment of the ipsilateral sacroiliac joint or the lumbar spine is presumed. The left ipsilateral kinetic test examines the ability of the left innominate to posteriorly rotate, the sacrum to left rotate, and the L5 vertebra to left rotate and right side-flex.

Extension Kinetic Test This test serves as a functional mobility test of the sacroiliac joint for the extension kinetic test, the clinician palpates under the ipsilateral PSIS with one thumb, and at the median sacral crest (S2) directly parallel with the opposite thumb (Figure 17–16). The patient extends the ipsilateral hip, with the knee extended into varying degrees of hip extension while the clinician notes the superior-lateral displacement of the posterior superior iliac spine (PSIS) relative to the sacrum. Both sides are tested. The right extension test examines the ability of the right innominate to anteriorly rotate, and the sacrum to left rotate and counternutate. The left extension test examines the ability of the left innominate to anteriorly rotate, and the sacrum to right rotate and counternutate.

The test can be repeated on both sides using hip flexion and knee extension to assess the ability of the innominates to posteriorly rotate and should confirm the findings from the ipsilateral flexion kinetic test.

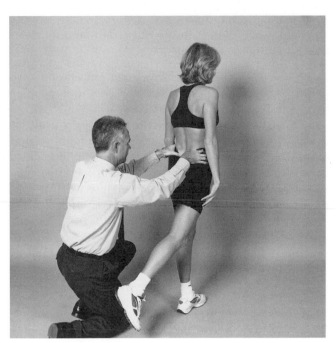

FIGURE 17–16   Patient and clinician position for the ipsilateral weight-bearing extension test.

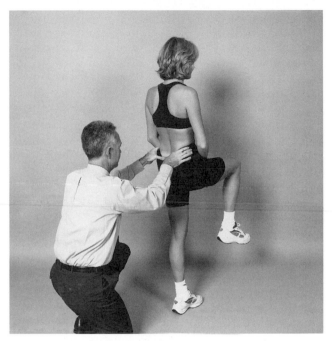

FIGURE 17–17   Patient and clinician position for the contralateral weight-bearing kinetic test.

The potential impairments within the pelvic girdle, which render the kinetic tests positive, include[111]:

1. An anteriorly or posteriorly rotated innominate of the ipsilateral side (intra-articular or extra-articular in origin).
2. A pubic symphysis impairment on the ipsilateral side.
3. An innominate flare on the ipsilateral side.
4. A subluxed innominate on the ipsilateral side (intra-articular in origin).

Contralateral Flexion Kinetic Test   The contralateral flexion kinetic test[111] evaluates the mobility of the long-arm of the auricular surface, and the ability of the sacrum to side-flex to the opposite side of the hip flexion. With the patient standing, the clinician places his or right thumb on the medial sacral crest of the sacrum (S2), and the left thumb on the left posterior superior iliac spine (PSIS). The patient is asked to flex the right hip to 90 degrees (Figure 17–17). During this movement, the right thumb, on the sacral crest, travels caudally initially, as a result of the posterior rotation of the right innominate, which produces a right side-flexion and left rotation of the sacrum (conjunct rotation). At about 75 degrees of hip flexion, all of the available motion of the sacrum is taken up and the movement then begins to take place at the right sacroiliac joint. The right hip continues to flex, producing lumbar spine flexion and left side-flexion of the sacrum on the fixed right sacroiliac joint. In addition, the lumbar vertebral

bodies of L5 and above will rotate to the right due to the influence of the iliolumbar ligament on L5.

When the contralateral kinetic test is positive, the right thumb travels either caudally or it does not move, indicating that the sacrum is unable to side-flex.

The potential sacroiliac impairments that render the test positive with right up flexion include[111]:

1. Left sacral torsion
2. Left sacral nutation and flexion

The ipsilateral and contralateral tests are evaluated on both sides for comparison.

Nonweight-Bearing (NWB) Kinetic Tests[120]

The patient is positioned in prone. The clinician palpates the posterior superior iliac spine on one side and the median sacral crest (S2), and asks the patient to flex the ipsilateral knee. During this maneuver, the clinician should feel an anterior rotation of the innominate (Figure 17–18). The test is repeated, except that the patient flexes the other knee. The clinician should feel a relative posterior rotation of the innominate during this maneuver. The test is repeated on the other side. The nonweight-bearing ipsilateral test examines the ability of the innominate to perform an anterior rotation, whereas the weight-bearing ipsilateral kinetic test examines the ability of the ilium to produce a posterior rotation.

Although, the weight-bearing kinetic tests demonstrate which movements of the sacrum and innominate are

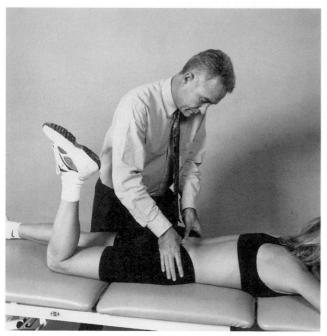

FIGURE 17–18 Patient and clinician position for the ipsilateral nonweight-bearing kinetic test.

abnormal, they will not, by themselves, determine the specific cause of the abnormality. The sacroiliac joint is presumably subject to the same types of impairments that affect other joints, that is pericapsular, myofascial, or subluxation hypomobilities. The weight-bearing tests highlight any hypomobility, however, they are much less sensitive for detecting hypermobilities or instabilities. If an unstable subluxation exists (that is, where the subluxation reduces spontaneously), it will be discernible as a hypomobility on the weight-bearing tests when body weight subluxes it, but will appear normal with the nonweight-bearing tests when it is reduced (Table 17–2).

A subluxation demonstrates:

- No motion in one direction, but full motion in the opposite direction.
- Consistency of the findings between the weight-bearing and nonweight-bearing tests.

TABLE 17–2 WEIGHT-BEARING VERSUS NONWEIGHT-BEARING TESTS[64]

WEIGHT BEARING	NONWEIGHT BEARING	INDICATION
+	+	Stable subluxation or significant hypomobility
+	−	Unstable subluxation
−	+	Mild to moderate hypomobility
−	−	Normal or hypermobile or unstable, but not subluxing

Short and Long Arm Tests

To confirm the findings in the kinetic tests, the short and long arm tests, are performed.

Short Arm Test The short arm test confirms the findings of the ipsilateral kinetic tests. The following description is for a test of the left side of the sacrum.

The patient lies supine with the legs straight, while the clinician stands on the left side of the patient. The clinician slides his or her right hand under the left side of the patient's lumbar spine, and palpates the left sacral base and sulcus with the index and long finger. With the left hand, the clinician, grasps the anterior aspect of the patient's left innominate/ASIS (Figure 17–19). From this position, the clinician stabilizes the left sacral base and sulcus with the right hand, and pushes the left innominate down toward the bed, using the left. Some motion should be felt before a ligamentous end feel is reached.

Long Arm Test The long arm test confirms the findings of the contralateral kinetic test. The following description is for a test of the right side of the sacrum.

The palpation and stabilization points are as for the short arm test. The patient's right hip is flexed to about 45 degrees with one hand. Using the heel of the right hand, the clinician pushes down the length of the flexed femur, while stabilizing the sacral base with the left hand (Figure 17–20). Again, slight motion should be felt (more than with the short arm test) before a solid ligamentous end feel is reached. There should be no pain.

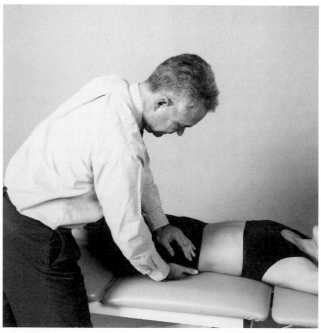

FIGURE 17–19 Patient and clinician position for the short arm test on the left.

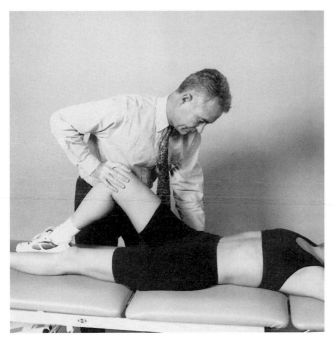

FIGURE 17–20 Patient and clinician position for the long arm test on the right.

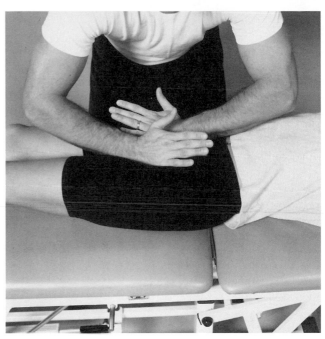

FIGURE 17–21 Patient and clinician position for the pubic stress test.

Following the weight-bearing and nonweight-bearing tests and the confirmatory long and short arm tests, the clinician should be able to determine the following.

- The side of the lesion
- The type of lesion

Having determined both the side and type of lesion, an intervention plan can be formulated. Ideally, the patient's condition can be categorized into one of the following.

- One side of the sacrum is nutated while the ipsilateral ilium is posteriorly rotated. The pubic tubercle is superior on the side of the posteriorly rotated ilium.
- One side of the sacrum is counternutated while the ipsilateral ilium is anteriorly rotated. The pubic tubercle is inferior on the side of the anteriorly rotated ilium.
- One side of the sacrum is nutated while the ipsilateral ilium is anteriorly rotated. The pubic tubercle is inferior on the side of the anteriorly rotated ilium.
- One side of the sacrum is counternutated while the ipsilateral ilium is posteriorly rotated. The pubic tubercle is superior on the side of the posteriorly rotated ilium.

However, if the tests just described proved negative, the source of the lesion lies elsewhere, and further investigation is required.

Pubic Stress Tests[120]

The patient is positioned in supine, and the clinician stands at the patient's side. With the heel of one hand, the clinician palpates the superior aspect of the superior ramus of one pubic bone, and with the heel of the other hand, palpates the inferior aspect of the superior ramus of the opposite pubic bone (Figure 17–21). Fixing one pubic bone, the clinician applies a slow, steady inferior-superior force to the other bone and, noting the quantity and end feel of motion, as well as the reproduction of any symptoms, the clinician then switches hands and repeats the test so that both sides are stressed superiorly and inferiorly.

In some cases of trauma, or occasionally with child bearing, the pubis can become destabilized. This is a very severe and painful impairment and one that is not easily missed. The pain is local to the pubic area with the patient quite disabled with all movements, and weight-bearing postures are very painful. The impairment generally shows up on one legged weight-bearing X-rays and often requires surgical intervention to stabilize the symphysis.

Ligament Stress Tests

Sacrotuberous and Interosseous Ligaments The sacrotuberous ligament can be stressed, with the patient in supine, by flexing the patient's hip to the ipsilateral shoulder (Figure 17–22), thus stressing the ligament and forcing

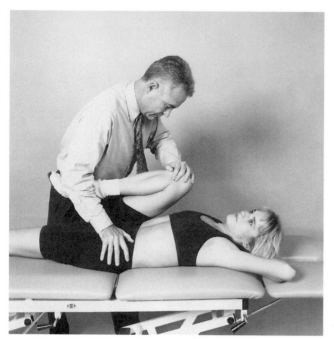

FIGURE 17–22   Patient and clinician position for the sacrotuberous ligament stress test.

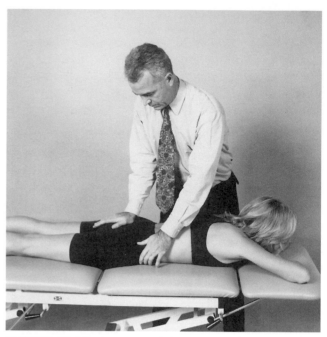

FIGURE 17–23   Patient and clinician position for the long dorsal ligament stress test.

the sacrum to nutate. This force is maintained for about 20 seconds, and any reproduction of symptoms is noted.

Long Dorsal Sacroiliac Ligament   The patient is positioned in prone and the clinician stands at the patient's side. With one hand, the clinician palpates the inferior aspect of the sacrum in the midline and places the heel of this hand over the area (Figure 17–23). The clinician then applies an anterior force to the sacrum, thus forcing the sacrum to counternutate. This force is maintained for about 20 seconds and the reproduction of symptoms is noted.

Iliolumbar Ligament   The patient is positioned in prone and the clinician stands at the patient's side. The clinician places a thumb over the transverse process of L5 on one side, to stabilize against rotation and pull up on the ipsilateral iliac crest, thereby producing a posterior rotation of the right innominate to stress the iliolumbar ligament (Figure 17–24). The clinician can also prevent the rotation by placing the thumb against the contralateral side of the spinous process to the iliac crest being lifted.

INTERVENTIONS

A number of interventions for the sacroiliac joint have been adopted by the various disciplines. These interventions consist of manual therapy, therapeutic exercises, orthoses, modalities, and education.

Manual Therapy

This has a very limited place in the intervention of the acutely inflamed joint. In almost every case, the presence of a positive primary stress test contraindicates the use of passive

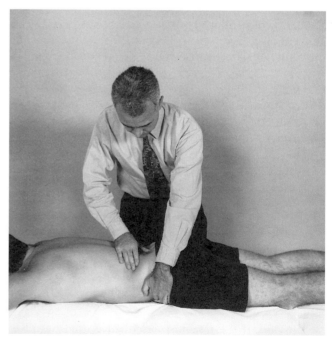

FIGURE 17–24   Patient and clinician position for the iliolumbar ligament stress test.

mobilization or manipulation for that joint. However, mobilization or manipulation of the contralateral joint can reduce the stress on the painful and inflamed articulation.

The majority of sacroiliac joint impairments comprise a number of structural changes that occur simultaneously. These structural changes can be treated individually or as part of a combined intervention strategy.

Muscle energy (active mobilization) techniques are most effective in cases of myofascial or mild pericapsular hypomobility, and less useful in cases of very stiff joints or subluxations. Among the individual conditions that are more amenable for this type of technique are the following.[113]

- Inferior or superior pubic symphysis
- Innominate flexion hypomobility (anterior rotation)
- Innominate extension hypomobility (posterior rotation)
- Forward sacral torsion (Left on Left or Right on Right)
- Backward sacral torsion (Left on Right or Right on Left)

Probably the least used technique in the sacroiliac joint is passive mobilization, but it can be more specific than muscle energy. The principles of mobilization, that pertain to other joints, also apply here.

Techniques to Restore Pubic Symphyseal Joint Dysfunction

Superior Pubic Symphyseal Joint (Left Side) The patient is positioned in supine near the left side of the bed and with the left lower extremity hanging off the edge of the bed. The clinician stands on the left side of the patient and supports the patient's left leg with one hand, and stabilizing the patient's right ASIS with the other. The clinician slowly guides the patient's left leg towards the floor while also slightly abducting it, until the motion barrier is reached. From this position, the patient is asked to lift their left knee "up and in", against the clinician's unyielding counterforce. The contraction is held for 3 to 5 seconds, and the maneuver is repeated 3–5 times, followed by a reevaluation.

Inferior Pubic Symphyseal Joint (Right Side) The patient is positioned in supine near to the right side of the bed. The clinician, standing to the patient's right, flexes the patient's hip and knee, and stabilizes the patient's left ASIS with the left hand, while placing the closed fist of the right hand under the patient's right ischial tuberosity, palm side down (Figure 17–25). From this position, the patient is asked to attempt to straighten their right leg against the clinician's unyielding counterforce, while the clinician applies a cranial force to the patient's right ischial tuberosity using the right fist. The contraction is held for 3 to 5 seconds, and the maneuver is repeated 3–5 times, followed by a re-evaluation.

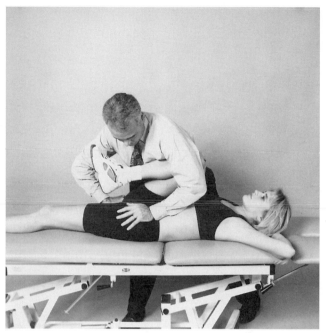

FIGURE 17–25 Patient and clinician position for pubic symphysis mobilization.

Inferior or Superior Pubic Symphyseal Joint (Modified Shot-gun) The patient is positioned in supine, with the knees and hips flexed so that the soles of their feet rest on the bed. The clinician sits at the patient's feet and holds the patient's knees together. The patient is asked to try and abduct, or open, their legs against the clinician's unyielding counterforce. The contraction is held for 3 to 5 seconds, and the maneuver is repeated 3–5 times, followed by a re-evaluation.

Next the clinician abducts the patient's legs, while keeping their feet together, and places a forearm between the patient's knees, so that the palm of the hand is on the medial aspect of one knee and the elbow rests against the medial aspect of the other knee. The patient is then asked to adduct, or close, their legs against the clinician's unyielding counterforce. The contraction is held for 3 to 5 seconds, and the maneuver is repeated 3–5 times, followed by a re-evaluation.

Home Exercise This technique can be performed at home using a strap, or belt for the abduction part and a rolled towel for the adduction part.

Techniques to Restore Anterior rotation of the Right Innominate

Passive Mobilization The patient is positioned in supine-lying, and the clinician stands on the right side of the patient. Sliding the left hand under the patient's back, the

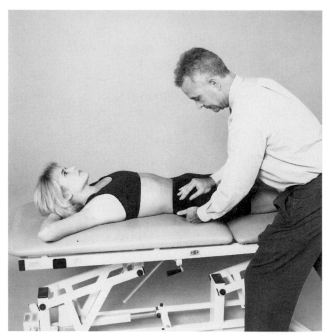

FIGURE 17–26 Patient and clinician position for passive mobilization into anterior rotation of the right innominate.

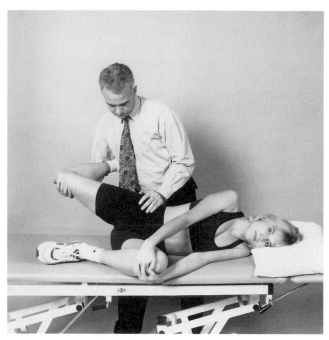

FIGURE 17–27 Patient and clinician position for active mobilization of the right innominate into anterior rotation.

clinician stabilizes the apex of the sacrum, and places the heel of the right hand on the patient's right iliac crest. Using a series of small oscillations, the clinician rotates the right innominate anteriorly (Figure 17–26). By altering the angle of the anterior rotation, the clinician can find the direction that is the most comfortable and efficient.

After a number of these oscillations, the patient is positioned in prone-lying with the right ASIS off the edge of the table. Ensuring that the motion of the patient's right ASIS into anterior rotation is not blocked by the table, the clinician passively rotates the right innominate anteriorly with a series of small oscillations. As more motion is gained, the clinician places a pillow under the right thigh of the patient, or the end of the table can be elevated, and the patient's left leg is lowered off the side of the bed. In this position, the clinician continues to mobilize the right innominate into anterior rotation.

Muscle energy can be incorporated into the technique. While the clinician stabilizes the apex of the sacrum, the patient is instructed to push the right hip into the pillow or table while keeping the right leg straight, thereby using the rectus femoris, sartorius, and iliopsoas muscles. By inserting a hand between the patient's thigh and the table, the force of the hip flexion can be monitored.

Active Mobilization: Method One The patient is positioned in left side-lying, facing the clinician and with the left hip fully flexed. Grasping the anterior aspect of the patient's right thigh, the clinician passively extends the right

hip, while monitoring the right posterior inferior iliac spine and S2 and ischial tuberosity with the other hand, until motion occurs. At the motion barrier, the patient performs an isometric contraction of right hip flexion against the clinician's resistance (Fig 17–27). The patient relaxes, and the right hip is extended to the new barrier.

Active Mobilization: Method Two The patient is positioned in left side-lying, facing the clinician and with the left hip flexed to about 90 degrees. The clinician stabilizes the patient's left leg using the thigh. The patient's right hip is passively extended to the motion barrier and is, both supported in this position, and prevented from moving into adduction. The clinician leans onto the patient, and places the heel of the right hand over the apex of the sacrum. The left arm of the clinician is placed between the patient's legs and the hands are clasped together (Figure 17–28). The patient is then instructed to push the right hip into flexion against the clinician's body. The patient then relaxes and the right hip is moved to the new barrier to hip extension and the process is repeated.

Active Mobilization: Method Three The patient is positioned in prone-lying, with the clinician standing on the patient's left side. With the right hand, the clinician supports the anterior aspect of the patient's right thigh, at a point just above the knee. The clinician places the heel of the left hand over the patient's right posterior inferior iliac spine. Extending the right hip until motion at the

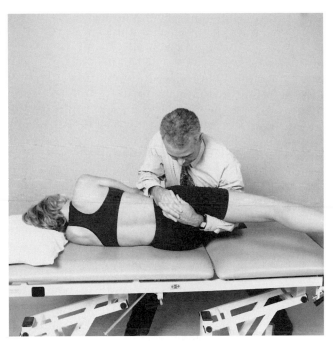

FIGURE 17–28   Patient and clinician position for active mobilization of the right innominate into anterior rotation.

lumbosacral junction is perceived, (Figure 17–29) the clinician localizes the motion barrier. The patient is instructed to flex the right hip against the clinician's resistance. This isometric contraction is held up to 5 seconds, following which, the patient is instructed to completely relax. The

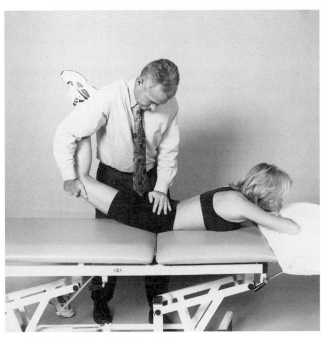

FIGURE 17–29   Active mobilization of the right innominate into anterior rotation.

new barrier to anterior rotation is achieved by further extension of the hip. The mobilization is repeated three times and followed by a reexamination of function.

Home Exercise to Produce Anterior Rotation of the Innominate   The patient is positioned in supine on a bed with the uninvolved extremity flexed to the chest and the involved leg close to the edge of the bed. The patient lowers the involved leg toward the floor producing a combined motion of hip extension and slight abduction until the motion barrier is reached. From this position the patient performs an isometric contraction of the hip adductor muscles for 3–5 seconds. The patient then initiates slight hip flexion and holds this position for 3–5 seconds. Following each contraction, the patient moves their involved leg into further hip extension to localize the new motion barrier. The exercise is repeated 2–3 times.

Techniques to Restore Posterior Rotation of the Right Innominate

Passive Mobilization   Patient lies supine with the knees and hips flexed, and the clinician stands at the patient's right side. With the long and ring finger of the left hand, the clinician palpates the right sacral sulcus, just medial to the posterior inferior iliac spine, to monitor motion between the right innominate bone and the sacrum. With the index finger of the same hand, the clinician palpates the lumbosacral junction to note any movement between the pelvic girdle and the L5 vertebra. The heel of the right hand is placed on the right ASIS and iliac crest (Figure 17–30). A grade II to IV posterior rotation force is applied to the right ASIS and iliac crest to produce an anterior-superior glide at the sacroiliac joint.

Active Mobilization: Method One   The patient is positioned in supine near the end of the bed, with the clinician standing on the right side of the patient. If necessary, a towel roll is placed under the patient's lumbar spine. With the index and middle fingers of the left hand, the clinician palpates the lumbosacral junction and the sacral sulcus. With the right hand, the clinician cups the right ischial tuberosity and, by leaning onto the patient's right leg, passively flexes the patient's right hip to the point of restriction (Figure 17–31). Further hip flexion rotates the innominate posteriorly, and this is applied until the motion at the lumbosacral junction is perceived. The sacroiliac joint motion barrier has then been reached. The patient is asked to extend the right hip against the clinician's chest. This isometric contraction is held for up to 5 seconds, following which, the patient is instructed to completely relax. The new barrier to posterior rotation is localized by further flexion of the hip joint. This mobilization is repeated three times and followed by a reexamination.

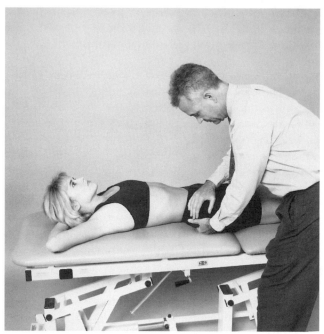

FIGURE 17–30   Active mobilization into nutation of the sacrum on the right.

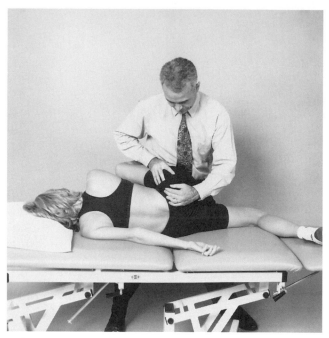

FIGURE 17–32   Active mobilization of the right innominate into posterior rotation, using the gluteus maximus.

Active Mobilization: Method Two   Patient left side-lying, facing the clinician. The patient's left leg is stabilized by the clinician, or by a belt. The patient's right leg is placed around the trunk of the clinician and the right hip is flexed to the barrier. The right leg must not be allowed to

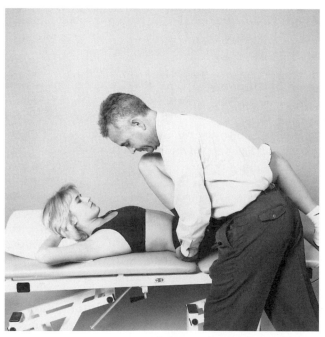

FIGURE 17–31   Patient and clinician position for passive mobilization of the right innominate into posterior rotation.

adduct. The right innominate is grasped by both hands (Figure 17–32). The patient is then instructed to extend their right hip against the clinician's trunk. If the patient keeps the right knee flexed (see Figure 17–32), only the gluteus maximus is used for the contraction. By keeping the right leg straight, the patient utilizes the hamstrings as well as the gluteus maximus (Figure 17–33). This isometric contraction is held for up to 5 seconds, following which, the patient is instructed to completely relax. The new barrier to posterior rotation is localized by further flexion of the hip joint. This mobilization is repeated three times and followed by a reexamination.

Active Mobilization: Method Three   The patient is positioned in prone-lying with their right hip and leg over the edge of the table. The clinician stands at the patient's right side. The patient's right foot is placed between the clinician's legs and held there. While monitoring the sacral sulcus with the index finger of the left hand, the clinician moves the patient's right leg to the barrier (Figure 17–34). The patient is asked to gently push the right foot toward the foot of the table. This movement is resisted by the clinician left leg, and after 3 to 5 seconds, the patient is told to relax. Once again, when full relaxation has occurred, the slack is taken up and the patient's right leg is moved in the direction of hip flexion until the monitoring finger indicates that the new barrier has been reached. This mobilization is repeated three times and followed by a reexamination.

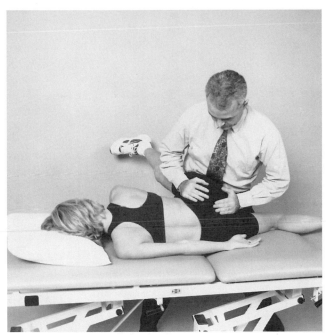

FIGURE 17–33 Patient and clinician position for active mobilization of the right innominate into posterior rotation, using the gluteus maximus and hamstrings.

Home Exercise to Produce Posterior Rotation of the Innominate The patient is positioned in supine on a bed with their uninvolved extremity hanging off the edge of the bed, while the involved extremity is positioned in flexion towards the chest. Once the motion barrier is engaged, the patient attempts to gently extend the hip of the involved side against an unyielding counterforce for about 3–5 seconds. Upon relaxation, the patient further flexes and posteriorly rotates their involved hip to localize the new motion barrier. The exercise is repeated 2–3 times.

Techniques to Correct a Counternutation of the Sacrum on the Right (R on L)
This is not a motion that occurs in normal walking. It can only occur when the lumbar spine is operating in nonneutral mechanics. It is always associated with a nonneutral impairment of the lumbar spine, often with a restriction of extension. The correction is thought to be produced by the combined action of the right piriformis, pulling the sacrum and the gluteus medius, with the tendon of fascia lata pulling on the ilium.

Active Mobilization: Method One The patient is positioned on the left side with the clinician facing the patient. The L5–S1 junction is palpated with the right hand. The clinician positions the patient using an upper lock of left rotation (see Chap 13). The clinician grasps the patient's left ankle, and moves the left hip into extension, until motion is felt to occur at the sacral base (Figure 17–35). The patient is asked to resist the clinician's attempt to move the hip into further extension. This is achieved by activation of the erector spinae and the left iliopsoas muscles. The patient relaxes and the clinician locates the new motion barrier.

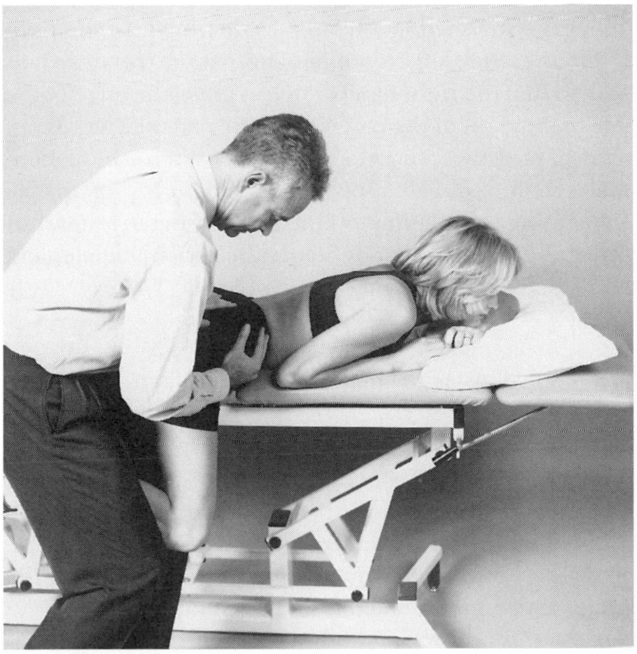

FIGURE 17–34 Active mobilization of the right innominate into posterior rotation (side-lying).

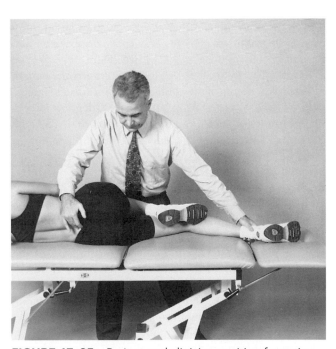

FIGURE 17–35 Patient and clinician position for active mobilization to correct a counternutation of the sacrum on the right.

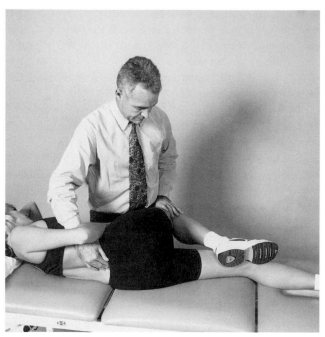

FIGURE 17–36 Active mobilization technique for a Right on Left correction.

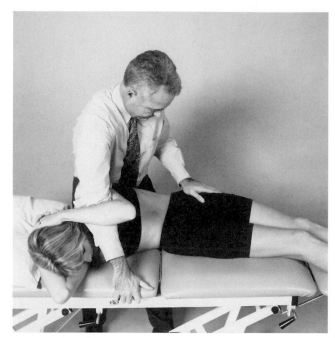

FIGURE 17–37 Patient and clinician position for thrust technique for a Right on Left correction.

Active Mobilization: Method Two   The patient is positioned on the left side with the clinician facing the patient. The L5–S1 junction is palpated with the right hand. The clinician locks down from above using an extension and right rotation lock of the lumbar spine. The clinician extends the patient's left leg until the sacral base is felt to move. The patient's right hip is passively flexed to about 90 degrees, producing a posterior rotation of the right innominate. The leg is positioned so that the right knee is off the edge of the bed (Figure 17–36). The patient is asked to abduct the right leg toward the ceiling against the resistance of the clinician. The piriformis is an abductor of the hip when the hip is flexed to 90 degrees. Its contraction produces a right nutation of the sacrum. The contraction and relaxation is repeated and the patient is reassessed.

Thrust Technique for a Right on Left   A thrust technique may also be used to correct a posterior sacral torsion. The patient lies supine and his or her fingers are laced together behind the neck with the elbows forward. The patient's pelvis should be close to the clinician (at the side of the table) and the patient's feet and upper trunk are moved to the opposite side of the table, producing a right side bend of the patient's trunk. Leaning over the patient, the clinician threads his or her right forearm, from the lateral side, through the gap between the patient's left arm and chest, and grasps the edge of the table, thereby rotating the patient's thorax away without losing the patient's right side-flexion until the patient's left ilium just begins to lift off the

table. The clinician holds the left ilium down, and takes up any slack by slightly increasing the rotation without losing the side-bend. The correction is made by a high-velocity, low-amplitude thrust using the left hand in a posterior direction (Fig 17–37). The patient is then reevaluated.

Home Exercise to Treat a Right on Left Sacral Torsion   The patient is positioned in left lateral side lying with the right leg off the edge of the table. The patient rotates their trunk so that the right hand is able to grasp the edge of the table to the right of the patient and the patient's face is oriented toward the ceiling. From this position, the patient inhales slightly and attempts to lift the right leg toward the ceiling using only slight movement. The isometric contraction is held for 3–5 seconds before the patient exhales and lowers their foot to the new motion barrier. The exercise is repeated 2–3 times.

Technique to Treat a Nutated Sacrum on the Right (L on L)

Active Mobilization   Because the ILA is both posterior and caudal on the left side, there are a number of muscles around the hip that are utilized to pull the sacrum into the correct position. With a nutated sacrum on the right, the right piriformis is often tight, so this technique attempts to relax the right piriformis and its antagonists, the right hip internal rotators, through a reciprocal inhibition of the right piriformis. At the same time, a pull from the left piriformis is encouraged to help pull the sacrum into its correct position.

The patient is positioned in left side-lying, facing the clinician. As the dysfunction is a nutated sacrum on the right (L on L), the patient is positioned to encourage a counternutation of the sacrum on the right (R on L). To produce a Right on Left motion of the sacrum, the lumbar spine is positioned in flexion (which extends the sacrum, pulling the right sacral base posteriorly) and right rotation (which will also pull the right sacral base posteriorly) by flexing the patient from below using the legs. The patient's trunk is placed into rotation into the table by placing the right arm over the edge of the table and the left arm behind them so that the chest is resting on the table. This position is accentuated by asking the patient to reach toward the floor with the right hand. The clinician flexes the patient's hips by grasping the patient's feet and ankles with his or her left hand, while palpating for motion at the patient's sacral base with the right hand. The patient's thighs are supported on the clinician's thighs.

With the patient's lower legs off the edge of the table (Figure 17–38), the patient's left piriformis is placed on stretch, producing a passive right rotation of the sacrum. The patient is asked to perform lateral rotation of the left hip and medial rotation of the right hip simultaneously. After each 3- to 5-second contraction, the slack is taken up and the new motion barrier is located while the L5–S1 junction is palpated. It is important that the L5–S1 junction remain in neutral throughout the whole procedure. At the new motion barrier, the clinician grasps the patient's ankles and raises them to the ceiling, until the sacral base begins to move. At this point, the patient is asked to either push the feet toward the ceiling against the clinician's resistance or to push the feet down toward the floor against the clinician's resistance. After a 3- to 5-second contraction, the patient relaxes and the clinician raises the patient's feet toward the ceiling.

Home Exercise to Treat a Left on Left Sacral Torsion The patient is positioned in left side lying, Sims position with both feet and knees positioned near the edge of the bed. The patient reaches toward the floor with the right hand to increase rotation of the lumbar spine to the left. From this position, both feet are lowered off the bed toward the floor, creating left side-flexion of the lumbar spine, to the motion barrier. The exercise involves the patient attempting to lift their feet toward the ceiling using only slight movement, while taking and holding a deep breath. The isometric contraction is held for 3–5 seconds before the patient exhales and lowers their feet to the new motion barrier. The exercise is repeated 2–3 times.

Therapeutic Exercise

No prospective trials have evaluated the effect of aerobic exercise, stabilization exercises, or restoration of range of motion in these interventions. Empirically, however, exercise has been an important aspect of intervention for musculoskeletal impairments, and general rehabilitation principles applied in a manner specific for the sacroiliac joint should be instituted.

For the most part, exercises are avoided in the acute stage as they tend to increase the symptoms. Intervention strategies should emphasize pelvic stabilization,[121] the elimination of trunk and lower extremity muscle imbalances, and the correction of gait abnormalities.[122] This includes stretching of the trunk and lower extremities, especially the piriformis, gluteus maximus, and hamstring, because of their attachment to the sacrotuberous ligament and potential influences on the sacroiliac joint.[29] Corrective exercises can be used to position the innominate bone in proper relation to the sacrum. Postural correction and the correction of compensatory movements need to be addressed. As symptoms are controlled, therapy should be advanced to activity-specific stabilization exercises to facilitate return to function at the patients' occupation, sport, or avocational activities.

No group of exercises are exclusive for the sacroiliac joint, so it is necessary to approach the rehabilitation of this region to include the lumbar spine and hip joints. The focus of the therapeutic exercises is to augment the force closure mechanism and to reduce any stress that could prove detrimental to the sacroiliac complex. The same principles

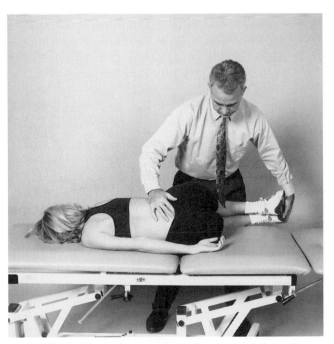

FIGURE 17–38 Patient and clinician position for active mobilization technique for a Left on Left correction.

apply here as elsewhere, stretch those muscles that are tight and shortened and strengthen those muscles that are found to be weak. The muscles to be stretched are usually the erector spinae, quadratus lumborum, hamstrings, rectus femoris, iliopsoas, tensor fascia lata, adductors, piriformis, and the deep external rotators of the hip.

The strengthening component of the exercises is aimed at improving the function of the muscles of the inner unit and outer unit. The appropriate muscles must be isolated and retrained to increase their strength and endurance, and to automatically recruit to support and protect the region. A four-stage program has been designed to isolate and retrain the inner unit.[123,124] The early stages are the most difficult to teach and often take the longest time to master. If limb motion is added or the load is increased beyond that which can be controlled by the inner unit, the pain will increase.

Inner Unit[33]

Stage 1   As a review, the inner unit consists of the four parts of the levator ani muscle, the multifidus, and the transversus abdominis, and the interrelationship between the pelvic floor and the abdominals.

● *Levator ani:* the patient is first taught the location of the levator ani. To strengthen the muscle, the patient is asked to shorten the distance between the coccyx and the pubic symphysis and to hold the contraction for 10 seconds. When the muscle contracts properly, the transverse abdominis muscle can be felt to contract at a point 2-cm medial and inferior to the ASIS, there is no contraction of the buttocks, and by carefully palpating the sacral apex, the sacrum is felt to counternutate as the levator ani contracts. The exercise is repeated 10 times.
● *Transversus abdominis and multifidus:* to test for isolation of the transversus abdominis, the patient is positioned in prone and a pressure biofeedback unit is placed underneath the abdomen.[123,124] The cuff is inflated to a base level of 70 mm Hg. The patient is asked to draw the navel up and in toward the chest (abdominal hollowing). When the muscle contracts properly, an increase in tension can be felt at a point 2-cm medial and inferior to the ASIS. If a bulging is felt at this point, the internal oblique is contracting. Simultaneously, the multifidus is palpated and should be felt to swell at a point just lateral to the spinous process.

If a pressure biofeedback unit is not available, an alternative technique can be used to test these muscles and involves the patient assuming the quadriped position on the hands and knees. The patient's shoulders and hips are centered over the hands and knees and the lumbar spine is in a neutral position. The patient is asked to take a deep breath in, breathe out, and then draw the navel up toward the spine (abdominal hollowing).[124] If performed correctly, the lower abdomen should elevate before the upper abdomen. There should be no expansion or contraction of the lower rib cage and the oblique muscles should not contract. The multifidus can be tested in this position by having the patient make the muscle harden under the clinician's fingers.

Outer Unit[33]

As a review, the outer unit consists of the following four systems.

● *Posterior oblique:* latissimus dorsi, gluteus maximus, and thoracodorsal fascia.
● *The deep longitudinal :* erector spinae muscle, deep lamina of thoracodorsal fascia, sacrotuberous ligament, and the biceps femoris muscle.
● *Anterior oblique:* oblique abdominals, contralateral adductor muscles of the thigh, and anterior abdominal fascia.
● *Lateral oblique:* gluteus medius and minimus and contralateral adductors of the thigh.

Stage 2   The stabilization program is progressed to the next stage with the introduction of lower or upper extremity motion, which changes the focus of the program to one of outer unit activation and control while maintaining the control over the inner unit.

In the supine position with the hips and knees flexed, the patient is asked to isolate the inner unit, while maintaining the lumbar spine in a neutral position. From this position, the patient is asked to slowly let the knee fall to one side. Alternatively, he or she may extend the leg with the foot supported on the table. The exercise can be made more difficult by asking the patient to lift the foot off the table while maintaining the hip and knee flexed.

The final progression involves asking the patient to slowly extend this leg (with the foot lifted) to 45 degrees above the table. This exercise is initially performed unilaterally, and is then progressed to alternate leg extensions. The same exercises can be performed sitting on a gym ball or lying supine on a long roll. By making the base unstable, the exercise becomes more difficult without having to progress into the next stage.

Exercising on a gym ball requires core stability (inner unit control), coordination, and appropriate reflexes. While sitting on the ball, the patient is asked to contract the muscles of the inner unit. This contraction is maintained while the patient moves forward and back and up and down on the ball. The patient is instructed to incorporate the cocontraction of the inner unit into his or her activities of daily living.

If the individual muscles of an outer unit system are weak or poorly recruited, the exercise program should include isolation and training at this time.

- *Posterior oblique system:* in the posterior oblique system, it is common to find the gluteus maximus both lengthened and weak.[33] Having the patient squeeze the buttocks together and sustain the contraction for 10 seconds isolates the gluteus maximus. A surface electromyography (EMG) unit can provide a useful biofeedback system for this muscle. The exercise is progressed by having the patient lie prone over a gym ball and asking him or her to initially recruit the inner unit and then extend the hip while the knee is flexed. Lifting the extended thigh increases the degree of difficulty.

Leg extension machines can help to strengthen the gluteal group. Initially, the patient exercises in the supine position with one or both feet on the foot plate.

Functional training is introduced by having the patient practice going from sitting to standing with a stabilized trunk, using primarily the gluteus maximus.

- *Lateral system:* In the lateral system, the posterior fibers of the gluteus medius are often weak, which can have a marked impact on walking and load transference through the hip joint.[63]

Isolation of the gluteus medius is taught in the sidelying position with a pillow placed between the knees. The exercise is progressed by asking the patient to lift the knee off of the pillow and then to extend the knee while maintaining the correct position of the trunk and hip. Resistance can be added using a theraband, or a cuff weight.

- *Anterior system:* isolation of the anterior oblique system involves training the specific contraction of the external and internal oblique abdominals. When the external obliques contract bilaterally, the infrasternal angle narrows, whereas when internal obliques contract bilaterally, the infrasternal angle widens. The patient is taught to palpate the lateral costal margin and to specifically widen and narrow the infrasternal angle through specific contraction of the oblique abdominals.

The progression includes activation of the anterior and posterior oblique systems and differentiation of trunk from thigh motion. To begin, the patient is supine with the hips and knees flexed. The patient is asked to bridge and then to rotate the trunk and pelvic girdle at the hip joints in the unsupported position, while maintaining the lumbar joints in a neutral position.

Stage 3 Stage-3 exercises involve controlled motion of "the unstable region."[123] Because this stage is much more advanced, it is only given when required by an individual's work or sport. The protocol includes concentric and eccentric work with variable resistance in all three planes.

Stage 4 Stage 4[123] of the protocol involves stabilization during high-speed motions. Very few people require stage-4 stabilization, particularly in view of the fact that high-speed exercise tends to reduce the ability of the trunk muscles to stabilize.[124]

In addition to the strengthening protocol outlined, the clinician must correct any muscle imbalances in the following muscles, or muscle groups:

- Hip adductors
- Hip flexors
- Hamstrings
- Tensor fascia lata
- Piriformis
- Lumbodorsal fascia
- Quadratus lumborum
- Abdominals

Orthoses

Various investigators have advocated the use of orthoses in the intervention of this region,[125–127] but no prospective studies have been done to evaluate the effectiveness of bracing. Clinicians often correct leg length discrepancies of greater than 0.5 inches, as such inequalities have been described as altering normal sacroiliac joint function.[127] Sacroiliac (S) joint and pelvic stabilization orthoses have been employed in an attempt to limit SI joint motion and improve proprioception.[128] Not much force is needed to be exerted by these belts (20 to 50 newtons) to afford relief to the patient.[128] The elastic ones tend to be better than the firm ones, but the sacrum-shaped patches are not very useful. The position of the belt, in terms of its height on the ilium, should be experimented with to find the optimal position for pain relief. The recommended position is just above the greater trochanter.[129] A bicycle inner tube can be used as an SI belt, as this is the right width and has the correct degree of elasticity. The following conditions appear to respond well to bracing.

1. Sacroiliitis
2. Sacroiliac hypermobility and instability (pre-and post-partum and microtraumatic)
3. Pubic instability (may afford some relief)

Electrotherapeutic Modalities and Physical Agents

The application of hot and/or cold packs, ultrasound, TENS, and so forth, are indicated when the joint has been demonstrated to be inflamed by the primary stress tests. Together with the external support, these modalities complete the rest, ice, compression, and elevation approach to acute inflammatory states.

Patient Education

This involves advice on what activities and postures to avoid, and what resting positions to adopt.

Case Study: Left-sided Low Back and Buttock Pain

Subjective

A 47-year-old male presented at the clinic who had developed left-sided low back and buttock pain while at work 2 weeks previously. When describing the mechanism of injury, the patient reported feeling something "pop" in his low back during a lifting maneuver that involved bending forward and twisting to the right. The pain was now localized to an area slightly inferior to the left posterior superior iliac spine (PSIS), which he reported as being very tender to the touch. The pain was also aggravated with forward bending and turning at the waist to the left in sitting. The patient reported sleeping well, provided that he remained prone, and there were no complaints of paresthesias or anesthesias. The patient denied any neurologic symptoms related to cauda equina or spinal cord involvement. The patient was in otherwise good health.

Questions
1. Given a distinct mechanism of injury, what structure(s) could be at fault with complaints of left-sided low back and buttock pain?
2. What does the region of localized tenderness tell the clinician?
3. Why do you think the patient is sleeping well in prone?
4. What is your working hypothesis at this stage? List the various diagnoses that could present with low back and buttock pain, and the tests you would use to rule out each one.
5. Does this presentation and history warrant a scan? Why or why not?

Examination
The patient had a specific mechanism of injury, and although the pain distribution initially was more widespread, the presence of a very localized area of pain, suggesting a musculoskeletal impairment, and so a lumbar and SI scan was not considered necessary. If this hypothesis proved incorrect, a lumbosacral scan would have been necessary.

His standing posture was unremarkable. Active range-of-motion testing for the lumbar spine revealed pain and restriction with forward flexion, right side-flexion, and left rotation. There was palpable tenderness along the S3–S4 level on the sacrum. However, a number of structures in this specific area are capable of producing pain. As a ligament sprain was suspected, the iliolumbar ligament was assessed but did not reproduce the pain. The anterior and posterior stress tests for the sacroiliac joint were also assessed. The anterior test was negative and, although the posterior test caused a slight increase in symptoms, it was not considered a positive test. The long dorsal ligament was assessed. The patient was positioned in prone, and the clinician, while palpating the tender area with one hand, pushed the sacral base anteriorly with the palm of the other hand, thereby producing a sacral nutation. The tenderness lessened according to the patient. To produce a counternutation, and therefore stress the long dorsal ligament, both ILA were pushed anteriorly. This maneuver immediately caused a significant increase in the patient's pain. It was decided to use a functional test for the long dorsal ligament to confirm the hypothesis.

The patient was positioned in supine with both legs straight. The patient was asked to perform a straight leg raise with the left leg and to hold the leg about 5 degrees off the bed. As the initial 5 degrees of a straight leg raise produces an anterior rotation of the ilium and a counternutation force of the sacrum on the ipsilateral side, a positive finding for this test is the reproduction of pain or weakness. Slight modifications to the test were used to help in the confirmation.

- The right knee was flexed and the patient was asked to perform a straight leg raise with the right leg. Flexing the contralateral knee to the straight leg raise has the effect of relaxing the lumbar spine while maintaining the counternutation on the ipsilateral side. If this decreases the pain, a muscle imbalance is probably present (quadratus lumborum, multifidus, etc.).
- The patient was asked to lift the right shoulder off bed against manual resistance from the clinician, while performing the straight leg raise on the right. This tests the ability of the anterior oblique system of force closure.
- The sacroiliac joint was manually compressed via the innominates as in the posterior stress test of the sacroiliac joint, while the patient performed a straight leg raise on the right. Compressing the innominates produces a slight counternutation of the sacrum.

All of the modifications produced an increase in the patient's symptoms, confirming the provisional diagnosis of a sprained left long dorsal sacroiliac ligament.

Questions

1. Having confirmed the diagnosis, what will be your intervention?
2. How would you describe this condition to the patient?
3. In order of priority, and based on the stages of healing, list the various goals of your intervention?
4. How will you determine the amplitude and joint position for the intervention?
5. What would you tell the patient about your intervention?
6. Estimate this patient's prognosis
7. What modalities could you use in the intervention of this patient?
8. What exercises would you prescribe?

Intervention

● *Electrotherapeutic modalities and thermal agents.* A moist heat pack was applied to the area over the long dorsal ligament when the patient arrived for each treatment session. Electrical stimulation with a medium frequency of 50 to 120 pulses per second was applied with the moist heat to aid in pain relief. Ultrasound at 1 MHz was administered following the moist heat. An ice pack was applied to the area at the end of the treatment session

● *Manual therapy.* Following the ultrasound, transverse frictional massage was applied to the tender aspect of the ligament

● *Therapeutic exercises.* To strengthen the opposite gluteus maximus, exercises for the ipsilateral latissimus dorsi and the erector spinae of both sides were prescribed. To achieve this, the following exercises were used.

1. Lunges. The patient grasped a weight in the right hand and was asked to perform a lunge, leading with the left leg, while swinging the right arm into shoulder extension.
2. To strengthen the erector spinae, the patient wore a rucksack containing cuff-weights on the front of the trunk throughout the therapeutic exercise session.
3. Lat pull downs were prescribed to strengthen the latissimus dorsi.
4. Seated rows were initiated to strengthen the latissimus dorsi.
5. Aerobic exercises using a stationary bike and upper body ergometer (UBE) were also prescribed.

● *Patient-related instruction.* Explanation was given as to the cause of the patient's symptoms. The patient was advised against bending forward and twisting to the right in standing, and forward bending and turning at the waist to the left in sitting. The patient was instructed to continue sleeping in the prone position.

The patient received instructions regarding correct lifting techniques. The patient was advised to continue the exercises at home, 3 to 5 times each day and to expect some postexercise soreness. The patient also received instruction on the use of heat and ice at home.

● *Goals and outcomes.* Both the patient's goals from the treatment and the expected therapeutic goals from the clinician were discussed with the patient. It was concluded that the clinical sessions would occur three times per week for a month, at which time, the patient would be discharged to a home exercise program. With adherence to the instructions and exercise program, it was felt that the patient would make a full return to function.

Case Study: Tail Bone Pain

Subjective

A 26-year-old female presented herself to the clinic after a fall down the stairs with her 3-month-old baby in her arms 2 weeks previously. While the baby was not hurt, the patient had landed in a sitting position. Immediately after the accident she was able to walk, but the pain persisted in the anal region.

Examination

On examination, the only positive finding was pain with sitting and palpable tenderness at the level of the sacrococcygeal joint. On rectal examination, a painful anterior displacement of the joint was confirmed.

Intervention

Correction for this impairment involves grasping the coccyx after inserting the index finger in the anal canal. The coccyx is distracted and pulled posteriorly, while pulling laterally on the medial surface of the ischial tuberosity.

Case Study: Right-sided Low Back Pain

Subjective

A 55-year-old male presented with right-sided low back pain that occurred while lifting a heavy object at work. The pain occasionally spread along the right iliac crest to the groin area and was aggravated with sustained postures, especially standing, sitting up straight, and twisting to the left. A recent x-ray was unremarkable.

Examination

No deviation was visible in the standing position.

● Demonstration of full range of motion in all planes, but with pain at the end ranges of flexion and extension, and side-flexion to the left.

- No dural or nerve root findings.
- Normal findings for the hip and sacroiliac joints.
- Positive anterior shear test for pain and slight increase in mobility.
- Positive iliolumbar ligament stress test.

Evaluation

One of the classic signs of an iliolumbar ligament sprain is a nonarticular pattern with the H and I tests (see Chap 13), and a subjective history of a lifting and twisting injury. Pain can be referred from this structure down to the foot, but more commonly into the buttocks.

Intervention

This is a difficult impairment to treat but it usually responds well to rest, transverse friction massage, and ultrasound. The ligament takes at least 12 weeks to recover. The use of tape to remind patients to avoid certain positions is useful.

Case Study: Right-sided Low Back and Buttock Pain

Subjective

A 22-year-old male soccer player presented at the clinic with complaints of right-sided low back and buttock pain that occurred after an over-zealous right-legged kick against a missed target about 2 weeks previously. Initially, the pain had been intense, but had now subsided to a dull ache that was aggravated with weight bearing on one limb, bending backward, walking, and supine-lying with the extremity in extension. The patient reported sleeping well, and there were no complaints of paresthesia or anesthesia. The patient denied any neurologic symptoms related to cauda equina or spinal cord involvement. The patient appeared in good health.

Questions

1. What structure(s) could be at fault with complaints of right-sided low back and buttock pain?
2. What does the history of the pain tell the clinician?
3. Why do you think the patient is sleeping well?
4. What information does the subjective history of no paresthesia or anesthesia give the clinician?
5. What questions would you ask to help rule out a cauda equina impairment?
6. What questions would you ask to help rule out a spinal cord impairment?
7. What is your working hypothesis at this stage? List the various diagnoses that could present with low back and buttock pain, and the tests you would use to rule out each one.
8. Does this presentation and history warrant a scan? Why or why not?

Examination

The patient has a specific mechanism of injury that suggests a musculoskeletal impairment, and so the lumbosacral scan was not performed. An observation of the patient's gait revealed a shortened stance phase and a marked vertical limp. His standing posture was unremarkable. The H and I tests (see Chap 13) were positive in the posterior right quadrant, but the tests were negative if sacral motion was prevented. Because of this finding, a sacroiliac examination was initiated, which revealed the following.

- The left iliac crest was inferior relative to the right in standing and sitting, but superior relative to the right in lying. This reversal in position of the crests from sitting and standing to lying is thought to be due to the release of tension from the iliopsoas and quadratus lumborum muscles which, in standing, were counteracting the effects of gravity. Relaxation of these muscles in the supine position allows the true position of the left iliac crest relative to the sacrum to be seen.
- The left ASIS was slightly anterior relative to the right in standing and sitting.
- The lumbar spine has a left convexity.
- Point tenderness was elicited on the crest of the left ilium at the origin of the lateral margin of the iliocostalis lumborum muscle, and the left iliotibial band.
- A trigger point was found deep in the buttock within the piriformis muscle.
- The weight-bearing ipsilateral kinetic test was positive on the right, but negative in the nonweight-bearing position.
- The corresponding short arm test was restricted.
- The contralateral kinetic test was positive on the left, but negative in the nonweight-bearing position.
- The corresponding long arm test was restricted.
- In prone, fullness was found posterior to the left transverse process of the fifth lumbar vertebra, the lumbar lordosis was accentuated, the sacral sulcus was deeper on the right than on the left, and the sacral lateral angle (ILA) was posterior and inferior on the left.
- With sacral stabilization through the left innominate, which was prevented from rotating anteriorly by the application of a caudal counter force against the inferior aspect of the ASIS, extension and medial rotation of the right innominate was passively induced and a hard capsular end feel was gained.
- With passive physiologic mobility testing, innominate motion was restricted on the right.

Questions

1. Why were the initial H and I tests positive?
2. Did the sacral examination confirm your working hypothesis? How?

3. What was the reason for the left convexity in the lumbar spine?
4. What information was gathered from the modified H and I tests?
5. Given the findings from the biomechanical examination of the sacroiliac joint, what is the diagnosis, or is further testing warranted in the form of special tests? What information would be gained with further testing?

Evaluation

It was deduced from the clinical findings that the patient had a loss of the anterior rotation of the right innominate and a loss of the counternutation of the sacrum on the right. This is also referred to as a type I left sacral torsion syndrome.[111]

Questions

1. Having confirmed the diagnosis, what will be your intervention?
2. How would you describe this condition to the patient?
3. In order of priority, and based on the stages of healing, list the various goals of your intervention?
4. How will you determine the amplitude and joint position for the intervention?
5. What would you tell the patient about your intervention?
6. Estimate this patient's prognosis.
7. What modalities could you use in the intervention of this patient?
8. What exercises would you prescribe?

Intervention

- *Electrotherapeutic modalities and thermal agents.* A moist heat pack was applied to the lumbar spine when the patient arrived for each treatment session. Electrical stimulation with a medium frequency of 50 to 120 pulses per second was applied with the moist heat to aid in pain relief. Ultrasound at 1 MHz was administered following the moist heat. An ice pack was applied to the area at the end of the treatment session.
- *Manual therapy.* Following the ultrasound, soft tissue techniques were applied to the area followed by a specific mobilization. The manual intervention for this condition involves the correction of the loss of the anterior rotation of the right innominate and a loss of the counternutation of the sacrum on the right. These asymmetries are treated separately using any one of the previously outlined techniques.
- *Therapeutic exercises.* To strengthen the abdominals, the gluteals, the multifidus, and the erector spinae, therapeutic exercises were prescribed. Aerobic exercises using a stationary bike and upper body ergometer (UBE) were also prescribed.
- *Patient-related instruction.* Explanation was given as to the cause of the patient's symptoms. Instructions to

sleep on the side were given. The patient received instructions regarding correct lifting techniques. The patient was advised to continue the exercises at home, 3 to 5 times each day and to expect some postexercise soreness. The patient also received instruction on the use of heat and ice at home.

- *Goals and outcomes.* Both the patient's goals from the treatment and the expected therapeutic goals from the clinician were discussed with the patient. It was concluded that the clinical sessions would occur three times per week for 1 month, at which time, the patient would be discharged to a home exercise program. With adherence to the instructions and exercise program, it was felt that the patient would make a full return to function.

Case Study: Right-sided Low Back, Buttock, and Posterior Thigh Pain

Subjective

A 35-year old pregnant female presented at the clinic with an insidious onset of right-sided low back, buttock, and right posterior thigh pain. She described the onset as occurring the previous month during the sixth month of her pregnancy, and could not remember any particular event that precipitated the pain. The pain was aggravated by bending forward, or to her left side, and was alleviated with sitting or supine-lying. The patient reported sleeping well, and there were no complaints of paresthesias or anesthesias. The patient denied any neurologic symptoms related to cauda equina or spinal cord involvement. The patient appeared in good health.

Questions

1. What structure(s) could be at fault with complaints of right-sided low back and posterior thigh pain?
2. What does the history of the onset tell the clinician?
3. What effect does pregnancy have on ligamentous structures?
4. What information does the subjective history of no paresthesia or anaesthesia give the clinician?
5. What is your working hypothesis at this stage? List the various diagnoses that could present with low back and buttock pain, and the tests you would use to rule out each one.
6. Does this presentation and history warrant a scan? Why or why not?

Examination

The patient appeared to be a healthy, pregnant female. However, due to the insidious onset of her symptoms and the fact that the patient was experiencing a potential radiculopathy, a lumbar and sacroiliac scan was performed, which revealed the following positive findings.

● Restriction of forward bending
● Restriction of left side-flexion

Both motions reproduced the posterior thigh pain and a "pulling sensation" over the right lower lumbar area. Due to the fact that the neurologic tests were negative, an assumption was made that the posterior thigh pain was referred, and a biomechanical examination was initiated. The H and I tests (see Chap 13) were positive in the anterior right quadrant, indicating a flexion and right side-flexion restriction, but the tests were negative if sacral motion was prevented. Because of this finding, a sacroiliac examination was initiated, which revealed the following.

● The left iliac crest was inferior relative to the right in standing, but superior relative to the right in sitting.[111,112]
● The left ASIS was considerably more ventral relative to the right in standing and sitting.[111,112]
● The lumbar spine demonstrated a left convexity.
● Point tenderness was elicited at the origin of the left iliocostalis on the left iliac crest and the left iliotibial band.
● The ipsilateral and contralateral kinetic tests were positive on the left, as were their corresponding short and long arm tests.[111,112]
● In supine, the right iliac crest was superior relative to the left.[111,112]
● In prone, there was fullness felt posterior to the right transverse process of the fifth lumbar vertebrae, the lumbar lordosis was decreased, the sacral sulcus was deeper on the right than on the left, the sacral ILA was posterior on the left, and the sacral ILA was inferior on the left.[111,112]
● With passive physiologic mobility testing, the sacrum was stabilized through the left innominate, which was prevented from rotating posteriorly, by the application of a caudal counter force against the superior aspect of the ASIS, and the right innominate was rotated passively into flexion and lateral rotation and a hard capsular end feel was gained.[111,112]

Questions

1. Did the sacral examination confirm your working hypothesis? How?
2. Why were the lumbar motions of forward bending and left side-flexion restricted?
3. Given the findings from the biomechanical examination of the sacroiliac joint, what is the diagnosis, or is further testing warranted in the form of special tests? What information would be gained with further testing?

Evaluation

Based on the clinical findings of a loss of the posterior rotation of the right innominate and a loss of the nutation of the sacrum on the right, the diagnosis of a type II left sacral torsion was made.

Questions

1. Having confirmed the diagnosis, what will be your intervention?
2. How would you describe this condition to the patient?
3. In order of priority, and based on the stages of healing, list the various goals of your intervention?
4. How will you determine the amplitude and joint position for the intervention?
5. How would you explain the rationale of your intervention to the patient?
6. Estimate this patient's prognosis.
7. What modalities could you use in the intervention of this patient?
8. What exercises would you prescribe?

Intervention

● *Electrotherapeutic modalities and thermal agents.* A moist heat pack was applied to the sacroiliac joint when the patient arrived for each treatment session. Due to the fact that the patient was pregnant, it was felt that the use of electrical stimulation and ultrasound was contraindicated. An ice pack was applied to the area at the end of the treatment session.
● *Manual therapy.* Following the moist heat, soft tissue techniques were applied to the area followed by a specific mobilization. The manual intervention for this condition involves the correction for the loss of the posterior rotation of the right innominate and a loss of the nutation of the sacrum on the right. These asymmetries are treated separately using any one of the previously outlined techniques.
● *Therapeutic exercises.* To strengthen the abdominals, the gluteals, the multifidus, and the erector spinae, therapeutic exercises were prescribed. Aerobic exercises using a stationary bike and upper body ergometer (UBE) were also prescribed.
● *Patient-related instruction.* Explanation was given as to the cause of the patient's symptoms. Instructions to sleep on the side were given. The patient received instructions regarding correct lifting techniques. The patient was advised to continue the exercises at home, 3 to 5 times each day and to expect some postexercise soreness. The patient also received instruction on the use of heat and ice at home.
● *Goals and outcomes.* Both the patient's goals from the treatment and the expected therapeutic goals from the clinician were discussed with the patient. It was

concluded that the clinical sessions would occur three times per week for 1 month, at which time, the patient would be discharged to a home exercise program. With adherence to the instructions and exercise program, it was felt that the patient would make a full return to function.

Case Study: Right Groin Pain[130]

Subjective

The patient was a 55-year-old woman who presented with a diagnosis of right hip pain. The patient reported injuring the right leg 3 months prior but was unable to recall any specific mechanism of injury. For the subsequent 2 months, the pain had worsened and the patient sought a medical consultation. X-rays were taken, and a diagnosis of early osteoarthritis was made. The patient was immediately referred to physical therapy.

The patient described the area of pain as the right groin area, radiating into the right anterior thigh. She also complained of right posterior low back pain. The pain was of a variable, intermittent-type ache, aggravated by walking and eased by rest in the supine position. On waking, the patient felt no pain. The pain was reduced on rising compared with the pain following prolonged weight bearing. During the day, the patient's job involved standing, walking, and sitting, and the patient's symptoms worsened as the day progressed. The patient reported sleeping well, and there were no complaints of paresthesias or anesthesias. The patient denied any neurologic symptoms related to cauda equina or spinal cord involvement. The patient was in good health.

Questions
1. What is your working hypothesis at this stage? List the various diagnoses of groin and anterior thigh pain that is aggravated by walking and relieved by rest.
2. Is the patient's condition irritable or nonirritable?
3. What part of the subjective history alludes to the fact that this is a musculoskeletal injury?
4. Does this presentation and history warrant a scan? Why or why not?
5. What special tests would you perform
6. By using active range of motion, how could you help confirm the diagnosis?

Discussion

A positive x-ray for early osteoarthritis and a vague diagnosis of right hip pain should not indicate to the clinician that the diagnosis of hip osteoarthritis is conclusive. Groin pain can be produced by a number of pathologies including muscle strain, prostatitis, orchitis, inguinal hernia, urolithiasis, ankylosing spondylitis, Reiter's syndrome, hyperparathyroidism, metastasis, osteitis pubis, stress fracture, and rheumatoid arthritis.[131] The anterior thigh pain could be lumbar in origin. The insidious onset, in addition to the other symptoms, warrants a scan.

The scan elicited the following findings.

- Capsular pattern of the lumbar spine
- Capsular pattern of the hips
- No neurologic deficits in terms of strength, sensation, or deep tendon reflexes
- Positive scour test of right hip

Questions
1. Did the scan confirm the working hypothesis? How?
2. Given the findings from the scan, what is the diagnosis, or is further testing warranted in the form of a biomechanical examination? What information would be gained with further testing?

Although the findings from the scan indicated a diagnosis of right hip osteoarthritis, a biomechanical examination should be performed to determine all of the impairments, and thus help formulate an intervention plan.

Examination

On observation, the patient walked with antalgic gait. Structural inspection revealed decreased weight bearing through the right leg, with a slight shift in the lumbar spine toward the left. There appeared to be a flattening of the right gluteal musculature. On palpation of the pelvic levels in standing, the right posterior inferior iliac spine was lower than the left. The levels of the greater trochanters, gluteal folds, and posterior knee creases appeared symmetrical. With passive range of motion, there was an abnormal capsular end feel limiting all ranges of hip motion. The accessory motions of the hip capsule were graded as having considerable restriction to motion. Directional glides at the hip joint do not occur and were not assessed. The lumbar spine and knee joints appeared normal.

Manual muscle testing was performed on the pelvic, hip, and knee musculature. On muscle length testing, there was tightness in the right iliopsoas, iliotibial band, and hamstring muscles. Extension of the right hip was measured as 5 degrees. The normal range of hip extension is 30 degrees.[132]

On evaluation of the patient's gait, she appeared to have a shorter stride length on the right and a decreased heel strike. There was an increased lumbar lordosis during midstance and push off. The patient ambulated with a cane.

Questions
1. Did the biomechanical examination confirm the working hypothesis? How?

2. Why was there a leg length discrepancy? List the potential causes of a leg length discrepancy.
3. Why was there a decreased heel strike and shorter stride length on the right?

Evaluation

As indicated earlier in this chapter, osteoarthritis (OA) is characterized by the deterioration of the cartilaginous weight-bearing surfaces of joints, sclerosis of subchondral bone, and proliferation of new bone at the joint margins.[133] Early osteoarthritis of the hip can have many manifestations in neighboring joints, particularly the lumbar spine and the foot. This is because the motion restrictions produced by the osteoarthritis process remove the amount of available rotation occurring at the hip. If the hip is unable to produce the rotation, the sacroiliac joint and lumbar spine are forced to absorb those forces.

Questions
1. Having confirmed the diagnosis, what will be your intervention?
2. In order of priority, and based on the stages of healing, what will be the goals of your intervention?

Intervention

Osteoarthritis is a common problem treated by physical therapists. In the involved joints, the intervention plan should address the decreased strength of the periarticular muscles,[132] the decreased flexibility, and the decreased aerobic capacity, which leads to decreased mobility and decreased activities of daily living.[133]

Recent guidelines set forth by the American College of Rheumatology (ACR) for the management of hip and knee OA highlight the importance of nonpharmacologic modes of therapy to relieve pain and improve joint biomechanics and overall function. These include local heat or ice, ultrasound, and stimulation with electrical devices (TENS).[134,135] Weight reduction in obese patients may also significantly relieve pain through a reduction of the biomechanical stress on weight-bearing joints. The use of proper orthotic devices and shock-absorbing shoes compensate for permanent functional deficits and are protective. The ACR guidelines also acknowledge the importance of exercise as an integral part of OA management.[135] Recent evidence indicates that joint loading and mobilization are essential for articular integrity.[136] In addition, quadriceps weakness develops early in OA, and may contribute to progressive articular damage.[137] Recent studies of community-residing older adults with symptomatic knee OA have shown improvements in physical performance, painful symptoms, and reports of disability after 3 months of aerobic or resistance exercise.[138] Others have shown that resistive strengthening and weight-bearing range of motion improves gait, strength, and overall function.[139,140] Low-impact or gravity-limiting activities, including water-resistive exercises or bicycle training, may achieve increased muscle tone and strength, neuromuscular function, and cardiovascular endurance without excessive force across, or injury to, joints.[138–143]

Intervention Stages

Early Stage (Acute)
- Rest and positioning of the hip in flexion, abduction, and external rotation. The patient can also sleep in this position.
- Home program of gluteal, quadriceps, and hamstring isometrics in varying parts of the range. Gentle, pain-free active and active assisted range-of-motion exercises.
- Distractive mobilization techniques are used.

Middle Stage (Subacute) Regaining muscle extensibility through hold and relax techniques followed by stretches.

- Inner quadrant flexion positional stretches to increase range into flexion. Patient can do the same exercise at home.
- FABERs positioning (flexion, abduction, and external rotation) with static and eccentric contract and relax techniques, while stabilizing the ilium.
- A home program is issued.

To determine the suitability of this patient for this home exercise protocol, a preliminary test is performed. The patient is instructed to sit on the floor, or a low stool, with the back against the wall and the legs crossed, so that the soles of the feet are facing each other. The patient allows the knees to drop to the side, toward the floor, and attempts to maintain this position for 5 minutes. If the patient is unable to tolerate the 5 minutes, the condition is probably too acute, and the patient is referred back to the physician for a course of nonsteroidals and/or injection.

If they are able to tolerate this, the distance between the lateral aspect of the knees and the floor is measured, and the patient is issued the following home program. During the next few weeks, the clinician calls the patient regularly to monitor progress.

- Using the above cross-legged position on the floor, stool, or a bed, the patient performs the position twice a day for 5 minutes. It is performed for 3 days.
- If the hip does not feel inflamed after the 3 days the patient adds 1 minute each day until he or she is able to tolerate a 10 minute session twice a day (this may take a while), at which point, the patient returns to the clinic.
- Following the reexamination, the protocol is continued at 10 minute sessions, twice a day, with the patient

adding 1 minute each day, until the position can be maintained for 15 minutes, twice a day. This progression is continued until the patient is able to tolerate this position for 20 minutes, twice a day.

Once at this level, the patient returns to the clinic for the initiation of a strengthening program and for mobilization techniques to mobilize the sacroiliac joint and/or lumbar spine if necessary.

- Contract-relax techniques into extension and internal rotation are initiated.
- Stretching of the adductors. The patient is positioned in prone, in the FABER position.
- Pendular swings. The patient stands on a step and swings the other leg in a pendular fashion.

Strengthening in nonweight-bearing and functional weight-bearing positions can take place as follows.

1. The patient sits erect with both hips flexed, abducted, and externally rotated. The patient is asked to rotate the trunk to the left then bring the left knee toward the chest. The procedure is repeated on the other side.
2. The patient is positioned in side-lying and the asymptomatic leg is placed in the knee to chest position, while the symptomatic hip is passively extended. The patient can perform a modification of this exercise at home by standing with the back against a wall, weight bearing through the symptomatic lower extremity, and bringing the asymptomatic one to the chest.
3. The patient stands in front of a chair and raises one leg to place a foot on the chair. While keeping the other leg extended, the patient leans toward the chair, increasing the flexion of the raised hip. The procedure is repeated on the other side. This functional weight-bearing exercise is safer to adopt than a full squat.
4. The patient is positioned in prone-lying. Russian electrical stimulation is applied to the gluteus maximus, while moist heat is placed over the buttocks.
5. The patient can perform side-stepping drills.
6. The patient can perform a hoopla-hoop motion at the hips and waist, while using both arms for support.

All of the exercises need to be done frequently, and for sustained periods.

Passive articular mobilizations are done as follows.

- The clinician emphasizes the regaining of the close packed position.
- Walking, if not antalgic, provides excellent mobilization.
- Joint distraction: these techniques are used if the pain is felt by the patient before the end feel. The patient is supine with the clinician sitting beside the patient. The

patient's leg is placed over the clinician's shoulder in the open pack, or resting, position. The clinician takes hold of the patient's thigh as high up as possible and applies traction through the line of the femoral neck. A belt can also be used for this technique. If the patient is unable to tolerate this position, he or she rests the thigh on a pillow, in the open pack position, while the traction is applied.

- Leg traction (inferior glide): the patient is positioned in supine, with the hip placed in the resting position. The clinician grasps the patient's ankle and applies gentle oscillations along the length of the leg. The patient can be stabilized using one belt around the waist and another from the head of the bed and around the patient's pelvic floor.
- Flexion quadrant mobilizations. Grade II mobilizations are applied perpendicular to the arc of the joint throughout.

The use of strengthening exercises for patients with osteoarthritis is well documented.[146] These patients have type II fiber atrophy (refer to Chapter 11) in muscles supporting the joints.[146] Strengthening exercises are used to gain increased muscle strength to provide better shock-absorbing capabilities to the joints and to maintain and improve the use of the joint(s) in functional activities. It has been shown that aerobic weight-bearing exercises are not detrimental to the patient with osteoarthritis of the hip and help to improve the aerobic capacity.[132] Stretching and range-of-motion exercises are frequently recommended for patients with osteoarthritis, but there are no studies to support this. There are a number of therapeutic techniques aimed at increasing tissue length including joint mobilization, stretches, and proprioceptive neuromuscular facilitation.[147] With this patient, prolonged hip joint stretches, joint mobilizations, and proprioceptive neuromuscular facilitation were all applied with the aim of increasing the range of motion of the hip. This patient had an abnormal capsular end feel of the hip, which Cyriax described as suggestive of nonacute arthritis.[148]

By using prolonged stretching, joint mobilizations, proprioceptive neuromuscular facilitation, strengthening, and aerobic exercises, this patient had a significant decrease in pain, an increase in range of motion of the hip, increased strength of the periarticular hip musculature, improved mobility, and functional abilities.

Case Study: Pubic Pain[131]

Subjective

A 44-year-old man came to the clinic complaining of worsening abdominal and midline pelvic pain. The pain had developed gradually, and there was no report of recent direct trauma or acute injury. The pain was aggravated with forced flexion at the waist and the Valsalva maneuver, but the patient reported no pain at rest. The pain, described as a sharp, "stabbing" sensation, remained fairly localized to his upper pelvis and lower abdominal area.

The patient had no history of abdominal or genitourinary diseases or surgeries, and he had not experienced similar symptoms in the past. A review of systems was unremarkable. He denied dysuria, hematuria, diarrhea, constipation, fever, chills, or weight change.

The patient frequently participated in physical activity and played soccer, averaging four games per week, an increase from his usual level of commitment. An inguinal hernia had been ruled out by his physician.

Questions

1. What structure(s) could be at fault when abdominal and midline pelvic pain is the major complaint?
2. What is the significance of the Valsalva maneuver?
3. Why are the questions with regard to dysuria, hematuria, diarrhea, constipation, fever, chills, or weight change pertinent?
4. What does no pain at rest suggest?
5. What is your working hypothesis at this stage? List the various diagnoses that could present with this pain and the tests you would use to rule out each one.
6. Does this presentation and history warrant a scan? Why or why not?

Examination

Given the location of the patient's symptoms, and the relatively insidious onset, a lumbosacral scanning examination was performed with the following findings.

- The patient demonstrated full range of motion of his lumbar spine without spasm.
- Straight leg raise testing was negative.
- His gait was moderately wide based, and he had full range of motion of knees and hips, though hip flexion, abduction, and external rotation (the FABER test) produced some pubic discomfort.
- Femoral pulses were 2+ bilaterally.
- Special tests revealed palpable tenderness of the pubic symphysis and inguinal ligament bilaterally. The sacroiliac kinetic tests and pubic stress tests were positive.

Questions

1. Did the scanning examination confirm the working hypothesis? How?
2. Why were the femoral pulses assessed?
3. Why were the kinetic tests performed?
4. Given the findings from the scanning examination, what is the diagnosis, or is further testing warranted in the form of special tests? What information would be gained with further testing?

Evaluation

The findings for this patient's symphysis tenderness were consistent with osteitis pubis.

Questions

1. Having confirmed the diagnosis, what will be your intervention?
2. In order of priority, and based on the stages of healing, list the various goals of your intervention.
3. Estimate this patient's prognosis.
4. What modalities could you use in the intervention of this patient?
5. What exercises would you initiate?

Intervention

Intervention for the inflammatory type of osteitis pubic is conservative. Most athletes return to their respective sports within a few days to weeks. Intervention for this area includes plenty of rest from weight-bearing activities, a course of nonsteroidal antiinflammatory medicine, and physical therapy to gently mobilize, stretch, and strengthen the muscles about the groin. This is usually all that is necessary.[149] Patients should be able to swim for exercise.

This is a condition that is traditionally slow to heal. If mobilization is used, only one direction needs to be chosen for correction, because the other direction occurs as a consequence of the osteokinematic motion. Improvement of position and decreased pain on palpating the inguinal ligament should be found if the technique has been successful. By restoring the posterior component of the impairment complex, the superior positional displacement is also corrected.

Alternatively, the modified shot-gun technique can be used for impairments that do not respond to the mobilization techniques. The short adductors cross the inferior aspect of the pubic articulation in a cruciate manner, and, when recruited, bring the joint into a level position. Since a slight "popping" noise is often elicited as the operator overcomes the muscle resistance by a short, high-velocity movement in the opposite direction, which can be of concern and surprise to the patient, a preliminary word of warning is necessary.

Following the intervention, the kinetic test and positional findings are reevaluated. If there is no improvement, a sacroiliac impairment is the probable cause.

Normally, pelvic impairments are presented as isolated entities when, in fact, clinically, they tend to occur in combination. Therefore, a sequence of treatment progression is necessary. The pelvic impairments should be treated in the following order.

1. Segmental restrictive faults of the lumbar spine
2. Pubic symphysis impairment

3. Sacral torsion syndrome
4. Innominate subluxation
5. Innominate rotation
6. Innominate flare
7. Any impairment of the lower limb and foot

REVIEW QUESTIONS

1. Name the three bones which fuse to form the innominate.
2. Which sacroiliac ligament resists counternutation of the sacrum?
3. Give five conditions that can produce groin pain.
4. Which two trunk motions produce a Left on Left motion at the sacrum?
5. Which two muscles have the potential to hold the innominate in an anteriorly rotated position?
6. Which sacroiliac ligament prevents nutation of the sacrum and counteracts against dorsal and cranial migration of the sacral apex during weight-bearing?
7. Which two-joint muscle group should be stretched in order to reduce a posteriorly rotated innominate caused by adaptive muscle shortening?
8. Which is the only muscle that can be considered as a prime mover of the sacrum?
9. Define what 'force closure' is
10. List the muscles that constitute the inner unit of the proposed sacroiliac stabilization system.

ANSWERS

1. Ilium, ischium, and pubis
2. The long dorsal sacroiliac ligament
3. Muscle strain, inguinal hernia, ankylosing spondylitis, osteitis pubis, pubic stress fracture, hip osteoarthritis, peripheral nerve entrapment
4. Backward bending and left rotation
5. Rectus femoris, iliopsoas
6. Sacrotuberous ligament
7. The hamstrings
8. The piriformis muscle
9. Force closure is the need for an extra force, or forces, to maintain the position of an object
10. Pelvic floor muscles, transverse abdominis, multifidus, the diaphragm

REFERENCES

1. Pettman, E. *Level One Course notes from North American Institute of Orthopedic Manual Therapy.* Portland, Or: Course notes 1990.
2. Mixter WJ, Barr JS. Rupture of the intervertebral disc. *New Eng J Med* 1934;211:210–215.
3. Albee FH. A study of the anatomy and the clinical importance of the sacroiliac joint. JAMA 1909;53:1273.
4. Grieve GP. *Common Vertebral Joint Problems.* 2nd ed. Edinburgh: Churchill Livingstone; 1988.
5. Basmajian JV. Deluca CJ. *Muscles Alive: Their Functions Revealed by Electromyography.* Baltimore: Williams & Wilkins; 1985.
6. Schwarzer AC, Aprill CN, Bogduk N. The sacroiliac joint in chronic low back pain. *Spine* 1995;20:31–37.
7. Duckworth JWA. The anatomy and movements of the sacroiliac joints. In: Wolff HD, ed. *Manuelle Medizin und ihre wissenschaftlichen Grundlagen.* Heidelberg: Physikalische Medizin; 1970:56.
8. Warwick R, Williams P. Gray's Anatomy. 35th ed, Philadelphia: Lippincott; 1978.
9. Solonen KA. The sacroiliac joint in the light of anatomical roentgenographical and clinical studies. *Acta Orthop Scand Suppl* 1957;26:9.
10. Schunke GB. The anatomy and development of the sacro-iliac joint in man. *Anat Rec* 1938;72:313.
11. MacDonald GR, Hunt TE. Sacro-iliac joint observations on the gross and histological changes in the various age groups. *Can Med Assoc J* 1951;66:157.
12. Resnick D, Niwayama G, Goergen TG. Degenerative disease of the sacroiliac joint. *Invest Radiol* 1975;10:608–621.
13. Vleeming A, Wingerden JP, van Dijkstra PF, Stoeckart R, Snijders CI, Stijnen T. Mobility in the SI-joints in old people: a kinematic and radiological study. *Clin Biomechan* 1992;7:170–176.
14. Bowen V, Cassidy JD. Macroscopic and microscopic anatomy of the sacroiliac joint from embryonic life until the eighth decade. *Spine* 1980;6:620–625.
15. Vleeming A, Stoeckart R, Volkers ACW, Snijders CJ. Relation between form and function in the sacroiliac joint. 1: Clinical anatomical aspects. *Spine* 1990;15:130–132.
16. Kissling RO, Jacob HAC. The mobility of the sacroiliac joints in healthy subjects. *Bull Hosp Joint Dis* 1996;54:158–164.
17. Vleeming A, Volkers ACW, Snijders CJ, Stoeckart R. Relation between form and function in the sacroiliac joint. 2: Biomechanical aspects. *Spine* 1990;15:133–136.
18. Weisl H. The articular surfaces of the sacro-iliac joint and their relation to the movements of the sacrum. *Acta Anat* 1954;22:1.
19. Kapandji IA. *The Physiology of the Joints II: The Lower Limb.* 2nd ed. Edinburgh: Churchill Livingstone; 1970.
20. Solonen KA. The sacroiliac joint in the light of anatomical roentgenographical and clinical studies. *Acta Orthop Scand Suppl* 1957;26:9.

21. Fryette HH. *Principles of Osteopathic Technique.* Academy of Applied Osteopathy, Carmel, California; 1954.

22. Erdmann H. Die Verspannung des Wirbelsockels im Beckenring. In: Junghanns H, *Wirbelsaule in Forschung und Praxis.* Vol. 1. Stuttgart: Hippokrates; 1956:51.

23. Mennel JB. *The Science and Art of Joint Manipulation: The Spinal Column.* London: Churchill; 1952.

24. Johnston TB, Whillis J, eds. *Gray's Anatomy: Descriptive and Applied.* London: Longmans, Green; 1944.

25. Vleeming A, Pool-Goudzwaard AL, Hammudoghlu D, Stoeckart R, Snijders, CJ, Mens, JMA. The function of the long dorsal sacroiliac ligament: its implication for understanding low back pain. *Spine* 1996; 21:556–562.

26. Willard FH. The muscular, ligamentous and neural structure of the low back and its relation to back pain. In: Vleeming A, Mooney V, Dorman T, Snijders C, Stoeckart R, eds. *Movement, Stability and Low Back Pain.* Edinburgh: Churchill Livingstone; 1997:3.

27. Fortin JD, Pier J, Falco F. Sacroiliac joint injection: pain referral mapping and arthrographic findings. In: Vleeming A, Mooney V, Dorman T, Snijders C, Stoeckart R, eds. *Movement, Stability and Low Back Pain.* Edinburgh: Churchill Livingstone; 1997:271.

28. Wingerden JP van, Vleeming A, Snijders CJ, Stoeckart R. A functional-anatomical approach to the spine-pelvis mechanism: interaction between the biceps femoris muscle and the sacrotuberous ligament. *Eur Spine J* 1993;2:140–144.

29. Vleeming A, Van Wingerden JP, Snijders CJ, Stoeckart R, Stijnen T. Load application to the sacrotuberous ligament. *Clin Biomech* 1989;4:204–209.

30. Vleeming A, Stoeckart R, Snijders CJ. The sacrotuberous ligament: a conceptual approach to its dynamic role in stabilizing the sacroiliac joint. *Clin Biomech* 1989;4:201–203.

31. Vleeming A, Mooney V, Dorman T, Snijders GJ, eds. *Second Interdisciplinary World Congress on Low Back Pain. The Integrated Function of the Lumbar Spine and Sacroiliac Joint.* Part 172. San Diego, CA: November 1995;9–11.

32. Kapandji IA. *The Physiology of the Joints III: The Trunk and Vertebral Column.* 2nd ed. Edinburgh: Churchill Livingstone; 1970.

33. Lee D. *The Pelvic Girdle: An Approach to the Examination and Treatment of the Lumbo-Pelvic-Hip Region.* 2nd ed. Edinburgh: Churchill Livingstone; 1999.

34. McQueen PM. The piriformis syndrome. *Physiother Soc Manip News* 1977;8:1.

35. Greenman PE. Clinical aspects of the sacroiliac joint in walking. In: Vleeming A, Mooney V, Dorman T, Snijders C, Stoeckart R, eds. *Movement, Stability and Low Back Pain.* Edinburgh: Churchill Livingstone; 1997;236.

36. Travell JG, Rinzler SH. The myofascial genesis of pain. *Postgrad Med* 1952;11:425.

37. Mennel JB. *The Science and Art of Joint Manipulation.* London: Churchill; 1952.

38. Macintosh JE, Valencia F, Bogduk N, Munro RR. The morphology of the human multifidus. *Clin Biomech* 1986;1:196–204.

39. McGill SM. Kinetic potential of the lumbar trunk musculature about three orthogonal orthopaedic axes in extreme postures. *Spine* 1991;16:809–815.

40. Vleeming A, Pool-Goudzwaard AI, Stoeckart R, Snijders CJ. The posterior layer of the thoracolumbar fascia: its function in load transfer from spine to legs. *Spine* 1995;20:753–758.

41. Dorman T. Pelvic mechanics and prolotherapy. In: Vleeming A, Mooney V, Dorman T, Snijders C, Stoeckart R, eds. *Movement, Stability and Low Back Pain.* Edinburgh: Churchill Livingstone; 1997: p507.

42. Bogduk N, Twomey LT. *Clinical Anatomy of the Lumbar Spine and Sacrum.* 3rd ed. New York: Churchill Livingstone; 1997.

43. Bogduk N. The sacroiliac joint. In: Bogduk N, ed. *Clinical Anatomy of the Lumbar Spine and Sacrum.* 3rd ed. New York: Churchill Livingstone; 1977:177–186.

44. Dreyfuss P, Michaelson M, Pauza K, et al. The value of medical history and physical examination in diagnosing sacroiliac joint pain. *Spine* 1996;21:2594–2602.

45. Pitkin HC, Pheasant HC. Sacrarthrogenic telalgia I: a study of referred pain. *J Bone Joint Surg* 1936;18:111–133.

46. Solonen KA. The sacroiliac joint in light of anatomical, roentgenological, and clinical studies. *Acta Orthop Scand* 1957;27:1–27.

47. Bradlay KC. The posterior primary rami of segmental nerves. In: Glasgow EF, Twomey LT, Scull ER, Kleyhans AM, eds. *Aspects of Manipulative Therapy.* 2nd ed. Melbourn : Churchill Livingstone; 1985:59.

48. Grob KR, Neuhuber WL, Kissling RO. Innervation of the sacroiliac joint of the human. *Zeitschrift für Rheumatologie* 1995;54:117–122.

49. Inman VT, Saunders JB. Referred pain from skeletal structures. *J Nerv Ment Dis* 1944;99:660–667.

50. Egund N, Olsson TH, Schmid H, et al. Movement of the sacroiliac joint demonstrated with roentgenstereophotogrammetry. *Acta Radiol* 1978;19:833–846.

51. Miller JAA, Schultz AB, Andersson GBJ Load displacement behavior of sacro-iliac joints. *J Orthop Res* 1987;5:92–101.

52. Sturesson B, Selvik G, Ude A. Movements of the sacroiliac joints: a roentgen stereophotogrammetric analysis. *Spine* 1989;14:162–165.

53. Smidt GL, Wei SH, McQuade K, et al. Sacroiliac motion for extreme hip positions. A fresh cadaver study. *Spine* 1997;22:2073–2082.

54. Weisl H. The movements of the sacroiliac joints. *Acta Ana* 1955;23:80–91.

55. Bakland O, Hansen JH. The axial sacroiliac joint. *Anat Clin* 1984;6:29–36.

56. Illi F, *The Vertebral Column: Lifeline of the Body*. Chicago: National College of Chiropractic; 1951.

57. Grice AS, Fligg DB. *Biomechanics of the Pelvis*. Denver Conference monograph. Des Moines: ACA Council of Technic; 1980.

58. Vleeming A, Mooney V, Dorman T, Snijders C, Stoeckart R, eds. *Movement, Stability and Low Back Pain*. Edinburgh: Churchill Livingstone; 1997.

59. Snijders CJ, Vleeming A, Stoeckart R, Mens JMA, Kleinrensink GJ. Biomechanics of the interface between spine and pelvis in different postures. In: Vleeming A, Mooney V, Dorman T, Snijders C, Stoeckart R, eds. *Movement, Stability and Low Back Pain*. Edinburgh: Churchill Livingstone; 1997:103.

60. Snijders CJ, Vleeming A, Stoeckart R, Transfer of lumbosacral load to iliac bones and legs. 2: Loading of the sacroiliac joints when lifting in a stooped posture. *Clin Biomech* 1993;8:295–301.

61. Richardson CA, Jull GA. Muscle control—pain control. What exercises would you prescribe? *Manual Ther* 1995;1:2–10.

62. Snijders CJ, Slagter AHE, van Strik R, Vleeming A, Stoeckart R, Stam HJ. Why leg-crossing? The influence of common postures on abdominal muscle activity. *Spine* 1995;20:1989–1993.

63. Lee DG. Instability of the sacroiliac joint and the consequences for gait. In: Vleeming A, Mooney V, Dorman T, Snijders C, Stoeckart R, eds. *Movement, Stability and Low Back Pain*. Edinburgh: Churchill Livingstone; 1997:231.

64. Meadows JTS. *Manual Therapy: Biomechanical Assessment and Treatment, Advanced Technique, Lecture and Video Supplemental Manual*. 1995.

65. Gracovetsky S, Farfan HF. The optimum spine. *Spine* 1986;11:543.

66. Pearcy M, Tibrewal SB. Axial rotation and lateral bending in the normal lumbar spine measured by three-dimensional radiography. *Spine* 1984;9:582.

67. Inman VT, Ralston HJ, Todd, F. *Human Walking*. Baltimore: Williams & Wilkins; 1981.

68. Gracovetsky S. Linking the spinal engine with the legs: a theory of human gait. In: Vleeming A, Mooney V, Dorman T, Snijders C, Stoeckart R, eds. *Movement, Stability and Low Back Pain*. Edinburgh: Churchill Livingstone; 1997:243.

69. Gladman DD. Clinical aspects of the spondyloarthropathies. *Am J Med Sci*. 1998;316:234–238.

70. Gladman DD. Psoriatic arthritis. In: Kelley WN, Harris ED, Ruddy S, Sledge CB, eds. *Textbook of Rheumatology*. 5th ed. Philadelphia: Saunders;1997:999–1005.

71. Buskila D, Langevitz P, Gladman DD, Urowitz S, Smythe H. Patients with rheumatoid arthritis are more tender than those with psoriatic arthritis. *J Rheumatol* 1992;19:1115–1119.

72. Gladman DD, Brubacher B, Buskila D, Langevitz P, Farewell VT. Differences in the expression of spondyloarthropathy: a comparison between ankylosing spondylitis and psoriatic arthritis: genetic and gender effects. *Clin Invest Med* 1993;16:1–7.

73. Gladman DD, Anhorn KB, Schachter RK, Mervart H. HL Anantigens in psoriatic arthritis. J Rheumatol 1986;13:586–592.

74. Gladman DD. The natural history of psoriatic arthritis. In: Wright V, Helliwell P, eds. *Psoriatic Arthritis (Baillière's Clinical Rheumatology: International Practice and Research)*. London: Baillières Tindall; 1994;379–394.

75. McClusky OE, Lordon RE, Arnett FC Jr. HL-A 27 in Reiter's syndrome and psoriatic arthritis: a genetic factor in disease susceptibility and expression. *J Rheumatol* 1974;1:263–268.

76. Arnett FC. Reactive arthritis (Reiter's syndrome) and enteropathic arthritis. In: Klippel JH, ed. *Primer on the Rheumatic Diseases*. 11th ed. Atlanta: Arthritis Foundation; 1997:184–188.

77. McEwen C, Di Tata D, Lingg C, et al. Ankylosing spondylitis accompanying ulcerative colitis, regional enteritis, psoriasis and Reiter's disease: a comparative study. *Arthritis Rheum* 1971;14:291.

78. Russel. AS, Davis B, Percy JS, et al. The sacroiliitis of acute Reiter's syndrome. *J Rheumatol* 1977;4:293–296.

79. Butler MJ, Russell AS, Percy JB, et al. A follow-up study of 48 patients with Reiter's syndrome. *Am J Med* 1979;67:808–810.

80. Ashby EC. Chronic obscure groin pain is commonly caused by enthesopathy tennis elbow of the groin. *Br J Surg* 1994;81:1632–1634.

81. Martens MA, Hansen L, Mulier JC. Adductor tendinitis and musculus rectus abdominis tendonopathy. *Am J Sports Med* 1987;15:353–356.

82. Zimmerman G. Groin pain in athletes. *Aust Fam Physician* 1988;17:1046–1052.

83. Bradshaw C, McCrory P, Bell S, Bruckner P. Obturator neuropathy a cause of chronic groin pain in athletes. *Am J Sports Med* 1997;25:402–408.

84. Kopell HP, Thompson WAL, Postel AH. Entrapment neuropathy of the ilioinguinal nerve. *N Engl J Med* 1962;266:16–19.

85. Westman M. Ilioinguinalis—och genitofemoralis-neuralgi. *Lakartidningen* 1970;67:47.

86. Yukawa Y, Kato F, Kajino G, Nakamura S, Nitta H. Groin pain associated with lower lumbar disc herniation. *Spine* 1997;22:1736–1739.

87. Murphey F. Sources and patterns of pain in disc disease. *Clin Neurosurg* 1968;15:343–51.

88. Edger MA, Nundy S. Innervation of the spinal dura matter. *J Neurol Neurosurg Psychiatry* 1966;29:530–534.

89. Groen GJ, Baljet B, Drukker J. Nerves and nerve plexuses of the human vertebral column. *Am J Anat* 1990;188:282–296.

90. Spiera H. Osteoarthritis as a misdiagnosis in elderly patients. *Geriatrics* 1987;42:37–42.

91. Schon L, Zuckerman JD. Hip pain the elderly: evaluation and diagnosis. *Geriatrics* 1988;43:48–62.

92. Guralnik J, Ferrucci L, Simonsick EM, et al. Lower-extremity function in persons over the age of 70 years as a predictor of subsequent disability. *N Engl J Med* 1995;332:556–560.

93. Fried LP, Guralnik JM. Disability in older adults: evidence regarding significance, etiology, and risk. *J Am Geriatr Soc* 1997;45:92–100.

94. Ettinger WH Jr, Fried LP, Harris T, et al. Self-reported causes of physical disability in older people: the cardiovascular health study. *J Am Geriatr Soc* 1994;42:1035–1044.

95. Hochberg MC, Kaspar J, Williamson J, et al. The contribution of osteoarthritis to disability: preliminary data from the women's health and aging study. *J Rheumatol* 1995;(suppl) 43:16–18.

96. Gibbs J, Hughes S, Dunlop D, et al. Joint impairment and ambulation in the elderly. *J Am Geriatr Soc* 1993;41:1205–1211.

97. Ensrud K, Nevitt M, Yunis C, et al. Correlates of impaired function in older women. *J Am Geriatr Soc* 1994;42:481–489.

98. Hughes SL, Gibbs J, Edelman P, et al. Joint impairment and hand function in the elderly. *J Am Geriatr Soc* 1992;40:871–877.

99. Baron M, Dutil E, Berkson L, et al. Hand function in the elderly: relation to osteoarthritis. *J Rheumatol* 1987;14:815–819.

100. Sudarsky L. Current concepts—geriatrics: gait disorders in the elderly. *N Engl J Med* 1990;322:1441–1445.

101. Cambell AJ, Borrie MJ, Spears GF. Risk factors for falls in a community-based prospective study of people 70 years and older. *J Gerontol Med Sci* 1989;44:M112–M117.

102. Tinetti ME, Speechley M, Ginter SF. Risk factors for falls among elderly persons living in the community. *N Engl J Med* 1988;319:1701–1707.

103. Henderson DSCL. Osteitis pubis with five case reports. *Br J Urol* 1950;22:30–50.

104. Beer E. Periostitis of the symphysis and descending rami of the pubes following suprapubic operations. *Int J Med Surg* 1924;37:224–225.

105. Middleton R, Carlisle R. The spectrum of osteitis pubis. *Compr Ther* 1993;19:99–105.

106. Wiley JJ. Traumatic osteitis pubis: the gracilis syndrome. *Am J Sports Med* 1983;11:360–363.

107. Fricker PA, Tauton JE, Ammann W. Osteitis pubis in athletes. Infection, inflammation, or injury? *Sports Med* 1991;12:266–279.

108. Grace JN, Sim FH, Shives TC, Coventry MB. Wedge resection of the symphysis pubis for the treatment of osteitis pubis. *J Bone Joint Surg Am* 1989;71:358–364.

109. Barry NN, McGuire JL. Acute injuries and specific problems in adult athletes. *Rheum Dis Clin North Am* 1996;22:531–549.

110. Lynch FW. The pelvic articulation during pregnancy, labor and the puerperium. An x-ray study. *Surg Gynecol Obstet* 1920;30:575–580.

111. Fowler C. Muscle energy techniques for pelvic dysfunction. In: Grieve GP, ed. *Modern Manual Therapy of the Vertebral Column.* Edinburgh: Churchill Livingstone; 1986:781.

112. Lee DG. Clinical manifestations of pelvic girdle dysfunction. In: Boyling JD, Palastanga N, eds. *Grieve's Modern Manual Therapy: The Vertebral Column.* 2nd ed. Edinburgh: Churchill Livingstone; 1994:453–462.

113. Mitchell F, Moran PS, Pruzzo NA. *An Evaluation and Treatment Manual of Osteopathic Muscle Energy Procedures.* Mitchell, Moran Pruzzo Associates, 1979, Valley Park, MO.

114. Kirkaldy-Willis WH, Hill RJ. A more precise diagnosis for low back pain. *Spine* 1979;4:102–109.

115. Potter NA, Rothstein JM. Intertester reliability for selected clinical tests of the sacroiliac joint. *Phys Ther* 1985;11:1671–1675.

116. McCombe PF, Fairbank JCT, Cockersole BC, Pynsent PB. Reproducibility of physical signs in low back pain. *Spine* 1989;14:908–918.

117. Sturesson B, Uden A, Vleeming A. A radiostereometric analysis of movements of the sacroiliac joints during the standing hip flexion test. *Spine* 2000;25:364–368.

118. Levangie PK. The association between static pelvic asymmetry and low back pain. *Spine* 1999;24:1234–1242.

119. Kirkaldy-Willis WH. Managing low back pain 2nd Ed p. 135. New York. Churchill Livingstone, 1988.

120. Lee DG, Walsh MC. *A Workbook of Manual Therapy Techniques for the Vertebral Column and Pelvic Girdle.* 2nd ed. Vancouver: Nascent; 1996.

121. DonTigney RL. Function and pathomechanics of the sacroiliac joint. A review. *Phys Ther* 1985;65:35–44.

122. Greenman PE. Clinical aspects of sacroiliac function in walking. J Man Med 1990;5:125–129.

123. Richardson CA, Jull GA, Hodges P, Hides J. *Therapeutic Exercise for Spinal Segmental Stabilization in Low Back Pain*. London: Churchill Livingstone; 1999:79–145.

124. Richardson, CA, Jull, GA. Muscle control—pain control. What exercises would you prescribe? *Manual Therapy* 1995;1:2–10.

125. Fitch RR. Mechanical lesions of the sacroiliac joints. *Am J Orthop Surg* 1908;6:693–698.

126. Fortin JD. Sacroiliac joint dysfunction. A new perspective. *J Back Musculoskel Rehab* 1993;3:31–43.

127. Cibulka MT, Koldehoff RM. Leg length disparity and its effect on sacroiliac joint dysfunction. *Clin Manage* 1986;6:10–11.

128. Vleeming A, Buyruk HM, Stoeckart R, et al. An integrated therapy from peripartum pelvic instability: A study of the biomechanical effects of pelvic belts. Am J Obstet Gynecol 1992;166:1243–1247.

129. Huston C. The sacroiliac joint. In: Gonzalez EG, ed. *The Nonsurgical Management of Acute Low Back Pain*. New York: Demos Vermande; 1997:137–150.

130. King L. Case study: physical therapy management of hip osteoarthritis prior to total hip arthroplasty. *J Orthop Sports Phys Ther* 1997;26:35–38.

131. Andrews SK, Carek PJ. Osteitis pubis: a diagnosis for the family physician. *J Am Board Fam Pract* 1998;11:291–295.

132. American Academy of Orthopaedic Surgeons. *Joint Motion: Method of Measuring and Recording*. Chicago: American Academy of Orthopaedic Surgeons; 1965.

133. Beals CA, Lampman MR, Figley Banwell B, Braunstein EM, Alders JW, Castor CW. Measurement of exercise tolerance with patients with rheumatoid and osteoarthritis. *J Rheumatol* 1985;12:458–461.

132. Minor MA, Hewett JE, Webel RR, Anderson SK, Kay DR. Efficiency of physical conditioning exercises in patients with rheumatoid arthritis and osteoarthritis. *Arthritis Rheum* 1989;32:1369–1405.

133. Yelen E, Lubeck D, Holman H, Epstein W. The impact of rheumatoid arthritis and osteoarthritis: the activities of patients with rheumatoid arthritis and osteoarthritis compared to controls. *J Rheumatol* 1987; 14:710–717.

134. Hochberg MC, Altman RD, Brandt KD, et al. Guidelines for the medical management of osteoarthritis. Part 1. Osteoarthritis of the hip. *Arthritis Rheum* 1995; 38:1535–1540.

135. Hochberg MC, Altman RD, Brandt KD, et al. Guidelines for the medical management of osteoarthritis. Part II. Osteoarthritis of the knee. *Arthritis Rheum* 1995;38:1541–1546.

136. Palmoski MJ, Bolyer RA, Brandt KD. Joint motion in the absence of normal loading does not maintain normal articular cartilage. *Arthritis Rheum* 1980;23:325–334.

137. Brandt KD, Heilman DK, Mazzuca S, et al. Quadriceps weakness and osteoarthritis of the knee. *Ann Intern Med* 1997;127.97–104.

138. Ettinger WH Jr, Burns R, Messier SP, et al. A randomized trial comparing aerobic exercise and resistance exercise with a health education program in older adults with knee osteoarthritis: The Fitness Arthritis and Seniors Trial (FAST). *JAMA* 1997;277:25–31.

139. Schilke JM. Effects of muscle-strength training on the functional status of patients with osteoarthritis of the knee joint. *Nurs Res* 1996;45:68–72.

140. Judge JO, Underwood M, Gennosa T. Exercise to improve gait velocity in older persons. *Arch Phys Med Rehabil* 1993;74:400–406.

141. Gerber LH. Exercise and arthritis. *Bull Rheum Dis* 1990;39:1–9.

142. Puett D, Griffin M. Published trials of nonmedicinal and noninvasive therapies for hip and knee osteoarthritis. *Ann Intern Med* 1994;121:133–140.

143. Kovar PA, Allegrante JP, MacKenzie CR, et al. Supervised fitness walking in patients with osteoarthritis of the knee. A randomized, controlled trial. *Ann Intern Med* 1992;116:529–534.

145. Province MA, Hadley EC, Hornbrook, MC, et al. The effects of exercise on falls in elderly patients. *JAMA* 1995;273:1341–1347.

146. Semble EL, Loeser RF, Wise CM. Therapeutic exercise for rheumatoid arthritis and osteoarthritis. *Semin Arthritis Rheum* 1990;20:32–40.

147. Sullivan PE, Marcos PD. *Clinical Decision Making in Therapeutic Exercise*. East Norwalk, CT: Appleton & Lange; 1995.

148. Cyriax J. *Textbook of Orthopaedic Medicine (Volume 1). Diagnosis of Soft Tissue Lesions*. London: Balliere Tindall; 1978.

149. Holt MA, Keene JS, Graf BK, Helwig DC. Treatment of osteitis pubis in athletes. *Am J Sports Med* 1995; 23:601–606.

CHAPTER EIGHTEEN

THE CRANIOVERTEBRAL JUNCTION

Chapter Objectives

At the completion of this chapter, the reader will be able to:

1. Describe the anatomy of the vertebra, ligaments, muscles, and blood and nerve supply that comprise the craniovertebral segments.
2. Describe the biomechanics of the craniovertebral joints, including coupled movements, normal and abnormal joint barriers, kinesiology, and reactions to various stresses.
3. Perform a detailed objective examination of the craniovertebral musculoskeletal system, including palpation of the articular and soft tissue structures, specific passive mobility and passive articular mobility tests for the joints, and stability tests.
4. Perform and interpret the results from combined motion testing.
5. Analyze the total examination data to establish the definitive biomechanical diagnosis.
6. Apply active and passive mobilization techniques and combined movements to the craniovertebral joints, using the correct grade, direction, and duration, and explain the mechanical and physiologic effects.
7. Describe intervention strategies based on clinical findings and established goals.
8. Evaluate intervention effectiveness to progress or modify intervention.
9. Plan an effective home program, and instruct the patient in same.
10. Develop self-reliant examination and intervention strategies.

OVERVIEW

Because of its distinct anatomic structure, the craniovertebral region is generally considered separately and is deemed to consist of the occipitoatlantal (OA) joint, the atlantoaxial (AA) joint and ligaments, and the suboccipital muscles.

This occipitoatlantoaxial segment is a single functional unit with a distinct embryology, which many consider to be the most complex joint of the axial skeleton, anatomically and kinematically.

The upper portion of the cervical spine accounts for approximately 25% of the vertical height of the entire cervical spine. It is the muscles and ligaments that restrain motion in this area, and not the discs and capsule, as occurs elsewhere.

Most of the movement in the cervical spine (approximately 50%) occurs between the upper two joints—at the occipitoatlantal and atlantoaxial joints. Motion at the atlantoaxial joint occurs relatively independently. Below C2, normal motion is a combination of other levels.

ANATOMY

Articulations

One of the functions of an intervertebral disc is to both facilitate motion and provide stability. In the absence of a disc in this region, the supporting soft tissues of the joints of the upper cervical spine must be lax to permit motion, while being subjected to great mechanical stresses.[1]

Articular facet asymmetry of the human upper cervical spine has been recognized for more than 30 years.[2,3] The implications of this anatomic observation in the human spine has been considered in relation to joint disease.[4–6] Specifically, facet tropism is linked with subsequent degenerative joint disease. Thus, those clinicians who rely on joint palpation to determine joint function need to acknowledge the effects of the aforementioned joint asymmetry in the interpretation of their findings.

The joints in the craniovertebral segment are all positioned anterior to those of the lower cervical region, so the motion above C2 occurs anterior to that below C2.[7]

Occipitoatlantal Joint

The occipitoatlantal joint is formed between the convex occipital condyles and the concave superior articular facets of C1, and represents the most superior zygapophysial joint of the vertebral column.

The smaller anterior region of the foramen magnum is defined by a pair of tubercles to which the alar ligaments attach. The posterior portion houses the brain stem and spinal cord junction. The separation of the two regions is marked by a pair of tubercles to which the transverse ligament of the atlas attaches.

The shape of the atlas is that of a ring (Figure 18–1) and is formed by two lateral masses that are interconnected by anterior and posterior arches. It has a smaller vertical dimension than any vertebra and is considerably wider than any other cervical vertebra.[1] Since it has no spinous process, there is no bone posteriorly between the occipital bone and the spinous process of C2, which increases the potential for extension in the upper cervical spine.

The superior-lateral aspects of the posterior arches accommodate the vertebral arteries.

The articular surface of the inferior facet is circular, relatively flat, and slopes inferiorly from medial to lateral, while the upper articular facets of C1 are elongated from front to back. The anterior ends curve upward to a greater extent than the posterior ends, resulting in the availability of much more extension than flexion at this joint.[8]

Even though these surfaces appear to be reciprocal in shape, they are not, and bony stability is only minimal. The primary motion that occurs at this joint is flexion and extension of the occipital bone on the vertebra of C1. One cadaveric study found the range of flexion and extension to have a combined range of 13 degrees,[9] while another cadaveric study,[10] using radiographic imaging, found the mean ranges to be:

- Flexion-extension: 18.6 degrees ($\pm$ 0.6)
- Axial rotation: 3.4 degrees ($\pm$ 0.4)
- Lateral flexion: 3.9 degrees ($\pm$ 0.6)

Pure rolling occurs on the convex posterior surface (preventing cord impingement). On the concave anterior surface, gliding occurs from extension to neutral. By necessity, the joint capsules are loose to permit motion.

It is generally agreed that rotation and side-flexion occur to opposite sides at this joint when they are combined, and this can be demonstrated by palpating and observing the head's motion during these movements. During occiput rotation, the atlas is felt to translate and side-flex to the opposite side.

The results from a study by Werne[11] have since been validated with cadaveric investigations, using radiographic markers and CT scanning, indicating side-flexion ranges at an average of a little over 9 degrees to both sides, and rotation ranges of 2 degrees[12] to 10 to 25 degrees,[13] although the latter study involved patients with suspected instability. Clinical studies suggested that hypermobility of this joint should only be considered as a diagnosis if the range of rotation exceeds 8 degrees, necessitating rotational mobility and stability testing at this articulation.

Atlantoaxial Joint

This is a fairly complex, biconvex articulation that consists of:

- Two lateral zygapophysial joints between the articular surfaces of the inferior articular processes of the atlas, and the superior processes of the axis.
- Two medial joints between the anterior surface of the dens of the axis and the anterior surface of the atlas, and

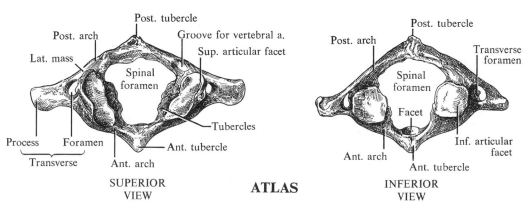

FIGURE 18–1 The Atlas *(Reproduced, with permission from Pansky B: Review of Gross Anatomy, 6/e. McGraw-Hill, 1996)*

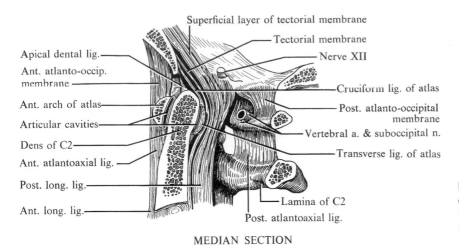

Apical dental lig.
Ant. atlanto-occip. membrane
Ant. arch of atlas
Articular cavities
Dens of C2
Ant. atlantoaxial lig.
Post. long. lig.
Ant. long. lig.

Superficial layer of tectorial membrane
Tectorial membrane
Nerve XII
Cruciform lig. of atlas
Post. atlanto-occipital membrane
Vertebral a. & suboccipital n.
Transverse lig. of atlas
Lamina of C2
Post. atlantoaxial lig.

MEDIAN SECTION

FIGURE 18–2 The relationship of the dens and the anterior arch of the atlas. *(Reproduced, with permission from Pansky B: Review of Gross Anatomy, 6/e. McGraw-Hill, 1996)*

the posterior surface of the dens and the anterior hyalinated surface of the transverse ligament[1] (Figure 18–2).

The axis (Fig. 18–3) is a transitional vertebra in several ways. The unique features of the axis are located on its superior aspect. Of these features, the most interesting is the odontoid process, or dens. This process extends superiorly from the body before tapering to a blunt point. The dens and a part of the axis body develop from an ossification center that could have become the centrum of the atlas.[14] The anterior aspect of the dens has a hyaline cartilage-covered mid-line facet for articulation with the anterior tubercle of the atlas (the median atlantoaxial joint). The posterior aspect of the dens is usually marked with a groove where the transverse ligament passes. The dens functions as a pivot for the upper cervical joints, and as the center of rotation for the atlantoaxial joint.

The relatively large superior articular facets of the axis lie lateral and anterior to the dens. These facets slope considerably downward from medial to lateral in line with the zygapophysial facets of the mid-low cervical spine.[15] As the lateral atlantoaxial joints function to convey the entire

weight of the atlas and head to lower structures, the laminae and pedicles of this vertebra are quite robust. The stout, moderately long, spinous process serves as the uppermost attachment for muscles that are essentially lower cervical in function, and for muscles that act specifically on the cranioverterbral region. The spinous process is the first palpable midline structure below the occiput.

Kapandji[16] describes both articular surfaces of the lateral atlantoaxial joints as being convex, resulting in an incongruent joint. It could be argued that the reason for this arrangement is to allow the atlas to descend on the axis during rotation, thereby slackening the alar ligament and allowing rotation to occur at this joint. The major motion that occurs at all three of the atlantoaxial articulations is axial rotation, and averages about 40 to 47 degrees to both sides.[17,18]

As the atlas rotates, the ipsilateral facet moves posteriorly, while the contralateral facet moves anteriorly, so that each facet of the atlas slides inferiorly along the convex surface of the axial facet, telescoping the head downward.

This joint is provided with strong support by the transverse ligament and the two alar ligaments (see later).

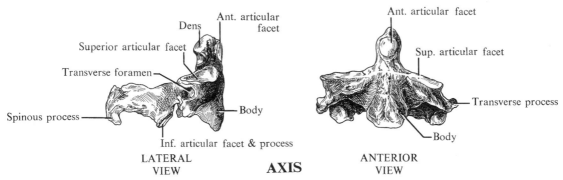

Dens
Ant. articular facet
Superior articular facet
Transverse foramen
Spinous process
Body
Inf. articular facet & process
LATERAL VIEW

AXIS

Ant. articular facet
Sup. articular facet
Transverse process
Body
ANTERIOR VIEW

FIGURE 18–3 The Axis *(Reproduced, with permission from Pansky B: Review of Gross Anatomy, 6/e. McGraw-Hill, 1996)*

The first 25 degrees of head rotation (60%) occur primarily at the atlantoaxial articulations.[19] However, the axial rotation of the atlas is not a pure motion, as it is coupled with a significant degree of extension (14 degrees), and in some cases, flexion.[20]

The large amounts of rotation that occur at the C1–2 articulation can cause problems with the vertebral artery. Selecki[21] found that at 30 degrees of rotation, there is kinking of the contralateral artery, and at 45 degrees of rotation, kinking occurs at the ipsilateral artery.[22]

Flexion and extension movements of the atlantoaxial joint amount to a combined range of 10 to 15 degrees[23] and are associated with small translational movements (2 to 3 mm in adults and 4.5 mm in the child). During flexion, the arch of the atlas glides inferiorly on the dens until it abuts against it, and at the lateral articulations, the atlas surfaces glide posteriorly and roll anteriorly. In atlantoaxial extension, the opposite occurs. Coupling at this joint is commonly cited as contralateral side-flexion during rotation. However, palpation of the axis during side-flexion or rotation tends to argue against this.

If the length of the spinous process is palpated with two fingers, while the subject rotates the head to the left (it holds just as well for right rotation), the superior finger is felt and seen to move to the right while the inferior finger moves to the left. This would indicate that the vertebra of the axis has side-flexed to the right under the atlas, placing the atlantoaxial joint into left side-flexion. In this case, rotation and side-flexion occur to the same side, as is generally held. However, if the spinous process is palpated while the head is side-flexed to the left, it will be felt to move to the right, indicating that the axis is rotating to the left. During side-flexion, the atlas does not rotate, but translates contralaterally. This means that the axis rotates under the atlas. As the position of the joint is described by the relative motion of the superior vertebra (e.g., L4–5 flexion when L4 flexes on L5, as in forward bending, or L5 extends under L4, as in posterior pelvic tilting) the atlantoaxial joint is actually in right rotation. Therefore, left side-flexion of the occiput results in right rotation of the joint.

The direction of the conjunct rotation, therefore, appears to be dependent on the initiating movement. If the initiating movement is side-flexion (latexion), the conjunct rotation (rotation) of the joint is to the opposite side. If the initiating movement is rotation (rotexion), the conjunct motion (side-flexion) is to the same side. This principle can be exploited in the assessment of the craniovertebral joints.

Rotexion Rotation of the head to the right (rotexion) produces:

- Left side-flexion and right rotation of the occipitoatlantal joint, accompanied by a translation to the right.

- Right side-flexion and right rotation of the atlantoaxial joint and at C2–3.

In other words, if the head motion is initiated with rotation, ipsilateral side-flexion of the atlantoaxial joint and C2–3 occurs, while at the occipitoatlantal joint, contralateral side-flexion occurs.

Latexion Side-flexion of the head to the right produces:

- Left rotation of the occipitoatlantal joint, accompanied by a translation to the left.
- Left rotation of the atlantoaxial joint.
- Right rotation of C2–3.

In other words, if head motion is initiated with side-flexion, contralateral rotation of the occipitoatlantal and atlantoaxial joints occurs, but ipsilateral rotation occurs at C2–3.

It is postulated by some that to fully protect the vertebral artery from impingement, the atlantoaxial joint behaves in the following manner.

- *Extreme flexion*: the atlas (C1) rotates in one direction and side-flexes in the opposite direction on the axis.
- *Extreme extension*: the atlas rotates and side-flexes to the same side on the axis.

Osteoarthrosis of the atlantoaxial joints, unrelated to trauma, is a rare cause of pain in the occipitocervical region, and an even more uncommon cause of atlantoaxial instability. Indeed, osteoarthrosis of the atlantoaxial articulations has only fairly recently been described in the literature,[24] while degenerative osteoarthrosis of the subaxial cervical spine is common in elderly patients,[25] and is typically characterized by neck, shoulder, and arm pain, rather than occipitocervical pain.[26] However, osteoarthrosis of the atlantoaxial joints may be overlooked when the patient has occipitocervical pain associated with degenerative changes in the subaxial spine. Halla and Hardin[27] reported a 4% prevalence of osteoarthrosis of the atlantoaxial lateral mass articulations in 705 consecutive outpatients who had peripheral osteoarthrosis or degenerative joint disease of the spine. Fielding et al[28] found that the stability of the atlantoaxial joints depends greatly on the ligamentous structures. When the anterior atlantoodontoid interval is more than 3 millimeters, there is disruption of the transverse ligament.[29] As the anterior atlantoodontoid interval increases further, additional ligamentous damage occurs.[29] It could be argued that as osteoarthrosis of the lateral mass articulations progresses, the synovitis gradually involves the ligamentous structures, thereby weakening them, and rendering them prone to rupture.[30]

Nerve Supply

The dorsal ramus of spinal nerve C1 is larger than the anterior ramus. It exits from the spinal canal by passing posteriorly between the posterior arch of the atlas and the rim of the foramen magnum, along with the vertebral artery. It then enters the suboccipital triangle and supplies most of the muscles that form that triangle. It typically has no cutaneous distribution.

The posterior ramus of spinal nerve C2, larger than the anterior ramus, is called the greater occipital nerve. This nerve is the largest of the cervical posterior rami and is primarily a cutaneous nerve. It supplies most of the posterior aspect of the scalp, extending anteriorly to a line across the scalp that extends from one external auditory meatus to the other.[31] It exits from the vertebral canal by passing through the slit between the posterior arch of the atlas and the lamina of the axis. Since this nerve has an extensive cutaneous distribution, it has a very large dorsal root ganglion. This ganglion is commonly located in a vulnerable location almost directly between the posterior arch of C1 and the lamina of C2. The interval between these two bony structures is small, and is reduced with extension of the upper cervical spine. Given the greater sensitivity of the dorsal root ganglion to compression, as compared to the nerve roots,[32] the possible relationship between the forward head position and occipital headaches is apparent. Support for this theory is provided by a study[33] of 383 patients diagnosed as having migraines, which found that 184 (48%) were suffering from headaches due to irritation of the greater occipital nerve.

Craniovertebral Ligaments

The controlling ligaments for these segments that must be considered together are the:

- Capsule
- Accessory capsular
- Apical (Figure 18–4)
- Vertical and transverse bands of the cruciform (Figure 18–4)
- Alar (Figure 18–4)
- Accessory alar
- Anterior atlanto-occipital membrane (Figure 18–4)

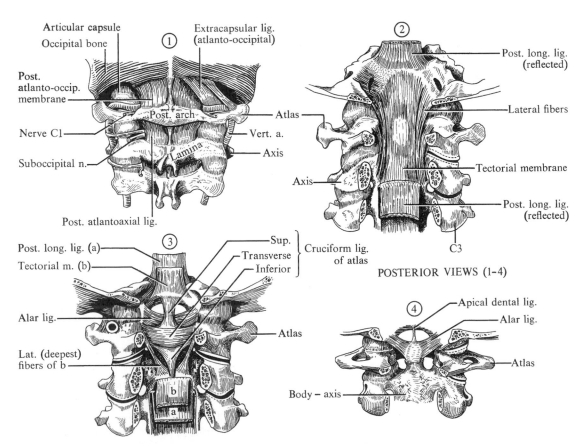

FIGURE 18–4   The craniovertebral ligaments. *(Reproduced, with permission from Pansky B: Review of Gross Anatomy, 6/e. McGraw-Hill, 1996)*

- Posterior atlanto-occipital membrane (Figure 18–4)
- Tectorial membrane (Figure 18–4)
- Anterior longitudinal

The anterior occipitoatlantal membrane is thought to be the superior continuation of the anterior longitudinal ligament. It extends from the anterior arch of vertebra C1 to the anterior aspect of the foramen magnum.

The posterior occipitoatlantal membrane, which interconnects the posterior arch of the atlas and the posterior aspect of the foramen magnum, forms part of the posterior boundary of the vertebral canal.[1]

The lateral capsular ligaments (anterior-lateral occipitoatlantal ligament) of the occipitoatlantal joints are typical of synovial joint capsules. They run obliquely from the basiocciput to the transverse process of the atlas. To permit maximal motion, they are quite lax, so they provide only moderate support to the joints in contralateral head rotation.

Atlantoaxial Ligaments

The anterior longitudinal (anterior atlantoaxial) ligament is continuous with the anterior occipitoatlantal membrane above.[34,35,36]

The posterior atlantoaxial ligament interconnects the posterior arch of the atlas and the laminae of the axis.

Occipitoaxial Ligaments

The occipitoaxial ligaments are very important to the stability of the upper cervical spine.[37]

The apical ligament of the dens (see Figure 18–4) extends from the apex of the dens to the anterior rim of the foramen magnum. The ligament is short and thick, running from the top of the dens to the basiocciput and is thought to be a remnant of the notochord. It appears to be only a moderate stabilizer of the dens relative to both the atlas and occipital bone.

The alar ligaments (see Figure 18–4) connect the superior part of the dens to fossae on the medial side of the occipital condyles, although they can also attach to the lateral masses of the atlas.[38,39]

In a study of 44 cadavers,[40] the researchers found the ligament's orientation to be superiorly, posteriorly and laterally, and that the fiber direction of the alar ligament was divided into three types: caudacranial type, horizontal type, and craniocaudal type.

In another study,[38] 19 upper cervical spine specimens were dissected to examine the macroscopic and functional anatomy of alar ligaments. The researchers found that the most common orientation (10/19), was caudacranial, followed by transverse (5/19), and the classical

craniocaudal the least common (4/19). In two of the specimens, they found a previously undescribed ligamentous connection between the dens and the anterior arch of the atlas, the anterior atlantodental ligament. In 12 specimens, the ligament also attached via caudal fibers to the lateral mass of the atlas. The posterior-anterior orientation of the ligaments in seventeen of the nineteen subjects was either directly lateral from the dens to the occipital attachment or somewhat posterior, 150 to 170 degrees.

The function of the ligament is to resist flexion, side-flexion, and rotation.[41] Combined cervical flexion and rotation proves to be the most stressful force applied to the ligament. Due to their connections, side-flexion of the head produces an ipsilateral rotation of C2.[42]

Functional loss of the alar ligaments indicates a potential for instability which, however, must be determined in conjunction with other clinical findings, such as neurologic impairment, pain, and deformity. If the tests for this ligament are positive, indicating a laxity, but the patient is asymptomatic, intervention is not indicated. However, if the laxity is symptomatic and produces suboccipital pain, nausea, headache, and other symptoms, additional stability can be provided through the nuchal ligament by incorporating a sustained chin-tuck during activities of daily living. Cervical proprioceptive neuromuscular facilitation (PNF) and stabilization exercises should also be utilized.

The tectorial membrane (see Figure 18–4) is the most posterior of the three ligaments interconnecting the occipital bone and axis. This ligament is described as the superior continuation of the posterior longitudinal ligament, and it extends from the body of vertebra C2 to the anterior rim of the foramen magnum. This bridging ligament is an important limiter of upper cervical flexion, and holds the occiput off the atlas.

The horizontal transverse ligament of the atlas interconnects two parts of the atlas. The transverse ligament, connecting the atlas with the dens of the axis, is, in fact, part of the cruciform ligament, however, it is so distinct and important that it is often considered as a ligament in it so own right.

The transverse ligament runs between tubercles on the medial aspects of the lateral masses of the atlas. As it crosses behind the dens, it is separated from it by a small bursa, which facilitates motion between the dens and the ligament. The vertical components of this "cross-shaped" ligament attach to the posterior aspect of the body of the dens and the anterior rim of the foramen magnum (see Figure 18–4). Its major responsibility is to maintain the position of the dens relative to the anterior arch of the atlas.[43] The transverse ligament functions to counteract anterior translation of the atlas relative to the axis, and to limit flexion between the atlas and axis.[44] Generally, tears in upper central region will allow an anterior translation of the atlas. These limiting functions are of extreme importance because excessive movement of either type could result in the dens compressing the spinal cord, epipharynx, vertebral artery, and superior cervical ganglion, and produce cranial nerve signs, pins and needles, and a sensation of having a lump in throat (hematoma of epipharynx).

The importance of the ligament is reflected in its physical properties. The ligament is comprised almost entirely of collagen, with a parallel orientation close to the atlas and the dens, but with an approximately 30-degrees obliquity at other points in the ligament. Dvorak and co-workers[45] found the transverse ligament to be almost twice as strong as the alar ligaments, and to have a tensile strength of 330 newtons (73 lb). Transverse ligament rupture was only thought to occur secondary to other disease processes, or by spontaneous rupture,[46] but recent studies have shown that a rupture can occur in the absence of dens fractures.[29]

The integrity of the transverse ligament is not only pertinent to acute ligamentous injuries but is also essential to the stability of atlas fractures; degenerative, inflammatory, and congenital disorders; and other abnormalities that affect the craniovertebral junction.

Injuries to the transverse ligament are classified as follows.

- *Type I injuries*: disruptions of the substance of the transverse ligament, without an osseous component.
- *Type II injuries*: fractures or avulsions involving the tubercle for insertion of the transverse ligament on the C1 lateral mass, without disruption of the ligament substance.

The medical literature that is available in the English language supports the conclusion that a type I injury is incapable of healing without surgery for internal fixation, but that most type II injuries heal when treated with an orthosis.[46]

Craniovertebral Muscles

Anterior Suboccipital Muscles

Rectus Capitis Anterior   This muscle runs deep to the longus capitis from the anterior aspect of the lateral mass of the atlas vertically to the inferior surface of the base of the occiput, anterior to the occipital condyle. A tight right rectus capitis anterior will produce a decreased left translation in extension during mobility testing of the occipitoatlantal joint. The rectus capitis anterior flexes and minimally rotates the head, and is supplied by the ventral rami of C1 and C2.

Rectus Capitis Lateralis   This muscle arises from the superior surface of the C1 transverse process and inserts into the inferior surface of the jugular process of the occiput. It is homologous to the posterior intertransverse muscle of the spine. The rectus capitis lateralis side-flexes the head ipsilaterally, and is supplied by the ventral rami of C1 and C2.

Posterior Suboccipital Muscles

The posterior suboccipitals function to control segmental sliding at C1 and C2. They are highly innervated, having more muscle spindles than any other muscle for their size, and are also strongly linked with the trigeminal nerve. They receive their blood supply from the vertebral artery. To palpate these structures, it is necessary to go through the splenius capitis, trapezius, and, in older men, a fat pad.

Rectus Capitis Posterior Major   The largest muscle of the group, it runs from the C2 spinous process, widening as it runs cranially, to attach to the lateral part of inferior nuchal line (Figure 18–5). Found inferior and lateral to the occipital protuberances, the rectus capitis posterior majors, when working together, extend the head. When working individually, the muscles produce ipsilateral side-flexion and rotation. The muscles are supplied, in common with the other posterior suboccipitals, by the posterior ramus of C1.

Rectus Capitis Posterior Minor   A small unisegmental muscle, it runs from the posterior arch tubercle of the atlas, to the medial part of the inferior nuchal line (see Figure 18–5). Because of the shortness of the atlantean tubercle, the muscle is very horizontal, running almost parallel with the occiput. It is located inferior medial to occipital protuberances and may be impossible to palpate. The muscle functions to extend the head and provides minimal support during ipsilateral side-flexion of the head.

Inferior Oblique   This muscles is the larger of the two oblique muscles, and runs from the spinous process and lamina of the axis superior-laterally to the transverse process of the atlas (see Figure 18–5). It is found between the spinous process of C2 and the transverse process of C1. Laxity of the transverse ligament can produce spasm in this muscle. A tight right inferior oblique exerts an inferior and posterior pull on the right transverse process of the atlas, producing a right rotated atlantoaxial joint. This results in a gross limitation of left rotation while in cervical flexion, but no limitation of left rotation in extension. Other conditions that can produce a decrease in upper cervical left rotation include a left occipitoatlantal joint impairment or a right atlantoaxial joint impairment. The muscle works to produces ipsilateral rotation of the atlas and skull, and to control anterior translation of C1 (atlas).

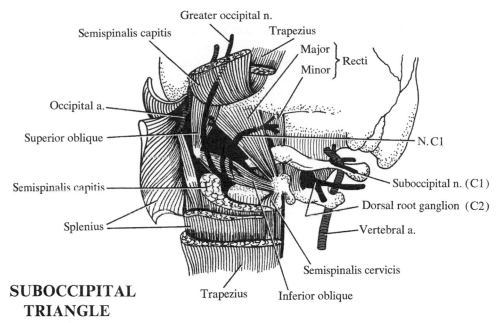

Greater occipital n.

Semispinalis capitis

Trapezius

Major
Minor
} Recti

Occipital a.

Superior oblique

Semispinalis capitis

Splenius

N. C1

Suboccipital n. (C1)

Dorsal root ganglion (C2)

Vertebral a.

Semispinalis cervicis

SUBOCCIPITAL TRIANGLE

Trapezius

Inferior oblique

FIGURE 18–5 The suboccipital muscles *(Reproduced, with permission from Pansky B: Review of Gross Anatomy, 6/e. McGraw-Hill, 1996)*

Superior Oblique From the transverse process of the atlas, the superior oblique runs superior-posterior-medially to the bone between the superior and inferior nuchal lines lateral to the attachment of rectus capitis posterior major (see Figure 18–5). The muscle runs parallel with the occiput and is a common cause of chronic headaches. It functions to provide contralateral rotation due to its posterior-medial orientation, ipsilateral side-flexion of the occipitoatlantal joint when acting unilaterally, and head extension when working bilaterally.

These muscles are probably more important as segmental controllers, either acting concentrically with the larger extensors and rotators, or eccentrically, controlling the action of the flexors. As two of these muscles parallel the occiput, their effect could be more linear than angular, producing or controlling the arthrokinematic, rather than the osteokinematic.

Blood Supply to the Spinal Cord

The cervical cord is supplied by two arterial systems, central and peripheral, which overlap but are discrete. The first is dependent entirely on the single anterior spinal artery (ASA). The second, without clear-cut boundaries, receives supplies from the ASA and both posterior spinal arteries.[47] Because the ASA is medial and dominant, unilateral cord infarctions are very rare. They may occur in the perfusion territory supplied by the ASA[48,49] as a result of the

obstruction of either a duplicated ASA,[48] or the obstruction of one of the sulcal arteries, which arise from the ASA and turn alternatively left or right, to supply one side of the central cord.[50] Peripheral hemicord infarction may result from ischemia in the territory of the ASA[49] or posterior spinal artery.[51]

BIOMECHANICAL EXAMINATION

In addition to the vertebral artery and the transverse ligament tests, the craniovertebral scan, outlined as follows, should be used on any patient with a history of trauma to this area.

The biomechanical examination follows the flow diagram in Figure 18–6. Unless the results from the active motion differentiation test are definitive, both of the joints will probably need to be assessed separately. The OA joint is examined and treated first, otherwise the findings from a combined test of both joints would be confusing. Once the OA joint is cleared, the examination of the AA complex can proceed using the same flow diagram.

The scan is terminated if any serious signs are demonstrated by the patient (drop attack, lip paresthesia,[52] nystagmus, distal extremity paresthesias), which would indicate a compromise to the blood supply of the brain stem or cerebellum, or a spinal cord compression.

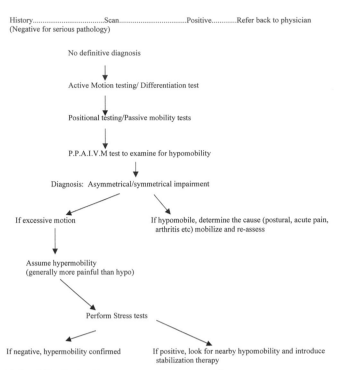

History.................................Scan.............................Positive............Refer back to physician
(Negative for serious pathology)

No definitive diagnosis

Active Motion testing/ Differentiation test

Positional testing/Passive mobility tests

P.P.A.I.V.M test to examine for hypomobility

Diagnosis: Asymmetrical/symmetrical impairment

If excessive motion

If hypomobile, determine the cause (postural, acute pain, arthritis etc) mobilize and re-assess

Assume hypermobility
(generally more painful than hypo)

Perform Stress tests

If negative, hypermobility confirmed

If positive, look for nearby hypomobility and introduce stabilization therapy

FIGURE 18–6 Examination sequence for the craniovertebral region.

The Craniovertebral Scan

Because of its association with the trigeminal nerve, a quick screening examination of the TMJ is performed to rule out pain referral from this joint.

While the clinician palpates over the head of the mandible, the patient is asked to perform active range of motion of opening and closing of the mouth, lateral deviation, protrusion, and retrusion. Overpressure and resistance is applied at the end of range of each of these motions. The amount of mouth opening is measured grossly using the PIP joints. Two to three of the PIP joints should fit comfortably. If the TMJ screen is negative, the clinician can proceed with the craniovertebral scan. If, however, pain is reproduced with the TMJ screen, a full examination of the TMJ must be performed.

1. The patient is asked to perform active neck flexion. If the neck is unstable secondary to a dens fracture and/or transverse ligament tear, the patient will be unable to flex the neck in the traditional manner and will substitute with a chin protrusion. If this occurs, a modified version of the Sharp-Purser test can be used.

    The patient is asked to segmentally flex the head and relate any signs or symptoms that this might evoke to the clinician. Local symptoms, such as soreness, are ignored for the purposes of evaluating the test. If no

cardinal signs or symptoms are provoked, the test is discontinued. However, if cardinal symptoms are provoked, a provisional assumption is made that they are caused by excessive translation of the atlas compromising one or more of the sensitive structures listed previously. The test is considered positive and the examination is terminated. If the neck flexion produces symptoms of nausea and/or dizziness, a cervical fracture may be present and the examination is terminated.[52] Thus, if a patient is able to flex the neck, a cervical fracture or a transverse ligament compromise can be provisionally ruled out.

2. The patient is asked to perform active neck rotation, which is the functional movement of the craniovertebral joints. Some of the possible symptoms and their causes could be:

    ● Facial tingling (C4–5 instability)
    ● Tingling of the tongue (C2–3 impairment)
    ● Lip paresthesia[52] (indicative of vertebrobasilar compromise).

    If dizziness occurs with rotation before the end of range, the head is passively rotated further. If the dizziness increases, then there is a vascular compromise and further cervical testing should cease. This motion also helps to rule out the presence of a fracture (dens, hangman's) as the patient will refuse to, or be unable to, move.

Differentiation Test

Given the fact that the clinician is faced with a biomechanical impairment, a screening test can be used to focus the examination on a particular segment. In the following example used to illustrate the screen, the patient presented with complaints of retro-orbital pain that is provoked when turning the head to the right. Generally speaking, pain originating from the craniovertebral joints tends to refer to the neck, head, or face.

The patient is seated and the clinician stands behind. The clinician induces right side-flexion to the patient's head and neck. This right side-flexion produces the biomechanics of latexion—a left rotation of the occipitoatlantal and atlantoaxial, but a right rotation of C2–3.

● If this motion reproduces the patient's pain, the C2–3 joint is implicated. To confirm this, the clinician passively moves the patient's neck into left side-flexion. If C2–3 is at fault, this movement should have no effect on the symptoms, as left side-flexion of the neck produces a right rotation of both the occipitoatlantal and atlantoaxial, but a left rotation of C2–3.

- If the eye pain is reproduced by the right side-flexion and:

    1. Increased if right rotation is superimposed, then the C2–3 joint/joint capsule is implicated.
    2. Is not increased with the right rotation, left rotation is superimposed on the right side-flexion (Figure 18–7). If the left rotation increases the eye pain, the upper two joints are implicated. However, if the left rotation provokes pain in another area in the neck, then a subchondral/zygapophysial joint crack fracture may be present at the C2–3 level.

- If the right side-flexion with right rotation did not change the patient's symptoms, the upper two joints are implicated. To confirm, the clinician places the patient's neck into left side-flexion. This should reproduce the symptoms. A differentiation between the occipitoatlantal and atlantoaxial now has to be made.

The patient remains seated and the clinician locates the patient's external occipital protuberance, which can be palpated on the posterior-inferior aspect of the occipital bone as a prominent midline elevation. Passing laterally from the external protuberance, the superior nuchal line leads directly to the mastoid process, and just inferior and anterior to the mastoid process, the transverse process of C1 is palpable. Palpation of the transverse process of the atlas can also be accomplished by gliding the palpating fingers inferiorly along the anterior aspect of the mastoid bilaterally, then directly inferior to the mastoid, and, finally, posterior to the mastoid. Having located the transverse process of C1, the clinician stabilizes the patient's head in a position of left mid to low cervical rotation and right craniovertebral rotation. The atlas has very few ligaments attaching to it, except the transverse ligament, and, thus, by stabilizing the patient's head, the clinician is also stabilizing C2 because of the number of ligaments that attach between the head and C2. The clinician passively rotates the atlas (C1) to the left by applying gentle manual pressure to the posterior aspect of the right C1 transverse process (Figure 18–8). This left rotation of C1 produces a relative right rotation of the occipitoatlantal joint, but a left rotation of the atlantoaxial joint.

If the left rotation of C1 produces an increase in eye pain, the occipitoatlantal joint is at fault. This can be confirmed by passively rotating C1 to the right, which should decrease the pain. If the left rotation of C1 produces no change, the clinician introduces right rotation of C1. If this is positive, it will indicate involvement of the atlantoaxial joint.

If the results from this screen are inconclusive, resistance can be applied. The clinician rotates the patient's head and neck to the right and to the point of pain. Resistance is applied in both directions of rotation. An increase in pain with resistance could indicate a contractile, articular, or a ligamentous impairment. Further differentiation can be

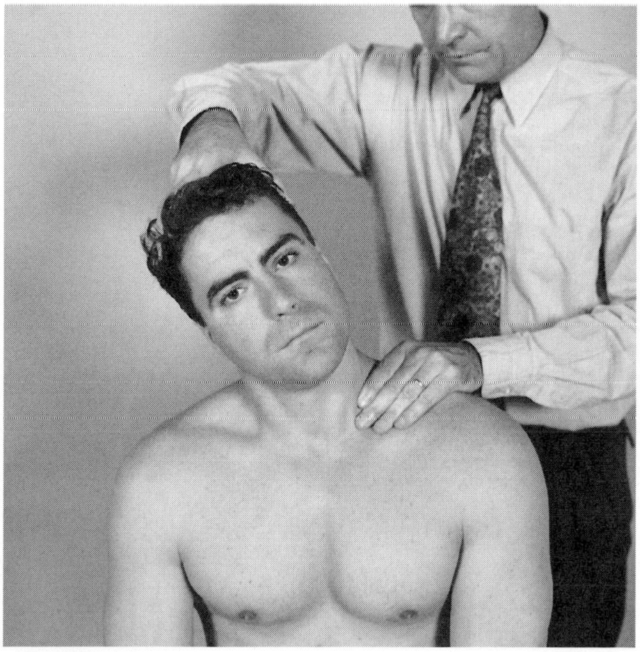

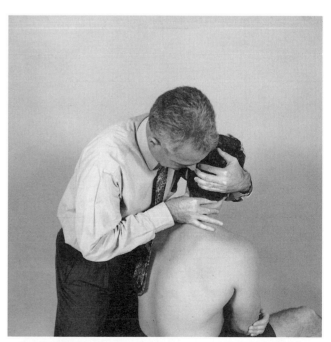

FIGURE 18–7 Testing position of passive right side flexion and left rotation of the cervical spine.

FIGURE 18–8 Testing position of passive right side flexion and left rotation of the cervical spine and left rotation of the atlas.

made using traction and compression. The rotation is maintained and a traction and compression force is applied.

1. Application of gentle traction: if the pain decreases, then this may implicate a subchondral fracture, zygapophysial joint fracture, or traumatic arthritis. If the pain increases, a ligamentous or capsular structure is implicated. However, due to its vertical orientation, the traction would also stretch the superior oblique, producing pain if it is injured.
2. Application of gentle compression: if the pain increases, then this may implicate a subchondral fracture, zygapophysial joint fracture, or traumatic arthritis. If the pain decreases, then this would confirm a ligamentous or superior oblique impairment.

Positional Tests

The patient is sitting. The clinician is standing behind the patient. With the index and middle finger of both hands, the clinician palpates the distance between the transverse processes of the atlas and the mastoid processes of the temporal bones.

Flexion

Occipitoatlantal Joint With the index and long finger of one hand, the clinician palpates the mastoid process and the transverse process of C1 (Figure 18–9). The patient is asked to flex the OA joint complex and the clinician assesses the position of the occiput relative to the atlas. The other side is then tested and a comparison is made. The side to which the occiput is side-flexed in flexion is the side of the shortest distance.

Atlantoaxial Joint Positional testing of this joint is performed by bilaterally palpating the posterior arch of the atlas in the suboccipital gutter and the lamina of the axis with the index and middle finger of both hands (Figure 18–10). The joint is flexed around its axis and the clinician assesses the position of the C1 vertebra relative to C2 by noting the position of the posterior arch relative to the corresponding lamina of C2. The other side is then tested and a comparison is made. A posterior left posterior arch of C1 relative to the left lamina of C2 is indicative of a left rotated position of the C1–2 joint complex in flexion.

Extension

Occipitoatlantal Joint The OA joint complex is flexed around the appropriate axis and the clinician assesses the position of the occiput relative to the atlas by comparing the left with the right side, the side to which the occiput is side-flexed in extension is the side of the shortest distance.

Atlantoaxial Joint Positional testing of this joint is performed by bilaterally palpating the posterior arch of the atlas in the suboccipital gutter and the lamina of the axis with the index and middle finger of both hands. The joint is extended around the appropriate axis and the clinician

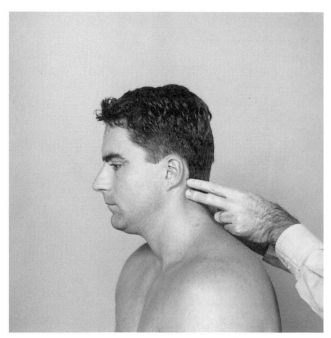

FIGURE 18–9 Patient and clinician position for position testing of the occipital-atlantal joint.

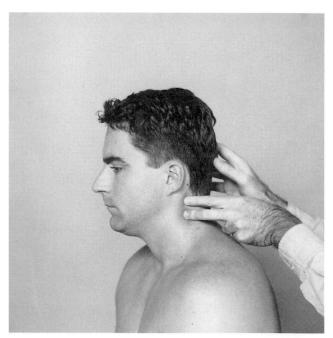

FIGURE 18–10 Patient and clinician position for position testing of the atlanto-axial joint (shown on left side).

assesses the position of the C1 vertebra relative to C2 by noting the position of the posterior arch relative to the corresponding lamina of C2. A posterior left posterior arch of C1 relative to the left lamina of C2 is indicative of a left rotated position of the C1–2 joint complex in extension.

Active Mobility of the Occiput, Atlas, and Axis

The patient is sitting with the clinician standing behind. Using the thumbs and index fingers of both hands, the clinician palpates each mastoid process of the temporal bones and the transverse processes of the atlas. With the middle fingers of each hand, the clinician palpates the transverse processes of the axis (Figure 18–11). The clinician notes the quantity and quality of the motions.

For flexion, the patient is asked to flex the head around the appropriate axis. The mastoid processes should travel posteriorly along a curved path at equal distance. When interpreting the mobility findings, the position of the joint at the beginning of the test should correlate with the subsequent mobility noted because alterations in joint mobility may merely be a reflection of an altered starting position.[53]

To assess extension, the patient is asked to extend the head around the appropriate axis. The mastoid processes should travel anteriorly along a curved path at equal distance. When interpreting the mobility findings, the position of the joint at the beginning of the test should be correlated with the subsequent mobility noted because alterations in

joint mobility may merely be a reflection of an altered starting position.[53]

To assess side-flexion, the patient is asked to side-flex the head around the appropriate axis. As conjunct contralateral rotation is usually combined with side-flexion at this joint, the mastoid process should be felt to approximate the ipsilateral transverse process in the coronal plane during side-flexion.[53]

Passive Mobility Testing of Occiput, Atlas, and Axis

Seated Technique

The patient is sitting, with a clinician standing beside. Using the index and middle finger of the posterior hand, the clinician palpates the occipitoatlantal joints and palpates the lateral atlantoaxial joints with the thumb and ring finger of the posterior hand. The ulnar border of the fifth finger of the anterior hand is applied to the occiput (Figure 18–12). Fixation of the cranium should not occur.

The clinician passively flexes, extends, side-flexes, and rotates the occipitoatlantal joint around the appropriate axis and, with the index finger and the middle finger of the posterior hand, notes the quantity, quality, and the end feel of motion at the occipitoatlantal joint.

Supine Techniques

Occipitoatlantal Joint When mobility testing this joint, the first point to remember is that the joint is capable of

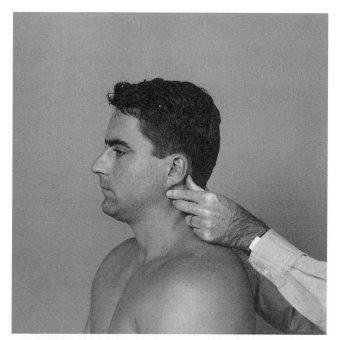

FIGURE 18–11 Patient and clinician position to assess the active mobility of the occipito-atlantal joint and atlanto-axial joint start position.

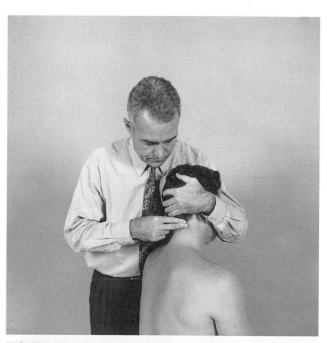

FIGURE 18–12 Passive mobility testing.

flexion, extension, and a coupling of side-flexion and rotation, albeit slight. The second point to keep in mind is that the arthrokinematics of this joint are the reverse of those occurring in the other zygapophysial joints, and that they occur in a different plane (horizontal).

With the patient in supine, the head is extended around the axis for the occipitoatlantal joint (an approximately common axis with that of the atlantoaxial joint that runs through the external auditory meatus) (Figure 18–13). The head is then side-flexed left, and right, around a common cranivertebral axis that runs roughly through the nose. As the side-flexion is carried out, a gradual translation force is applied in the opposite direction to the side-flexion. The range of movement of the side-flexion is assessed from side to side as is the end feel of the translation. This procedure is then repeated for flexion.

Extension of the occipitoatlantal glides the occipital condyles anteriorly to the limit of their symmetrical extension range. During left side-flexion and right translation in extension, the coupled right rotation is produced. This rotation causes the right occipital condyle to retreat toward a neutral position, while the left condyle advances further into the extension barrier. If left side-flexion in extension is limited, then the limiting factor is on the left joint of the segment, that is, ipsilateral to the side-flexion, which is preventing the advance of the condyle into its normal position. Thus, extension and right translation tests the anterior glide of the left occipitoatlantal joint, whereas extension and

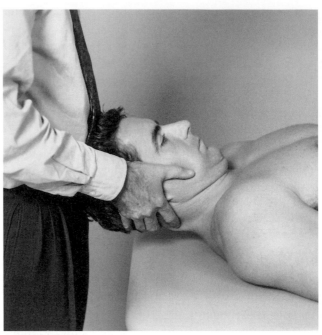

FIGURE 18–14 Patient and clinician position to assess the passive mobility of the occipito-atlantal joint in flexion.

left translation stresses the anterior glide of the right occipitoatlantal joint.

In flexion, the occipital condyles move posteriorly (Figure 18–14). The right rotation associated with left side-flexion causes the left condyle to move away from the flexion barrier toward the neutral position while the right condyle is moved posteriorly further into the flexion barrier. Thus, flexion and translation to the right tests the posterior glide of the right occipitoatlantal joint, whereas flexion and left translation tests the posterior glide of the left occipitoatlantal joint.

It is apparent that the arthrokinematic and osteokinematic are tested simultaneously. However, in this region, the arthrokinematic does not afford much information concerning the type of hypomobility, as it does elsewhere. This is due to the orientation of some of the suboccipital muscles, which are positioned such that they can restrict the glide of the joint. As a consequence, the cause of the hypomobility can only be determined from the end feel. If a hypomobility is detected, the superior oblique, which commonly restricts motion at this joint, is assessed first and then treated, if necessary.

The following patterns of impairment are more or less commonly seen, and the causes of the impairments can be deduced (Table 18–1). However, it must be remembered that deductions are only of value if the resultant intervention is successful.[37]

1. A patient who has a subluxation into flexion on the right occipitoatlantal joint should demonstrate decreased

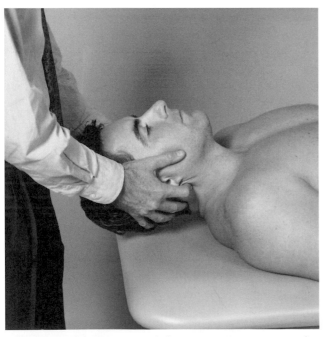

FIGURE 18–13 Patient and clinician position to assess the passive mobility of the occipito-atlantal joint in extension.

TABLE 18–1 MOVEMENT RESTRICTIONS AND PROBABLE CAUSES[37]

MOVEMENT RESTRICTED	POSSIBLE REASON
Flexion and right side-flexion	Left flexion hypomobility
	Left extensor muscle tightness
	Left posterior capsular adhesions
	Left subluxation (into extension)
Extension and right side-flexion	Right extension hypomobility
	Right flexor muscle tightness
	Right anterior capsular adhesions
	Right subluxation (into flexion)
Flexion and right side-flexion > extension and left side-flexion	Left capsular pattern
	Arthritis
	Arthrosis
Flexion and right side-flexion = extension and left side-flexion	Left arthrofibrosis (very hard) capsular end feel
Right side-flex in flexion and extension	Probably an anomaly

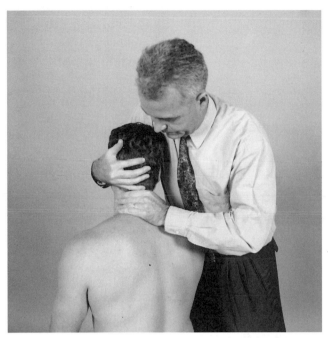

FIGURE 18–15 Patient and clinician position to assess atlanto-axial joint rotexion.

extension, decreased right side-flexion and right rotation, and a jammed end feel with translation to left.

2. A patient with a periarticular restriction of the left occipitoatlantal joint into flexion should demonstrate decreased flexion, decreased right side-flexion and right rotation, and a capsular end feel with translation to left.

3. A patient with a fibrous adhesion of the right occipitoatlantal joint should demonstrate decreased extension and right side-flexion and decreased flexion and left side-flexion, with a hard capsular end feel at both extremes.

4. With motion testing, a decreased flexion and right side-flexion, with a pathomechanic end feel, indicates a left occipitoatlantal joint subluxed into flexion.

5. With motion testing, a decreased flexion and right side-flexion limitation indicates a capsular pattern of the left occipitoatlantal joint. A decreased extension and left side-flexion limitation, with a spasm end feel in both directions (flexion with greater range), indicates traumatic arthritis.

6. A decreased right translation of the occipitoatlantal in flexion would indicate a right posterior occipitoatlantal joint problem or an impaired or tight right superior oblique.

7. Limited extension of the left atlantoaxial joint would indicate that the left occipitoatlantal joint cannot glide posteriorly, or there is an impaired or tight right inferior oblique.

Atlantoaxial Joint

There are a number of documented methods to assess the passive mobility of the atlantoaxial joint. The most common involves the patient lying supine and the clinician applying full cervical flexion and then introducing cervical rotation.

This joint can also be tested with either latexion or rotexion. There is speculation that the joint can be damaged differently depending on whether the traumatic force produces latexion or rotexion.

Rotexion

The patient sits with the clinician standing to one side. C2 (in line with base of hairline/the biggest spinous process) is stabilized in a wide lumbrical pinch grip, and the clinician's other hand reaches around the head to hold the occiput and the C1 neural arch with the little finger (Figure 18–15). The head is held against the clinician's chest and a compressive force is applied as the head is rotated toward the clinician. The compression force allows the telescoping that normally occurs as the C1 facets descend on C2. The range of motion is assessed and the end feel evaluated.

Latexion

With the patient seated, the clinician stabilizes C2 with one hand while holding the top of the patient's head with the other. The clinician side-flexes the head and neck around the craniovertebral axis, and then rotates the head in the direction opposite to the side-flexion (Figure 18–16). The clinician assesses the amount of range available and then assesses the other side. Due to the fact that the alar ligament is

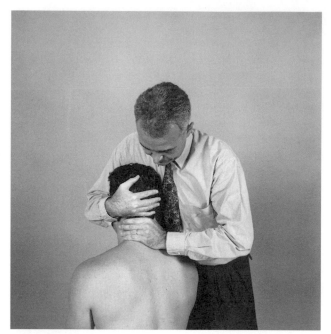

FIGURE 18–16 Patient and clinician position to assess atlanto-axial joint latexion.

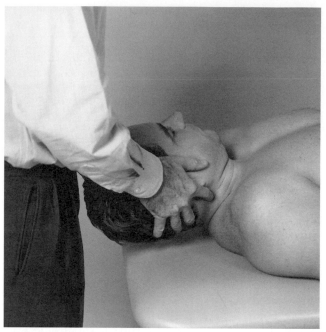

FIGURE 18–17 Patient and clinician position to assess the anterior glide of the atlanto-axial joint on the right.

slackened with the side-flexion, the amount of available atlantoaxial rotation should be increased as compared to that found with the rotexion test. It is advisable to first assess the C2–3 segment before drawing any conclusions from this test to prevent any false positives about the status of C1–2.

Anterior and Posterior Glides

The patient is supine and the head and neck is placed into full side-flexion. The craniovertebral joints are then flexed or extended before being rotated. For example, right cervical side-flexion (Figure 18–17), followed by craniovertebral flexion and left rotation, tests the ability of the right atlantoaxial joint to move maximally anteriorly, whereas left cervical side-flexion, followed by extension and left rotation of the craniovertebral joints, tests the ability of the left atlantoaxial joint to move posteriorly maximally.

Muscle Testing

Before specifically testing the musculature of this area, it is worthwhile to check the muscle groups as a whole in terms of the cardinal plane motions.

Gross Motions

As the focus for these tests is to detect muscle tears, the short muscles to be tested need to be placed on stretch, so that a minimum amount of force will be required to produce a positive finding. The long muscles have to be positioned in

their shortened positions so that they are not able to assist during the motions.

Flexors

The patient is positioned in supine while the head is cradled by the clinician. The clinician lifts the patient's head into the forward head position, placing the long neck flexors in a shortened position, and the short flexors in a lengthened position. The patient is asked to resist the clinician using the following command: "Don't let me lift your chin up to the ceiling."

Extensors

The patient is positioned in supine while the head is cradled by the clinician. The clinician places the patient's head into a craniovertebral chin tuck (chin on Adam's apple). This places the long extensors in a shortened position and the short extensors in a lengthened position. The patient is asked to resist the clinician using the following command: "Don't let me pull the back of your head up toward the ceiling."

Right Side-Flexors

The patient is positioned in supine while the head is cradled by the clinician. The clinician performs a right lateral glide of the patient's head and neck, keeping the patient's eyes horizontal. This positions the short right side-flexors in a lengthened position and the long right side-flexors in a shortened position. The patient is asked to resist the clinician using the following command: "Don't let me pull your right ear up towards the top of your head."

Left Rotators

The patient is positioned in supine while the head is cradled by the clinician. Using the principles of craniovertebral biomechanics, right side-flexion occurs with left rotation. Thus, if the right side-flexors are on stretch, so are the left rotators, although primarily at the occipitoatlantal joint. Therefore, the patient is positioned as for testing the right side-flexors. The patient is asked to resist the clinician using the following command: "Don't let me turn your head to the right."

Rectus Capitis Anterior

The anterior major and minor are tested by positioning the patient's head into craniovertebral extension and lower cervical flexion, with one hand under the occiput and the other under the mandible. The patient is asked to resist the clinician pulling the chin to the ceiling.

Rectus Capitis Posterior Major

To palpate this muscle, the clinician slides the palpating finger caudally from the occipital condyle into the space between the C2 spinous process and the condyle. The patient is asked to look up and down rapidly using eye movements only.

The muscle is tested by placing the patient's head and neck into flexion and opposite side-flexion and rotation. The patient is asked to resist the clinician using the following command: "Don't let me take you further."

To stretch this muscle, the patient is positioned in supine. The clinician fixes C2 into flexion. To stretch the left one, a right side-flexion and left rotation motion is added and the patient is instructed to not let the head drop back.

Rectus Capitis Posterior Minor

Very difficult to palpate and to isolate, but this muscle is tested along with the rectus capitis posterior major.

Inferior Oblique

The patient is positioned in supine while the head is cradled by the clinician. The clinician places a palpating finger in the space between the transverse process of C1 and the spinous process of C2, while the patient is asked to look to the same side, using eye movement only. Alternatively, the clinician can localize to the atlantoaxial by extending the occipitoatlantal joint and then rotating C1 in the appropriate direction, while C2 is stabilized.

The patient can also be positioned in side-lying with the affected side up, and the head supported underneath by the clinician's forearm. The muscle is stretched by placing the patient's head and neck into occipitoatlantal flexion, left side-flexion, and right rotation. A massage to the muscle can be applied by stroking the muscle from the C1 transverse process to the C2 spinous process, applying a force in the direction of less pain.

Superior Oblique

This muscle is located in the soft dip, just behind the mastoid process. If the right muscle is contracted, there is a decrease in flexion, left side-flexion and right rotation, and right translation of the occipitoatlantal joint. To stretch the right superior oblique, the patient's head and neck must be placed in flexion, left side bend and right rotation. The patient is positioned in sitting. The clinician places a thumb over the posterior aspect of the right transverse process of C1. The other hand wraps around the head, and the patient's head is positioned into craniovertebral flexion, left side bend and right rotation. Hold and relax or contract and relax commands can be used.

Craniovertebral Stress Testing

In the mid-cervical region, there are essentially no muscles that protect against forced cervical extension such that occurs in a whiplash injury. Most of the extension forces in the mid-cervical region are resisted by the disc and the zygapophysial joints, resulting in compression and subchondral crack fractures (subchondral). Forced flexion, on the other hand, is heavily guarded against by muscles, the ligaments, and the sternum. A posterior dislocation of the occipitoatlantal joint is the most common cervical cause of death. If the head hits an object during a cervical trauma, there is a high chance that a crack fracture through the lamina and pedicle occurred in the cervical region. Subjective reports of immediate post-trauma symptoms are of serious concern, especially if they include loss of balance.

The craniovertebral region demonstrates a lot of mobility but little stability. What ligaments there are, afford little protection during a high-velocity injury. Even a lax ligament with a small degree of trauma can have dire consequences. The craniovertebral joints are adiscal and synovial. Their zygapophysial joints facilitate motion. In the peripheral joints and the craniovertebral joints, it is the muscles that restrain angular motion, while the ligaments, bony opposition, or intra-articular congruence restrain against accessory or linear motion. Consequently, it is possible for a patient to exhibit an angular hypomobility of craniovertebral motion (through a protective muscle spasm) while simultaneously exhibiting linear or accessory hypermobility and instability (through ligamentous laxity or intra-articular attrition).

Stress tests of the whole cervical region will not be affected by muscle spasm and can, therefore, highlight the presence of instability. However, in weight bearing, the muscles can often splint an area of instability, making the joint appear normal. Although a very small percentage of the population will have a craniovertebral instability, everyone needs to be checked, especially if a history of trauma is involved.

The ligaments involved in resisting motion in this region area are a series of strong ligaments from the occiput to the first and second cervical vertebrae, which maintain the normal osseous relationship. Instability of this region can result from a number of causes.

- Trauma (especially a hyperflexion injury).
- Rheumatoid arthritis, psoriatic arthritis, and ankylosing spondylitis. Nontraumatic hypermobility or frank instability of the occipitoatlantal joint has been reported in association with rheumatoid arthritis.[54]
- Gout is the most common form of inflammatory arthritis in men over the age of 40 years and appears to be on the increase.[55] In the United States, the self-reported prevalence of gout almost trebled in men aged 45 to 64 years between 1969 and 1981.[56] Reasons for the rising prevalence of gout are thought to stem from dietary changes, environmental factors, increasing longevity, subclinical renal impairment, and the increased use of drugs causing hyperuricemia, particularly diuretics.[57–59] The usual presentation of acute gout is a monoarticular arthritis usually affecting the great toes, feet, or ankles. Less commonly the knee, elbow, and wrist are affected.[60] Its occurrence in the vertebral axis is distinctly uncommon; when reported, the neurologic symptoms range from radiculopathy to frank spinal cord compression.[61,62] In a report by Kersley and colleagues,[63] the autopsy findings in a 21-year-old man who had had severe polyarticular gout were described. The patient had a history of neck pain that was probably due to partial destruction of the odontoid process and of the body of the second cervical vertebra with subluxation of the first cervical vertebra. It was not clear if there were any neurologic symptoms, and death was attributed to pneumonia. In 1987, in a letter to the editor, Van de Laar and co-workers[64] reported on a 69-year-old man in whom progressive neurologic symptoms had developed. The symptoms resolved after operative removal of an intradural tophus at the occipital-first cervical junction. The patient had had no previous symptoms to suggest gout; but synovial aspiration of a first metatarsophalangeal joint revealed sodium urate crystals. There were no peripheral tophi. The disease process itself is a rare cause of complications, but the medications used to treat it can have serious side effects. In particular,

systemic corticosteroid therapy can weaken collagen tissue.

- Corticosteroid use. As just mentioned, prolonged exposure to this class of drug can produce a softening of the dens and transverse ligament by deteriorating the Sharpey fibers that attach the ligament to the bone. Steroid use also promotes osteoporosis.
- Recurrent upper respiratory tract infections (UTRI)/ chronic sore throats in children. Maladie de Grisel syndrome[65] is a spontaneous atlantoaxial dislocation affecting children between 6 and 12 years. The outstanding symptom is a spontaneously arising torticollis. The most likely etiology seems to be an inflammation of the retropharyngeal space caused by upper respiratory tract infections or by adenotonsillectomy, producing pharyngeal hyperemia and bone absorption.
- Congenital. Nontraumatic hypermobility or frank instability of the occipitoatlantal joint has been reported in association with congenital bony malformations.[66]
- Down's syndrome. Nontraumatic hypermobility or frank instability of the occipitoatlantal joint has been reported in association with Down's syndrome.[67–69] Gabriel and associates[70] demonstrated a high prevalence of occipitoatlantal hypermobility in children and adolescents with Down's syndrome. Harris and co-workers[71] noted that the tectorial membrane plays an essential role in maintaining upper cervical stability. As it is recognized that Down's syndrome is associated with generalized soft tissue laxity, laxity of the tectorial membrane may play a role in the occipitoatlantal hypermobility.
- Patient's under the age of 12 years, who can often have an immature or absent dens.
- Osteoporosis.

Indications for Stress Testing:[52]

- Post trauma
- Patient reports that their neck feels unstable
- Subjective history of the above. Biomechanical pain should improve in the recumbent position.

The positive signs and symptoms for these tests are:

- The presence of any serious signs, results from ischemia or insult to the brain stem or cerebellum.
- The presence of the following signs and symptoms: lump in the throat, nausea and vomiting, severe headache and muscle spasm, soft end feel, and dizziness.

The patient is laid supine to remove any muscular influences. If the patient is unable to lie down, the clinician may need to reconsider the appropriateness of performing these tests.

Longitudinal Stability

This is the opening test. Initially, general traction is applied to the whole cervical region with the patient supine or seated. If this is negative, C2 is stabilized and craniovertebral traction is applied in neutral, flexion, and extension (tectorial membrane).

Anterior Shear—Transverse Ligament[52]

The patient is positioned in supine, the head cradled in the clinician's hands. Holding the occiput, C1, and placing both thumbs on the cheeks of the patient, the clinician lifts the patient's head, keeping the patient's face parallel to the ceiling (Figure 18–18). The patient is instructed to keep the eyes open and to count backward aloud. The position is held for approximately 15 seconds or until an end feel is perceived.

The transverse ligament (Figure 18–19) can be tested more specifically in the following manner. The patient is positioned in supine with the head cradled in the clinician's hands. The clinician locates the anterior arches of C2 by following around the vertebra from the back to the front using the thumbs. Once located, the clinician pushes down on the anterior arches of C2 with the thumbs towards the table, while the patient's occiput and C1, cupped in the clinician's hands, is lifted, keeping the head parallel to the ceiling, but in slight flexion.

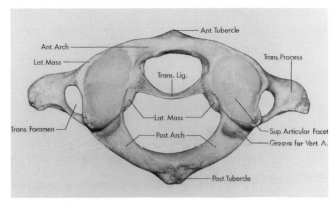

FIGURE 18–19 Transverse ligament. *(Reproduced, with permission from Wilkins RH (editor): Neurosurgery, 2e. McGraw-Hill, 1996).*

Coronal (Lateral Occipitoatlantal Test)—Alar Ligament

Rotation and side-flexion tighten the contralateral alar (rotation or side-flexion to the right tightens the left alar), whereas flexion tightens both alar ligaments (approximately 1/20 of them tighten with extension). The integrity of the alar ligaments can be tested in a number of ways.

Kinetic Test This test does not involve fixating one bone while moving the other, but it seems to give accurate results. The patient's head is rotated passively while the C2 spinous process is palpated for motion (Figure 18–20). If

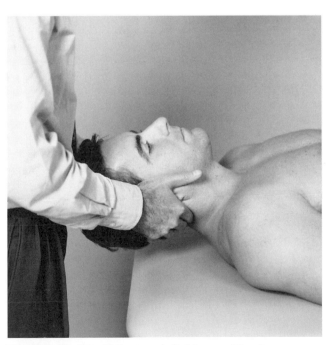

FIGURE 18–18 Patient and clinician position to assess the integrity of the transverse ligament.

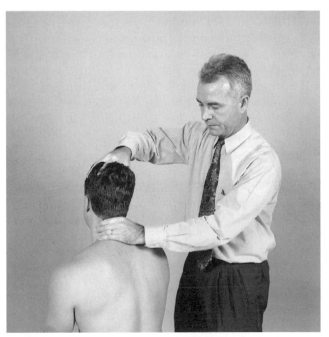

FIGURE 18–20 Patient and clinician position for the kinetic alar ligament test.

the C2 spinous process does not move immediately when the head is rotated, laxity of the ligament should be suspected.

The same test can be performed using passive side-flexion of the patient's head.

Stress Test The patient is positioned in sitting or supine. The clinician stabilizes C2 with a lumbrical grip, pushing down on its posterior neural arch with the thumb on the side opposite to the side-flexion (to block the rotation), and the index finger is placed over the other posterior neural arch of C2 (to block the side bend of C2) (see Figure 18–20). The patient's head is side-flexed with the neck in the following positions, flexion (chin tuck), neutral, and then extension.[52] With the exception of the neutral position, when the ligament will be fairly lax, the clinician should encounter a firm end feel. A test demonstrating laxity in all three positions would implicate the following.

- An insufficient ligament
- An arthrotic instability
- Differentiating alignment
- Cranioverteberal arthrosis
- Incorrect technique

To help differentiate between a ligamentous and arthrotic instability, rotation is used. As the alar ligament restricts motion in both the contralateral side-flexion and rotation directions, if side-flexion to the left, which tests the right alar, has a lax end feel, then rotation to the left should also have a lax end feel, if the right alar is the cause of the instability. However, if rotation to the left is normal, but rotation to the right has a lax end feel, an arthrotic instability should be suspected.

If the left side-flexion is slack in all three positions of flexion, neutral, and extension, the patient is seated and left rotation is assessed. The left rotation will be slack if the right alar ligament is lax. If when rotating the patient's head to the left, a block occurs at around 20 to 30 degrees of rotation (normal), right rotation is assessed. If right rotation is excessive, then an arthrotic instability is present, not an alar ligament insufficiency. Alternatively, with the patient seated, the clinician rotates the patient's head to the left, which should be blocked at about 20 to 30 degrees if the alar is intact. The head is then side-flexed to the right, and then rotated to the left. If the rotation movement is still blocked at 20 to 30 degrees, then the restriction is occurring at the cranioverteberal joints, in particular, the atlantoaxial joint, as the addition of the right side-flexion before the left rotation, should slacken the right alar ligament, allowing for more rotation to the left to occur. Until cranioverteberal

motion has been fully restored, the alar cannot be accurately assessed, as full rotation at those joints is necessary to stress it.

If the ligament is lax but asymptomatic, it should not be treated. If the ligament is symptomatic (suboccipital pain, nausea, headache, etc.), the patient can be instructed on the use of a sustained chin tuck to provide nuchal ligament support during activities of daily living.

Segmental Stability Tests for the Occipitoatlantal Joint

An initial indication that there is a segmental instability present occurs when the alar ligament stress test demonstrates movement but a normal end feel. More direct testing is needed.

Sagittal Stress Tests

Posterior Stability of the Occipitoatlantal Joint [52] The patient is supine. The sides of the patient's cranium are gently compressed with the palms of both hands. With the pads of both index fingers over each arch of the axis, the clinician uses a lumbrical muscle action, in an attempt to translate anteriorly the axis and atlas under a fixed occiput (Figure 18–21). This has the affect of moving C1–2 anteriorly on the occiput (in a similar fashion

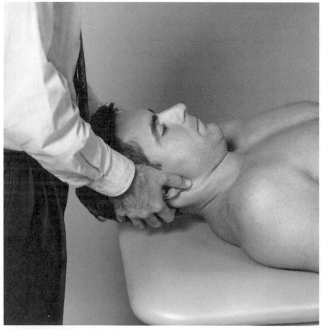

FIGURE 18–21 Posterior stability test of the occipitoatlantal joint.

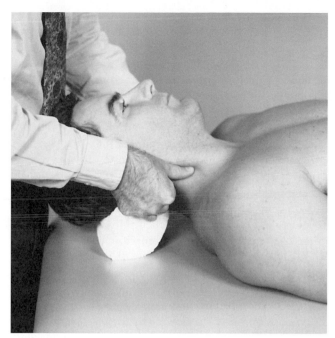

FIGURE 18–22 Anterior stability test of the occipito-atlantal joint.

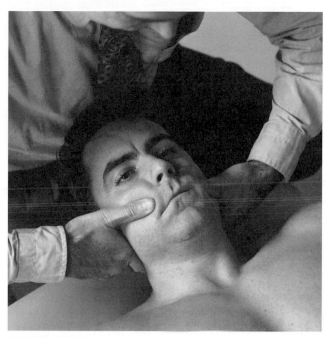

FIGURE 18–23 Patient and clinician position for the translational shear test of the occipito-atlantal joint.

as that of the transverse ligament test but with the occiput stabilized).

Anterior Stability of the Occipitoatlantal Joint[52] The patient is supine. The clinician, using the pads of fingers 2 through 5, gently cradles the occiput. The pads of the thumbs are turned medially to gently fix the anterior-lateral aspect of the transverse masses of the atlas and axis (Figure 18–22). By simultaneously and bilaterally producing a lumbrical action at the metacarpopha-langeal joints of 2 through 5, together with flexion at the thenar metacarpophalangeal joint, an anterior translatory force will occur at the occipitoatlantal joint. This has the affect of moving the occiput anteriorly on C1–2.

Transverse Shear[52] Transverse shearing of the joint, without allowing the normal curved path of translation, or rotation and side-flexion, tests the medial side of the ipsilateral joint and the lateral side of the contralateral joint. This is performed with the patient supine. Stabilizing the mastoid, C1 is moved in a transverse direction, using the soft part of the metacarpophalangeal joint of the index finger (Figure 18–23). If the instability can be demonstrated in every direction, the problem is a true segmental instability. However, if the instability is just unilateral or bilateral, the more probable cause is a capsular tear.

Segmental Stability Tests for the Atlantoaxial Joint

It must be remembered that the atlantoaxial joint complex consists of three joints. Although it has no weight bearing function, it is the median joint that is extremely important in maintaining stability, while at the same time, facilitating motion within this joint complex. Stability of this joint, in turn, is dependent on a normal and intact dens. On occasion, the integrity of the dens can be compromised:[52]

A. Anomalies of the dens.
1. *Os odontoidium*: a condition where the intervertebral disc between the developing bodies of axis and atlas does not ossify.
2. Congenital absence of the dens.
3. Underdeveloped dens with a lack of height that renders it unchecked by the transverse ligament.

B. Pathologies affecting the dens.
1. Demineralization or resorption of the dens: maladie de Grisel syndrome,[65] rheumatoid arthritis.
2. Old, undisplaced fractures (especially of the dens) that originally escaped diagnosis and subsequently, formed a pseudoarthrosis. It must be emphasized that stress tests are contraindicated if a recent dens fracture is suspected.

C. Developmental considerations.
1. The body of the dens is not of sufficient size to be retained in the osseoligamentous ring of the atlas until

a child is approximately 12 years old. It must be assumed, therefore, that the atlantoaxial joint of a child under this age is naturally unstable. Great care and justification is needed with any cranioverbral mobilization or manipulative technique with this age group.

D. Postural changes.
   1. Cadaver studies have indicated that those patients with a marked forward head posture in life, have had anatomic changes in the dens and transverse ligament. Therefore, extreme care should be undertaken when using high-velocity thrust techniques on elderly patients, especially those who exhibit a marked forward head posture.

Transverse Shear (Lateral Stability)

The transverse shear test of the atlantoaxial joint is used with a history of maladie de Grisel syndrome.[65] The soft aspect of each second metacarpal head is placed on the opposite transverse processes and laminae of C1 and C2, with the palms facing each other. Stabilize C1 and attempt to move C2 transversely, using the soft part of MCPs (Figure 18–24). Observe for movement (of which there should be none).

Modified Sharp-Purser—Anterior Stability of Atlantoaxial Joint

The Sharp-Purser test was originally designed to test sagittal stability of the atlantoaxial segment in rheumatoid

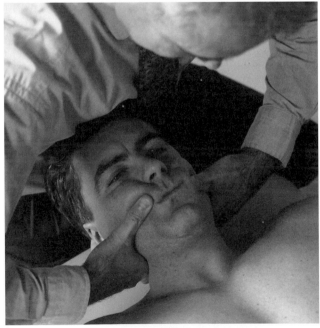

FIGURE 18–24 Patient and clinician position for the translational shear test of the atlantoaxial joint.

arthritic patients. In these patients, a number of pathologic conditions can affect the stability of the osseoligamentous ring of the median joints of the atlantoaxial segment. The articular cartilage between the odontoid and the anterior arch of atlas can degenerate and thin, the dens can become softened, and the ligament's collagen affected so that it becomes lax. There can even be ossification of the ligament. The aim of the original test was to determine whether the patient's central nervous system's signs and/or symptoms were being caused by such an instability.

The patient is asked to flex the head and to report any signs or symptoms evoked. If no cardinal symptoms are provoked, the test is discontinued. However, if cardinal symptoms are provoked, the assumption is made that they are caused by excessive translation of the atlas. The assumption is tested when the examiner employs one of two methods of reducing the potential anterior translation. With the flexed position maintained, either the forehead can be stabilized and the axis manually translated anteriorly, or, the axis can be stabilized and the head translated posteriorly with pressure against the forehead.

In reality, one should question the wisdom of investigating the cause of the cardinal symptoms as, for the physical therapist, the mere presence of those symptoms should be sufficient to return the patient to their physician.

INTERVENTIONS

Manual Therapy

Mobilization

The following mobilization techniques for the restriction of extension, right side-flexion, and left rotation of the left atlantooccipital joint can be performed. The reader is expected to extrapolate the information to produce the necessary techniques for an anterior glide restriction of the left joint.

Techniques to Increase Extension, Right Side-Flexion, and Left Rotation of the Left Atlantooccipital Joint

Specific Traction[72] Specific traction is used here, as elsewhere in the spine, to apply a gentle degree of mechanical stimulation. It is typically used with acute conditions.

Traction for the atlantooccipital joint is performed with the patient seated. True distraction at this level cannot effectively be carried out because of the alar ligaments. In order to gain any separation of the joint surfaces, the alar ligament must first be slackened off. This is most easily accomplished by the introduction of cranioverbral side-flexion. The clinician stands to one side of the patient and stabilizes the C1 vertebra using a wide pinch grip, while the other arm reaches around the patient's head and stabilizes it against the clinician's chest, while the hand cradles the occiput (Fig 18–25). A traction force is then applied, utilizing a graded cranial force (I–II) by the occipital hand and the chest.

Supine Axial Technique   The patient is supine with the head supported. The clinician grasps the head from its vertex toward the ears with both hands. The head is extended by counter-nodding it around an axis through the ears and then right side-flexed by taking the ear to the neck around an axis through the nose. As the side-flexion is being carried out, the head is also translated to the left until the extension barrier for the right joint is reached, in a manner similar to the joint assessment. Mobilization is then carried out by graded force against the translation barrier.

Specific Seated Technique[72]   The patient is in seated with the clinician standing on the left side. C1 is stabilized anteriorly using a wide pinch grip by the right hand and wrapping the pads of the index finger and thumbs around the front of the transverse process. The left arm stabilizes the patient's head against the clinician's chest and the left hand grasps the occiput. The patient's head is then extended and right side-flexed around the appropriate axes, with left translation being produced with the side-flexion until the extension barrier is reached. Mobilization is then carried out by graded force against the translation barrier.

As an alternative to stabilizing below the atlantooccipital joint, the whole cervical spine is placed in a position of full chin protrusion (Figure 18–26). From this position, the head is extended and side-flexed to the right and translated to the left, allowing for the congruent left rotation to occur. The right condyle is then mobilized anteriorly.

Active participation from the patient can be introduced. From the motion barrier, the patient is asked to gently meet the clinician's resistance. The direction of resistance is that which facilitates further extension, right lateral bending, and left rotation. The isometric contraction is held for up to 5 seconds and followed by a period of complete relaxation. The joint is then passively taken to the new motion barrier. The technique is repeated three times and followed by a reexamination.

Distraction Techniques   For the first technique, the patient is positioned in supine, the clinician at the head of the table, seated to the patient's right. Contact is made by the clinician's right hand, using the web space between the thumb and the forefinger, on the inferior and right aspect of C0 (the right mastoid process). The clinician's right hand is positioned parallel to the patient's sternum and his or her left forearm wraps around the patient's head so that the hand cups the patient's chin. The patient's head is then side-flexed toward the clinician (to the right) around the appropriate axis (through the nose),

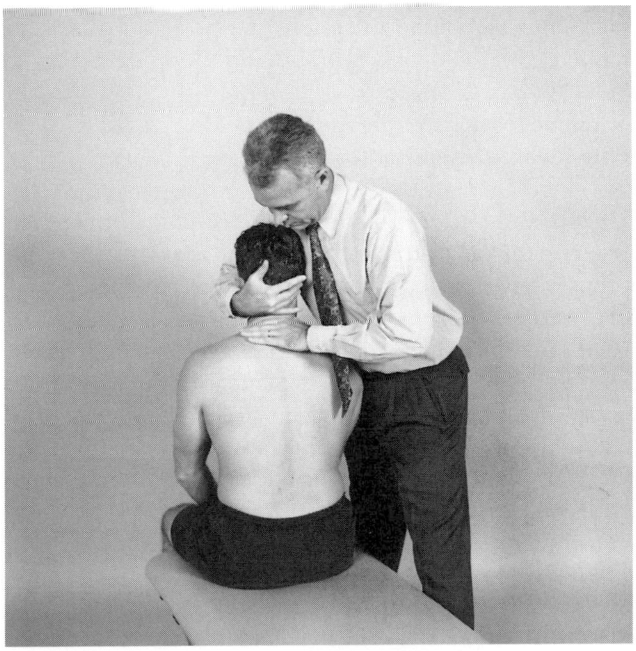

FIGURE 18–25   Patient and clinician position to apply specific traction to the occipitoatlantal joint.

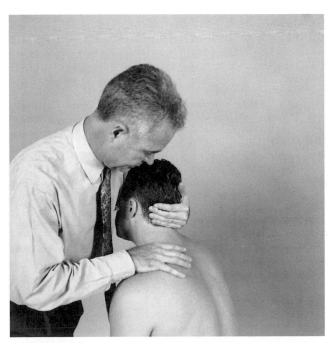

FIGURE 18–26   Patient and clinician position to mobilize the occipitoatlantal joint into extension, right side-flexion, and left rotation. Note how the clinician positions the patient's cervical spine in flexion.

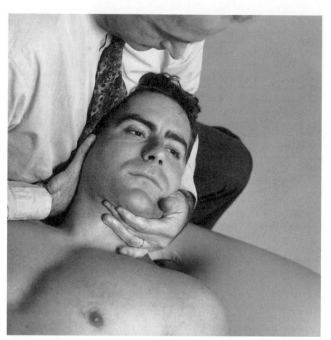

FIGURE 18–27 Patient and clinician position for the distraction technique for the occipitoatlantal joint.

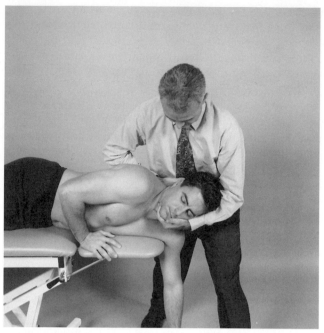

FIGURE 18–28 Distraction thrust technique for the occipitoatlantal joint with the patient positioned in left side-lying.

allowing for the conjunct rotation to the left to occur (Figure 18–27). Having taken up the slack with the right hand, a mobilizing force of I–V is then applied to the mastoid in a superior direction (by the right hand), while the other hand and arm help to guide the intended movement.

The second technique begins with the patient is positioned in left side-lying, so that the left axilla is at the head of the bed and the bottom arm is hanging off the end of the bed (Fig 18–28). The clinician stands behind the patient and cradles the patient's head with their left arm, while the left hand cups the patient's chin. Using the left hand and arm, the clinician side-flexes the patient's neck toward the ceiling, around the appropriate axis, allowing for the conjunct rotation to the left to occur. Contact is made with the inferior aspect of C0 (mastoid process) by the clinician's right hand, using the MCP joint of the index finger. The clinician's right forearm is positioned parallel to the patient's vertebral column. Having taken up the slack with the right hand, a high-velocity, low-amplitude thrust is then applied to the mastoid in a superior and anterior direction. Care must be taken not to be overly aggressive with this technique.

To restore the left rotation of the right atlantoaxial joint, the clinician can either perform a technique to increase the anterior glide of the right atlantoaxial joint, or a technique to increase the posterior glide of the left atlantoaxial joint, or apply both at the same time. In this joint, the side of the impairment is not often considered to be an

issue. It is felt that regardless of the side of impairment, an asymmetrical impairment will always lead to a loss of either rotexion or latexion, and that this hypomobility can be addressed grossly. However, anatomically and biomechanically, it can be seen that there are different consequences associated with the loss of the anterior glide versus a loss of the posterior glide. From a clinical safety perspective, an overzealous technique to restore the posterior glide can threaten both the vertebral artery and the spinal cord.

Technique to Increase the Anterior Glide of the Right Atlantoaxial Joint

Distraction Technique Apart from the point of contact, the set up for the distraction technique is exactly the same as that of the first occipitoatlantal distraction technique just described (Fig 18–27). The patient is positioned in supine, and the clinician is at the head of the table, seated to the patient's right. Contact is made with the inferior aspect of C1 (atlas) by the clinician's right hand, using the MCP joint of the index finger. The clinician's right forearm is positioned parallel to the patient's sternum. The patient's neck is side-flexed to the right around the cranioverbetral axis (through the nose), allowing for the conjunct rotation (to the left) to occur. Having taken up the slack with the right hand, a high-velocity, low-amplitude thrust is applied to C1 in a superior direction, parallel to the patient's sternum. Care must be taken not to be overly aggressive with this technique.

Technique 2 The patient is positioned in supine, the clinician at the head of the table. The clinician supports the patient's head in his or her hands and the posterior aspect of C1 on the right is monitored, using the index finger of the right hand. The thumbs of both hands rest on the patient's jaw and cheeks. Gripping the patient's jaw and cheeks, the patient's head is then side-flexed to the right, either throughout the whole cervical spine (the patient's right ear is passively taken to their ipsilateral shoulder), or around the craniovertebral axis (through the nose). The head is then rotated to the left to the end of the available range (Figure 18–29). After the slack has been taken up into right side-flexion and left rotation, a high-velocity, low-amplitude thrust is then applied into left rotation by the right hand while the left hand guides the movement. Care must be taken not to be overly aggressive with this technique.

Posterior Glide of Left Atlantoaxial Joint It is the author's opinion that restoration of the posterior glide is more safely achieved using a mobilization technique.

The patient is seated, the clinician standing on the left side of the patient. Using a wide lumbrical pinch grip of the right hand, the clinician stabilizes the axis (C2) and the vertebra below. The clinician reaches around the patient's face with his or her left arm and forearm. Using the little finger of that hand, the right facet joint of C1 is stabilized against anterior motion. The patient's head is then side-flexed to the right around the craniovertebral axis (through the nose), allowing for the conjunct rotation (to the left) to occur. Using his or her left shoulder, the clinician leans against the patient's left forehead and applies a backward and downward mobilization force into left rotation, thereby mobilizing the left joint of C1 posteriorly (Figure 18–30).

Soft Tissue Techniques[73]

Soft tissue techniques are generally applied before performing the local segmental examination and in preparation for a mobilization or manipulation treatment. Soft tissue techniques are capable of producing a strong analgesic and relaxing effect. With a reduction in cervical muscle tension, or spasm, it becomes much easier for the clinician to palpate and register movement.

Suboccipital Massage[72] There are a number of sites in the cervical region where transverse friction can be performed. In principle, every tender site can be treated, even though it usually involves areas of referred pain or tenderness. Temporary pain relief results, allowing for more effective performance of the segmental examination and/or segmental treatment.

The patient lies in a prone position on the treatment table with the forehead resting on the hands. The head is positioned in slight flexion, without rotation. The clinician stands on the opposite side to be treated, at the head of the bed. While one hand supports the head, the other hand

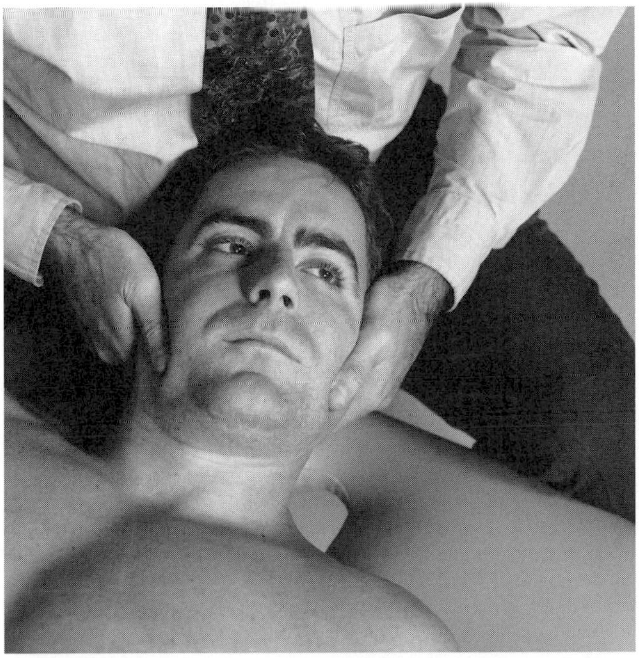

FIGURE 18–29 Supine rotational thrust technique to restore the anterior glide of the atlantoaxial joint on the right.

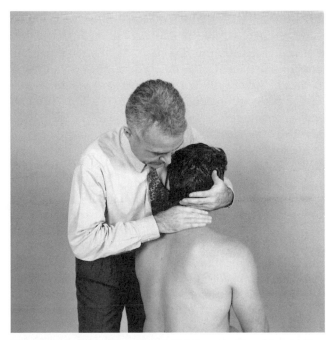

FIGURE 18–30 Patient and clinician position for mobilization technique to restore the posterior glide of the atlantoaxial joint on the left.

palpates the suboccipital muscles. The sternocleidomastoid (SCM) may need to be displaced laterally in order to palpate the muscles attaching to the transverse process of C1. The clinician locates the most tender area, which is often found just caudal to the lateral third of the inferior linea nuchae. The clinician places the index finger, reinforced by the middle finger, directly lateral to the tender spot. The thumb rests on the other side of the patient's head, at a level slightly cranial to the index finger. During the "friction" phase, the index finger moves from laterally to medially and slightly cranially. At the same time, pressure is exerted in a anterior-medial-superior direction (toward the thumb). Pain arising during this technique is likely due to pressure on the greater occipital nerve. In this instance, the transverse friction is performed in an area just medial or lateral to that spot.

A similar technique is used in a combination of upper cervical traction and soft tissue mobilization of the suboccipital muscles. While one hand grasps the patient's head, the clinician uses the fingers of the other hand to press gently into the muscles between two vertebrae. While maintaining the pressure on the muscles, a slight traction force is applied and sustained for several seconds, before being released. The procedure is repeated in a rhythmical manner.

The paravertebral muscles can be treated in a similar fashion. With one hand, the clinician stabilizes the patient's head at the forehead. If the right side is to be treated, the clinician positions the patient's head and upper cervical spine in slight left side-flexion. With the index and/or middle fingers of the right hand, the clinician "hooks" just medial to the paravertebrals musculature between the atlas and axis. The musculature is then "pulled" in a lateral and ventral direction. At the same time, the hand on the patient's forehead rotates the patient's head toward the side bending treated. The end position is held for 2 to 3 seconds before returning to the initial position. The clinician repeats this technique for several seconds, or minutes, in a rhythmic manner.

Rhythmic Flexion C2 to C7   The patient is positioned in supine and the clinician stands at the head of the bed. The clinician cradles the patient's head in his or her hands. After first performing craniovertebral flexion, a flexion movement in the rest of the cervical spine is performed. Simultaneously, the thumb and fingers push toward each other, through the musculature, and pull in a dorsal direction. The clinician begins at the level of C2–3, and the flexion motion is performed no further than this point. The end position is held for 2 to 3 seconds, before returning to the initial position. The clinician repeats this technique several times in a rhythmic manner.

The same procedure can then be performed per segment, by shifting the dorsal hand caudally. As the successive caudal segments are localized, increasingly more flexion is performed. This technique can be used to treat the segments C2–7.

In the same way, coupled movements in flexion can also be performed. After first performing an upper cervical flexion, the clinician brings the patient's head simultaneously, into flexion, ipsilateral rotation, and side-flexion. In this instance, pressure is emphasized on the convex side of the cervical spine.

General Kneeding   General kneeding can also be applied to the soft tissues of the craniovertebral region. This technique is especially useful prior to performing a specific mobilization or manipulation.

Electrotherapeutic Modalities and Physical Agents

Therapeutic Exercise

All exercises should be performed at an intensity level that achieves an improvement without a regression of status. The following exercises have been found to be useful, providing that correct stabilization is used by the patient.

1.   Chin tuck: The patient is seated in the correct posture. The patient is instructed to attempt to move the head as a unit in a posterior direction while maintaining eye level. As mentioned in other chapters, the clinician should limit the number of chin tucks the patient performs so as to remove any potential for harm to the cervical structures from overuse.

2.   C2–3 side-flexion/rotation: The pattern of limitation for this area is usually one of a closing restriction. The patient is seated in the correct posture. The patient places both hands behind the neck, with the ulnar border of the little finger just below the C2 spinous process, and the rest of the hand covering as much of the mid-cervical region as possible. The patient is then instructed to simultaneously side bend and rotate the head in the direction of the restriction by attempting to look downward and backward (for a closing restriction). This technique can be used for all mid-cervical levels, provided that the correct localization is used.

3.   AA rotation: The patient is seated in the correct posture. The patient places both hands behind the neck, with the ulnar border of the little finger at the level of the C2 spinous process, and the rest of the hand covering as much of the mid-cervical region as possible. The patient is then instructed to gently turn the head in the direction of the restriction. If the patient has a restriction with right rotation, emphasize right rotation and left side-flexion.

4. OA flexion: The patient is seated in the correct posture. The patient performs a chin tuck and is then instructed to place the tips of the index and middle fingers of both hands over the anterior aspect of the chin. The finger tips provide resistance for an attempted extension movement of the head on the neck. The patient then attempts to look upward while resisting the motion with the fingertips. This is followed by relaxation and another chin tuck.

Case Study: Headache and Neck Pain

Subjective

A self-employed 42-year old man presented to the clinic complaining of posterior upper neck pain and right suboccipital and occipital headache that began 2 months earlier after a diving accident. He denied being knocked unconscious and could remember everything about the accident, except for a few minutes after it. The posterior neck pain was felt immediately, but was much worse the next morning upon waking. The occipital headaches started, a few days later that became worse with fatigue or exertion. The patient also reported difficulty concentrating and sleeping, and had occasional bouts of dizziness, especially when turning his head to the left, during which he would become unsteady, but denied vertigo. When the neck and occipital pain flared up, it spread from the occipital region over the head to the right eye. Previous interventions included physical therapy in the form of ultrasound, massage, spray, and stretch; myofascial release; and cranial sacral therapy, which had provided no relief. The patient had no history of back or neck pain, apart from the occasional ache and his medical history was unremarkable.

Questions

1. List the concerns the clinician should have following this history.
2. Using the flow diagram outlined in this chapter, describe how would you proceed with this patient following the subjective history.
3. What special tests should be considered at this point?
4. Are additional questions needed with regard to the subjective reports?

Examination

Given the subjective history, it is likely that the patient was concussive, even though he denies being unconscious. The reports of dizziness appear related to a specific movement, but because that movement is rotation of the head, further testing will be needed to rule out a vertebral artery or head injury. Some of the more insidious reasons for the headache, such as a slow intracranial bleed, can be excluded, as the symptoms are not progressing and the condition is 2 months old. The type of headache associated with the patient is the typical cervical headache in the occiput with occasional spread occipitofrontally and orbitally when exacerbated, and is usually related to head and neck movements and postures. However, the neck pain and occipital headache should have responded to physical therapy. The fact that it did not suggests that inappropriate therapy may have been given.

With this type of history, it would be prudent to perform a scanning examination with the addition of a cranial nerve, and vertebral artery examination. The scanning examination and additional tests revealed the following findings.

- The patient had no obvious postural deficits or deformities.
- Cranial nerve testing was negative except that during the tracking tests for the third, fourth, and sixth nerves, he experienced mild, short-duration vertigo and longer lasting nausea.
- Craniovertebral ligament stress testing was negative for both instability and symptomatology.
- Dizziness was not reproduced with the vertebral artery tests.

  As the vertebral artery appeared to be normal (given the lack of cranial nerve signs and the negative tests), the Hallpike-Dix test was performed. The Hallpike-Dix test, a clinical test for vestibular impairment, involves having the patient suddenly lie down from a sitting position with the head rotated in the direction the examiner feels is the provocative position. The end-point of the test is where the head overhangs the end of the bed so that the neck is extended. This reproduced his dizziness when his head was in left rotation and extension. The dizziness came on almost immediately and disappeared within a minute. No cranial nerve signs were discovered on testing while he was dizzy.

- The patient had full range cervical movements except for extension, left rotation, and right side-flexion.
- There were no signs of neurologic deficit. All neuromeningeal (dural and neural tension) tests were negative.
- The compression and traction tests were negative.
- Posterior-anterior pressure over the spinous process of C2 and over the back of C1 neural arch reproduced his headache and local tenderness.
- The posterior suboccipital muscles were hypertonic and tender to moderate palpation.

Questions

1. Given these findings, what is your working hypothesis?
2. List some of the possible reasons for the dizziness.
3. How would you proceed?

Evaluation

It seems probable that the occipital headache is due to an impairment in the craniovertebral joints,[74,75] but exactly where cannot be ascertained as yet from the examination. A biomechanical examination is required.

Passive physiologic and accessory (arthrokinematic) movement testing of the craniovertebral area determined that there was decreased anterior glide of the right occipitoatlantal joint with a hard end feel and a decreased anterior glide of the right atlantoaxial joint. There was also some point tenderness over the right levator scapular and right upper trapezius.

Questions

1. Given the findings from the biomechanical examination, how would you explain your intervention to the patient?
2. Explain the correlation between the loss of the glides and the loss of active range of motion.
3. How would you proceed?

Intervention

There is every likelihood that the patient's dizziness is from a musculoskeletal dysfunction within the craniovertebral area. However, to confirm this, once the two restrictions have been corrected and are functioning normally, the patient should be reassessed.

● *Electrotherapeutic modalities and thermal agents.* A moist heat pack was applied to the upper cervical spine when the patient arrived for each treatment session. Electrical stimulation with a low frequency was applied with the moist heat to aid in for pain and edema reduction. Ultrasound at 3 MHz was administered following the moist heat. An ice pack was applied to the area at the end of the treatment session

● *Manual therapy.* Following the ultrasound, generalized soft tissue techniques were applied to the area followed by a specific mobilization and manipulation to increase the anterior glide of the right occipitoatlantal joint, and a separate technique to increase the glide of the right atlantoaxial joint.

● *Therapeutic exercises* were prescribed to maintain the mobility gained into extension, left rotation, and right side-flexion. The patient performed OA extension and AA rotation to the left in a slow and controlled manner, stooping at the point in the range when symptoms were produced.

● *Patient-related instruction.* Explanation was given as to the cause of the patient's symptoms. The patient was advised against sudden or repetitive turning of the head to the left. Sustained positions of the head were to be avoided unless the head was supported.

Instructions to sleep on the right side were given. The patient was advised to continue the exercises at home, 3 to 5 times each day. The patient also received instruction on the use of heat and ice at home.

● *Goals and outcomes.* Both the patient's goals from the treatment and the expected therapeutic goals from the clinician were discussed with the patient. It was concluded that the clinical sessions would occur three times per week for 1 month, at which time, the patient would be discharged to a home exercise program. However, after only six sessions, the patient was symptom free.

REVIEW QUESTIONS

1. Describe the articular anatomy of the craniovertebral region.
2. What are the unique structures providing stability in the craniovertebral region?
3. What essential structures are vulnerable to craniovertebral instability?
4. What pathologic conditions are likely to lead to an instability of the craniovertebral region?
5. What signs and symptoms would you expect to find in a patient with an acute undisplaced fracture of the dens?
6. What clinical tests would you carry out in a patient whom you suspected had a fractured dens?
7. What investigations would you suggest to the physician when you suspected a dens fracture?
8. List four *symptoms* suggestive of severe CNS compromise that would cause you to return the patient to the physician for further investigation.
9. List six *signs* of severe CNS compromise that would cause you to return the patient to the physician for further investigation.
10. Discuss and demonstrate a test for craniovertebral instability.
11. Which of the following is not a suboccipital muscle: rectus capitis lateralis, rectus capitis posterior major, rectus capitis posterior minor, obliquus capitis inferior, obliquus capitis superior?
12. What is the extension of the posterior longitudinal ligament called?
13. Where does the extension of the posterior longitudinal ligament attach?
14. What is the action of the rectus capitis posterior major?
15. What is the action of the rectus capitis posterior minor?
16. Which muscle produces side-flexion of the OA to the same side, as well as extension and contralateral rotation of the OA.

17. A decreased anterior glide of the right occiput condyle would produce which movement deficits at the OA joint?
18. Approximately, how many degrees of side-flexion occur at the OA joint?
19. Approximately, how many degrees of rotation occur at the OA joint?
20. Side-flexion of the OA joint is limited by which ligament?
21. Right side-flexion at the OA joint involves an anterior glide of the occiput condyle on which side?
22. With the OA joint tested in extension, a decreased left side glide would indicate a impairment on which side of the OA joint?
23. A tight rectus capitis anterior would produce a decreased translation to which direction while in craniovertebral extension?
24. What is the function of the transverse ligament?
25. At the AA joint, if rotation occurs first (rotexion), in which direction do the side-flexion and rotation occur?

ANSWERS

1. OA joint. Occipital condyles are biconvex and articulate with the superior facets of the atlas, which are biconcave. The AA joint has two lateral and two median articulations. The lateral articulations are biconvex with lax capsular ligaments allowing for good mobility. The median articulations are formed between the posterior surface of the dens and the anterior aspect of the transverse ligament.
2. The dens, alar ligament, transverse ligament, and tectorial membrane.
3. Vertebral artery, transverse ligament (tear), dens (fracture).
4. Trauma (hyperflexion), systemic arthritis (RA, Reiter's), Down's producing adensia, microdensia, and maladie de Grisel's syndrome (juvenile upper respiratory tract infection).
5. Inability to flex or compensate flexion and will protrude the chin in an effort to achieve flexion. Nausea, dizziness, drowsy, and reluctance to move the head.
6. None.
7. An open mouth X-ray.
8. Paresthesia: bilateral or quadrilateral, dysphasia, dysarthria, ataxia.
9. Neurogenic bladder, saddle paresthesia, hypo- or anesthesia—bilateral or quadrilateral, drop attacks, Babinski, Hoffmann, or Oppenheim; paresis—bilateral or quadrilateral.
10. Transverse ligament stress test. Look for abnormal end feel and CNS symptoms. If movement does occur or end feel is softer than it should be, but there are no CNS

symptoms, maintain position for 15 seconds in order to look for possible signs and symptoms of ischemia.
11. Rectus capitis lateralis.
12. Tectorial membrane.
13. The body of C2.
14. Ipsilateral side-flexion, contralateral rotation, and extension of the OA joint.
15. Ipsilateral side-flexion, contralateral rotation, and extension of the OA joint.
16. Obliquus capitis superior.
17. Decreased extension, right side-flexion, and left rotation.
18. 5.
19. 8.
20. Alar.
21. Right.
22. Right.
23. Left translation.
24. Prevents anterior translation of C1 on C2.
25. To the same side.

REFERENCES

1. Williams PL, Warwick R, Dyson M, Bannister LH. *Gray's Anatomy*. 37th ed. Edinburgh: Churchill Livingstone; 1989.
2. Singh S. Variations of the superior articular facets of atlas vertebrae. *J Anat* 1965;99:565–571.
3. Tulsi RS. Some specific anatomical features of the atlas and axis: dens, epitransverse process and articular facets. *Aust N Z J Surg* 1978;48:570–574.
4. Cassidy JD, Loback D, Yong-Hing K, Tchang S. Lumbar facet joint asymmetry: Intervertebral disc herniation. *Spine* 1992;17:570–574.
5. Malmavaara A, Videman T, Kuosma E, Troup JDG. Facet joint orientation, facet and costovertebral joint osteoarthritis, disc degeneration, vertebral body osteophytosis, and Schmorl's nodes in the thoracolumbar junctional region of cadaveric spines. *Spine* 1987;12:458–463.
6. Noren R, Trafimow J, Andersson GBJ, Huckman MS. The role of facet joint tropism and facet angle in disc degeneration. *Spine* 1991;16:530–532.
7. Pratt N. Anatomy of the cervical spine. *APTA Orthopedic Physical Therapy Home Study Course*. Orthopedic Section, APTA; La Crosse, WI; Jan 1996.
8. Panjabi M, Dvorak J, Duranceau J, et al. Three-dimensional movement of the upper cervical spine. *Spine* 1988;13:727.
9. White AA, Panjabi MM. *Clinical Biomechanics of the Spine*. 2 ed. Philadelphia: Lippincott Co; 1990.
10. Worth DR, Selvik G. Movements of the craniovertebral joints. In: Grieve G. (ed): Modern Manual Therapy of

the Vertebral Column. Edinburgh: Churchill Livingstone; 1986:53.

11. Werne S. The possibilities of movements in the craniovertebral joints. *Acta Orthop Scand* 1959;28:165–173.

12. Penning L, Wilmink JT. Rotation of the cervical spine. A CT study in normal subjects. *Spine* 1987;12:732–738.

13. Dvorak J, Hayek J, Zehender R. CT—functional diagnosis of the rotary instability of the upper cervical spine—2. An evaluation on healthy adults and patients with suspected instability. *Spine* 1987;12:726–731.

14. Schaffler MB, Alkson MD, Heller JG, Garfin SR. Morphology of the dens: a quantitative study. *Spine* 1992;17:738.

15. Ellis JH, Martel W, Lillie JH, Aisen AM. Magnetic resonance imaging of the normal craniovertebral junction. *Spine* 1991;16:105.

16. Kapandji IA: *The Physiology of the Joints, Vol 3: The Trunk and Vertebral Column.* New York: Churchill Livingstone; 1974.

17. Braakman R, Penning L. *Injuries of the Cervical Spine.* Amsterdam: Excerpta Medica; 1971:3–30.

18. Werne S. Studies in spontaneous atlas dislocation. *Acta Orthop Scand* 1957;23(suppl):23–28.

19. White AA, Panjab MM. The clinical biomechanics of the occipitoatlantoaxoid complex. *Orthop Clin N Am* 1975;9:867–878.

20. Mimura M, Moriya H, Watanabe T, et al. Three-dimensional motion analysis of the cervical spine with special reference to the axial rotation. *Spine* 1989;14:1135.

21. Selecki BR. The effects of rotation of the atlas on the axis: experimental work. *Med J Aust,* 1969;1:1012.

22. Fielding JW. Cineroentgenography of the normal cervical spine. *J Bone Joint Surg,* 1957;39A:1280.

23. Hohl M, Baker HR. The atlanto-axial joint. *J Bone Joint Surg* 1964;46A:1739–1752.

24. Harata S, Tolmo S, Kawagish T. Osteoarthritis of the atlanto-axial joint. *Intl Orthop* 1981;5:277–282.

25. Bohlman HH. Degenerative arthritis of the lower cervical spine. McC. Evarts, C. ed. 2. In: *Surgery of the Musculoskeletal System,* 2nd ed. New York: Churchill Livingstone; 1990;1857–1886.

26. Emery SE, Bohlman HH. Osteoarthritis of the cervical spine. In: *Osteoarthritis Diagnosis and Medical/Surgical Management,* 2nd ed. Moskowitz RW, Howell DS, Goldberg VM, Mankin HJ, eds. Philadelphia: Saunders; 1992;651–668.

27. Halla JT, Hardin JG, Jr. Atlantoaxial facet joint osteoarthritis: a distinctive clinical syndrome. *Arthr Rheumatol* 1987;30:577–582.

28. Fielding JW, Hawkins RJ, Ratzan SA. Spine fusion for atlanto-axial instability. *J Bone Joint Surg* 1976;58-A:400–407.

29. Fielding JW, Cochran GV, Lawsing JF, III, Hohl M. Tears of the transverse ligament of the atlas. A clinical and biomechanical study. *J Bone Joint Surg,* 1974;56-A:1683–1691.

30. Ghanayem AJ, Leventhal M, Bohlman HH. Osteoarthrosis of the atlanto-axial joints. Long-term follow-up after treatment with arthrodesis. *J Bone Joint Surg* [Am] 1996;78:1300–1307.

31. Bogduk N. The rationale for patterns of neck and back pain. *Patient Management* 1984;8:13.

32. Howe JF, Loeser JD, Calvin WH. Mechanosensitivity of dorsal root ganglia and chronically injured axons: a physiological basis for the radicular pain of nerve root compression. *Pain* 1977;3:25–41.

33. Anthony M. Headache and the greater occipital nerve. *Clin Neurol Neurosurg* 1992;94:297–301.

34. Hollinshead WH. Anatomy for Surgeons: Vol 3, The Back and Limbs. Philadelphia: Lippincott; 1982.

35. Boden SD, Wiesel SW, Laws ER, et al. *The Aging Spine.* Philadelphia: Saunders; 1991.

36. Yoganandan N, Pintar F, Butler J, et al. Dynamic response of human cervical spine ligaments. *Spine* 1989;14:1102.

37. Meadows J. Manual Therapy: Biomechanical Assessment and Treatment-Advanced Technique. Swodeam Consulting Calgary, AB,1995.

38. Dvorak J, Panjabi MM. Functional anatomy of the alar ligaments. *Spine* 1987;12:183.

39. Dvorak J, Panjabi MM, Gerber M, Wichmann W. CT functional diagnostics of the rotary instability of the upper cervical spine and experimental study in cadavers. *Spine* 1987;12:197–205.

40. Okazaki K. [Anatomical study of the ligaments in the occipito-atlantoaxial complex]. [Japanese] *Nippon Seikeigeka Gakkai Zasshi* [Journal of the Japanese Orthopaedic Association] 1995;69:1259–1267.

41. Panjabi M, Dvorak J, Crisco J, et al. Flexion, extension, and lateral bending of the upper cervical spine in response to alar ligament transections. *J Spinal Dis* 1991;4:157–167.

42. Vangilder JC, Menezes AH, Dolan KD. *The Craniovertebral Junction and Its Abnormalities.* Mount Kisco, NY: Futura Publishing Co; 1987.

43. Pal GP, Sherk HH. The vertical stability of the cervical spine. *Spine* 1988;13:447.

44. White AA, Johnson RM, Panjabi MM, et al: Biomechanical analysis of clinical stability in the cervical spine. *Clin Orthop* 1975;109:85–96.

45. Dvorak J, Schneider E, Saldinger P, et al. Biomechanics of the craniocervical region: the alar and transverse ligaments. *J Orthop Res* 1988;6:452–461.

46. Werne S. Studies in spontaneous atlas dislocation. *Acta Orthop Scand* 1957;23.

46. Lipson SJ. Fractures of the atlas associated with fractures of the odontoid process and transverse ligament ruptures. *J Bone Joint Surg Am* 1977;59:940–943.

47. Lazorthes G. Pathology, classification and clinical aspects of vascular diseases of the spinal cord. In: Vinken PJ, Bruyn GW, (eds). *Handbook of Clinical Neurology.* vol 12. Oxford: Elsevier; 1972:494–506.

48. Wells CEC. Clinical aspects of spinovascular disease. Proceedings of the Royal Society of Medicine 1966; 59:790–796.

49. Baumgartner RW, Waespe W. ASA syndrome of the cervical hemicord. *Eur Arch Psychiatry Clin Neurosci* 1992;241:205–209.

50. Decroix JP, Ciaudo-Lacroix C, Lapresle J. Syndrome de Brown-Sequard du a un infarctus spinal *Rev Neurol* 1984;140:585–586.

51. Gutowski NJ, Murphy RP, Beale DJ. Unilateral upper cervical posterior spinal artery syndrome following sneezing. *J Neurol Neurosurg Psychiatry* 1992;55:841–843.

52. Pettman E. In: Boyling JD, Palastanga N, (eds). *Grieve's Modern Manual Therapy: The Vertebral Column,* 2nd ed. Edinburgh: Churchill Livingstone; 1994.

53. Lee DG, Walsh MC. *A Workbook of Manual Therapy Techniques for the Vertebral Column and Pelvic Girdle.* 2nd ed. Vancouver: Nascent; 1996.

54. Martel W. The occipito-atlanto-axial joints in rheumatoid arthritis. *AJR Am J Roentgenol* 1961;86:223–240.

55. Roubenoff R. Gout and hyperuricaemia. *Rheum Dis Clin North Am* 1990;16:539–550.

56. Lawrence RC, Hochberg MC, Kelsey JL, et al. Estimates of the prevalence of selected arthritic and musculoskeletal diseases in the United States. *J Rheumatol* 1989;16:427–441.

57. Isomaki H, von Essen R, Ruutsalo H-M. Gout, particularly diuretics-induced, is on the increase in Finland. *Scand J Rheumatol* 1977;6:213–216.

58. Currie WJC. Prevalence and incidence of the diagnosis of gout in Great Britain. *Ann Rheum Dis* 1979;38: 101–106.

59. Rigby AS, Wood PHN. Serum uric acid levels and gout: what does this herald for the population? *Clin Exp Rheumatol* 1994;12:395–400.

60. Cornelius R, Schneider HJ. Gouty arthritis in the adult. *Radiol Clin North Am* 1988;26:1267–1276.

61. Varga J, Giampolo C, Goldenberg DL. Tophaceous gout of the spine in a patient with no peripheral tophi:

case report and review of the literature. *Arthr Rheumatol* 1985;28:1312–1315.

62. Fenton P, Young S, Prutis K. Gout of the spine: two case reports and a review of the literature. *J Bone Joint Surg* [Am] 1995;77:767–771.

63. Kersley GD, Mandel L, Jeffrey MR. Gout: an unusual case of softening and subluxation of the first cervical vertebra and splenomegaly. *Ann Rheumat Dis* 1950;9: 282–303.

64. Van de Laar MA, Van Soesbergen RM, Matricali B. Tophaceous gout of the cervical spine without peripheral tophi (letter). *Arthr Rheumatol* 1987;30:237–238.

65. Parke WW, Rothman RH, Brown MD: The pharyngovertebral veins: an anatomical rationale for Grisel's syndrome. J Bone Joint Surg 1984;66A:568.

66. Georgopoulos G, Pizzutillo PD, Lee MS. Occipitoatlantal instability in children. *J Bone Joint Surg* [Am] 1987;69:429–436.

67. Brooke DC, Burkus JK, Benson DR. Asymptomatic occipito-atlantal instability in Down's syndrome. *J Bone Joint Surg* [Am] 1987;69:293–295.

68. El-Khoury GY, Clark CR, Dietz FR, Harre RG, Tozzi JE, Kathol MH. Posterior atlantooccipital subluxation in Down syndrome. *Radiology* 1986;159:507–509.

69. Ishida Y, Yamada H, Yamanaka H, Shinoda T. Atlantoaxial instability in Down's syndrome. *Seikeigeka* 1989;40:1297–1308.

70. Gabriel KR, Manson DE, Carango P. Occipito-atlantal translation in Down's syndrome. *Spine* 1990;15:997–1002.

71. Harris MB, Duval MJ, Davison Jr JA, Bernini PM. Anatomical and roentgenographic features of atlantooccipital instability. *J Spinal Disord* 1993;6:5–10.

72. Kaltenborn F. The Spine: Basic Evaluation and Mobilization Techniques. Wellington: New Zealand University Press; 1993.

73. Winkel D, Omer Matthijs, Valerie Phelps et al. *Diagnosis and Treatment of the Spine; Non-operative Orthopaedic Medicine and Manual Therapy.* Gaithersburg, Maryland; Aspen; 1996.

74. Adeboye KA, Emerton, DG, Hughe T. Cervical sympathetic chain dysfunction after whiplash injury. *J R Soc Med.* 2000;93:378–379.

75. Evans RW. The postconcussion syndrome and the sequelae of mild head injury. *Neurol Clin* 1992;10:815–847.

CHAPTER NINETEEN

WHIPLASH-ASSOCIATED DISORDERS

Chapter Objectives

At the completion of this chapter, the reader will be able to:

1. Define the term whiplash-associated disorders (WAD).
2. List the various mechanisms of injury for whiplash associated disorders.
3. Describe the types and causes of injuries sustained in whiplash associated disorders.
4. List the major areas of involvement associated with whiplash associated disorders, their pertinent anatomy, and presentation.
5. Perform a detailed objective examination of the musculoskeletal system following a motor vehicle accident, paying particular attention to the signs that could indicate a compromise to the central nervous system (CNS) or vertebrobasilar system.
6. Analyze the total examination data to establish the definitive biomechanical diagnosis.
7. Apply a variety of tests and techniques that assess for dizziness or injury to the temporomandibular joint, and demonstrate an awareness for the caution needed with this type of patient.
8. Develop self-reliant examination and intervention strategies, based on the stage of healing.
9. Describe the intervention based on clinical findings and established goals.

OVERVIEW

The term whiplash injury was introduced in 1928 by the American orthopedist H. E. Crowe.[1] It was defined as the effects of sudden acceleration–deceleration forces on the neck and upper trunk due to external forces exerting a "lash-like effect." Crowe emphasized that the term whiplash "describes only the manner in which a head was moved suddenly to produce a sprain in the neck." In 1953, Gay and Abbott[2] described common whiplash injuries of the neck in the *Journal of the American Medical Association*. Since then, whiplash injury incidence has risen and, according to the editors of a 1998 text, is still rising.[3]

Despite significant medical resources for both diagnostic examination and intervention, whiplash associated disorders (WAD) remain poorly understood. A lack of thorough understanding of whiplash is, in part, a result of the nature of the disease. The subjective nature of the symptoms and their high prevalence have led to controversy over the determination of their cause, and appropriate financial compensation.[4–6] The subjective complaints are most often characterized by reports of neck pain in the absence of focal physical findings and positive imaging studies.[7] Although most patients have spontaneous resolution of symptoms within 6 months of their onset, there is a small subgroup of patients who are symptomatic beyond 1 year.[7] Aggressive imaging and diagnostic testing routinely fails to identify the specific source of the symptoms, and therapeutic interventions are often unsuccessful. It is experience with this group of patients with chronic symptoms where the need for a better understanding of the risk factors, pathophysiology, natural history, and effectiveness of intervention options becomes apparent.[7]

Despite attention from a profusion of health care professionals and conferences, the whiplash injury remains an enigma. Part of the confusion lies in its definition.[8]

Definition

Some authors of whiplash articles, such as Gay and Abbott[2] do not define whiplash clearly. Neither Gotten[9] nor Macnab[10,11] offered definitions, although Macnab noted that "a significant soft tissue injury can result from the application of an extension strain to the neck by sudden acceleration."[11] Farbman[12] classed whiplash injury as a simple musculoligamentous neck sprain, which excluded nerve root damage, fractures, and other complications. Nordhoff[13] describes the whiplash injury in equally simplistic terms, as injuries which occur as a result of occupant motions within a vehicle that is rapidly decelerating or accelerating, without reference to the body parts involved. Radanov[14] did not initially define whiplash, but later he described it as a simple musculoligamentous sprain, excluding fractures, head injuries, and alteration in consciousness.[15] Even the definition provided by The Quebec Task Force on Whiplash-associated Disorders,[7] offered the following definition that, for whatever reason, did not include front end collisions.

> Whiplash is an acceleration-deceleration mechanism of energy transfer to the neck. It may result from rear-end or side-impact motor vehicle collisions, but can also occur through diving and other mishaps. The impact may result in bony or soft-tissue injuries (whiplash injury), which in turn may lead to a variety of clinical manifestations.

Finally, it is worth remembering that although "neck sprains" from motor vehicle accidents usually involve the cervical spine, one of the upper eight thoracic spinal joints is sometimes found to be affected; so injuries of this sort could be included in a definition of whiplash.[16] Whiplash is thus best defined as a traumatic event involving high acceleration–deceleration forces that act on the spine, producing an excursion of the head and neck without a direct blow to the head.

Causes

- Motor vehicle accidents
- Sporting injuries
- Blows to the neck or body
- Pulls and thrusts on the arms
- Falls, landing on the trunk or shoulder

Mechanism

Eighteen percent of motor vehicle accidents involving passenger cars in the United States in 1994 were rear-end impacts, and resulted in injury to 500,000 people.[17] Pure extension injuries seem to be uncommon.[18] A more likely mechanism, in a rear-end collision, is a rotational force on the neck, resulting from a turned position on impact. Examining the effects of low-impact rear-end collisions in seven volunteers, McConnell and co-workers[19] observed the first movement to be head rotation, then forward translation of the entire head; hyperextension was not seen. None of these volunteers, nor Severy's two, 40 years earlier,[20] reported any relevant symptoms after the tests.

Head rests also appear to play a part with drivers often setting their head rests too low or sitting too far forward to obtain adequate support from the head rests.[21,22]

Experiments on healthy volunteers have indicated the most likely sites of injury and their mechanism.[23] During the early phase of a rear-end collision, the trunk is forced upward toward the head, and the cervical spine undergoes a sigmoid deformation.[24] During this motion, at about 100 msec after impact, the lower cervical vertebrae undergo extension, but without translation.[24] This motion causes the vertebral bodies to separate anteriorly, and the zygapophysial joints to impact posteriorly.[24] The impairments likely to result from such motion are tears of the anterior anulus fibrosus and fractures or contusions of the zygapophysial joints,[23] and these impairments are found postmortem in victims of fatal motor vehicle crashes.[25,26]

EPIDEMIOLOGY

According to reports of data in other studies, more than 1 million whiplash injuries occur each year in the United States.[5] In addition to the subjective distress resulting from neck and upper extremity pain, absenteeism from work and subsequent costs to society are also incurred.

A recent study[15] examined a group of 117 consecutive patients, who were followed on a regular basis from shortly after the initial injury through 2 years, to determine whether preinjury status, mechanism of injury, physical examination, and somatic, radiologic, or neuropsychologic factors could be used to predict eventual outcome. At 2 years, those patients with persistent symptoms were found to be older at the time of injury than the asymptomatic group, and had a higher incidence of pretraumatic headache. There was a higher incidence of a rotated, or inclined, head position at the time of impact as well as a higher intensity of initial neck pain and headache, a higher incidence of initial radicular symptoms, a greater number of initial overall symptoms, as well as a higher average score on a multiple-symptom analysis.[15]

Financial compensation, which is determined by the continued presence of pain and suffering, appears to provide a barriers to recovery, and may promote persistent illness and disability. The incidence of insurance claims for whiplash is about 1 per 1000 population per year,[27] yet not all persons involved in motor vehicle crashes develop symptoms, and not all symptomatic patients experience chronic injury. After an acute injury, most patients rapidly recover, with some 80% being asymptomatic by 12 months.[15] After 12 months, between 15% and 20% of patients remain symptomatic, and only about 5% are severely affected. The latter group of patients however, constitute the major burden to insurance companies and to health care resources.

While neck pain and headache are the two most common symptoms,[28] other symptoms, such as visual disturbances, balance disorders, and altered cerebral function, are reported. Postmortem studies reveal that many injuries occur that are undetectable by plain X-rays.[29]

Injury

Damage can occur to the following types of structures.

- Soft tissue (tears)[30]
- Bone (fractures)
- Joint (capsule and ligament tears)
- Central and/or peripheral neurologic systems (secondary to traction, impingement, hemorrhage, avulsion, and/or concussion)
- Dorsal root ganglia[26]
- Vascular (vertebrobasilar arteries)
- Vestibular (otolithic avulsion, endolymph leaks)
- Visceral (secondary to ruptures or contusions)

The degree of damage done in an accident depends, in part, on the position of the head at the point of impact, the amount of force involved, and the direction of those forces.

As many as 57% of persons sustaining whiplash injury with symptoms persisting 2 years after collisions, reported having their heads rotated out of the anatomic position at the time of impact.[15,50] In fact, head position has been reported as the only accident feature of a collision event that has a statistically significant correlation with symptom duration.[50]

The amount of force applied to the neck is approximately equal to the weight of the head and the speed that the head moves. Consequently, the heavier the head or the faster it moves, the greater the stress that is put through the neck. However, it is well recognized by clinicians with any experience with post-MVA patients, that some patients who have survived high velocity accidents do better than many who appear to have been involved in trivial impacts. The third factor, force direction, must, therefore, play a significant role in the degree of damage sustained by the patient. The direction of the forces depends on:[62]

- Where the car is hit, that is, front end, rear end, or side.
- The symmetry of the impact, that is, directly head on or rear end, or the forward or backward side.
- Whether the car is pushed ahead into another vehicle, the curb, or other stationary object.
- The position of the victim (looking straight ahead, sideways, or backward at the passengers) and whether

the accident was expected or unexpected. If the head was rotated, it is possible that the alar ligaments were irreversibly overstretched or even ruptured.[51]

Hyperextension forces result in the head being moved upward and backward initially, and this is the most damaging motion, and can lead posterior dislocations.[10,52,53] The reason for the greater severity of hyperextension injuries over other force directions is believed to be related to a number of factors including:[13]

- Whether the seat back breaks
- Whether the occupant hits the front of the occupant space
- The differential motion between the seat back and occupant
- Hyperextension of the neck over the head restraint
- Rebound neck flexion as the head rebounds off the head rest

However, the fatal accidents involving hyperextension appear to occur in the absence of a head restraint where there is no structural limitation to the head movement except anatomical structure. Hyperflexion injuries are typically less severe because the amount of head excursion is limited by the chin striking the chest. With side-flexion injuries, the head can strike the window if closed or, if moving in the other direction, the trunk is free to move with it, attenuating the force on the neck and, in addition, the head can only go as far as the shoulder before it is stopped thereby sustaining disc injuries, and strains and sprains from side-flexion and rotation of the head and neck.

The subject of seatbelts is controversial. The seatbelt is responsible for producing more injuries than any other contact source in the car, albeit minor ones. This is in part due to their design which restrains only one shoulder and also to the fact that the belt acts as a fulcrum for energy concentration on the occupant.[13]

As of 1997, federal law has required all passenger vehicles to have airbags and although early indications appear to suggest a decrease in neck injuries with airbags, they may merely change the distribution of injuries.[13]

MacNab's[54] research on the effects of hyperextension forces in primates revealed the following impairments.

- Minor to major tears of the sternomastoid, longus colli.
- Retropharyngeal hematomas (always present if longus colli torn).
- Esophageal hemorrhaging.
- Horner's syndrome.
- Anterior longitudinal ligament tearing. However, studies on humans, using scintigraphy and MRI, have not been able to verify this occurring in humans.[34,55] An

explanation for the divergent findings might be that the animals were exposed to a more severe trauma, enough to result in the described impairments.

● Separation of the disc from the vertebral body.

Even the most severe of these impairments, the disc separation, did not show up on X-ray.[54] These and other impairments, including fractures and dislocations, many causing cord damage, have been demonstrated on human victims of hyperextension injuries who had no radiographic evidence of such severe impairments.[56,62]

A number of other variables also determine the type, and extent, of the injury.[13]

● Seat position
● Occupant size, height and posture
● Vehicle interior design
● Size of vehicle
● Sex of driver. Women generally position their seats more forward than men, which places their bodies closer to the front car structures, and therefore at higher risk of impacting the front interior.

Thus, other than perhaps to screen for possible fractures, there is no valid indication for medical imaging after whiplash unless the patient has neurologic signs.[7] Findings on plain films are typically normal, and magnetic resonance imaging reveals nothing but age-related changes with the same prevalence as in asymptomatic individuals.[34-36] An enticing, but small, recent study suggests that in patients with persisting acute neck pain, single photon emission computed tomography at 4 weeks after injury can reveal occult, small fractures of the vertebral rims or the synovial joints of the neck.[37]

It is, therefore, obvious that a meticulous examination of the traumatized patient by the physical therapist is of paramount importance.[38] Signs and symptoms to alert the clinician include:

● Central nervous system signs
● Periodic loss of consciousness
● Patient does not move the neck, even slightly (fractured dens)
● Painful weakness of the neck muscles (fracture)
● Gentle traction and compression are painful (fracture)
● Severe muscle spasm (fracture)
● Complaints of dizziness

SOURCE OF SYMPTOMS

As in the lumbar spine, the outer layers of the cervical anulus are innervated,[39] and are, therefore, a reasonable

TABLE 19–1   PAIN DISTRIBUTION FROM CERVICAL STRUCTURES

STRUCTURE	PAIN AREA
Occipital condyles	Frontal
Occipitocervical tissues	Frontal
C1 dorsal ramus	Orbit, frontal, and vertex
C1–2	Temporal, sub to occipital
C3 dorsal ramus	Occiput, mastoid, and frontal

source of pain, a possibility demonstrated by discography.[40] Zygapophysial joint pain is the only basis for chronic neck pain after whiplash that has been subjected to scientific scrutiny.[32-33] However, it cannot be diagnosed clinically, or by medical imaging. The diagnosis relies on fluoroscopically guided, controlled diagnostic blocks of the painful joint. Although there is uncertainty about the exact pathway that elicits neck pain, the cervical zygapophysial joint has been identified as a site of neck pain in between 25% and 65% of people with neck pain.[41-47] Specifically, the prevalence of lower cervical facet joint pain has been reported to be 49%.[42] Both mechanoreceptors and nociceptors have been identified in the human cervical joint capsule[48] and ligaments,[49] indicating a neural input in pain sensation and proprioception.(Table 19–1)

Although the same amount of research on the muscles, bone, dura, and ligaments has not been forthcoming, it seems likely that these have the potential for pain production.

OUTCOMES

Preexisting symptoms, such as headache and radiologic degenerative changes, are important predictors for an unfavorable outcome.[59] Experimental and clinical studies have consistently demonstrated how poorly and slowly disc impairments heal after a hyperextension trauma. An experiment, using surgically caused rim lesions in the discs of sheep, found that those lesions reached a depth of 5 mm ($\frac{1}{20}$ inch) and did not heal for a period of at least 18 months.[60] Other autopsy studies[26] support this finding.

A study averaging a review time of nearly 11 years[61] found that 40% of patients were still having intrusive or severe symptoms (12% severe and 28% intrusive). The same study also found that in general, the symptoms did not alter after 2 years postaccident.

As the underlying injury is often hidden from the physical examination, and almost invariably from plain radiographs, the clinician must be careful, not only with the intervention, but also with the examination, to not cause more damage. Where possible, the examination, and the intervention, must be very gentle until the acute healing phase is over.

INDICATIONS FOR A GENTLE APPROACH[62]

- Recent Trauma of 6 weeks or less
- An acute capsular pattern
- Severe movement loss, whether capsular or noncapsular
- Strong spasm
- Paresthesia
- Segmental paresis
- Segmental or multisegmental hypo-or areflexia
- Other neurologic signs and/or symptoms
- Constant or continuous pain
- Moderate to severe radiating pain
- Moderate to severe headaches
- Dizziness

MAJOR AREAS OF INVOLVEMENT

Over recent years, the role of the manual clinician in the intervention of the consequences of whiplash has increased dramatically. It is imperative that the manual clinician have a strong understanding of the mechanisms that produce the myriad of symptoms that these patients can present with so as to improve the understanding behind the various intervention protocols and rationale. The following systems, regions, conditions, or symptoms occur frequently in the whiplash population.

1. Alteration in the central nervous system
2. Temporomandibular impairment
3. Cervical impairment
4. Vertebral artery insufficiency

Central Nervous System Trauma

Mild brain injury or concussion is not an uncommon occurrence following a motor vehicle accident and, as such, is frequently part of the history related to the clinician. Most of these traumatic episodes do not produce profound neurologic damage and are termed concussions (contusions). Concussion is not always associated with some degree of loss of consciousness, and typically involves a sudden acceleration (or deceleration) force which causes the brain to move within the skull. For a loss of consciousness to occur, these forces must disconnect the alerting system in the brain stem, after which, there is temporary lack of activity in the reticular formation, probably secondary to hypoxia resulting from induced ischemia. It is estimated that a velocity of only 20 mph can cause

concussion from inertial loading (no head impact) for most healthy adults.[13]

Temporomandibular Dysfunction

Although the temporomandibular joint is afforded its own chapter, for the sake of completeness, its relation to whiplash associated disorders is included here.

Dental malocclusion and temporomandibular joint impairments have been inculpated in the production of pain and dizziness. Although the exact mechanism is unclear, postural influences, alteration in the position of the jaw by the malocclusion, and the subsequent mismatching between the cervical muscles, might be enough to produce the symptoms. The temporomandibular joint should, therefore, always be considered in patients complaining of jaw pain and dizziness, following a motor vehicle accident.

Cervical Spine

From the perspective of the manual clinician, cervical pain is a very common finding, but one that is potentially fraught with difficulties.[62] The intervention for an inappropriate patient, or an inappropriate intervention of the cervical spine, could result in severe consequences. Planning the intervention is made more complicated in the presence of cervicogenic dizziness.

It is not always an easy task for the manual clinician to determine if the dizziness, experienced by the patient is a result of disturbed afferent input from the cervical spine, which can be extremely rewarding to treat, or if the cause is more serious, and contraindicates any intervention.

Among those cervical causes, that must be carefully considered by the clinician, are cervical articular vertigo and vertebral artery disease. Of interest is that some manual practitioners believe that if a patient's vertebral artery symptoms are as the result of a hypermobility of C1–2 (produced by a hypomobility of C2–3), the C2–3 segment should be mobilized. Although this appears to be good rationale, this decision should only be undertaken by the most experienced practitioner.

Cervical Vertigo

Cervical vertigo is a diagnosis/disorder that seems to be poorly understood. Ryan and Cope[63] coined the term "cervical vertigo" in 1955 for this syndrome, which involves vertigo, in addition to tinnitus, hearing loss, and neck pain. It would appear that this form of dizziness results from a disturbed sensory input from the mechano-receptors of the neck. The syndrome often results from trauma, such as a whiplash injury, but in one article on the subject, only 50%

of the cervical vertigo patients in the group had experienced trauma.[64] Macnab[65] argued that the 575 patients he studied exhibited little evidence of overt neck damage, or of neurologic damage, and proposed that areas other than the neck itself, such as the brain, the brain stem, the cranial nerves, the cervical nerve roots, or the inner ear, might be responsible for the symptoms. Biesinger,[66] on the other hand, proposed three possible origins.

1. A participant of the sympathetic plexus surrounding the vertebral arteries
2. Vertebral artery occlusion
3. Functional disorders of proprioceptive in segments C1–2.

Biesinger thought that some historical data was needed to support the theory that the neck was the source of the vertigo in (1) neck pain following trauma, (2) vertigo provoked by certain positions or movements of the head, and (3) provoked vertigo of short duration.

Certainly, clinical experience tends to confirm the clinical study of Wing and Hargrave Wilson,[64] that dizziness is also a result of more acute trauma, both major and minor, that is correctable by appropriate intervention regimens.[62]

It would seem likely that those patients who sustain direct damage to the vestibular apparatus, or severe damage to the vertebral artery, would report immediate dizziness, whereas dizziness arising from the cervical joints, or a less severe vertebral artery lesion, would not occur until the joints themselves became abnormal, or until the ischemia had time to make itself felt.

The physical examination of such patients usually reveals some neck muscle spasm and limited neck mobility. Cervicogenic dizziness is demonstrated best by rotational movements of the body, with the head stationary.

As early as 1926, Barré[67] described a syndrome involving suboccipital pain, and vertigo, that was usually precipitated by turning the head, and not accompanied by any other vestibular functions, and tinnitus along with visual symptoms. These symptoms appear to result from an alteration to proprioceptive spinal afferents. Several investigators have shown nystagmus and disorientation when local anesthetics were injected into the neck muscles, or when experimental animals underwent transection of cervical sensory roots. These alterations in the neck were signaled to the brain stem through spinovestibular pathways. In 1927, Klein and Nieuwenhuyse[68] first demonstrated that simple rotation of the patient's neck while the head was maintained fixed, caused vertigo and nystagmus. In 1976, Toglia[69] reported objective electronystagmography (ENG) abnormalities in 57% percent of 309 patients with whiplash injuries. Wing and Hargrave Wilson[64] reported that 100% of their 80 patients showed nystagmus in ENG

records with the head flexed, extended, or rotated to the right and left. In 1991, Chester reported finding abnormal peripheral vestibular function using platform posturography in 90% of 48 patients examined.[70]

The intervention for cervical vertigo generally begins with conservative physical therapy and antiinflammatory medications, once testing rules out an active inner ear disorder. With time and therapy, most patients with abnormal ENGs end up having normal ENGs at follow-up testing.[62]

Vertebral Artery

Vertebral artery compromise (see Chap 5) can produce a number of neurologic symptoms, including vertigo which is discussed here.[71,72] Although isolated vertigo can be assigned a benign cause, a number of studies indicate that this is rarely the case.[73,74] The pathogenesis of this isolated vertigo must be considered in the context of the vascular anatomy and physiology of the vestibular system. At the level of the brain stem, the vestibular nuclei are supplied by penetrating and short circumferential arterial branches of the basilar artery. In turn, the internal auditory artery, arising either directly from the basilar artery or from the anterior inferior cerebellar artery (AICA), supplies the vestibulocochlear nerve, the cochlea, and the labyrinth.[75,76] Because the labyrinthine branches are small and receive less collateral flow, it is possible that the labyrinth becomes a more prominent target of the effects of atherosclerosis of the vertebrobasilar system.[77] In contrast, the cochlea receives collateral flow from branches of the internal carotid artery that supply the adjacent portions of the petrous bone and, thus, may have more protection against vascular insufficiency.

EXAMINATION OF THE WHIPLASH PATIENT

The examination of the acute and recently traumatized neck is necessarily different from the routine examination, because of the potential for the examination itself to be harmful.

Where possible, the patient should be examined for central and peripheral neurologic deficit, neurovascular compromise, and serious skeletal injury, such as fractures or craniovertebral ligamentous instability. The examination must be discontinued at the first signs of serious pathology.[62]

It must also be remembered that every post-MVA patient, especially the ones with a history of hyperextension, are at potential risk for serious head and neck injuries. The following signs and symptoms are ascribable to head injury (but, of course, could have other causes) and demand a cautious approach to the examination of the patient.

- Headache
- Dizziness or tinnitus
- Loss of concentration
- Memory loss or forgetfulness
- Difficulties with problem solving
- Apathy
- Fatiguability
- Reduced motivation
- Irritability
- Anxiety and/or depression
- Insomnia

Although there is conflicting evidence of the prevalence of vertebrobasilar ischemia from vertebral artery damage,[54,78] the possibility of such damage cannot be ignored and the patient must be safeguarded as much as possible from the possibility of causing a vertebrobasilar infarction. To this end, the arterial system should preferably be left unstressed for at least 6 weeks.[62]

Extensive tissue damage has been demonstrated both experimentally and clinically. Tissue damage in monkeys subjected to comparable experimental insults in the early 1960s and 1970s[79–82] was found to be almost exactly the same as that found in humans in hyperextension injuries.[26,58,81,83]

Three precautions that the clinician can take are:

1. Listen and observe carefully for central nervous system signs or symptoms including the following.

   - Hemiplegia or quadriplegia of the trunk or extremities
   - Paralysis or paresis of the face
   - Spasticity or rigidity
   - Sensory loss
   - Nystagmus
   - Ataxic gait
   - Dysphasia
   - Dysphagia
   - Dysarthria
   - Blurred vision
   - Nausea and/or vomiting
   - Anesthesia of the lip (perioral)—suspected to be secondary to a impairment of the trigeminal thalamic tract from thalamus and/or the superior cerebral branch of vertebral artery.
   - Hypoacousia
   - Diplopia
   - Horner's syndrome
   - Atrial fibrillation

   - Vertigo
   - Drop attacks

2. Make a thorough examination.
3. Avoid extension and rotation as part of the intervention as these are a common feature of manipulation-induced strokes.

The examination should include:

- Range of motion in straight planes, as well as rotation out of flexion and extension to assess the function of the upper and lower cervical spine separately.[84]
- Comparison of active and passive range of motion.
- Cranioverterbral instability. Any indication that there is a loss of integrity of the atlantoaxial osseoligamentous ring should demand immediate immobilization of the neck with the hardest collar available, while the patient is left lying on the treatment table until a physician or ambulance arrives.[62] No further intervention should be undertaken.

Partial or complete tears of the alar ligament, generally, are not an immediate serious danger to the patient's life and a less drastic approach can be taken. The intervention can be continued, but should not be such that it exacerbates the symptoms ascribable to damage of this ligament.

The following screen is a useful tool to aid in determining the cause of a patient's dizziness. It must not, of course, take the place of a full neurologic screen. In this example, the patient reports dizziness when turning the head to the left.

1. The patient attempts to follow the clinician's finger, using the eyes only. If dizziness is reproduced, it is the result of ocular incoordination. Oscillopsia can also be tested for by having the patient focus on a distant object. The clinician moves a hand rapidly in front of the patient's eyes. The patient should report a blurring of the hand but the distant object should remain in focus. The patient then focuses on the same distant object while the clinician places a hand in front of the face. The patient now rotates the head from side to side. If the patient perceives the hand to be moving, there is a lesion in one of the balance centers.
2. The patient closes the eyes and rotates the head to the left. If this reproduces the dizziness, there is a problem with either the patient's inner ear or the craniovertebral joints.
3. The patient is asked to close the eyes and keep the head still. The clinician rotates the patient's trunk and shoulders to the right. If this reproduces the symptoms, the

craniovertebral joints are at fault. If this test is negative, then the inner ear is at fault.

- *Vertebrobasilar insufficiency:* if the examination of the patient suggests the possibility of vertebrobasilar artery insufficiency, manipulation must be considered absolutely contraindicated.

  Dvŏrák and Orelli[85] have suggested that manipulative techniques be abandoned totally in the neck and other less forceful manual techniques substituted.

- *Central nervous system involvement:* long tract tests. Nociception, proprioception, thermoception, and mechanoception may be tested to ensure that all pathways are functioning at least grossly normally.[62] As pain, temperature, and light and crude touch are carried by essentially the same pathways and can be tested simultaneously, pin prick and/or light touch should ensure that these pathways are sufficiently assessed.

Stretch Reflexes

- *Deep tendon:* the deep tendon reflexes are carried out looking for hyperreflexia. The best reflexes to use for this purpose are those easiest to elicit, biceps brachia, quadriceps, and Achilles.

- *The scapulohumeral reflex is a test of high cervical neurologic compromise.* The spine of the scapular and/or the acromion is tapped with the reflex hammer and a positive test is one where there is elevation of the shoulder girdle or abduction of the arm. A long reflex hammer has been recommended for the test rather than a small lightweight one.[62] A positive test is believed to be indicative of an upper motor neuron impairment between the C1–3 levels.[86]

- *Clonus:* the dynamic stretch reflex that assesses how well the central nervous system inhibits the reflex.

- *Nocioceptive spinal:* Babinski, Oppenheim, and Hoffmann tests.

INTERVENTION

The following discussion on intervention is based on what has clinically seemed to work best, and is grounded on the stages of healing and biomechanical principles. It should also be noted that the significantly injured post-MVA patient is one of the most difficult and challenging, yet potentially rewarding patients that the clinician can work with.

The goals of the intervention should be aimed at:

1. Promotion and progression of healing and preventing further damage. This is a vital component as a considerable percentage of these patients become chronic pain sufferers.

2. Control of pain and inflammation with antiinflammatory modalities (RICE) and a soft cervical collar (until capsular pattern subsides).

3. Patient education

4. Preventing a dependence on health care practitioners.

5. Restoring motion and strength as well as neuromuscular function through:

   - Early, but gentle, mobilization exercises[87]
   - Nonweight-bearing, progressing to weight-bearing, mid-range active exercises, and then careful full-range active movement exercises.
   - Gentle isometric exercises.
   - Treat specific articular impairments with mobilizations providing these do not threaten the vertebral artery.[62]
   - Electromuscular stimulation if no muscle tearing has occurred.

6. Restoring maximal function.

The chosen intervention techniques should be specific, low amplitude, and nonrotational.

The intervention of the significantly injured post-MVA patient will generally follow the stages of healing and will consist of: the acute, phase; the sub-acute, phase and the chronic phase.

The Acute Phase

Patient Education
The clinician must discuss diagnosis, prognosis, and the intervention with the patient. Expectations must be set out both from the patient and from the clinician. The patient must realize at the outset that he or she is responsible for his or her own recovery, and must participate actively in treatment.

It is important that the clinician describes the basic anatomy and function of the cervical spine in a terminology that the patient can relate to.

Rest
The patient should be encouraged to perform as many activities of daily living as possible. Rest is advocated in the first 72 hours to give healing a chance, or recovery from the acute phase is delayed. The patient is told that rest means just that. Pillows should be adjusted so that the head remains in a neutral position when sleeping in side-lying or supine. The patient should be cautioned about prone-lying.

Collar

The collar has a number of functions including:

1. Providing support in maintaining the cervical spine in the erect position.
2. Reminding the patient that the neck is injured and, thereby, preventing the patient from engaging in unguarded movements, or excessive movements.
3. Allowing the patient to rest the chin thereby offsetting the weight of the head.

Although several studies have concluded that the wearing of a cervical collar results in delayed recovery, these studies looked at the use of collars and other passive modalities versus other more active forms of intervention such as early patient activation and exercise.

While it is true that prolonged reliance on the collar may induce stiffness and weakness, this can be avoided by recommending a time-limited use of the collar, which is based on specific factors such as the patient's condition and function. Certain situations warrant the use of a collar including long drives in a vehicle, or prolonged standing or sitting. However, patients should be weaned off the collar as their recovery progresses.

The patient is allowed to wear the collar as much as he or she wants, including in bed, but it must be worn whenever vertical. The collar should be removed when there is significant improvement in the range of motion and pain levels. This will normally be 3 or 4 weeks postaccident if the patient is compliant.

Exercises[88]

Mealy and Colleagues[89] found that early active physical therapy using the active mobilization technique improved pain reduction and increased mobility compared with a control group receiving 2 weeks of rest with a soft cervical collar and gradual mobilization thereafter. McKinney and co-workers[90] found physical therapy or exact instructions in self-mobilization to be better than 2 weeks of rest with a soft collar at 1 and 2 months of follow-up. A similar result was found at the 2-year follow-up.[91] Borchgrevink and associates[92] found that patients encouraged to continue with daily activities had a better outcome than patients prescribed sick leave and immobilization.

In the first part of the acute phase, usually the first few days or so, any exercises should be nonweight bearing. The main three reasons for the exercises are:

1. Patient involvement
2. Mechanoreceptor stimulation
3. Increased vascularization

The exercises are not intended to increase range of movement. Consequently, they are gentle repetitions, well within the pain-free range. Usually, the easiest and most comfortable exercise is rotation in supine with the head comfortable and supported. The Occipital Float (OPTP, Winnetonka, Minnesota) is a device which is extremely effective in providing support for the head and neck in the supine position. The head is gently rolled from side to side without lifting it from the pillow. To relieve muscle tension, it can be done in conjunction with breathing, whereby the patient reaches the easy end of range (where the neck is about to leave its neutral zone and some tissue resistance is first being felt).[62] The patient then takes a moderate breath in and then releases it. At the end of the release, the relaxation of the muscles allows a slight increase in range without stressing any tissues and without causing pain. Once the non-weight-bearing range of motion can be performed, active range of motion exercises into rotation can be initiated in the seated and then standing positions.

Mild resistance exercises are introduced very early in the recovery phase. Although these exercises should not cause sharp pain, they may produce mild delayed-onset muscle soreness. Minimal resistance is used in the neutral position to aid in venous return, stimulate the mechanoreceptors in the muscle, and allay any concerns regarding weakening of the neck from disuse or the collar.[62]

Shoulder shrugging and circumduction exercises, hip and knee flexion and extension exercises in nonweight bearing, toe dorsiflexion (to help move the dura), and isometric hip, shoulder, and abdominal (using the Valsalva, not pelvic tilting or sit ups) exercises are helpful in keeping the patient active and involved, maintaining some level of musculoskeletal fitness, and reducing the build up of stressors in the system.[62]

The following treatment protocol was presented at a course in mechanical diagnosis and therapy in Sweden by Laslett in May 1993 (Part B, Mechanical Diagnosis and Therapy: The Cervical and Thoracic Spine). The early and repeated movement concept comes from Laslett's interpretation of Salter's work on continuous passive motion[93] and Laslett's clinical experience in whiplash injuries.

Patients perform gentle, active, small-range and amplitude rotational movements of the neck, first in one direction, then the other. The movements are repeated 10 times in each direction every waking hour. The movements are performed up to a maximum comfortable range. Patients are instructed to perform these home exercises in the sitting position if symptoms are not too severe. The unloaded supine position is used when the sitting position is too painful. Guidelines are provided for safe home exercising by teaching the patient to identify warning signs that could lead to exacerbation or recurrence of symptoms. In the event of an increase of symptoms, treatment is adjusted by either reducing the amplitude of the movements, by reducing the number of movements, or both. If symptoms persist 20 days after the motor vehicle collision, the patient is examined by a dynamic mechanical evaluation consistent with the McKenzie protocol.[94] An individual treatment program, also based on McKenzie principles and further developed by Laslett,[95] is added to the initial program of rotational movements. These movements could be cervical retraction, extension, flexion, rotation, side-flexion, or a combination of these, depending on which movements are found to be beneficial during the assessment.

Modalities

While passive modalities have their uses with this patient type, the clinician should remember that they must only be used as an adjunct to the more active program, and with a specific goal in mind (reduce inflammation, control pain).

Ultrasound   Ultrasound should be used precisely. It can be applied to the posterior aspects of the zygapophyseal joints to control pain and reduce inflammation, or to a torn muscle. In the acute phase, care must be taken not to overheat the tissues with the ultrasound.

Thermal Agents   Theoretically ice is the preferred choice in the acute phase. However, ice can often increase pain that arises from a trigger point. In these cases, the application of heat, with its ability to relax muscles and stimulate vasodilation may be advocated.

Electrical Muscle Stimulation[62]   Providing that none of the muscles stimulated are torn, electromuscle stimulation used in the early stages acts as both an effective pain reliever and, presumably, as a venous pump. The most effective way is with the patient supine. A small electrode is placed on each of the left and right suboccipital muscles, and a large common electrode is placed along the upper thoracic spinous process. The channels are made to stimulate asynchronously with a long "on" ramp, and a contraction length of 2 or 3 seconds (certainly, no longer than 5, as this becomes uncomfortable). The intervention session can last anywhere from a few minutes to 30 minutes, once it is established that there are no adverse effects from the intervention.

The Subacute Phase

The intervention during this phase can be progressed based on the patients response to treatment. The patient should be weaned off the use of modalities and the focus of the exercise program is to maintain the newly attained ranges, and to provide neuromuscular feedback.

Exercises

Segmental proprioceptive neuromuscular facilitation (PNF) techniques are particularly useful in the achievement of the latter.[62]

Activities

The patient is further encouraged to take up, or resume a regular activity, such as walking or, later in this phase, swimming and, perhaps, running, or anything else that will get them back to a normal mind set about function without reinjuring the area.[62]

The Chronic Phase

Any residual joint hypomobilities are addressed by mobilization or manipulation.

By this time, the patient should be engaged in normal activities based on a 1990 study by Gargan and Bannister,[61] it would appear that the patient's condition at the 2-year mark is the final condition that he or she is likely to achieve, at least in the immediate (10 years) future, which would indicate that patients coming for treatment after the 2-year period have a very limited capacity for improvement.[62]

REFERENCES

1. Crowe H. Injuries to the cervical spine. In: *Presentation to the Annual Meeting of the Western Orthopaedic Association.* San Francisco: 1928.
2. Gay JR, Abbott KH. Common whiplash injuries of the neck. *JAMA* 1953;152:1698–1704.
3. Gunzberg R, Spalski M, eds. *Whiplash Injuries: Current Concepts in Prevention, Diagnosis, and Treatment of the Cervical Whiplash Syndrome.* Philadelphia: Lippincott-Raven; 1998.
4. Reilly PA, Travers R, Littlejohn GO. Epidemiology of soft tissue rheumatism: the influence of the law. *J Rheumatol* 1991;18:1448–1449.
5. Evans RW. Some observations on whiplash injuries. *Neurol Clin* 1992;10:975–997.
6. Ferrari R, Russell AS. Epidemiology of whiplash: an international dilemma. *Ann Rheum Dis* 1999;58:1–5.
7. Spitzer WO, Skovron ML, Salmi LR, et al. Scientific monograph of the Quebec Task Force on Whiplash-Associated Disorders: redefining "whiplash" and its management. *Spine* 1995;20:suppl:1S–73S. [Erratum, *Spine* 1995;20:2372.]
8. Livingston M. Whiplash injury: why are we achieving so little? [Article] *J R Soc Med* 2000;93:526–529.
9. Gotten N. Survey of 100 cases of whiplash injury after settlement of litigation. *JAMA* 1956;162:854–857.
10. MacNab I. Acceleration injuries of the cervical spine. *J Bone Joint Surg Am* 1964;46:1797–1799.
11. Macnab I. The whiplash syndrome. *Orthop Clin North Am* 1971;2:389–403.
12. Farbman AA. Neck sprain. Associated factors. *JAMA* 1973;223:1010–1015.

13. Nordhoff LS Jr. Cervical trauma following motor vehicle collisions. In: Murphy, DR, ed. *Cervical Spine Syndromes*. New York: McGraw-Hill; 2000.

14. Radanov BP, DiStephano G, Schnidrig A, Ballinari P. Role of psychosocial stress in recovery from common whiplash. *Lancet* 1991;338:712–715.

15. Radanov BP, Sturzenegger M, DiStephano G. Long-term outcome after whiplash injury. A 2 year follow-up considering features of injury mechanism and somatic, radiologic, and psychosocial findings. *Medicine* 1995;74:281–297.

16. Livingston M. *Common Whiplash Injury: A Modern Epidemic*. Springfield IL: Charles C Thomas; 1999.

17. National Highway Traffic Safety Administration. *Traffic Safety Facts 1994: A Compilation of Motor Vehicle Crash Data from the Fatal Accident Reporting System and the General Estimates System*. Washington DC: National Highway Traffic Safety Administration; 1995.

18. Pennie B, Agambar L. Patterns of injury and recovery in whiplash. *Injury* 1991;22:57–60.

19. McConnell WE, Howard RP, Vanpoppel J, Krause RR. Human head and neck kinematics after low velocity rear-end impacts-understanding "whiplash," 1995, Society of Automotive Engineers paper 952724.

20. Severy DM, Mathewson JH, Bechtol CO. Controlled automobile rear end collisions, an investigation of related engineering and medical phenomena. *Can Serv Med J* 1955;11:727–759.

21. Maimaris C, Barnes MR, Allen MJ. Whiplash injuries of the neck: a retrospective study. *Injury* 1988;19:393–396.

22. Morris F. Do headrests protect the neck from whiplash injuries? *Arch Emerg Med* 1989;6:17–21.

23. Kaneoka K, Ono K, Inami S, Hayashi K. Motion analysis of cervical vertebrae during whiplash loading. *Spine* 1999;24:763–769; (discussion 770).

24. Nikolai MD, Teasell R, Whiplash: the evidence for an organic etiology. *Arch Neurol*. 2000;57:590–591.

25. Jonsson H, Cesarini K, Sahlstedt B, Rauschning W. Findings and outcomes in whiplash-type neck distortions. *Spine* 1994;19:2733–2743.

26. Taylor JR, Twomey LT. Acute injuries to cervical joints: an autopsy study of neck sprain. *Spine* 1993;9:1115–1122.

27. Barnsley L, Lord S, Bogduk N. The pathophysiology of whiplash. In: Malanga GA, ed. *Cervical Flexion-Extension/Whiplash Injuries. Spine: State of the Art Reviews*. vol 12. Philadelphia: Hanley & Belfus; 1998: 209–242.

28. Bovim G, Schrader H, Sand T. Neck pain in the general population. *Spine* 1994;19:1307–1309.

29. Rauschning W, McAfee P, Jónsson H Jr. Pathoanatomical and surgical findings in cervical spine injuries. *J Spinal Disord* 1989;2:213–222.

30. Hohl M. Soft-tissue injuries of the neck in automobile accidents. *J Bone Joint Surg* [Am] 1974;56-A:1675–1682.

31. Bogduk N, Lord SM. Cervical zygapophysial joint pain. *Neurosurg Q.* 1998;8:107–117.

32. Lord SM, Barnsley L, Bogduk N. Cervical zygapophysial joint pain in whiplash injuries. In: Malanga GA, ed. *Cervical Flexion-Extension/Whiplash Injuries. Spine: State of the Art Reviews*. vol 12. Philadelphia: Hanley & Belfus; 1998:301–344.

33. Winkelstein B, Nightingale RW, Richardson WJ, Myers BS. The cervical facet capsule and its role in whiplash injury: a biomechanical investigation. *Spine* 2000;25: 1238–1246.

34. Borchgrevink GE, Smevik O, Nordby A, Rinck PA, Stiules TC, Lereim I. MR imaging and radiography of patients with cervical hyperextension-flexion injuries after car accidents. *Acta Radiol* 1995;36:425–428.

35. Ellertsson AB, Sigurjonsson K, Thorsteinsson T. Clinical and radiographic study of 100 cases of whiplash injury [abstract]. *Acta Neurol Scand* 1978;57(suppl 67): 269.

36. Ronnen HR, de Korte PJ, Brink PRG, van der Bijl HJ, Tonino AJ, Franke CL. Acute whiplash injury: is there a role for MR imaging? A prospective study of 100 patients. *Radiology* 1996;201:93–96.

37. Seitz JP, Unguez CE, Corbus HF, Wooten WW. SPECT of the cervical spine in the evaluation of neck pain after trauma. *Clin Nucl Med* 1995;20:667–673.

38. Grob D. Posterior surgery. In: Gunzburg R, Szpalski M, eds. *Whiplash Injuries: Current Concepts in Prevention, Diagnosis and Treatment of the Cervical Whiplash Syndrome*. Philadelphia: Lippincott-Raven; 1998; 241–246.

39. Mendel T, Wink CS. Neural elements in cervical intervertebral discs. *Anat Record* 1989;223:78A.

40. Cloward RB. Cervical diskography. A contribution to the etiology and mechanism of neck pain. *Ann Surg* 1959;150:1052.

41. Deans GT, Magalliard K, Rutherford WH. Neck sprain: a major cause of disability following car accidents. *Injury* 1987;18:10–12.

42. Lord SM, Barnsley L, Wallis BJ, Bogduk N. Chronic cervical zygapophysial joint pain after whiplash: a placebo-controlled prevalence study. *Spine* 1996;21: 1737–1744.

43. Aprill C, Bogduk N. The prevalence of cervical zygapophysial joint pain: a first approximation. *Spine* 1992;17:744–747.

44. Barnsley L, Lord S, Bogduk N. Comparative local anaesthetic blocks in the diagnosis of cervical zygapophysial joint pain. *Pain* 1993;55:99–106.

45. Barnsley L, Lord SM, Wallis BJ, Bogduk N. The prevalence of chronic cervical zygapophysial joint pain after whiplash. *Spine* 1995;20:20–26.

46. Bogduk N. Neck pain. *Aust Fam Phys* 1984;13:26–30.

47. Bogduk N, Marsland A. The cervical zygapophysial joints as a source of neck pain. *Spine* 1988;13:610–617.

48. McLain RF. Mechanoreceptor endings in human cervical facet joints. *Spine* 1994;19:495–501.

49. Dwyer A, Aprill C, Bogduk N. Cervical zygapophysial joint pain patterns 1: a study in normal volunteers. *Spine* 1990;15:453.

50. Sturzenegger M, Radanov BP, DiStefano G. The effect of accident mechanisms and initial findings on the long-term course of whiplash injury. *J Neurol* 1995;242:443–449.

51. Ommaya AR. The head: kinematics and brain injury mechanisms. In: Aldman B, Chapon A, eds. *The Biomechanics of Impact Trauma:* Amsterdam: Elsevier;1984;117–138.

52. Forsyth HF. Extension injury of the cervical spine *J Bone Joint Surg* 1964;46A:1792–1797.

53. Barne R. Paraplegia in cervical spine injuries. *J Bone Joint Surg* 1948;30B:234.

54. MacNab I. The whiplash syndrome. *Clin Neurosurg* 1973;20:232.

55. Jónsson H, Cesarini K, Sahlstedt B, Rauschning W. Findings and outcome in whiplash-type neck distortions. *Spine* 1994;19:2733–2743.

56. Edeiken-Monroe B, Wagner LK, Harris JH Jr. Hyperextension dislocation of the cervical spine. *AJR* 1986;146:803–808.

57. McKenzie JA, Williams JF. The dynamic behaviour of the head and cervical spine during "whiplash." *J Biomech* 1971;4:477–490.

58. Taylor J, Kakulas B, Margolius K. Road accidents and neck injuries. *Proc Australas Soc Hum Biol* 1992;5:211–216.

59. Radanov B, Sturzenegger M, Di Stefano G, Schnidrig A, Aljinovic M. Factors influencing recovery from headache after common whiplash. *Br Med J* 1993;307:652–655.

60. Osti OI, Vernon-Roberts B, Frazer RD. Annulus tears and intervertebral disc degeneration: a study using an animal model. *Spine* 1990;15:762.

61. Gargan MF, Bannister GC. Long term prognosis of soft tissue injuries of the neck. *J Bone Joint Surg* 1990;72B:901.

62. Meadows J. Manual therapy: biomechanical assessment and treatment—a rationale and complete approach to the acute and sub-acute post-MVA cervical patient. *Supplement to Swodeam Consulting Video Series.* Swodeam Consulting Calgary, AB; 1995.

63. Ryan GMS, Cope S. Cervical vertigo. *Lancet* 1955;2:1355–1361.

64. Wing LW, Hargrave-Wilson W. Cervical vertigo. *Aust N Z J Surg* 1974;44:275.

65. Macnab I. Acceleration extension injuries of the cervical spine. In: Rothman RH, Simeoni FA, (eds). *The Spine,* vol. 2, Philadelphia: Saunders; 1982;515–527.

66. Biesinger E. Vertigo caused by disorders of the cervical vertebral column. *Adv Otorhinolaryngol* 1988;39:44–51.

67. Barré M. Surun syndrome sympathetique cervical posterieur et sa cause frequente: l'arthrite cervicale Rev. Neurol, 1926,33:1246–1248.

68. Klein de A, Nieuwenhuyse AC. Schwindelanfaalle und Nystagumus bei einer bestimmeten Lage des Kopfes. *Arch Otolaryngol* 1927;11:155–160.

69. Toglia JU. Acute flexion-extension injury of the neck. *Neurology* 1976;26:808–814.

70. Chester JB Jr. Whiplash, postural control, and the inner ear. *Spine* 1991;16:716–720.

71. Fisher CM. Vertigo in cerebrovascular disease. *Arch Otolaryngol* 1967;85:529–534.

72. Troost BT. Dizziness and vertigo in vertebrobasilar disease. *Stroke* 1980;11:413–415.

73. Fife TD, Baloh RW, Duckwiler GR. Isolated dizziness in vertebrobasilar insufficiency: clinical features, angiography, and follow-up. *J Stroke Cerebrovasc Dis* 1994;4:4–12.

74. Gomez CR, Cruz-Flores S, Malkoff MD, Sauer CM, Burch CM. Isolated vertigo as a manifestation of vertebrobasilar ischemia. *Neurology* 1996;47:94–97.

75. Grad A, Baloh RW. Vertigo of vascular origin. Clinical and electronystagmographic features in 18 patients. *Arch Neurol* 1989;46:281–284.

76. Oas JG, Baloh RW. Vertigo and the anterior inferior cerebellar artery syndrome. *Neurology* 1992;42:2274–2279.

77. Mazzoni A. Internal auditory artery supply to the petrous bone. *Ann Otol Rhinol Laryngol* 1974;81:13–21.

78. Davis D, Bohlman H, Walker AE, Fisher R, Robinson R. The pathological findings in fatal craniospinal injuries. *J Neurosurgery* 1971;34:603–613.

79. Macnab I. Whiplash injuries of the neck. *Manitoba Med Rev* 1966;46:172–174.

80. McCullough D, Nelson KM, Ommaya AK. The acute effects of experimental head injury on the vertebrobasilar circulation: angiographic observations. *J Trauma-Injury Infect Crit Care* 1971;11:422–428.

81. Ommaya AK, Yarnell P. Subdural haematoma after whiplash injury. *Lancet* 1969;2:237–239.

82. Ommaya AK, Faas F, Yarnell P. Whiplash injury and brain damage: an experimental study. *JAMA* 1968;204:285–289.

83. Davis SJ, Teresi LM, Bradley WG Jr, Ziemba MA, Bloze AE. Cervical spine hyperextension injuries: MR findings. *Radiology* 1991;180:245–251.

84. Dvořák J, Dvořák V, Schneider W, Tritschler T, Spring H, (eds). *Manuelle medizin: diagnostik.* Stuttgart: Thieme Verlag; 1997.

85. Dvořák J, von Orelli F. [The frequency of complications after manipulation of the cervical spine (case report and epidemiology (author's transl)]. [German] *Schweizerische Rundschau fur Medizin Praxis* 1982;71:64–69.

86. Shimizu T, Shimada H, Shirakura K. Scapulohumeral reflex (Shimizu). Its clinical significance and testing maneuver. *Spine* 1993;18:2182–2190.

87. Nordin M. Education and return to work. In: *Whiplash Injuries: Current Concepts in Prevention, Diagnosis and Treatment of the Cervical Whiplash Syndrome.* Gunzburg R, Szpalski M (eds). Philadelphia: Lippincott-Raven; 1998;199–210.

88. Rosenfeld M, Gunnarsson R, Borenstein P. Early intervention in whiplash-associated disorders: a comparison of two treatment protocols. *Spine* 2000;25:1782–1787.

89. Mealy K, Brennan H, Fenelon GC. Early mobilization of acute whiplash injuries. *BMJ* 1986;292:656–657.

90. McKinney LA, Dornan JO, Ryan M. The role of physiotherapy in the management of acute neck sprains following road-traffic accidents. *Arch Emerg Med* 1989; 6:27–33.

91. McKinney LA. Early mobilisation and outcome in acute sprains of the neck. *BMJ* 1989;299:1006–1008.

92. Borchgrevink GE, Kaasa A, McDonagh D, et al. Acute treatment of whiplash neck sprain injuries. *Spine* 1998;23:25–31.

93. Salter RB. The physiologic basis of continuous passive motion for articular cartilage healing and regeneration. *Hand Clin* 1994;10:211–219.

94. McKenzie R. *The Cervical and Thoracic Spine, Mechanical Diagnosis and Therapy.* Waikane, New Zealand: Spinal Publications; 1990.

95. Laslett M. *Mechanical Diagnosis and Therapy.* Waikane, New Zealand: Mark Laslett; 1996.

CHAPTER TWENTY

THE TEMPOROMANDIBULAR JOINT

Chapter Objectives

At the completion of this chapter, the reader will be able to:

1. Describe the anatomy of the temporomandibular joint, and the ligaments, muscles, blood, and nerve supply that comprise the temporomandibular joint.
2. Describe the biomechanics of the temporomandibular joint, including the movements, normal and abnormal joint barriers, kinesiology, and reactions to various stresses.
3. List the causes of temporomandibular impairment.
4. Perform a detailed objective examination of the temporomandibular musculoskeletal system, including palpation of the articular and soft tissue structures, specific passive mobility, passive articular mobility tests, and stability tests.
5. Analyze the total examination data to establish the definitive biomechanical diagnosis.
6. Apply active and passive mobilization techniques to the temporomandibular joint, using the correct grade, direction, and duration, and explain the mechanical and physiologic effects.
7. Describe intervention strategies based on clinical findings and established goals.
8. Evaluate intervention effectiveness in order to progress or modify intervention.
9. Plan an effective home program and instruct the patient in same.
10. Develop self-reliant examination and intervention strategies.

OVERVIEW

The temporomandibular joint (TMJ), the masticatory systems, the related organs and tissues, such as the salivary glands, and muscles of facial expression, all function as an integrated whole that is called the stomatognathic system. The components of this stomatognathic system are the bones of the skull, the mandible, the hyoid, the masticatory muscles and ligaments; the dentoalveolar (joints of the teeth) and temporomandibular joint; the vascular neurological and lymphatic systems; and the teeth themselves.[1]

Temporomandibular disorders (TMD) is a collective term used to describe a number of related disorders affecting the temporomandibular joints, masticatory muscles, and associated structures, all of which have common symptoms such as pain and limited mouth opening.[2] The diagnosis of TMD, like "whiplash syndrome," remains controversial.[3] Indeed, the relationship between TMD and cervical trauma is, not surprisingly, an area of great controversy. Although this relationship has been in debate for many years, there is an apparent paucity of studies regarding the incidence, course, management, and prognosis of claimed TMDs after traumas.[4,5]

Pain in the temporomandibular region is present in more than 10% of adults at any given time, and in 1 of every 3 adults at some time during their lives.[6,7] Persistent or recurrent pain is considered to be the main reason that more than 90% of patients with temporomandibular disorders (TMD) seek an intervention.[8,9] The large variability in TMD pain severity and suffering remains unexplained, inasmuch as such pain relates poorly with the nature and extent of the pathophysiologic findings.[10,11] Scientific understanding of many aspects of TMD is rapidly progressing but has been only slowly incorporated into clinical practice,[12,13] resulting in a gap between science-based TMD diagnostic and management methodology and many clinical practices.[12]

Most cases of TMD consist of a group of mild, self-limiting disorders that resolve without active intervention.[14] The most common TMD by far, comprising 90% to 95% of all TMD cases, involves multiple complaints of musculoskeletal facial pain and a variety of jaw impairments, for which there is no identified structural cause.[15] A correct diagnosis of TMD, therefore, requires a subset of specific diagnoses in order to appreciate the individual patient's condition,[15,16] and must include consideration of all of the following: jaw muscles; bone and cartilage joint structures; soft tissue joint structures; joint function; the cervical spine and an analysis of the pain disorder, including patient behaviors. Appropriate diagnoses could include the following.

1. Rheumatoid arthritis with synovitis, arthralgia, condylar degenerative disease.
2. Chronic pain with a behavioral disorder.
3. Myofascial pain and impairment.
4. Internal disk derangement with displacement.

The term TMJ in association with jaw and facial symptoms has been discontinued because it is inaccurate and misleading, implying structural conditions when none—or when many other, more important factors—are involved.[17]

ANATOMY

The temporomandibular joint (Figure 20–1) is a synovial, compound modified ovoid bicondylar joint, formed between the articular eminence of the temporal bone, the intra-articular disc and the head of the mandible. It can be differentiated from other freely movable synovial joints by the fact that the articulating surfaces of the bones are covered, not by hyaline cartilage, but by fibrocartilage.[18,19] The presence of this fibrocartilage indicates that the joint is designed to withstand

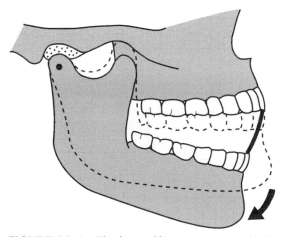

FIGURE 20–1   The hinge-like temporomandibular joint.

large and repeated stresses.[20] The fibrocartilage covers the articulating surfaces of the mandible as well as the articular eminence of the temporal bone.[21,22] The load-bearing surface of the joint is the eminence where the fibrocartilage is the thickest. At the roof of the fossa, where the fibrocartilage is at its thinnest, little or no load bearing should occur.[23]

The mandible works like a class-three lever, with its joint as the fulcrum (see Figure 20–1). There is no agreement among the experts concerning force transmission through the joint. However, there is agreement that postural impairments of the cervical and upper thoracic spine can produce both pain and impairment of the temporomandibular joint.[24]

Fibrocartilaginous Disc

Located between the under surface of the temporal bone and the mandibular condyle is a fibrocartilaginous disc. Although, both the disc and the lateral pterygoid muscle develop from the first branchial arch, it is not known whether the lateral pterygoid muscle contributes to the formation of the disc,[25] but there is very little differentiation between the muscle, the disc, and the joint capsule. Blood vessels and nerves are found only in the thickened periphery of this disc, with its thinner center being avascular and aneural.[23] The size and shape of the disc are both determined by the shape of the condyle, and the articular eminence.

The attachment of the articular disc to the capsular ligament anteriorly and posteriorly, and the attachment of the disc to the medial and lateral poles of the condyle divides the temporomandibular joint into two distinct compartments (Figure 20–2).

- *Mandibulomeniscal (inferior) compartment*: this compartment, bordered by the mandibular condyle and the inferior surface of the articular disc, is where the osteokinematic spin of the condyle occurs.
- *Meniscotemporal (superior) compartment*: this compartment, bordered by the mandibular fossa and the superior surface of the articular disc, primarily allows translation of the disc and condyle along the fossa, and onto the articular eminence.

Rees has described the fibrocartilaginous disc as having three clearly defined transverse, ellipsoidal zones that are divided into three regions: posterior band, intermediate zone, and anterior band.[19] The intermediate zone, avascular and aneural (pars gracilis), is considerably thinner (1 millimeter) than the posterior (pars posterior) and anterior (pes meniscus) bands, and the posterior band is generally thicker (3 millimeter) than the anterior band

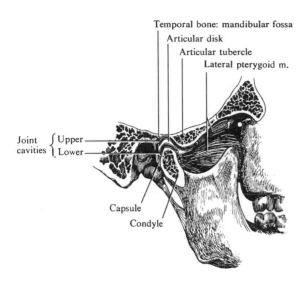

Temporal bone: mandibular fossa
Articular disk
Articular tubercle
Lateral pterygoid m.

Joint cavities { Upper — Lower —

Capsule
Condyle

SAGITTAL SECTION OF ARTICULATION

FIGURE 20–2 The superior and inferior joint cavities.

(2 millimeter).[26] It is the intermediate zone that comes into contact with the articular surface of the condyle, and the upper surface of the disc adapts to the contours of the fossa and eminence of the temporal bone.[33]

Medially and laterally, the fibrocartilaginous disc is firmly attached to the medial and lateral poles of the condyle, by way of collateral, discal ligaments.[27,28] These ligaments permit anterior and posterior rotation of the disc on the condyle. The disc is attached posteriorly by fibroelastic tissue to the posterior mandibular fossa and the back of the mandibular condyle by nonelastic tissue.[27,28] Its circumference is attached to the joint capsule and the mandibular condyle. Anteriorly, the disc is attached to the upper part of the tendon of the lateral pterygoid muscle.[27,28]

As the disc is not directly attached to the temporal bone, the disc has liberty to move with the condyle as the condyle translates in relation to the articular eminence.[29] The disc, which envelopes the condyle, follows the condyle closely in normal function, being pulled anteriorly during mouth opening, and posteriorly, by the elasticity of its posterior attachment, changing shape as it does so.[30] The thicker posterior margin of the disc prevents linear displacement of the disc anteriorly. Likewise, the thicker anterior margin prevents excessive posterior displacement.

Masticatory System

Three components make up the masticatory system: the maxilla and the mandible, which support the teeth, and the temporal bone, which supports the mandible at its articulation with the skull. The sphenoid bone and the

hyoid bone must also be included as, they provide important anatomical and functional links to the temporomandibular joint.

Maxilla

The borders of the maxillae extend superiorly to form the floor of the nasal cavity as well as the floor of each orbit. Inferiorly, the maxillary bones form the palate and the alveolar ridges, which support the teeth.

Mandible

The mandible, or jaw (Fig. 20–3) supports the lower teeth and is the largest, strongest, and lowest bone in the face. It has external and internal surfaces, separated by upper and lower borders, and is suspended below the maxillae by muscles and ligaments that provide mobility and stability. The medial surface receives the medial pterygoid and the digastric muscles, while on the lateral aspect, the platysma, mentalis, and buccinator attach. Two broad, vertical rami extend upward, the condylar and the coronoid. The anterior of the two processes, the coronoid, serves as the attachment for the temporalis and massester muscles.[31] The posterior process articulates with the temporal bone.

The mandibular condyles are elliptical, with their long axes oriented medial-lateral, and at right angles to the plane of the mandibular ramus, with each condyle measuring about 20 millimeter medial and laterally and approximately 10 millimeter anterior-posterior.[23]

Temporal Bone

The articulating surface of the temporal bone is situated anterior to the tympanic plate in the squamous portion of the temporal bone, and is made up of a concave mandibular, or glenoid, fossa, and a convex bony prominence called the articular eminence.[23]

The articular tubercle situated anterior to the glenoid fossa serves as an attachment for the temporomandibular ligament (Figure 20–5).[31]

Sphenoid Bone

The greater wings of the sphenoid bone form the boundaries of the anterior part of the middle cranial fossa. From these greater wings, the pterygoid laminae serve as the attachment for the medial and lateral pterygoid muscles.

Hyoid Bone

The hyoid bone (Fig. 23–10) is a U-shaped bone, also known as the skeleton of the tongue. The hyoid is involved with the mandible to provide reciprocal stabilization during swallowing. This is best appreciated when one attempts to swallow and feels the tongue held against the palate. The hyoid also serves as the attachment for the infrahyoid muscles and some of the extrinsic tongue muscles.

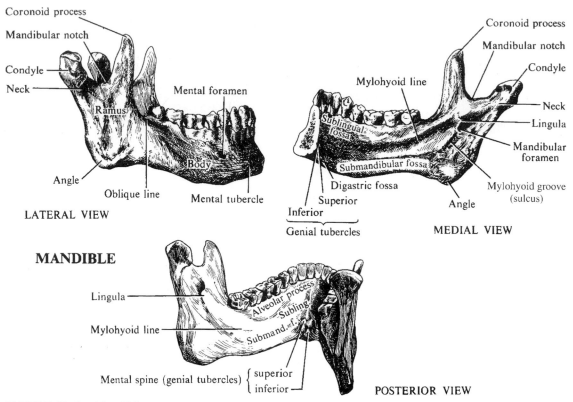

FIGURE 20–3 Mandible.

Synovial Membrane

The synovial membrane of the temporomandibular joint is a highly vascularized layer of connective tissue that lines the fibrous capsule and covers the loose connective tissue between it and the posterior border of the disc.[23]

Supporting Structures

The ligaments of the temporomandibular joint, serving the role of all ligaments, protect and support the joint structures and act as passive restraints to joint movement. Two strong ligaments provide joint stability.

1. The joint capsule, or capsular ligament
2. The temporomandibular ligament (see Figure 20–5).

Two other ligaments assist the above ligaments:

1. Stylomandibular
2. Sphenomandibular

Capsular Ligament

This thin structure surrounds the entire joint.[23] The capsular ligament functions to maintain the synovial fluid

and is highly innervated. While it provides proprioceptive feedback regarding joint position and movement,[32,33] it is also a common pain generator after abrupt trauma to the jaw.[27]

All synovial joints of the body are provided with an array of corpuscular (mechanoreceptors) and noncorpuscular (nociceptors) receptor endings with varying characteristic behaviors and distributions depending on articular tissue.

In the temporomandibular joint, type I receptors are most numerous in the posterior region of the joint capsule. Type I mechanoreceptors contribute to reflex regulation of postural tone, coordination of muscle activity, and perceptional awareness of mandibular position.[23,32,33]

Type II receptors operate as low-threshold, rapidly adapting mechanoreceptors that fire off brief bursts of impulses only at the onset of changes in tension in the joint capsule. Their behavior suggests their role as a control mechanism to regulate motor-unit activity of the prime movers of the temporomandibular joint.[23]

Type III mechanoreceptors, regarded as high threshold, only evoke charges during strong capsular tension.

The type IV receptor system is activated when its nerve fibers are depolarized by the generation of high mechanical or chemical stresses in the joint capsule.

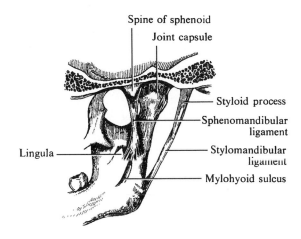

MEDIAL VIEW

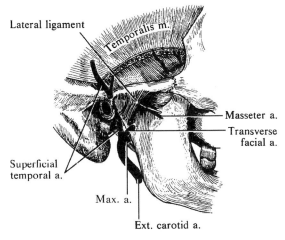

LATERAL VIEW

FIGURE 20–4   The sphenomandibular and stylomandibular ligaments.

Temporomandibular Ligament

The capsule of the temporomandibular joint is reinforced laterally by the two divisions of the temporomandibular ligament (Figure 20–5).[23] These two divisions, an outer oblique portion and an inner horizontal portion, function as the suspensory mechanism of the mandible during moderate opening movements, and resist rotation, and posterior displacement of the mandible.

Stylomandibular Ligament

The stylomandibular ligament is a specialized band of deep cervical fascia that splits away from the superficial lamina of the deep cervical fascia to run deep to both pterygoid muscles (see Figure 20–4).[23] This ligament becomes taut and acts as a guiding mechanism for the mandible, keeping the condyle, disc and temporal bone firmly opposed.

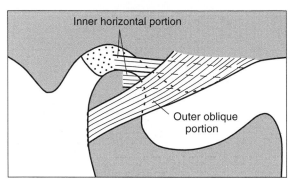

FIGURE 20–5   The two portions of the temporomandibular ligament.

Sphenomandibular Ligament

The sphenomandibular ligament, an accessory ligament, is a thin band that runs from the spine of the sphenoid bone to a small bony prominence on the medial surface of the ramus of the mandible, called the lingula (see Figure 20–4). This ligament acts to check the angle of the mandible from sliding as far forward as the condyles during the translatory cycle, and serves as a suspensory ligament of the mandible during wide opening. It is this ligament that hurts with any prolonged jaw opening, such as that which occurs at the dentist.

Another ligament in this area worth a mention is the anterior ligament of the malleus or Pinto's ligament.

Pinto's ligament[34] which is a vestige of embryological tissue, arises from the neck of the malleus of the inner ear and runs in a medial-superior direction to insert into the posterior aspect of the temporomandibular joint capsule and disc. While the role of this ligament in mandibular mechanics is thought to be neglible, its relationship to the middle ear and the temporomandibular joint could be a basis for the middle ear symptoms which are often present with TMD.

Muscles

The masticatory muscles are the key muscles when discussing TMD. Masticatory muscles contain all three of the muscle fiber types (type I, II and IIa).

Three of these muscles, the masseter, medial pterygoid, and temporalis, exert their power in a vertical direction, and function to raise the mandible during mouth closing. The digastric and geniohyoid muscles retrude and depress the mandible by pulling it in a posterior and inferior direction.

Although these muscles work most efficiently in groups, an understanding of the specific action(s) of the individual muscles is necessary for an appreciation of their coordinated function during masticatory activity.

Temporalis

The temporalis muscle arises from the cranial fossa that bears its name (Figure 20–6), and inserts by way of a tendon into the medial surface, the apex, the anterior and posterior border of the coronoid process, and the anterior border of the mandibular ramus. This muscle can move the jaw in many directions, and is responsible for forceful mouth closing and side to side grinding movements. It provides a good deal of stability to the joint. The temporalis muscle is supplied by the anterior and posterior deep temporal nerves, which branch from the anterior division of the mandibular branch of the trigeminal nerve.

Masseter

The masseter, a quadrilateral muscle, consists of three layers which blend anteriorly. The deep and superficial fibers form a raphe with the medial pterygoid (Figure 20–7). The multipennate effect of the alternating muscle fibers and layers of tendons serves to shorten the average of length of the contractile elements and to increase the total number of fibers in the muscle, making the masseter the most powerful muscle in the body with a relatively short contractile range.[23]

The major function of the masseter is to elevate the mandible thereby occluding the teeth during mastication.

Medial Pterygoid

The medial pterygoid muscle is a thick quadrilateral muscle with a deep origin on the medial aspect of the mandibular ramus. (Figure 20–8). Bilaterally, the muscles, together with the masseter and temporalis, assist in elevation of the

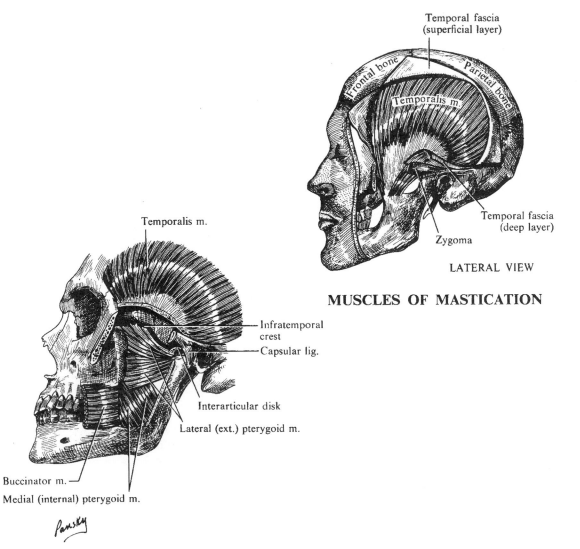

Temporal fascia
(superficial layer)

Frontal bone

Parietal bone

Temporalis m.

Temporal fascia
(deep layer)

Zygoma

LATERAL VIEW

MUSCLES OF MASTICATION

Temporalis m.

Infratemporal crest

Capsular lig.

Interarticular disk

Lateral (ext.) pterygoid m.

Buccinator m.

Medial (internal) pterygoid m.

FIGURE 20–6 Temporalis muscle.

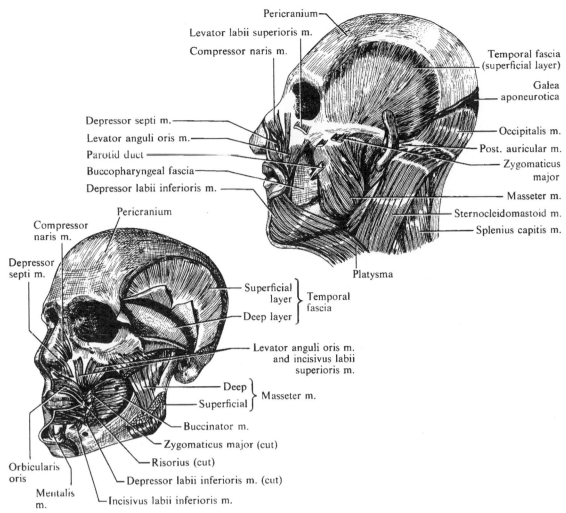

Pericranium

Levator labii superioris m.

Compressor naris m.

Temporal fascia (superficial layer)

Galea aponeurotica

Depressor septi m.

Levator anguli oris m.

Parotid duct

Buccopharyngeal fascia

Depressor labii inferioris m.

Occipitalis m.

Post. auricular m.

Zygomaticus major

Masseter m.

Sternocleidomastoid m.

Splenius capitis m.

Platysma

Pericranium

Compressor naris m.

Depressor septi m.

Superficial layer } Temporal fascia

Deep layer }

Levator anguli oris m. and incisivus labii superioris m.

Deep } Masseter m.
Superficial }

Buccinator m.

Zygomaticus major (cut)

Risorius (cut)

Depressor labii inferioris m. (cut)

Orbicularis oris

Mentalis m.

Incisivus labii inferioris m.

FIGURE 20–7 Muscles of mastication.

mandible. Each medial pterygoid muscle is capable of deviating the mandible toward the opposite side. This muscle also acts as an assist to the lateral pterygoid for protrusion of the mandible.

Lateral Pterygoid

Despite several investigations,[36–39] no consensus has been reached regarding the insertion of the lateral pterygoid muscle (Figure 20–8).

The two divisions of the lateral pterygoid muscles are functionally and anatomically two separate muscles. The inferior lateral pterygoid muscle exerts a forward, inward, and downward pull on the mandible, thereby opening the jaw, protruding the mandible, and deviating the mandible to the opposite side by the action of one muscle functioning unilaterally.

The superior lateral pterygoid muscle is involved mainly with chewing and functions to anteriorly rotate the disc on the condyle during mouth closing.[40,41]

Both divisions of this muscle are innervated by the lateral pterygoid nerve from the anterior division of the mandibular branch of the trigeminal nerve.

Infrahyoid or "Strap" Muscles

The infrahyoid muscles consist of the sternohyoid, omohyoid, sternothyroid, and thyrohyoid muscles. (Figure 20–9). The sternohyoid muscle is a strap-like muscle which functions to depress the hyoid as well as assist in speech and mastication.

The omohyoid muscle is situated lateral to the sternohyoid and consists of two bellies. The omohyoid functions to depress the hyoid and has been speculated to tense the inferior aspect of the deep cervical fascia in prolonged inspiratory efforts, thereby releasing tension on the apices of the lungs and on the internal jugular vein, which are attached to this fascial layer.[23]

Deep to the sternohyoid muscle are the sternothyroid and thyrohyoid muscles. Both of these muscles are

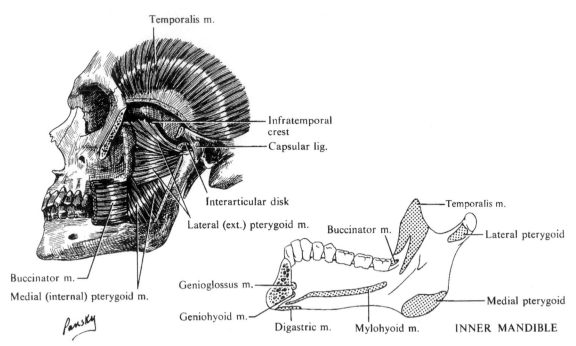

FIGURE 20–8 Medial and lateral pterygoid muscles.

involved with moving the larynx and altering the pitch of the voice.

These infrahyoid muscles are innervated by fibers from the upper cervical nerves. The nerves to the lower part of these muscles are given off from the ansa cervicalis (cervical loop).[23]

Suprahyoid Muscles

The supra- and infrahyoid muscles play a major role in co-ordinating mandibular function, by providing a firm base on which the tongue and mandible can be moved.

Geniohyoid

The geniohyoid muscle is a narrow muscle situated under the mylohyoid muscle (Figure 20–10).

The geniohyoid muscle, which functions to elevate the hyoid bone, is innervated by fibers from the ventral rami of the lesser occipital nerve (C1).

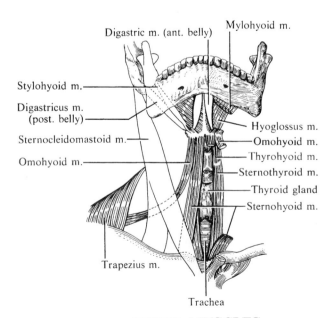

HYOID MUSCLES

FIGURE 20–9 Digastric, stylohyoid, and infrahyoid muscles.

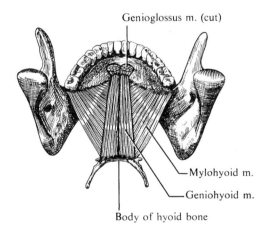

FLOOR OF MOUTH

FIGURE 20–10 Geniohyoid and mylohyoid muscles.

Digastric

The two bellies of the digastric muscle are joined by a rounded tendon that attaches to the body and greater cornu of the hyoid bone through a fibrous loop or sling (see Figure 20–9).[23]

The posterior belly is innervated by the facial nerve. The anterior belly is supplied by the mylohyoid nerve from the inferior alveolar branch of the posterior division of the mandibular nerve.

Bilaterally, the digastrics assist in forced mandibular depression. The posterior bellies are especially active during coughing and swallowing.

Mylohyoid

This flat, triangular muscle receives its innervation from the mylohyoid nerve, from the inferior alveolar branch of the mandibular division of the trigeminal nerve (see Figure 20–10). The mylohyoid is functionally a muscle of the tongue, stabilizing or elevating the tongue during swallowing, and elevating the floor of the mouth in the first stage of deglutition.

Stylohyoid

The stylohyoid muscle is innervated by the facial nerve. (see Figure 20–9). Its role in speech, mastication, and swallowing has yet to be determined.

Nerve Supply

The temporomandibular joint is primarily supplied from three nerves that are part of the mandibular division of the trigeminal nerve (Table 20–1).

The nerve is named trigeminal due to its tripartite division into the maxillary, ophthalmic, and mandibular branches. All three contain sensory cells, but the ophthalmic and maxillary are exclusively sensory, the latter supplying the soft and hard palate, maxillary sinuses, upper teeth, upper lip, and the mucous membrane of the pharynx. The mandibular branch carries sensory information but is the motor component of the nerve supplying the muscles of mastication, both pterygoids, the anterior belly of digastric, tensor tympani, tensor veli palatini, and mylohyoid.

The spinal nucleus and tract of the trigeminal cannot be distinguished either histologically or on the basis if afferent reception from the cervical nerves. Consequently, the entire column can be viewed as a single nucleus and may be legitimately called the trigeminocervical nucleus.[42]

BIOMECHANICS OF THE TEMPOROMANDIBULAR JOINT

The temporomandibular joint can assume three relative positions when the mandible is not in motion. These

TABLE 20–1 THE TRIGEMINAL NERVE

Motor nucleus	Anterior-lateral upper pons and forms, the mandibular branch of the trigeminal.
Sensory nucleus	There are two nuclei, the chief sensory nucleus in the dorsal-lateral pons, and the mesencephalic nucleus, which extends from the chief sensory upward through the pons to the mid-brain. The chief sensory nucleus receives all sensory input, except that from the muscles supplied by the mandibular branch.
Spinal nucleus	The spinal tract consists of small- and medium-sized myelinated nerve fibers and runs caudally to reach the upper cervical segments of the spinal cord. The lowest nerve fibers in the tract mix with the spinal fibers in the tract of Lissauer.
Nerves	Mandibular Maxillary Ophthalmic
Termination	The muscles of mastication, both pterygoids, tensor veli palatini, tensor tympani, mylohyoid, and the anterior belly of digastric. The skin of the vertex, temporal area, forehead and face, the mucosa of the sinus, nose, pharynx, anterior two-third of the tongue, and the oral cavity. The lacrimal, parotid, and lingual glands and the dura of the anterior and middle cranial fossae. The external aspect of the tympanic membrane and the external auditory meatus, temporomandibular joint, teeth. Dilator pupillae and probably the proprioceptors of the extraocular muscles. Sensation from the upper three or four cervical levels.

mandibular postures are the rest position, occlusal position, and hinge position.

Rest Position

The residual tension of the muscles at rest is termed resting tonus. The rest position of the tongue is up against the palate of the mouth.[43] In this position, the most anterior-superior tip of the tongue lies in the area against the palate, just posterior to the back side of the upper central incisors. No occlusal contact occurs between maxillary and mandibular teeth in this position. The significance of the rest position is that it permits the tissues of the stomatognathic system to rest and repair.[44] This rest position is entirely dependent on the mandibular musculature, soft tissue, and gravity, and because of the variations in muscle tonus, this position is not constant. A normal resting position for the tongue is necessary for correct nasal and diaphragmatic breathing. It is proposed that if the tongue comes away from the roof of the mouth, the vagus nerve is stimulated. This results in a stimulation of the vagal muscles (trapezius and sternocleidomastoid (SCM)) that act to pull the head into extension. This extended head position is the position of least airway resistance and maximum airflow (it is the position that athletes adopt before and after an event to maximally aerate their lungs). In essence, the position changes the airflow angle from 90 degrees to 180 degrees. People who develop a forward head posture, also develop a malposition of the tongue as the tongue cannot remain in contact with the roof of the mouth in this position. However, because the forward head posture puts the airway in a more efficient flow position, this posture soon becomes habitual and becomes the new resting posture.

Occlusal Position

This position is defined as the point at which contact between some or all of the teeth occur. The maximum intercuspated position is the median occlusal position in which all the teeth are fully interdigitated.[18] This position, considered the start position for all mandibular motions, is dependent on the presence, shape, and position of the teeth. Absent or abnormally shaped teeth can displace the mandible from this position, creating an imbalance.

The Hinge Position

The hinge position is the position of the mandible from which a pure hinge opening and closing can occur.[18] In this position, the condyles are in the most retruded position that the muscles of the jaw can accomplish.

MANDIBULAR MOVEMENTS

Mandibular movements guided by the temporomandibular joint and muscle activity occur as a series of interrelated three-dimensional rotational and translational activities which depend on four factors: (1) initiating position, (2) types of movements, (3) direction of movement, and (4) degree of movement.[23] The temporomandibular joint has three degrees of freedom, and each of the degrees of freedom is associated with a separate axis of rotation.[45]

Movements of this joint are extremely complex— opening and closing, protrusion and retrusion, and lateral motions. The two basic motions required for functional motion, rotation and translation, occur around three planes, sagittal, horizontal, and frontal.

● Rotation: the mandible has three axes of rotation: medial-lateral (x), anterior-posterior (y), and longitudinal (z).[23] The rotation occurs in a hinge motion around a medial-lateral axis and produces opening and closing. Mandibular movement, around an anterior-posterior

axis (y) produces a depression of the mandible on the moving side. The longitudinal, or vertical, axis (z) of rotation results in a unilateral protrusive-retrusive movement.

● Translation: translation, or gliding movements, occur in the superior compartment between the inferior surface of the articular fossa and eminence of the temporal bone and the superior surface of the articular disc during the downward and forward movement of the disc-condyle complex, a protrusive movement.[23] A return of this complex in the upward and backward position is called a retrusive movement.

Opening and Closing

Opening and closing movements of the jaw are a combination of rotary and translatory movements of the mandible and disc. Opening also involves a lateral deviation and protrusion—an inferior, anterior, and a lateral glide. Closing involves the opposite, a superior and posterior glide and a medial glide, that is, the mandible head moves up, back, and inward.

Protrusion

Protrusion is a forward movement of the mandible occurring at the superior joint compartments. If the movement occurs unilaterally, it is called lateral translation, or lateral deviation. For example, if only the left temporomandibular joint protrudes, the jaw deviates to the right. Protrusion consists of the disc and condyle moving downward and forward.

Retrusion

Retrusive range is limited by the taut temporomandibular ligaments, and rarely amounts to more than 3 mm.[23]

The angle of the joint is oriented in an anterior and lateral direction, resulting in maximal lateral motion occurring with full opening. The capsular pattern of the temporomandibular joint is one of deviation of motion to the same side as the affected joint, with a loss of functional opening. Its close-packed position is difficult to determine as the position for maximal muscle tightness is also the position of least joint surface congruity and vice versa.[16]

TEMPOROMANDIBULAR DISORDERS

Temporomandibular disorders (TMD) are also referred to as craniomandibular disorders and arthrosis temporomandibularis.[46] It is generally thought that the modern concepts of temporomandibular disorders began with three publications by Costen, an otolaryngologist, and his theory that temporomandibular disorders were the result of "bony erosions" of the temporomandibular joint and the tympanic plate of the temporal bone.[47–49]

Anatomic investigations in the 1940s disproved Costen's theories,[50–52] and over the past half century, much attention was directed toward defining four "gold standard" diagnostic symptoms and signs of temporomandibular disorders.[53]

1. Facial or jaw pains.
2. Tenderness of the muscles of mastication.
3. Sounds (clicks or pops) that originate in the temporomandibular joint, often with jaw deviations.
4. Restricted jaw opening (defined in the adult as opening less than about 40 mm).

Clinicians often see patients who present with either persistent or recurrent lateral facial pain. Having eliminated the possibility of ear or sinus problems, the next step is to consider the possibility of temporomandibular joint pain and impairment, particularly if the pain is accompanied by clicking jaw joints and limited mouth opening.[53]

Displacement of the temporomandibular joint disc is by far the most common finding among patients who seek treatment for temporomandibular disorders symptoms. A consecutive study of unselected adult patients with temporomandibular disorders symptoms, verifying the temporomandibular joint disc position arthrographically, showed a prevalence of disc displacement of 64%.[54] In adult patients with temporomandibular joint pain and impairment who were referred for arthrographic or magnetic resonance imaging (MRI) of the temporomandibular joint, the prevalence of disc displacement varied between 78% and 84%.[55–57] Similar findings were found in juvenile patients.[58,59]

About 60 to 70% of the general population has at least one sign of a temporomandibular disorder, yet only around one in four people with signs is actually aware of, or reports any, symptoms.[8,24, 60–64] Furthermore, only about 5% of people with one or more signs of a temporomandibular disorder will actually seek an intervention.[8,60–62] Most of those who seek an intervention for temporomandibular disorders are female, outnumbering male patients by at least four to one.[8,61,63] Although temporomandibular disorders may occur at any age, the disorder cannot be considered a disease of aging, as patients most commonly present in early adulthood.[8,60–64]

Etiology

The etiology of the most common types of temporomandibular disorders is complex and is still largely unresolved.

Many clinicians over the years have described numerous conditions that share features, such as fatigue, pain, and other symptoms, in the absence of objective findings. These include illnesses such as chronic fatigue syndrome (CFS), fibromyalgia (FM), temporomandibular disorder (TMD).

Although often labeled "psychosomatic" or "functional" disorders, similarities in clinical manifestations among these conditions, such as increased pain sensitivity, suggest a possible common alteration in central processing mechanisms.[65]

CFS, FM, and TMD are all associated with poor functional status[66–68] and psychiatric illness.[69–72] Some literature on relationships between CFS, FM, and TMD supports the possibility that these syndromes may represent "overlapping" conditions. In this regard, it has been estimated that between 20 and 70% of patients with FM meet criteria for CFS and, conversely, 35 to 70% of those with CFS also have FM.[69,73–75] Studies investigating the relationship between FM and TMD have demonstrated that 18% of patients with TMD meet FM criteria, and 75% of patients with FM satisfy the Research Diagnostic Criteria for TMD (myofascial type).[76,77] Although psychogenic factors have also been implicated, these are often considered as exacerbating factors rather than the primary cause of temporomandibular disorders.[24,60]

Schwartz,[78,79] a dentist, headed a multidisciplinary temporomandibular disorders clinic where over 500 patients were treated. He hypothesized that temporomandibular disorder symptoms originated in mandibular muscles that went through three pathologic phases.

1. Early incoordination of muscles producing joint clicking and recurrent subluxation.
2. A middle phase of limitation of mandibular movements by muscle spasm.
3. A final phase of muscle shortening and fibrosis, often irreversible. Psychogenic causes were the most common.

Over the next 35 years, the Schwartz supporters studied other large temporomandibular disorders cohorts and drew these conclusions.[24,60]

1. Over 85% of subjects were women, 80% of whom had histories of stress, depression, daytime tooth clenching, and nocturnal bruxism.
2. The largest number of patients had other psychogenic disorders, along with atypical pain syndromes and low pain thresholds.
3. Antidepressant medications were far superior to placebo or bite guard prostheses.
4. Prognosis was more favorable in those with recent stress and no operations.

5. Psychological counseling gave excellent result.
6. Those examined a year after diagnosis showed 90% improvement, with loss of abnormal jaw sounds in over 80%.
7. Patients with temporomandibular disorders and normal temporomandibular joints have higher psychometric scores denoting pain, chronic disability, and depression.[80–84]

Malocclusion has not been determined as an important factor in TMD,[85–87] as very few patients with malocclusion actually go on to develop temporomandibular pain and impairment.[64]

Previous reports have shown an increased prevalence of traumas and injuries in the TMD population in comparison with the non-TMD population.[88–90] Direct injury to the masticatory structure is thought to cause certain temporomandibular joint (TMJ) disorders, such as disc displacements.[91,92] However, the transition from acute temporomandibular joint problems to chronic TMD problems and the role of trauma in the etiology of chronic TMD remain unclear.[93] Injuries to nerves and soft and hard tissues as a result of repeated traumas have been reported to produce persistent pain because of sensitization of both peripheral and central neurons.[94] The sensitization process has been shown to influence subsequent pain experience. Increased postoperative pain resulting from insufficient preemptive analgesia, such as incomplete use of local anesthetics and/or pain medication before surgery, has been well documented.[94–96] Poorly managed postoperative or posttraumatic pain is also considered to play a role in pain persistence.[94,97] Sensitization has also been implicated in the mechanism of TMD pain.[98]

Other causes of TMD range from immune-mediated systemic disease to neoplastic growths to neurobiologic mechanisms.[99] Less common, but better recognized, causes of TMD are:

1. A wide range of direct injuries to the joint, such as fractures of the mandibular condyle
2. Systemic diseases, such as rheumatoid arthritis
3. Growth disturbances
4. Psychological overlay

Some nonfunctional movements of the mandible (bruxing) and tooth-clenching habits have been associated with a variety of jaw muscle symptoms, but are associated less with internal joint disc derangements.[100] Chronic parafunctional clenching, however, has been shown experimentally to cause acute TMD in human beings.[101]

There is conflicting evidence that health care manipulations, orthodontic, or surgical intervention increase the chances of developing TMD.[102–107] Changes of the mandibular condyle range from remodeling to resorption, are probably associated with biomechanical loading and altered jaw position and mechanics, and are related to the inherent adaptive capacity of the temporomandibular joint.[107]

There are no scientifically established anatomic risk factors for developing TMD. While anatomic variations in temporomandibular joint structure, jaw relationships, and dental relationships are wide; none of these appear to predispose a person to TMD.[108,109] Although a common relationship between TMD and parafunctional jaw and tooth habits has been noticed clinically, this does not necessarily predispose the patient to TMD, although parafunctional jaw habits do seem to propagate TMD symptoms already established and may be associated with TMD, rather than as an external factor.[110] A wide range of associated factors, such as depression, anxiety, and gum chewing, may propagate TMD symptoms on the basis of physical, emotional, and/or neurobiologic factors.[66] Pain, muscle tension headache, and chronic pain in the head, neck, and jaws, may predispose to TMD via neuroanatomic and neurobiologic mechanisms.[66,111,112]

The role of cervical whiplash injuries secondary to motor vehicle accidents (MVAs) in such disorders, is somewhat controversial, and is questioned by some authors.[113–116] Others,[117–120] however, believe that trauma from cervical whiplash injuries[93,121–124] is important. "Cervical strain" as a cause of TMD was described by Roydhouse.[123] Brooke and Stenn[125] reported that patients with posttraumatic TMD have a poor prognosis for recovery compared with nontraumatic TMD, stating reasons of the consequence of litigation and the personality of the patient. Some researchers reported that some patients claimed the onset of symptoms days or weeks after the professed whiplash incident with diagnoses and intervention beginning even later.[120,126,127]

Mechanisms have been proposed to explain how a MVA trauma could cause TMDs.[121,128,129] In a prospective study of 155 post-MVA whiplash injuries, Heise and associates[130] found that masticatory muscle and temporomandibular joint pain were initially present in 12.7% of patients with positive radiologic findings and 15.2% of patients with negative radiologic findings of cervical skeletal injury. Pain symptoms had diminished within 1 month. One year after the injury, pain symptoms had resolved in all patients. No new cases of pain symptoms and clicking were reported.

In addition to the involvement of the masticatory muscles just mentioned, the anterior muscles of the neck are often injured with the whiplash mechanism. It seems plausible that an injury to the suprahyoid and infrahyoid muscles would affect the function of the mandible, thereby setting up the joint for dysfunction.

To assess the relationship between various crash variables, including vehicular and postural characteristics, and TMDs, Burgess and co-worker[117] studied 219 patients who identified MVAs as the cause of signs and symptoms suggesting TMDs. They found that the amount of jaw opening was significantly less for the subgroup whose vehicles had been "totaled" than for the subgroup with less than $1000 worth of vehicle damage, and the group with speeds of impact of 40 mph or greater had greater overall pain intensity than the group with speeds of impact of less than 40 mph. Facial injury, such as bruising, appeared significantly more likely to be reported when impact was not from the side, and there was an interaction between facial pain and front or rear impact. Looking right or left at the time of impact has been associated with significantly greater overall pain and significantly greater masticatory muscle tenderness.

The probable reason for these symptoms depends on the mechanism. During the initial backwards movement, the jaw could be forced open, stretching and, possibly, tearing the anterior joint capsule and intra-articular disc. On the flexion phase, the jaw is snapped shut by the stretch reflex of the masticatory muscles and, in the presence of malocclusion, damages the posterior and temporal attachments of the articular cartilage and disc.

However, thorough acceleration-deceleration studies on human volunteers concluded that the force of a low velocity extension-flexion injury is less than the forces exerted by normal mastication.[128] Similar extensive experiments on human subjects sponsored by the Society of Automotive Engineers concluded, " · · · no jaw motion relative to the cranium was seen for any human subject during rear-end impacts."[131,132]

In 1993, The American Academy of Orofacial Pain published their official opinion of mandibular whiplash, "Thus, the condition of mandibular strain at the time of a motor vehicular accident, without a direct blow to the mandible, resulting in hyperextension of the mandibular capsule, ligaments, and masticatory muscles is questionable."[60] Skeptical neurologists suspect that "temporomandibular joint whiplash" is often a clinical manifestation of malingering.

The term internal derangement describes a temporomandibular disorder in which the articular disc is in an abnormal position, resulting in mechanical interference and restriction of the normal range of mandibular activity. The theory of internal derangement of the temporomandibular joint (TMJ) involves the anterior (and medial) displacement of the disc, which is thought to be brought about by the action of the upper head of the lateral pterygoid muscle.[133–135] It has been suggested that in normal function of the craniomandibular complex,

the upper head of the lateral pterygoid muscle plays an important role in stabilizing and controlling the movements of the disc. In abnormal function, excessive action or hyperactivity of the upper head of the lateral pterygoid muscle loads the disc leading to its eventual anterior and medial displacement. A recent study by Wongwatana and colleagues[136] reported that the upper head of the lateral pterygoid muscle contributed to the anterior-medial displacement of the disc only in cases of prior damage to the disc. However, the lateral pterygoid muscle has a variable attachment to the disc, confirmed by a postmortem study of 40 individuals, which found that in 65% of the specimens, the upper head of the lateral pterygoid muscle was attached to the medial aspect of the capsule, disc, and to the pterygoid fovea of the condyle. In 27.5% of specimens, the upper head was attached solely to the condyle; in the remaining 7.5% of cases, there were other types of attachments of the lateral pterygoid muscle to the disc.[137]

Osteoarthrosis is a localized degenerative disorder that affects mainly the articular cartilage of the temporomandibular joint and is often seen in older people.

Pigmented villonodular synovitis (PVNS), is a proliferative but nonneoplastic disorder that affects the synovial membranes of joints,[138,139] is generally thought to be a benign, inflammatory process, although it may develop as an aggressive local process. Pigmented villonodular synovitis was first reported in detail by Jaffe and colleagues[140] in 1941. It was described as expressing multiple manifestations of a histologic lesion characterized by a fibrous stroma, multinucleated giant cells, spindlelike cells, and histiocytic cells, with hemosiderin and lipid inclusions occurring in the synovial membrane of joints. The pathogenesis of PVNS is unknown.

Pigmented villonodular synovitis is subdivided into diffuse and localized forms, depending on the extent of synovial involvement. Although typical PVNS has a shaggy villous appearance, the diffuse form usually does not have grossly discernible patterns.[139] Pigmented villonodular synovitis may extend into bone, and, in most instances, the diffuse form probably represents aggressive extra-articular extension and occasional recurrence after surgical intervention.[139] According to site, 80% of cases involve the knee, followed in order of frequency by the hip, ankle, and shoulder.[139,141] Although any joint can be affected, involvement of the temporomandibular joint (TMJ) is very rare.[142–144]

The symptoms for temporomandibular joint PVNS vary, but typically include, swelling in the preauricular area, progressive temporomandibular joint pain during mastication, and a history of progressive difficulty in opening of the mouth.[145] The recommended intervention for PVNS lesions involves wide synovectomy at all sites involved.[139–141]

Epidemiology

Epidemiologic studies on nonpatient populations in the early 1970s reported that the prevalence of temporomandibular disorders signs and symptoms were similar for females and males.[146–148] Studies of temporomandibular disorders signs and symptoms in nonpatients revealed either no gender difference,[149,150] or a somewhat greater prevalence among females.[151,152] A recent longitudinal study,[153] however, showed that the course of temporomandibular disorders symptoms differed significantly with respect to gender: women who had reported symptoms during adolescence consistently reported symptoms one decade later, whereas the figure for men was only 60%.

In contrast to studies of nonpatient populations, studies of temporomandibular disorders patients have shown a strong preponderance of females, with female to male ratios of 2:1 and 4:1.[54,154] In patients referred for radiographic imaging of the temporomandibular joint, the female to male ratio was between 5:1 and 9:1.[57,155] In patients with radiographically verified temporomandibular joint disc displacement, the female predominance was significant; the prevalence was four to six times greater for females,[57,155] and four times more joints with disc displacement occurred in women than in men.[156] In addition, disc displacement in asymptomatic joints is twice as frequent in females as in males, both for juveniles[59,157] and adults.[57]

The reason for the higher prevalence of temporomandibular joint disc displacement in women and the over-representation of females at orofacial pain clinics remains obscure. A hypothesis has been put forward that women more readily seek treatment for illness than do men.[158] A recent literature review on pain ended with a recommendation to researchers and health professionals to give gender more detailed attention in pain research.[159]

The higher prevalence of temporomandibular joint disc displacement in adults than in juveniles could be due to a cumulative effect, but there are few studies on the incidence of disc displacement relative to age. One investigation revealed a statistically significant peak in incidence of symptomatic temporomandibular joint disc displacement during puberty for both females and males.[160]

Clinical Features

There are three cardinal features of temporomandibular disorders—orofacial pain, joint noise, and restricted jaw function. Pain is the most common presenting complaint and is by far the most difficult problem to evaluate.[161–163] Joint noise is of little clinical importance in the absence of pain.[163,164]

Restricted jaw function encompasses a limited range of mandibular movements in all directions. Like pain, restricted jaw function causes considerable anxiety for the patient, who faces difficulties in everyday activities such as eating and speaking. Patients describe either a generalized tight feeling, which is probably a muscular disorder, or the sensation that the jaw suddenly "catches" or "gets stuck," which is usually related to internal derangement.

Headaches, earaches, tinnitus, and neck and shoulder pains are just a few of a number of nonspecific symptoms that are often reported by patients with temporomandibular disorders. However, since these symptoms are not considered to be specific for temporomandibular disorders, other possible causes should be sought and ruled out.[165–167]

A growing understanding of the natural history of TMD and some of the physical changes associated with TMD has played an important role in the intervention and management of TMD.[66] Many of the signs and symptoms of TMD are present and detected in significant portions of the normal nonpatient population; for example, approximately 33% of humans have a temporomandibular joint click without pain or significant impairment.[168–171] Current research indicates that biochemical mechanisms and biomechanical adaptive mechanisms play a major role in the natural course of DJD, a self-limiting and nonprogressive course usually being expected in the absence of systemic disease and/or iatrogenesis.

Most instances of TMD involve masticatory muscle pains that vary in location and intensity with time; the majority of these resolve without intervention. Masticatory muscle pain TMD does not appear to progress in severity with age,[172] and facial pain is less prevalent in older persons than younger persons, thus distinguishing TMD from many other chronic diseases associated with increasing age.

Well-established associations have been made between TMD and other disorders, such as headache and neck pain.[14]

- Headache. Temporal muscle tendinitis (TMT), an overuse disorder, is a common but frequently overlooked disorder that mimics a headache.[173] TMT symptoms usually include pain near the temporomandibular joint and ear, ear fullness, temporal headaches, and facial pain. Treatment primarily includes cessation of the offending activity, such as gum chewing or teeth clenching.
- Neck pain.[173] In 1962, Moss[174] proposed the "functional matrix theory," which attempted to build an association between craniofacial changes and nasal airway obstruction. These craniofacial changes

TABLE 20–2 THE CONSEQUENCES OF THE FORWARD HEAD[274–277]

DEFICIT	IMPAIRMENT	EFFECT

Cervical hyperlordosis	Overclosing of TMJ
	    Posterior compression
	    Capsular ligament injury
	    Meniscal derangement
		Trigeminal facilitation
		    Suboccipital hypertonicity
		    Scalene hypertonicity with first rib impairment

	Craniovertebral hyperextension
	    AO flexion hypomobility
	    AA rotation hypomobility
	    AO extension hypermobility
	    Craniovertebral instability
		Trigeminal facilitation
		    Masticator hypertonicity
		    TMJ impairment

	Mid-cervical hyperextension
	    Flexion hypomobility
	    Extension hypermobility
	    Anterior instabilities
		C4 facilitation
		    Levator scapulae hypertonicity
		    with adduction of scapula and overuse
		    of supraspinatus
		C5 facilitation
		    Rotator cuff hypertonicity
		    Tennis elbow

Shoulder protraction	Glenohumeral instability Acromioclavicular instability	Supraspinatus tendonitis Infraspinatus tendonitis Acromioclavicular sprain

Cervicothoracic hyperkyphosis	Extension hypomobilities	Shoulder girdle hypomobility
		    Glenohumeral instability
		    Acromioclavicular instability
		    Supraspinatus tendonitis

included a "clockwise" rotation of the mandible in a more vertical and posterior direction, elongation of the lower face height, open bite, crosbite, retrognathia, and the forward head posture. One of the most prevalent postural deviations is the forward head position. The habitual placement of the head anterior to the body's center of gravity has been suggested by many as a component in the etiology of numerous musculoskeletal and neurovascular impairments.[175–181] (Table 20–2) When the number of occupations that require the head to be bent forward and the arms to be carried in front of the body is considered, it is not surprising that this posture frequently develops.

The anteriorly displaced line of gravity induced by the forward head has an effect on respiration. This change in posture is postulated to have the following consequences.[182]

● Open-mouth breathing.[183] Initially a normal response in a baby, it becomes abnormal if it persists into the 5- to 7-year-old age range. A child with a long bout of sinus infections and blockages is forced to use mouth breathing as his or her primary method of breathing. With the development of the teeth and tongue, this abnormal pattern is accentuated, as both serve to block the oral passageway, forcing the child to open

the mouth further in order to breathe. It is postulated that this can result in the following.[183,184–186]

1. A failure to filter inspired air of pathogens and particles. These particles go directly into the alveoli producing an inflammatory reaction in the lungs resulting in bronchospasm and asthma, and stimulating a future hypersensitivity to any new particles.
2. A failure to humidify inspired air, so that the air entering the lungs is dry.
3. A failure to warm the inspired air. Cold or cool air entering the lungs stimulates an increased presence of white blood cells, increasing the hypersensitivity of the lungs.

Early intervention with mouth breathers is essential, and it is recommended that the child be encouraged to keep the tongue against the roof of the mouth while breathing.

Although only theoretical, the thoracic compensation is necessary to counteract the backward tilting of the head and to return the eyes to a horizontal position. This produces:

1. A reduction in thoracic extension.
2. A reduced ability of the ribs to elevate during inspiration due to a reduced ability of the thoracic cavity to expand during inspiration[184–187]
3. An increase in the respiratory rate.[184–186]

4. A flattening of the lumbar lordosis resulting in a posterior pelvic tilt. This leads to a decrease in hip extension and an increase in flexion forces at the only joint in the lumbar spine that cannot flex, the L5–S1 segment. These forces may eventually produce an instability at this level.

Stages of Healing

Acute

Acute injuries to the temporomandibular joint most frequently have a traumatic origin, but may be associated with a systemic arthritis. The patient demonstrates a capsular pattern of restriction (decreased ipsilateral opening), with pain and tenderness on the same side. There may be ligamentous damage, which will be demonstrated on the stress tests, or muscular damage, which will become apparent on isometric testing.

In the early stages, the patient is preoccupied with the local pain, which can be severe. If allowed to undergo adaptive shortening, the hypomobile joint can, and usually will, result in hypermobility on the opposite side.[16] The range of motion may be normal, with pain experienced when the patient tries to force opening. Passively, spasm is experienced as the end feel on depression and protrusion on that side, whereas the hypomobility is discovered on the other.

Nonacute

Chronic impairment frequently occurs from an inadequately treated arthritis that has resulted in adaptive shortening, or from a fixed head forward posture, abnormal stress levels, or from the patient suffering from chronic pain syndrome. Prolonged pain is frequently due to a secondary hypermobility.

CLINICAL EXAMINATION OF THE TEMPOROMANDIBULAR JOINT

Diagnosis in TMD consists of (1) patient history, (2) physical examination, and, in most chronic cases, (3) behavioral or psychologic examination.[16,17,66,100,188–190] This examination should include a detailed pain and jaw function history as well as objective measurements of such jaw functions as interincisal opening, opening pattern, and range of eccentric jaw motions (Figure 20–11).

Temporomandibular joint sounds should be described and related to symptoms.

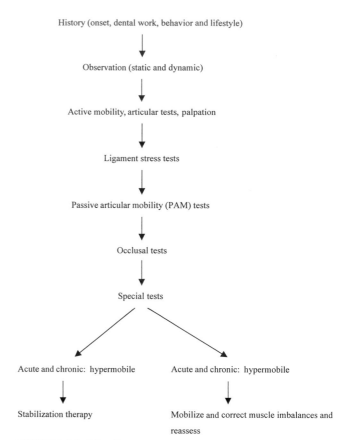

History (onset, dental work, behavior and lifestyle)

↓

Observation (static and dynamic)

↓

Active mobility, articular tests, palpation

↓

Ligament stress tests

↓

Passive articular mobility (PAM) tests

↓

Occlusal tests

↓

Special tests

Acute and chronic: hypermobile   Acute and chronic: hypermobile

↓   ↓

Stabilization therapy   Mobilize and correct muscle imbalances and reassess

FIGURE 20–11 Examination sequence.

History

The symptoms, which can be local or remote, can include orofacial pain, headaches, joint noises, restricted mouth opening, or a combination of these, in addition to other less specific, and seemingly unrelated, problems. Questions should focus on any history of trauma during birth or childhood as well as more recently. The clinician should attempt to clarify any emotional factors in the patient's background that may provoke habitual protrusion or muscular tension.[1]

Pain should be evaluated carefully in terms of its onset, nature, intensity, site, duration, aggravating and relieving factors, and, especially, how it relates to the other features, such as joint noise and restricted mandibular movements. The distribution of pain is useful in that the temporomandibular joint and the upper three cervical joints all refer to the head, whereas the mid to low cervical spine typically refers to the shoulder and arm.[191–193] Pain that is centered immediately in front of the tragus of the ear and projects to the ear, temple, cheek, and along the mandible is highly diagnostic for temporomandibular disorder. One study demonstrated that 50% of patients with a mandibular impairment complained of headaches and pain in the neck, back, and shoulders.[194]

A history of limited mouth opening, which may be intermittent or progressive, is also a key feature of temporomandibular disorders.

The patient may report clicking in the ear as the jaw is opened and/or closed or may relate symptoms of crepitus. These noises may not be audible to the clinician and a stethoscope may be required. Clicking, whether painful or not, is postulated to be caused by a movement of the disc on the condyle. A click is pathological if the condyle subluxes off the disc. Generally, articular instability will produce a clunk at the end of opening and the patient will have to provide a strong contraction to "clunk the jaw back" again.[16] Crepitus is usually associated with articular surface damage or with severe disc degeneration.[195]

Due to the wide distribution of the trigeminal nerve, temporomandibular joint symptoms can be widespread. In addition to supplying the sensory and motor control of the joint, the nerve also supplies the following.[16]

● Skin of the face
● Paranasal, frontal sinuses
● Mucosa of the nose, mouth, tongue, external auditory meatus
● Tympanic membrane
● Muscles of mastication
● Anterior digastric, lateral pterygoid, mylohyoid
● Tensor veli palatines
● Tensor tympani

The result of this widespread distribution is a variety of symptoms, which may include[16]:

● Otalgia, which may be mechanical due to over-closing and compression of the bone by the condyle, or may be due mucosal hypersensitivity from a facilitated nerve.
● Tinnitus secondary to increased tympanic membrane tension from a facilitatory hypertonicity of the tensor tympani.
● Facial pain and hyperesthesia.
● Conjunctival or retro-ocular pain.
● Cervical pain.

In general, the longer the duration of the symptoms and the greater the number of interventions, and in particular "failed" interventions, the smaller the likelihood that the patient will respond well to further intervention.[196]

Static Observation

The position of the head on the neck is examined. The typical patient with a temporomandibular disorder has a posture of forward head, stiff neck and back, and has shallow, restricted breathing,[200] due to the functional relationship between the temporomandibular joint, and the cervical spine. The neuromuscular influence of the cervical and masticatory region actively participate in the function of the mandibular movement and cervical positioning.[33,201–203] Many factors influence the masticatory muscles and affect the rest position and the mechanism of mandibular closure.[23,205–207] A change in head position caused by cervical muscles changes the mandibular position.[205,208–211] This change affects the occlusion and masticatory muscles.[193,212]

The face is observed for symmetry, noting any jaw deviation, flattening of the cheek, hypertonicity of the muscles, dryness of the lips, jaw position, and changes in eye position.

Dynamic Observation

The clinician observes the patient as they open and close their mouth, observing both the range and quality of movement. The opening of the mouth is the most revealing and diagnostic maneuver for TMD. The patient with the unstable subluxing condyle will avoid opening the jaw into the unstable range unless specifically asked to do so. Overpressure is thus applied, ensuring that the jaw is maximally depressed to detect the presence of these instabilities. If there is a hypomobility on one side, the jaw deviates towards the less mobile side during opening. A normal joint can appear to be hypomobile if the other joint is hypermobile, so the clinician must observe the full range of opening. An early deviation during opening indicates a hypomobility, whereas a late deviation suggests a hypermobility.

Articular Tests

The passive ranges are assessed for quantity, end feel, and the reproduction of pain. Isometrics at the end ranges are used to test for contractile impairments, and stress tests are performed to rule out ligamentous tears. The following motions are assessed first with overpressure, and then with resistance applied at the ends of range.

● Elevation of mandible (mouth closing): the clinician applies overpressure by placing his or her fingers under the patient's chin (Figure 20–12).
● Depression of mandible (mouth opening): using a lumbrical grip placed on the patient's chin, under the bottom lip, overpressure of mouth opening is applied (Figure 20–13).
● Protrusion of mandible: the clinician stands in front of patient, with index and middle fingers behind the mandible angles and thumbs on the patient's cheeks.

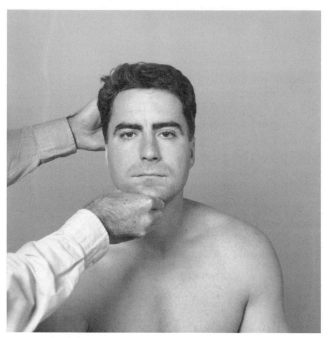

FIGURE 20–12   Patient and clinician position for over-pressure into elevation.

The clinician gently pulls anteriorly to apply over pressure (Figure 20–14).

● Retrusion of the mandible: using a lumbrical grip positioned under the patient's bottom lip, the mandible is pushed posteriorly (Figure 20–15).

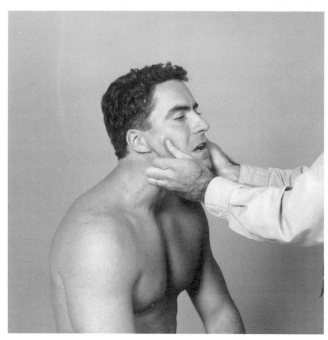

FIGURE 20–14   Patient and clinician position for over-pressure into protrusion.

● Deviation of the mandible to both sides, with mouth closed.

The clinician measures the amount of mouth opening using the patient's PIP joints. The maximum amount of

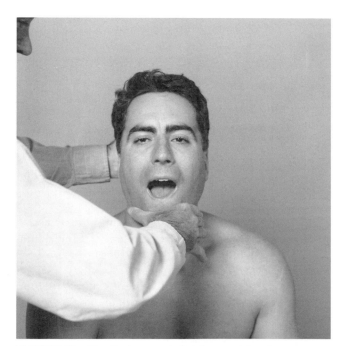

FIGURE 20–13   Patient and clinician position for over-pressure into depression.

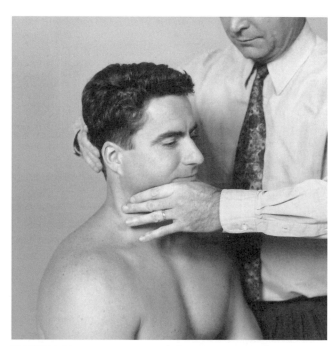

FIGURE 20–15   Patient and clinician position for over-pressure into retrusion.

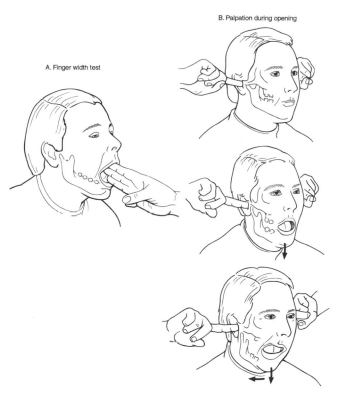

FIGURE 20–16 Mouth opening test, and palpation during opening.

opening should not exceed two and a half to three finger widths (males, 2; females, 3) at the PIP joints (Figure 20–16A).

The clinician palpates over the mandible heads during opening and closing to determine that they move together (see Figure 20–16).

If all of the above motions are normal and pain free, the problem is not from the temporomandibular joint. However, if the motion is restricted, then the surrounding muscles are probably at fault, and an examination of the accessory glides is necessary.

Palpation

The medial and lateral pterygoids, the masseters, temporalis, and perihyoid muscles are palpated for hypertonicity and tenderness. In addition, the lateral aspect of the joint capsule and the lateral temporomandibular joint ligament are palpated. The clinician feels for abnormal motions on opening and closing (Figure 20–16B), which would indicate hypermobility, a posterior meniscal ligament problem, or a meniscal derangement especially if they are accompanied by pain.

Medial Pterygoid
The patient is asked to move the tongue to the opposite side. The clinician slides a thumb onto the medial aspect of the lower gum and toward the back of the patient's mouth/angle of the mandible. The thumb is maintained at the bottom of the mouth to prevent the patient from gagging. The insertion site is on the medial aspect of the mandible angle.

Lateral Pterygoid
The clinician slides a thumb back to the medial aspect of the base of the upper molars. The patient is asked to open the mouth wider and the clinician slides the thumb back and up at an angle of 45 degrees. Does pressure in this area reproduce any pain?

The following structures should also be located.

- Angle of mandible
- Prearticular eminence
- Head of mandible (anterior aspect, can only feel the posterior aspect with the jaw opened)
- Coronoid process (between the tip of the zygoma and the angle of the mandible)
- Articular eminence

Ligamentous Stress Tests

The patient is seated.

- *Lateral temporomandibular*: the clinician cradles and stabilizes the patient's head. The patient's mandible is positioned slightly open. The clinician, placing the thumb of the mobilizing hand on the tongue of the patient, depresses the mandible with a caudal shear (Figure 20–17A).

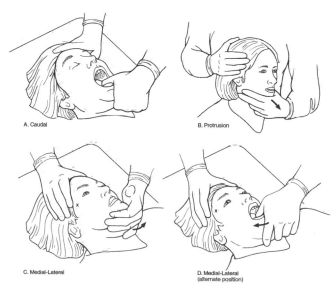

FIGURE 20–17 Caudal traction, protrusion, medial and lateral glides.

- Stylomandibular and sphenomandibular: the clinician stands in front of the patient. The patient's mandible is closed. The clinician, placing each hand on the ramus and angle of each side, applies an anterior-inferior shear at a 45-degree angle (see Figure 20–17B).
- Capsular: the clinician stands in front of the patient. The patient's mandible is closed. The clinician, placing one hand on the top of the patient's head and the other on the ramus and angle of one side, applies a contralateral protrusion and ipsilateral deviation (see Figure 20–17C/D).

Passive Articular Mobility (PAM) Testing

From the rest position (or as close as possible, given that the clinician's thumb is in the patient's mouth) and on each side, the following is carried out assessing for range and end feel. The clinician should remove the thumb from the patient's mouth about every 15 seconds to allow him or her to swallow. The following movements are performed.

- Distraction (caudal)—the lateral ligament becomes vertical with mouth opening
- Inferior glide (Figure 20–18)
- Anterior glide (see Figure 20–18)
- Posterior glide—with lateral deviation for the posterior ligaments (Figure 20–19)
- Lateral glide (see Figure 20–17)
- Medial glide (see Figure 20–17)
- Superior glide (compression)

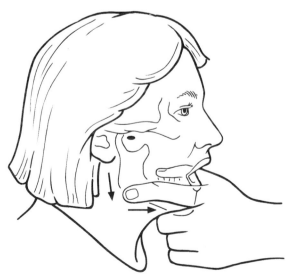

FIGURE 20–18 Inferior glide and anterior glide.

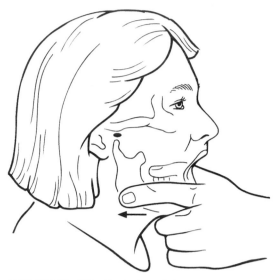

FIGURE 20–19 Posterior glide.

It is important to check the glides that are related to the loss of active motion. For example, if a patient's mouth deviates to the left during opening, this would indicate that either the left joint cannot open fully (go down, forward, and out), or the right joint cannot deviate to the right (go up, back, and in).

Occlusal Tests

Although malocclusion is common in asymptomatic patients and should only be evaluated by a specialist, three simple tests can be used to determine if the malocclusion is relevant to the presenting symptoms.[16]

1. *Passive repeated closing*: The patient sits, with the clinician standing behind, with his or her head resting against the clinician. The clinician holds the jaw with one hand and taps the teeth together while the patient is asked if the two sides are contacting simultaneously.
2. *External auditory meatus palpation*: The external auditory meatus is palpated as the patient closes the mouth and the simultaneity of the condylar movement is assessed (Figure 20–16B).
3. Incisor relationships: The superior and inferior incisors are assessed for any deviation of the jaw laterally (crossbite) or anterior-posterior (overbite).

Special Tests

Trigeminal Tests

Sensation The skin near the midline (there is overlap from the ventral rami of C2 and C3 if tested too laterally) of the forehead and face can be stroked with cotton wool or tissue paper or can be tested for pinprick sensation. It is best if the testing is carried out bilaterally and simultaneously.

Reflex The jaw jerk can be used to test trigeminal function where a lesion superior to the pons would produce hyperreflexia, and below hypo-or areflexia.[16]

IMAGING STUDIES

Many reports question the utility of temporomandibular joint imaging studies because 30% of normal people have disc displacements and joint arthrosis (degenerative processes affecting the temporomandibular joint) is usually benign.[60,213,214] Postmortem examinations of a total of 140 persons (dental histories unknown) showed that 40 to 80% had joint pathology or disc displacements.[213] The relevance of bony joint arthrosis was also disputed by evidence that patients with temporomandibular joint rheumatoid arthritic pathology actually had fewer symptoms than normal subjects.[215]

INTERVENTION

Nonsurgical intervention[216,217] of temporomandibular disorders continues to be the most effective way of managing over 80% of patients. There are numerous nonsurgical interventions for temporomandibular disorders. These involve not one but a number of different specialist practitioners who come together under the umbrella of a multidisciplinary team. Although each intervention will be discussed separately, for optimal success, they are best used in combination, depending on the patient's needs.[60,218]

Explanation and Reassurance

Probably the most important part of the intervention of temporomandibular disorders is to explain to the patient the cause and nature of the disorder, and to reassure them of the benign nature of the condition. Many patients will benefit from the reassurance that the symptoms of the temporomandibular disorder they are experiencing is not an indication of a life-threatening condition, although a thorough examination is needed to effectively rule out the more sinister causes.

Patient Education and Self-care

A self-care routine should include the following: limitation of mandibular function, habit awareness and modification, a home exercise program, and avoidance of stress.

Voluntary limitation of mandibular function is encouraged to promote rest or immobilization of muscular and articular structures. Hence, the patient is advised to eat soft foods and avoid those that need a lot of chewing, and is discouraged from wide yawning, singing, chewing gum, and any other activities that would cause excessive jaw movement. The rest position of the tongue is taught. Massaging the affected muscles and applying moist heat will promote muscle relaxation and help soothe aching or tired muscles. Patients should also be advised to identify the source(s) of stress and try to change his or her lifestyle accordingly. Posture education should form the cornerstone of any plan of care for temporomandibular dysfunction.

Drug Intervention

The patient's physician may prescribe medications. If used properly as part of a comprehensive management program, drugs can be a valuable help in relieving symptoms,[219,220] although no single drug has been proved to be effective for all cases of temporomandibular disorders.

The analgesic effects of nonsteroidal antiinflammatory drugs is specific only in cases of temporomandibular disorders where pain is the result of an inflammatory process, such as synovitis or myositis. For moderate to severe pain, opiates are best prescribed for a short period because of the risks of addiction. At the doses usually prescribed clinically, opiates are more effective in dampening the patient's emotional response to pain than eliminating the pain itself.[216]

Occlusal Therapy

The most common form of intervention provided by dentists for temporomandibular disorders is occlusal appliance therapy. This may be referred to as a bite-raising appliance, occlusal splint, or a biteguard. It is a removable device, usually made of hard acrylic, that is custom made to fit over the occlusal surfaces of the teeth. Although occlusal appliance therapy has been shown clinically to alleviate symptoms of temporomandibular disorders in over 70% of patients, the physiologic basis of the response to treatment has never been well understood.[221,222]

Surgical Intervention

Between 1887 and 1929, surgical meniscectomies began to be performed to relieve temporomandibular disorders pain and jaw locking.[223–226] Researchers in several postmortem studies ascribed temporomandibular joint pain to perforations of the articular disc that were traumatized by backward pressure from the mandibular condyle.[224,227]

Published reports show that about 5% of patients undergoing an intervention for temporomandibular disorders require surgery.[8,228] A range of surgical procedures is currently used to treat temporomandibular disorders, ranging from temporomandibular joint arthrocentesis and arthroscopy to the more complex, open-joint surgical procedures, referred to as arthrotomy.[228] Oral and maxillofacial surgeons with a special interest in this area often prefer patients to have undergone a period of nonsurgical treatment before seeking a surgical opinion. The benefits and limitations of each of the surgical procedures are readily determined on an individual case basis.[229,230]

The proximity of the medial aspect of the temporomandibular joint (TMJ) to the structures of the infratemporal fossa raises the possibility of complications associated with temporomandibular joint surgery on the medial aspect of the Joint. Weinberg and co-workers[231] demonstrated a 4% involvement of the inferior alveolar and lingual nerves after arthroscopic surgery. Moses and colleagues[232] reported an unusual arteriovenous fistula associated with arthroscopic temporomandibular joint surgery. Loughner and associates[233] demonstrated risk to the auriculotemporal nerve, which is interposed between the medial pole of the mandibular condyle and an elongated wall of the glenoid fossa. A number of studies have examined complications associated with temporomandibular joint surgery.[231,234–236] One study found that the location of such vital structures as the middle meningeal artery, the carotid artery, the internal jugular vein, and the trigeminal nerve, varied, increasing the likelihood of significant intraoperative or postoperative complications.[237]

Behavioral Therapy

In a controlled historical cohort study in Lithuania,[238] none of more than 200 subjects who had been involved in rear-end collisions 1 to 3 years earlier had persistent and disabling complaints of jaw pain or headache due to their accidents. (This has been confirmed in a recent prospective study.[239]) It has been postulated that several cultural and psychosocial factors may in fact be more relevant than the injury to the explanation of why accident victims in some other societies report chronic symptoms.[240,241]

Where persistent habits exacerbate, or maintain, the temporomandibular disorder and these cannot be modified easily by simple patient awareness, a structured program of cognitive behavioral therapy may be required. Behavioral modification strategies can include counseling on lifestyle, relaxation therapy, hypnosis, and biofeedback.[242]

Psychotherapy

Occasionally, temporomandibular disorders may be the somatic expression of an underlying psychological or psychiatric disorder, such as depression or a conversion disorder.[243,244] The best clue to this possibility is when a patient's suffering seems to be excessive or persistent, beyond what would be normal for that condition. In these patients, referral to a psychiatrist or clinical psychologist is a mandatory part of the overall management strategy.

Postural Education

Posture appears to be a uniquely human concern. During evolution, humans have adopted an upright posture requiring bipedal gait. The advantages of an erect posture are numerous but there are disadvantages too. Those disadvantages are mainly centered around the spine, temporomandibular joint, and the lower limbs, and the increased stresses placed upon them.

The focus of the intervention should be to educate the patient on correct posture so as to help minimize their symptoms. Often, the education consists of getting the patient to reduce the times spent in habitual positions during work and recreation. These positions, which cause an alteration in the tensile properties of the muscles, and adaptive shortening of the joint capsule and ligaments, result in a variety of problems including joint strain and improper weight bearing through the joint.[245–247] The pathologic posture then becomes associated with, or the precursor of, other deformities.

Because these postural deviations do not always cause symptoms,[248] and the corrected positions require effort to maintain, patients need reassurance that changing their posture will be beneficial.

In the past, the postural correction for a forward head has involved having the patient retract the head, flatten the lumbar spine, and hold this position. However, over a prolonged period, it is possible that this can lead to a hypermobility in the mid-cervical spine if all of the joints, particularly in the craniovertebral and upper thoracic region, are hypomobile, as the stress of the exercise would tend to fall on the mobile joint. Therefore, all of the segments should be examined for mobility and segmental mobilizations applied as necessary. Table 20–2 highlights some of the more common syndromes associated with the fixed forward head posture.

Manual Therapy

The aim of manual therapy is to restore normal mandibular function by a number of physical techniques that serve to relieve musculoskeletal pain and promote healing of tissues.[249] The clinician needs to be well versed in the management of musculoskeletal disorders of the head and neck.

Physical therapies for TMD are commonly used,[250,251] although there appears to be little evidence that passive modalities alone can cause long-lasting reductions in the signs or symptoms of TMD.[252,253] However, the present state of knowledge indicates that during the time they are treated, patients with TMD are helped with most forms of physical therapy, and that patients receiving multiple forms of physical therapy may do better than patients with single therapies.[252,253]

Moist Heat Packs and Cold Packs

Hecht and co-workers[254] compared the effectiveness of local applications of cold and heat in conjunction with exercise, versus exercise alone, on postsurgical pain of the knee. The application of cold with exercise was rated as providing significantly greater relief than the application of heat plus exercise or exercise alone, and swelling was also significantly decreased in the group that received the cold therapy. No other significant differences between groups were found. Chapman[255] concluded that local application of cold can provide short-term relief of pain, possibly because of its analgesic effects and ability to reduce inflammation.

When combined with the short-term effects of cold to decrease pain, passive exercise and stretching may be useful in increasing range of motion.[254]

Low-intensity Laser

A study by Gam and colleagues[256] concluded that laser therapy was not efficacious. However, another study by Beckerman and associates[257] was more positive. Bertolucci and Grey[258] reported that laser therapy reduced pain and tenderness associated with degenerative disease of the temporomandibular joint more than placebo.

Hi-volt Electric Stimulation

High-voltage stimulators deliver a monophasic, twin peak waveform. Because of the short duration of the twin peak wave, high voltages with high peak current but low average current can be achieved. These characteristics provide patient comfort and safety in application. In addition, in contrast to low voltage direct current devices, thermal and galvanic effects are minimized.[259–261]

High-voltage stimulators have been applied clinically to reduce or eliminate muscle spasm and soft tissue edema, as well as for muscle reeducation (noncentral nervous system-produced muscle contraction), trigger point therapy, and increasing blood flow to tissues with decreased circulation.[198,259,261–263]

Transcutaneous Electrical Nerve Stimulation

Transcutaneous electrical nerve stimulation (TENS) was introduced in the early 1950s to determine the suitability of patients with pain as candidates for the implantation of dorsal column electrodes. One study suggesting that there may be some beneficial effect of transcutaneous electrical nerve stimulation comes from Graff-Radford and co-workers,[264] who applied four different forms of TENS to "active" trigger points of myofascial pain subjects. Pain ratings were gathered before and after 10 minutes of treatment. Pain decreased for all groups, and post treatment pain was significantly less in three of the TENS treatment groups than in the placebo and the fourth TENS group.

Exercise

Some evidence also suggests that exercise of the specific painful area is effective in strengthening the muscles, improving function, and reducing pain. Tegelberg and Kopp[265] ran parallel studies of jaw exercise versus a no-treatment control in subjects with rheumatoid arthritis and ankylosing spondylitis. Significant differences were detected for both conditions in mean maximal opening, but no between-group differences were detected for change in the subjective symptoms (pain, stiffness). However, the results of Dao and colleagues[266] suggest that exercise must be used with caution. They measured pain levels of patients with TMDs before and after 3 minutes of chewing on wax and found that exercise gave relief to those whose pain levels were high but exacerbated low-level pain.

The strongest evidence of efficacy comes from studies of exercise to improve general fitness, no matter what the condition under study.[267–270]

Biofeedback

The use of muscle relaxation techniques assisted by electromyographic biofeedback has been demonstrated to be useful in treating chronic musculoskeletal pain; and it may be useful in TMD.[271,272] Close cooperation with a clinician who is well versed in the management of musculoskeletal disorders of the head and neck is essential.

The outlines below incorporate a combination of the interventions described, and relate them to two stages of healing.

ACUTE STAGE

The common methods of decreasing inflammation (rest and ice), should be initiated as soon as possible. The rest position for the tongue should be taught as early as possible, as well as instructions on the types of food to avoid. Usually, the softer the food, the better. The patient should avoid the extremes of jaw motions, whether that be excessive opening, or sustained clenching (it is very difficult to close the mouth fully if the tongue is in the rest position). The sleeping position must also be addressed. If the patient has damage to the capsule and/or lateral ligaments, he or she should sleep in the fetal position with the mouth closed. Care must be taken to ensure that the patient does not sleep in the prone position, especially if they are in the habit of placing a hand under the pillow. If the hand placement is such that it is positioned under the mandible, the jaw is placed in a position of lateral deviation. If the intrinsic ligaments are injured, sleeping on the back with the mouth open is advised. The mouth must also be protected against yawning. Yawning is theorized to be the result of an increase in the CO_2 levels in the body or an unsuppressed tonic neck reflex. Yawning can be prevented if the patient tucks and holds the chin onto the chest.

Very gentle active exercises, well within the pain-free range, should be performed frequently (every hour or so) to help stimulate the mechanoreceptors and modulate pain, as well as improve vascularization.[16]

The use of modalities should include ultrasound over the joint, TENS at the angle of the mandible (2 Hz seems to work well for cranial nerves; 4 Hz for peripheral nerves; 7.5 Hz for muscles; 9.5 Hz for the circulatory system; 8 to 13 Hz for the sympathetic system; and 8 to 10 Hz for the articular joints) and interferential currents.

Manual therapy should be applied gently, as this joint tends to be very reactive and can flare up easily.[16]

If the patient is unable to open the mouth sufficiently to allow the clinician to place their thumbs in the mouth, manual techniques should not be considered.

The hypermobile joint is treated by reducing the stress placed upon it with mobilizations to the hypomobile joint, and having the patient avoid full opening.[16]

CHRONIC STAGE

If the joint is still quite painful, a shift from ice to heat might be beneficial with the patient using ice-filled towels soaked in warm water, applied all around the jaw.[16] The patient should be encouraged to begin full active range-of-motion exercises (the 6 × 6 series; see discussion later).[212] However, if jaw deviation is occurring, the exercises should only be performed in the range that the patient can control the deviation. To control this, the patient with the deviating jaw is asked to practice opening and closing in front of a mirror. Manual therapy in this stage consists of restoring the glides.[16]

Postural correction may also be necessary as an habitual and excessive head forward posture adversely alters the occlusal relationship and may lead to continual stressing of the temporomandibular joint.

The cervical spine, particularly the suboccipital joints, often requires intervention. The hypomobile cervical joint is mobilized and normal movements reeducated.

If the examination shows that the restriction of movement is due to shortened muscles (or other structures), then the following manual techniques may be used.

Technique 1[273]

To increase the anterior and inferior movement of the mandible for the patient that can only achieve slight opening of the mouth (Figure 20–18), the patient is positioned in sitting and the clinician stands to the patient's left side. The clinician grips the patient's head, using his or her right forearm and hand, fingers against the patient's forehead. The clinician stabilizes the patient's head between his or her right hand, arm, and chest. With a medical gloved hand, the clinician's left thumb is placed on the patient's lower molars on the right side, as far back in the mouth as possible. The clinician's index and middle fingers grip the angle of the patient's mandible on right side with the ring and/or little fingers held under the patient's mandible (depending on the size of the clinician's hand and patient's mandible). Using this grip, the clinician applies light traction inferiorly to patient's right TMJ by pressing his or her thumb inferiorly against the lower molars, while gradually and maximally, pulling anteriorly to produce an anterior glide of the right head of the mandible at the TMJ. To stimulate the antagonists, the clinician retains the grip with right hand, places the left hand on the left side of the patient's chin, and asks patient to look to the left and downward, and then move the patient's mandible inferiorly and to the left (in the direction of stretching). The clinician resists the movements to stimulate the patient's antagonists. Note: if the restriction of movement is bilateral, the same intervention can be performed on the patient's opposite side. The procedure must be performed gradually. The clinician combines the inferior traction with an anterior glide. The patient is again asked to open his or her mouth as much as possible. The procedure is repeated until the patient is able to fully open his or her mouth, or considerable improvement is attained.

Technique 2[273]

To increase posterior movement of the mandible (retraction) for the patient with an inability to fully close the mouth (Figure 20–19), the patient is positioned in sitting and the clinician stands to the patient's left side. The clinician, using his or right forearm, grips the patient's head from behind, fingers against the patient's forehead. The clinician stabilizes the patient's head between his or her right hand, arm, and chest. The clinician's left hand holds the patient's chin. Using this grip, the clinician gradually and maximally pushes posteriorly against the patient's mandible to produce a posterior glide of the head of the mandible at the TMJ. To stimulate the antagonists, the clinician's left hand is placed over the patient's right mandible, fingers behind the angle. The clinician then asks the patient to look to the right and move the mandible to the right (in the direction of stretching). The clinician resists that movement to stimulate the patient's antagonists. Note: during the procedure, the patient's mandible should be completely relaxed, and the patient should not attempt to open his or her mouth. If the restriction of movement is bilateral, the same intervention can be performed on the patient's opposite side. The procedure is used when the patient cannot close his or her mouth. It may also be tried when patient cannot fully open his or her mouth and the previous technique is ineffective.

6 × 6 Exercise Protocol

The patient should be instructed to perform the following exercises 6 times each at a frequency of 6 times per day.[212]

1. Tongue rest position and nasal breathing. The patient places the tip of the tongue on the roof of the mouth, just behind the front teeth. In this position, the patient makes a "clucking" sound and gently holds the tongue against the palate with slight pressure. With the tongue in this position, the patient is asked to breathe through the nose and to use the stomach muscles for expiration.
2. Controlled opening. The patient positions the tongue in the rest position and practices opening the mouth to the point where the tongue begins to leave the roof of the mouth. The patient can monitor the joint rotation by placing an index finger over the TMJ region. The patient is encouraged to chew with this technique.
3. Rhythmic stabilization. The patient positions the tongue in the rest position and grasps the chin with one or both hands. The patient applies a resistance sideways to the right, and then to the left. The patient then applies a resistance toward opening and closing. Throughout all of these exercises, the patient must maintain the jaw position at all times and excessive force is cautioned against.

4. Stabilized head flexion. The patient places both hands behind the neck and interlaces the fingers. The neck is kept upright while the patient nods forward.
5. Axial neck extension. In one motion, the patient is asked to glide the neck backward and stretch the head upward. This exercise needs to be monitored closely to prevent a hypermobility of the cervical segments.
6. Shoulder retraction. In one motion, the patient is asked to pull the shoulders back and downward while squeezing the shoulder blades together.

REVIEW QUESTIONS

1. List the components of the stomatognathic system.
2. What type of cartilage lines the joint surfaces of the temporomandibular joint?
3. In which direction does the fibrocartilaginous disc move during normal mouth opening?
4. Which muscles elevate the mandible?
5. Which 3 nerves primarily supply the temporomandibular joint?
6. Describe the rest position for the stomatognathic system.
7. True or False: Mouth opening involves a lateral deviation and retrusion of the mandible.
8. What is capsular pattern of the temporomandibular joint?
9. Which sleeping position is recommended for the patient with an injury to the intrinsic ligaments of the temporomandibular joint?
10. Which frequency of TENS (Hz) is recommended for injured muscles?

ANSWERS

1. Bones of the skull, the mandible, the hyoid, the masticatory muscles and ligaments, the teeth and their respective joints, the temporomandibular joint, and the vascular, neurological and lymphatic systems.
2. Fibrocartilage
3. Anteriorly
4. Temporalis, masseter, and medial pterygoid
5. The maxillary, ophthalmic, and mandibular branches of the trigeminal nerve
6. The rest position of the stomatognathic system involves placing the tongue up against the palate of the mouth, with its tip placed behind the top incisors.
7. False
8. Deviation of motion to the same side as the affected joint, with a loss of functional opening.
9. Supine with the mouth open.
10. 7.5 Hz

REFERENCES

1. Hertling D, Kessler RM. *Management of Common Musculoskeletal Disorders: Physical Therapy Principles and Methods.* 2nd ed. Philadelphia: J Lippincott, 1990.

2. McNeill C. Temporomandibular disorders: guidelines for diagnosis and management. *CDA J* 1991;19:15–26.

3. Moses AJ. Good science, bad science, and scientific double-talk. *J Craniomandib Pract* 1996;14:170–172.

4. Kolbinson DA, Epstein JB, Burgess JA. Temporomandibular disorders, headaches, and neck pain following motor vehicle accidents and the effects of litigation review of the literature. *J Orofac Pain* 1996;10:101–125.

5. Ferrari R, Leonard M. Whiplash and temporomandibular disorders: a critical review. *J Am Dent Assoc* 1998;129:1739–1745.

6. Von Korff M, Dworkin SF, Le Resche L, Kruger A. An epidemiological comparison of pain complains. *Pain* 1988;32:173–183.

7. Morgan DH, Hall WP, Vamvas SJ (eds): *Disease of the Temporomandibular Apparatus: A Multi-disciplinary Approach.* 2nd ed. St. Louis: CV Mosby, 1982.

8. Dworkin SF, Huggins KH, Le Resche L, et al. Epidemiology of signs and symptoms in temporomandibular disorders: clinical signs in cases and controls. *J Am Dent Assoc* 1990;120:273–281.

9. Von Korff M, Wagner EH, Dworkin SF, Saunders KW. Chronic pain and use of ambulatory health care. *Psychosom Med* 1991;53:61–79.

10. Rudy TE, Turk DC, Zaki HS. An empirical taxonomic alternative to traditional classification of temporomandibular disorders. *Pain* 1989;36:311–320.

11. Ohrbach R, Dworkin SF. Five-year outcomes in TMD: relationship of changes in pain to changes in pain to changes in physical and psychological variables. *Pain* 1998;74:315–324.

12. Mohl ND, Ohrbach R. The dilemma of scientific knowledge versus clinical management of temporomandibular disorders. *J Prosthet Dent* 1992;67:113–120.

13. Raphael K, Marbach JJ. Evidence-based care of musculoskeletal facial pain: implications for the clinical science of dentistry. *J Am Dent Assoc* 1997;128:73–79.

14. Carlsson GE, LeResche L. Epidemiology of temporomandibular disorders. In: Sessle, B J, Bryant, PS, Dionne, RA, eds. *Temporomandibular Disorders and Related Pain Conditions, Progress in Pain Research and Management.* Vol 4. Seattle: IASP Press; 1995;211–226.

15. Stohler CS. Clinical perspectives on masticatory and related muscle disorders. In: Sessle BJ, Bryant PS, Dionne RA, eds. *Temporomandibular Disorders and Related Pain Conditions, Progress in Pain Research and Management.* Vol 4. Seattle: IASP Press; 1995;3–29.

16. Meadows JTS. Manual Therapy: Biomechanical Assessment and Treatment, Advanced Technique. Lecture and Video Supplemental Manual. Swodeam Consulting Calgary, Alberta, 1995.

17. Okeson JP. Current terminology and diagnostic classification schemes. *Oral Surg Oral Med Oral Pathol Oral Radiol Endod* 1997;83:61–66.

18. Sicher H, Du Brul EL. *Oral Anatomy.* 8th ed. St. Louis: CV Mosby; 1988.

19. Rees LA. The structure and function of the mandibular joint. *Br Dent J* 1954;96:125.

20. Mohl DN. Functional anatomy of the temporomandibular joint. In: *The President's Conference on the Examination, Diagnosis and Management of Temporomandibular Disorders.* Chicago: American Dental Association; 1983;20–57.

21. Glineburg RW, Laskin DM, Blaustein DI. The effects of immobilization on the primate temporomandibular joint. *J Oral Maxillofac Surg* 1982;40:3.

22. DeBont LGM, Boering G, Havinga P, et al. Spatial arrangement of collagen fibrils in the articular cartilage of the mandibular condyle: a light microscopic and scanning electron microscopic study. *J Oral Maxillofac Surg* 1984;42:306.

23. Kraus SL, ed. *TMJ Disorders: Management of the Craniomandibular Complex, Clinics in Physical Therapy* (vol 18). New York: Churchill Livingstone;1988.

24. Bell WE. *Orofacial Pains: Classification, Diagnosis, Management.* 3rd ed. Chicago: New Year Medical Publishers; 1985.

25. Naidoo LCD. The development of the temporomandibular joint: a review with regard to the lateral pterygoid muscle. *J Dent Assoc S Africa* 1993;48:189–194.

26. Dolwick MF, Katzberg RW, Helms CA, Bales DJ. Arthrotomographic evaluation of the temporomandibular joint. *J Oral Surg* 1979;11:793.

27. Skaggs CD. Diagnosis and treatment of temporomandibular disorders. In: Murphy DR(ed). *Cervical Spine Syndromes.* New York: McGraw-Hill, 2000;579–592.

28. Juniper RD. The pathogenesis and investigation of TMJ dysfunction. *Br J Oral Maxillofac Surg* 1987;25:105–112.

29. Kraus SL. Physical therapy management of TMJ dysfunction. In: Kraus SL, ed. *TMJ Disorders: Management of the Craniomandibular Complex.* New York: Churchill Livingstone; 1988;139–173.

30. Hargreaves A. Dysfunction of the temporomandibular joints. *Physiotherapy* 1986;72:209–212.

31. Williams P.L, Warwick R, eds. *Gray's Anatomy.* 38th ed. Edinburgh: Churchill Livingstone; 1995.

32. Clark R, Wyke B. Contributions of temporomandibular articular mechanoreceptors to the control of mandibular posture: an experimental study. *J Dent* 1974;2:121–129.

33. Wyke BD. Neuromuscular mechanisms influencing mandibular posture: a neurologist's review of current concepts. *J Dent* 1972;2:111–120.

34. Pinto OF. A new structure related to the temporomandibular joint and the middle ear. *J Prosthet Dent* 1962;12:95–103.

35. Ermshar CB. Anatomy and neuroanatomy. In: Morgan DH, Hall WP, Vamvas SV, eds. *Disease of the Temporomandibular Apparatus: A Multidisciplinary Approach.* St. Louis: CV Mosby; 1977.

36. Meyenberg K, Kubick S, Palla S. Relationship of the muscles of mastication to the articular disk of the temporomandibular joint. *Helv Odont Acta* 1986;30: 815–834.

37. Carpentier P, Yung J-P, Marguelles-Bonnet R, Meunisser M. Insertions of the lateral pterygoid muscle: an anatomic study of the human temporomandibular joint. *J Oral Maxillofac Surg* 1988;46: 477–482.

38. Bittar GT, Bibb CA, Pullinger AG. Histological characteristics of the lateral pterygoid muscle insertion into the temporomandibular joint. *J Orofac Pain* 1994;8:243–249.

39. Honée GLJM. The anatomy of the lateral pterygoid muscle. *Acta Morphol Need Scand* 1972;10: 331–340.

40. Luschei ES, Goodwin GM. Patterns of mandibular movement and muscle activity during mastication in the monkey. *J Neurophysiol* 1974;35:954–966.

41. McNamara JA. The independent function of the two heads of the lateral pterygoid muscle. *Am J Anat* 1973;138:197–205.

42. Bogduk N. Innervation and pain patterns of the cervical spine. In: Grant R ed. *Physical Therapy of the Cervical and Thoracic Spine.* New York: Churchill Livingstone; 1988;65–76.

43. Fish F. The functional anatomy of the rest position of the mandible. *Dent Prac* 1961;11:178–183.

44. Atwood DA. A critique of research of the rest position of the mandible. *J Prosthet Dent* 1966;16:848–854.

45. Viener AF. Oral surgery. In: Garliner D, ed. *Myofunctional Therapy.* Philadelphia: Saunders; 1976.

46. Shore MA. *Temporomandibular Joint Dysfunction and Occlusal Equilibration.* Philadelphia: Lippincott; 1976.

47. Costen JB. A syndrome of ear and sinus symptoms dependent upon disturbed function of the temporomandibular joint. *Ann Otol Rhinol Laryngol* 1934;43: 1–15.

48. Costen JB. Some features of the mandibular articulation as it pertains to medical diagnosis, especially otolaryngology. *J Am Dent Assoc Dent Cosmos* 1937;24: 1507–1511.

49. Costen JB. Correlation of x ray findings of the mandibular joint with clinical signs, especially trismus. *J Am Dent Assoc* 1939;26:405–407.

50. Dingman RO. Diagnosis and treatment of lesions of temporomandibular joint. *Am J Orthodont* 1940;26: 374–390.

51. Sicher H. Temporomandibular articulation in mandibular overclosure. *J Am Dent Assoc* 1948;36: 131–139.

52. Shapiro HH, Truex RC. The temporomandibular joint and the auditory function. *J Am Dent Assoc* 1943;30:1147–1168.

53. Laskin DM. Etiology of the pain-dysfunction syndrome. *J Am Dent Assoc* 1969;79:147–153.

54. Isacsson G, Linde C, Isberg A. Subjective symptoms in patients with temporomandibular disk displacement versus patients with myogenic craniomandibular disorders. *J Prosthet Dent* 1989;61:70–77.

55. Katzberg RW, OMara RE, Tallents RH, Weber DA. Radionuclide skeletal imaging and single photon emission computed tomography in suspected internal derangements of the temporomandibular joint. *J Oral Maxillofac Surg* 1984;42:782–787.

56. Paesani D, Westesson P-L, Hatala M, Tallents RH, Kurita K. Prevalence of temporomandibular joint internal derangement in patients with craniomandibular disorders. *Am J Orthod Dentofac Orthop* 1992;101: 41–47.

57. Katzberg RW, Westesson P-L, Tallents RH, Drake CM. Orthodontics and temporomandibular joint internal derangement. *Am J Orthod Dentofac Orthop* 1996;109: 515–520.

58. Sanchez-Woodworth RE, Katzberg RW, Tallents RH, Guay JA. Radiographic assessment of temporomandibular joint pain and dysfunction in the pediatric age-group. *J Dent Children* 1988;55: 278–281.

59. Ribeiro RF, Tallents RH, Katzberg RW, et al. The prevalence of disc displacement in symptomatic and asymptomatic volunteers aged 6 to 25 years. *J Orofac Pain* 1997;11:37–47.

60. McNeill C, ed. *Temporomandibular Disorders–Guidelines for Classification, Assessment and Management.* 2nd ed. Chicago: Quintessence Books; 1993.

61. Salonen L, Hellden L. Prevalence of signs and symptoms of dysfunction in the masticatory system: an

epidemiological study in an adult Swedish population. *J Craniomandib Disord Fac Oral Pain* 1990;4: 241–250.

62. Hannson T, Milner M. A study of occurrence of symptoms of diseases of the temporomandibular joint, masticatory musculature, and related structures. *J Oral Rehabil* 1975;2:313–324.

63. Pullinger A, Seligman DA, Solberg W. Temporomandibular joint disorders. Part 1: functional status, dentomorphologic features and sex differences in a non patient population. *J Prosthet Dent* 1988;59: 228–235.

64. Greene CS, Marbach JJ. Epidemiologic studies of mandibular dysfunction: a critical review. *J Prosthet Dent* 1982;48:184–190.

65. Clauw DJ, Schmidt M, Radulovic D, Singer A, Katz P, Bresette J. The relationship between fibromyalgia and interstitial cystitis. *J Psychiatr Res* 1997;31:125–131.

66. Goldstein BH, Temporomandibular disorders: A review of current understanding. *Oral Surg Oral Med Oral Pathol*, 1999;88:379–385.

67. Aaron LA, Bradley LA, Alarcon GS, et al. Perceived physical and emotional trauma as precipitating events in fibromyalgia: associations with health care seeking and disability status but not pain severity. *Arthritis Rheum* 1997;40:453–460

68. Bombardier CH, Buchwald D. Chronic fatigue, chronic fatigue syndrome, and fibromyalgia: disability and health-care use. *Med Care* 1996;34:924–930.

69. Buchwald D, Garrity D. Comparison of patients with chronic fatigue syndrome, fibromyalgia, and chemical sensitivities. *Arch Intern Med* 1994;154:2049–2053.

70. DeLuca J, Johnson SK, Ellis SP, Natelson BH. Sudden versus gradual onset of chronic fatigue syndrome differentiates individuals on cognitive and psychiatric measures. *J Psychiatr Res* 1997;31:83–90.

71. Aaron LA, Bradley LA, Alarcon GS, et al. Psychiatric diagnoses in patients with fibromyalgia are related to health care-seeking behavior rather than to illness. *Arthritis Rheum* 1996;39:436–445.

72. Schulte JK, Anderson GC, Hathaway KM, Will TE. Psychometric profiles and related pain characteristics of temporomandibular disorder patients. *J Orofac Pain* 1993;7:247–253.

73. Hudson JI, Goldenberg DL, Pope HG, Keck PE, Schlesinger L. Comorbidity of fibromyalgia with medical and psychiatric disorders. *Am J Med* 1992;92: 363–367.

74. Wysenbeek AJ, Shapira Y, Leibovici L. Primary fibromyalgia and the chronic fatigue syndrome. *Rheumatol Int* 1991;10:227–229.

75. Goldenberg DL, Simms RW, Geiger A, Komaroff AK High frequency of fibromyalgia in patients with chronic fatigue seen in a primary care practice. *Arthritis Rheum* 1990;33:381–387.

76. Hedenberg-Magnusson B, Ernberg M, Kopp S. Symptoms and signs of temporomandibular disorders in patients with fibromyalgia and local myalgia of the temporomandibular system: a comparative study. *Acta Odontol Scand* 1997;55:344–349.

77. Plesh O, Wolfe F, Lane N. The relationship between fibromyalgia and temporomandibular disorders: prevalence and symptom severity. *J Rheumatol* 1996; 23:1948–1952.

78. Schwartz LL. Pain associated with temporomandibular joint. *J Am Dent Assoc* 1955;51:393–397.

79. Schwartz LL. A temporomandibular joint pain-dysfunction syndrome. *J Chronic Dis* 1956;3:284–293.

80. Brooke RI, Stenn PG, Mothersill KJ. The diagnosis and conservative treatment of myofascial pain dysfunction syndrome. *Oral Surg* 1977;44:844–852.

81. Alling CC III. The diagnosis of chronic maxillofacial pain. *Alabama J Med Sci* 1982;19:242–246.

82. Malow RM, Olson RE, Greene CS. Myofascial pain dysfunction syndrome: a psychophysiological disorder. In: Golden C, Alcaparras S, Strider F, et al, eds. *Applied Techniques in Behavioral Medicine*. New York: Grune and Stratton; 1981:101–133.

83. Feinmann C, Harris M, Cawley R. Psychogenic facial pain: presentation and treatment. *BMJ* 1984;288: 436–468.

84. Kinney RK, Gatchel RJ, Ellis E, et al. Major psychological disorders in chronic temporomandibular disorders patient: implications for successful management. *J Am Dent Assoc* 1992;123:49–54.

85. Seligman DA, Pullinger AG. The role of intercuspal occlusal relationships in temporomandibular disorders: a review. *J Craniomandib Disord Fac Oral Pain* 1991;5:96–106.

86. Seligman DA, Pullinger AG. The role of functional occlusal relationships in temporomandibular disorders: a review. *Craniomandib Disord Fac Oral Pain* 1991;5:265–279.

87. Bales JM, Epstein JB. The role of malocclusion and orthodontics in temporomandibular disorders. *J Can Dent Assoc* 1994;60:899–905.

88. Harkins SJ, Marteney JL. Extrinsic trauma: a significant precipitating factor in temporomandibular dysfunction. *J Prosthet Dent* 1985;54:271–272.

89. Pullinger AG, Monteiro AA. History factors associated with symptoms of temporomandibular disorders. *J Oral Rehabil* 1988;15:117–124.

90. Pullinger AG, Seligman DA. Trauma history in diagnostic groups of temporomandibular disorders. *Oral Surg Oral Med Oral Pathol* 1991;71:529–534.

91. Stenger J. Whiplash. Basal facts. *J Prosthet Dent* 1977;2: 5–12.

92. Weinberg LA, Larger LA. Clinical report on the etiology and diagnosis of TMJ dysfunction-pain syndrome. *J Prosthet Dent* 1980;44:642–653.

93. Schneider K, Zerneke RF, Clark G. Modeling of jaw-head-neck dynamics during whiplash. *J Dent Res* 1989;68:1360–1365.

94. Coderre TJ, Katz J, Vaccarino AL, Melzack R. Contribution of central neuroplasticity to pathological pain: review of clinical and experimental literature. *Pain* 1993;52:259–285.

95. Trowskoy M, Cozacov C, Ayache M, Bradley EL, Kassin I. Postoperative pain after inguinal herniorraphy with different types of anesthesia. *Anesth Analg* 1990;70:29–35.

96. McQuay J. Pre-emptive analgesia. *Br J Anesth* 1992; 69:1–3.

97. Cousins M. Acute and postoperative pain. In: Wall PD, Melzack R, eds. *Textbook of Pain.* Edinburgh: Churchill Livingstone; 1994;357–385.

98. Sessle BJ. Masticatory muscle disorders: basic science perspective. In: Sessle BJ, Bryant PS, Dionne RA, eds. *Temporomandibular Disorders and Related Pain Conditions: Progress in Pain Research and Management.* Vol. 4. Seattle: IASP Press; 1995:47–61.

99. Milam SB, Schmitz JP. Molecular biology of temporomandibular joint disorders: proposed mechanisms of disease. *J Oral Maxillofac Surg* 1998;56:89–191.

100. Okeson JP. Orofacial pain: guidelines for assessment, diagnosis, and management. Chicago: Quintessence Publishing; 1996.

101. Glaros AG, Tabacchi KN, Glass EG. Effect of parafunctional clenching on TMD pain. *J Orofac Pain* 1998;12:145–152.

102. McNamara JA, Turp JC. Orthodontic treatment and temporomandibular disorders: is there a relationship? 1: Clinical studies. *J Orofac Orthop* 1997;58:74–89.

103. Turp JC, McNamara JA. Orthodontic treatment and temporomandibular disorders: is there a relationship? 2: Clinical implications. *J Orofac Orthop* 1997;58: 136–143.

104. Tucker MR, Thomas PM. *Temporomandibular Disorders and Dentofacial Skeletal Deformities: Selected Readings in Oral and Maxillofacial Surgery.* Vol 4, no 5. Dallas: University of Texas Southwestern Medical Center at Dallas; 1996.

105. Hoppenreijs TJM, Freihofer HPM, Stoelinga PJW, Tuinzing DB, van't Hof MA. Condylar remodeling and resorption after Le Fort I and bimaxillary osteotomies in patients with anterior open bite: a clinical and radiological study. *Int J Oral Maxillofac Surg* 1998;27:81–91.

106. Arnett GW, Milam SB, Gottesman L. Progressive mandibular retrusion—idiopathic condylar resorption, 1. *Am J Orthod Dentofac Orthop* 1996;110:8–15.

107. Arnett GW, Milam SB, Gottesman L. Progressive mandibular retrusion—idiopathic condylar resorption, 2. *Am J Orthod Dentofac Orthop* 1996;110: 117–127.

108. McNamara JA, Seligman DA, Okeson JP. The relationship of occlusal factors and orthodontic treatment to temporomandibular disorders. In: Sessle BJ, Bryant PS, Dionne RA, eds. *Temporomandibular Disorders and Related Pain Conditions, Progress in Pain Research and Management.* Vol 4. Seattle: IASP Press; 1995:399–427.

109. Pullinger AG, Seligman DA, Gornbein JA. A multiple regression analysis of the risk and relative odds of temporomandibular disorders as a function of common occlusal features. *J Dent Res* 1993;72:968–979.

110. Rugh JD, Harlan J. Nocturnal bruxism and temporomandibular disorders. *Adv Neurol* 1988;49:329–341.

111. Dubner R. Neural basis of persistent pain: sensory specialization, sensory modulation, and neuronal plasticity. In: Jensen TS, Turner JA, Weisenfeld-Hallin Z, eds. *Proceedings of the 8th World Congress on Pain, Progress in Pain Research and Management.* Vol. 8. Seattle: IASP Press; 1997:243–257.

112. Hu JW, Tsai C-M, Bakke M, et al. Deep craniofacial pain: involvement of trigeminal subnucleus caudalis and its modulation. In: Jensen TS, Turner JA, Weisenfeld-Hallin Z, eds. *Proceedings of the 8th World Congress on Pain, Progress in Pain Research and Management.* Vol 8. Seattle: IASP Press; 1997: 497–506.

113. Heise AP, Laskin DM, Gervin AS. Incidence of temporomandibular joint symptoms following whiplash injury. *J Oral Maxillofac Surg* 1992;50:825–828.

114. Probert TCS, Wiesenfeld D, Reade PC. Temporomandibular pain dysfunction disorder resulting from road traffic accidents: an Australian study. *Int J Oral Maxillofac Surg* 1994;23:338–341.

115. Dornan R, Clark GT. Incidence of trauma induced disease in a TMD clinic population. *J Dent Res* 1991;70:441.

116. Locker D, Slade G. Prevalence of symptoms associated with temporomandibular disorders in a Canadian population. *Commun Dent Oral Epidemiol* 1988;16:310–313.

117. Burgess JA, Kolbinson DA, Lee PT, Epstein JB. Motor vehicle accidents and TMDs: assessing the relationship. *J Am Dent Assoc* 1996;127:1767–1772.

118. Seligman DA, Pullinger AG. A multiple stepwise logistic regression analysis of trauma history and 16 other history and dental cofactors in females with temporomandibular disorders. *J Orofa Pain* 1996;10: 351–361.

119. Bakland LK, Christiansen EL, Strutz JM. Frequency of dental and traumatic events in the etiology of temporomandibular disorders. *Endodont Dent Traumatol* 1988;4:182–185.

120. Burgess J. Symptom characteristics in TMD patients reporting blunt trauma and/or whiplash injury. *J Craniomandib Disord: Fac Oral Pain* 1991;5:251–257.

121. Weinberg S, Lapointe H. Cervical extension-flexion injury (whiplash) and internal derangement of the temporomandibular joint. *J Oral Maxillofac Surg* 1987;45:653–656.

122. Kronn E. The incidence of TMJ dysfunction in patients who have suffered a cervical whiplash injury following a traffic accident. *J Orofac Pain* 1993;7:209–213.

123. Roydhouse RH. Whiplash and temporomandibular dysfunction. *Lancet* 1973;1:1394–1395.

124. Kolbinson DA, Epstein JB, Senthilselvan A, Burgess JA. A comparison of TMD patients with or without prior motor vehicle accident involvement: initial signs, symptoms and diagnostic characteristics. *J Orofac Pain* 1997;11:206–214.

125. Brooke RI, Stenn PG. Postinjury myofascial dysfunction syndrome: its etiology and prognosis. *Oral Surg Oral Med Oral Pathol* 1978;45:846–850.

126. Mannheimer J, Attanasio R, Cinotti WR, et al. Cervical strain and mandibular whiplash: effects upon the craniomandibular apparatus. *Clin Prevent Dent* 1989;11:29–32.

127. Schellhas KP. Temporomandibular joint injuries. *Radiology* 1989;173:211–216.

128. Howard RP, Benedict JV, Raddin JH, Smith HL. Assessing neck extension-flexion as a basis for temporomandibular joint dysfunction. *J Oral Maxillofac Surg* 1991;49:1210–1213.

129. Howard RP, Hatsell CP, Guzman HM. Temporomandibular joint injury potential imposed by the low-velocity extension-flexion maneuver. *J Oral Maxillofac Surg* 1995;53:256–262.

130. Heise AP, Laskin DM, Gervin AS. Incidence of temporomandibular joint symptoms following whiplash injury. *J Oral Maxillofac Surg* 1992;50:825–828.

131. Welcher JB, Szabo TJ. Relationships between seat properties and human subject kinematics in rear impact tests. Accident analysis and prevention 2001;33(3):289–304.

132. Ward CC, Szabo TJ, Welcher JB. Recent research on rear impact collisions. SAE technical paper series 3104540924 1994:1–8.

133. Juniper RP. Temporomandibular joint dysfunction: a theory based upon electromyographic studies of the lateral pterygoid muscle. *Br J Oral Maxillofac Surg* 1984;22:1–8.

134. Porter MR. The attachment of the lateral pterygoid muscle to the meniscus. *J Prosthet Dent* 1970;24:555–562.

135. Osborn JW. The disk of the human temporomandibular joint: design, function, and failure. *J Oral Rehabil* 1985;12:279–293.

136. Wongwatana S, Kronman JH, Clark RE, Kabani S, Mehta S. Anatomic basis for disk displacement in temporomandibular joint (TMJ) dysfunction. *Am J Orthod Dentofac Orthop* 1994;105:257–264.

137. Naidoo LC. Lateral pterygoid muscle and its relationship to the meniscus of the temporomandibular joint. *Oral Surg Oral Med Oral Pathol Oral Radiol Endodont* 1996;82:4–9.

138. Goldman AB, DiCarlo EF. Pigmented villonodular synovitis: diagnosis and differential diagnosis. *Radiol Clin North Am* 1988;26:1327–1347.

139. Enzinger FM, Weiss SW. Benign tumors and tumor-like lesions of synovial tissue. In: *Soft Tissue Tumors.* 3rd ed. St Louis: Mosby-Year Book; 1995:735–755.

140. Jaffe HL, Lichtenstein L, Sutro CJ. Pigmented villonodular synovitis, bursitis and tenosynovitis. *Arch Pathol* 1941;31:731–765.

141. Goldman AB, DiCarlo EF. Pigmented villonodular synovitis: diagnosis and differential diagnosis. *Radiol Clin North Am* 1988;26:1327–1347.

142. Barnard JDW. Pigmented villonodular synovitis in the temporomandibular joint: a case report. *Br J Oral Surg* 1975;13:183–187.

143. Takagi M, Ishikawa G. Simultaneous villonodular synovitis and synovial chondromatosis of the temporomandibular joint: report of case. *J Oral Surg* 1981;39:699–701.

144. O'Sullivan TJ, Alport EC, Whiston HG. Pigmented villonodular synovitis of the temporomandibular joint. *J Otolaryngol* 1984;13:123–126.

145. Tanaka K, Suzuki M, Nameki H, Sugiyama H. Pigmented villonodular synovitis of the temporomandibular joint. *Arch Otolaryngol Head Neck Surg* 1997;123:536–539.

146. Agerberg G, Carlsson GE. Functional disorders of the masticatory system, I: distribution of symptoms according to age and sex as judged from investigation by questionnaire. *Acta Odont Scand* 1972;30:597–613.

147. Helkimo M. Studies on function and dysfunction of the masticatory system, IV: age and sex distribution of symptoms of dysfunction of the masticatory system in Lapps in the north of Finland. *Acta Odont Scand* 1974;32:255–267.

148. Helkimo M. Epidemological surveys of dysfunction of the masticatory system. *Oral Sci Rev* 1976;7:54–69.

149. Gazit E, Lieberman M, Eini R, et al. Prevalence of mandibular dysfunction in 10–18 year old Israeli schoolchildren. *J Oral Rehab* 1984;11:307–317.

150. Glass RH, McGlynn FD, Glaros AG, Melton K, Romans K. Prevalence of temporomandibular disorder symptoms in a major metropolitan area. *J Craniomandib Prac* 1993;11:217–220.

151. Solberg WK, Woo ME, Houston JB. Prevalence of mandibular dysfunction in young adults. *J Am Dent Assoc* 1979;98:25–34.

152. Pullinger AG, White SC, Efficacy of TMJ radiographs in terms of expected versus actual findings. *Oral Surg Oral Med Oral Pathol Oral Radiol Endod* 1995;79: 367–374.

153. Wänman A. Longitudinal course of symptoms of craniomandibular disorders in men and women: a 10-year follow-up study of an epidemiologic sample. *Acta Odontol Scand* 1996;54:337–342.

154. Ishigaki S, Bessette RW, Maruyama T. The distribution of internal derangement in patients with temporomandibular joint dysfunction: prevalence, diagnosis and treatments. *J Craniomand Pract* 1992;10: 289–296.

155. Paesani D, Westesson P-L, Hatala M, Tallents RH, Kurita K. Prevalence of temporomandibular joint internal derangement in patients with craniomandibular disorders. *Am J Orthod Dentofacial Orthop* 1992;101: 41–47.

156. Tasaki MM, Westesson P-L, Isberg AM, Ren Y-F, Tallents RH. Classification and prevalence of temporomandibular joint disk displacement in patients and symptom-free volunteers. *Am J Orthod Dentofac Orthop* 1996;109:249–262.

157. Hans MG, Liberman J, Goldberg J, Rozencweig G, Bellon E. A comparison of clinical examination history and magnetic resonance imaging for identifying orthodontic patients with temporomandibular joint disorders. *Am J Orthod Dentofac Orthop* 1992;101: 54–59.

158. Bush FM, Harkins SW, Walter GH, Price DD. Analysis of gender effects on pain perception and symptom presentation in temporomandibular pain. *Pain* 1993; 53:73–80.

159. Unruh AM. Gender variations in clinical pain experience. *Pain* 1996;65:123–167.

160. Isberg A, Hagglund M, Paesani D. The effect of age and gender on the onset of symptomatic temporomandibular joint disk displacement. *Oral Surg Oral Med Oral Pathol Oral Radiol Endod* 1998;85: 252–257.

161. Ohrbach R, Gale EN. Pressure pain thresholds, clinical assessment and differential diagnosis: reliability and validity in patients with myogenic pain. *Pain* 1989;39:157–169.

162. Dworkin SF, LeResche LR, DeRouen T, Von Korff M. Assessing clinical signs of temporomandibular disorders: reliability of clinical examiners. *J Prosthet Dent* 1990;63:574–579.

163. Dolwick MF. Clinical diagnosis of temporomandibular joint internal derangement and myofascial pain and dysfunction. *Oral Maxillofac Surg Clin North Am* 1989;1:1–6.

164. Green CS, Laskin DM. Long term status of TMJ clicking in patients with myofascial pain dysfunction. *J Am Dent Assoc* 1988;117:461–465.

165. Clark GT, Seligman DA, Solberg WK, Pullinger AG. Guidelines for the examination and diagnosis of temporomandibular disorders. *J Craniomandib Disord Fac Oral Pain* 1989;3:7–14.

166. Keith DA. Differential diagnosis of facial pain and headache. *Oral Maxillofac Surg Clin North Am* 1989;1: 7–12.

167. Duinkerke AS, Luteijn F, Bouman TK, de Jong HP. Relations between TMJ pain dysfunction syndrome (PDS) and some psychological and biographical variables. *Commun Dent Oral Epidemiol* 1985;13:185–189.

168. Davant TS, Greene CS, Perry HT, Lautenschlager EP. A quantitative computer-assisted analysis of disc displacement in patients with internal derangement using sagittal view magnetic resonance imaging. *J Oral Maxillofac Surg* 1993;51:974–979.

169. Dolwick MF. Temporomandibular joint disc displacement: clinical perspectives. In: Sessle BJ, Bryant PS, Dionne RA, eds. *Temporomandibular Disorders and Related Pain Conditions, Progress in Pain Research and Management.* Vol 4. Seattle: IASP Press; 1995;79–87.

170. Morrow D, Tallents RM, Katzberg RW, Murphy WC, Mart TC. Relationship of other joint problems and anterior disc position in symptomatic TMD patients and in asymptomatic volunteers. *J Orofac Pain* 1996;10:15–20.

171. Katzberg RW, Westesson P-L, Tallents RH, Drake CM. Anatomic disorders of the temporomandibular joint disc in asymptomatic subjects. *J Oral Maxillofac Surg* 1996;34:147–153.

172. Stohler CS. Phenomenology, epidemiology, and natural progression of the muscular temporomandibular disorders. *Oral Surg Oral Med Oral Pathol Oral Radiol Endod* 1997;83:77–81.

173. Murphy DR. *Conservative Management of Cervical Spine Disorders.* New York: McGraw-Hill; 2000:245–246.

174. Moss ML. The functional matrix: functional cranial components. In: Krauss BS, Reidel WL, eds. *Vistas in Orthodontics.* Philadelphia: Lea & Febiger; 1962:85–90.

175. Cailliet R. *Neck and Arm Pain,* 3rd ed. Philadelphia: F.A. Davis, 1991:1–4, 72–79.

176. Darnell MW. A proposed chronology of events for forward head posture. *J Craniomandib Pract* 1983;1: 49–54.

177. Kendall FP, McCreary EK, Provance PG. *Muscles Testing and Function,* 4th ed. Baltimore: Williams & Wilkins; 1993.

178. Mannheimer JS, Rosenthal RM. Acute and chronic postural abnormalities as related to craniofacial pain and temperomandibular disorders. *Dent Clin North Am* 1991;35:185–208.

179. Kisner CK, Colby LA. *Therapeutic Exercise. Foundations and Techniques,* 2nd ed Philadelphia: F.A. Davis; 1990:437–445.

180. Kraus SL. Cervical spine influences on the craniomandibular region. In: *TMJ Disorders: Management of the Craniomandibular Complex.* New York: Churchill Livingstone; 1988:367–396.

181. Travell JG, Simons DG. *Myofascial Pain and Dysfunction. The Trigger Point Manual.* Baltimore: Williams & Wilkins; 1983:219–318.

182. Lewit K. Chain reactions in disturbed function of the motor system. *J Manual Med* 1987;3:27.

183. Vig PS, Sarver DM, Hall DJ, Warren DW. Quantitative evaluation of nasal airflow in relation to facial morphology. *Am J Orthod* 1981;79;263–272.

184. Lewit K. Relation of faulty respiration to posture, with clinical implications. *J Amer Osteopath Assoc* 1980;79:525–529.

185. Bolton PS. The somatosensory system of the neck and its effects on the central nervous system. In: *Proceedings of the Scientific Symposium.* World Federation of Chiropractic; 1997:32–49.

186. Chaitow L, Monro R, Hyman J, Witt P. Breathing dysfunction. *J Bodywork Mov Ther* 1997;1:252–261.

187. Kuchera M, et al. Athletic functional demand and posture. *J Amer Osteopath Assoc* 1990;90:843–844.

188. Fricton J, Schiffman E. Reliability of a craniomandibular index. *J Dent Res* 1986;65:1359–1364.

189. Fricton J, Schiffman E. The craniomandibular index: validity. *J Prosthet Dent* 1987;58:222–228.

190. LeResche L, Von Korff MR, eds. Research diagnostic criteria. *J Craniomandib Disord Fac Oral Pain* 1992;6: 327–334.

191. Cyriax J. Rheumatic headache. *Br Med J* 1982;2: 1367–1368.

192. Feinstein B, Lanton NJK, Jameson RM, Schiller F. Experiments on pain referred from deep somatic tissues. *J Bone Joint Surg* 1954;36(A):981–997.

193. Friedman MH, Weisberg J. *Temporomandibular Joint Disorders: Diagnosis and Treatment. Chicago: Quintessence Publishing;* 1985.

194. Berry DC. Mandibular dysfunction pain and chronic minor illness. *Br Dent J* 1969;127:170–175.

195. Gelb H. The craniomandibular syndrome. In: Garliner D, ed. *Myofunctional Therapy.* Philadelphia: Saunders; 1976.

196. Dimitroulis G, Dolwick MF, Gremillion HA. Temporomandibular disorders. 1. Clinical evaluation. *Aust Dent J* 1995;40:301–305.

197. Day LD. History taking. In: Morgan DH, Hall WP, Vamvas SJ, eds. *Diseases of the Temporomandibular Apparatus: A Multidisciplinary Approach.* St. Louis: Mosby; 1977.

198. Shore MA. *Temporomandibular Joint Dysfunction and Occlusal Equilibration.* Philadelphia: Lippincott; 1976;

199. Morgan DH, Rosen LM. Interpretation of radiograph. In: Morgan DH, Hall WP, Vamvas SJ, eds. *Diseases of the Temporomandibular Apparatus: A Multidisciplinary Approach.* 2nd ed. St. Louis: Mosby; 1982:

200. Heiberg AN, Heloe B, Krogstad BS. The myofascial pain dysfunction: dental symptoms and psychological and muscular function: an overview. *Psychother Psychosom* 1978;30:81–97.

201. Halbert R. Electromyographic study of head position. *J Can Dent Assoc* 1958;23:11–23.

202. Perry C. Neuromuscular control of mandibular movements. *J Prosthet Dent* 1973;30:714–720.

203. Thompson JR, Brodie AG. Factors in the position of the mandible. *J Am Dent Assoc* 1942;29:925–941.

204. Mintz VW. The orthopedic influence. In: Morgan DH, Hall WP, Vamvas SJ, eds. *Diseases of the Temporomandibular Apparatus: A Multidisciplinary Approach.* 2nd ed. St. Louis: Mosby; 1982:

205. Mohl ND. Head posture and its role in occlusion. *N Y State Dent J* 1976;42:17–23.

206. Prieskel HW. Some observations on the postural position of the mandible. *J Prosthet Dent* 1965;15:625–633.

207. Ramfjord SP. Dysfunctional temporomandibular joint and muscle pain. *J Prosthet Dent* 1961;11:353–374.

208. Cohen S. A cephalometric study of rest position in edentulous persons: Influences of variations head position. *J Prosthet Dent* 1957;7:467–472.

209. Darling DW, Kraus S, Glasheen-Wray MB. Relationship of head posture and the rest position of the mandible. *J Prosthet Dent* 1984;52:111–115.

210. Goldstein DF, Kraus SL, Williams WB, Glasheen-Wray M. Influence of cervical posture on mandibular movement. *J Prosthet Dent* 1984;52:421–426.

211. Robinson MJ. The influence of head position on TMJ dysfunction. *J Prosthet Dent* 1966;16:169–172.

212. Rocabado M. Management of the temporomandibular joint. Presented at a course on physical therapy in dentistry. Vail, Colorado, 1978.

213. Solberg WK, Hansson TL, Nordstrom B. The temporomandibular joint in young adults at autopsy: a morphologic classification and evaluation. *J Oral Rehab* 1985;12:303–321.

214. Kircos LT, Ortendahl DA, Mark AS, et al. Magnetic resonance imaging of the TMJ disk in asymptomatic volunteers. *J Oral Maxillofac Surg* 1987;45:852–854.

215. Ettala-Ylitalo UM, Syrjanen S, Halonen P. Functional disturbances of the masticatory system related to temporomandibular joint involvement by rheumatoid arthritis. *J Oral Rehabil* 1987;14:415–427.

216. Goldstein BH. Temporomandibular disorders: a review of current understanding. *Oral Surg Oral Med Oral Pathol Oral Radiol Endod* 1999;88:379–385.

217. Truelove EL, Sommers EE, LeResche L, Dworkin SF, Von Korff M. Clinical diagnostic criteria for TMD. *J Am Dent Assoc* 1992;143:47–54.

218. Dimitroulis G, Gremillion HA, Dolwick MF, Walter JH. Temporomandibular disorders. 2. Non-surgical treatment. *Aust Dent J* 1995;40:372–376.

219. Gangarosa LP, Mahan PE. Pharmacologic management of TMJ-MPDS. *Ear Nose Throat J* 1982;61:30–41.

220. Ready LB, Hare B. Drug problems in chronic pain patients. *Anesthesiol Rev* 1979;6:28–31.

221. Clark GT. A critical evaluation of orthopedic interocclusal appliance therapy. Design theory and overall effectiveness. *J Am Dent Assoc* 1984;108:359–364.

222. Clark GT, Adler RC. A critical evaluation of occlusal therapy. Occlusal adjustment procedures. *J Am Dent Assoc* 1885;110:743–750.

223. Annandale T. On displacement of the inter-articular cartilage of the lower jaw, and its treatment by operation. *Lancet* 1887;i:411.

224. Summa R. The importance of the inter-articular fibrocartilage of the temporo-mandibular articulation. *The Dental Cosmos* 1918;60:512–514.

225. Pringle JH. Displacement of the mandibular meniscus and its treatment. *Br J Surg* 1918;6:385–389.

226. Wakeley CPG. The causation and treatment of displaced mandibular cartilage. *Lancet* 1929;ii:543–545.

227. Prentiss HJ. A preliminary report upon the temporomandibular articulation in the human type. *The Dental Cosmos* 1918;60:505–514.

228. Salonen L, Hellden L. Prevalence of signs and symptoms of dysfunction in the masticatory system: an epidemiological study in an adult Swedish population. *J Craniomandib Disord Faci Oral Pain* 1990;4:241–250.

229. Dimitroulis G, Dolwick MF. Temporomandibular disorders. 3. Surgical treatment. *Aust Dent J* 1996;41:16–20.

230. Dolwick MF, Dimitroulis G. Is there a role for temporomandibular surgery? *Br J Oral Maxillofac Surg* 1994;32:307–313.

231. Weinberg S, Kryshtalskyj B. Analysis of facial and trigeminal nerve function after arthroscopic surgery of the temporomandibular joint. *J Oral Maxillofac Surg* 1996;54:40–43.

232. Moses JJ, Topper DC. Arteriovenous fistula: an unusual complication associated with arthroscopic temporomandibular joint surgery. *J Oral Maxillofac Surg* 1990;48:1220–1222.

233. Loughner BA, Gremillion HA, Mahan PE, Watson RE. The medial capsule of the human temporomandibular joint. *J Oral Maxillofac Surg* 1997;55:363–369.

234. Westesson PL, Eriksson L, Liedberg J. The risk of damage to facial nerve, superficial temporal vessels, disk, and articular surfaces during arthroscopic examination of the temporomandibular joint. *Oral Surg Oral Med Oral Pathol* 1986;62:124–127.

235. Nellestam P, Eriksson L. Preauricular approach to the temporomandibular joint: a postoperative follow-up on nerve function, hemorrhage and esthetics. *Swed Dent J* 1997;21:19–24.

236. Carls FR, Engelke W, Lochler MC, Sailer HF. Complications following arthroscopy of the temporomandibular joint: analysis covering a 10-year period (451 arthroscopies). *J Craniomaxillofac Surg* 1996;24:12–15.

237. Talebzadeh N. Rosenstein TP. Pogrel MA. Anatomy of the structures medial to the temporomandibular joint. *Oral Surg Oral Med Oral Pathol Oral Radiol Endod* 1999;88:674–678.

238. Schrader H, Obelieniene D, Bovim G, et al. Natural evolution of late whiplash syndrome outside the medicolegal context. *Lancet* 1996;347:1207–1211.

239. Obelieniene D, Schrader H, Bovim G, Miseviciene I, Sand T. Pain after whiplash: a controlled prospective inception cohort study. *J Neurol Neurosurg Psychiatry* 1999;66:279–284.

240. Ferrari R, Russell AS. Epidemiology of whiplash: an international dilemma. *Ann Rheum Dis* 1999;58:1–5.

241. Ferrari R, Schrader H, Obelieniene D. Prevalence of temporomandibular disorders associated with whiplash injury in Lithuania. *Oral Surg Oral Med Oral Pathol Oral Radiol Endod* 1999;87:653–657.

242. Carlsson SG, Gale EW. Biofeedback in the treatment of long-term temporomandibular joint pain: an outcome study. *Biofeedback Self Regul* 1977;2:161–165.

243. Rugh JD. Psychological components of pain. *Dent Clin North Am* 1987;31:579–594.

244. Moss RA, Adams HE. The class of personality, anxiety and depression in mandibular pain dysfunction subjects. *J Oral Rehabil* 1984;11:233–237.

245. Kendall FP, McCreary EK, Provance PG. *Muscles Testing and Function.* 4th ed. Baltimore: Williams & Wilkins; 1993.

246. Mannheimer JS, Rosenthal RM. Acute and chronic postural abnormalities as related to craniofacial pain and temperomandibular disorders. *Dent Clin North Am* 1991;35:185–208.

247. Sahrmann S. *Diagnosis and Treatment of Movement Disorders.* Mosby Year Book, St. Louis, 2001.

248. Griegel-Morris P, Larson K, Mueller-Klausk K, Oatis CA. Incidence of common postural abnormailities in the cervical, shoulder, and thoracic regions and their association with pain in two age groups of health subjects. *Phys Then* 1992;72:425–430.

249. Clark GT, Adachi NY, Dornan MR. Physical medicine procedures affect temporomandibular disorders: a review. *J Am Dent Assoc* 1990;121:151–161.

250. Glass EG, McGlynn FD, Glaros AG. A survey of treatments for myofascial pain dysfunction. *J Craniomandib Pract* 1991;9:165–168.

251. Glass EG, Glaros AG, McGlynn FD. Myofascial pain dysfunction: treatments used by ADA members. *J Craniomandib Pract* 1993;11:25–29.

252. Feine JS, Widmer CG, Lund JP. Physical therapy: a critique. *Oral Surg Oral Med Oral Pathol Oral Radiol Endod* 1997;83:123–127.

253. Feine JS, Lund JP. An assessment of the efficacy of physical therapy and physical modalities for the control of chronic musculoskeletal pain. *Pain* 1997;71: 5–23.

254. Hecht PJ, Bachmann S, Booth RE Jr, Rothman RH. Effects of thermal therapy on rehabilitation after total knee arthroplasty: a prospective randomized study. *Clin Orthop* 1983;178:198–201.

255. Chapman CE. Can the use of physical modalities for pain control be rationalized by the research evidence? *Can J Physiol Pharmacol* 1991;69:704–712.

256. Gam AN, Thorsen H, Lannberg F. The effect of low-level laser therapy on musculoskeletal pain: a meta-analysis. *Pain* 1993;52:63–66.

257. Beckerman H, de Bie RA, Bouter LM, De Cuyper HJ, Oostendrop RAB. The efficacy of laser therapy for musculoskeletal and skin disorders: a criteria-based meta-analysis of randomized clinical trials. *Phys Ther* 1992;72:13–21.

258. Bertolucci LE, Grey T. Clinical analysis of mid-laser versus placebo treatment of arthralgic TMJ degenerative joints. *J Craniomandibular Pract* 1995;13: 27–29.

259. Wolf SL. *Electrotherapy: Clinics in Physical Therapy.* New York: Churchill Livingstone; 1981:1–24, 99–121.

260. Nelson RM, Currier DD. Clinical Electrotherapy. Norwalk (CN): Appleton & Lange; 1987:166–182.

261. Murphy GJ. Electrical Physical therapy in treating TMJ patients. *J Craniomandib Pract* 1983;2:67–73.

262. Okeson JP. *Management of Temporomandibular Disorders and Occlusion.* St. Louis: Mosby-Year Book; 1993: 345–378.

263. Talley RL, Murphy GJ, Smith SD, Baylin MA, Haden JL. Standards for the history, examination, diagnosis and treatment of temporomandibular disorders (TMD): a position paper. *J Craniomandib Pract* 1990;1: 60–70.

264. Graff-Radford SB, Reeves JL, Baker RL, Chiu D. Effects of transcutaneous electrical nerve stimulation on myofascial pain and trigger point sensitivity. *Pain* 1989;37:1–5.

265. Tegelberg A, Kopp S. Short-term effect of physical training on temporomandibular joint disorder in individuals with rheumatoid arthritis and ankylosing spondylitis. *Acta Odontol Scand* 1988;46:49–56.

266. Dao TTT, Lund JP, Lavigne GJ. Pain responses to experimental chewing in myofascial pain patients. J Dent Res 1994;73:1163–7.

267. Spitzer WO, Leblanc F, Dupuis M, Abenham L, Belanger AY, Bloch R, et al. Scientific approach to the assessment and management of activity-related spinal disorders: Report of the Quebec Task Force on Spinal Disorders. Spine 1987;12(7S):S1-S59.

268. Fordyce WE. Back pain in the workplace management of disability in nonspecific conditions: Report of the Task Force on Pain in the Workplace of the Interaction. Seattle: IASP Press, 1995.

269. Minor MA, Hewett JE, Webel RR, Anderson SK, Kay DR. Efficacy of physical conditioning exercise in patients with rheumatoid arthritis and osteoarthritis. Arthritis Rheum 1989;32:1396–1405.

270. Timm KS. A randomized-control study of active and passive treatments for chronic low back pain following L5 laminectomy. J Orthop Sports Phys Ther 1994;20:276–286.

271. Mohl ND, Ohrbach RK, Crow HC, Gross AJ. Devices for the diagnosis and treatment of temporomandibular disorders, III: thermography, ultrasound, electrical stimulation, and electromyographic biofeedback. J Prosthet Dent 1990;63:472–477.

272. NIH Technology Assessment Panel on Integration of Behavioral and Relaxation Approaches to the Treatment of Chronic Pain and Insomnia. Integration of behavioral and relaxation approaches into the treatment of chronic pain and insomnia. JAMA 1996;276: 313–318.

273. Evjenth O, Hamberg J. *Muscle Stretching in Manual Therapy; A Clinical manual, Vol 1; The Extremities; Vol 2, The Spinal Column and the TMJ.* Alfta, Sweden, Alfta rehab Forlag, 1980.

274. Jull GA, Janda V. Muscle and motor control in low back pain. In: Twomey LT, Taylor JR, eds. *Physical*

Therapy of the Low Back: Clinics in Physical Therapy. New York: Churchill Livingstone; 1987:259–276.

275. Pettman E. Level III *Course Notes from North American Institute of Orthopedic Manual Therapy* Portland, Course notes, OR: 1990.

276. Troyanovich SJ, Harrison DE, Harrison DD. Structural rehabilitation of the spine and posture: ration-

ale for treatment beyond the resolution of symptoms. *J Manip Phys Ther* 1998;21:37–50.

277. Mannheimer JS. Prevention and restoration of abnormal upper quarter posture. In: Gelb H, Gelb M, eds. *Postural Considerations in the Diagnosis and Treatment of Cranio-Cervical-Mandibular and Related Chronic Pain Disorders.* St. Louis: Ishiyaku EuroAmerica; 1991:93–161.

Index